P9-CMO-897

AACN

Procedure Manual *for* High Acuity, Progressive, *and* Critical Care

Edited by

Debra L. Wiegand, RN, PhD, CCRN, CHPN, FAHA, FPCN, FAAN

Associate Professor
University of Maryland School of Nursing
Baltimore, Maryland;
Staff Nurse
Surgical Cardiac Care Unit
Thomas Jefferson University Hospital
Philadelphia, Pennsylvania

7th EDITION

AMERICAN
ASSOCIATION
of CRITICAL-CARE
NURSES

ELSEVIER

ELSEVIER

3251 Riverport Lane
St. Louis, Missouri 63043

AACN PROCEDURE MANUAL FOR HIGH ACUITY, PROGRESSIVE, ISBN: 978-0-323-37662-4
AND CRITICAL CARE, SEVENTH EDITION
Copyright © 2017 by Elsevier, Inc. All rights reserved.

No part of this publication may be reproduced or transmitted in any form or by any means, electronic or mechanical, including photocopying, recording, or any information storage and retrieval system, without permission in writing from the publisher. Details on how to seek permission, further information about the Publisher's permissions policies and our arrangements with organizations such as the Copyright Clearance Center and the Copyright Licensing Agency, can be found at our website: www.elsevier.com/permissions.

This book and the individual contributions contained in it are protected under copyright by the Publisher (other than as may be noted herein).

> **Notices**
>
> Knowledge and best practice in this field are constantly changing. As new research and experience broaden our understanding, changes in research methods, professional practices, or medical treatment may become necessary.
>
> Practitioners and researchers must always rely on their own experience and knowledge in evaluating and using any information, methods, compounds, or experiments described herein. In using such information or methods they should be mindful of their own safety and the safety of others, including parties for whom they have a professional responsibility.
>
> With respect to any drug or pharmaceutical products identified, readers are advised to check the most current information provided (i) on procedures featured or (ii) by the manufacturer of each product to be administered, to verify the recommended dose or formula, the method and duration of administration, and contraindications. It is the responsibility of practitioners, relying on their own experience and knowledge of their patients, to make diagnoses, to determine dosages and the best treatment for each individual patient, and to take all appropriate safety precautions.
>
> To the fullest extent of the law, neither the Publisher nor the authors, contributors, or editors, assume any liability for any injury and/or damage to persons or property as a matter of products liability, negligence or otherwise, or from any use or operation of any methods, products, instructions, or ideas contained in the material herein.

Previous editions copyrighted 2011, 2005, 2001, 1994, 1985.

Library of Congress Cataloging-in-Publication Data

Names: Wiegand, Debra J. Lynn-McHale, editor. | American Association of Critical-Care Nurses, issuing body.
Title: AACN procedure for high-acuity, progressive, and critical care / edited by Debra Lynn-McHale Wiegand.
Other titles: AACN procedure manual for critical care (Wiegand) | Procedure for high-acuity, progressive, and critical care
Description: Seventh edition. | St. Louis, Missouri : Elsevier, [2017] | Preceded by: AACN procedure manual for critical care / edited by Debra Lynn-McHale Wiegand. 6th ed. C2011. | Includes bibliographical references and index.
Identifiers: LCCN 2016010545 | ISBN 9780323376624 (pbk. : alk. paper)
Subjects: | MESH: Critical Care Nursing—methods | Critical Illness—nursing | Handbooks
Classification: LCC RT120.I5 | NLM WY 49 | DDC 616/.028—dc23 LC record available at http://lccn.loc.gov/2016010545

Executive Content Strategist: Lee Henderson
Content Development Manager: Jean Sims Fornango
Senior Content Development Specialist: Laura Selkirk
Publishing Services Manager: Jeff Patterson
Project Manager: Lisa A. P. Bushey
Designer: Ryan Cook

Printed in the United States of America

Last digit is the print number: 9 8 7 6 5 4 3 2 1

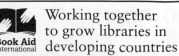

Section Editors

Michael W. Day, RN, MSN, CCRN, TCRN
Clinical Practice Specialist
Trauma and Acute Care Surgery
Northeast Georgia Medical Center
Gainesville, Georgia

Eleanor Fitzpatrick, RN, MSN, ACNP-BC, AGCNS-BC, CCRN
Clinical Nurse Specialist
Surgical Critical Care
Thomas Jefferson University Hospital
Philadelphia, Pennsylvania

Mary Beth Flynn Makic, RN, PhD, CNS, CCNS, CCRN-K, FAAN, FNAP
Associate Professor
University of Colorado College of Nursing
Aurora, Colorado

Debra L. Wiegand, RN, PhD, CCRN, CHPN, FAHA, FPCN, FAAN
Associate Professor
University of Maryland School of Nursing
Baltimore, Maryland;
Staff Nurse
Surgical Cardiac Care Unit
Thomas Jefferson University Hospital
Philadelphia, Pennsylvania

Contributors

Richard B. Arbour, MSN
Clinical Faculty, School of Nursing
LaSalle University
Philadelphia, Pennsylvania
Procedure 88: *Bispectral Index Monitoring*

Jane V. Arndt, MS, RN, CWOCN, ACNS-BC
Clinical Nurse Specialist
Surgical and Support Services
Poudre Valley Hospital
Fort Collins, Colorado
Procedure 135: *Fecal Containment Devices and Bowel Management System*

Sonia M. Astle, RN, MS
Clinical Nurse Specialist
Critical Care
Inova Fairfax Medical Campus
Falls Church, Virginia
Procedure 119: *Continuous Renal Replacement Therapies*
Procedure 120: *Hemodialysis*
Procedure 121: *Peritoneal Dialysis*
Procedure 123: *Apheresis and Therapeutic Plasma Exchange (Assist)*

John C. Bazil, RN, BSN, BSEE
Staff Nurse
Neurological Intensive Care Unit
UT Southwestern Medical Center
Dallas, Texas
Procedure 98: *Pupillometer*

Marcia Belcher, MSN, BBA, RN, CCRN-CSC, CCNS
Clinical Nurse Specialist
The Ohio State University Wexner Medical Center Richard M. Ross Heart Hospital
Columbus, Ohio
Procedure 17: *Extracorporeal Life Support (ECLS) and Extracorporeal Membrane Oxygenation (ECMO)*

Cameron Bell, MS, RN, CCNS, CCRN
Associate Nurse Manager, Burn Center
University of Colorado Hospital
Aurora, Colorado
Procedure 126: *Burn Wound Care*
Procedure 127: *Donor-Site Care*

Tracey M. Berlin, MSN-Ed, RN, CCRN, CNRN
Nursing Education Consultant
Eagleville, Pennsylvania
Procedure 90: *Cerebral Blood Flow Monitoring*

Kathleen Berns, MS, APRN, CNS, CFRN
Clinical Nurse Specialist
Mayo Clinic Medical Transport
Mayo Clinic
Rochester, Minnesota
Procedure 79: *Thenar Tissue Oxygen Saturation Monitoring*

Angela Bingham, MSN, RN
Clinical Educator, Critical Care
Providence St. Vincent Medical Center
Portland, Oregon
Procedure 53: *Ventricular Assist Devices*

Cynthia Blank-Reid, RN, MSN, CEN
Trauma Clinical Nurses Specialist
Department of Trauma and Surgical Critical Care
Temple University Hospital
Philadelphia, Pennsylvania
Procedure 109: *Focused Assessment with Sonography in Trauma*

Stephen Both, CRNA-MAE
Premiere Anesthesia
Brooks Memorial Hospital
Dunkirk, New York
Procedure 8: *Laryngeal Mask Airway*

Joel M. Brown II, RRT, FAARC
Director, Respiratory Care and Sleep Medicine
Nemours-Al DuPont Hospital for Children
Wilmington, Delaware
Procedure 81: *Arterial Puncture*

Shelley Burcat, RN, MSN
Clinical Nurse Specialist, Nursing
Thomas Jefferson University
Philadelphia, Pennsylvania
Procedure 141: *Calculating Doses, Flow Rates, and Administration of Continuous Intravenous Infusions*

Justin Burleson, BSN
Charge Nurse, Burn ICU
University of Colorado Hospital
Aurora, Colorado
Procedure 137: *Wound Management with Excessive Drainage*

Mary G. Carey, PhD, RN
Associate Director, Clinical Nursing Research Center
University of Rochester Medical Center Strong Memorial Hospital
Associate Professor, School of Nursing
University of Rochester
Rochester, New York
Procedure 54: *Cardiac Monitoring and Electrocardiographic Leads*
Procedure 56: *ST-Segment Monitoring (Continuous)*

Roger Casey, MSN, CEN, TCRN, FAEN
Staff Nurse
Kadlec Regional Medical Center/Freestanding Emergency
  Department
Kennewick, Washington
Procedure 11: *Surgical Cricothyrotomy (Perform)*
Procedure 12: *Surgical Cricothyrotomy (Assist)*

Sandy Cecil, BA, AA Nursing
Nurses Manager, Neuro Trauma Intensive Care Unit
Legacy Emanuel Medical Center
Portland, Oregon
Procedure 91: *Cerebral Microdialysis*

Alice Chan, RN, MN, CNS, CCRN
Manager, Critical Care
Cedars-Sinai Medical Center
Los Angeles, California
Procedure 39: *Emergent Open Sternotomy (Perform)*
Procedure 40: *Emergent Open Sternotomy (Assist)*

Susan Chioffi, MSN
Nurse Practitioner, Advanced Practice
Duke University Medical Center
Durham, North Carolina
Procedure 96: *Lumbar Puncture (Perform)*
Procedure 97: *Lumbar Puncture (Assist)*

Kathleen M. Cox, DNP, APRN, ACNP-BC, CCNS
Director, Adult-Gerontologic Acute Care Nurse Practitioner
  Program
School of Nursing Graduate Studies
University of Texas El Paso
El Paso, Texas
Procedure 42: *Pericardiocentesis (Perform)*
Procedure 43: *Pericardiocentesis (Assist)*
Procedure 62: *Blood Sampling from a Central Venous Catheter*
Procedure 63: *Blood Sampling from a Pulmonary Artery Catheter*
Procedure 78: *Pericardial Catheter Management*

Stephanie Cox, MS
Quality Improvement Specialist
Clinical Excellence and Patient Safety
University of Colorado Hospital
Aurora, Colorado
Procedure 94: *Intraventricular Catheter with External Transducer
  for Cerebrospinal Fluid Drainage and Intracranial Pressure
  Monitoring*

Hillary Crumlett, BSN, MS
Clinical Director of Critical Care
Northwestern Medicine-Central DuPage Hospital
Winfield, Illinois
Procedure 58: *Arterial Catheter Insertion (Perform)*
Procedure 59: *Arterial Catheter Insertion (Assist), Care, and
  Removal*
Procedure 61: *Blood Sampling from an Arterial Catheter*
Procedure 68: *Esophageal Cardiac Output Monitoring: Perform*
Procedure 69: *Esophageal Cardiac Output Monitoring: Assist,
  Care, and Removal*

Janice Y. Dawson, BSN
Staff Nurse Nurse, Noninvasive Cardiology
Lankenau Hospital
Wynnewood, Pennsylvania
Procedure 80: *Transesophageal Echocardiography (Assist)*

Michael W. Day, RN, MSN, CCRN, TCRN
Clinical Practice Specialist
Trauma and Acute Care Surgery
Northeast Georgia Medical Center
Gainesville, Georgia
Procedure 85: *Intraosseous Devices*

Kate Deis, MSN, RN, CEN, ACNS-BC
Clinical Nurse Specialist, Emergency Department
Thomas Jefferson University Hospital
Philadelphia, Pennsylvania
Procedure 117: *Peritoneal Lavage (Perform)*
Procedure 118: *Peritoneal Lavage (Assist)*

Anne Delengowski, RN, MSN, AOCN
Oncology Clinical Nurse Specialist, Nursing
Thomas Jefferson University Hospital
Philadelphia, Pennsylvania
Procedure 84: *Implantable Venous Access Device: Access,
  Deaccess, and Care*

Coleen Dever, MSN, AGCNS-BC
Trauma Program Coordinator
Christiana Care Health System
Newark, Delaware
Procedure 122: *Use of a Massive Infusion Device and a Pressure
  Infusor Bag*

Cara Diaz, RN, BSN, MS, CRNP
Acute Care Nurse Practitioner, Trauma Neurosurgery
R. Adams Cowley Shock Trauma Center
Baltimore, Maryland
Procedure 103: *Halo Ring and Vest Care*
Procedure 104: *Pin-Site Care: Cervical Tongs and Halo Pins*

Sharon Dickinson, MSN
CNS, Nursing
University of Michigan
Ann Arbor, Michigan
Procedure 19: *Pronation Therapy*

Joni L. Dirks, MSN, RN-BC, CCRN-K
Manager Clinical Educators & ICU Educator
Department of Educational Services
Providence Health Care
Spokane, Washington
Procedure 16: *Continuous Venous Oxygen Saturation Monitoring*

Julia E. Dunning, BSN, MSN
Senior Nurse Practitioner, Shock Trauma Orthopedics
University of Maryland Shock Trauma Center
Baltimore, Maryland
Procedure 129: *Intracompartmental Pressure Monitoring*

Margaret M. Ecklund, MS, RN, CCRN-K, ACNP-BC
Clinical Nurse Specialist, Clinical Practice Support
Legacy Health
Portland, Oregon
Procedure 138: *Percutaneous Endoscopic Gastrostomy (PEG), Gastrostomy, and Jejunostomy Tube Care*
Procedure 139: *Small-Bore Feeding Tube Insertion and Care*

Joanna C. Ellis, CRNP, MSN, ACNP-BC
Trauma Nurse Practitioner
Division of Traumatology, Surgical Critical Care and Emergency Surgery
Penn Presbyterian Medical Center
Philadelphia, Pennsylvania
Procedure 131: *Wound Closure*

Eleanor Fitzpatrick, BSN, RN, MSN, ACNP-BC, AGCNS-BS, CCRN
Clinical Nurse Specialist, Surgical Critical Care
Thomas Jefferson University Hospital
Philadelphia, Pennsylvania
Procedure 111: *Endoscopic Therapy*
Procedure 115: *Paracentesis (Perform)*
Procedure 116: *Paracentesis (Assist)*

Susan K. Frazier, PhD, RN, FAHA
Associate Professor, Director, PhD Program Co-Cirector RICH Heart Program
University of Kentucky, College of Nursing
Lexington, Kentucky
Procedure 30: *Noninvasive Positive Pressure Ventilation: Continuous Positive Airway Pressure (CPAP) and Bilevel Positive Airway Pressure (BiPAP)*
Procedure 33: *Weaning Mechanical Ventilation*

John Gallagher, DNP, RN, CCNS, CCRN, RRT
Trauma Program Coordinator/Clinical Nurse Specialist
Division of Trauma, Surgical Critical Care and Emergency Surgery
Penn Presbyterian Medical Center
Philadelphia, Pennsylvania
Procedure 29: *Invasive Mechanical Ventilation (Through an Artificial Airway): Volume and Pressure Modes*

Kyle Gibson, MSN, RN, CEN, TCRN, EMT-P
Shock Trauma Nurse, Emergency Department
Northeast Georgia Medical Center-Gainesville
Gainesville, Georgia
Procedure 1: *Combitube Insertion and Removal*
Procedure 7: *King Airway Insertion and Removal*

Karen A. Gilbert, RN, MSN, CNSC, CRNP
Nutrition Support Clinical Nurse Specialist, Specialist
Thomas Jefferson University Hospital
Philadelphia, Pennsylvania
Procedure 140: *Small-Bore Feeding Tube Insertion Using an Electromagnetic Guidance System (CORTRAK 2 Enteral Access System EAS)*

Cindy Goodrich, RN, MSN, CCRN
Clinical Educator and Flight Nurse
Airlift Northwest
Seattle, Washington
Procedure 2: *Endotracheal Intubation (Perform)*
Procedure 3: *Endotracheal Intubation (Assist)*
Procedure 26: *Needle Thoracostomy (Perform)*

Cynthia Hambach, MSN, RN, CCRN
Assistant Clinical Professor
College of Nursing and Health Professions
Drexel University
Philadelphia, Pennsylvania
Procedure 35: *Cardioversion*
Procedure 36: *Defibrillation (External)*

Jillian Hamel, MS, ACNP-BC
Nurse Practitioner, Cardiology
Western Washington Cardiology
Everett, Washington
Procedure 45: *Atrial Overdrive Pacing (Perform)*
Procedure 65: *Central Venous Catheter Removal*
Procedure 66: *Central Venous Catheter Site Care*

John P. Harper, MSN -BC
Clinical Educator, Critical Care
Nursing Education
Corzer-Chester Medical Center
Upland, Pennsylvania
Procedure 52: *Intraaortic Balloon Pump Management*

Julie Lynn Henderson, RN, MSN, ANP, FNP-BC
Nurse Practitioner
Little People's Clinic
Highlands Ranch, Colorado
Procedure 133: *Débridement: Pressure Ulcers, Burns, and Wounds*

Kiersten Henry, RN, DNP
Chief Medicine Advanced Practice Provider
Cardiology
MedStar Montgomery Medical Center
Olney, Maryland
Procedure 34: *Automated External Defibrillation*
Procedure 41: *External Wearable Cardioverter-Defibrillator*
Procedure 47: *Implantable Cardioverter-Defibrillator*

Linda Hoke, PhD, RN, CCNS, ACNS-BC, CCRN
Clinical Nurses Specialist
Cardiac Intermediate Care Unit
Hospital of the University of Pennsylvania
Philadelphia, Pennsylvania
Procedure 80: *Transesophageal Echocardiography (Assist)*

Nathan W. Howard, RN, BSN, CCRN
Staff Nurse, Cardiac Intensive Care Unit
Providence Sacred Heart Medical Center
Spokane, Washington
Procedure 32: *Peripheral Nerve Stimulators*

Alexander Johnson, MSN, RN, CCNS, ACNP-BC, CCRN
Clinical Nurse Specialist, Critical Care
Cadence Health—Northwestern Medicine
Winfield, Illinois
Procedure 58: *Arterial Catheter Insertion (Perform)*
Procedure 59: *Arterial Catheter Insertion (Assist), Care, and Removal*
Procedure 61: *Blood Sampling from an Arterial Catheter*
Procedure 68: *Esophageal Cardiac Output Monitoring: Perform*
Procedure 69: *Esophageal Cardiac Output Monitoring: Assist, Care, and Removal*

Renee Johnson, APRN, MSN, CCRN, CCNS
Critical Care Clinical Nurse Specialist, Critical Care
Gwinnett Medical Center
Lawrenceville, Georgia
Procedure 13: *Tracheostomy Cuff and Tube Care*

Maribeth Kelly, MSN, RN, PCCN
Clinical Nurse Specialist, Medical Telemetry
Thomas Jefferson University Hospital
Philadelphia, Pennsylvania
Procedure 141: *Calculating Doses, Flow Rates, and Administration of Continuous Intravenous Infusions*

Peggy Kirkwood, RN, MSN, ACNCP, CHF, AACC
Cardiovascular Nurse Practitioner
Mission Hospital
Mission Viejo, California
Procedure 23: *Chest Tube Removal (Perform)*
Procedure 24: *Chest Tube Removal (Assist)*

Lisa Koser, DNP, ACNP-BC, CPNP-AC
Trauma and Acute Care Surgery Nurse Practitioner
The Ohio State University Wexner Medical Center
Columbus, Ohio;
Flight Nurse Practitioner
The Cleveland Clinic Foundation
Cleveland, Ohio
Procedure 5: *Extubation/Decannulation (Perform)*
Procedure 6: *Extubation/Decannulation (Assist)*

Teri M. Kozik, RN, PhD, CNS, CCRN
Clinical Nurse Specialist—Research Supervisor
Clinical Research
St. Joseph's Medical Center
Stockton, California
Procedure 54: *Cardiac Monitoring and Electrocardiographic Leads,*

Thomas Lawson, MS
Nurse Practitioner, Neurocritical Care
The Ohio State University Wexner Medical Center
Columbus, Ohio
Procedure 17: *Extracorporeal Life Support (ECLS) and Extracorporeal Membrane Oxygenation (ECMO)*

Donna Barge Lee, MSN
Trauma Education & Outreach Coordinator
Northeast Georgia Medical Center
Gainesville, Georgia
Procedure 18: *Oxygen Saturation Monitoring with Pulse Oximetry*

Rosemary Lee, DNP, ARNP, ACNP-BC, CCNS, CCRN
Clinical Nurse Specialist, Critical Care
Homestead Hospital
Homestead, Florida;
Adjunct Faculty, College of Nursing
Nova Southeastern University
Palm Beach Garden, Florida
Procedure 108: *Esophagogastric Tamponade Tube*
Procedure 112: *Intraabdominal Pressure Monitoring*

Thomas Levins, BSN, RN, CCRN, CFRN
Clinical Coordinator, PennSTAR Flight
University of Pennsylvania Health System
Philadelphia, Pennsylvania
Procedure 31: *Manual Self-Inflating Resuscitation Bag-Valve Device*

Karen A. Lovett, MS, CNS, CCNS
Director Patient Services
University of Colorado Hospital
Aurora, Colorado
Procedure 100: *Thermoregulation: External and Intravascular Warming/Cooling Devices*

Paul Luehrs, BSEd, BSRT, RRT, ACCS
Adult Critical Care Supervisor, Respiratory Care
CoxHealth
Springfield, Missouri
Procedure 14: *Continuous End-Tidal Carbon Dioxide Monitoring*

Jennifer MacDermott, MS
Clinical Care Specialist, Critical Care
Columba, Ohio
Procedure 15: *Continuous Lateral Rotation Therapy*

Mary Beth Flynn Makic, RN, PhD, CNS, CCNS, CCRN-K, FAAN, FNAP
Associate Professor, College of Nursing
University of Colorado
Aurora, Colorado
Procedure 99: *RotoRest Lateral Rotation Surface*
Procedure 134: *Drain Removal*

Eileen Maloney Wilensky, MSN, ACNP-BC
Director, Clinical Research, Quality & Safety Program
Neurosurgery
Penn Medicine
Philadelphia, Pennsylvania
Procedure 89: *Brain Tissue Oxygen Monitoring: Insertion (Assist), Care, and Troubleshooting*

Carrie Marvill, MSN, RN, AOCNS
Clinical Nurse Education Specialist
Penn Medicine
Philadelphia, Pennsylvania
Procedure 124: *Bone Marrow Biopsy and Aspiration (Perform)*
Procedure 125: *Bone Marrow Biopsy and Aspiration (Assist)*

Jennifer Massetti, BSN, MS, ACNP-BC
ACNP-BC, Trauma Neurosurgery
R Adams Cowley Shock Trauma Center
University of Maryland
Baltimore, Maryland
Procedure 101: *Cervical Tongs or Halo Ring: Application for Use in Cervical Traction (Assist)*
Procedure 102: *Cervical Traction Maintenance*

Carol McGinnis, DNP, CNS, RN, CNSC
Clinical Nurse Specialist
Sanford USD Medical Center
Sioux Falls, South Dakota
Procedure 113: *Nasogastric and Orogastric Tube Insertion, Care, and Removal*

Kelly McGinty, BSN, MSN, FNP
Spokane Emergency Physicians
Sacred Heart Medical Center
Spokane, Washington
Procedure 20: *Autotransfusion*

Marion E. McRae, RN, MScN, ACNP-BC, CCRN-CSC-CMC
AACC Nurse Practitioner
Guerin Family Congenital Heart Program
Cedars-Sinai Medical Center
Clinical Instructor
David Geffen School of Medicine
University of California at Los Angeles
Los Angeles, California
Procedure 37: *Defibrillation (Internal) Perform*
Procedure 38: *Defibrillation (Internal) Assist*
Procedure 44: *Atrial Electrogram*
Procedure 46: *Epicardial Pacing Wire Removal*

Reba McVay, MSN, RN, CNS-BC, CCRN
Director of Cardiovascular Service Line
WellStar Atlanta Medical Center & AMC South
Atlanta, Georgia
Procedure 67: *Central Venous/Right Atrial Pressure Monitoring*
Procedure 72: *Pulmonary Artery Catheter Insertion (Assist) and Pressure Monitoring*
Procedure 74: *Pulmonary Artery Catheter and Pressure Lines, Troubleshooting*
Procedure 75: *Single-Pressure and Multiple-Pressure Transducer Systems*

Lorie Ann Meek, MSN, RN
Duke Telestroke Coordinator, Network Services
Duke Health
Durham, North Carolina
Procedure 106: *Patient-Controlled Analgesia*

Megan T. Moyer, MSN
Acute Care Nurse Practitioner, Neurosurgery
Hospital of the University of Pennsylvania
Philadelphia, Pennsylvania
Procedure 89: *Brain Tissue Oxygen Monitoring: Insertion (Assist), Care, and Troubleshooting*

Theresa Nino, RN, MSN, CCRN
Instructor, College of Nursing
University of Colorado
Critical Care Trauma Nurse
Burn Trauma Intensive Care Unit
University of Colorado Hospital
Aurora, Colorado
Procedure 99: *RotoRest Lateral Rotation Surface*

DaiWai M. Olson, PhD, RN, CCRN, FNCS
Neurology & Neurotherapeutics
UT Southwestern Medical Center
Dallas, Texas
Procedure 98: *Pupillometer*

Michele M. Pelter, RN, PhD
Assistant Professor, Director of the ECG Monitoring Research Lab
Physiological Nursing
University of California, San Francisco
San Francisco, California
Procedure 54: *Cardiac Monitoring and Electrocardiographic Leads*
Procedure 56: *ST-Segment Monitoring (Continuous)*

Glen Peterson, DNP, ACNP
Assistant Professor, Clinical Director, APP Education and Quality
Blood Cancer and Bone Marrow Transplant Program
University of Colorado Hospital, University of Colorado Health
Aurora, Colorado
Procedure 124: *Bone Marrow Biopsy and Aspiration (Perform)*
Procedure 125: *Bone Marrow Biopsy and Aspiration (Assist)*

Joya D. Pickett, PhD, RN, ARNP-CNS, CCNS, ACNS-BC, CCRN
Critical Care Clinical Nurse Specialist, Intensive Care
Swedish Medical Center
Adjunct Faculty, Biobehavioral Nursing
University of Washington
Seattle, Washington
Procedure 25: *Closed Chest-Drainage System*

Ann Will Poteet, MS, RN, CNS
Clinical Nurse Specialist, College of Nursing
University of Colorado
Aurora, Colorado
Procedure 110: *Gastric Lavage in Hemorrhage and Overdose*

Jan Powers, PhD, RN, CCNS, CCRN, CNRN, NE-BC, FCCM
Clinical Nurse Specialist
Indianapolis, Indiana
Procedure 19: *Pronation Therapy*

Mark Puhlman, RN, MSN
Left Ventricular Assist Device Coordinator
Center for Advanced Heart Disease
Providence St. Vincent Medical Center
Portland, Oregon
Procedure 53: *Ventricular Assist Devices*

Barbara Quinn, RN, MSN, ACNS-BC
Clinical Nurse Specialist, Quality Services
Sutter Medical Center
Sacramento, California
Procedure 4: *Endotracheal Tube Care and Oral Care Practices for Ventilated and Non-ventilated Patients*

Marylou V. Robinson, PhD, FNP-C
Associated Professor, College of Nursing
University of Colorado
Aurora, Colorado
Procedure 132: *Cleaning, Irrigating, Culturing, and Dressing an Open Wound*

Thomas A. Santora, RN, BSN, CCRN
Professor of Surgery
Vice Chair, Department of Surgery
Temple University Hospital
Philadelphia, Pennsylvania
Procedure 109: *Focused Assessment With Sonography in Trauma*

Brian D. Schaad, BSN, BA
Charge Nurse, Burn/Trauma ICU
University of Colorado Hospital
Aurora, Colorado
Procedure 130: *Suture and Staple Removal*
Procedure 134: *Drain Removal*

Nicolle Schraeder, RN, MSN, ACNPC-AG
Acute Care Nurse Practitioner, Neurosciences
Littleton Adventist Hospital
Littleton, Colorado
Procedure 95: *Lumbar Subarachnoid Catheter Insertion (Assist) for Cerebrospinal Fluid Drainage and Pressure Monitoring*

Susan S. Scott, MSN
Clinical Educator, MICU/SICU
Baystate Medical Center
Springfield, Massachusetts
Procedure 60: *Arterial Pressure–Based Cardiac Output Monitoring*
Procedure 64: *Cardiac Output Measurement Techniques (Invasive)*
Procedure 70: *Noninvasive Cardiac Output Monitoring*

Dawn Sculco, BSN, MS
Clinical Nurse Specialist
Critical Care Unit and Emergency Department
Valley View Hospital
Glenwood Springs, Colorado
Procedure 128: *Skin-Graft Care*

Maureen A. Seckel, RN, APRN, MSN, ACNS-BC, CCNS, CCRN, FCCM
Clinical Nurse Specialist Medical Pulmonary Critical Care and Sepsis Coordinator
Christiana Care Health System
Affiliated Instructor, College of Health Sciences, School of Nursing
University of Delaware
Newark, Delaware
Procedure 10: *Suctioning: Endotracheal or Tracheostomy Tube*

Rose B. Shaffer, RN, MSN, ACNP-BC, CCRN, FAHA
Cardiology Nurse Practitioner, Nursing
Thomas Jefferson University Hospital
Philadelphia, Pennsylvania
Procedure 76: *Femoral Arterial and Venous Sheath Removal*
Procedure 77: *Radial Arterial Sheath Removal*

Tess Slazinski, RN, MN, CCRN, CNRN, SCRN, CCNS
Neuroscience/Critical Care Clinical Nurse Specialist
Critical Care Services
Cedars-Sinai Medical Center
Pacific Palisades, California
Procedure 92: *Fiberoptic Catheter Insertion (Assist), Intracranial Pressure Monitoring, Care, Troubleshooting, and Removal*
Procedure 93: *Intraventricular/Fiberoptic Catheter Insertion (Assist), Monitoring, Nursing Care, Troubleshooting, and Removal*

Mary Lou Sole, PhD, RN, CCNS, FAAN, FCCM
Dean and Professor; Orlando Health Endowed Chair
College of Nursing
University of Central Florida
Nurse Scientist, Center for Nursing Research
Orlando Health
Orlando, Florida
Procedure 4: *Endotracheal Tube Care and Oral Care Practices for Ventilated and Non-ventilated Patients*

Valerie Spotts, BSN, RN
Educational Nurse Coordinator, Nursing-Inpatient Cardiology
University of Michigan
Ann Arbor, Michigan
Procedure 48: *Permanent Pacemaker (Assessing Function)*
Procedure 49: *Temporary Transcutaneous (External) Pacing*
Procedure 51: *Temporary Transvenous and Epicardial Pacing*

Jamie St. Clair, MS, RN, ACNS-BC, CCRN
Clinical Nurse Specialist
The Ohio State University Wexner Medical Center
Columbus, Ohio
Procedure 15: *Continuous Lateral Rotation Therapy*

Mary D. Still, BSN, MSN, APRN, ACNS
Clinical Nurse Specialist Critical Care/Transplant
Nursing/Critical Care
Emory Healthcare
Atlanta, Georgia
Procedure 114: *Molecular Adsorbent Recirculating System (MARS)*

Nikki Taylor, MS, BSN, RN
Clinical Nurse Level D, Cardiology
University of Michigan Health System
Ann Arbor, Michigan
Procedure 50: *Temporary Transvenous Pacemaker Insertion (Perform)*
Procedure 71: *Pulmonary Artery Catheter Insertion (Perform)*
Procedure 73: *Pulmonary Artery Catheter Removal*

Kathleen Vollman, MSN, RN, CCNS, FCCM, FAAN
Clinical Nurse Specialist/Consultant
Advancing Nursing LLC
Northville, Michigan
Procedure 4: *Endotracheal Tube Care and Oral Care Practices for Ventilated and Non-ventilated Patients*
Procedure 19: *Pronation Therapy*

Julie Waters, RN, MS, CCRN
Clinical Nurse Educator for Critical Care
Providence Health Care
Spokane, Washington
Procedure 21: *Chest Tube Placement (Perform)*
Procedure 22: *Chest Tube Placement (Assist)*

Debra L. Wiegand, RN, PhD, CCRN, CHPN, FAHA, FPCN, FAAN
Associate Professor, School of Nursing
University of Maryland
Baltimore, Maryland;
Staff Nurse
Surgical Cardiac Care Unit
Thomas Jefferson University Hospital
Philadelphia, Pennsylvania
Procedure 86: *Midline Catheters*
Procedure 87: *Peripherally Inserted Central Catheter*

Kimberly Williams, BSN, RN-BC
Clinical Manager, Plain Service
University of Louisville
Louisville, Kentucky
Procedure 105: *Epidural Catheters: Assisting with Insertion and Pain Management*
Procedure 107: *Peripheral Nerve Blocks: Assisting with Insertion and Pain Management*

Lisa Woods, MSN, BSN, BA
Wound, Ostomy, and Continence Nurse
Lutheran Medical Center
Wheat Ridge, Colorado
Procedure 136: *Negative-Pressure Wound Therapy*

Patricia H. Worthington, RN, MSN, CNSC
Nutrition Support Clinical Specialist, Nursing
Jefferson University Hospital
Philadelphia, Pennsylvania
Procedure 140: *Small-Bore Feeding Tube Insertion Using an Electromagnetic Guidance System (CORTRAK 2 Enteral Access System EAS),*

Kimberly Wright, MSN, RN, CEN, TCRN
Director of Trauma Services
Lawnwood Regional Medical Center & Heart Institute
Fort Pierce, Florida
Procedure 9: *Nasopharyngeal and Oral Airway Insertion*

Shu-Fen Wung, PhD, RN, ACNP, FAAN
Associate Professor, College of Nursing
The University of Arizona
Tucson, Arizona
Procedure 55: *Extra Electrocardiographic Leads: Right Precordial and Left Posterior Leads*
Procedure 57: *Twelve-Lead Electrocardiogram*

Susan Yeager, MS, RN, CCRN, ACNP-BC, FNCS
Neurocritical Care Nurse Practitioner–Lead
The Ohio State University Wexner Medical Center
Clinical Instructor, Acute Care Nurse Practitioner Program
The Ohio State University College of Nursing
Columbus, Ohio
Procedure 27: *Thoracentesis (Perform)*
Procedure 28: *Thoracentesis (Assist)*
Procedure 82: *Central Venous Catheter Insertion (Perform)*
Procedure 83: *Central Venous Catheter Insertion (Assist)*

Reviewers

Lillian Aguirre, MSN, CNS, CCRN, CCNS
Clinical Nurse Specialist
Orlando Health
Orlando, Florida

Bim Akintade, PhD, MBA, MHA, ACNP-BC, CCRN
Specialty Director, Trauma, Critical Care, ED, AGACNP/CNS
Assistant Professor, OSAH
University of Maryland School of Nursing
College Park, Maryland

Anna M. Alvarez, MSN, CNS, CCNS, CWOCN
Wound Ostomy Continence Nurse
Orlando Health
Orlando, Florida

Suzanne Ashworth, CNS, MSN, CCRN, CCNS
Neuroscience Clinical Nurse Specialist
Orlando Health
Orlando, Florida

Mary Kay Bader, RN, MSN, CCNS, CNRN, CCRN, SCRN, FAHA, FNCS
Neuro/Critical Care CNS
Mission Hospital
Mission Viejo, California

Tracey M. Berlin, MSN-Ed, RN, CCRN, CNRN
Nursing Education Consultant and Clinical Applications Specialist
Eagleville, Pennsylvania

Bryan Boling, DNP, AGACNP-BC, CCRN-CSC, CEN
Advanced Practice Provider
Division of Critical Care, Department of Anesthesiology
University of Kentucky
Lexington, Kentucky

Lindsay Brookhart, RN, BSN, CCRN
General Staff RN, Adult Intensive Care Unit
Providence Sacred Heart Medical Center
Spokane, Washington

Kathy Bunzli RN, MS, ACNS-BC, CCRN, ACHPN
St. Anthony Hospital
Lakewood, Colorado

Shelley Burcat, MSN, RN, AOCNS
Clinical Nurse Specialist, Blood and Marrow Transplant
Thomas Jefferson University Hospital
Philadelphia, Pennsylvania

Kimberly Bush, MSN, RN
Staff Nurse/Clinical Nurse Educator, ISICU
Thomas Jefferson University Hospital
Philadelphia, Pennsylvania

Jaime Byrne, MSN, RN, CRNP, CCRN
Clinical Nurse Specialist, Cardiovascular Intensive Care Unit
Thomas Jefferson University Hospital
Philadelphia, Pennsylvania

Christina M. Canfield, MSN, RN, ACNS-BC, CCRN
Clinical Nurse Specialist
Cleveland Clinic
Cleveland, Ohio

Mary Centinaro, MSN, RN, CCRN
Clinical Nurse Specialist ICU/PCU
Thomas Jefferson University Medical Center, Methodist Campus
Philadelphia, Pennsylvania

Cheryl Ciocca, RN, MS
Nurse Manager, Medical Intensive Care Unit
Philadelphia Veterans Affairs Medical Center
Philadelphia, Pennsylvania

Kathleen Colfer, MSN, RN-DC
Clinical Nurse Specialist, Manager, Staff Nurse
Acute Pain Management
Jefferson Hospital
Philadelphia, Pennsylvania

James D. Colquitt, Jr., PhD, RRT, RCP
Director of Clinical Education
Middle Georgia State College
Macon, Georgia

Leigh Dangerfield, MSN, PCCN, RN-BC
Nursing Professional Development Facilitator
Medical University of South Carolina
Charleston, South Carolina

Michele DeFilippis, MSN, RN, CCRN, CNRN
Nurse Manager
Morristown Medical Center
Morristown, New Jersey

Karlene Dewar, RN, MBA, CNN
Facility Administrator
DaVita, Inc.
Philadelphia, Pennsylvania

Joni L. Dirks, RN-BC, MSN, CCRN-K
Manager, Clinical Educators and ICU Educator
Providence Health Care
Spokane, Washington

Jenna Dziedzic, BSN, RN, CCRN
Educational Coordinator—Nursing (Cardiac ICU)
University of Michigan Health System
Ann Arbor, Michigan

Andrea Efre, DNP, ARNP, ANP, FNP
Nurse Practitioner and Consultant
Healthcare Education Consultants
Tampa, Florida

Nancy Eksterowicz, MSN, RNBC
Clinical Nurse Pain Specialist
University of Virginia Health System
Charlottesville, Virginia

Myra F. Ellis, MSN, RN, CCRN-CSC
Clinical Nurse IV
Duke University Hospital
Durham, North Carolina

Andrea Evans-Davis, BSN, RN, CCRN
Staff RN, CCU
Providence Sacred Heart Medical Center
Spokane, Washington

Kathleen Flarity, DNP, PhD, CEN, CFRN, FAEN
Emergency CNS/Nurse Scientist
University of Colorado Health, Memorial Hospital
Colorado Springs, Colorado

John J. Gallagher, MSN, RN, CCNS, CCRN, RRT
Clinical Nurse Specialist/Trauma Program Manager
Division of Traumatology, Surgical Critical Care and Emergency
  Surgery
Penn Presbyterian Medical Center
Philadelphia, Pennsylvania

Dawn Gambrill, RN, CRNI
PICC Nurse
Thomas Jefferson University Hospital
Philadelphia, Pennsylvania

Lisa A. Gorski, MS, RN, HHCNS-BC, CRNI, FAAN
Clinical Nurse Specialist
Wheaton Franciscan Home Health & Hospice
Milwaukee, Wisconsin

Aimee D. Goss, RN, BSN, CCRN
University of Michigan Health System
Ann Arbor, Michigan

Carrol Graves, RN, MSN, CCRN, CNL
Clinical Nurse Leader
Medical Intensive Care Unit
NF/SG Veterans Health System
Gainesville, Florida

Jane Guttendorf, DNP, RN, CRNP, ACNP-BC, CCRN
Assistant Professor, Adult-Gerontology Acute Care Nurse
  Practitioner Program
University of Pittsburgh, School of Nursing
Acute Care Nurse Practitioner, Department of Critical Care
  Medicine
UPMC Presbyterian
Pittsburgh, Pennsylvania

Linda Hale, RN, CNSC
Nurse Clinician, Nutrition Support Service
William Beaumont Hospital
Royal Oak, Michigan

Tonja M. Hartjes, DNP, ACNP/FNP-BE, CCRN, CSC
Clinical Associate Professor, University of Florida
Adult-Gerontology Acute Care CNP Track Coordinator
UF Health Surgical Critical Care ARNP
Gainesville, Florida

Amy Howell, CNRN
Staff Nurse
Providence Sacred Heart Medical Center
Spokane, Washington

Flerida Imperial-Perez, MN, RN, CNS-BC, CCNS
Clinical Manager
Children's Hospital Los Angeles
Los Angeles, California

Tina Johnson, RN-BSN, CFRN, CEN, CPEA, CMTE
Assistant Manager Critical Care Transport
Children's Healthcare of Atlanta
Atlanta, Georgia

Tamara M. Kear, PhD, RN, CNN
Assistant Professor of Nursing
Villanova University College of Nursing
Villanova, Pennsylvania

Alyson Dare Kelleher, BSN, RN, CCRN
Chest Pain Coordinator
Froedtert Hospital
Milwaukee, Wisconsin

Bridget Kelly, MSN, RN-BC, CCTN
Clinical Nurse Specialist
Jefferson University Hospital
Philadelphia, Pennsylvania

Lynn A. Kelso, MSN, APRN, FCCM, FAANP
Assistant Professor; Acute Care Nurse Practitioner
University of Kentucky
Lexington, Kentucky

Debra Kitchens, RN, BSN, CEN, NRP-P
Trauma Program Manager
Greenville Health System
Greenville, South Carolina

Janet A. Kloos, RN, PhD, CCNS, CCRN
CNS, Cardiology
University Hospitals Case Medical Center
Cleveland, Ohio

Lisa K. Koser, DNP, ACNP-BC, CPNP-AC
Trauma and Acute Care Surgery Nurse Practitioner
The Ohio State University Wexner Medical Center
Columbus, Ohio;
Flight Nurse Practitioner
The Cleveland Clinic Foundation
Cleveland, Ohio

Sara Knippa, MS, RN, CCRN, PCCN, ACCNS-AG
Clinical Nurse Specialist/Educator, Cardiac ICU
University of Colorado Hospital
Aurora, Colorado

Cathleen Lindauer, RN, MSN, CEN
Clinical Outcomes Management Analyst
Department of Emergency Medicine
Johns Hopkins Hospital
Baltimore, Maryland

Karen Lovett, RN, MS, ACNS-BC, CCNS
Clinical Nurse Specialist – Critical Care
St. Anthony Hospital
Lakewood, Colorado

Patricia Marcelle, MSN, RN, CCRN-K
Nurse Educator
Monmouth Medical Center
Long Branch, New Jersey

Isagani I. Marquez, Jr., RN, BSN
Administrative Nurse II, Apheresis Program
University of California – San Diego
San Diego, California

Michelle A. McKay, RN, MSN, CCRN
Clinical Charge RN
Thomas Jefferson University Hospital
Philadelphia, Pennsylvania

Patricia A. McQuade, DEd, MSN, CCRN
Critical Care Nursing Educator
Chilton Memorial Hospital, Atlantic Health System
Pompton Plains, New Jersey

Kathy Meloche, BSN, RN-BC
Pain Management Coordinator
Harper University Hospital, Hutzel Women's Hospital
Detroit, Michigan

Britt M. Meyer, PhD, RN, CRNI, VA-BC, NE-BC
Nurse Manager of Operations, Vascular Access Team
Duke University Hospital
Durham, North Carolina

Nicole Taylor Moulder, MSN, BSN, ACNP-BC
Trauma and Acute Care Surgery ACNP
Northeast Georgia Medical Center
Gainesville, Georgia

CPT Mark R. Oherrick, MSN, ACNP/FNP-BC, CEN, AN
Advanced Practice RN
UPMC Bedford Memorial Hospital, Department of Emergency Medicine, U.S. Army Reserves
Everett, Pennsylvania

DaiWai M. Olson, PhD, RN, CCRN, FNCS
Neurology and Neurotherapeutics
UT Southwestern Medical Center
Dallas, Texas

Amy Della Penna, RN, CCRN, MSN
Clinical Specialist
Thomas Jefferson University Hospital
Philadelphia, Pennsylvania

Lynelle N. B. Pierce, MS, RN, CCRN, CCNS
Clinical Nurse Specialist, Critical Care
University of Kansas Hospital
Kansas City, Kansas

Anne Pirzadeh, RN, BSN, CWOCN
Certified Wound Ostomy Continence Nurse
Centura Health, Porter Adventist Hospital
Denver, Colorado

Patricia Radovich, PhD, CNS, FCCM
Director, Nursing Research
Loma Linda University Medical Center
Loma Linda, California

Paul C. Reid, Sr., RN, MSN
Lung Transplant Nurse Coordinator
Temple University Hospital
Philadelphia, Pennsylvania

Becky Reidy, ARNP, FNP, MSN
Providence Sacred Heart Medical Center
Spokane, Washington

Lori Renaud, RN, BSN, CCRN, SCRN
Charge Nurse
Mission Hospital
Mission Viejo, California

David Ricke, RN, BSN, CCRN, CNRN, SCRN
Permanent Charge Registered Nurse; Level IV Clinical RN
University of Colorado Hospital
Aurora, Colorado

Louise Rose, RN, BN, ICU Cert, Adult Ed Cert, MN, PhD
TD Nursing Professor in Critical Care Research
Sunnybrook Health Sciences Centre and the University of Toronto
Toronto, Ontario, Canada

Carol L. Ross, BSN, RN, CCRN
Staff RN
Presbyterian/St. Luke's Medical Center
Denver, Colorado

Erin Sarsfield, MSN, RN
Clinical Nurse Specialist, Adult ICUs
Penn State Milton S. Hershey Medical Center
Hershey, Pennsylvania

Hildy Schell-Chaple, PhD, RN, CCRN, CCNS
Clinical Nurse Specialist, Adult Critical Care
University of California, San Francisco Medical Center
San Francisco, California

Ashley Heath Seawright, DNP, ACNP-BC
Instructor, Department of Surgery
Division of Transplant and Hepatobiliary Surgery
University of Mississippi Medical Center
Jackson, Mississippi

Pol-Andre Senecal, MSN, CNS, NP, CCNS, ACNP, BC
Instructor, Pulmonary Sciences and Critical Care Medicine
University of Colorado School of Medicine
Aurora, Colorado

Rose Shaffer, RN, MSN, ACNP-BC, CCRN, FAHA
Cardiology Nurse Practitioner, Nursing
Thomas Jefferson University Hospital
Philadelphia, Pennsylvania

Tammy M. Slater, DNP, MS, ACNP
Johns Hopkins, School of Nursing
Baltimore, Maryland

Michelle D. Smeltzer, MSN, RN, CEN
Clinical Educator
Einstein Medical Center Montgomery
Norristown, Pennsylvania

Traci B. Smith, RN, BSN
Registered Nurse
Northeast Georgia Medical Center
Gainesville, Georgia

Susan L. Smith, DHSe, MSN, FNP, ACNP, FAANP
Senior Acute Core Nurse Practitioner
Orlando Health
Orlando, Florida

Christine L. Sommers, MN, RN, CNE, CCRN Emeritus
Executive Dean, Faculty of Nursing
Universitas Pelita Harapan
Lippo Karawaci, Tangerang, Indonesia

Linda Staubli, RN, BSN, CCRN
Clinical Nurse Educator
University of Colorado Hospital
Aurora, Colorado

Rosemary A. Timmerman, DNP, RN, CCNS, CCRN-CSC-CMC
Clinical Nurse Specialist
Providence Alaska Medical Center
Anchorage, Alaska

Jo Ann Valent, RN, BSN, BC, CWOCN, COS-C
CWOCN
Chilton Medical Center
Pompton Plains, New Jersey

Jeremy Yves Vergara, MSN, RN, CNL
Clinical Nurse Manager for the MS-ICU, CCU, and TCU
California Pacific Medical Center - Pacific Campus
Stanford, California

Brooke Wagner, RN, MSN, AGCNS-BC, CNRN
Neurosciences Clinical Nurse Specialist, Evidence Based
  Practice Coordinator
Banner, University Medical Center Phoenix
Phoenix, Arizona

David Waters, RN, BA, MA
Senior Lecturer, Critical Care Nursing
Uxbridge Campus
Buckinghamshire New University
Uxbridge, United Kingdom

Whitney L. Watson, MSN, APRN, AGCNS-BC, CCRN
Nurse Manager
Medical/Transplant ICU
The University of Kansas Hospital
Kansas City, Kansas

Anita J. White, MSN, APRN, ACNS-BC, CCRN
Clinical Nurse Specialist, Medical Intensive Care Unit
Cleveland Clinic
Cleveland, Ohio

John Weisbrod, CRNA, MAE
Clinical Director, Gonzaga University/Providence
Gonzaga University/Providence Sacred Heart Medical Center
  Master of Anesthesiology Education Program
Spokane, Washington

Kimberly S. Wright, MSN, RN, CEN, TCRN
Trauma Program Director
Lawnwood Regional Medical Center & Heart Institute
Fort Pierce, Florida

Susan Yale-Mancini, RN
Chilton Medical Center
Pompton Plains, New Jersey

Susan Yeager, MS, RN, CCRN, ACNP-BC, FNCS
Neurocritical Care Nurse Practitioner–Lead
The Ohio State University Wexner Medical Center;
Clinical Instructor, Acute Care Nurse Practitioner Program
The Ohio State University College of Nursing
Columbus, Ohio

Amy Young, MSN, RN, ACCNS-AG
Clinical Nurse Specialist
Cleveland Clinic
Cleveland, Ohio

Preface

The seventh edition of the *Procedure Manual* has a new title: the *AACN Procedure Manual for High Acuity, Progressive, and Critical Care*. The title has been changed to reflect the expanding use of the procedures in diverse settings. I have worked closely with the section editors, clinical experts, and key AACN and Elsevier staff members to revise and update this edition. We have removed procedures no longer common and added procedures for new technologies, devices, and interventions. Although every attempt was made to capture current clinical practice, we recognize that high acuity, progressive, and critical care clinical practice is dynamic and therefore that any resource to support that practice must be considered a work in progress.

AACN is dedicated to the care of patients with critical illness or injury and their families. AACN's vision is of a healthcare system driven by the needs of patients and their families in which critical care nurses make their optimal contribution. Toward that vision, our hope is that this edition of the *AACN Procedure Manual for High Acuity, Progressive, and Critical Care* will be a useful resource for nurses in providing quality patient care.

The seventh edition of the *AACN Procedure Manual for High Acuity, Progressive, and Critical Care* will be an asset for nurses across the spectrum of acute and critical care practice. The manual includes a comprehensive review of state-of-the-art information on acute and critical care procedures. The following procedures related to new and emerging trends have been added:

- King Airway Insertion and Removal (AP)
- Extracorporeal Life Support (ECLS) and Extracorporeal Membrane Oxygenation (ECMO)
- Defibrillation (Internal) Assist
- External Wearable Cardioverter Defibrillator
- Esophageal Cardiac Output Monitoring (Perform and Assist)
- Noninvasive Cardiac Output Monitoring
- Radial Arterial Sheath Removal
- Thenar Tissue Oxygen Saturation Monitoring
- Midline Catheters
- Cerebral Blood Flow Monitoring
- Cerebral Microdialysis
- Pupilometer
- Focused Assessment with Sonography in Trauma (FAST)
- Nasogastric and Orogastric Tube Insertion, Care, and Removal
- Molecular Adsorbents Recirculation System (MARS)

All procedures have been revised to reflect changes in practice. As with the last edition, this edition of the *AACN Procedure Manual for High Acuity, Progressive, and Critical Care* contains not only procedures commonly performed by critical care nurses but also procedures performed by advanced practice nurses. Each advanced practice procedure has an AP designation in the Table of Contents and a special AP icon and explanatory footnote on the first page of the procedure.

Because we recognize that the procedures included in this manual are only a portion of the repertoire needed by today's critical care practitioners to skillfully care for critically ill patients, we recommend that it be used in conjunction with the *AACN Core Curriculum for High Acuity, Progressive, and Critical Care Nursing, the Certification and Core Review for High Acuity and Critical Care,* and *AACN Advanced Critical Care Nursing.*

The *AACN Procedure Manual for High Acuity, Progressive, and Critical Care* is designed so that information within each procedure can be found quickly. To provide high-quality care to seriously ill patients, we need resources that provide us with readily available, need-to-know information. The book is organized into units, with most of the units having several sections. All procedures are designed in the same style and begin with the following:

- Purpose of the procedure
- Prerequisite Nursing Knowledge, which includes information the nurse needs before performing the procedure
- Equipment list, which includes equipment necessary to perform the procedure (some of the procedures identify additional equipment that may be necessary based on individual situations)
- Patient and Family Education, which identifies essential information that should be taught to patients and their families
- Patient Assessment and Preparation, which includes specific assessment criteria that should be obtained before the procedure and describes how the patient should be prepared for the procedure

Each step-by-step procedure includes the following:

- Steps, Rationales, and, for some steps, Special Considerations
- Associated research and appropriate figures and tables
- Expected Outcomes, including the anticipated results of the procedure
- Unexpected Outcomes, including potential complications or untoward outcomes of the procedure
- Patient Monitoring, which includes information related to assessments and interventions that should be completed (the rationale for each item is described, and conditions that necessitate notification of an advanced practice nurse, physician, or other healthcare professional are identified)
- Documentation that describes what should be documented after the procedure is performed
- References are included, and the majority of procedures also include Additional Readings

This edition of the *AACN Procedure Manual for High Acuity, Progressive, and Critical Care* includes several icons that are common to many of the procedures. These icons include the following:

AP A procedure with the AP icon should be performed only by physicians, advanced practice nurses, and other healthcare professionals (including critical care nurses) with additional knowledge, skills, and demonstrated competence per professional licensure or institutional standard.

HH A procedure step with the HH icon designates that hand hygiene should be performed. This step is essential to reduce the transmission of microorganisms and is part of Standard Precautions.

PE A procedure step with the PE icon designates that personal protective equipment should be applied. Personal protective equipment may include gloves, protective eyeglasses, masks, gowns, and any additional equipment needed to protect the nurse or provider performing the procedure. The application of personal protective equipment reduces the transmission of microorganisms, minimizes splash, and is part of Standard Precautions.

This edition of the *AACN Procedure Manual for High Acuity, Progressive, and Critical Care* uses AACN's current levels of evidence system. Therefore, whenever it is available, this research-based information is provided to indicate the strength of recommendation for various interventions. AACN's level of evidence system includes:

Level A: Meta-analysis of quantitative studies or meta-synthesis of qualitative studies with results that consistently support a specific action, intervention, or treatment (including systematic review of randomized controlled trials).

Level B: Well-designed, controlled studies with results that consistently support a specific action, intervention, or treatment .

Level C: Qualitative studies, descriptive or correlational studies, integrative reviews, systematic reviews, or randomized controlled trials with inconsistent results.

Level D: Peer-reviewed professional and organizational standards with the support of clinical study recommendations.

Level E: Multiple case reports, theory-based evidence from expert opinions, or peer-reviewed professional organizational standards without clinical studies to support recommendations.

Level M: Manufacturer's recommendations only.

The references and additional readings for the seventh edition are now provided online. To access the references and additional readings for each Procedure, simply use your smartphone's QR code reader and camera to scan the QR code found at the end of the procedure. QR code reader apps are freely available on the Apple App Store and Google Play. Alternatively, you can access the references by going to http://booksite.elsevier.com/9780323376624.

Finally, many of the included procedures use electrical equipment. This manual makes the assumption that all equipment is maintained by the institution's bioengineering department according to accepted national and state regulations for the individual piece of equipment.

I hope that you find this book an essential resource for clinical practice.

Debra L. Wiegand

Acknowledgments

This edition of the *AACN Procedure Manual for High Acuity, Progressive, and Critical Care* could not have been published without the help of numerous hardworking people. I would like to thank AACN for giving me the opportunity to edit this edition. This has been the first time I have had the opportunity to work with Michael Muscat, Publishing Director for AACN. Michael's expertise has greatly contributed to the successful development of the book. I would like to thank Michael for his advice and support.

I want to extend a huge thank you to each of the section editors: Michael Day, Eleanor Fitzpatrick, and Mary Beth Makic. The section editors coordinated the development and revision of each of the procedures within their sections. They worked with the contributors and reviewers as each procedure was developed, reviewed, revised, and edited. I am very appreciative of their hard work and commitment to a quality product. I tremendously enjoyed working with such an expert team.

This book would not be possible without the hard work and commitment from the contributors. The contributors are the staff nurses and advanced practice nurses who developed new procedures and revised existing procedures. Each contributor worked very hard to ensure that each procedure included all of the information needed so that acute and critical care nurses would have the most helpful information at their fingertips. I cannot thank each of the contributors enough for their commitment to this book.

I also want to thank the staff nurses and advanced practice nurses who reviewed each of the procedures. At least two reviewers critiqued each procedure and provided important feedback to the contributors. The reviewers' critiques improved the quality of each procedure.

In addition I would like to thank Paula Lusardi for helping with this edition of the book. Paula reviewed every procedure in the book and provided important feedback. I am grateful for her hard work, time, and expertise.

I am very grateful that I had the opportunity to work with the talented, hard-working, and dedicated editorial staff at Elsevier. I want to extend a special thank you to Lee Henderson, my editor. Lee provided essential leadership, guidance, and support throughout the entire publication process. I also want to thank Laura Selkirk, Senior Developmental Editor, for coordinating the day-to-day progress of the book. She provided important behind-the-scenes help as figures were drawn, permissions were obtained, and all of the key aspects of the book were pulled together. She worked closely with Lisa Bushey, Project Manager, as individual procedures, figures, tables, and additional key components of the book were produced. Laura and Lisa provided important timelines and did their best to keep the production of the book moving forward. I also want to thank Scott Henson, Copyeditor; Ryan Cook, Designer; and Jeff Patterson, Publishing Services Manager for all of their time, hard work, and dedication to the process of producing this book. The Elsevier team worked very hard to produce this quality textbook.

Contents

PROCEDURE

1

Combitube Insertion **AP** and Removal

Kyle Gibson

PURPOSE: A Combitube may be used to provide an emergency airway during resuscitation of a profoundly unconscious patient who needs artificial ventilation when endotracheal intubation is not readily available or has failed in successfully establishing an airway.

PREREQUISITE NURSING KNOWLEDGE

- Anatomy and physiology of the upper airway should be understood.
- The Combitube does not require direct visualization of the airway for insertion and is inserted in a "blind" fashion, as an adjunct when endotracheal intubation attempts fail or trauma makes visualization of the airway difficult.[1,10] The Combitube (Fig. 1-1) is available in two sizes, determined by patient height.
  - ❖ The 37F size is used for patients 48 to 66 inches tall (122 to 168 cm).
  - ❖ Either size 37F or size 41F is applicable in patients 60 to 66 inches tall (152 to 168 cm).
  - ❖ For patients ≥66 inches (168 cm), the 41F size should be used.
- The Combitube has a unique design that includes:
  - ❖ A double-lumen, semirigid airway
    - ○ Blue lumen opening to the perforations between the cuffs
    - ○ White lumen opening distal to the distal cuff
    - ○ Each lumen fitted with a 15-mm male adapter
  - ❖ Two cuffs for occlusion
    - ○ Proximal cuff (85 mL or 100 mL, depending on tube size) to occlude the hypopharynx
    - ○ Distal cuff (12 mL or 15 mL, depending on tube size) to occlude either the esophagus or the trachea
    - ○ Each cuff connected to a pilot balloon and valve: blue for proximal (No. 1), white for distal (No. 2)

- ❖ The two black lines located on the Combitube identify proper depth placement when aligned with the patient's teeth or gum line.
- The correct placement of a Combitube in the airway is as follows:
  - ❖ Esophageal insertion (Figs. 1-2 and 1-3), in which the distal cuff occludes the esophagus and the proximal balloon occludes the hypopharynx, allows ventilation via the blue lumen.
  - ❖ Tracheal insertion (Fig. 1-4), in which the distal cuff occludes the trachea and the proximal balloon occludes the hypopharynx, allows ventilation through the white lumen.
- Before the insertion of a Combitube, adequate ventilation of an unconscious patient with a mouth-to-mask or a bag-valve-mask device is necessary.
- In simulations, the Combitube has been successfully superior in situations of trismus, tongue edema, limited mobility of the cervical spine, or a combination of the above.[14]
- Use of the Combitube is contraindicated for airway management[10] in the following cases:
  - ❖ Patients with an intact gag reflex
  - ❖ Patients with known esophageal disease
  - ❖ Patients who have ingested caustic substances
  - ❖ Patients with a known or suspected foreign body in the hypopharynx
- The Combitube contains latex and may cause an allergic reaction in patients or in personnel who handle the device with sensitivity to latex.
- The Combitube is supplied either in a complete kit (with all of the necessary components for insertion), in soft or rigid packaging, or as a single individual device (without any of the necessary components for insertion). If the single individual device is used, additional components are necessary for insertion. See equipment list below.
- Initial and ongoing training is needed to maximize insertion success and minimize complications.[8]

AP This procedure should be performed only by physicians, advanced practice nurses, and other healthcare professionals (including critical care nurses) with additional knowledge, skills, and demonstrated competence per professional licensure or institutional standard.

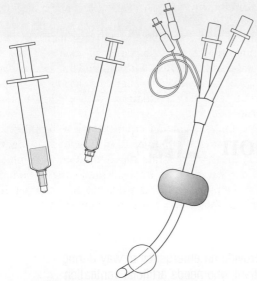

Figure 1-1 Components of the combitube.

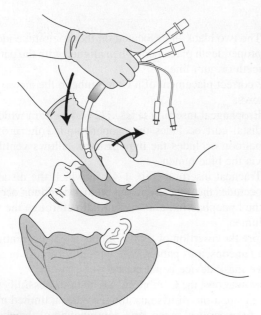

Figure 1-2 Esophageal insertion of a combitube.

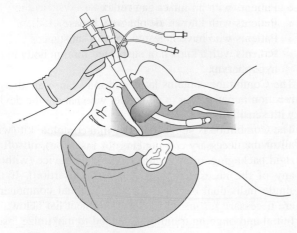

Figure 1-3 Combitube in esophageal position.

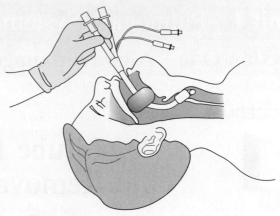

Figure 1-4 Combitube in tracheal position.

- Medications delivered via endotracheal tube cannot be used with a Combitube in the esophageal position. Medications may not reach the alveolar surfaces of the lung for absorption.
- The Combitube is intended for use up to 8 hours only.

EQUIPMENT

- Gloves, mask, gown, and eye protection
- Suction equipment (suction canister with control head, tracheal suction catheters, Yankauer suction tip)
- Combitube, of the appropriate size for the patient's height
- Large (100-mL) Luer-tip syringe
- Small (20-mL) Luer-tip syringe
- Water-soluble lubricant
- Oxygen source and tubing
- Mouth-to-mask or self-inflating manual resuscitation bag-valve-mask device and mask attached to a high-flow oxygen source
- Fluid deflector elbow
- Colormetric carbon dioxide (CO_2) device or end-tidal CO_2 detector with waveform capnography if available

PATIENT AND FAMILY EDUCATION

- If time allows, provide the family with information about the Combitube and the reason for insertion. ***Rationale:*** This information assists the family in understanding why the procedure is necessary and decreases their anxiety.

PATIENT ASSESSMENT AND PREPARATION
Patient Assessment

- Assess level of consciousness and responsiveness. ***Rationale:*** In an emergency situation, the Combitube should be inserted only into a patient who is profoundly unconscious, unresponsive, and unable to maintain adequate ventilation. Administration of neuromuscular blocking agents and sedation may be needed to ensure that the patient's gag reflex does not return while the Combitube is in place.[11]

- Assess history and patient information for possibility of esophageal disease or caustic substance ingestion. **Rationale:** A Combitube is contraindicated in patients with these conditions.[10]
- Assess patient's height. **Rationale:** This assessment allows the selection of an appropriately sized Combitube.
- Assess risk for hypertensive bleeding and take precautions if increased catecholamine stress response is likely. **Rationale:** Combitube insertion may cause pronounced catecholamine response.[6,12]

Patient Preparation

- Verify correct patient with two identifiers. **Rationale:** Prior to performing a procedure, the nurse should ensure the correct identification of the patient for the intended intervention.
- Ensure adequate ventilation and oxygenation with either a mouth-to-mask or a self-inflating manual resuscitation bag-valve-mask device. **Rationale:** The patient is nonresponsive and unable to maintain adequate ventilation without assisted ventilation before the Combitube insertion.
- Ensure that the suction equipment is assembled and in working order. **Rationale:** The patient may regurgitate during insertion or while the Combitube is in place and need oropharyngeal or tracheal suctioning or both.
- Perform a preprocedure verification and time out, if nonemergent. **Rationale:** Ensures patient safety.

Procedure	for Combitube Insertion	
Steps	**Rationale**	**Special Considerations**
1. 🔲HH		
2. 🔲PE		
3. Open the package and test the integrity of both cuffs. **(Level M*)**	Ensures that the device is not defective and will work as indicated.	
A. Pull the plunger back on the large syringe to the appropriate volume for the size of the tube and attach it to the proximal (blue) valve, marked "No. 1."	Readies the syringe for inflating the cuff.	Use 85-mL volume for the 37F size and 100-mL volume for the 41F size.
B. Inflate the proximal cuff with the appropriate volume and assess for leaks.	Ensures that the device is not defective and will work as indicated.	If a leak is found, discard the device and secure another.
C. Actively deflate the proximal cuff, leaving the syringe attached to the valve.	Provides for smoother insertion and readies the syringe for inflation after insertion.	
D. Pull the plunger back on the small syringe to the appropriate volume for the size of the tube and attach it to the distal (white) valve, marked "No. 2."	Readies the syringe for inflating the cuff.	Use 12-mL volume for the 37F size and 15-mL volume for the 41F size.
E. Inflate the distal cuff with the appropriate volume and assess for leaks.	Ensures that the device is not defective and will work as indicated.	If a leak is found, discard the device and secure another.
F. Actively deflate the distal cuff, leaving the syringe attached to the valve.	Provides for smoother insertion and readies the syringe for inflation after insertion.	
4. Lubricate the device with water-soluble lubricant. **(Level M)**	Facilitates and eases insertion.	
5. Attach a fluid deflector to the clear lumen marked "No. 2." **(Level M)**	Diverts any fluid that may be regurgitated through the tube during insertion away from the person inserting the device.	A fluid deflector is included in the kits but not in the single individual devices.

*Level M: Manufacturer's recommendations only.

Procedure continues on following page

Procedure for Combitube Insertion—*Continued*

Steps	Rationale	Special Considerations
6. Grasp the patient's jaw with one hand and pull up (or forward if the patient is in a sitting position), maintaining the head in a neutral position (see Fig. 1-4).[11] **(Level M*)**	Pulls the tongue forward and away from the hypopharynx.	With facial trauma, assess for the presence of broken teeth (real or artificial) and remove loose fragments. Maintain cervical spine precautions with suspected or known spine trauma. A Combitube used during airway management causes cervical spine movement less or equal to conventional laryngoscopes.[9] Use extreme caution to avoid puncturing the balloons during insertion.
7. Grasp the Combitube in the other hand so that it curves toward the patient's feet. **(Level M)**	Places the Combitube in the appropriate position for insertion.	
8. Insert the tip of the Combitube into the patient's mouth and advance it in a downward curving motion, maintaining a midline position, until the teeth or gum line is between the two black marks on the device. **(Level M)**	Allows the Combitube to follow the patient's hypopharynx until it is in the correct position.	***Do not force the Combitube.*** If it does not easily advance, attempt to redirect or remove and reinsert.
9. Inflate the proximal cuff with the appropriate volume, using the blue valve, marked "No. 1." **(Level M)**	Inflates and seats the proximal cuff into the posterior hypopharynx and seals it.	Use 85-mL volume for the 37F size and 100-mL volume for the 41F size. Significant resistance is felt as the cuff is inflated. Keep the syringe plunger depressed while removing it from the valve to prevent air escaping from the cuff.[4] If an air leak develops, add 10 mL of air at a time until the leak seals. Volumes of 150 mL may be needed for some individuals.[4]
10. Inflate the distal cuff with the appropriate volume, using the white valve, marked "No. 2." **(Level M)**	Inflates the distal cuff and seals the esophagus (or trachea) depending on location. Both locations allow the establishment of an effective airway.	Use 12-mL volume for the 37F size and 15-mL volume for the 41F size.
11. Connect the self-inflating manual resuscitation bag-valve device to the 15-mm adapter on the blue lumen, marked "No. 1," and ventilate. **(Level M)**	Most of the time, the distal balloon is in the esophagus.[2] With both cuffs inflated, the only place the ventilation can go is into the trachea.	

*Level M: Manufacturer's recommendations only.

Procedure   for Combitube Insertion—*Continued*

Steps	Rationale	Special Considerations
12. Assess for tube placement. **(Level M*)**	Determines placement of the tube and which lumen should be used to ventilate.	
A. Assess for gurgling over the epigastrium, chest rise and fall, and breath sounds in the lung fields with each ventilation.	If the distal cuff is in the esophagus, no gurgling is heard over the epigastrium and the ventilation expands the lungs, causing the chest to rise and fall and breath sounds to be heard over the lung fields. **Go to Step 13.** If the distal cuff is in the trachea, gurgling is heard over the epigastrium and no rise and fall of the chest is seen or breath sounds heard over the lung fields. **Go to Step 12B.** If no gurgling or breath sounds are noted with ventilation, the Combitube may have been advanced too far into the esophagus, blocking the perforations from the blue lumen. **Go to Step 12C.**	Listening over the epigastrium initially provides rapid determination that the ventilation is going into the esophagus.[1] When assessing for the presence of breath sounds, always consider the possibility of a pneumothorax. This condition can change the breath sounds presentation and lead the inserter to believe that the Combitube is misplaced.
B. Immediately switch the self-inflating manual resuscitation bag-valve device to the clear lumen, marked "No. 2," and attempt to ventilate, assessing for gurgling over the epigastrium, chest rise and fall, and breath sounds in the lung fields with ventilation.	If the distal cuff is in the trachea, no gurgling is heard over the epigastrium and the ventilation expands the lungs, causing the chest to rise and fall and breath sounds to be heard over the lung fields. **Go to Step 13.**	Listening over the epigastrium initially provides rapid determination that the ventilation is going into the esophagus.[1] When assessing for the presence of breath sounds, always consider the possibility of a pneumothorax. This condition can change the breath sounds presentation and lead the inserter to believe that the Combitube is misplaced.
C. Deflate the proximal cuff, using a syringe on the blue valve, marked "No. 1," withdraw the Combitube approximately 2 to 3 cm, and reinflate the "No. 1" cuff.	Allows for the repositioning of the Combitube so that the soft tissue of esophagus no longer occludes the blue lumen perforations. **Return to Step 9.**	If repositioning of the Combitube does not establish an effective airway, remove the device and establish an airway with alternative means.
13. Secure the Combitube with either tape or a manufactured tube holder (see Fig. 2-10).	Prevents the possibility of dislodgement.[3]	
14. Further assess device placement with an end-tidal carbon dioxide device,[2,13] or an esophageal detector device.[2,13] **(Level E*)**	Confirms proper placement with two additional methods.[4,5]	
15. Continue ventilation through whichever lumen provides the airway. **(Level M)**	Adequate ventilation can be achieved with the distal cuff of the Combitube in either the esophagus or the trachea.	

*Level E: Multiple case reports, theory-based evidence from expert opinions, or peer-reviewed professional organizational standards without clinical studies to support recommendations.
*Level M: Manufacturer's recommendations only.

Procedure continues on following page

Procedure	for Combitube Insertion—*Continued*	
Steps	Rationale	Special Considerations
16. Remove and discard PE.		
17. HH		
18. Document the procedure in the patient's record.		

Procedure	for Combitube Removal	
Steps	Rationale	Special Considerations
1. HH		
2. PE		
3. To remove the Combitube:	Removal is indicated within 8 hours of insertion or when skilled personnel can manage the patient's airway.	A fiber-optic scope may be used to replace a Combitube with an endotracheal tube. If the Combitube has been placed in the trachea, cricoid pressure should be established and maintained until the new airway is established.
A. Decompress the stomach.	Removes any contents from the stomach, which makes regurgitation less likely with removal of the device.	If the Combitube is placed in the esophagus, a small suction catheter may be inserted through the white "No. 2" lumen to decompress the stomach.
B. Attach a 100-mL syringe to the blue valve, marked "No. 1," and deflate the cuff.	Deflates the proximal cuff and allows suctioning of the hypopharynx.	
C. Suction the hypopharynx.	Removes secretions that may have accumulated in the hypopharynx.	
D. Attach a 20-mL syringe to the white valve, marked "No. 2," and deflate the cuff.	Deflates the distal cuff and allows the Combitube to be withdrawn.	
E. Withdraw the Combitube from the airway, and administer supplemental oxygen.	Allows the patient to breathe on his or her own and supplies supplemental oxygen to counter any hypoxia.	
4. Remove and discard PE.		
5. HH		
6. Document the procedure in the patient's record.		

Expected Outcomes

- Establishment of an effective airway in an emergency situation
- Maintenance of adequate ventilation and oxygenation
- Recovery of spontaneous ventilation

Unexpected Outcomes

- Complications from use of the Combitube related to insertion technique or excessive cuff pressures
- Sore throat[7]
- Dysphagia[7]
- Bleeding[15]
- Pharyngeal perforation[15]
- Esophageal lacerations[15]
- Esophageal rupture[15]
- Improper placement, resulting in hypoventilation

Patient Monitoring and Care

Steps	Rationale	Reportable Conditions
		These conditions should be reported if they persist despite nursing interventions.
1. Monitor ventilation effectiveness while the Combitube is in place by monitoring: A. Difficulty of ventilation. B. SpO_2. C. $PetCO_2$.	Determines that the Combitube is functioning correctly and providing adequate ventilation and oxygenation.	• Increased difficulty in ventilation • Unexplained decreases in oxygen saturation (SpO_2) or end-tidal carbon dioxide ($PetCO_2$) levels
2. Monitor for return of spontaneous attempts at breathing.	May indicate need either to remove the device or use medications (sedatives or nondepolarizing neuromuscular blockade) to prevent the gag reflex.[7]	

Documentation

Documentation should include the following:

- Assessment findings that indicate the need to insert a Combitube
- Confirmation of adequacy of ventilation, with auscultation of gastric area and lung fields with $PetCO_2$
- Any difficulties with placement of the Combitube
- $PetCO_2$ levels
- Need for sedation or neuromuscular blockade or both
- Assessment findings on removal of the Combitube, including work of breathing, breath sounds, and SpO_2 levels

- Assessment findings after insertion of the Combitube that indicate which lumen ventilates the patient
- Secondary confirmation of adequacy of ventilation, or an esophageal detection device, in conjunction with SpO_2 levels with ventilation
- Ongoing monitoring of difficulty or ease of ventilation
- SpO_2 levels
- Assessment findings that indicate the need to remove the Combitube or replace it with an endotracheal tube

References and Additional Readings

For a complete list of references and additional readings for this procedure, scan this QR code with any freely available smartphone code reader app, or visit http://booksite.elsevier.com/9780323376624.

2 Endotracheal Intubation AP (Perform)

Cindy Goodrich

PURPOSE: Endotracheal intubation is performed to establish and maintain a patent airway, facilitate oxygenation and ventilation, reduce the risk of aspiration, and assist with the clearance of secretions.

PREREQUISITE NURSING KNOWLEDGE

- Anatomy and physiology of the pulmonary system should be understood.
- Indications for endotracheal intubation include the following[15,20]:
  - Inadequate oxygenation and ventilation
  - Altered mental status (e.g., head injury, drug overdose) for airway protection
  - Anticipated airway obstruction (e.g., facial burns, epiglottitis, major facial or oral trauma)
  - Upper airway obstruction (e.g., from swelling, trauma, tumor, bleeding)
  - Apnea
  - Ineffective clearance of secretions (i.e., inability to maintain or protect airway adequately)
  - High risk of aspiration
  - Respiratory distress, respiratory failure
- Pulse oximetry should be used during intubation so that oxygen desaturation can be quickly detected and treated (see Procedure 18).[3,14]
- Proper positioning of the patient is critical for successful intubation.
- Two types of laryngoscope blades exist: straight and curved. The straight (Miller) blade is designed so that the tip extends below the epiglottis, to lift and expose the glottic opening. The straight blade is recommended for use in obese patients, pediatric patients, and patients with short necks because their tracheas may be located more anteriorly. When a curved (Macintosh) blade is used, the tip is advanced into the vallecula (the space between the epiglottis and the base of the tongue), to expose the glottic opening.
- Laryngoscope blades are available with bulbs or with a fiberoptic light delivery system. Fiberoptic light delivery systems provide a brighter light. Bulbs are prone to becoming scratched or covered with secretions.

- Videolaryngoscopy is gaining increased popularity as a method for oral intubation. This involves using fiberoptics or a micro video camera encased in the laryngoscope that provides a wide-angle view of the glottic opening while attempting oral intubation. Emerging literature supports this highly effective tool as a method to increase first-pass success by providing a superior view of the glottis compared with traditional direct laryngoscopy.[5,7,16] This method also requires minimal lifting force, resulting in less movement of the cervical spine during intubation.[13]
- Endotracheal tube size reflects the size of the internal diameter of the tube. Tubes range in size from 2 mm for neonates to 9 mm for large adults. Endotracheal tubes that range in size from 7 to 7.5 mm are used for average-sized adult women, whereas endotracheal tubes that range in size from 8 to 9 mm are used for average-sized adult men (Fig. 2-1).[9,10,20] The tube with the largest clinically acceptable internal diameter should be used to minimize airway resistance and assist in suctioning.
- Double-lumen endotracheal tubes are used for independent lung ventilation in situations with bleeding of one lung or a large air leak that would impair ventilation of the good lung.
- The patient's airway should be assessed before intubation. The LEMON[©] mnemonic can be used to determine whether a difficult intubation is anticipated.[3]
  - L = Look Externally: look for features associated with a difficult intubation such as a short neck, prominent incisors, broken teeth, a large protruding tongue, a narrow or abnormally shaped face, a receding jaw, or a prominent overbite.[3]
  - E = Evaluate using the 3-3-2 rule: These three rules help to determine whether there will be alignment of the pharyngeal, laryngeal, and oral axes.[3]
    - Three fingers: distance between upper and lower incisors in the mouth opening
    - Three fingers: distance between tip of chin and chin-neck junction (hyoid bone)
    - Two fingers: distance between thyroid cartilage and mandible
  - M = Mallampati Grade: This scoring system provides an estimate of the space available for oral intubation using direct laryngoscopy. It relates the amount of mouth opening to the size of the tongue. Classes 1 and

AP This procedure should be performed only by physicians, advanced practice nurses, and other healthcare professionals (including critical care nurses) with additional knowledge, skills, and demonstrated competence per professional licensure or institutional standard.

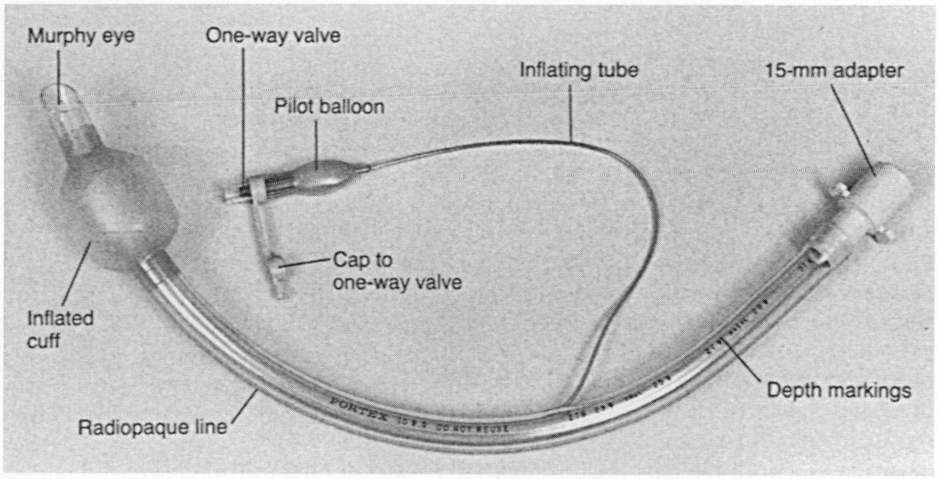

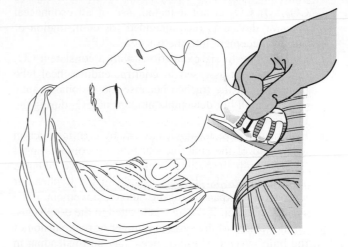

Murphy eye   One-way valve

Pilot balloon

Inflating tube   15-mm adapter

Cap to
one-way valve

Inflated
cuff

Depth markings

Radiopaque line

Figure 2-1 Parts of the endotracheal tube (Soft-Cuffed Tube by Smiths Industries Medical Systems, Co, Valencia, CA). *(From Kersten LD: Comprehensive respiratory nursing, Philadelphia, 1989, Saunders, 637.)*

2 predict a routine laryngoscopy, class 3 predicts difficulty, and class 4 predicts extreme difficulty. The patient is asked to open his or her mouth as wide as possible, sticking the tongue out. Look into the mouth using a light to assess the amount of hypopharynx that is visible.[3]

❖ O = Obstruction: Look for causes that might interfere with intubation, such as tonsillar abscess, epiglottitis, trauma, tumors, swollen tongue, and obesity.[3]

❖ N = Neck Mobility: Look for conditions that might limit neck range of motion such as a hard cervical collar (trauma), ankylosing spondylitis, previous neck surgery, and rheumatoid arthritis. If trauma is not suspected, ask the patient to touch his or her chin to his or her chest and extend the neck to the ceiling.[3]

• Visualization of the vocal cords can be aided by using laryngeal manipulation. This is accomplished by applying backward, upward, and rightward pressure (BURP) on the thyroid cartilage to move the larynx to the right while the tongue is displaced to the left by the laryngoscope blade.[3]

• Application of cricoid pressure (Sellick maneuver) may increase the success of the intubation as long as it does not interfere with ventilation or placement of the endotracheal tube. This procedure is accomplished by applying firm downward pressure on the cricoid ring, pushing the vocal cords downward so that they are visualized more easily (Fig. 2-2). When applied correctly it may protect against insufflation of the stomach and aspiration of the lungs. If applied incorrectly it may interfere with ventilation and make laryngoscopy intubation more difficult. *Once begun, cricoid pressure must be maintained until intubation is completed* unless there is difficulty intubating or ventilating the patient. The routine use of cricoid pressure is not recommended during cardiac arrest.[14]

• Endotracheal intubation can be done via nasal or oral routes. The route selected will depend on the skill of the practitioner performing the intubation and the patient's clinical condition.

• Nasal intubation requires a patient who is breathing spontaneously and is relatively contraindicated in trauma

Figure 2-2 Cricoid pressure. Firm downward pressure on the cricoid ring pushes the vocal cords downward toward the field of vision while sealing the esophagus against the vertebral column.

patients with facial fractures or suspected fractures at the base of the skull, and after cranial surgeries, such as transnasal hypophysectomy.[3]

• Improper intubation technique may result in trauma to the teeth, soft tissues of the mouth or nose, vocal cords, and posterior pharynx.

• In trauma patients with suspected spinal cord injuries and those not completely evaluated, manual in-line cervical immobilization of the head must be maintained during endotracheal intubation to keep the head in a neutral position. An assistant should be directed to manually immobilize the head and neck by placing his or her hands on either side of the patient's head, with thumbs along the mandible and fingers behind the head on the occipital ridge. Gentle but firm stabilization should be maintained throughout the procedure.[3,10]

• Confirmation of endotracheal tube placement should be done immediately after intubation to protect against unrecognized esophageal intubation. This includes using both clinical findings and end-tidal carbon dioxide(CO_2).[3,4,14]

❖ Clinical findings consistent with tracheal placement include visualization of the tube passing through the vocal cords, absence of gurgling over the epigastric area, auscultation of bilateral breath sounds, bilateral chest rise and fall during ventilation, and mist in the tube.[14,15]

❖ End-tidal CO_2 detectors assist in confirming proper placement of the endotracheal tube into the trachea (see Procedure 14). The presence of CO_2 in the expired air indicates that the airway has been successfully intubated, but does not ensure the correct position of the endotracheal tube.

❖ Disposable end-tidal CO_2 detectors are chemically treated with a nontoxic indicator that changes color in the presence of CO_2.

❖ Continuous end-tidal CO_2 (capnography) assists in confirming proper placement of the endotracheal tube into the trachea as well as allowing for detection of future tube dislodgment.

❖ During cardiac arrest (nonperfusing rhythms), low pulmonary blood flow may cause insufficient expired CO_2.[22] If CO_2 is not detected, use of an esophageal detector device is recommended for confirmation of proper placement into the trachea.[2,3,14,18,23]

❖ At least five to six exhalations with a consistent CO_2 level must be assessed to confirm endotracheal tube placement in the trachea because the esophagus may yield a small but detectable amount of CO_2 during the first few breaths.[15]

❖ Esophageal detector devices work by creating suction at the end of the endotracheal tube by compressing a flexible bulb or pulling back on a syringe plunger. When the tube is placed correctly in the trachea, air allows for reexpansion of the bulb or movement of the syringe plunger. If the tube is located in the esophagus, no movement of the syringe plunger or reexpansion of the bulb is seen. These devices may be misleading in patients who are morbidly obese, in status asthmaticus, late in pregnancy, or in patients with large amounts of tracheal secretions.[14]

• Endotracheal tube cuff pressure should be checked after verifying correct endotracheal tube position. The cuff pressure recommended for assistance in preventing both microaspiration and tracheal damage is 20 to 30 cm H_2O.[11,17,19]

• Intubation attempts should take no longer than 15 to 20 seconds. If more than one intubation attempt is necessary, ventilation with 100% oxygen using a self-inflating manual resuscitation bag device with a tight-fitting face mask should be performed for 3 to 5 minutes before each attempt. If intubation is not successful after three attempts, consider using another airway adjunct, such as a laryngeal mask airway (LMA), Combitube, or King LT Airway (see Procedures 1, 7, and 8).

• It is important to have a clearly defined difficult/failed airway plan and alternative airway equipment available at the bedside in case of unsuccessful intubation. This may consist of a gum elastic bougie, LMA, and videolaryngoscope. Surgical airway equipment such as that needed for a cricothyroidotomy should be available at the bedside in case of a failed airway.[15]

• This procedure should be performed only by physicians, advanced practice nurses, and other healthcare professionals (including critical care nurses) with additional knowledge, skills, and demonstrated competence per professional licensure and institutional standard.

EQUIPMENT

• Personal protective equipment, including eye protection
• Endotracheal tube with intact cuff and 15-mm connector (women, 7-mm to 7.5-mm tube; men, 8-mm to 9-mm tube)
• Laryngoscope handle with fresh batteries
• Laryngoscope blades (straight and curved)
• Spare bulb for laryngoscope blades
• Flexible stylet
• Magill forceps (to remove foreign bodies obstructing the airway if present)
• Self-inflating manual resuscitation bag-valve-mask device with tight fitting face mask connected to supplemental oxygen (15 L/min)
• Oxygen source
• Luer-tip 10-mL syringe for cuff inflation
• Water-soluble lubricant
• Rigid pharyngeal suction-tip (Yankauer) catheter
• Suction apparatus (portable or wall)
• Suction catheters
• Bite-block or oropharyngeal airway
• Endotracheal tube–securing apparatus or appropriate tape
  ❖ Commercially available endotracheal tube holder
  ❖ Adhesive tape (6 to 8 inches long)
• Stethoscope
• Monitoring equipment: cardiac monitor, pulse oximetry, and sphygmomanometer
• Disposable end-tidal CO_2 detector, continuous end-tidal CO_2 monitoring device, and esophageal detection device
• Drugs for intubation as indicated (induction agent, sedation, paralyzing agents, lidocaine, atropine)
• Assortment of oropharyngeal airways and nasopharyngeal airways
• Rescue airways such as LMA, King LT, or Combitube
• Failed airway equipment: gum elastic bougie, videolaryngoscope, optical stylet fiberoptic scope, and cricothyroidotomy kit

Additional equipment, to have available as needed, includes the following:

• Anesthetic spray (nasal approach)
• Local anesthetic jelly (nasal approach)
• Ventilator

PATIENT AND FAMILY EDUCATION

• If time permits, assess the patient's and the family's level of understanding about the condition and rationale for endotracheal intubation. **Rationale:** This assessment identifies the patient's and the family's knowledge deficits concerning the patient's condition, the procedure, the expected benefits, and the potential risks. It also allows time for questions to clarify information and voice concerns. Explanations decrease patient anxiety and enhance cooperation.

- Explain the procedure and the reason for intubation, if the clinical situation permits. If not, explain the procedure and reason for the intubation after it is completed. **Rationale:** This explanation enhances patient and family understanding and decreases anxiety.
- If indicated and the clinical situation permits, explain the patient's role in assisting with insertion of the endotracheal tube. **Rationale:** This explanation elicits the patient's cooperation, which assists with insertion.
- Explain that the patient will be unable to speak while the endotracheal tube is in place but that other means of communication will be provided. **Rationale:** This information enhances patient and family understanding and decreases anxiety.
- Explain that the patient's hands are often immobilized to prevent accidental dislodgment of the tube. **Rationale:** This information enhances patient and family understanding and decreases anxiety.

PATIENT ASSESSMENT AND PREPARATION

Patient Assessment

- Verify correct patient with two identifiers. **Rationale:** Prior to performing a procedure, the nurse should ensure the correct identification of the patient for the intended intervention.
- Assess for recent history of trauma with suspected spinal cord injury or cranial surgery. **Rationale:** Knowledge of pertinent patient history allows for selection of the most appropriate method for intubation, which helps reduce the risk of secondary injury.
- Assess nothing-by-mouth status, the use of a self-inflating manual resuscitation bag-valve device with mask before intubation, and for signs of gastric distention. **Rationale:** Increased risk of aspiration and vomiting occurs with accumulation of air (from the use of a self-inflating manual resuscitation bag-valve-mask device), food, or secretions.
- Assess level of consciousness, level of anxiety, and respiratory difficulty. **Rationale:** This assessment determines the need for sedation or the use of paralytic agents and the patient's ability to lie flat and supine for intubation.
- Assess oral cavity for presence of dentures, loose teeth, or other possible obstructions and remove if appropriate. **Rationale:** Ensures that the airway is free from any obstructions.
- Assess vital signs and assess for the following: tachypnea, dyspnea, shallow respirations, cyanosis, apnea, altered level of consciousness, tachycardia, cardiac dysrhythmias, hypertension, and headache. **Rationale:** Any of these conditions may indicate a problem with oxygenation or ventilation or both.
- Assess patency of nares (for nasal intubation). **Rationale:** Selection of the most appropriate naris facilitates insertion and may improve patient tolerance of the tube.
- Assess need for premedication. **Rationale:** Various medications provide sedation or paralysis of the patient as needed.

Patient Preparation

- Perform a preprocedure verification and time out. **Rational:** Ensures patient safety.
- Ensure that the patient understands preprocedural teaching, if appropriate. Answer questions as they arise, and reinforce information as needed. **Rationale:** Understanding of previously taught information is evaluated and reinforced.
- Before intubation, initiate intravenous or intraosseous access. **Rationale:** Readily available intravenous or intraosseous access may be necessary if the patient needs to be sedated or paralyzed or needs other medications because of a negative response to the intubation procedure.
- Position the patient appropriately.
  - Positioning of the nontrauma patient is as follows: place the patient supine with the head in the sniffing position, in which the head is extended and the neck is flexed. Placement of a small towel under the occiput elevates it several inches, allowing for proper flexion of the neck (Fig. 2-3). **Rationale:** Placement of the head in the sniffing position allows for better visualization of the larynx and vocal cords by aligning the axes of the mouth, pharynx, and trachea.
  - Positioning of the trauma patient is as follows: manual in-line cervical spinal immobilization must be maintained during the entire process of intubation. **Rationale:** Because cervical spinal cord injury must be suspected in all trauma patients until proved otherwise, this position helps prevent secondary injury should a cervical spine injury be present.
- Premedicate as indicated. **Rationale:** Appropriate premedication allows for more controlled intubation, reducing the incidence of insertion trauma, aspiration, laryngospasm, and improper tube placement.
- As appropriate, notify the respiratory therapy department of impending intubation so that a ventilator can be set up. **Rationale:** The ventilator is set up before intubation.

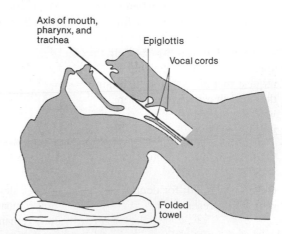

Figure 2-3 Neck hyperextension in the sniffing position aligns the axis of the mouth, pharynx, and trachea before endotracheal intubation. (*From Kersten LD: Comprehensive respiratory nursing, Philadelphia, 1989, Saunders, 642.*)

Procedure for Performing Endotracheal Intubation

Steps	Rationale	Special Considerations
General Setup		
1. ⬛ **HH**		
2. ⬛ **PE**		
3. Establish intravenous or intraosseous access if not present.	Provides access to deliver indicated medications.	
4. Attach patient to monitoring equipment including cardiac and blood pressure monitor and pulse oximeter.	Provides continuous patient monitoring during intubation.	
5. Set up suction apparatus, and connect rigid suction-tip catheter to tubing.	Prepares for oropharyngeal suctioning as needed.	
6. Check equipment.		
A. Choose appropriate-sized endotracheal tube.	Appropriate-sized endotracheal tubes facilitate both intubation and ventilation.	Generally a 7–7.5-mm internal diameter tube is used for adult females and an 8–9-mm internal diameter for adult males.[9,10,14,20]
B. Use 10-mL syringe to inflate cuff on tube, assessing for leaks. Completely deflate cuff.	Verifies that equipment is functional and that tube cuff is patent without leaks; prepares tube for insertion.	Once the endotracheal tube cuff has been checked for leaks and it is completely deflated, place back into its packaging to avoid contamination.
C. Insert the stylet into the endotracheal tube, ensuring that the tip of the stylet does not extend past the end of the endotracheal tube.	Provides structural support for the flexible endotracheal tube during insertion. Maintaining the tip of the stylet within the lumen of the endotracheal tube prevents damage to the vocal cords and trachea.	Stylet must be recessed by at least 0.5 inch from the distal end of the tube so that it does not protrude beyond the end of the tube.
D. Connect the laryngoscope blade to the handle, and ensure the blade's bulb is securely seated.	Verifies that the equipment is functional.	Check the bulb for brightness. Replace bulb if dull or burnt out.
7. Assess patient's airway to determine whether a difficult intubation is anticipated. **(Level D*)**	Use of LEMON© mnemonic can assist in determination of difficult intubation.[3]	
8. Position the patient's head by flexing the neck forward and extending the head, in sniffing position (only if neck trauma is not suspected; see Fig. 2-3). If spinal trauma is suspected, request that an assistant maintain the head in a neutral position with in-line spinal immobilization.	Allows for visualization of the vocal cords with alignment of the mouth, pharynx, and trachea.	The ear (external auditory meatus) and sternal notch should be aligned when patient is examined from the side. This allows for flexion of the cervical spine.[15] Placement of a small towel under the occiput elevates it, allowing for proper neck flexion. *Do not flex or extend neck of patient with suspected spinal cord injury; the head must be maintained in a neutral position with manual in-line cervical spine immobilization.*[3]
9. Check the mouth for dentures and remove if present.	Dentures should be removed before oral intubation is attempted but may remain in place for nasal intubation.	

*Level D: Peer-reviewed professional and organizational standards with the support of clinical study recommendations.

Procedure for Performing Endotracheal Intubation—*Continued*

Steps	Rationale	Special Considerations
10. Suction the mouth and pharynx as needed if copious secretions are visualized.	Provides for a clear view of the posterior pharynx and larynx.	
11. Insert oropharyngeal airway if indicated (see Procedure 9).	Assists in maintenance of upper airway patency. Helps to improve ability to ventilate during bag-valve-mask ventilation.	Use only in unconscious patients with an absent gag reflex.
12. Preoxygenate for 3–5 minutes, with 100% oxygen via a nonrebreather mask if ventilations are adequate or via a self-inflating manual resuscitation bag-valve-mask device (see Procedure 31) if ventilations are inadequate. **(Level D*)**	Helps prevent hypoxemia. Gentle breaths reduce incidence of air entering stomach (leading to gastric distention, aspiration), decrease airway turbulence, and distribute ventilation more evenly within the lungs. Preoxygenation ensures that nitrogen is washed out of the lungs and will extend the allowable apneic time until the oxygen in the lungs is used up.[4,15]	Bag-valve-mask ventilation may not be needed in the spontaneous breathing patient. Avoid aggressive positive-pressure ventilation with a self-inflating manual resuscitation bag because this may increase the risk for gastric vomiting.
13. Premedicate patient as indicated.	Sedates and relaxes the patient, allowing easier intubation.	
14. Remove oropharyngeal airway if present. For nasotracheal intubation, proceed to Step 35	Clears the airway for advancement of the laryngoscope blade and endotracheal tube.	
Orotracheal Intubation		
15. Grasp laryngoscope (with blade in place and illuminated light on) in left hand.	Prepares for efficient blade placement.	Grasp handle as low as possible and keep wrist rigid to prevent using upper teeth as a fulcrum.
16. Use fingers of right hand to open the mouth.	Provides access to oral cavity.	Use a scissor-like motion with thumb and second finger of right hand to gently open the mouth. Hold the tips of the thumb and middle finger of the right hand together. Insert them between the upper and lower incisors. Using a scissor-like motion move fingers past one another by flexing each finger.[15]
17. Using a controlled motion, slowly insert the blade into the right side of the patient's mouth, using it to push the tongue to the left (Fig. 2-4). Advance the blade inward and toward midline past the base of the tongue.	Displaces the tongue to the left, increasing visualization of the glottic opening (Fig. 2-5).	Avoid pressure on the teeth and lips. Inserting the blade smoothly and quickly obtaining an optimal view of the glottis opening will help to increase first-pass success.[15] If the patient's chest is obstructing placement of the laryngoscope handle, consider placing blankets or towels under the head and upper back to elevate the head relative to the chest. Do not do this if cervical spine injury is suspected.[15] In trauma victims, consider turning the handle 90 degrees to insert the blade into the mouth and rotate to midline as the blade is advanced.

*Level D: Peer-reviewed professional and organizational standards with the support of clinical study recommendations.

Procedure continues on following page

Procedure   **for Performing Endotracheal Intubation—*Continued***

Steps	Rationale	Special Considerations

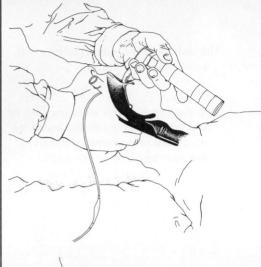

Figure 2-4 Technique of orotracheal intubation. The laryngoscope blade is inserted into the oral cavity from the right, pushing the tongue to the left as it is introduced.

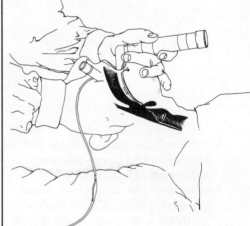

Figure 2-5 The blade is advanced into the oropharynx, and the laryngoscope is lifted to expose the epiglottis.

18. Visually identify the epiglottis and vocal cords.

Identification of anatomical landmarks provides landmarks for successful intubation

External laryngeal manipulation (BURP) may assist with visualization of the vocal cords.[3] Apply BURP on the thyroid cartilage to move the larynx to the right while the tongue is displaced to the left by the laryngoscope blade.[3] This may be done by the intubator or by an assistant.

Cricoid pressure (Sellick maneuver) may provide increased visualization of the vocal cords by moving the trachea posteriorly. This is accomplished by applying firm downward pressure on the cricoid ring, pushing the vocal cords downward so that they are visualized more easily (see Fig. 2-1). *Once cricoid pressure is applied, it must be maintained until the intubation is completed.* The routine use of cricoid pressure is not recommended during cardiac arrest.[14]

Procedure | **for Performing Endotracheal Intubation—*Continued***

Steps	Rationale	Special Considerations
19. Carefully advance the blade toward the epiglottis in a well-controlled manner.	Identification of the epiglottis is key for successful direct laryngoscopy intubation.	
A. With a curved blade, advance tip into vallecula (area between the base of the tongue and the epiglottis) and exert outward and upward gentle traction at a 45-degree angle (decreases the risk of teeth inadvertently being used as a fulcrum). Lift the laryngoscope in the direction of the handle to lift the tongue and posterior pharyngeal structures out of the way, allowing for exposure of the glottis opening. Do not allow the handle to lever back, causing the blade to hit the teeth.	Exposes the glottic opening. This lifting motion elevates the epiglottis, keeping the tongue out of the way, allowing for maximal exposure of the glottis.	Keep left arm and back straight when pulling upward, allowing for use of shoulders when lifting patient's head to the bed (Fig. 2-6). Levering back on the laryngoscope handle will impair the view and may damage the teeth. Touching the teeth indicates excessive levering or ineffective lift.[15]

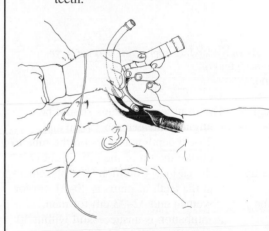

Figure 2-6 The tip of the blade is placed in the vallecula, and the laryngoscope is lifted further to expose the glottis. The tube is inserted through the right side of the mouth.

Steps	Rationale	Special Considerations
B. With a straight blade, advance tip just beneath the epiglottis and exert gentle traction outward and upward at a 45-degree angle to the bed. Blade may be inserted to the right of the tongue into the natural gutter between the lower molars (paraglossal technique) or midline.[15] Do not allow the handle to lever back, causing the blade to hit the teeth.	Exposes the glottic opening. Using the paraglossal technique allows for a better view by displacing the tongue with minimal effort.[15]	Keep left arm and back straight when pulling upward, allowing for use of shoulders when lifting patient's head (decreases use of teeth as a fulcrum). Using a straight blade may provide a better view when the larynx is more anterior or in those with a receding chin.[15] Midline insertion of the blade often results in difficulty in controlling the tongue which may obscure the view, particularly in unconscious adults.
20. Lift the laryngoscope handle up and away from the operator (at a 45- to 55-degree angle from the trachea) until the vocal cords are visualized.	Allows for correct placement of tube into trachea (Fig. 2-7).	Do not use the blade as a pry bar; this may result in damage to the teeth or mouth.[15] BURP may assist with visualization of the vocal cords.[3]

Procedure continues on following page

Procedure for Performing Endotracheal Intubation—*Continued*

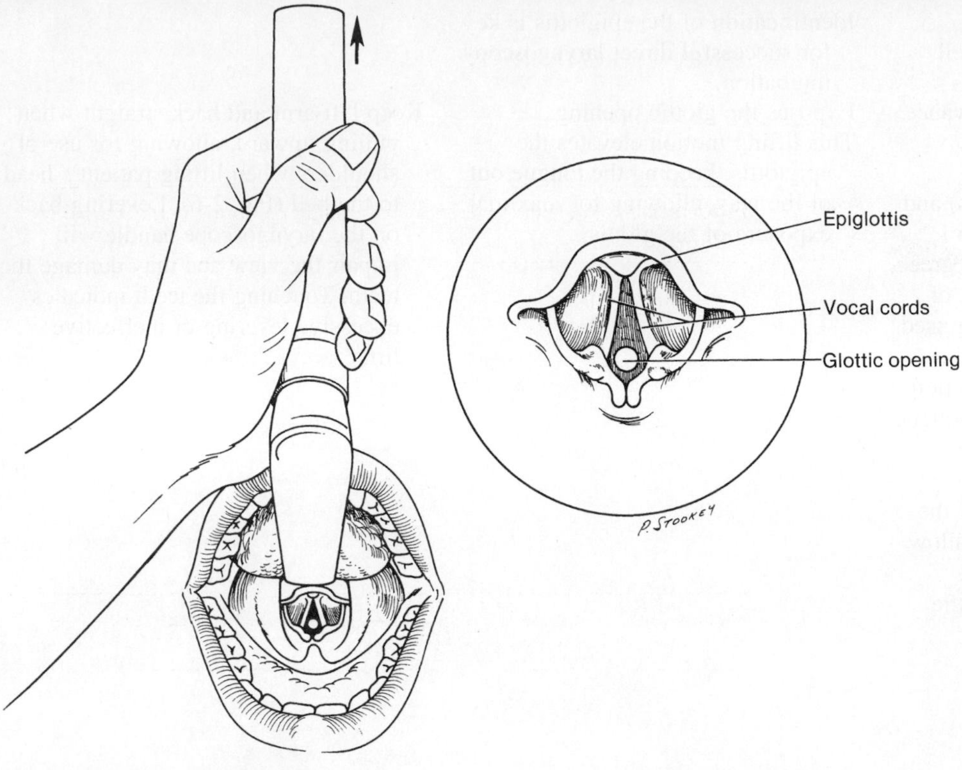

Steps	Rationale	Special Considerations

Epiglottis

Vocal cords

Glottic opening

Figure 2-7 The endotracheal tube is passed through the vocal cords. (*From Flynn JM, Bruce NP: Introduction to critical care skills, St Louis, 1993, Mosby, 56.*)

Steps	Rationale	Special Considerations
21. Hold end of tube in right hand with curved portion downward.	Tube is placed with the right hand.	
22. With use of direct vision, gently insert tube from right corner of mouth through the vocal cords (Fig. 2-8) until the cuff is no longer visible and has passed through the vocal cords (Fig. 2-9). Do not apply pressure on the teeth or oral tissues.	Tube must be seen passing through the vocal cords to ensure proper placement. Advance tube 1.25–2.5 cm farther into the trachea. When correctly positioned, the tip of the tube should be halfway between the vocal cords and the carina.[4,14]	The front teeth or gums should be aligned between the 19-cm and 23-cm depth markings on the tube to ensure the tip of the tube is above the carina.[4] Common tube placement at the teeth or gums is 20–21 cm for women and 22–23 cm for men.[10,15] If intubation is unsuccessful within 30 seconds, or the patient's oxygen saturations falls below 90% during the attempt, remove the tube.[15] Ventilate with 100% oxygen with a bag-valve-mask device before another intubation attempt is made (repeat Steps 13 through 20). Before reattempting intubation, correct problems related to positioning, procedure, or equipment.

Procedure **for Performing Endotracheal Intubation—*Continued***

Steps	Rationale	Special Considerations

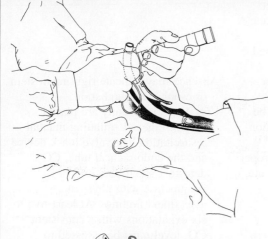

Figure 2-8 The tube is advanced through the vocal cords into the trachea.

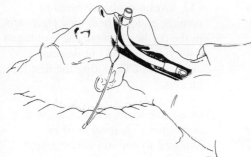

Figure 2-9 The tube is positioned so that the cuff is below the vocal cords, and the laryngoscope is removed.

Steps	Rationale	Special Considerations
23. When the tube is correctly placed, continue to hold it securely in place at the lips with right hand while first withdrawing the laryngoscope blade and then the stylet with left hand.	Firmly holding tube at the lips provides stabilization and prevents inadvertent extubation.	An assistant may remove the stylet while the intubator firmly holds the endotracheal tube in place, preventing dislodgement of the tube.
24. Inflate cuff with 5–10 mL of air depending on the manufacturer's recommendation. Do not overinflate the cuff. **(Level M*)**	Inflation volumes vary depending on manufacturer and size of tube. Keep cuff pressure between 20 and 30 mm Hg to decrease risk of aspiration and prevent ischemia and decreased blood flow.[11,14]	In adults, decreased mucosal capillary blood flow (ischemia) results when pressure is greater than 40 mm Hg.[4,14] Consider using manometer to measure cuff pressure and increase or decrease pressure as indicated to achieve cuff pressure of 20–30 mm Hg.[11,14]
25. Confirm endotracheal tube placement while manually bagging with 100% oxygen.	Ensures correct placement of endotracheal tube.	
A. Auscultate over epigastrium. **(Level D*)**	Allows for identification of esophageal intubation.[4,14]	If air movement or gurgling is heard, esophageal intubation has occurred. The tube must be removed and intubation reattempted. Improper insertion may result in hypoxemia, gastric distention, vomiting, and aspiration.

*Level D: Peer-reviewed professional and organizational standards with the support of clinical study recommendations.
*Level M: Manufacturer's recommendations only.

Procedure continues on following page

Procedure   for Performing Endotracheal Intubation—*Continued*

Steps	Rationale	Special Considerations
B. Auscultate lung bases and apices for bilateral breath sounds. **(Level D)**	Assists in verification of correct tube placement into the trachea. A right main-stem bronchus intubation results in diminished left-sided breath sounds.[3,4]	
C. Observe for symmetrical chest wall movement. **(Level D)**	Assists in verification of correct tube placement.[3,4,14]	Absence may indicate right main stem or esophageal intubation.
D. Attach disposable end-tidal CO_2 detector. Watch for color change, which indicates the presence of CO_2. **(Level B*)**	Disposable CO_2 detectors may be used to assist with identification of proper tube placement.[6,9,18,21] Detection of CO_2 confirms proper endotracheal tube placement into the trachea.[3,4,14]	CO_2 detectors usually are placed between the self-inflating manual resuscitation bag-valve mask device and the endotracheal tube. CO_2 detectors should be used in conjunction with physical assessment findings. At least five to six exhalations with a consistent CO_2 level must be assessed to confirm endotracheal tube placement in the trachea because the esophagus may yield a small but detectable amounts of CO_2 during the first few breaths.[15]
or Attach continuous end-tidal CO_2 monitor and watch for detection of CO_2 (see Procedure 14). **(Level B)**	Continuous end-tidal CO_2 is a reliable indicator of proper tube placement and also allows for detection of future tube dislodgment.[14]	At least five to six exhalations with a consistent CO_2 level must be assessed to confirm endotracheal tube placement in the trachea since the esophagus may yield small but detectable amounts of CO_2 during the first few breaths.[15]
or Consider use of esophageal detection device in cardiac arrest. **(Level B)**	During cardiac arrest (nonperfusing rhythms), low pulmonary blood flow may cause insufficient expired CO_2.[22] If CO_2 is not detected, use of an esophageal detector device is recommended.[2,8,12,18,23]	
E. Evaluate oxygen saturation (Spo_2) with noninvasive pulse oximetry. (see Procedure 18). **(Level D)**	Spo_2 decreases if the esophagus has been inadvertently intubated. The value may or may not change in a right main-stem bronchus intubation.[4,14]	Spo_2 findings should be used in conjunction with physical assessment findings.
26. If CO_2 detection, assessment findings, or Spo_2 reveals that the tube is not correctly positioned, deflate cuff and remove tube immediately. Ventilate and hyperoxygenate with 100% oxygen for 3–5 minutes, then reattempt intubation, beginning with Step 13.	Esophageal intubation results in gas flow diversion and hypoxemia.[4,14]	

*Level B: Well-designed, controlled studies with results that consistently support a specific action, intervention, or treatment.
*Level D: Peer-reviewed professional and organizational standards with the support of clinical study recommendations.

Procedure	for Performing Endotracheal Intubation—*Continued*	
Steps	**Rationale**	**Special Considerations**
27. If breath sounds are absent on the left, deflate the cuff and withdraw tube 1-2 cm. Reevaluate for correct tube placement (Step 25).	Absence of breath sounds on the left may indicate right main-stem intubation, which is common because of the anatomical position of the right main-stem bronchi.[2]	When correctly positioned, the tube tip should be halfway between the vocal cords and the carina.
28. Connect endotracheal tube to oxygen source via self-inflating manual resuscitation bag-valve device, or mechanical ventilator, using swivel adapter.	Reduces motion on tube and mouth or nares.	
29. Insert a bite-block or oropharyngeal airway (to act as a bite-block) along the endotracheal tube, with oral intubation if indicated.	Prevents the patient from biting down on the endotracheal tube.	The bite-block should be secured separately from the tube to prevent dislodgment of the tube.
30. Secure the endotracheal tube in place (according to institutional standard). **(Level B*)**	Prevents inadvertent dislodgment of tube.[1,4,9,14]	Commercial tube holder or tape should not cause compression on sides or front of the neck, which may result in impaired venous return to the brain.[14] Consider manually holding the endotracheal tube when moving the patient to prevent inadvertent dislodgement of the tube.
Use of Commercially Available Endotracheal Tube Holder		
A. Apply according to manufacturer's directions. **(Level M*)**	Allows for secure stabilization of the tube, decreasing the likelihood of inadvertent extubation.	Commercially available tube holders are often more comfortable for patients and easier to manage if the endotracheal tube is manipulated.[15]
Use of Adhesive Tape		
A. Prepare tape as shown in Fig. 2-10.	Use of a hydrocolloid membrane on the patient's cheeks helps protect the skin.	

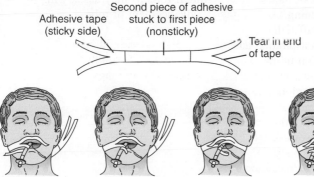

Adhesive tape (sticky side)
Second piece of adhesive stuck to first piece (nonsticky)
Tear in end of tape

Figure 2-10 Methods of securing adhesive tape. Example protocol for securing the endotracheal tube with adhesive tape. 1. Clean the patient's skin with mild soap and water. 2. Remove oil from the skin with alcohol and allow to dry. 3. Apply a skin adhesive product to enhance tape adherence. (When the tape is removed, an adhesive remover is necessary.) 4. Place a hydrocolloid membrane over the cheeks to protect friable skin. 5. Secure with adhesive tape as shown. *(From Henneman E, Ellstrom K, St John RE: AACN protocols for practice: Care of the mechanically ventilated patient series, Aliso Viejo, CA, 1999, American Association of Critical-Care Nurses, 56.)*

*Level B: Well-designed, controlled studies with results that consistently support a specific action, intervention, or treatment.
*Level M: Manufacturer's recommendations only.

Procedure continues on following page

Procedure for Performing Endotracheal Intubation—*Continued*

Steps	Rationale	Special Considerations
B. Secure tube by wrapping double-sided tape around patient's head and torn tape edges around endotracheal tube.	Secures the endotracheal tube in place.	Tape should not cause compression on sides or front of the neck, which may impair venous return to the brain.[14]
31. Reevaluate for correct tube placement (Step 25).	Verifies that the tube was not inadvertently displaced during the securing of the tube.	
32. Note position of tube at teeth or gums (use centimeter markings on tube).	Establishes a baseline for future assessment of possible endotracheal tube migration, in or out.	Common tube placement at the teeth or gums is 20–21 cm for women and 22–23 cm for men.[10,15]
33. Hyperoxygenate and suction endotracheal tube and pharynx (see Procedure 10) as needed.	Removes secretions that may obstruct tube or accumulate on the top of the cuff.	
34. Confirmation of correct tube position should be verified with a chest radiograph. (**Level D***)	Chest radiograph documents actual tube location (distance from the carina).	Because a chest radiograph is not immediately available, it should not be used as the primary method of tube assessment.[3,10,14]
Nasotracheal Intubation		
35. Follow Steps 1 through 14.	Steps necessary to initiate nasal intubation.	Dentures may be left in place for nasotracheal intubation.
36. Spray nasal passage with anesthetic and vasoconstrictor, as indicated or ordered.	Anesthetizes and vasoconstricts nasal mucosa to decrease incidence of trauma and bleeding.	
37. Lubricate tube with local anesthetic jelly.	Allows for smooth passage of tube.	
38. Slowly insert tube into selected naris, and guide tube up from the nostril, then backward and down into the nasopharynx.	Tube is introduced into airway channel.	
39. Gently advance the tube until maximal sound of moving air is heard through the tube.	Tube is located at opening of trachea.	Breath sounds become maximal just before entering the glottis.
40. While listening, continue to advance tube during inspiration.	Facilitates movement of tube through glottic opening.	Magill forceps may assist with advancement of tube.
41. When endotracheal tube is placed, inflate cuff. (See Step 24)	A properly inflated cuff will minimize secretion aspiration and facilitate stabilization in the trachea.	
42. Follow Steps 25-28 and 30-34 to evaluate tube placement and secure tube in place.	For nasotracheal intubation note position of tube at nare.	
43. Remove PE.	Reduces transmission of microorganisms and body secretions; Standard Precautions.	
44. HH		

---

*Level D: Peer-reviewed professional and organizational standards with the support of clinical study recommendations.

Expected Outcomes	Unexpected Outcomes
• Placement of patent artificial airway • Properly positioned and secured airway • Improved oxygenation and ventilation • Facilitation of secretion clearance	• Intubation of esophagus or right main-stem bronchus (improper tube placement) • Accidental extubation • Cardiac dysrhythmias because of hypoxemia and vagal stimulation • Broken or dislodged teeth • Leaking of air from endotracheal tube cuff • Oral or nasal trauma with bleeding • Tracheal injury at tip of tube or at cuff site • Laryngeal edema • Vocal cord trauma • Suctioning of gastric contents or food from endotracheal tube (aspiration) • Obstruction of endotracheal tube

Patient Monitoring and Care

Steps	Rationale	Reportable Conditions
		These conditions should be reported if they persist despite nursing interventions.
1. Auscultate breath sounds on insertion, with every manipulation of the endotracheal tube and every 2–4 hours and as needed.	Allows for detection of tube movement or dislodgment.	• Absent, decreased, or unequal breath sounds
2. Maintain tube stability, with use of specially manufactured holder, twill tape, or adhesive tape.	Reduces risk of movement and dislodgment of tube.	• Unplanned extubation
3. Monitor and record position of tube at teeth, gums, or nose (in reference to centimeter markings on tube).	Provides for identification of tube migration.	• Tube movement from original position
4. Maintain endotracheal tube cuff pressure of 20–30 mm Hg.[11,14]	Provides adequate inflation to decrease aspiration risk and prevents overinflation of cuff to avoid tracheal damage.[11,14]	• Cuff pressure less than 20 or higher than 30 mm Hg that persists despite nursing interventions.
5. Hyperoxygenate and suction endotracheal tube, as needed (see Procedure 10).	Prevents obstruction of tube and resulting hypoxemia.	• Inability to pass a suction catheter • Copious, frothy, or bloody secretions • Significant change in amount or character of secretions
6. Assess for pain and inadequate sedation.	Allows identification of pain and/or discomfort related to the intubation.	• Pain not controlled by medications or nursing interventions • Observed ventilator dyssynchrony
7. Inspect nares or oral cavity once per shift while patient is intubated.	Allows for the detection of skin breakdown and necrosis.	• Redness, necrosis, skin breakdown

Procedure continues on following page

Documentation

Documentation should include the following:
- Patient and family education
- Vital signs before, during, and after intubation, including oxygen saturation and end-tidal CO_2.
- Size of endotracheal tube
- Type of intubation: oral or nasal
- Type and size of blade used
- Depth of endotracheal tube insertion in centimeters at teeth, gums, or naris
- Confirmation of tube placement, including chest radiograph, end-tidal CO_2 detector, and capnography (method of placement confirmation)
- Clinical confirmation of tube placement including assessment of breath sounds
- Measurement of cuff pressure
- Number of intubation attempts
- Use of any medications
- Patient response to procedure
- Occurrence of unexpected outcomes
- Pain assessment, interventions, and effectiveness

References and Additional Readings

For a complete list of references and additional readings for this procedure, scan this QR code with any freely available smartphone code reader app, or visit http://booksite.elsevier.com/9780323376624.

3 Endotracheal Intubation (Assist)

Cindy Goodrich

PURPOSE: Endotracheal intubation is performed to establish and maintain a patent airway, facilitate oxygenation and ventilation, reduce the risk of aspiration, and assist with the clearance of secretions.

PREREQUISITE NURSING KNOWLEDGE

- Anatomy and physiology of the pulmonary system should be understood.
- Indications for endotracheal intubation include the following[15,20]:
  - Inadequate oxygenation and ventilation
  - Altered mental status (e.g., head injury, drug overdose) for airway protection
  - Anticipated airway obstruction (e.g., facial burns, epiglottitis, major facial or oral trauma)
  - Upper airway obstruction (e.g., from swelling, trauma, tumor, bleeding)
  - Apnea
  - Ineffective clearance of secretions (i.e., inability to maintain or protect airway adequately)
  - High risk of aspiration
  - Respiratory distress, respiratory failure
- Pulse oximetry should be used during intubation so that oxygen desaturation can be quickly detected and treated (see Procedure 18).[3,14]
- Proper positioning of the patient is critical for successful intubation.
- Two types of laryngoscope blades exist: straight and curved. The straight (Miller) blade is designed so that the tip extends below the epiglottis to lift and expose the glottic opening. The straight blade is recommended for use in obese patients, pediatric patients, and patients with short necks because their tracheas may be located more anteriorly. When a curved (Macintosh) blade is used, the tip is advanced into the vallecula (the space between the epiglottis and the base of the tongue) to expose the glottic opening.
- Laryngoscope blades are available with bulbs or with a fiberoptic light delivery system. Fiberoptic light delivery systems provide a brighter light. Bulbs are prone to becoming scratched or covered with secretions.
- Video laryngoscopy is gaining increased popularity as a method for oral intubation. This involves using fiberoptics or a micro video camera encased in the laryngoscope that provides a wide-angle view of the glottic opening while attempting oral intubation. Emerging literature supports this highly effective tool as a method to increase first-pass success by providing a superior view of the glottis, compared with traditional direct laryngoscopy.[5,7,16] This method also requires minimal lifting force, resulting in less movement of the cervical spine during intubation.[13]
- Endotracheal tube size reflects the size of the internal diameter of the tube. Tubes range in size from 2 mm for neonates to 9 mm for large adults. Endotracheal tubes that range in size from 7 to 7.5 mm are used for average-sized adult women, whereas endotracheal tubes that range in size from 8 to 9 mm are used for average-sized adult men (see Fig. 2-2).[9,10,20] The tube with the largest clinically acceptable internal diameter should be used to minimize airway resistance and assist in suctioning.
- Double-lumen endotracheal tubes are used for independent lung ventilation in situations with bleeding of one lung or a large air leak that would impair ventilation of the good lung.
- Visualization of the vocal cords can be aided by using laryngeal manipulation. This is accomplished by applying backward, upward, and rightward pressure (BURP) on the thyroid cartilage to move the larynx to the right while the tongue is displaced to the left by the laryngoscope blade.[3]
- Application of cricoid pressure (Sellick maneuver) may increase the success of the intubation as long as it does not interfere with ventilation or placement of the endotracheal tube. This procedure is accomplished by applying firm downward pressure on the cricoid ring, pushing the vocal cords downward so that they are visualized more easily (see Fig. 2-1).When applied correctly it may protect against insufflation of the stomach and aspiration of the lungs. If applied incorrectly it may interfere with ventilation and make laryngoscopy intubation more difficult. *Once begun, cricoid pressure must be maintained until intubation is completed* unless there is difficulty intubating or ventilating the patient. The routine use of cricoid pressure is not recommended during cardiac arrest.[14]
- Endotracheal intubation can be done via nasal or oral routes. The route selected will depend on the skill of the practitioner performing the intubation and the patient's clinical condition.
- Nasal intubation requires a patient who is breathing spontaneously and is relatively contraindicated in trauma patients with facial fractures or suspected fractures at the

base of the skull and after cranial surgeries, such as trans-nasal hypophysectomy.[3]

- Improper intubation technique may result in trauma to the teeth, soft tissues of the mouth or nose, vocal cords, and posterior pharynx.
- In trauma patients with suspected spinal cord injuries and those not completely evaluated, manual in-line cervical immobilization of the head must be maintained during endotracheal intubation to keep the head in a neutral position. An assistant should be directed to manually immobilize the head and neck by placing his or her hands on either side of the patient's head, with thumbs along the mandible and fingers behind the head on the occipital ridge. Gentle, but firm stabilization should be maintained throughout the procedure.[3,10]
- Confirmation of endotracheal tube placement should be done immediately after intubation to protect against unrecognized esophageal intubation. This includes using both clinical findings and end-tidal carbon dioxide (CO_2).[3,4,14]
  - Clinical findings consistent with tracheal placement include visualization of the tube passing through the vocal cords, absence of gurgling over the epigastric area, auscultation of bilateral breath sounds, bilateral chest rise and fall during ventilation, and mist in the tube.[14,15]
  - End-tidal CO_2 detectors assist in confirming proper placement of the endotracheal tube into the trachea (see procedure 14). The presence of CO_2 in the expired air indicates that the airway has been successfully intubated, but does not ensure the correct position of the endotracheal tube.
  - Disposable end-tidal CO_2 detectors are chemically treated with a nontoxic indicator that changes color in the presence of CO_2.
  - Continuous end-tidal CO_2 (capnography) assists in confirming proper placement of the endotracheal tube into the trachea as well as allowing for detection of future tube dislodgment.
  - During cardiac arrest (nonperfusing rhythms), low pulmonary blood flow may cause insufficient expired CO_2.[22] If CO_2 is not detected, use of an esophageal detector device is recommended for confirmation of proper placement into the trachea.[2,3,14,18,23]
  - At least five to six exhalations with a consistent CO_2 level must be assessed to confirm endotracheal tube placement in the trachea because the esophagus may yield a small but detectable amount of CO_2 during the first few breaths.[15]
  - Esophageal detector devices work by creating suction at the end of the endotracheal tube by compressing a flexible bulb or pulling back on a syringe plunger. When the tube is placed correctly in the trachea, air allows for reexpansion of the bulb or movement of the syringe plunger. If the tube is located in the esophagus, no movement of the syringe plunger or reexpansion of the bulb is seen. These devices may be misleading in patients who are morbidly obese, in status asthmaticus, late in pregnancy, or in patients with large amounts of tracheal secretions.[14]

- Endotracheal tube cuff pressure should be checked after verifying correct endotracheal tube position. The cuff pressure recommended for assistance in preventing both microaspiration and tracheal damage is 20 to 30 cm H_2O.[11,17,19]
- Intubation attempts should take no longer than 15 to 20 seconds. If more than one intubation attempt is necessary, ventilation with 100% oxygen using a self-inflating manual resuscitation bag device with a tight-fitting face mask should be performed for 3 to 5 minutes before each attempt. If intubation is not successful after three attempts, consider using another airway adjunct, such as a laryngeal mask airway (LMA), Combitube, or King LT Airway (see Procedures 1, 7, and 8).
- It is important to have a clearly defined difficult/failed airway plan and alternative airway equipment available at the bedside in case of unsuccessful intubation. This may consist of a gum elastic bougie, LMA, and video laryngoscope. Surgical airway equipment such as that needed for a cricothyroidotomy should be available at the bedside in case of a failed airway.[15]
- Those assisting with intubation should have additional knowledge, skills, and demonstrated competence per professional licensure and institutional standard.

EQUIPMENT

- Personal protective equipment, including eye protection
- Endotracheal tube with intact cuff and 15-mm connector (women, 7-mm to 7.5-mm tube; men, 8-mm to 9-mm tube)
- Laryngoscope handle with fresh batteries
- Laryngoscope blades (straight and curved)
- Spare bulb for laryngoscope blades
- Flexible stylet
- Magill forceps (to remove foreign bodies obstructing the airway if present)
- Self-inflating manual resuscitation bag-valve-mask device with tight fitting face mask connected to supplemental oxygen (15 L/min)
- Oxygen source
- Luer-tip 10-mL syringe for cuff inflation
- Water-soluble lubricant
- Rigid pharyngeal suction-tip (Yankauer) catheter
- Suction apparatus (portable or wall)
- Suction catheters
- Bite-block or oropharyngeal airway
- Endotracheal tube–securing apparatus or appropriate tape
  - Commercially available endotracheal tube holder
  - Adhesive tape (6 to 8 inches long)
- Stethoscope
- Monitoring equipment: cardiac monitor, pulse oximetry, and sphygmomanometer
- Disposable end-tidal CO_2 detector, continuous end-tidal CO_2 monitoring device, and esophageal detection device
- Drugs for intubation as indicated (induction agent, sedation, paralyzing agents, lidocaine, atropine)
- Assortment of oropharyngeal airways and nasopharyngeal airways
- Rescue airways such as LMA, King LT, or Combitube

- Failed airway equipment: gum elastic bougie, video laryngoscope, optical stylet fiberoptic scope, and cricothyroidotomy kit

Additional equipment, to have available as needed, includes the following:

- Anesthetic spray (nasal approach)
- Local anesthetic jelly (nasal approach)
- Ventilator

PATIENT AND FAMILY EDUCATION

- If time permits, assess the patient's and the family's level of understanding about the condition and rationale for endotracheal intubation. *Rationale:* This assessment identifies the patient's and the family's knowledge deficits concerning the patient's condition, the procedure, the expected benefits, and the potential risks. It also allows time for questions to clarify information and voice concerns. Explanations decrease patient anxiety and enhance cooperation.
- Explain the procedure and the reason for intubation, if the clinical situation permits. If not, explain the procedure and reason for the intubation after it is completed. *Rationale:* This explanation enhances patient and family understanding and decreases anxiety.
- If indicated and the clinical situation permits, explain the patient's role in assisting with insertion of the endotracheal tube. *Rationale:* This explanation elicits the patient's cooperation, which assists with insertion.
- Explain that the patient will be unable to speak while the endotracheal tube is in place but that other means of communication will be provided. *Rationale:* This information enhances patient and family understanding and decreases anxiety.
- Explain that the patient's hands are often immobilized to prevent accidental dislodgment of the tube. *Rationale:* This information enhances patient and family understanding and decreases anxiety.

PATIENT ASSESSMENT AND PREPARATION

Patient Assessment

- Verify correct patient with two identifiers. *Rationale:* Prior to performing a procedure, the nurse should ensure the correct identification of the patient for the intended intervention.
- Assess for recent history of trauma with suspected spinal cord injury or cranial surgery. *Rationale:* Knowledge of pertinent patient history allows for selection of the most appropriate method for intubation, which helps reduce the risk of secondary injury.
- Assess nothing-by-mouth status, the use of a self-inflating manual resuscitation bag-valve device with mask before intubation, and for signs of gastric distention. *Rationale:* Increased risk of aspiration and vomiting occurs with accumulation of air (from the use of a self-inflating manual resuscitation bag-valve-mask device), food, or secretions.

- Assess level of consciousness, level of anxiety, and respiratory difficulty. *Rationale:* This assessment determines the need for sedation or the use of paralytic agents and the patient's ability to lie flat and supine for intubation.
- Assess oral cavity for presence of dentures, loose teeth, or other possible obstructions and remove if appropriate. *Rationale:* Ensures that the airway is free from any obstructions.
- Assess vital signs and assess for the following: tachypnea, dyspnea, shallow respirations, cyanosis, apnea, altered level of consciousness, tachycardia, cardiac dysrhythmias, hypertension, and headache. *Rationale:* Any of these conditions may indicate a problem with oxygenation or ventilation or both.
- Assess patency of nares (for nasal intubation). *Rationale:* Selection of the most appropriate naris facilitates insertion and may improve patient tolerance of the tube.
- Assess need for premedication. *Rationale:* Various medications provide sedation or paralysis of the patient as needed.

Patient Preparation

- Perform a preprocedure verification and time out. *Rational:* Ensures patient safety.
- Ensure that the patient understands preprocedural teaching, if appropriate. Answer questions as they arise, and reinforce information as needed. *Rationale:* Understanding of previously taught information is evaluated and reinforced.
- Before intubation, initiate intravenous or intraosseous access. *Rationale:* Readily available intravenous or intraosseous access may be necessary if the patient needs to be sedated or paralyzed or needs other medications because of a negative response to the intubation procedure.
- Position the patient appropriately.
  - ❖ Positioning of the nontrauma patient is as follows: Place the patient supine with the head in the sniffing position, in which the head is extended and the neck is flexed. Placement of a small towel under the occiput elevates it several inches, allowing for proper flexion of the neck (see Fig. 2-3). *Rationale:* Placement of the head in the sniffing position allows for better visualization of the larynx and vocal cords by aligning the axes of the mouth, pharynx, and trachea.
  - ❖ Positioning of the trauma patient is as follows: Manual in-line cervical spinal immobilization must be maintained during the entire process of intubation. *Rationale:* Because cervical spinal cord injury must be suspected in all trauma patients until proved otherwise, this position helps prevent secondary injury should a cervical spine injury be present.
- Premedicate as indicated. *Rationale:* Appropriate premedication allows for more controlled intubation, reducing the incidence of insertion trauma, aspiration, laryngospasm, and improper tube placement.
- As appropriate, notify the respiratory therapy department of impending intubation so that a ventilator can be set up. *Rationale:* The ventilator is set up before intubation.

Procedure   for Performing Endotracheal Intubation

Steps	Rationale	Special Considerations
General Setup		
1. **HH**	Reduces the transmission of microorganisms and body secretions. Standard Precautions.	Protective eyewear should be worn by all individuals involved in the intubation, including those who are assisting, to avoid exposure to secretions.
2. **PE**		
3. Establish intravenous or intraosseous access if not present.	Provides access to deliver indicated medications.	
4. Attach patient to monitoring equipment, including cardiac and blood pressure monitor and pulse oximeter.	Provides continuous patient monitoring during intubation.	
5. Set up suction apparatus, and connect rigid suction-tip catheter to tubing.	Prepares for oropharyngeal suctioning as needed.	
6. Check equipment as directed by individual performing the intubation.		
A. Gather appropriate-sized endotracheal tube.	Appropriate-sized endotracheal tubes facilitate both intubation and ventilation.	Generally a 7–7.5-mm internal diameter tube is used for adult females and an 8–9-mm internal diameter for adult males.[9,10,14,20]
B. Use 10-mL syringe to inflate cuff on tube, assessing for leaks. Completely deflate cuff.	Verifies that equipment is functional and that tube cuff is patent without leaks; prepares tube for insertion.	Once the endotracheal tube cuff has been checked for leak and it is completely deflated, place back into its packaging to avoid contamination.
C. Insert the stylet into the endotracheal tube, ensuring that the tip of the stylet does not extend past the end of the endotracheal tube.	Provides structural support for the flexible endotracheal tube during insertion. Maintaining the tip of the stylet within the lumen of the endotracheal tube prevents damage to the vocal cords and trachea.	Stylet must be recessed by at least 0.5 inch from the distal end of the tube so that it does not protrude beyond the end of the tube.
D. Connect the laryngoscope blade to the handle, and ensure the blade's bulb is securely seated.	Verifies that the equipment is functional.	Check the bulb for brightness. Replace bulb if dull or burnt out.
7. Assist in positioning the patient's head by flexing the neck forward and extending the head, into the sniffing position (only if neck trauma is not suspected; see Fig. 2-3). If spinal trauma is suspected, assist in maintaining the head in a neutral position with in-line spinal immobilization. *This is performed by manually immobilizing the head and neck by placing your hands on either side of the patient's head, with thumbs along the mandible and fingers behind the head on the occipital ridge. Use gentle but firm stabilization throughout the procedure.*[3,10] (**Level D***)	Allows for visualization of the vocal cords with alignment of the mouth, pharynx, and trachea.	The ear (external auditory meatus) and sternal notch should be aligned when patient is examined from the side. This allows for flexion of the cervical spine.[15] Placement of a small towel under the occiput elevates it, allowing for proper neck flexion. *Do not flex or extend neck of patient with suspected spinal cord injury; the head must be maintained in a neutral position with manual in-line cervical spine immobilization.*[3]

*Level D: Peer-reviewed professional and organizational standards with the support of clinical study recommendations.

Procedure for Performing Endotracheal Intubation—*Continued*

Steps	Rationale	Special Considerations
8. Check the mouth for dentures and remove if present.	Dentures should be removed before oral intubation is attempted but may remain in place for nasal intubation.	
9. Suction the mouth and pharynx as needed if copious secretions are visualized.	Provides for a clear view of the posterior pharynx and larynx.	
10. Insert oropharyngeal airway if indicated (see Procedure 9).	Assists in maintenance of upper airway patency. Helps to improve ability to ventilate during bag-valve-mask ventilation.	Use only in unconscious patients with an absent gag reflex.
11. Preoxygenate for 3–5 minutes, with 100% oxygen via a nonrebreather mask if ventilations are adequate or via a self-inflating manual resuscitation bag-valve-mask device (see Procedure 31) if ventilations are inadequate. (**Level D***)	Helps prevent hypoxemia. Gentle breaths reduce incidence of air entering stomach (leading to gastric distention, aspiration), decrease airway turbulence, and distribute ventilation more evenly within the lungs. Preoxygenation ensures that nitrogen is washed out of the lungs and will extend the allowable apneic time until the oxygen in the lungs is used up.[4,15]	Bag-valve-mask ventilation may <u>not</u> be needed in the spontaneous breathing patient. Avoid aggressive positive-pressure ventilation with a self-inflating manual resuscitation bag because this may increase the risk for gastric vomiting.
12. Premedicate patient as directed by the practitioner intubating the patient.	Sedates and relaxes the patient, allowing easier intubation.	This may require a second assistant to administer and document medications given before, during, and after intubation.
13. Remove oropharyngeal airway if present.	Clears the airway for advancement of the laryngoscope blade and endotracheal tube.	
14. Have self-inflating manual resuscitation bag-valve-mask device connected to 100% oxygen source and face mask ready for hyperoxygenation and manual ventilation.	Intubation attempts should not take longer than 30 seconds. Patients need to be hyperoxygenated and ventilated between intubation attempts.[3,4]	If intubation is unsuccessful within 30 seconds, or the patient's oxygen saturations falls below 90% during the attempt, remove the tube.[15] Ventilate with 100% oxygen with a bag-valve-mask device before another intubation attempt is made. Before reattempting intubation, correct problems related to positioning, procedure, or equipment
15. Apply external laryngeal manipulation (BURP) and/or cricoid pressure **ONLY** as directed by the practitioner performing the intubation.	External laryngeal manipulation (BURP) may assist with visualization of the vocal cords.[3] Apply BURP on the thyroid cartilage to move the larynx to the right while the tongue is displaced to the left by the laryngoscope blade.[3] Cricoid pressure moves the trachea toward the posterior, which may provide better visualization of the vocal cords by the practitioner.	In some cases, the intubator may perform BURP manipulation by him- or herself to initially visualize the vocal cords. The assistant should be prepared to take over for the intubator once the cords are visualized. Once cricoid pressure (Sellick maneuver) is applied, it must be maintained until the intubation is completed. The intubator may request the assistant to retract the corner of the patient's right lip to increase the field of view.

*Level D: Peer-reviewed professional and organizational standards with the support of clinical study recommendations.

Procedure continues on following page

Procedure for Performing Endotracheal Intubation—*Continued*

Steps	Rationale	Special Considerations
16. Once the tube has been correctly placed, assist with cuff inflation as directed. Inflate cuff with 5–10 mL of air depending on the manufacturer's recommendations. Do not overinflate the cuff.	Inflation volumes vary depending on manufacturer and size of tube. Keep cuff pressure between 20 and 30 mm Hg to decrease risk of aspiration and prevent ischemia and decreased blood flow.[11,14]	In adults, decreased mucosal capillary blood flow (ischemia) results when pressure is greater than 40 mm Hg.[4,14] Consider using a manometer to measure cuff pressure and increase or decrease pressure as indicated to achieve cuff pressure of 20–30 mm Hg.
17. Once endotracheal tube has been placed, assist with confirmation of tube placement as directed by the intubator. Continue ventilating with 100% O_2 self-inflating manual resuscitation bag.	Ensures correct placement of endotracheal tube into trachea.	If requested, hold the endotracheal tube securely at the lip, making note of how far tube has been placed into trachea by noting markings on endotracheal tube. Avoid hyperventilation; gently ventilate with 10–12 breaths per minute watching for visible chest rise.[4,14]
A. Auscultate over epigastrium. **(Level D*)**	Allows for identification of esophageal intubation.[4,14]	If air movement or gurgling is heard, esophageal intubation has occurred. The tube must be removed and intubation reattempted. Improper insertion may result in hypoxemia, gastric distention, vomiting, and aspiration.
B. Auscultate lung bases and apices for bilateral breath sounds. **(Level D)**	Assists in verification of correct tube placement into the trachea. A right main-stem bronchus intubation results in diminished left-sided breath sounds.[3,4]	
C. Observe for symmetrical chest wall movement. **(Level D)**	Assists in verification of correct tube placement.[3,4,14]	Absence may indicate right main-stem or esophageal intubation.
D. Attach disposable end-tidal CO_2 detector. Watch for color change, which indicates the presence of CO_2. **(Level B*)**	Disposable CO_2 detectors may be used to assist with identification of proper tube placement.[6,9,18,21] Detection of CO_2 confirms proper endotracheal tube placement into the trachea.[3,4,14]	CO_2 detectors usually are placed between the self-inflating manual resuscitation bag-valve device and the endotracheal tube. CO_2 detectors should be used in conjunction with physical assessment findings. At least five to six exhalations with a consistent CO_2 level must be assessed to confirm endotracheal tube placement in the trachea because the esophagus may yield small but detectable amounts of CO_2 during the first few breaths.[15]
or		
Attach continuous end-tidal CO_2 monitor and watch for detection of CO_2 (see Procedure 14). **(Level B)**	Continuous end-tidal CO_2 is a reliable indicator of proper tube placement and also allows for detection of future tube dislodgment.[14]	At least five to six exhalations with a consistent CO_2 level must be assessed to confirm endotracheal tube placement in the trachea because the esophagus may yield small but detectable amounts of CO_2 during the first few breaths.[15]

*Level B: Well-designed, controlled studies with results that consistently support a specific action, intervention, or treatment.
*Level D: Peer-reviewed professional and organizational standards with the support of clinical study recommendations.

Procedure | for Performing Endotracheal Intubation—*Continued*

Steps	Rationale	Special Considerations
Or Consider use of esophageal detection device in cardiac arrest. **(Level B*)**	During cardiac arrest (nonperfusing rhythms), low pulmonary blood flow may cause insufficient expired CO_2.[22] If CO_2 is not detected, use of an esophageal detector device is recommended.[2,8,12,18,23]	
E. Evaluate oxygen saturation (SpO_2) with noninvasive pulse oximetry (see Procedure 18). **(Level D*)**	SpO_2 decreases if the esophagus has been inadvertently intubated. The value may or may not change in a right main-stem bronchus intubation.[4,14]	SpO_2 findings should be used in conjunction with physical assessment findings.
18. If CO_2 detection, assessment findings, or SpO_2 reveals that the tube is not correctly positioned, deflate cuff and assist with tube removal as directed by the intubator. Ventilate and hyperoxygenate with 100% oxygen for 3–5 minutes, then assist with reattempt at intubation, beginning with Step 11.	Esophageal intubation results in gas flow diversion and hypoxemia.[4,11]	
19. If breath sounds are absent on the left, cuff should be deflated and withdrawn by 1–2 cm. Reevaluate for correct tube placement (Step 17) as directed by the intubator.	Absence of breath sounds on the left may indicate right main-stem intubation, which is common because of the anatomical position of the right main-stem bronchi.	When correctly positioned, the tube tip should be halfway between the vocal cords and the carina.[2]
20. Connect endotracheal tube to oxygen source via self-inflating manual resuscitation bag-valve device, or mechanical ventilator, using swivel adapter.	Reduces motion on tube and mouth or nares.	
21. Insert a bite-block or oropharyngeal airway (to act as a bite-block) along the endotracheal tube, with oral intubation if indicated.	Prevents the patient from biting down on the endotracheal tube.	The bite-block should be secured separately from the tube to prevent dislodgment of the tube.
22. Secure the endotracheal tube in place as directed (according to institutional standard). **(Level B)**	Prevents inadvertent dislodgment of tube.[1,4,9,14]	Commercial tube holder or tape should not cause compression on sides or front of the neck, which may impair venous return to the brain.[14] Consider manually holding the endotracheal tube when moving the patient to prevent inadvertent dislodgement of the tube.
Use of Commercially Available Endotracheal Tube Holder		
A. Apply according to manufacturer's directions. **(Level M*)**	Allows for secure stabilization of the tube, decreasing the likelihood of inadvertent extubation.	Commercially available tube holders are often more comfortable for patients and easier to manage if the endotracheal tube is manipulated.[15]

*Level B: Well-designed, controlled studies with results that consistently support a specific action, intervention, or treatment.

*Level D: Peer-reviewed professional and organizational standards with the support of clinical study recommendations.

*Level M: Manufacturer's recommendations only.

Procedure continues on following page

Procedure for Performing Endotracheal Intubation—*Continued*

Steps	Rationale	Special Considerations
Use of Adhesive Tape A. Prepare tape as shown in Fig. 2-10.	Use of a hydrocolloid membrane on the patient's cheeks helps protect the skin.	
B. Secure tube by wrapping double-sided tape around patient's head and torn tape edges around endotracheal tube.	Secures the endotracheal tube in place.	Tape should not cause compression on sides or front of the neck, which may impair venous return to the brain.[14]
23. Reevaluate for correct tube placement (**Step 17**).	Verifies that the tube was not inadvertently displaced during the securing of the tube.	
24. Note position of tube at teeth or gums (use centimeter markings on tube).	Establishes a baseline for future assessment of possible endotracheal tube migration, in or out.	Common tube placement at the teeth or gums is 20–21 cm for women and 22–23 cm for men.[10,15]
25. Hyperoxygenate and suction endotracheal tube and pharynx (see Procedure 10) as needed.	Removes secretions that may obstruct tube or accumulate on the top of the cuff.	
26. Confirmation of correct tube position should be verified with a chest radiograph. (**Level D***)	Chest radiograph documents actual tube location (distance from the carina). Because a chest radiograph is not immediately available, it should not be used as the primary method of tube assessment.[3,10,14]	
27. Remove **PE**.	Reduces transmission of microorganisms and body secretions; Standard Precautions.	
28. **HH**		

*Level D: Peer-reviewed professional and organizational standards with the support of clinical study recommendations.

Expected Outcomes

- Placement of patent artificial airway
- Properly positioned and secured airway
- Improved oxygenation and ventilation
- Facilitation of secretion clearance

Unexpected Outcomes

- Intubation of esophagus or right main-stem bronchus (improper tube placement)
- Accidental extubation
- Cardiac dysrhythmias because of hypoxemia and vagal stimulation
- Broken or dislodged teeth
- Leaking of air from endotracheal tube cuff
- Oral or nasal trauma with bleeding
- Tracheal injury at tip of tube or at cuff site
- Laryngeal edema
- Vocal cord trauma
- Suctioning of gastric contents or food from endotracheal tube (aspiration)
- Obstruction of endotracheal tube

Patient Monitoring and Care

Steps	Rationale	Reportable Conditions
		These conditions should be reported if they persist despite nursing interventions.
1. Auscultate breath sounds on insertion, with every manipulation of the endotracheal tube and every 2–4 hours.	Allows for detection of tube movement or dislodgment.	• Absent, decreased, or unequal breath sounds
2. Maintain tube stability, with use of specially manufactured holder, twill tape, or adhesive tape.	Reduces risk of movement and dislodgment of tube.	• Unplanned extubation
3. Monitor and record position of tube at teeth, gums, or nose (in reference to centimeter markings on tube).	Provides for identification of tube migration.	• Tube movement from original position
4. Maintain endotracheal tube cuff pressure of 20–30 mm Hg.[11,14]	Provides adequate inflation to decrease aspiration risk and prevents overinflation of cuff to avoid tracheal damage.[11,14]	• Cuff pressure less than 20 or higher than 30 mm Hg that persists despite nursing interventions.
5. Hyperoxygenate and suction endotracheal tube, as needed (see Procedure 10).	Prevents obstruction of tube and resulting hypoxemia.	• Inability to pass a suction catheter • Copious, frothy, or bloody secretions • Significant change in amount or character of secretions
6. Assess for pain and inadequate sedation.	Allows identification of pain and/or discomfort related to the intubation.	• Pain not controlled by medications or nursing interventions • Observed ventilator dyssynchrony
7. Inspect nares or oral cavity once per shift while patient is intubated.	Allows for the detection of skin breakdown and necrosis.	• Redness, necrosis, skin breakdown

Documentation

Documentation should include the following:
- Patient and family education
- Vital signs before, during, and after intubation, including oxygen saturation and end-tidal CO_2
- Size of endotracheal tube
- Type of intubation: oral or nasal
- Type and size of blade used
- Depth of endotracheal tube insertion centimeters at teeth, gums, or naris
- Confirmation of tube placement, including chest radiograph, end-tidal CO_2 detector, capnography (method of placement confirmation)
- Clinical confirmation of tube placement including assessment of breath sounds
- Measurement of cuff pressure
- Number of intubation attempts
- Use of any medications
- Patient response to procedure
- Occurrence of unexpected outcomes
- Pain assessment, interventions, and effectiveness

References and Additional Readings

For a complete list of references and additional readings for this procedure, scan this QR code with any freely available smartphone code reader app, or visit http://booksite.elsevier.com/9780323376624.

4

Endotracheal Tube Care and Oral Care Practices for Ventilated and Non-ventilated Patients

Kathleen Vollman, Mary Lou Sole, and Barbara Quinn

PURPOSE: Endotracheal tube (ETT) management and oral care are performed to prevent buccal, oropharyngeal, and tracheal trauma from the tube and cuff; to provide oral hygiene; to promote ventilation; and to decrease the risk of ventilator-associated pneumonia (VAP) and hospital-acquired pneumonia.

PREREQUISITE NURSING KNOWLEDGE

- Anatomy and physiology of the pulmonary system should be understood.
- ETTs are used to maintain a patent airway or to facilitate mechanical ventilation. The presence of artificial airways, especially ETTs, prevents effective coughing and secretion removal, necessitating periodic removal of pulmonary secretions with suctioning; serves as a direct portal for microorganisms; and significantly increases the risk for pneumonia. They also increase the risk for the development of VAP.[22,31,56]
- Suctioning of airways should be performed only for clinical indications and not as a routine fixed-schedule treatment (see Procedure 10). In acute-care situations, suctioning is performed as a sterile procedure to prevent healthcare-acquired pneumonia.[55]
- Adequate systemic hydration and supplemental humidification of inspired gases assist in thinning secretions for easier aspiration from airways.[31,57] The oropharynx and the upper gastrointestinal tract are the main reservoirs for pathogens associated with VAP and hospital-acquired pneumonia (HAP). Micro aspiration of this oral bacteria can result in VAP and HAP.[16,18,19,31,42]
- Appropriate cuff management (see Procedure 13) helps prevent major aspirations of pulmonary secretions, prepares for tracheal extubation, and decreases the risk of iatrogenic infections.[31]
- Constant pressure from the ETT on the mouth or nose can cause skin breakdown.
- If the patient is anxious or uncooperative, use of two caregivers for retaping and/or repositioning the ETTs may help prevent accidental dislodgment of the tube.

- VAP and HAP increase not only ventilator and intensive care unit (ICU) days and hospital length of stay, but also overall morbidity and mortality of the patient.[3,10,31,39,64]
- Oral hygiene:
  - Anatomy and physiology of the oral cavity and the importance of evidence-based oral hygiene procedures on a regular basis should be understood.[4,17,18,20,34,53,60]
  - The oral cavity is a significant source of bacterial colonization. Within 48 hours of admission to the hospital, the normal oral flora changes to include respiratory pathogens not normally found in healthy individuals.[24]
  - Salivary flow is a natural host defense in facilitating the removal of plaque and microorganisms. The major immune factor in saliva is immunoglobulin A (IgA). Its role is to protect the upper airway by limiting the absorption and penetration of microorganisms.[18]
  - Mechanical ventilation often promotes dry mouth or reduced salivary flow, contributing to plaque accumulation and decreased production of salivary immune factors.[11]
  - Certain medications as well as withholding food and oral fluids may also contribute to dry mouth in all patients, including those not on a ventilator.
  - The equipment used to remove oral secretions as well as suctioning of the ETT may contribute to the colonization of the oral cavity.[5,52]
- Oral care practices for ventilator patients:
  - Tooth brushing is an essential component of an effective oral care program; however, evidence related to prevention of VAP is not conclusive.[1]
  - Foam swabs are limited in their ability to remove plaque from sheltered areas or between teeth. Brushing is able to clean the proximal sites and crevices.[43]

❖ Mouthwashes while having beneficial antibacterial properties, frequently contain alcohol which can dry the oral tissues.[18]

❖ Use of chlorhexidine oral rinse (CHG) twice daily should be part of a comprehensive oral care program for ventilated patients to reduce the incidence of VAP.[33,50]

❖ Effect of povidone-iodine as an oral cleanser to reduce VAP remains unclear.[33]

❖ Oral care given every 2 to 4 hours appears to provide a greater improvement in oral health. If oral care is not provided for 4 to 6 hours, previous benefits are thought to be lost.[13]

- Oral care practices for non-ventilated patients:

❖ Patients not on a ventilator are still at risk for pneumonia, and studies indicate that oral care can reduce this risk. Currently, non-ventilator HAP occurs more often than VAP, with similar mortality rates, costing more lives and dollars than VAP.[10]

❖ Brushing teeth after each meal and a weekly review by a dentist or hygienist can reduce the incidence of pneumonia in elderly patients, resulting in fewer days with fever and lower mortality rates.[63]

❖ Not only can enhanced oral care reduce pneumonia in nursing home residents, it may also improve swallow and cough reflex sensitivities, factors that could also help to prevent pneumonia.[62]

❖ Increased frequency of oral care for non-ventilated adult patients in an acute-care hospital reduced non-ventilated HAP by 37% over 12 months.[45]

❖ There are no documented studies that show the optimal frequency of oral care for non-ventilated patients. For the general public, the American Dental Association recommends brushing twice daily with a soft-bristled toothbrush using therapeutic toothpaste, and rinsing with an antiseptic rinse.[2]

❖ If a non-ventilated patient cannot manage oral secretions and is at high risk for aspiration, the caregiver may consider using a suction toothbrush, similar to those used in the ventilated-patient setting.[46]

EQUIPMENT

- Goggles or glasses and mask
- Bite-block or oral airway if needed
- Adhesive or twill tape; commercial ETT holder (design must ensure ability to provide oral care and suctioning)
- 2 × 2 gauze or cotton swab for cleaning around the nares
- Normal saline solution
- Soft pediatric/adult toothbrush or suction toothbrush
- Foam oral swab or oral suction swab
- Oral cleansing solution (c.g., 1.5% H_2O_2,[7,18,28,38,49,51] chlorhexidine,[7,12,21,26,27,30,32,33,50,58,59] cetylpyridinium chloride,[7,37,48,56] toothpaste[13,29,32,43])

Additional equipment, to have available as needed, includes the following:

- Suction catheter for oral and nasal suctioning (single-use Yankauer, covered Yankauer, disposable oral saliva ejector)

- Two sources of suction or a bifurcated connection device attached to a single suction source
- Connecting tube(s) (4 to 6 feet)
- Nonsterile gloves
- Stethoscope

PATIENT AND FAMILY EDUCATION

- Explain the procedure to the patient and family, including the purpose of ETT care and the importance of comprehensive oral care in prevention of infection in both intubated and non-intubated patients.[1] *Rationale:* This step identifies patient and family knowledge deficits concerning patient condition, procedure, expected benefits, and potential risks and allows time for questions to clarify information and voice concerns. Explanations decrease patient anxiety and enhance cooperation.

- If indicated, explain the patient's role in assisting with ETT care. *Rationale*: Eliciting the patient's cooperation assists with care.

- Explain that the patient will be unable to speak while the ETT is in place but that other means of communication will be provided. *Rationale*: This information enhances patient and family understanding and decreases anxiety.

- Explain that the patient's hands may be immobilized to prevent accidental dislodgment of the tube. *Rationale*: This information enhances patient and family understanding and decreases anxiety.

PATIENT ASSESSMENT AND PREPARATION

Patient Assessment

- Verify correct patient with two identifiers. *Rationale*: Prior to performing a procedure, the nurse should ensure the correct identification of the patient for the intended intervention.

- Assess for signs and symptoms that indicate that oral cavity and ETT care is necessary. *Rationale*: Assessment provides for early recognition that oral or ETT care is needed.

❖ Excessive secretions (oral or tracheal)

❖ Dry oral mucosa

❖ Debris in the oral cavity

❖ Plaque buildup on teeth

❖ Soiled tape or ties or commercial device

❖ Patient biting or kinking tube

❖ Pressure areas on nares, corner of mouth, or tongue

❖ ETT moving in and out of mouth

❖ Patient able to verbalize or audible air leak around ETT

- Assess level of consciousness and level of anxiety. *Rationale:* This assessment determines the need for pain medication or sedation during ETT care and the number of care providers needed to perform the activities.

Patient Preparation

- Ensure that the patient understands preprocedural teachings. Answer questions as they arise and reinforce information as needed. *Rationale*: This process evaluates and reinforces understanding of previously taught information.

- Maintain the patient in a semi-Fowler's (≥30 degrees) position during mechanical ventilation to reduce the risk of aspiration.[15,31,59] Assist the patient to a high Fowler's (≥60 degrees) position or the most comfortable position for both the patient and nurse before performing the care. *Rationale*: This position promotes comfort and reduces physical strain and maintains head of bed elevation to reduce risk of aspiration.[15,31,59]

Procedure	for Endotracheal Tube and Oral Care for Ventilated Patients	
Steps	Rationale	Special Considerations
1. HH		
2. PE		
3. Ensure that ETT is connected to the ventilator with a swivel adapter.	Decreases pressure exerted by ventilator tubing on the ETT, thereby minimizing risk of pressure ulceration.	
4. Support the ETT and tubing as needed.	Prevents inadvertent displacement or dislodgement of the tube.	If the patient is at risk for inadvertent or sudden movements, obtain an assistant to manually support the ETT and tubing.
5. If suctioning is clinically indicated,[55] hyperoxygenate via the ventilator before ETT suction and between attempts (see Procedure 10).	Removes secretions that may obstruct tube.	Suctioning of airways should be performed only for a clinical indication and not as a routine fixed-schedule treatment.[55]
6. If patient is nasally intubated, clean around ETT with saline solution–soaked gauze or cotton swabs.	Removes secretions that could cause pressure and subsequent skin breakdown.	The Society for Healthcare Epidemiology of America (SHEA) compendium and The Centers for Disease Control and Prevention (CDC) guidelines for prevention of VAP recommend that patients intubated nasally be reintubated orally as soon as possible to reduce the risk of VAP.[31,57]
7. If patient is intubated orally, remove bite-block or oropharyngeal airway (acting as bite-block) before proceeding with oral hygiene.	The bite-block or oropharyngeal airway prevents the patient from biting down on the ETT and occluding airflow.	The bite-block should be secured separately from the tube to prevent dislodgment of the ETT. The bite-block or ETT securing mechanism may be a barrier to providing good oral care.
8. Initiate oral hygiene with a pediatric or adult (soft) toothbrush, at least twice a day. Gently brush patient's teeth to clean and remove plaque from teeth. Suction oropharyngeal secretions after brushing. Use toothpaste or a cleansing solution that assists in the breakdown of debris **(Level C*)**.[4,9,23,25,28,35,45,54,58]	Mechanical cleansing and oral hygiene reduce oropharyngeal colonization and dental plaque, which is associated with VAP.[16,35,36,43,45,47,48] Toothpaste or cleansing solution should contain additives that assist in the breakdown of mucus in the mouth. Sodium bicarbonate assists in removal of debris accumulation on oral tissue and teeth.[18]	Pediatric or soft-bristle toothbrushes may be easier to use in adult intubated patients.[39,45,60]

*Level C: Qualitative studies, descriptive or correlational studies, integrative reviews, systematic reviews, or randomized controlled trials with inconsistent results.

Procedure	for Endotracheal Tube and Oral Care for Ventilated Patients—*Continued*	
Steps	**Rationale**	**Special Considerations**
9. In addition to brushing twice daily, use oral swabs with a 1.5% hydrogen peroxide solution to clean mouth every 2–4 hours.	Oral cleansing, suctioning, and moisturizing every 2–4 hours is a part of comprehensive oral care that has shown to improve oral health and reduce the risk of healthcare-acquired pneumonia.[13,18,45,49,51,54,58,60] Studies support the safety and efficacy of greater than 1% and less than 3% H_2O_2 as a cleanser for plaque removal and maintaining overall gingival health.[20,42,43]	Foam swabs are effective in stimulating mucosal tissue but less effective in plaque removal.[13,43]
10. Suction oropharyngeal secretions after cleansing. After each cleansing, apply a mouth moisturizer to the oral mucosa and lips to keep tissue moist. **(Level C*)**	Saliva serves a protective function. Mechanical ventilation causes drying of the oral mucosa, affecting salivary flow and contributing to mucositis and regions for bacterial deposits and growth.[18,39,44]	Implementation of a comprehensive oral care program is recommended by the CDC, SHEA, and the Institute for Health Care Improvement to reduce VAP.[27,31,57] Use of mouthwash as a cleansing agent is not recommended.[18]
11. Suction oral cavity and pharynx at a minimal frequency of every 4 hours.[54] **(Level C)** (Continuous subglottic suctioning: **Level A***) (Intermittent suctioning: **Level C**)	Removes secretions that may accumulate on top of the cuff and cause microaspiration.[8,49,54] Continuous subglottic suctioning with a specially designed ETT has been shown to reduce VAP.[31,41,60] Intermittent deep oral cleansing with a disposable or covered catheter as a part of a comprehensive oral care program has been shown to reduce VAP in a quality-improvement project.[18,28,49]	Oral suction equipment and suction tubing should be changed every 24 hours. Nondisposable, noncovered oral suction apparatus has been shown to be colonized with microorganisms present in the oral cavity.[52] Nondisposable oral suction apparatus should be rinsed with sterile isotonic sodium chloride solution after each use and placed on a paper towel if not disposable or covered.[18,49,52,63] Covered oral suction apparatus should be rinsed with sterile or distilled water and cover put back in place.[18,28,49,52] Placement of tonsil suction back into the package is associated with greater colonization.[18,39,52] Disconnection of a closed suction system to provide oral suctioning may contribute to increased bacterial colonization at the point of the disconnection.[18,39,52]

*Level A: Meta-analysis of quantitative studies or metasynthesis of qualitative studies with results that consistently support a specific action, intervention, or treatment (including systematic review of randomized controlled trials).

*Level C: Qualitative studies, descriptive or correlational studies, integrative reviews, systematic reviews, or randomized controlled trials with inconsistent results.

Procedure continues on following page

Procedure	for Endotracheal Tube and Oral Care for Ventilated Patients—*Continued*	
Steps	**Rationale**	**Special Considerations**
12. Application of antiseptic oral rinses (chlorhexidine, cetylpyridinium chloride, added after brushing or done in conjunction with comprehensive oral care, can help reduce VAP.[33,50,58] **(Level B*)**	Twice a day application of 2% and 0.12% chlorhexidine gluconate to the oral cavity within a 2-hour time period from brushing has reduced VAP rates.[7,12,21,26,27,50,58] Cetylpyridinium chloride has been shown to be an effective solution in the removal of plaque and prevention of gingivitis.[7,37,48,55] Povidone-iodine effectiveness as a rinse to reduce VAP remains unclear.[33]	More frequent use of antiseptics than recommended may result in greater discoloration of the teeth.[18,37,47]
13. Move oral tube to the other side of the mouth. Replace bite-block or oropharyngeal airway (to act as bite-block) along the ETT if necessary to prevent biting. If deflation of the cuff is necessary to move from one side of the mouth to the other, deep oral suctioning should be performed before deflation. **(Level C*)**	Prevents or minimizes pressure areas on lips, tongue, and oral cavity. Deep oral suctioning above the cuff before deflation or position change can reduce the risk of colonized oral secretions being aspirated.[8,54]	
14. After oral hygiene is completed, change the ETT securing mechanism with new tape, ties, or commercial device, as needed, according to institutional standard (see Fig. 2-10). **(Level C)**	The securing mechanism should be changed if using tape and/or moved at least once daily to provide an opportunity for assessment and repositioning of the ETT to reduce the risk of a pressure skin injury. If the securing mechanism loosens, more frequent change may be necessary.[44,53] When tape was compared with commercially available devices, tape was superior to three of four devices in withstanding high external forces and was the most cost effective.[6,40]	If the method to secure the ETT obstructs the ability to provide effective oral care, consider changing the securement method.
15. Ensure proper cuff inflation (see Procedure 13).	Helps in preventing air leaks during ventilation and aspiration.	
16. Reconfirm tube placement (see Procedure 2), and note position of tube at teeth, gumline, or nares.	Common tube placement at the teeth is 21 cm for women and 23 cm for men.	
17. Remove **PE** and discard supplies.		
18. **HH**		

*Level B: Well-designed, controlled studies with results that consistently support a specific action, intervention, or treatment.
*Level C: Qualitative studies, descriptive or correlational studies, integrative reviews, systematic reviews, or randomized controlled trials with inconsistent results.

Procedure | for Oral Care: Non-ventilated Patients

Steps	Rationale	Special Considerations
Independent Self-Care		
1. Instruct patient to brush gently for 1–2 minutes and swish with oral rinse. Moisturize lips and mouth as needed for dryness.	Promotes good oral hygiene.	Consider using the following tools: soft-bristled toothbrush, therapeutic toothpaste, alcohol-free antiseptic oral rinse, and non–petroleum-based moisturizer.[45,46]
2. Encourage brushing four times a day (i.e., after each meal and before bedtime).[45,46] (Level C*)	Promotes good oral hygiene.	
Dependent, Unable to Manage Own Oral Care or Secretions Safely		
1. ▨ HH		
2. ▨ PE		
3. Brush with a suction toothbrush and toothpaste or gel for 1–2 minutes, suctioning frequently.	Promotes good oral hygiene.	Consider using the following tools: suction toothbrush, therapeutic toothpaste or gel, alcohol-free antiseptic oral rinse, and non–petroleum-based moisturizer.
4. Remove ▨ PE and discard supplies.		
5. ▨ HH		
Edentulate Patients, Dentures		
1. ▨ HH		
2. ▨ PE		
3. If no teeth or dentures, gently brush gums, tongue four times a day (i.e., after each meal and before bedtime). If patient is allowed nothing by mouth or is on tube feedings, oral care can be performed every 6 hours. Apply antiseptic oral rinse with moistened swab and suction. Apply moisturizer with swab.[45,46] (Level C)	Promotes good oral hygiene.	Consider using the following tools: soft-bristled toothbrush, therapeutic toothpaste/gel, alcohol-free antiseptic oral rinse, and non–petroleum-based moisturizer.[45,46]
4. If patient is wearing dentures, soak at night in denture cleanser. During the daytime, rinse/swab with antiseptic rinse after each meal and apply moisturizer, prn.[45,46] (Level C)	Promotes good oral hygiene.	
5. Remove ▨ PE and discard supplies.		
6. ▨ HH		

*Level C: Qualitative studies, descriptive or correlational studies, integrative reviews, systematic reviews, or randomized controlled trials with inconsistent results.

Expected Outcomes

- Patent airway
- Secured ETT
- Removal of oral secretions
- Intact oral and nasal mucous membranes
- Reduced oral colonization
- Moist pink oral cavity

Unexpected Outcomes

- Dislodged ETT
- Occluded ETT
- ETT cuff leak
- Pressure ulcers in mouth or on the lip or nares
- VAP

Procedure continues on following page

Patient Monitoring and Care

Steps	Rationale	Reportable Conditions
		These conditions should be reported if they persist despite nursing interventions.
1. Keep head of bed elevated at least 30 degrees, unless contraindicated.[8,15,31,59,60] (**Level C***)	Maintaining the head of the bed in an elevated position decreases the risk of aspiration. Contraindications include hemodynamic instability, decreased cerebral perfusion pressure, and patient in the prone position.	
2. Suction ETT if clinically indicated.	Maintains patent airway.	• Inability to pass suction catheter
3. Monitor amount, type, and color of secretions.	Monitors for signs of infection.	• Change in quantity or characteristics of secretions
4. If patient is nasally intubated, recommend reintubation in the oral cavity. (**Level C**)	Nasal intubation is associated with an increased risk for sinusitis and the potential development of VAP.[31]	• Purulent drainage from the nares or present in the back of the throat
5. Assess oral cavity and lips every 2 hours, and perform oral care (as outlined in **Steps 7–12**) every 2–4 hours and as needed. (**Level C**)	If oral care is omitted for an extended period, previous benefits are lost.[13,18,28,49,61] Early recognition of pressure or drainage allows for prompt intervention. Promotes good oral hygiene.	• Breakdown of lip, tongue, or oral cavity • Presence of mouth sores • Bleeding of the gums during brushing
6. For non-vented patients, assess oral cavity and lips every 2 hours and perform oral care outlined in **Steps 1–4** based on patient type. (**Level C**)		
7. With oral care, assess for buildup of plaque on teeth or potential infection related to oral abscess.	Assessment and removal of plaque decreases bacteria in the mouth.	• Continued plaque buildup on teeth, presence of an abscess
8. Avoid reusing devices unless covered or protected (i.e., in-line suction or covered Yankauer).	Apparatuses exposed to the oral cavity or secretions in the lungs when left unprotected within the environment have been shown to be colonized with bacteria in the oral cavity.[52]	
9. Reconfirm tube placement (see Procedure 2), and note position of tube at teeth or nares.	Ensures secured tube.	• Tube movement in and out of mouth
10. Retape or secure ETT every 24 hours and as needed for soiled or loose securing devices.		
11. With subglottic secretion drainage ETT in place, if tube becomes clogged irrigate with air per manufacturer's instructions but do not increase suction pressure beyond what is recommended by the manufacturer. (**Level M***)	Damage to the tracheal mucosa was noted with the use of subglottic secretion drainage. In one study in patients whose ETT was clogged, patients were reintubated and their clogged tubes were examined. In 17 of 19 subglottic suction ports, the clogging was caused by tracheal mucosa versus secretions.[14] Consider routine irrigation with air to prevent clogging.	• Clogged subglottic suction port

*Level C: Qualitative studies, descriptive or correlational studies, integrative reviews, systematic reviews, or randomized controlled trials with inconsistent results.
*Level M: Manufacturer's recommendations only.

Documentation

Documentation should include the following:

- Patient and family education
- Patient tolerance to suctioning
- Aspirate amount, type, and color
- Presence of nasal drainage
- Repositioning of ETT and new position
- Retaping of ETT
- Oral care, moisturization, and oral suctioning

- Condition of lips, mouth, and tongue
- Absence of a cuff leak
- Pressure in the cuff (2–30 mm Hg)
- Centimeter mark on ETT and placement position in the oral cavity
- Which naris ETT is in

References and Additional Readings

For a complete list of references and additional readings for this procedure, scan this QR code with any freely available smartphone code reader app, or visit http://booksite.elsevier.com/9780323376624.

5 Extubation/Decannulation AP (Perform)

Lisa Koser

PURPOSE: To remove the artificial airway, allowing the patient to breathe through the upper airway.

PREREQUISITE NURSING KNOWLEDGE

- *Extubation refers to removal of a translaryngeal endotracheal tube, whereas decannulation refers to removal of a tracheostomy tube.*
- Indications for extubation and decannulation include the following[1,3]:
  - ❖ The underlying condition that led to the need for an artificial airway is reversed or improved.
  - ❖ Hemodynamic stability is achieved, with no new reasons for continued artificial airway support.
  - ❖ The patient is able to effectively clear pulmonary secretions.
  - ❖ Adequate muscle strength is achieved.
  - ❖ The ability to protect airway and minimal risk for aspiration exist.
  - ❖ Mechanical ventilatory support is no longer needed (i.e., adequate spontaneous ventilation and oxygenation is achieved, or palliative extubation is planned).
- Most extubations and decannulations are planned. Planning allows for preparation of the patient physically and emotionally, decreasing the likelihood of reintubation* and hypoxic sequelae. Unintentional or unplanned extubation complicates a patient's overall recovery and increases risk of inpatient death.[2]
- Extubation may occur in a rapid fashion when the previous indications are met, whereas decannulation generally occurs in a stepwise fashion. The patient with a tracheostomy tube may be weaned gradually from the tracheostomy tube, including downsizing the tube diameter, using fenestrated tubes and inner cannulas, and capping the tracheostomy tube. The tracheostomy tube is removed when the patient is able to breathe comfortably, maintain adequate ventilation and oxygenation, and manage secretions through the normal anatomical airway.

EQUIPMENT

- Personal protective equipment (including eye protection)
- Self-inflating manual resuscitation bag-valve device connected to 100% oxygen source
- Oxygen delivery device (i.e., face mask) connected to humidified oxygen
- Suctioning equipment with sterile suction catheter or kit
- Rigid pharyngeal suction-tip (Yankauer) catheter
- Scissors (for tape or ties)
- 10-mL syringe (if cuff present)
- Sterile dressing for tracheal stoma
- Endotracheal intubation supplies and emergency cart

PATIENT AND FAMILY EDUCATION

- Explain the purpose of and procedure for removing the endotracheal or tracheostomy tube. *Rationale:* Identifies knowledge deficits of the patient and family concerning the patient's condition, the procedure, and the expected benefits. This step also allows time for questions to clarify information and voice concerns. Explanations decrease patient anxiety and enhance cooperation.
- Explain the suctioning process and the importance of coughing and deep breathing after the tube is removed. *Rationale:* Understanding therapy encourages cooperation with the follow-up procedures necessary to maintain a patent airway.
- Explain that the patient's voice may be hoarse after extubation or decannulation. Following the removal of the tracheostomy tube, occlusion of the stoma may be necessary to facilitate normal speech and coughing. *Rationale:* Knowledge minimizes the patient's and family's fear and anxiety.
- Explain that the patient may need continued oxygen or humidification support. *Rationale:* Many patients continue to need supplemental oxygen for some time after extubation. Continued humidification often helps decrease hoarseness and liquefies secretions.
- Explain that reinsertion of the endotracheal tube or cannula may be necessary if the patient develops respiratory failure. *Rationale:* Patients may require mechanical ventilation if respiratory failure develops after extubation or decannulation.

AP *This procedure should be performed only by physicians, advanced practice nurses, and other healthcare professionals (including critical care nurses) with additional knowledge, skills, and demonstrated competence per professional licensure or institutional standard.

- After extubation, a swallow evaluation is often necessary. *Rationale:* Assess the ability to swallow and prevent aspiration with oral intake.

PATIENT ASSESSMENT AND PREPARATION
Patient Assessment

- *Rationale:* Assesses patient's readiness for extubation. Desired level of consciousness has been achieved (most patients are awake and able to follow commands).[2]
- Assess the stability of the patient's respiratory status.[2,4]
  - *Rationale:* Assesses patient's readiness for extubation. Absence of respiratory distress and no other indication for intubation
  - Negative inspiratory pressure less than or equal to -20 cm H_2O
  - Positive expiratory pressure greater than or equal to $+30$ cm H_2O
  - Spontaneous tidal volume greater than or equal to 5 mL/kg ideal body weight
  - Fraction of inspired oxygen (Fio_2) less than or equal to 50%
  - Normal or baseline $Paco_2$

- Positive end-expiratory pressure <8 cm H_2O
- Hemodynamic stability and absence of serious cardiac dysrhythmias
- Assess the patient's ability to cough. *Rationale:* The ability to cough and clear secretions is important for successful airway management after extubation.

Patient Preparation

- Verify correct patient with two identifiers. *Rationale:* Prior to performing a procedure, the nurse should ensure the correct identification of the patient for the intended intervention.
- Ensure that the patient and family understand preprocedural teachings. Answer questions as they arise and reinforce information as needed. *Rationale:* This process evaluates and reinforces understanding of previously taught information.
- Place the patient in the high Fowler's (>60 degrees) or semi-Fowler's (>30 degrees) position if not contraindicated and does not contribute to restriction of breathing (i.e., obesity). *Rationale:* Respiratory muscles are more effective in an upright position versus a supine or prone position. This position facilitates coughing and minimizes the risk of vomiting and consequent aspiration.

Procedure	**for Performing Extubation and Decannulation**	
Steps	**Rationale**	**Special Considerations**
1. HH		
2. PE		
3. Hyperoxygenate and suction endotracheal tube or tracheostomy (see Procedure 10).	Removes secretions in artificial airway and oral cavity.	
4. Cut twill tape or remove tape or securement device to free tube.	Frees the tube for removal.	
5. Insert syringe into one-way valve of pilot balloon.	Prepares for cuff deflation.	
6. Suction the oral cavity.	Removes secretions that may be aspirated upon extubation.	Alternative methods to facilitate removal of secretions while an endotracheal tube is removed include application of positive pressure while the cuff is deflated, insertion of suction catheter 1–2 inches (5 cm) below distal end of tube, and application of suction while cuff is deflated and tube removed.[2]
7. Deflate the tube cuff (if it is inflated).	Readies the tube for removal.	
8. Ask the patient to take a deep breath and remove the tube on inspiration, while monitoring and supporting the patient.	Promotes hyperinflation. Vocal cords are maximally abducted at peak inspiration. Assists in a smooth, quick, less traumatic removal. Vocal cords are maximally abducted at peak inspiration. In addition, initial cough response expected after extubation should be more forceful if started from maximal inspiration versus expiration.	A self-inflating manual resuscitation bag-valve device can assist in hyperinflation (see Procedure 31).

Procedure continues on following page

Procedure for Performing Extubation and Decannulation—*Continued*

Steps	Rationale	Special Considerations
9. Encourage the patient to cough and breathe deeply.	Promotes hyperinflation; helps remove secretions.	
10. Suction the oral pharynx.	Removes secretions.	
11. Apply supplemental oxygen and aerosol, as appropriate.	Promotes moisture and prevents oxygen desaturation.	Cool humidification is usually preferred after extubation to help minimize upper airway swelling.[4]
12. Decannulation ONLY: place a dry, sterile, 4 × 4 dressing over stoma when tracheostomy tube is removed.	Contains secretions that may leak out of stoma.	Tracheostomy stoma closure usually occurs within a few days but may take longer with a long-term tracheostomy.
13. Discard used supplies and remove PE.		
14. HH		

Expected Outcomes

- Smooth atraumatic extubation or decannulation
- Stable respiratory status
- Stable hemodynamics
- Stable neurological status

Unexpected Outcomes

- Fatigue and respiratory failure
- Persistent hoarseness
- Tracheal stoma narrowing
- Aspiration
- Laryngospasm
- Trauma to soft tissue
- Upper airway obstruction
- Neurological decline

Patient Monitoring and Care

Steps	Rationale	Reportable Conditions
		These conditions should be reported if they persist despite nursing interventions.
1. Monitor vital signs, respiratory status, oxygenation, neurological status, and phonation immediately after extubation, within 1 hour, and per institutional standard.	Change in vital signs and oxygenation after extubation or decannulation may indicate respiratory compromise, which necessitates reintubation.	• Tachycardia • Tachypnea • Blood pressure significantly greater than baseline • Oxygen saturation (Spo_2) less than or equal to 90% (unless otherwise ordered) • Stridor • Breathing difficulty • Respiratory dyssynchrony
2. Provide supplemental oxygen as needed.	Decreases incidence of oxygen desaturation immediately after extubation.	• Spo_2 less than or equal to 90% (unless otherwise ordered) • Decreased level of consciousness (high $Paco_2$) • Inability to auscultate adequate air exchange
3. Monitor for aspiration related to pooled secretions.	Failure to suction or ineffective suctioning of the pharynx allows accumulated secretions to advance farther into the trachea on cuff deflation.	• Inability to handle secretions
4. Encourage frequent coughing and deep breathing and use of an incentive spirometer.	Prevents atelectasis and secretion accumulation.	• Ineffective cough

Patient Monitoring and Care —*Continued*

Steps	Rationale	Reportable Conditions
5. Frequent oral care (see Procedure 4).	Maintains oral mucosa and keeps oral cavity clear of dried secretions.	
6. Assess swallowing ability. Facilitate swallow study as indicated by institutional standard.	Presence of tube over extended periods may result in impaired swallowing ability.	• Inability to handle secretions • Inability to swallow without coughing
7. Follow institution standard for assessing pain. Administer analgesia as prescribed.	Identifies need for pain interventions.	• Continued pain despite pain interventions

Documentation

Documentation should include the following:
- Patient and family education
- Respiratory and vital signs assessment before and after procedure
- Date and time when procedure is performed
- Breath sounds and upper airway sounds
- Neurological status

- Patient response to procedure
- Unexpected outcomes and complications
- Nursing interventions taken
- Pain assessment, interventions, and effectiveness
- Ability to phonate

References and Additional Readings

For a complete list of references and additional readings for this procedure, scan this QR code with any freely available smartphone code reader app, or visit http://booksite.elsevier.com/9780323376624.

6

Extubation/Decannulation (Assist)

Lisa Koser

PURPOSE: To remove the artificial airway, allowing the patient to breathe through the upper airway.

PREREQUISITE NURSING KNOWLEDGE

- *Extubation refers to removal of a translaryngeal endotracheal tube, whereas decannulation refers to removal of a tracheostomy tube.*
- Indications for extubation and decannulation include the following[1,4]:
  - ❖ The underlying condition that led to the need for an artificial airway is reversed or improved.
  - ❖ Hemodynamic stability is achieved, with no new reasons for continued artificial airway support.
  - ❖ The patient is able to effectively clear pulmonary secretions.
  - ❖ Adequate muscle strength is achieved.
  - ❖ The ability to protect the airway and minimal risk for aspiration exist.
  - ❖ Mechanical ventilatory support is no longer needed (i.e., adequate spontaneous ventilation and oxygenation are achieved or palliative extubation is planned).
- Most extubations and decannulations are planned. Planning allows for preparation of the patient physically and emotionally, decreasing the likelihood of reintubation and hypoxic sequelae. Unintentional or unplanned extubation complicates a patient's overall recovery and increases risk of inpatient death.[2,3]
- Extubation may occur in a rapid fashion when the previous indications are met, whereas decannulation generally occurs in a stepwise fashion. The patient with a tracheostomy tube may be weaned gradually from the tracheostomy tube, including downsizing the tube diameter, using fenestrated tubes and inner cannulas, and capping the tracheostomy tube. The tracheostomy tube is removed when the patient is able to breathe comfortably, maintain adequate ventilation and oxygenation, and manage secretions through the normal anatomical airway.

EQUIPMENT

- Personal protective equipment (including eye protection)
- Self-inflating manual resuscitation bag-valve device connected to 100% oxygen source
- Oxygen delivery device (i.e., face mask) connected to humidified oxygen
- Suctioning equipment with sterile suction catheter or kit
- Rigid pharyngeal suction-tip (Yankauer) catheter
- Scissors (for tape or ties)
- 10-mL syringe (if cuff present)
- Sterile dressing for tracheal stoma
- Endotracheal intubation supplies and emergency cart

PATIENT AND FAMILY EDUCATION

- Explain the purpose of and procedure for removing the endotracheal tube or tracheostomy. *Rationale:* This step identifies knowledge deficits of the patient and family concerning the patient's condition, the procedure, and the expected benefits. This step also allows time for questions to clarify information and voice concerns. Explanations decrease patient anxiety and enhance cooperation.
- Explain the suctioning process and the importance of coughing and deep breathing after the tube is removed. *Rationale:* Understanding therapy encourages cooperation with the follow-up procedures necessary to maintain a patent airway.
- Explain that the patient's voice may be hoarse after extubation or decannulation. Following the removal of the tracheostomy tube, occlusion of the stoma may be necessary to facilitate normal speech and coughing. *Rationale:* Knowledge minimizes the patient's and family's fear and anxiety.
- Explain that the patient may need continued oxygen or humidification support. *Rationale:* Many patients continue to need supplemental oxygen for some time after extubation or decannulation. Continued humidification often helps decrease hoarseness and liquefies secretions.
- Explain that reinsertion of the endotracheal tube or cannula may be necessary if the patient develops respiratory failure. *Rationale:* Patients may require mechanical ventilation if respiratory failure develops after extubation or decannulation.
- After extubation, a swallow evaluation is often necessary. *Rationale:* Assess the ability to swallow and prevent aspiration with oral intake.

PATIENT ASSESSMENT AND PREPARATION

Patient Assessment

- *Rationale:* Assesses patient's readiness for extubation. Desired level of consciousness has been achieved (most patients are awake and able to follow commands).[2]
- Assess the stability of the patient's respiratory status. *Rationale:* Assesses patient's readiness for extubation.[2,5]
  - ❖ Absence of respiratory distress
  - ❖ Negative inspiratory pressure less than or equal to −20 cm H_2O
  - ❖ Positive expiratory pressure greater than or equal to +30 cm H_2O
  - ❖ Spontaneous tidal volume greater than or equal to 5 mL/kg ideal body weight
  - ❖ Fraction of inspired oxygen (FiO_2) less than or equal to 50%
  - ❖ Normal or baseline $PaCO_2$
  - ❖ Positive end-expiratory pressure <8 cm H_2O
  - ❖ Hemodynamic stability and absence of serious cardiac dysrhythmias

- Assess the patient's ability to cough. *Rationale:* The ability to cough and clear secretions is important for successful airway management after extubation.

Patient Preparation

- Verify correct patient with two identifiers. *Rationale:* Prior to performing a procedure, the nurse should ensure the correct identification of the patient for the intended intervention.
- Ensure that the patient and family understand preprocedural teachings. Answer questions as they arise and reinforce information as needed. *Rationale:* This process evaluates and reinforces understanding of previously taught information.
- Place the patient in the high Fowler's (>60 degrees) or semi-Fowler's (>30 degrees) position if not contraindicated and does not contribute to restriction of breathing (i.e., obesity). *Rationale:* Respiratory muscles are more effective in an upright position versus a supine or prone position. This position facilitates coughing and minimizes the risk of vomiting and consequent aspiration

---

Procedure   for Assisting with Extubation and Decannulation

Steps	Rationale	Special Considerations
1. **HH**		
2. **PE**		
3. Assist with hyperoxygenating and suctioning the tube (see Procedure 10).	Removes secretions in artificial airway and oral cavity.	
4. Manually stabilize the tube until the other healthcare provider is ready to remove it from the patient.	Prevents inadvertent removal or dislodgement of the tube.	
5. Encourage the patient to cough and breathe deeply.	Promotes hyperinflation; helps remove secretions.	
6. Suction the oral pharynx.	Removes secretions.	
7. Apply supplemental oxygen and aerosol, as appropriate.	Promotes moisture and prevents oxygen desaturation.	Cool humidification is usually preferred after extubation to help minimize upper airway swelling.[5]
8. Decannulation ONLY: place a dry, sterile, 4 × 4 dressing over stoma when tracheostomy tube is removed.	Contains secretions that may leak out of stoma.	Tracheostomy stoma closure usually occurs within a few days but may take longer with a long-term tracheostomy.
9. Discard used supplies and remove **PE**.		
10. **HH**		

Expected Outcomes

- Smooth atraumatic extubation or decannulation
- Stable respiratory status
- Stable hemodynamics
- Stable neurological status

Unexpected Outcomes

- Fatigue and respiratory failure
- Persistent hoarseness
- Tracheal stoma narrowing
- Aspiration
- Laryngospasm
- Trauma to soft tissue
- Upper airway obstruction
- Neurological decline

Procedure continues on following page

Patient Monitoring and Care

Steps	Rationale	Reportable Conditions
		These conditions should be reported if they persist despite nursing interventions.
1. Monitor vital signs, respiratory status, oxygenation, neurological status, and phonation immediately after extubation, within 1 hour, and per institutional standard.	Change in vital signs and oxygenation after extubation or decannulation may indicate respiratory compromise, which necessitates reintubation.	• Tachycardia • Tachypnea • Blood pressure significantly greater than baseline • Oxygen saturation (Spo_2) less than or equal to 90% (unless otherwise ordered) • Stridor • Breathing difficulty • Respiratory dyssynchrony
2. Provide supplemental oxygen as needed.	Decreases incidence of oxygen desaturation immediately after extubation.	• Spo_2 less than or equal to 90% (unless otherwise ordered) • Decreased level of consciousness (high $Paco_2$) • Inability to auscultate adequate air exchange
3. Monitor for aspiration related to pooled secretions.	Failure to suction or ineffective suctioning of the pharynx allows accumulated secretions to advance farther into the trachea on cuff deflation.	• Inability to handle secretions
4. Encourage frequent coughing and deep breathing, and use of an incentive spirometer.	Prevents atelectasis and secretion accumulation.	• Ineffective cough
5. Frequent oral care (see Procedure 4).	Maintains oral mucosa and keeps oral cavity clear of dried secretions.	
6. Assess swallowing ability. Facilitate swallow study as indicated by institutional standard.	Presence of tube over extended periods may result in impaired swallowing ability.	• Inability to handle secretions • Inability to swallow without coughing
7. Follow institution standard for assessing pain. Administer analgesia as prescribed.	Identifies need for pain interventions.	• Continued pain despite pain interventions

Documentation

Documentation should include the following:
- Patient and family education
- Respiratory and vital signs assessment before and after procedure
- Date and time when procedure is performed
- Breath sounds and upper airway sounds
- Neurological status
- Patient response to procedure
- Unexpected outcomes and complications—listed previously
- Nursing interventions taken
- Pain assessment, interventions, and effectiveness
- Ability to phonate

References and Additional Readings

For a complete list of references and additional readings for this procedure, scan this QR code with any freely available smartphone code reader app, or visit http://booksite.elsevier.com/9780323376624.

7

King Airway Insertion **AP**
and Removal

Kyle Gibson

PURPOSE: A King Airway, a type of supraglottic airway, can provide an emergency airway during resuscitation without the need for direct laryngoscopy. The King Airway may be used for a patient who is unconscious without a gag reflex and needs artificial ventilation when a definitive or alternative airway is not available or has failed.

PREREQUISITE NURSING KNOWLEDGE

- Anatomy and physiology of the upper airway should be well understood.
- The King Airway does not require direct laryngoscopy and may be inserted blindly.[3]
- The King Airway may act as an airway bridge when definitive airway control is not available or has failed.[7]
- The King Airway LT-D (Fig. 7-1) is manufactured in five sizes based on height or weight[4]:
  - ❖ Size 2 is used for patients 35 to 45 inches tall (90 to 115 cm) or 12 to 25 kg and has a green connector for identification.
  - ❖ Size 2.5 is used for patients 41 to 51 inches tall (105 to 130 cm) or 25 to 35 kg and has an orange connector for identification.
  - ❖ Size 3 is used for patients 4 to 5 feet tall (122 to 155 cm) and has a yellow connector for identification.
  - ❖ Size 4 is used for patients 5 to 6 feet tall (155 to 180 cm) and has a red connector for identification.
  - ❖ Size 5 is used for patients greater than 6 feet tall (>180 cm) and has a purple connector for identification.
- The King Airway LTS-D (Fig. 7-2) is manufactured to include a second lumen, allowing gastric access for a suction catheter up to 18 Fr. The King Airway LTS-D is not available in sizes 2 or 2.5.
- The King Airway allows for positive pressure ventilation over 30 mm H_2O.[4]
- The King Airway is supplied in either a complete kit (with all the necessary equipment for insertion) or as an indi-

vidual device. If the individual device is used, additional components are necessary for insertion.
- The latex-free King Airway has a unique design that includes the following:
  - ❖ A proximal and distal cuff that is inflated through a single inflation port with a pilot balloon
  - ❖ A 15-mm connector color coded for easy sizing identification and able to connect to bag-valve devices and ventilator circuits
  - ❖ A blue orientation line on the lumen to allow correct handling and placement of the King Airway
  - ❖ Black lines on the lumen indicating the position of the patient's teeth or gumline for tube-depth identification
  - ❖ Two cuffs for occlusion (cuff volume is 25 to 90 mL with a goal cuff pressure of 60 mm H_2O)
    - ○ Proximal cuff stabilizes the tube and occludes the oropharynx
    - ○ Distal cuff occludes the esophagus and decreases gastric ventilation
  - ❖ Two ventilation outlets laying in between the two cuffs, allowing passage of a fiberoptic bronchoscope or a tube-exchange device (gum elastic bougie) for both LTD and LTS-D models
- Upon insertion, the distal tip of the King Airway occludes the esophagus (Fig. 7-3).
- Before insertion of the King Airway, adequate ventilation and oxygenation needs to be performed by either mouth-to-mask or bag-valve mask connected to high-flow oxygen.
- The King Airway is contraindicated in the following cases[5]:
  - ❖ Patients with an intact gag reflex
  - ❖ Patients with a known esophageal disease, such as esophageal varices or esophageal trauma
  - ❖ Patients who have ingested caustic substances
  - ❖ Patients with a foreign body in the trachea
  - ❖ Patients with a tracheostomy or stoma
- Medications delivered via endotracheal tube cannot be used with the King Airway. Medications may not reach

AP   This procedure should be performed only by physicians, advanced practice nurses, and other healthcare professionals (including critical care nurses) with additional knowledge, skills, and demonstrated competence per professional licensure or institutional standard.

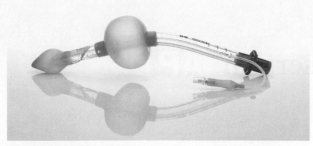

Figure 7-1   King Airway LT-D

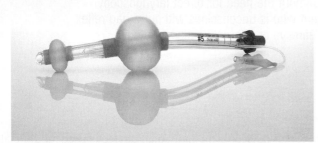

Figure 7-2   King Airway LTS-D

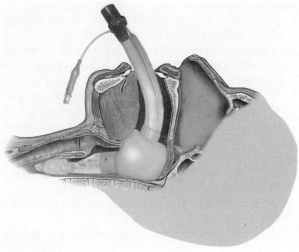

Figure 7-3   Properly placed King Airway, with the proximal cuff stabilizing the tube and occluded the oropharynx and the distal tip occluding the esophagus.

the alveolar surfaces of the lung for absorption due to the distal end of the King Airway being in the esophagus.
• Initial and continued education on and practice with insertion of the King Airway is essential to maximize insertion success and minimize complications.[6]

EQUIPMENT

• Personal protectant equipment
• Suction equipment including regulator, canister, tubing, and suctioning device
• Mouth-to-mask or self-inflating resuscitation bag-valve mask connected to high-flow oxygen
• King Airway of the appropriate size based on height for adult patients and either height or weight for pediatric patients

• Appropriate syringe for inflation of cuffs: this may be a 60- to 80-mL syringe for adult patients or a small 20-mL syringe for pediatric patients
• Water-soluble lubricant
• Colorimetric carbon dioxide (CO_2) device or end-tidal CO_2 device with monitor
• Appropriate-size gastric tube if using LTS-D model
Additional equipment, to have available as needed, includes the following:
• Laryngoscope or a tongue depressor

PATIENT AND FAMILY EDUCATION

• If time permits, provide the family or guardian with information about the King Airway and the reason for insertion. *Rationale*: Educating the family or guardian with information about the King Airway and the need for insertion is necessary. It may alleviate anxiety.

PATIENT ASSESSMENT AND PREPARATION
Patient Assessment

• Assess the level of consciousness of the patient. *Rationale:* The King Airway should only be inserted into a patient who is unconscious, unresponsive without a gag reflex, and unable to maintain adequate ventilation. Administration of paralytics and/or sedation may be needed to ensure the patient's gag reflex does not return after the King Airway is in place.
• Assess the patient for any type of esophageal injury, such as a clothesline injury. *Rationale:* The King Airway is contraindicated in esophageal trauma.
• Assess history and patient information from bystanders, if available, for possibility of esophageal disease or caustic substance ingestion. *Rationale:* A King Airway is contraindicated in patients with these conditions.
• Assess the patient's height or weight. *Rationale:* The King Airway is sized based on the patient's height for the adult population and based on height or weight for the pediatric population.

Patient Preparation

• Verify correct patient with two identifiers. *Rationale:* Prior to performing a procedure, the nurse should ensure the correct identification of the patient for the intended intervention.
• Ensure that suction equipment is assembled and readily available. *Rationale:* The patient may regurgitate during insertion or while the King Airway is in place and will ultimately need suctioning to prevent aspiration.
• Perform preprocedure verification and time out, if not emergent. *Rationale:* Ensures patient safety.
• Ensure adequate ventilation and oxygenation are being performed before insertion of the King Airway via a mouth-to-mask or a self-inflating bag-valve-mask device. *Rationale:* The patient is usually unresponsive and cannot adequately maintain ventilation without assistance.

Procedure for King Airway Insertion

Steps	Rationale	Special Considerations
1. **HH**		
2. **PE**		
3. Using the information provided, choose the correct King Airway size, based on patient height or weight.		The King Airway LTS-D is only manufactured for sizes 3–5.
4. Open the package and test the integrity of both cuffs. **(Level M*)** A. Pull the plunger back on the syringe to the appropriate volume for the size of the King Airway and attach it to the inflation port. B. Inflate the proximal and distal cuffs and assess for leaks. C. Deflate the cuffs, leaving the syringe attached.	Ensures that the device is not defective and will work as manufactured. Readies the syringe for inflating the cuffs upon insertion.	If a leak is found, discard the device and secure another.
5. Lubricate the King Airway with water-soluble lubricant.	Provides for smoother insertion.	Make sure that the ventilation holes are not covered with lubricant. **(Level M)**
6. Have a spare King Airway ready and prepared for immediate use if failure or damage occurs with the first one.	This allows no delay in initiating an airway if the first King Airway fails or becomes damaged while inserting.	
7. Preoxygenate the patient when possible.	Prevents hypoxia.	Provider must be aware of preventing anoxia during the procedure, especially if multiple attempts are made.
8. If no spinal injury is suspected, extend the neck and position the head in a "sniffing position."	Pulls the tongue forward, away from the posterior pharynx.	Maintain manual cervical spinal immobilization with suspected or known spine trauma.
9. Hold the King Airway at the connector with dominant hand. With nondominant hand, hold mouth open and apply chin lift. **(Level M)**	Readies the King Airway for insertion and opens the airway for insertion.	With facial trauma, assess for the presence of broken teeth and remove loose fragments.
10. With the King Airway rotated laterally such that the blue orientation line is touching the corner of the mouth, introduce tip of the King Airway into mouth and advance behind base of the tongue. **(Level M)**	Allows the King Airway to follow the patient's pharynx until it is in the correct position.	A laryngoscope or a tongue depressor can be used to lift the tongue anteriorly to allow easy advancement.[3]
11. As the King Airway passes under the tongue, rotate tube back to the midline so that blue orientation line faces the chin. **(Level M)**	Proper placement of the King Airway occurs when distal tip of the lumen is in the esophagus. Tracheal intubation does not occur.[8]	Do not force the King Airway. If it does not easily advance, attempt to redirect or remove and reinsert.
12. Without exerting excessive force, advance tube until base of connector is aligned with teeth or gums. **(Level M)**	Places the King Airway in the correct anatomical location for ventilation.	Depth of insertion is key to providing a patent airway.

*Level M: Manufacturer's recommendations only.

Procedure continues on following page

Procedure   for King Airway Insertion—*Continued*

Steps	Rationale	Special Considerations
13. Using the syringe provided, inflate the cuffs of the King Airway with the appropriate predetermined volume.	Inflates and seals the proximal and distal cuffs. This stabilizes the tube and reduces the possibility of gastric return.	The King Airway may rise out of the mouth during inflation of cuffs so that the teeth or gums are between the black lines on the lumen of the tube.
14. Attach bag-valve device to the 15-mm color-coded connector. While gently bagging the patient to assess ventilation, simultaneously withdraw the King Airway until ventilation is easy and free flowing. **(Level M*)**	With successful placement, the distal balloon is in the esophagus. With both cuffs inflated, the only place artificial ventilation can flow is into the trachea.	
15. Depth markings are provided at the proximal end of the King Airway lumen that refer to the distance from the distal ventilatory opening.	Determines placement of the King Airway.	During spontaneous ventilation, the epiglottis or other tissue can be drawn into the distal ventilatory opening, resulting in obstruction.[3] Advancing the King Airway 1–2 cm, or initiating deeper placement, normally eliminates this obstruction.
16. Confirm proper position by auscultation. A. Assess for gurgling over the epigastrium, equal chest rise and fall, and bilateral breath sounds. B. If available, use colorimetric CO_2 detector or end-tidal CO_2 (capnography).	Confirms proper placement of the King Airway.	When assessing for the presence of breath sounds, always consider the possibility of a pneumothorax, especially in the trauma patient. Absent breath sounds may lead the provider to believe that the King Airway is misplaced.
17. Readjust cuff inflation to just seal volume and prevent air leaks. **(Level M)**	Cuffs are inflated with minimum volume necessary to seal the airway at the peak ventilatory pressure employed.	
18. Secure the King Airway to the patient using either tape or a premanufactured tube holder.	Reduces the chance of dislodgment.	A bite-block may also be used, if desired, to provide greater tube security.
19. If using the King Airway LTS-D and a gastric tube is indicated, lubricate before insertion into gastric lumen.	May reduce gastric distention and may increase the ease of ventilation.	
20. Discard supplies and remove **PE**.		
21. **HH**		
22. Document the procedure in the patient's record.		

*Level M: Manufacturer's recommendations only.

Procedure | for King Airway Removal

Steps	Rationale	Special Considerations
1. **HH**		
2. **PE**		
3. Have suction readily available.	Allows suctioning of the airway preprocedure and postprocedure.	
4. Remove the King Airway.	Removal is indicated when airway can be managed by skilled personnel.	A fiberoptic scope or manufactured intubation catheter[1] or gum elastic bougie may be used to replace the King Airway with an endotracheal tube.
A. If King LTS-D is in place, decompress the stomach by inserting a gastric tube through the gastric access lumen.	Removes any content in the stomach, which makes regurgitation less likely upon removal.	Regurgitation is always a possibility upon removal of a King Airway.
B. Attach appropriate syringe to the pilot balloon and deflate the cuffs.	Deflates both proximal and distal cuffs and allows suctioning of pharynx to occur.	
C. Suction the pharynx.	Removes secretions from pharynx.	Suction no more than 10 seconds at a time.
D. Withdraw the King Airway from the airway.	Allows the patient to breathe on his or her own.	
5. Apply supplemental oxygen.	Reduces hypoxia postremoval.	
6. Discard supplies and remove **PE**.		
7. **HH**		
8. Document the procedure in the patient's record.		

Expected Outcomes

- Establishment of an effective airway in an emergent situation or a failed nonemergent situation
- Maintains adequate ventilation and oxygenation
- Recovery of spontaneous ventilation

Unexpected Outcomes

- Laryngospasm[3]
- Coughing[3]
- Sore throat[2,3]
- Dysphagia[3]
- Dysphonia[3]
- Gagging
- Vomiting

Patient Monitoring and Care

Steps	Rationale	Reportable Conditions
		These conditions should be reported if they persist despite nursing interventions.
1. Monitor ventilations and oxygenation while the King Airway is in place. A. Difficulty of ventilation. B. Oxygen saturation (Spo₂). C. End-tidal carbon dioxide (ETco₂).	Determines that the King Airway is functioning correctly and providing adequate ventilation and oxygenation.	• Increase difficulty in ventilation. • Decrease oxygen saturation. • Increase end-tidal carbon dioxide. • Absent breath sound[s].
2. Monitor for return of spontaneous attempts at breathing.	May indicate the need either to remove the device or chemically sedate the patient using sedatives or neuromuscular blockade to prevent the gag reflex.	• High-pressure alarms. • High minute volume.

Procedure continues on following page

Documentation

Documentation should include the following:

- Assessment findings that indicate the need to insert a King Airway
- Size of the King Airway used
- Confirmation of adequacy of ventilation, with auscultation of gastric area and lung fields
- Any difficulties with placement of the King Airway
- Number of attempts it took to place the King Airway
- What marking the King Airway is at via teeth or lips
- End-tidal CO_2 levels
- Need for sedation or neuromuscular blockade
- Assessment findings after the insertion of the King Airway
- Ongoing monitoring of difficulty or ease of ventilation
- SpO_2 levels
- If insertion of gastric tube, chart output of gastric contents.
- Assessment findings that indicate the need to remove the King Airway or replace it with an endotracheal tube

References and Additional Readings

For a complete list of references and additional readings for this procedure, scan this QR code with any freely available smartphone code reader app, or visit http://booksite.elsevier.com/9780323376624.

Laryngeal Mask Airway [AP]

Stephen Both

PURPOSE: Despite the wide adoption and use of the laryngeal mask airway (LMA) for routine surgery, this procedure focuses on this device's utility as an emergency airway device involving a lost or compromised airway in the unconscious patient when endotracheal intubation is not readily available or has failed (e.g., cardiac arrest, prehospital airway management, failed intubation/difficult airway, conduit for intubation). Although second-generation LMAs offer better protection against aspiration, it should be understood that the LMA is not a definitive airway.[1,2,4,7]

PREREQUISITE NURSING KNOWLEDGE

- The requirements for rapid airway management in an unconscious patient should be understood.
- The anatomy and physiology of the upper airway should be understood.
- The design of the LMA available should be understood (Figs. 8-1 and 8-2):
  - ❖ An airway tube connects the mask and the 15-mm male adapter.
  - ❖ The mask's cuff, when inflated, conforms to the contours of the hypopharynx, with the opening of the air tube positioned directly over the laryngeal opening.
  - ❖ A cuff inflation line with a valve and a pilot balloon leads to the mask's cuff.
- Benefits of second-generation LMAs over first generation LMAs should be understood (Table 8-1).
- The final placement of an LMA in the airway should be understood (Fig. 8-3).
- The ability to ventilate an unconscious patient adequately with a mouth-to-mask or bag-valve-mask device is necessary.
- The underlying risks of the LMA should be understood.
  - ❖ Due to the potential risk of regurgitation and aspiration, do not use the LMA as a "first-choice airway" in the following elective or difficult airway patients on a non-emergency pathway[9]:
    - ○ Patients who have not fasted, including patients whose fasting cannot be confirmed.[5]
    - ○ Patients who are morbidly obese, who are more than 14 weeks pregnant, who have multiple or massive injury or acute abdominal or thoracic injury, who have any condition associated with delayed gastric emptying, or who have used opiate medication

before fasting. However, in all these clinical scenarios, the LMA Supreme (second-generation supraglottic device) is ideally suited to serve as an "airway rescue device" in preference to the LMA Classic or the LMA Unique (first-generation supraglottic device).[3,5]

- ❖ LMA Supreme is contraindicated in the following:
  - ○ Patients with fixed decreased pulmonary compliance, such as in pulmonary fibrosis due to inadequate seal around the larynx[5]
  - ○ Adult patients who have had radiotherapy to the neck involving the hypopharynx (risk of trauma, failure to seal effectively)[5]
  - ○ Patients with a mouth opening inadequate to permit insertion[8]
  - ○ Patients with suspected acute intestinal obstruction or ileus or patients having been injured shortly after ingesting a substantial meal[8]
  - ○ Patients who have ingested caustic substances[5]
- ❖ LMA Supreme usage precautions include the following:
- ❖ The LMA Supreme is a single use–only device.[5]
  - ○ Due to oropharyngeal tissue being specifically prone to swelling and bleeding with mild to moderate traumatic forces (potentially resulting in dire consequences), excessive force should not be used at any time during insertion of the LMA Supreme or insertion of a gastric tube through the drain tube of the LMA Supreme.[5]
  - ○ Never overinflate the cuff after insertion. An appropriate intracuff pressure is 60 cm H_2O. Excessive intracuff pressure can result in malposition and sore throat, dysphagia, or nerve injury.[5,6,8]
  - ○ If airway problems persist or ventilation is inadequate, the LMA Supreme should be removed and an airway established by some other means.[9]
  - ○ The LMA Supreme is made of medical grade polyvinyl chloride that can be torn or perforated. Avoid contact with sharp or pointed objects at all times. Do not insert the device unless the cuff is fully deflated as described in the instructions for insertion.[5]

[AP]   This procedure should be performed only by physicians, advanced practice nurses, and other healthcare professionals (including critical care nurses) with additional knowledge, skills, and demonstrated competence per professional licensure or institutional standard.

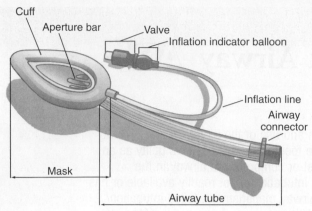

Figure 8-1 Components of the first-generation laryngeal mask airway (LMA; LMA Classic pictured). *(From the Laryngeal Mask Company Limited:* Instruction manual: LMA-Classic. *San Diego, 2005, Laryngeal Mask Company Limited.)*

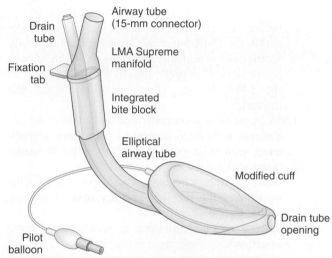

Figure 8-2 Components of a second-generation laryngeal mask airway (LMA; LMA Supreme pictured): Manifold with an integral bite block, an anatomically shaped airway tube enclosing a drain tube, a modified cuff through which a cuff inflation line with pilot tube. *(From Hagberg C:* Benumof and Hagberg's Airway Management, *ed 3, Philadelphia, 2013, Elsevier.)*

- ○ Gloves should be worn during preparation and insertion to minimize contamination of the airway.[5]
- ○ Store device in a dark, cool environment, avoiding direct sunlight or extremes of temperature.[5,9]
- • The LMA may provide a more viable means of ventilation than a bag-valve-mask device in patients with a beard or without teeth.[3]
- • Initial and ongoing training is necessary to maximize insertion success and minimize complications.[3–5,7]
- • This procedure refers specifically to the LMA Supreme, a second-generation LMA. Other types of second-generation LMA devices are available and provide additional features, such as use as a conduit for endotracheal intubation through the LMA (e.g., LMA Fastrach).
- • An understanding of the different models now available will aid in LMA selection (Table 8-2).
- • Understand the advantages and disadvantages of LMAs compared with facemask ventilation and endotracheal tube intubation (Table 8-3).

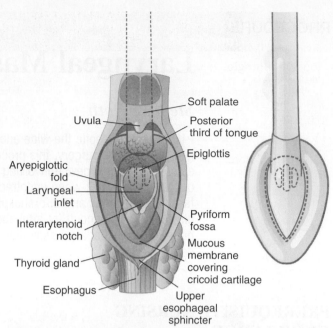

Figure 8-3 Dorsal view of the laryngeal mask airway (LMA) showing position in relation to pharyngeal anatomy (LMA Classic pictured.) *(From The Laryngeal Mask Company Limited:* Instruction manual: LMA-Classic. *San Diego, 2005, Laryngeal Mask Company Limited.)*

TABLE 8-1	Improvements to Second-Generation Supraglottic Airway Devices Compared With First Generation
Design Improvements	**Rationale**
Improved pharyngeal seal	Controlled ventilation at higher airway pressures (and hence in a wider range of patients and clinical situations)
Increased esophageal seal	Lessens the likelihood of regurgitant fluids entering the pharynx and leading to aspiration
Integrated bite block	Impedes patient's ability to bite and potentially occlude the airway, risking hypoxia and negative pressure pulmonary edema
Gastric port	May be used to confirm correct device positioning, enable access to the stomach, alert the user to the presence of regurgitation, and enable gastric contents to safely bypass the oropharynx and exit the patient (e.g., Laryngeal Mask Airway [LMA] Supreme and LMA Proseal)

From Cook T, Woodall N, Frerk C: Major complications of airway management in the UK: The Fourth National Audit Project of the Royal College of Anaesthetists, 2011, available at www.rcoa.ac.uk/nap4.

TABLE 8-2	Type of Laryngeal Mask Airway (LMA) With Corresponding Generation and Features	

Type of Supraglottic Device (LMA)	Generation LMA	Features
LMA Classic	1st	Early prototype nondisposable LMA
LMA Unique	1st	Disposable standard LMA
LMA Proseal	2nd	Inflatable cuff with improved pharyngeal seal = ventilation tolerances, gastric port, and an integrated bite block
LMA Supreme	2nd	
I-Gel LMA	2nd	Noninflatable gel cuff rather than inflatable cuff for pharyngeal seal, gastric channel, and integrated bite block
Air-Q LMA	2nd	Designed to facilitate endotracheal intubation through the LMA device; no gastric port
AMBU Aura-I LMA	2nd	
LMA Fastrach	2nd	
LMA CTrach	2nd	Incorporates a camera to facilitate passage of an endotracheal tube; no gastric port

From Hagberg C: Benumof and Hagberg's Airway Management, ed 3, Philadelphia, 2013, Elsevier; Butterworth J, Mackey DC, Wasnick J: Morgan & Mikhail's Clinical Anesthesiology, ed 5, New York, 2013, McGraw Hill; Nagelhout JJ, Plaus KL: Nurse anesthesia, ed 5, St. Louis, 2014, Elsevier.

TABLE 8-3	Advantages and Disadvantages of the Laryngeal Mask Airway (LMA) Compared With Facemask Ventilation and Tracheal Intubation	

	Advantages	Disadvantages
LMA compared with facemask	• Hands-free operation • Better seal in bearded patients • Often easier to maintain airway • Protects against airway secretions • Less facial nerve and eye trauma	• More invasive • More risk of airway trauma • Requires new skill • Multiple contraindications
LMA compared with tracheal intubation	• Less invasive • Very useful in difficult intubations • Less tooth and laryngeal trauma • Less laryngospasm and bronchospasm • Does not require neck mobility • No risk of esophageal or endobronchial intubation	• Increased risk of gastrointestinal aspiration • Limits maximum positive pressure ventilation • Less secure airway • Can cause gastric distention • Not designed for prolonged use; maximum time period of 10–24 hours has been studied without adverse effects[4]

From Butterworth J, Mackey DC, Wasnick J: Morgan & Mikhail's Clinical Anesthesiology, ed 5, New York, 2013, McGraw-Hill.

TABLE 8-4	Laryngeal Mask Airways (LMA) Supreme Selection Guide			

Airway Size	Patient Weight	Maximum Size Nasogastric Tube	Recommended Maximum Inflation Volume	Optimum Intra-Cuff Pressure (Do Not Exceed)
1	<5 kg	6 Fr	5 mL	60 cm H_2O
1.5	5–10 kg	6 Fr	8 mL	
2	10–20 kg	10 Fr	12 mL	
2.5	20–30 kg	10 Fr	20 mL	
3	30–50 kg	14 Fr	30 mL	
4	50–70 kg	14 Fr	45 mL	
5	70–100 kg	14 Fr	45 mL	

From Teleflex Medical Incorporated, Morrisville, NC.

EQUIPMENT

- LMA Supreme size selection (Table 8-4)
  ❖ For normal adults, use the size 4 device as a first choice.[5]
- Water-soluble lubricant
- Gloves, mask, and eye protection
- Suction equipment (suction canister with control head, tracheal suction catheters, Yankauer suction tip)
- Mouth-to-mask or bag-valve-mask device attached to a high-flow oxygen source
- Tape
- 60-cm^3 syringe

Additional equipment, to have available as needed, includes the following:

- Nasogastric (NG) tube (for sizing see Table 8-4). The drain port of the LMA Supreme can facilitate the passage of an appropriately sized NG tube after correct positioning of an LMA Supreme.

PATIENT AND FAMILY EDUCATION

- If time allows, provide the family with information regarding the LMA and the reason for insertion. *Rationale:* This information assists the family in understanding why the procedure is necessary and decreases family anxiety.

PATIENT ASSESSMENT AND PREPARATION

Patient Assessment

- Assess the level of consciousness and responsiveness. *Rationale:* In an emergency situation, the LMA should be inserted only into a patient who is profoundly unconscious and unresponsive.[5] Laryngospasm and/or vomiting may result, causing the inability to ventilate if an LMA is introduced into a conscious or semiconscious patient.
- Assess history and patient information for the possibility of delayed gastric emptying (e.g., hiatal hernia, recent food ingestion, poorly controlled diabetes). *Rationale:* In a patient with delayed gastric emptying, the benefits of LMA insertion must be weighed against the possibility of regurgitation.[5]
- Assess history and patient information for possibility of decreased pulmonary compliance (i.e., pulmonary fibrosis, obesity). *Rationale:* The high pressures needed to

ventilate a patient with decreased pulmonary compliance may override the occlusive pressure of the LMA.[5]

- Assess predictors of difficult LMA insertion.[10] Consider the mnemonic "RODS":
  - ❖ R = restricted mouth opening
  - ❖ O = obstruction/obesity
  - ❖ D = disrupted or distorted airway
  - ❖ S = stiff, as in asthma, pulmonary fibrosis, or pulmonary edema[10]

Patient Preparation

- If time permits, assess the patient's and family's level of understanding about the condition and rationale for use of the LMA. *Rationale:* This assessment identifies the patient's and family's knowledge deficits concerning the patient's condition.
- Ensure adequate ventilation and oxygenation with either a mouth-to-mask or bag-valve-mask device (see Procedure 31). *Rationale:* The patient is nonresponsive and apneic without assisted ventilation before the LMA insertion.[5]
- Ensure that the suction equipment is assembled and in working order. *Rationale:* The patient may regurgitate during the insertion or while the LMA is in place and may require oropharyngeal or tracheal suctioning.[5]
- Anything that is not permanently affixed in the patient's mouth (e.g., dentures, partials, jewelry) should be removed. *Rationale:* Inadvertent dislodgment and aspiration might occur with the placement of the LMA.[5] Significant time should not be wasted in removing such oral appliances if significant hypoxia is being experienced.
- Placement is most successful with the patient positioned supine with the head in the neutral or sniffing position.[5] *Rationale:* Proper head positioning facilitates successful placement of an LMA.

Procedures	for Laryngeal Mask Airway (LMA Supreme) Insertion	
Steps	**Rationale**	**Special Considerations**
1. **HH**		
2. **PE**		
3. Ensure that a spare LMA of the same type is immediately available. **(Level M*)**	Provides for a "backup" device should the initial device fail.	
4. Remove the LMA from the package and inspect. **(Level M)**	Ensures that the device is not defective and will work as indicated.	
A. Inspect the exterior of the mask for any cuts, tears, or scratches.	Ensures that the exterior surface of the device has not been damaged in any way.	
B. Inspect the interior of the airway tube for any particles	Particles in the airway tube may be inhaled when the device is used.	Discard the device if any evidence of damage is found and open the backup device
C. Examine the 15-mm male connector at the end of the airway tube and ensure that it fits tightly into the tube.	The 15-mm male connector is essential for ventilation with a bag-valve device or ventilator.	Discard the device if any particles cannot be removed from the tube and open the backup device

*Level M: Manufacturer's recommendations only.

Procedures	**for Laryngeal Mask Airway (LMA Supreme) Insertion—*Continued***	
Steps	**Rationale**	**Special Considerations**

5. Perform the deflation and inflation tests. **(Level M*)**

	Rationale	**Special Considerations**
A. Expel the air from the 60-mL syringe and connect it to the pilot balloon valve.	Ensures that the device is not defective and will work as indicated.	
B. Pull back the syringe plunger to deflate the cuff fully.	The appropriate-size syringe is needed to inflate the cuff to the proper test level.	Discard the device if the connector does not fit tightly into the airway tube and open the backup device.[5]
C. Examine the cuff to ensure that it remains fully deflated (Fig. 8-4).	Full deflation of the cuff helps ensure its patency.	Discard the device if the cuff does not remain fully deflated and open the backup device.[5]
D. Obtain a 60-ml syringe and pull back on the syringe to the volume required for each LMA size, reattach to the valve, and inflate the cuff with the appropriate volume for the size (see Table 8-4).	Ensures that the device is not defective and will work as indicated.	Discard the device if the cuff does not remain fully deflated and open the backup device.[5]
E. Examine the inflated cuff to ensure that it is symmetrical without bulges.	Ensure that the device is not defective and will work as indicated.	Discard the device if the cuff bulges asymmetrically and open the backup device.[5]
F. Examine the pilot balloon to ensure that its inflated shape is elliptical.	Ensures that the device is not defective and will work as indicated.	Discard the device if the pilot balloon is spherical or bulges and open the backup device.[5]

Insertion Technique

(If possible, preoxygenate patients with 100% oxygen for several minutes before the insertion of any advanced airway adjunct intervention) **(Level E*)**.[4,6,7]	Facilitates replacing nitrogen with oxygen in the lungs. Increases the duration of apnea without desaturation, which facilitates more time to place airway adjunct and improves patient safety	Conditions that increase oxygen demand (e.g., sepsis, pregnancy) and decrease functional residual capacity (e.g., morbid obesity, pregnancy) reduce the apnea period before desaturation ensues.[6]

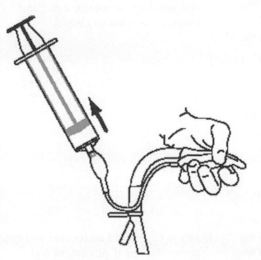

Figure 8-4 Laryngeal Mask Airway (LMA) Supreme deflation technique. After firmly connecting a syringe of at least 50 mL to the inflation port, hold the syringe and the LMA Supreme exactly as shown. Compress the distal end of the device in between the index finger and thumb while withdrawing air until a vacuum has been obtained. While deflating, hold the device so that the distal end is curled slightly anteriorly. Deflate the device until the tension in the syringe indicates that a vacuum has been created in the mask. Keep the syringe under tension while rapidly disconnecting it from the inflation port. *(From Teleflex Medical Incorporated, Morrisville, NC.)*

*Level E: Multiple case reports, theory-based evidence from expert opinions, or peer-reviewed professional organizational standards without clinical studies to support recommendations.
*Level M: Manufacturer's recommendations only.

Procedure continues on following page

Procedures   **for Laryngeal Mask Airway (LMA Supreme) Insertion—*Continued***

Steps	Rationale	Special Considerations
6. Fully deflate the cuff by holding the device so that the distal end is curled slightly anteriorly, as shown in Fig. 8-4. Attach a syringe. Compress the distal tip of the mask with thumb and index finger. **(Level M*)**	Facilitates smooth insertion and avoids deflection of the epiglottis.	
7. Lubricate the posterior surface of the cuff and airway tube with a small amount of water-soluble lubricant (Fig. 8-5, Step 2). **(Level M)**	Facilitates smooth insertion.	Avoid excessive lubrication on the anterior portion (aperture side) of the cuff because it may be aspirated or occlude lumen. Do not use lidocaine lubricants because they may delay the return of protective reflects and may cause an allergic reaction.[9]
8. Stand behind or besides the patient's head. Place the patient's head in the neutral or sniffing position (see Fig. 8-5, Step 3). **(Level E*)**	Facilitates proper body position for the person inserting the device and the patient's head during insertion.	The patient's head may be left in a neutral position if cervical spine injury is possible.[5] If cervical instability is suspected, manual stabilization should be maintained by the assistant during the placement procedure.
9. Hold the device exactly as shown in Fig. 8-5. Press the distal tip against the inner aspect of the upper teeth or gums (see Fig. 8-5, Step 3).	Facilitates smooth insertion.	
10. Slide inwards using a slightly diagonal approach (direct the tip away from the midline). Continue to slide inwards, rotating the hand in a circular motion so that the device follows the curvature behind the tongue (see Fig. 8-5, Step 4).	Assists in maneuvering the LMA into the proper position	Do not use force. If the LMA does not advance, remove, reventilate, and reinsert.[9] The mask must be pressed up against the hard palate to be inserted correctly.[9] If the cuff becomes obstructed by the tonsils, a diagonal maneuver is often successful.[5,9]
11. Resistance should be felt when the distal end of the device meets the upper esophageal sphincter. The device is now fully inserted (see Fig. 8-5, Step 5).	Continues moving the LMA into the proper final position.	
12. Inflate with the minimal amount of air needed to achieve an effective seal. For further details on a successful insertion, see Box 8-1.	The recommended intracuff pressure should not exceed 60 cm H_2O.	
Securing the LMA (Fixation)[5]		
13. Use a piece of adhesive tape 30–40 cm long, holding it horizontally by both ends	Facilitates the approximate length necessary to secure the LMA.	
14. Press the adhesive tape transversely across the fixation tab (if present) or an area 2–3 cm above the lips on the LMA airway tube.	The fixation tab is located above the bite block on LMA Supreme. Other first- and second-generation devices *do not* possess fixation tabs.	Fixation tab should be located 1–2 cm above the lips if placement and sizing is appropriate. Fixation tab should not be applied with downward pressure to lips/teeth nor be located >3 cm above the lips (may indicate improper sizing or improper placement of LMA).

*Level E: Multiple case reports, theory-based evidence from expert opinions, or peer-reviewed professional organizational standards without clinical studies to support recommendations.
*Level M: Manufacturer's recommendations only.

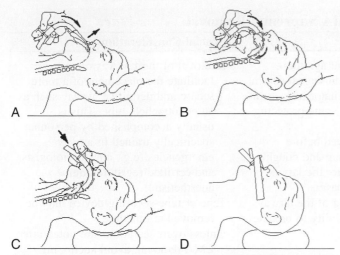

A _____   B _____

C _____   D _____

Figure 8-5 Insertion of second-generation Laryngeal Mask Airway (LMA) Supreme. (*From Teleflex Medical Incorporated, Morrisville, NC.*)

BOX 8-1	Successful Insertion of a Laryngeal Mask Airway Depends Upon Attention to Several Details

1. Choose the appropriate size (see Table 8-4) and check for leaks before insertion.
2. The leading edge of the deflated cuff should be wrinkle free and face away from the aperture.
3. Lubricate the back side of the cuff.
4. The patient must be vastly unresponsive and relaxed before attempting insertion.
5. Place the patient's head in sniffing position (see Fig. 8-5).
6. Correct positioning can be aided by using your index finger to guide the cuff along the hard palate and down into the hypopharynx until an increased resistance is felt.
7. Inflate with the correct amount of air (see Table 8-4).
8. Obstruction after insertion is usually due to a down-folded epiglottis or transient laryngospasm.
9. Avoid pharyngeal suction, cuff deflation, or laryngeal mask removal until the patient is awake (e.g., opening mouth on command) unless removing to facilitate a more secure airway.

From Butterworth J, Mackey DC, Wasnick J: Morgan & Mikhail's Clinical Anesthesiology, *ed 5, New York, 2013, McGraw-Hill.*

Procedures for Laryngeal Mask Airway (LMA Supreme) Insertion—*Continued*

Steps	Rationale	Special Considerations
15. Continue to press downward so that the ends of the tape adhere to each of the patient's cheeks and the device itself is gently pressed inwards by the tape.	Secures the LMA with slight inward pressure. This assists in maintaining LMA seal.	Without securing the LMA in place, displacement or migration of device from airway is probable.
16. Bite block may be considered if utilizing a first-generation LMA.	The patient may bite down on a first-generation LMA airway, collapsing the tube and thus compromising airway.	Second-generation LMAs incorporate bite blocks within the device.
17. Dispose of supplies.		
18. 🖐		

Procedures for Laryngeal Mask Airway (LMA Supreme) Correct Position

Steps	Rationale	Special Considerations
1. Correct placement should produce a leak-free seal against the glottis, with the mask tip at the upper esophageal sphincter	Maintenance of low ventilator pressures prevents overriding the pressure in the cuff, creating a leak, or forcing air into the stomach.	If sounds are heard in the epigastrium on auscultation, remove the device and manually ventilate the patient with a bag-valve mask.
2. The bite-block portion of the LMA Supreme should lie between the teeth.	Helps confirm correct depth with primary assessment.	Limit tidal volumes to <8 mL/kg.
3. A drop of water-soluble lubricant (1–2 mL) can be placed on the proximal end of the gastric drainage tube port.	Confirms proper placement with tip of LMA sealed in esophagus.	Observe a slight up-down meniscus movement of the lubricant following the application and release of gentle pressure on the suprasternal notch,[5] aka "suprasternal notch test."[5] This is
4. Observe a slight up-down meniscus movement of the lubricant following the application and release of gentle pressure on the suprasternal notch	Indicates that the distal end of the drain tube is correctly placed so that it seals around the upper esophageal sphincter	more important if the rescuer plans to pass an NG tube of appropriate size down the LMA for gastric decompression purposes. Increased risk of laryngospasm and airway occlusion can result if the LMA is mal-positioned, resulting in NG placement down the bronchi.

Procedure continues on following page

Procedures for Laryngeal Mask Airway (LMA Supreme) Removal

Steps	Rationale	Special Considerations

1. **HH**
2. **PE**
3. Remove the LMA as follows:
  A. Gently assist with ventilations when the patient begins spontaneously breathing.
  B. Observe for signs of swallowing. When the patient can open his or her mouth on command, deflate the cuff and remove the LMA.[5]
  C. Continue to assess for airway and breathing effectiveness:
    i. Establishment of an effective airway in an emergency situation
    ii. Maintenance of adequate ventilation
    iii. Recovery of spontaneous ventilation
4. Dispose of supplies.
5. **HH**
	Removal may prevent agitation, regurgitation, and laryngeal spasm.
	Prevents excess ventilator pressures.
	Indicates a return of some protective reflexes.
	If the LMA is removed before effective swallowing and coughing, secretions may enter the larynx, causing bronchospasm.
	Maintains monitoring of the airway and the patient's ability to breathe on his or her own.
		Removal of the LMA is often to facilitate the placement of a more secure and definitive airway such as an endotracheal tube. This is usually accomplished by personnel specifically trained in airway emergencies (e.g., anesthesiologists and certified registered nurse anesthetists).
		Tape or tube-securing device may be removed at this time.
		Unless overt secretions are noted after LMA removal, avoid suctioning because it may cause laryngeal spasm. The cuff should remove excess secretions when removed and prevent aspiration.[5]
		Potential complications related to the use of the LMA appear inversely proportional to the experience and skill level of the operator and patient-related factors (e.g., placement in semiconscious individual, patients with full stomachs, etc.).[4,8]
		• Regurgitation
		• Aspiration
		• Laryngospasm
		• Gagging
		• Retching
		• Trauma to tissues
		• Damage to various nerves
		• Sore or dry mouth
		• Hoarseness, stridor

Expected Outcome

• Placement of patent artificial Airway
• Properly positioned and secured airway
• Improved oxygenation and ventilation

Unexpected Outcomes

• Aspiration of gastric contents
• Trauma to oral and pharyngeal tissue potentially leading to worsening ventilation, nerve damage, and aspiration of blood
• Inability to ventilate lungs effectively secondary to:
  1. Improper sizing or position of LMA
  2. High airway and thoracic pressures (e.g.: Obese and Asthmatic patients)
  3. Obstruction: secretion or foreign body
  4. Pt semi-conscious
  5. Poor seal of LMA cuff (over or under inflated)
  6. Anatomical mismatch of patient and device (uncommon anatomical airway variants can result in a poor seal and fit of the LMA)[4,6,7]

Patient Monitoring and Care

Steps	Rationale	Reportable Conditions
		These conditions should be reported if they persist despite nursing interventions.
1. Monitor the patient and LMA during ventilation for potential problems.	Ensures proper ventilation and airway management.	• Inability to ventilate patient
A. Attach a pulse oximeter and monitor for trends.	Pressure-controlled and volume-controlled ventilation may be used but should be minimized or avoided because LMAs are not designed for long-term airway management.	• Decreased oxygen levels despite adequate oxygen delivery
B. Watch for air leaks around the cuff that may be caused by malposition. If suspected, assess for normal smooth oval swelling around cricothyroid membrane. If absent, in conjunction with prolonged expiratory phase, remove the LMA, reventilate, and reinsert.[9]	Pressure-controlled ventilation may require lower peak airway pressures.[4,5,9] Efforts should be made to secure a definitive airway (endotracheal intubation) as soon as possible. With mechanical ventilation, tidal volume, respiratory rate, and inspiratory-to-expiratory ratios need to be adjusted to prevent high peak airway pressures.[4,5,9]	• Indications of an air leak, especially with a prolonged expiratory phase or lack of normal smooth oval swelling around the cricothyroid membrane[4,5]
C. If regurgitation occurs, as indicated by fluid in the airway tube, immediately tilt the patient's head down and turn the patient's body to one side, remove bag-valve device, and suction through the airway tube.	Monitors adequate oxygenation. May indicate problems with the LMA position. Do not add more air to the cuff because it may force the soft cuff off the larynx.[5,9] Allows drainage and clearance of fluid from the airway tube. If airway problems, difficulty with ventilation, or regurgitation continue, remove the LMA and establish an airway by other means.[9]	• The LMA's cuff pressures may need to be adjusted during ascent and descent portions of air transport for unpressurized cabins
		• Monitor for signs of excessive or deficient LMA cuff pressures, namely, ventilation difficulties and excessive air leaks
		• Airway problems, difficulty with ventilation, or regurgitation

Documentation

Documentation should include the following:
- Initial patient assessment that indicates a need for LMA insertion
- Performance of visual inspection, inflation and deflation tests
- After insertion, assessment of end-tidal carbon dioxide and chest rise and fall
- Before removal, presence of swallowing and ability to open mouth
- Any complications while the LMA is in place (e.g., regurgitation or air leaks)

- Preoxygenation and ventilation before LMA insertion
- Insertion technique
- Initial cuff inflation pressure
- Signs of correct placement and cuff inflation
- Securing of the LMA
- After removal, patency of airway, effectiveness of breathing, pulse oximetry and vital sign readings, patient symptoms, or signs of complications

References and Additional Readings

For a complete list of references and additional readings for this procedure, scan this QR code with any freely available smartphone code reader app, or visit http://booksite.elsevier.com/9780323376624.

9 Nasopharyngeal and Oral Airway Insertion

Kimberly Wright

PURPOSE: Nasopharyngeal and oral airways are used to provide short-term airway maintenance and to facilitate the removal of tracheobronchial secretions.

PREREQUISITE NURSING KNOWLEDGE

Nasopharyngeal Airway

- Nasopharyngeal airways are inserted into a single naris and passed into the posterior oropharynx to the base of the tongue (Fig. 9-1).[2]
- The nasopharyngeal airway has three parts: the flange, cannula, and bevel or tip. The flange is the wide trumpet-like end that prevents further slippage into the airway. The hollow shaft of the cannula permits airflow into the hypopharynx. The bevel or tip is the opening at the distal end of the tube. When the correct size is properly inserted, the flange will rest against the patient's naris[3] and the tip can be seen resting posterior to the base of the tongue.
- The external diameter of the nasopharyngeal airway should be slightly smaller than the patient's external nares opening. The length of the nasopharyngeal airway is determined by measuring the distance between the tip of the patient's nose and the tip of the patient's earlobe (Fig. 9-2).[3] Improperly sized nasopharyngeal airways may result in increased airway resistance, limited airflow (if the airway is too small), kinking, mucosal trauma, gagging, vomiting, and gastric distention (if the airway is too large).[5]
- The advantages of the nasopharyngeal airway include ease and rapidity of insertion, increased comfort and tolerance in a conscious patient, decreased incidence of gag reflex stimulation, minimal incidence of mucosal trauma during frequent suctioning, and the ability to be inserted when the patient's teeth are clenched.[1,5]
- In selected patient situations, a nasopharyngeal airway may be used to facilitate the passage of a fiberoptic bronchoscope and to tamponade small bleeding blood vessels in the nasal mucosa.
- Most available nasopharyngeal airways are designed to be placed into the right naris. Therefore, when inserted in the left naris, the airway adjunct must be rotated until the bevel is facing the nasal septum.[3]
- Contraindications to the use of a nasopharyngeal airway are as follows:
  - Patients undergoing anticoagulation or antiplatelet therapy[5]
  - Patients prone to epistaxis
  - Patients with obstructed nasal passageways[5]
  - Patients with suspected basilar skull or cribriform plate fracture[5]
  - Patients with facial trauma that prevents the safe insertion or use of the airway[3,5]

Oropharyngeal Airway

- Oropharyngeal airways are typically disposable, curved, plastic or hard rubber devices with an opening or channel to facilitate suctioning.[1]
- The oropharyngeal airway is placed over the tongue. The curvature or body of the airway displaces the tongue forward from the posterior pharyngeal wall, a common site of airway obstruction.
- An oropharyngeal airway has four parts: the flange, body, tip, and channel (Fig. 9-3). The flange rests against the lips. This design protects against aspiration into the airway. The body of the airway curves over the tongue. The tip is the distal-most part of the airway toward the base of the tongue.
- Oral airways are manufactured in a variety of sizes for adults, children, and infants. Sizing depends on the age and size of the patient (Table 9-1). An alternative method used to select the size of an oral airway is to place the oropharyngeal airway on the space between the patient's ear lobe and the corner of the patient's mouth (Fig. 9-4).[3]
- Improperly sized airways can cause airway obstruction (if they are too small) and tongue displacement against the oropharynx (if they are too large).[3]
- Oropharyngeal airways are contraindicated in a conscious patient as they may stimulate a gag reflex and further put the airway at risk for compromise due to vomiting.[2]
- An oropharyngeal airway may be used in conjunction with an oral endotracheal tube to facilitate artificial ventilation, acting as a bite-block and preventing damage to the endotracheal tube, tongue, and soft tissues of the mouth.
- Oropharyngeal airway placement should never be attempted in a patient who is actively demonstrating seizure activity.

EQUIPMENT

- Appropriately sized nasal or oral airway
- Nonsterile gloves

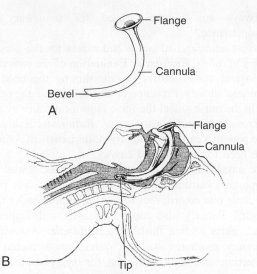

Figure 9-1 Nasopharyngeal Airway. **A,** Airway parts. **B,** Proper placement. *(From Eubanks DH, Bone RC: Comprehensive respiratory care: A learning system, St. Louis, 1990, Mosby, 518.)*

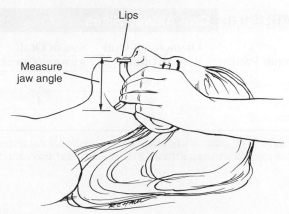

Figure 9-4 Alternative Method for Selecting the Size of an Oropharyngeal Airway. *(From Eubanks DH, Bone RC: Comprehensive respiratory care: A learning system, St. Louis, 1990, Mosby, 552.)*

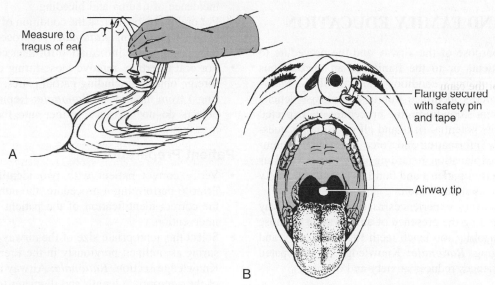

Figure 9-2 **A,** Estimating nasopharyngeal airway size. **B,** Nasopharyngeal position after insertion. *(From Eubanks DH, Bone RC: Comprehensive respiratory care: A learning system, St. Louis, 1990, Mosby, 552.)*

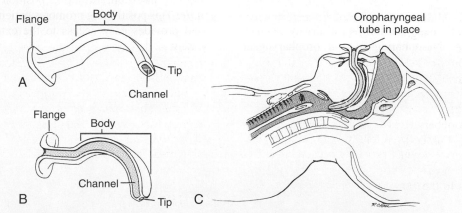

Figure 9-3 Oropharyngeal Airways. **A,** Guedel airway. **B,** Berman airway. **C,** Properly inserted oropharyngeal tube. *(From Eubanks DH, Bone RC: Comprehensive respiratory care: A learning system, St. Louis, 1990, Mosby, 518.)*

TABLE 9-1 Oral Airway Sizes

Size of Patient	Diameter of Oral Airway (mm)	Size of Oral Airway (Guedel)
Large adult	100	5
Medium adult	90	4
Small adult	80	3

From Cummins RO, editor: Airway, airway adjuncts, oxygenation, and ventilation. In ACLS: principles and practice, Dallas, 2003, American Heart Association, 145.

- Tongue depressor
- Water-soluble lubricant (nasopharyngeal airway)
- Tape (nasopharyngeal airway)

Additional equipment, to have available as needed, includes the following:
- Goggles, glasses, or face mask
- Suction equipment

PATIENT AND FAMILY EDUCATION

- Explain the purpose of the airway and the procedure to conscious patients or to the family of an unconscious patient, if the patient's condition and time allow. *Rationale:* This process identifies family knowledge deficits about the patient's condition, the procedure, its expected benefits, and its potential risks and allows time for questions to clarify information and voice concerns. Communication and explanation regarding therapy are cited as important needs of patients and families to relieve anxiety and encourage communication.
- Discuss the sensory experiences associated with airway insertion, including the presence of an airway in the nose (nasal), the inability to clench teeth together (oral), and possible gagging. *Rationale:* Knowledge of anticipated sensory experiences reduces anxiety and distress.

PATIENT ASSESSMENT AND PREPARATION

Patient Assessment

- Assess the patient's need for long-term airway maintenance. *Rationale:* Nasopharyngeal and oropharyngeal airways are generally used for temporary airway maintenance.[2]
- Assess neurological status and assess for the presence of the gag reflex. *Rationale:* Evaluation of the patient's neurological status assists in determining the need for an artificial airway. Presence or absence of the gag reflex can help the nurse select the most appropriate airway adjunct.
- Assess cardiopulmonary status. *Rationale:* Evaluation of the patient's cardiopulmonary status assists in determining the need for an artificial airway.
- For nasal insertion, assess the nasal passageway for any apparent obstruction or deformity.[3] With finger pressure, occlude one nostril; feel for air movement under the open nostril. Patency also can be assessed with inspection of each naris with a flashlight. *Rationale:* Assessment of patency promotes smooth, quick, unobstructed airway insertion, and reduces the risk for injury or bleeding.
- For nasal insertion, consider contacting the practitioner for an order to apply a topical anesthetic to coat the nasal passageway. *Rationale:* Topical anesthetics with a vasoconstrictor help shrink nasal mucosa and decrease the incidence of trauma and bleeding.
- For oral insertion, assess the condition of the oral mucosa, dentition, and gums. *Rationale:* Preprocedural assessment provides baseline information for later comparison.
- For oral insertion, remove loose-fitting dentures and any foreign objects (including partial plates, tongue studs, lip rings) from the mouth. *Rationale:* Removal ensures that objects do not advance further into the airway during insertion.

Patient Preparation

- Verify correct patient with two identifiers. *Rationale:* Prior to performing a procedure, the nurse should ensure the correct identification of the patient for the intended intervention.
- Select the appropriate size of the airway adjunct by measuring as outlined previously in the Prerequisite Nursing Knowledge section. *Rationale:* Airway adjuncts must be of the appropriate length and diameter to achieve airway patency.
- Position the patient. For nasal insertion, unless contraindicated, a supine or high Fowler's position is acceptable. For oral insertion, the supine position is preferred. *Rationale:* This positioning promotes patient and nurse comfort and provides easy access to the external nares or oral cavity.

Procedure   for Nasopharyngeal Airway Insertion

Steps	Rationale	Special Considerations
1. **HH**		
2. **PE**		To reduce the risk of exposure to exhaled or coughed secretions, consider donning protective eyewear and face mask.
3. Assess the airway for the need to suction blood or secretions.	Facilitates visualization of nasal structures and potential obstacles to insertion.	Suction should always be available to clear the airway of any visible secretions or foreign bodies.[6] **(Level D*)**
4. Generously lubricate the tip and outer cannula of the airway with water-soluble lubricant.[2-4] **(Level D)**	Facilitates passage of the device into the correct position while reducing friction-related trauma.	
5. Elevate the tip of the nose and gently slide airway into nostril. Guide it posteriorly and toward the ear, along the nasal passage until the flange rests against the nostril.[2] **(Level D)**	Following the natural contour of the nasal passage decreases the incidence of trauma.	If resistance is encountered, rotate the tube and continue gentle forward pressure. Do not force the tube. If resistance continues, withdraw the tube and try the other nostril. During tube insertion, if the patient has increasing dyspnea or respiratory distress, consider removing the tube.
6. Visualize the oropharynx and tip of the nasopharyngeal airway to ensure effective positioning has been achieved (see Fig. 9-2).	Verifying the location of the airway in the pharynx confirms proper airway positioning and allows for inspection of posterior pharynx for excessive bleeding or mucus.	
7. Reassess airway patency.[3] Feel for air movement over the flange. Listen for snoring or other sounds concerning for upper airway obstruction. **(Level D)**	Optimal airway positioning allows for forward airflow, removal of secretions, and possible prevention of airway occlusion.	
8. Suction secretions as needed.	Maintains patent airway.	Recheck flange for proper position.
9. Consider the need for bag-mask ventilation or the need for placement of a definitive airway.[3] **(Level D)**	If respiratory effort is insufficient or copious secretions threaten airway patency, additional measures are required to maintain adequate ventilation.	Nasopharyngeal airways are intended for short-term use to temporarily facilitate ventilation.
10. Follow institution standard for assessing pain. Administer analgesia as prescribed.	Identifies need for pain interventions.	Continued pain despite pain interventions.
11. Discard used supplies and equipment.		
12. Remove gloves and perform hand hygiene		

*Level D: Peer-reviewed professional and organizational standards with the support of clinical study recommendations.

Procedure continues on following page

Procedure for Oropharyngeal Airway Insertion

Steps	Rationale	Special Considerations

1. HH
2. PE

		Protective eyewear or face masks should be worn in the presence of copious secretions.

3. Suction the mouth and pharynx with a rigid pharyngeal suction tip (Yankauer) catheter, if blood or secretions are present.

Clears airway of secretions, blood, and vomit so that they do not enter the airway with airway insertion.[6] **(Level D*)**

4. Open the patient's mouth with the chin-lift maneuver crossed-finger technique (Fig. 9-5).[3] **(Level D)**

Provides access to oral cavity.

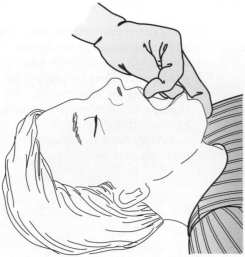

Figure 9-5 Crossed-Finger Technique for Opening the Mouth. *(From Eubanks DH, Bone RC: Comprehensive respiratory care: A learning system, St. Louis, 1990, Mosby, 631.)*

5. Remove poorly fitted or broken dentures, if present.

Poorly fitted or broken dentures can hinder the insertion of the airway adjunct and can pose additional risk for airway obstruction.

Consider leaving well-fitted dentures in place to maintain structure and support for the oropharyngeal airway.

6. Insert oral airway with curved end up (Fig. 9-6A), or lateral to tongue.[4] A tongue depressor may assist in tongue control during insertion. **(Level D)**

Prevents posterior tongue displacement.

Remove the airway immediately if the patient gags, gasps for air, or begins breathing irregularly. The airway should never be inserted end-up in children, as this poses increased risk for damage to the soft palate.

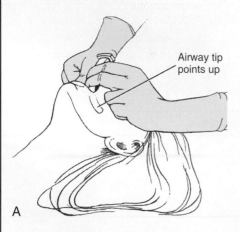

Airway tip points up

A

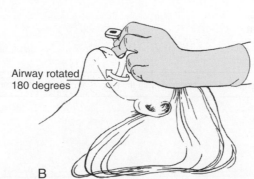

Airway rotated 180 degrees

B

Figure 9-6 Insertion of an Oropharyngeal Airway. **A,** Advance airway with curved end up. **B,** Rotate airway 180 degrees. *(From Eubanks DH, Bone RC: Comprehensive respiratory care: A learning system, St. Louis, 1990, Mosby, 551.)*

*Level D: Peer-reviewed professional and organizational standards with the support of clinical study recommendations.

Procedure for Oropharyngeal Airway Insertion—*Continued*

Steps	Rationale	Special Considerations
7. Advance oral airway over the base of the tongue until the flange is parallel with the patient's nose.	Prevents posterior tongue displacement.	
8. Gently rotate the tip to point down (see Fig. 9-6*B*); the flange should rest against the patient's lips.	Positions the airway adjunct to hold the tongue in the normal anatomical position.[3] **(Level D*)**	When the oral airway is properly sized, the flange should rest against the patient's lips (see Fig. 9-4).
9. Verify airway patency by ventilating the patient with a bag-mask device and carefully assessing for resistance or obstruction.	Proper placement and size are essential for securing and maintaining a patent airway.[2,3] **(Level D)**	
10. Suction pharynx as needed.	Maintains patent airway; pooled secretions provide a medium for bacterial growth.	
11. Reassess the patient's respiratory status.	Validates the effectiveness of the oral airway.	
12. Consider the need for placement of a definitive airway.[3] **(Level D)**	If respiratory effort is insufficient or copious secretions threaten airway patency, additional measures are required to maintain adequate ventilation.	Oropharyngeal airways are intended for short-term use to temporarily facilitate ventilation in the unconscious patient.[3]
13. Discard used supplies and equipment.		
14. Remove **PE** and perform hand hygiene.		

*Level D: Peer-reviewed professional and organizational standards with the support of clinical study recommendations.

Expected Outcomes

- Airway patency maintained
- Effective removal of tracheobronchial secretions
- Effective positioning of airway and displacement of tongue away from hypopharynx

Unexpected Outcomes

- Pulmonary aspiration
- Inability to insert airway due to patient condition
- Airway obstruction
- Nasal or oral mucosal trauma or ulceration
- Epistaxis

Patient Monitoring and Care

Steps	Rationale	Reportable Conditions
		These conditions should be reported if they persist despite nursing interventions.
1. In the rare event the adjunct must remain in place for a prolonged period of time, assess skin and mucosa in contact with airway adjunct every 8–12 hours.	Allows for more complete inspection of the mucosa, cavity, and surrounding tissues; enables complete hygiene.	• Redness • Swelling • Drainage • Bleeding • Skin breakdown
2. Consider removing and reinserting a new nasal airway in the opposite naris each assessment to prevent skin breakdown.		

Procedure continues on following page

Patient Monitoring and Care —*Continued*

Steps	Rationale	Reportable Conditions
3. Provide meticulous oral care every 2–4 hours and as needed.	Decreases secretions, encrustations, oral infections, and airway port occlusions.	• Lacerations • Ulcerations • Areas of necrosis • Drainage
4. Oxygenate and suction as necessary, per assessment.	Retained secretions increase the potential for airway obstruction and pulmonary infections.	• Change in character or amount of secretions
5. Monitor respiratory status every 2–4 hours.	Change in respiratory status may indicate displacement of airway or worsening respiratory condition.	• Change in respiratory status not corrected with repositioning of airway or suctioning • Stridor • Crowing • Gasping respirations • Snoring
6. Follow institution standard for assessing pain. Administer analgesia as prescribed.	Identifies need for pain interventions.	• Continued pain despite pain interventions

Documentation

Documentation should include the following:
- Patient and/or family education
- Insertion of nasopharyngeal or oropharyngeal airway
- Size of airway adjunct inserted
- Any difficulties with insertion or unexpected outcomes
- Use of lubrication and/or topical anesthetics
- Patient tolerance, including respiration, vital signs, and pain assessments before and after procedure

- Verification of proper placement
- Method of adjunct securement, if any
- Appearance and character of airway secretions, if present
- Tissue integrity around airway adjunct

References and Additional Readings

For a complete list of references and additional readings for this procedure, scan this QR code with any freely available smartphone code reader app, or visit http://booksite.elsevier.com/9780323376624.

10 Suctioning: Endotracheal or Tracheostomy Tube

Maureen A. Seckel

PURPOSE: Endotracheal or tracheostomy tube suctioning is performed to maintain the patency of the artificial airway and to improve gas exchange, decrease airway resistance, and reduce infection risk by removing secretions from the trachea and main-stem bronchi. Suctioning also may be performed to obtain samples of tracheal secretions for laboratory analysis.

PREREQUISITE NURSING KNOWLEDGE

- Endotracheal and tracheostomy tubes are used to maintain a patent airway and to facilitate mechanical ventilation. The presence of these artificial airways, especially endotracheal tubes, prevents effective coughing and secretion removal, necessitating periodic removal of pulmonary secretions with suctioning. In acute-care settings, suctioning is always performed as a sterile procedure to prevent hospital-acquired infections.
- Suctioning is performed with one of two basic methods. In the open-suction technique, after disconnection of the endotracheal or tracheostomy tube from any ventilatory tubing or oxygen sources, a single-use suction catheter is inserted into the open end of the tube. In the closed-suction technique, also referred to as in-line suctioning, a multiple-use suction catheter inside a sterile plastic sleeve is inserted through a special diaphragm attached to the end of the endotracheal or tracheostomy tube (Fig. 10-1). The closed-suction technique allows for the maintenance of oxygenation and ventilation support, which may be beneficial in patients with moderate to severe pulmonary insufficiency. In addition, the closed-suction technique decreases the risk for aerosolization of tracheal secretions during suction-induced coughing and may reduce some hand and equipment cross contamination. Use of the closed-suction technique is preferred in patients who experience cardiopulmonary instability during suctioning with the open technique, who have high levels of positive end-expiratory pressure (PEEP; >10 cm H_2O) or inspired oxygen (>80%),who are at risk for derecruitment, who have grossly bloody pulmonary secretions, or in whom airborne transmission of disease with risk to the healthcare worker, such as active pulmonary tuberculosis, is suspected.
- Indications for suctioning include the following:
  - ❖ Secretions in the artificial airway
  - ❖ Suspected aspiration of gastric or upper-airway secretions
  - ❖ Auscultation of adventitious lung sounds (rhonchi) over the trachea or main-stem bronchi or both
  - ❖ Increase in peak airway pressures when the patient is on mechanical ventilation
  - ❖ Increase in respiratory rate or frequent coughing or both
  - ❖ Gradual or sudden decrease in arterial blood oxygen (PaO_2), arterial blood oxygen saturation (SaO_2), or arterial saturation via pulse oximetry (SpO_2) levels
  - ❖ Sudden onset of respiratory distress, when airway patency is questioned
- Suctioning of airways should be performed only for a clinical indication and not as a routine fixed-schedule treatment.[28,29]
- Hyperoxygenation should always be provided before and after each pass of the suction catheter into the endotracheal tube, whether with the open- or closed-suctioning method. Use of the ventilator to hyperoxygenate is preferred over manual ventilation to hyperoxygenate and is more effective at delivering a fraction of inspired oxygen (FiO_2) of 1.0.[28,29] Note: Much of the research and guidelines regarding suctioning has been done with endotracheal or tracheostomy patients on mechanical ventilation. For tracheostomy patients who are not on mechanical ventilation, the need to preoxygenate or hyperventilate should be based on institutional protocol and individualized patient assessment including level of consciousness, ability to cough and manage secretions, SpO_2, and FiO_2.
- Suctioning is a necessary procedure for patients with artificial airways. When clinical indicators of the need for suctioning exist, there is no absolute contraindication to suctioning. In situations in which suctioning would be poorly tolerated by the patient, strong evidence of a clinical need for suctioning should exist and a specific plan for suctioning, developed with the healthcare team, should be implemented.
- Complications associated with suctioning of artificial airways include the following:
  - ❖ Hypoxemia
  - ❖ Respiratory arrest

- Cardiac arrest
- Cardiac dysrhythmias (premature contractions, tachycardias, bradycardias, heart blocks)
- Hypertension or hypotension
- Decreases in mixed venous oxygen saturation (Svo_2)
- Increased intracranial pressure
- Bronchospasm
- Pulmonary hemorrhage or bleeding
- Pain and anxiety
- Tracheal mucosal damage (epithelial denudement, hyperemia, loss of cilia, edema) occurs during suctioning when tissue is pulled into the catheter tip holes. These areas of damage increase the risk of infection and bleeding. Use of special-tipped catheters, low levels of suction pressure, or intermittent suction pressure has not been shown to decrease tracheal mucosal damage with suctioning.
- Postural drainage and percussion may improve secretion mobilization from small to large airways in chronic respiratory diseases with large mucus production (e.g., cystic fibrosis, bronchiectasis) but has not been shown in the literature to be effective for routine use in all patients.[34]

- Adequate systemic hydration and supplemental humidification of inspired gases assist in thinning secretions for easier aspiration from airways. Instillation of a bolus of normal saline solution does not thin secretions, may cause decreases in arterial and mixed venous oxygenation, and may contribute to lower-airway contamination from the mechanical dislodgment of bacteria within the artificial airway or from contamination of saline solution during instillation.[28,29]
- The suction catheter should not be any larger than half of the internal diameter of the endotracheal or tracheostomy tube (Table 10-1).

EQUIPMENT

- Open technique
  - Suction catheter of appropriate size (see Table 10-1)
  - Sterile saline or sterile water solution
  - Sterile gloves
  - Sterile solution container
  - Source of suction (wall mounted or portable)
  - Connecting tube, generally 4 to 6 ft.
  - Goggles and mask, or mask with eye shield

Additional equipment, to have available as needed, includes the following:
  - Manual self-inflating manual resuscitation bag-valve device connected to an oxygen flow meter, set at 15 L/min (not recommended for patients on mechanical ventilation as a routine method to deliver hyperoxygenation breaths)
  - Positive end expiratory pressure (PEEP) valve (for patients on >5 cm H_2O PEEP and who must be hyperoxygenated with a self-inflating manual resuscitation bag)
- Closed technique
  - Closed-suction setup with a catheter of appropriate size (see Table 10-1)
  - Sterile saline solution lavage containers (5 to 10 mL)
  - Obtain (individually packaged) suction catheters for oral care.
  - Source of suction (wall mounted or portable)
  - Connecting tube, generally 4 to 6 ft
  - Nonsterile gloves
  - Goggles and mask, or mask with eye shield

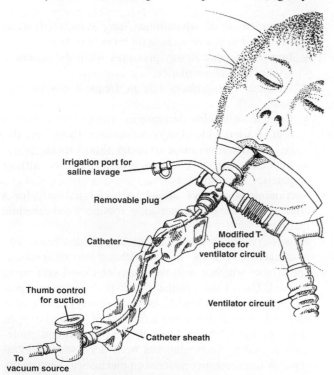

Irrigation port for saline lavage

Removable plug

Catheter

Modified T-piece for ventilator circuit

Thumb control for suction

Ventilator circuit

Catheter sheath

To vacuum source

Figure 10-1 Closed-suction technique. *(From Sills JR: The comprehensive respiratory therapist exam review: Entry and advanced levels, St. Louis, 2010, Elsevier, Mosby.)*

TABLE 10-1	**Guideline for Catheter Size for Endotracheal and Tracheostomy Tube Suctioning***

Patient Age	Endotracheal Tube Size (mm)	Tracheostomy Tube Size (mm, Inner Diameter)	Suction Catheter Size
Small child (2–5 years)	4.0–5.0	3.0–5.5	6F to 8F
School-age child (6–12 years)	5.0–6.0	4.0–6.5	8F to 10F
Adolescent to adult	7.0–9.0	5.0–9.0	10F to 16F

*This guide should be used as an estimate only. Actual sizes depend on the size and individual needs of the patient. Always follow manufacturer's guidelines.
Adapted from St John RE, Seckel M: Airway management. In AACN protocols for practice: care of the mechanically ventilated patient series, Sudbury, MA, 2007, Jones and Bartlett Publishers, 41.

PATIENT AND FAMILY EDUCATION

- Explain the procedure for endotracheal or tracheostomy tube suctioning to the patient and family. *Rationale:* The explanation reduces anxiety and allows for family members to step out if uncomfortable with the procedure.
- Explain that suctioning may be uncomfortable and could cause the patient to experience shortness of breath. *Rationale:* This information reduces anxiety and elicits patient cooperation.
- Explain the patient's role in assisting with secretion removal by coughing during the procedure. *Rationale:* This information encourages cooperation and facilitates removal of secretions.

PATIENT ASSESSMENT AND PREPARATION

Patient Assessment

- Assess for signs and symptoms of airway obstruction, including secretions in the airway, inspiratory wheezes, expiratory crackles, restlessness, ineffective coughing, decreased level of consciousness, decreased breath sounds, tachypnea, tachycardia or bradycardia, cyanosis, hypertension or hypotension, and shallow respirations. *Rationale:* Physical signs and symptoms result from inadequate gas exchange associated with airway obstruction.
- Note increased peak inspiratory pressures during volume ventilation or decreased tidal volume during pressure ventilation. *Rationale:* These pressure changes may indicate potential secretions in the airway, increasing resistance to gas flow.
- Evaluate SpO_2 and SaO_2 levels. *Rationale:* These values indicate potential secretions in the airway, impaired gas exchange.
- Assess signs and symptoms of inadequate breathing patterns, including dyspnea, shallow respirations, intercostal and suprasternal retractions, frequent triggering of ventilator alarms, and increased respiratory rate. *Rationale:* Respiratory distress is a late sign of lower-airway obstruction.

Patient Preparation

- Verify correct patient with two identifiers. *Rationale:* Prior to performing a procedure, the nurse should ensure the correct identification of the patient for the intended intervention.
- Ensure that the patient understands preprocedural teachings. Answer questions as they arise, and reinforce information as needed. *Rationale:* This communication evaluates and reinforces understanding of previously taught information.
- Assist the patient in achieving a position that is comfortable for the patient and nurse, generally semi-Fowler's or Fowler's, with the bed elevated to the nurse's waist level. *Rationale:* This positioning promotes comfort, oxygenation, and ventilation, and reduces strain.
- Secure additional personnel to assist with the self-inflating manual resuscitation bag-valve device to provide hyperoxygenation (open-suction technique only) if utilized. *Rationale:* Two hands are necessary to inflate the self-inflating manual resuscitation bag-valve device for adult tidal volume levels (>600 mL).

Procedure	for Endotracheal or Tracheostomy Tube Suctioning	
Steps	Rationale	Special Considerations
1. **HH**		
2. **PE**		
3. Turn on suction apparatus and set vacuum regulator to 80–120 mm Hg. **(Level D*)**	The amount of suction applied should be only enough to remove secretions effectively. High negative-pressure settings may increase tracheal mucosal damage.[1,13,15,29,37]	Follow manufacturer's directions for suction pressure levels with closed-suction catheter systems. **(Level M*)**
4. Secure one end of the connecting tube to the suction source and place the other end in a convenient location within reach.	Prepares suction apparatus.	

*Level D: Peer-reviewed professional and organizational standards with the support of clinical study recommendations.
*Level M: Manufacturer's recommendations only.

Procedure continues on following page

Procedure for Endotracheal or Tracheostomy Tube Suctioning—*Continued*		
Steps	**Rationale**	**Special Considerations**
5. Monitor the patient's cardiopulmonary status before, during, and after the suctioning period. **(Level B*)**	Observes for signs and symptoms of complications: decreased arterial and mixed venous oxygen saturation, cardiac dysrhythmias, bronchospasm, respiratory distress, derecruitment, cyanosis, increased blood pressure or intracranial pressure, anxiety, pain, agitation, or changes in mental status.[1,6,8,9,13–17,23–25,28,29,34,37–39]	Development of cardiopulmonary instability, particularly cardiac dysrhythmias or arterial desaturation, necessitates immediate termination of the suctioning procedure.
6a. Open-suction technique only.		
A. Open sterile catheter package on a clean surface, with the inside of the wrapping used as a sterile field.	Prepares catheter and prevents transmission of microorganisms.	
B. Depending on manufacturer, set up the sterile solution container or sterile field. Use prefilled solution container or open empty container, taking care not to touch the inside of the container. Fill with approximately 100 mL of sterile normal saline solution or sterile water.	Prepares catheter flush solution.	
C. Don sterile gloves.	Prevents contamination of the open sterile suction catheter.	In the event that one sterile glove and one nonsterile glove are used, apply the nonsterile glove to the nondominant hand and the sterile glove to the dominant hand. Handle all nonsterile items with the nondominant (nonsterile) hand.
D. Pick up suction catheter, with care to avoid touching nonsterile surfaces. With the nondominant hand, pick up the connecting tubing. Secure the suction catheter to the connecting tubing.	Maintains catheter sterility. Connects the suction catheter and connecting tubing.	The dominant (sterile) hand should not come into contact with the connecting tubing. Wrapping the suction catheter around the sterile dominant hand helps prevent inadvertent contamination of the catheter.
E. Check equipment for proper functioning by suctioning a small amount of sterile solution from the container. Proceed to **Step 7**	Ensures equipment function.	
6b. Closed-suction technique only.		
A. Connect the suction tubing to the closed system suction port or unlock the thumb valve according to manufacturer's guidelines.	Readies the suction setup for suctioning.	

*Level B: Well-designed, controlled studies with results that consistently support a specific action, intervention, or treatment.

Procedure for Endotracheal or Tracheostomy Tube Suctioning—*Continued*

Steps	Rationale	Special Considerations
7. Hyperoxygenate the patient for at least 30 seconds with one of the following three methods. **(Level B*)**	Hyperoxygenation with 100% oxygen is used to prevent a decrease in arterial oxygen levels during the suctioning procedure.[1,13,15,27–29,32,33]	Use of the ventilator to deliver the hyperoxygenation may be more effective in increasing arterial oxygen levels.[1,28,29]
A. Press the suction hyperoxygenation button on the ventilator with the nondominant hand.	Hyperoxygenation with 100% oxygen is used to prevent a decrease in arterial oxygen levels during the suctioning procedure.[1,13,15,27–29,33] **(Level B)**	
or		
B. Increase the baseline Fio_2 level on the mechanical ventilator.	Hyperoxygenation with 100% oxygen is used to prevent a decrease in arterial oxygen levels during the suctioning procedure.[1,13,15,27–29,33] **(Level B)**	With this method, caution must be used to return the Fio_2 to baseline levels after completion of suctioning.
or		
C. Disconnect the ventilator or gas-delivery tubing from the end of the endotracheal or tracheostomy tube, attach the self-inflating manual resuscitation bag-valvedevice to the tube with the nondominant hand, and administer five to six breaths over 30 seconds.	Attach a PEEP valve to the self-inflating manual resuscitation bag-valvedevice for patients on greater than 5 cm H_2O PEEP. Verify 100% oxygen delivery capabilities of manual resuscitation bag-valve device by checking manufacturer's guidelines or with direct measurement with an in-line oxygen analyzer when baseline ventilator oxygen delivery to the patient is greater than 60%. Some models of self-inflating manual resuscitation bag-valve device entrain room air and deliver less than 100% oxygen.	Use of a second person to deliver hyperoxygenation breaths with the self-inflating manual resuscitation bag-valvedevice significantly increases tidal volume delivery.[10–12,29] One handed bagging rarely achieves adult tidal volume breaths (>500 mL).

*Level B: Well-designed, controlled studies with results that consistently support a specific action, intervention, or treatment.

Procedure continues on following page

Procedure for Endotracheal or Tracheostomy Tube Suctioning—*Continued*

Steps	Rationale	Special Considerations
8. Remove the ventilator circuit or self-inflating manual resuscitation bag-valve device with the nondominant hand. With the control vent of the suction catheter open to air, gently but quickly insert the catheter with the dominant hand into the artificial airway until resistance is met, then pull back 1–2 cm before applying suction.[9,13,15,28–34] **(Level E*)**	Suction should be applied only as needed to remove secretions and for as short a time as possible to minimize decreases in arterial oxygen levels.	Directional catheters are available for selective right or left mainstem bronchus placement. Straight catheters usually enter the right mainstem bronchus.[18,20,33] Saline solution should not be instilled into the artificial airway before suctioning.[1,3,8,13,15,27,32–34] **(Level B*)** In adult patients, there is no conclusive evidence to support the practice of minimally invasive suctioning versus deep suctioning due to inconsistencies in the definitions. There are several definitions of minimally invasive or shallow suctioning in the literature, including the following examples: the combination of suctioning without hyperoxygenation or hyperinflation, without normal saline instillation, and without the suction catheter passing beyond the end of the endotracheal tube,[22,28] the insertion of the suctioning catheter to a predetermined length of the airway and connector,[1] or insertion of the suctioning catheter 2 cm beyond the endotracheal tube.[15] Deep suctioning has been defined as insertion of the suctioning catheter until resistance is felt[1,15] or the catheter is beyond the endotracheal tip.[9]
9. Place the nondominant thumb over the control vent of the suction catheter to apply continuous or intermittent suction. Place and maintain the catheter between the dominant thumb and forefinger as you completely withdraw the catheter for less than or equal to 10 seconds into the sterile catheter sleeve (closed-suction technique) or out of the open airway (open-suction technique).	Tracheal damage from suctioning is similar with intermittent or continuous suction.[6,19,21,26,28,33] **(Level C*)** Decreases in arterial oxygen levels during suctioning can be kept to a minimum with brief suction periods.[1,7,15,29,32,33] **(Level B)**	

*Level B: Well-designed, controlled studies with results that consistently support a specific action, intervention, or treatment.

*Level C: Qualitative studies, descriptive or correlational studies, integrative reviews, systematic reviews, or randomized controlled trials with inconsistent results.

*Level E: Multiple case reports, theory-based evidence from expert opinions, or peer-reviewed professional organizational standards without clinical studies to support recommendations.

Procedure	for Endotracheal or Tracheostomy Tube Suctioning—*Continued*	
Steps	**Rationale**	**Special Considerations**
10. Hyperoxygenate for 30 seconds as described in **Step 7.**	Hyperoxygenation with 100% oxygen is used to prevent a decrease in arterial oxygen levels during the suctioning procedure.[1,13,15,27–29,33] **(Level B*)**	
11. One or two more passes of the suction catheter, as delineated in **Steps 8 and 9,** may be performed if secretions remain in the airway and the patient is tolerating the procedure. Provide 30 seconds of hyperoxygenation before and after each pass of the suction catheter. **See Step 7.**	The number of suction passes should be based on the amount of secretions and the patient's clinical assessment due to the risk of complications including pain and discomfort.[1,27–31,33] **(Level E*)**	Consider allowing the patient rest and hemodynamic recovery time after several suction catheter passes. Discuss with the team the treatment plan for excessive secretions.
	Hyperoxygenation with 100% oxygen is used to prevent a decrease in arterial oxygen levels during the suctioning procedure.[1,13,15,21,27–29] **(Level B)**	
12. If the patient does not tolerate suctioning despite hyperoxygenation, try the following steps:	Use of a different suctioning technique may be physiologically less demanding.[33] **(Level E)**	
A. Ensure that 100% oxygen is being delivered.	Hyperoxygenation with 100% oxygen is used to prevent a decrease in arterial oxygen levels during the suctioning procedure.[1,13,15,27–29,33] **(Level B)**	
B. Maintain PEEP during suctioning. Check that the PEEP valve is attached properly to the self-inflating manual resuscitation bag-valve device with use of that method for hyperoxygenation.	Maintenance of PEEP prevents collapse of alveoli during suctioning.	
C. Switch to another method of suctioning (e.g., closed-suctioning technique).	Other methods of suctioning may be more effective and safer for the patient.	
D. Allow longer recovery intervals between suction passes.	Allows the patient to regain prior oxygenation levels.	
E. Hyperventilation may be used in situations in which the patient does not tolerate suctioning with hyperoxygenation alone, with either the self-inflating manual resuscitation bag-valve device or the ventilator.	Due to the possibility of barotrauma, hyperventilation should be used only if the patient does not tolerate suctioning with hyperoxygenation alone.	Hyperinflation should be delivered by the ventilator to control pressures and avoid disconnection.[1,28,29]

*Level B: Well-designed, controlled studies with results that consistently support a specific action, intervention, or treatment.

*Level E: Multiple case reports, theory-based evidence from expert opinions, or peer-reviewed professional organizational standards without clinical studies to support recommendations.

Procedure continues on following page

Procedure	for Endotracheal or Tracheostomy Tube Suctioning—*Continued*	
Steps	**Rationale**	**Special Considerations**
13. When the airway has been cleared adequately of secretions, perform oropharyngeal suctioning. **(Level D*)** A separate suction catheter must be opened for this step with the closed-suction technique.	Suctioning of the oropharyngeal area if secretions are present may enhance patient comfort and should be part of an oral hygiene program.[2,5,35,36] After oropharyngeal suctioning, the suction catheter is contaminated with bacteria present in the oral cavity, potentially gram-negative bacilli, and should not be used for lower-airway suctioning.[1,5,13,15,35,36] **(Level D)**	Care should be taken to avoid oropharyngeal tissue trauma and gagging during suctioning.
14. Rinse the catheter and connecting tubing with sterile saline or sterile water solution until clear. Open-suction technique: suction the unused sterile solution until tubing is clear. Closed-suction technique: instill sterile saline or water solution into side port of in-line suction catheter, taking care not to lavage down endotracheal tube, while applying continuous suction until catheter is clear.	Removes buildup of secretions in the connecting tubing and, with the closed-suction catheter system, in the in-line suction catheter.	
15. Open-suction technique only: on completion of upper-airway suctioning, wrap the catheter around the dominant hand. Pull glove off inside out. Catheter remains in glove. Pull off other glove in same fashion, and discard. Turn off suction device.	Reduces transmission of microorganisms.	
16. Suction collection tubing and canisters may remain in use for multiple suctioning episodes.	Solutions and catheters that come in direct contact with the lower airways during suctioning must be sterile to decrease the risks for hospital-acquired pneumonia. Devices that are not in direct contact with the lower airways have not been shown to increase infection risk.[5] **(Level D)**	Check institutional standards on the discarding of multiuse sterile solution containers and equipment removal.
17. Remove **PE** and discard used supplies.		
18. **HH**		

*Level D: Peer-reviewed professional and organizational standards with the support of clinical study recommendations.

Expected Outcomes

- Removal of secretions from the large airways
- Improved gas exchange
- Airway patency
- Amelioration of clinical signs or symptoms of need for suctioning (e.g., adventitious breath sounds, coughing, high airway pressures)
- Sample for laboratory analysis

Unexpected Outcomes

- Cardiac dysrhythmias (premature atrial or ventricular contractions, tachycardias, bradycardias, heart blocks, asystole)
- Hypoxemia
- Bronchospasm
- Excessive increases in arterial blood pressure or intracranial pressure
- Hospital-acquired infections
- Cardiopulmonary distress
- Decreased level of consciousness
- Airway obstruction
- Pain or discomfort

Patient Monitoring and Care

Steps	Rationale	Reportable Conditions
		These conditions should be reported if they persist despite nursing interventions.
1. Monitor the patient's cardiopulmonary status before, during, and after the suctioning period. **(Level B*)**	Observes for signs and symptoms of complications.[1,4,14,16,17,19,25,27,28,33,34,37,38,43,44]	<ul><li>Decreased arterial or mixed venous oxygen saturation</li><li>Cardiac dysrhythmias</li><li>Bronchospasm</li><li>Respiratory distress</li><li>Cyanosis</li><li>Increased blood pressure or intracranial pressure</li><li>Anxiety, agitation, pain, or changes in mental status</li><li>Diminished breath sounds</li><li>Decreased oxygenation</li><li>Increased peak airway pressures</li><li>Coughing</li><li>Increased work of breathing</li></ul>
2. Reassess the patient for signs of suctioning effectiveness.	Assesses effectiveness of intervention and the possible indications for further suctioning.	
3. Follow institution standard for assessing pain. Administer analgesia as prescribed.	Identifies need for pain interventions.	• Continued pain despite pain interventions.

*Level B: Well-designed, controlled studies with results that consistently support a specific action, intervention, or treatment.

Documentation

Documentation should include the following:
- Patient and family education
- Presuctioning assessment, including clinical indication for suctioning
- Suctioning of endotracheal or tracheostomy tube
- Size of endotracheal or tracheostomy tube and suction catheter
- Type of hyperoxygenation method used
- Pain assessment, interventions, and effectiveness
- Volume, color, consistency, and odor of secretions obtained
- Any difficulties during catheter insertion or hyperoxygenation
- Tolerance of suctioning procedure, including development of any unexpected outcomes during or after the procedure
- Nursing interventions
- Postsuctioning assessment

References and Additional Readings

For a complete list of references and additional readings for this procedure, scan this QR code with any freely available smartphone code reader app, or visit http://booksite.elsevier.com/9780323376624.

11 Surgical Cricothyrotomy AP (Perform)

Roger Casey

PURPOSE: Surgical cricothyrotomy is an emergent procedure that creates an opening in the cricothyroid membrane to facilitate placement of an endotracheal or tracheostomy tube to provide effective oxygenation and ventilation.

PREREQUISITE NURSING KNOWLEDGE

- Surgical cricothyrotomy is used only when the airway cannot be obtained or maintained by standard means such as bag-valve-mask device ventilation, the use of airway adjuncts (oropharyngeal or nasopharyngeal airways), endotracheal intubation, or rescue airways (King Airway, Combitube, or laryngeal mask airway [LMA]; Procedures 1, 7, and 8, respectively).[3]
- Surgical cricothyrotomy may be needed in patients with facial or neck trauma. Maintenance of the airway may be difficult in these patients because the injuries often disrupt the lower facial structures and may make an adequate seal with a bag-valve device difficult to obtain. The airway may also be obstructed or disrupted, making endotracheal intubation difficult or ineffective.
- Difficulty in obtaining or maintaining an airway may result from upper airway obstruction as a result of trauma, allergic reactions with swelling and angioedema, foreign bodies, anatomical variations, tumors, and bleeding.[2]
- The need for emergent surgical cricothyrotomy must be determined quickly. This intervention is potentially life-saving, and implementation cannot be delayed.
- Surgical cricothyrotomy requires specialized training and should be performed only by highly skilled medical providers[2] or nursing providers.[2]
- Commercially prepared kits, such as the Melker Emergency Cricothyrotomy Catheter (Cook Medical, Inc, Bloomington, Ind; www.cookmedical.com), are available and use a specially designed airway and a modified Seldinger (or percutaneous cricothyrotomy) technique for insertion.

Contraindications

Absolute

- Airway can be managed effectively with bag-valve-mask device, intubation, or rescue airway (King Airway, Combitube, or LMA)

- Complete transection of trachea
- Laryngotracheal disruption with retraction of distal trachea

Relative

- Anterior neck hematoma[5]—preexisting pathology of larynx or trachea including hematoma, infection, tumor, or abscess occurring at or near incision site[6]
- Coagulopathies
- Fractured larynx with inability to identify anatomical landmarks[3]
- Lacerations of the structures of the neck[3]
- Massive neck swelling[3]
- Children less than 12 years of age[5]

EQUIPMENT

- Personal protective equipment (mask, eye protection, gown)
- Sterile surgical gloves
- Sterile surgical drape
- Topical antiseptic solution
- No. 10 or 11 blade scalpel
- 4×4 gauze sponges
- Suction and suction catheter
- Curved hemostats
- Tracheal hook
- Tracheal (Trousseau) dilator or nasal speculum
- 5- to 6-mm cuffed endotracheal tube or No. 4 (Shiley) tracheostomy tube
- 10-mL syringe
- Cloth tracheostomy ties
- Bag-valve-mask device with oxygen source
- Stethoscope

Additional equipment, to have available as needed, includes the following:

- Commercially prepared kit which uses a specially designed airway and a modified Seldinger (or percutaneous cricothyrotomy) technique for insertion.

PATIENT AND FAMILY EDUCATION

- If time permits, assess the patient's and family's level of understanding about the condition and rationale for the procedure. ***Rationale:*** This assessment identifies the

AP This procedure should be performed only by physicians, advanced practice nurses, and other healthcare professionals (including critical care nurses) with additional knowledge, skills, and demonstrated competence per professional licensure or institutional standard.

patient's and family's knowledge deficits concerning the patient's condition, the procedure, the expected benefits, and the potential risks. It also allows time for questions to clarify information and voice concerns. Explanations decrease patient anxiety and enhance cooperation.

- Family members should be provided with a quick and concise explanation of the emergent need to obtain an airway. This information is often best explained by another member of the healthcare team rather than the provider performing the procedure to prevent delay in establishing the airway. If possible, obtain consent for the procedure from the family member. *Rationale:* This explanation enhances patient and family understanding and decreases anxiety.

- A patient who needs emergency surgical cricothyrotomy is likely unresponsive from the inability to maintain the airway and adequate oxygenation and ventilation; therefore, patient education may not be possible. If the patient is responsive, the airway and ventilatory efforts are adequate and surgical cricothyrotomy is not indicated. *Rationale:* The emergency nature of the procedure precludes patient education.

PATIENT ASSESSMENT AND PREPARATION

Patient Assessment

- Assess airway patency.
  - Open the airway with a jaw-thrust or chin-lift maneuver. If traumatic injury is suspected, maintain cervical stabilization. *Rationale:* Allows for visualization of the airway for any foreign bodies, secretions, or other obstructions.
  - Assess for presence of foreign bodies, secretions, or other obstructions. Use suction, basic life support (BLS) maneuvers, or Magill forceps to clear and maintain the airway. *Rationale:* Often airway patency can be achieved and maintained with simple maneuvers such as patient positioning, use of an airway maneuver, suction, or insertion of an oral or nasal pharyngeal airway. If the patient has potential for airway compromise (i.e., bleeding, swelling, or traumatic injuries) and is alert and able to maintain the airway, allow the patient to maintain a position of comfort and suction to maintain a patent airway.
  - Do not attempt to place the patient in a supine position because this may cause significant airway com-

promise. *Rationale:* If the patient has the ability to maintain an airway, allowing the patient to remain in an upright position, with suction provided if necessary, assists the patient in maintaining the airway. If the patient is placed in a supine position for packaging or transport, this may cause significant airway compromise.

- Assess respiratory effort.
  - Assess rate, depth of respirations, accessory muscle use, chest wall motion, and breath sounds. *Rationale:* This process is to identify inadequate respiratory efforts quickly and determine the optimal method for oxygenation and ventilation.
  - Monitor oxygen saturation and end tidal carbon dioxide ($ETco_2$). *Rationale:* This process is to identify inadequate respiratory efforts quickly and determine the optimal method for oxygenation and ventilation.
  - If respiratory efforts are inadequate, attempt ventilation with a bag-valve-mask device and supplemental oxygen. If an airway cannot be maintained or oxygenation and ventilation with a bag-valve-mask device are inadequate, prepare for endotracheal intubation. *Rationale:* This process is to identify inadequate respiratory efforts quickly and determine the optimal method for oxygenation and ventilation.
  - If intubation is not possible, prepare for emergent surgical cricothyrotomy. *Rationale:* This process is to identify inadequate respiratory efforts quickly and determine the optimal method for oxygenation and ventilation.

Patient Preparation

- Verify correct patient with two identifiers. *Rationale:* Prior to performing a procedure, the nurse should ensure the correct identification of the patient for the intended intervention.
- Perform a preprocedure verification and time out, if nonemergent. *Rationale:* Ensures patient safety.
- Position the patient supine and maintain cervical spine stabilization if indicated. *Rationale:* Patients who need emergent surgical cricothyrotomy often have traumatic injuries that necessitate cervical spine stabilization.
- Continue attempts to ventilate and oxygenate the patient with a bag-valve-mask device by any means possible if the patient is apneic or respiratory efforts are inadequate. *Rationale:* This action can prevent further hypoxia and hypercarbia.

Procedure	**for Surgical Cricothyrotomy**	
Steps	Rationale	Special Considerations
1. **HH**		
2. **PE**		Use of face mask and eye protection is recommended because of the increased risk of airborne blood or body fluids during this procedure.
3. Place the patient in a supine position, with head and neck in neutral position.	Position the patient to expose the neck and larynx.	Maintain manual cervical spine stabilization for patients with suspected cervical spine injury.

Procedure for Surgical Cricothyrotomy—*Continued*		
Steps	**Rationale**	**Special Considerations**
4. Identify the cricothyroid membrane (Fig. 11-1). First, identify the thyroid prominence, or Adam's apple. The cricothyroid membrane is palpated at the midline, approximately one fingerbreadth below the thyroid prominence.	Identifies the correct location for incision and endotracheal tube placement. The cricothyroid membrane is preferred over the trachea because it is more anterior than the lower trachea and less thyroid and soft tissue are found between the membrane and the skin. Additionally, there is less vascularity, leading to less significant chance of bleeding.	The incision is just inferior to the vocal cords and superior to the thyroid gland.

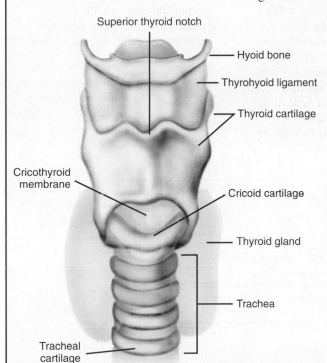

Superior thyroid notch

Hyoid bone

Thyrohyoid ligament

Thyroid cartilage

Cricothyroid membrane

Cricoid cartilage

Thyroid gland

Trachea

Tracheal cartilage

Figure 11-1 Anatomy of Neck and Location of Cricothyroid Membrane. *(Adapted from Patton KT, Thibodeau GA: Mosby's handbook of anatomy and physiology, ed. 2 St. Louis, 2014, Elsevier.)*

5. Prepare the skin with a topical antiseptic solution.	Decreases potential for wound infection.	
6. Immobilize the larynx by stretching the skin with the thumb and middle finger of the nondominant hand to make it taut and stabilize the larynx.	Allows for ease in creating an incision in the skin, and keeps the larynx from shifting.	Throughout the procedure the larynx must be immobilized.
7. Take the scalpel in the dominant hand and make a 2-cm vertical midline incision through the dermis, over the cricothyroid membrane.	Overly deep or long incisions risk damage to the larynx, cricoid cartilage, and trachea.	Avoid directing the scalpel toward the head, as this may cause laceration of the vocal cords.[3] Some references recommend a horizontal skin incision.[1,2]
8. Dab the wound with sterile gauze to control any bleeding from the incision.	Use a dabbing technique to minimize further tissue trauma and bleeding.	Use an assistant, if available, to control bleeding and minimize interruptions in the procedure.

Procedure continues on following page

Procedure | for Surgical Cricothyrotomy—*Continued*

Steps	Rationale	Special Considerations
9. Identify the cricothyroid membrane. Palpate the cricothyroid membrane through the skin incision with the index finger. If necessary, use the curved hemostats to bluntly dissect through the skin to locate and visualize the cricothyroid membrane.	Blunt dissection is preferred over sharp dissection to minimize further tissue trauma and bleeding.	The index finger can be placed on the inferior aspect of the thyroid cartilage to identify the superior border of the cricothyroid membrane.
10. Make a horizontal incision in the lower half of the cricothyroid membrane with the scalpel (Fig. 11-2).	Incising the lower half of the membrane is preferred to avoid the superior cricothyroid artery and vein. The opening needs to be large enough to accommodate a 5–6 mm cuffed endotracheal or No. 4 (Shiley) tracheostomy tube. A puncturing motion may also puncture the posterior wall of the trachea and lacerate the esophagus, and could lacerate or damage the vocal cords.	The incision should be approximately 1–1.5 cm in length. Do not attempt to puncture the cricothyroid membrane. Use the scalpel to gently incise only the membrane.

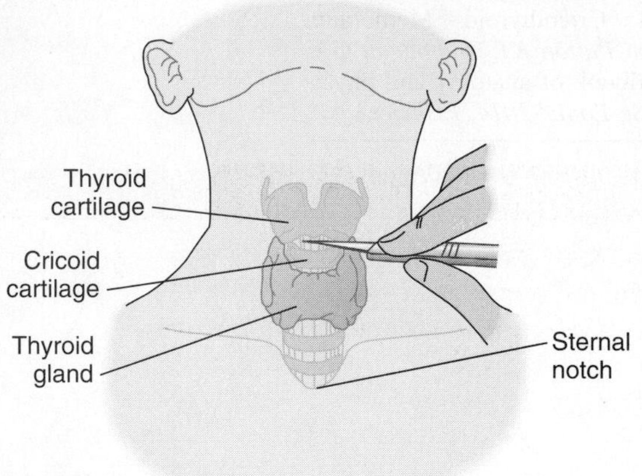

Figure 11-2 Surgical Cricothyrotomy. *(From Black JM, Hawks JH:* Medical-surgical nursing: Clinical management for positive outcomes, *ed 8, St. Louis, 2009, Elsevier.)*

Steps	Rationale	Special Considerations
11. Dab the wound with sterile gauze to control any bleeding from the incision.	Use a dabbing technique to minimize further tissue trauma and bleeding.	Use an assistant, if available, to control bleeding and minimize interruptions in the procedure.
12. Insert tracheal dilator or nasal speculum into the opening in the cricothyroid membrane. Direct the tip of the speculum toward the patient's feet.	Avoids further trauma to the cricothyroid membrane or vocal cords and guides the tube into the airway.	
13. Carefully spread the dilator or speculum vertically and advance the tube into the opening. If resistance is met, do not force the tube into the opening.	The dilator or speculum enlarges the opening vertically, but use caution to avoid further trauma to the cricothyroid membrane or vocal cords. Consider utilizing the tracheal hook to maintain the opening. Care must be undertaken to ensure there is an instrument in the airway at all times so as not to allow the cricothyroid incision to close.	The tube should advance easily into the tracheal opening.

Procedure | for Surgical Cricothyrotomy—*Continued*

Steps	Rationale	Special Considerations
14. Carefully remove the tracheal dilator or nasal speculum once the tube has been placed in the trachea.	Use caution to avoid inadvertent removal of the tube along with the dilator or speculum.	
15. Inflate the tube cuff with the syringe to a minimal occlusive pressure.	Prevents an air leak and optimizes oxygenation and ventilation.	A cuffed tube is preferred over an uncuffed tube to prevent an air leak and reduce the risk of aspiration.
16. Attach the bag-valve device to the tube and oxygenate and ventilate the patient.		
17. Auscultate for the presence of equal breath sounds and the absence of epigastric sounds with a stethoscope. Observe chest rise and fall.	Tube position may be confirmed with the same methods as oral or nasal endotracheal tube placement.	Primary confirmation relies on physical examination techniques to confirm correct tube placement.[2]
18. Confirm correct placement with secondary means such as an exhaled CO_2 detector or monitoring device. Obtain chest radiography.	Tube position may be confirmed with the same methods as oral or nasal endotracheal tube placement.	Secondary confirmation verifies correct tube placement.[2]
19. Secure the tube with tracheostomy ties.	Prevents dislodgment or movement of tube.	Use a square knot to secure the tracheostomy ties.
20. Dispose of supplies.		
21. **HH**		

Expected Outcomes

- Establishment of emergent surgical airway access
- Adequate oxygenation and ventilation
- Improved or stabilized patient condition

Unexpected Outcomes[1,2,5]

- Blood loss or hemorrhage
- Aspiration or asphyxia
- False passage of the endotracheal tube into subcutaneous tissue[4]
- Tracheal perforation
- Esophageal perforation
- Subcutaneous emphysema
- Mediastinal emphysema
- Vocal cord injury or paralysis
- Tracheal stenosis (delayed)

Patient Monitoring and Care

Steps	Rationale	Reportable Conditions
1. Monitor breath sounds, adequacy of oxygenation and ventilation, and oxygen saturation (SpO_2). Consider continuous capnography.	Monitors effectiveness of airway, oxygenation, and ventilation.	• Inability to ventilate • Decreased or absent breath sounds • Decrease in SpO_2 • Loss of $ETco_2$
2. Monitor endotracheal tube position.	Prevents movement or dislodgment of tube.	• Inadvertent dislodgment or removal of tube
3. Observe insertion site for bleeding, swelling, or subcutaneous air.	Identifies displacement of tube or significant air leak.	• Excessive bleeding from the site • Swelling or subcutaneous air at the insertion site
4. Follow institution standard for assessing pain. Administer analgesia as prescribed.	Identifies need for pain interventions.	• Continued pain despite pain interventions

Procedure continues on following page

Documentation

Documentation should include the following:

- Assessment findings to support the need for an emergent surgical airway
- Size and type of endotracheal/tracheostomy tube inserted and centimeter mark at skin opening
- Confirmation of proper tube placement with both primary and secondary means
- Pain assessment, interventions, and effectiveness
- Inability to obtain or maintain airway and provide oxygenation and ventilation by any other means
- Documentation of the procedure, to include date and time
- Any difficulties encountered during the procedure

References and Additional Readings

For a complete list of references and additional readings for this procedure, scan this QR code with any freely available smartphone code reader app, or visit http://booksite.elsevier.com/9780323376624.

12 Surgical Cricothyrotomy (Assist)

Roger Casey

PURPOSE: Surgical cricothyrotomy is an emergent procedure that creates an opening in the cricothyroid membrane to facilitate placement of an endotracheal or tracheostomy tube to provide effective oxygenation and ventilation.

PREREQUISITE NURSING KNOWLEDGE

- Surgical cricothyrotomy is used only when the airway cannot be obtained or maintained by standard means such as bag-valve-mask device ventilation, the use of airway adjuncts (oropharyngeal or nasopharyngeal airways), endotracheal intubation, or rescue airways (King Airway, Combitube, or laryngeal mask airway [LMA]; Procedures 1, 7, and 8, respectively).[3]
- Surgical cricothyrotomy may be needed in patients with facial or neck trauma. Maintenance of the airway may be difficult in these patients because the injuries often disrupt the lower facial structures and may make an adequate seal with a bag-valve device difficult to obtain. The airway may also be obstructed or disrupted, making endotracheal intubation difficult or ineffective.
- Difficulty in obtaining or maintaining an airway may result from upper airway obstruction as a result of trauma, allergic reactions with swelling and angioedema, foreign bodies, anatomical variations, tumors, and bleeding.[2]
- The need for emergent surgical cricothyrotomy must be determined quickly. This intervention is potentially life-saving, and implementation cannot be delayed.
- Surgical cricothyrotomy requires specialized training and should be performed only by highly skilled medical providers or nursing providers.[2]
- Commercially prepared cricothyrotomy kits are available and often use a modified Seldinger technique with a guidewire or dilator system.
- This procedure should be performed only by physicians, advanced practice nurses, and other healthcare professionals (including critical care nurses and trained transport personnel) with additional knowledge, skills, and demonstrated competence per professional licensure or institutional/organizational standards.

Contraindications
Absolute
- Airway can be managed effectively with bag-valve-mask device, intubation, or rescue airway (King Airway, Combitube, or LMA)
- Complete transection of trachea
- Laryngotracheal disruption with retraction of distal trachea

Relative
- Anterior neck hematoma[5]—preexisting pathology of larynx or trachea including hematoma, infection, tumor, or abscess occurring at or near incision site[6]
- Coagulopathies
- Fractured larynx with inability to identify anatomical landmarks[3]
- Lacerations of the structures of the neck[3]
- Massive neck swelling[3]
- Children less than 12 years of age[5]

EQUIPMENT

- Personal protective equipment (mask, eye protection, gown)
- Sterile surgical gloves
- Sterile surgical drape
- Topical antiseptic solution
- No. 10 or 11 blade scalpel
- 4 × 4 gauze sponges
- Suction device and suction catheter
- Curved hemostats
- Tracheal hook
- Tracheal (Trousseau) dilator or nasal speculum
- 5- to 6-mm cuffed endotracheal tube or No. 4 (Shiley) tracheostomy tube[4]
- 10-mL syringe
- Cloth tracheostomy ties
- Self-inflating manual resuscitation bag-valve-mask device with oxygen source
- Oxygen source and tubing
- Stethoscope
- Commercially prepared kits and use a specially designed airway and a modified Seldinger (or percutaneous cricothyrotomy) technique for insertion

PATIENT AND FAMILY EDUCATION

- If time permits, assess the patient's and family's level of understanding about the condition and rationale for the procedure. ***Rationale:*** This assessment identifies the patient's and family's knowledge deficits concerning the patient's condition, the procedure, the expected benefits, and the potential risks. It also allows time for questions to clarify information and voice concerns. Explanations decrease patient anxiety and enhance cooperation.

- Family members should be provided with a quick and concise explanation of the emergent need to obtain an airway. This information is often best explained by another member of the healthcare team rather than the provider performing the procedure to prevent delay in establishing the airway. If possible, obtain consent for the procedure from the family member. ***Rationale:*** This explanation enhances patient and family understanding and decreases anxiety.
- A patient who needs emergency surgical cricothyrotomy is likely unresponsive from the inability to maintain the airway and adequate oxygenation and ventilation; therefore, patient education may not be possible. If the patient is responsive, the airway and ventilatory efforts are adequate and surgical cricothyrotomy is not indicated. ***Rationale:*** The emergency nature of the procedure precludes patient education.

PATIENT ASSESSMENT AND PREPARATION

Patient Assessment

- Assess airway patency.
  - ❖ Open the airway with a jaw-thrust or chin-lift maneuver. If traumatic injury is suspected, maintain cervical stabilization. ***Rationale:*** Allows for visualization of the airway for any foreign bodies, secretions, or other obstructions.
  - ❖ Assess for presence of foreign bodies, secretions, or other obstructions. Use suction, basic life support (BLS) maneuvers, or Magill forceps to clear and maintain the airway. ***Rationale:*** Often airway patency can be achieved and maintained with simple maneuvers such as patient positioning, use of an airway maneuver, suction, or insertion of an oral or nasal pharyngeal airway. If the patient has potential for airway compromise (i.e., bleeding, swelling, or traumatic injuries) and is alert and able to maintain the airway, allow the patient to maintain a position of comfort and suction to maintain a patent airway.
  - ❖ Do not attempt to place the patient in a supine position because this may cause significant airway compromise. ***Rationale:*** If the patient has the ability to maintain an airway, allowing the patient to remain in an upright position, with suction provided if necessary, assists the patient in maintaining the airway. If the patient is placed in a supine position for packaging or transport, this move may cause significant airway compromise.
- Assess respiratory effort.
  - ❖ Assess rate, depth of respirations, accessory muscle use, chest wall motion, and breath sounds. ***Rationale:*** This process is to identify inadequate respiratory efforts quickly and determine the optimal method for providing oxygenation and ventilation.
  - ❖ If equipment is available, monitor oxygen saturation and end tidal carbon dioxide ($ETCO_2$). ***Rationale:*** This process is to identify inadequate respiratory efforts quickly and determine the optimal method for providing oxygenation and ventilation.
  - ❖ If respiratory efforts are inadequate, attempt ventilation with a self-inflating manual resuscitation bag-valve-mask device and supplemental oxygen. If an airway cannot be maintained or oxygenation and ventilation are adequate with a self-inflating manual resuscitation bag-valve-mask device, prepare for endotracheal intubation. ***Rationale:*** This process is to identify inadequate respiratory efforts quickly and determine the optimal method for providing oxygenation and ventilation.
  - ❖ If intubation is not possible, prepare for emergent surgical cricothyrotomy. ***Rationale:*** This process is to identify inadequate respiratory efforts quickly and determine the optimal method for providing oxygenation and ventilation.

Patient Preparation

- Verify correct patient with two identifiers. ***Rationale:*** Prior to performing a procedure, the nurse should ensure the correct identification of the patient for the intended intervention.
- Perform a preprocedure verification and time out, if nonemergent. ***Rationale:*** Ensures patient safety.
- Position the patient supine and maintain cervical spine stabilization if indicated. ***Rationale:*** Patients who need emergent surgical cricothyrotomy often have traumatic injuries that require cervical spine stabilization.
- Continue attempts to ventilate and oxygenate the patient with a self-inflating manual resuscitation bag-valve-mask device if the patient is apneic or respiratory efforts are inadequate. ***Rationale:*** This action can prevent further hypoxia and hypercarbia.

Procedure for Assisting with Surgical Cricothyrotomy		
Steps	Rationale	Special Considerations
1. HH		
2. PE		Use of face mask and eye protection is recommended because of the increased risk of airborne blood or body fluids during this procedure.
3. Place the patient in a supine position, with head and neck in neutral position.	Position the patient to expose the neck and larynx.	Maintain cervical spine stabilization for patients with suspected cervical spine injury.

Procedure for Assisting with Surgical Cricothyrotomy—*Continued*

Steps	Rationale	Special Considerations
4. If one assistant (assistant A) is available, continue attempts to oxygenate and ventilate the patient with a bag-valve-mask device.	Prevents further hypoxia and hypercarbia. Use of an assistant minimizes interruptions in the procedure.	Maintain sterile field and anticipate the needs of the person performing the procedure. Use caution when handling equipment to prevent contamination or inadvertent injury.
5. If a second assistant (assistant B) is available, assist the person performing the procedure.		
6. The person performing the procedure locates the cricothyroid membrane (see Fig. 11-1), prepares the skin with a topical antiseptic solution, and makes an incision through the skin.	Identifies the correct location for incision and tube placement. The cricothyroid membrane is preferred over the trachea because it is more anterior than the lower trachea and less thyroid and soft tissue are found between the membrane and the skin.	The incision is just inferior to the vocal cords and superior to the thyroid gland.
7. Assistant B uses gauze sponges and a dabbing technique to control any bleeding from the incision, when asked by the person performing the procedure.	A dabbing technique minimizes further tissue trauma and bleeding. Only assist with blood loss control when asked to avoid contact with the scalpel.	If a second assistant is not available, the primary assistant should continue to attempt to ventilate the patient.
8. The person performing the procedure incises the cricothyroid membrane with the scalpel (see Fig. 11-2). Assistant B prepares the curved hemostats that may be needed to bluntly dissect the skin to locate and visualize the cricothyroid membrane.	Discontinuing ventilations minimizes airborne contamination when the cricothyroid membrane is incised. Blunt dissection is preferred over sharp dissection to minimize further tissue trauma and bleeding.	Assistant A stops ventilations just before the incision is being made.
9. Assistant B prepares the endotracheal or tracheostomy tube and tracheal dilator or nasal speculum for the person performing the procedure.	Enlarging the opening in the cricothyroid membrane allows passage of the tube.	Assistant A continues to hold ventilation attempts until the tube is placed.
10. Assistant B uses the syringe to inflate the tube cuff to a minimal occlusive pressure once the tube is placed.	Prevents an air leak and optimizes oxygenation and ventilation.	A cuffed tube is preferred over an uncuffed tube to prevent an air leak and reduce the risk of aspiration.
11. Assistant A attaches the bag-valve device to the tube and oxygenates and ventilates the patient. Assistant B manually stabilizes the tube.	Prevents inadvertent movement or displacement of tube.	
12. Auscultate for the presence of equal breath sounds and the absence of epigastric sounds with a stethoscope. Observe chest rise and fall.	Tube position may be confirmed with the same methods as oral or nasal endotracheal tube placement.	Primary confirmation relies on physical examination techniques to confirm correct tube placement.[2]
13. Confirm correct placement with secondary means such as an exhaled CO_2 detector or monitoring device. Obtain chest radiography.	Tube position may be confirmed with the same methods as oral or nasal endotracheal tube placement.	Secondary confirmation verifies correct tube placement.[2]
14. Secure the tube with tracheostomy ties. Dress the site with gauze and tape.	Prevent dislodgment or movement of tube.	Use a square knot to secure the tracheostomy ties.
15. Dispose of supplies.		
16. 🖐		

Procedure continues on following page

Expected Outcomes

- Establishment of emergent surgical airway access
- Provision of adequate oxygenation and ventilation
- Improved or stabilized patient condition

Unexpected Outcomes[1,2,5]

- Blood loss or hemorrhage
- Aspiration or asphyxia
- False passage of the endotracheal tube into subcutaneous tissue[4]
- Tracheal perforation
- Esophageal perforation
- Subcutaneous emphysema
- Mediastinal emphysema
- Vocal cord injury or paralysis
- Tracheal stenosis (delayed)

Patient Monitoring and Care

Steps	Rationale	Reportable Conditions
		These conditions should be reported if they persist despite nursing interventions.
1. Monitor breath sounds, adequacy of oxygenation and ventilation, and oxygen saturation (SpO_2). Consider continuous capnography.	Monitors effectiveness of airway, oxygenation, and ventilation.	• Inability to ventilate • Decreased or absent breath sounds • Decrease in SpO_2 • Loss of $ETco_2$
2. Monitor endotracheal tube position.	Prevents movement or dislodgment of tube.	• Inadvertent dislodgment or removal of tube
3. Observe insertion site for bleeding, swelling, or subcutaneous air.	Identifies displacement of tube or significant air leak.	• Excessive bleeding from the site • Swelling or subcutaneous air at the insertion site
4. Follow institution standard for assessing pain. Administer analgesia as prescribed.	Identifies need for pain interventions.	• Continued pain despite pain interventions

Documentation

Documentation should include the following:
- Assessment findings to support the need for an emergent surgical airway
- Size and type of endotracheal/tracheostomy tube inserted and centimeter mark at skin opening
- Confirmation of proper tube placement by both primary and secondary means
- Pain assessment, interventions, and effectiveness
- Inability to obtain or maintain airway and provide oxygenation and ventilation by other means
- Documentation of the procedure, to include date and time
- Any difficulties encountered during the procedure

References and Additional Readings

For a complete list of references and additional readings for this procedure, scan this QR code with any freely available smartphone code reader app, or visit http://booksite.elsevier.com/9780323376624.

13

Tracheostomy Cuff and Tube Care

Renee Johnson

PURPOSE: Tracheostomy tube care includes care of the tracheal tube cuff, the inner and outer cannulas of the tracheal tube, and the tracheal dressing and ties. Proper care of the tracheostomy tube maintains an adequate airway seal and tracheal tube patency. Proper cuff inflation may decrease the risk of aspiration of some particles. The tracheal dressing and ties are changed to maintain skin integrity and decrease the risk of infection. Additionally, the tracheal ties help maintain stability of the tracheal tube and prevent tube dislodgement.

PREREQUISITE NURSING KNOWLEDGE

- *Tracheotomy* refers to the surgical procedure in which an incision is made below the cricoid cartilage through the second to fourth tracheal rings (Fig. 13-1). *Tracheostomy* refers to the opening, or the stoma, made by the incision. The tracheostomy tube is the artificial airway inserted into the trachea during the tracheotomy (Fig. 13-2).
- A tracheotomy is performed as either an elective or emergent procedure for a variety of reasons (Box 13-1). There is no standard time when a tracheotomy should be performed. The decision is based on the projected length of time that mechanical ventilation or an artificial airway is required to remain in place. A tracheostomy tube is the preferred method of airway maintenance in patients who may require mechanical ventilation for more than 14 to 21 days.[4-6,20,23,25] Further studies need to be done to help predict which mechanically ventilated patients may benefit from early tracheostomy.[2,3,11-13]
- Compared with endotracheal tubes, tracheostomy tubes provide added benefits to patients, including the following: prevention of further laryngeal injury from the translaryngeal tube; improved patient comfort, acceptance, and tolerance; ease of oral care; decreased work of breathing due to decreased airflow resistance; facilitation of weaning from mechanical ventilation; decreased requirements for sedation; provision of a speech mechanism which enhances communication; increased patient mobility; facilitation of removal of secretions; and reduced risk for unintentional airway loss.
- Elective tracheotomy is generally performed in the operating room but may be performed at the bedside; percutaneous tracheotomy is commonly performed at the bedside on ventilated patients. Emergent surgical cricothyrotomy may occur before the patient arrives in the critical care unit or at the bedside (for additional information on cricothyrotomy refer to Procedure 11).
- Surgical placement is performed under general anesthesia. Using an open surgical technique, a stoma is created. The trachea is visualized by the surgeon. Landmarks are

identified by the surgeon, and an incision is made below the cricoid cartilage. The isthmus of the thyroid gland is exposed, cross-clamped, and ligated. A Bjork flap may be created. The flap is created when a small portion of the tracheal cartilage is pulled down and sutured to the skin. The flap helps facilitate reinsertion of the tracheostomy tube if it is dislodged, especially in patients who may be obese or have difficult anatomy.[14] Percutaneous tracheotomy has been proven to be a safe alternative to surgical tracheostomy on mechanically ventilated patients.[8,13] Unlike surgical tracheotomy, percutaneous tracheotomy can be performed without direct visualization of the trachea.[14] A bronchoscope may or may not be used to assist with visualization during the procedure. A needle is passed into the trachea. A J-tipped guidewire is placed into the trachea, the incision is then the dilated, and the tracheostomy tube is placed.
- Tracheostomies are not without complications. Common complications include infection, bleeding, tracheomalacia, skin breakdown, and transesophageal fistula. Common postoperative tracheostomy emergencies are hemorrhage, tube obstruction, and dislodgement. Hemorrhage can occur at the stoma site or into the trachea. A small amount of bleeding is expected postprocedure and is limited to a short period of time. Bleeding that continues or is moderate to large in volume could be due to a bleeding vessel or a tracheoinnominate artery fistula. Bleeding vessels may need to be ligated by a physician.
- Tracheoinnominate artery fistula is a rare complication with high mortality indices. In this complication the innominate artery has eroded into the trachea, which can result in exsanguination and is more common when a tracheostomy tube is subject to traction to one side or the other, away from the midline. Any concerns over bleeding should be reported to the physician immediately. Tube obstruction can occur from occlusion due to secretions or from the tracheostomy tube being displaced into the anterior portion of the trachea within a false passage. If the tube is obstructed from secretions, it should be suctioned. If the tube is felt to be dislodged into a false passage, treatment depends on how mature the stoma is. If the

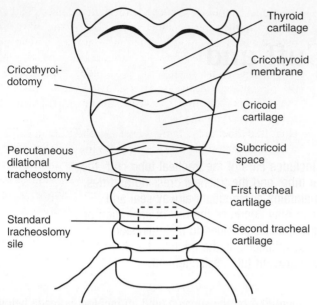

Figure 13-1 Sites for tracheostomy insertion. *(From Serra A: Tracheostomy care, Nurs Stand 14:42,45–52, 2000.)*

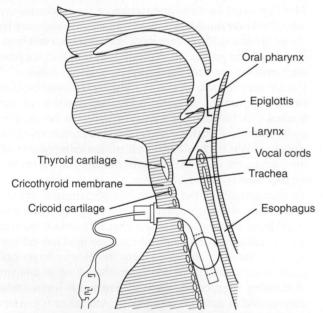

Figure 13-2 A tracheostomy (sometimes called a tracheotomy) is created surgically by making an opening through the skin of the neck into the trachea. *(From Serra A: Tracheostomy care, Nurs Stand 14:42,45–52, 2000.)*

BOX 13-1   **Indications for Tracheostomy**

- Bypass acute upper airway obstruction
- Prolonged need for artificial airway
- Prophylaxis for anticipated airway problems
- Reduction of anatomical dead space
- Prevention of pulmonary aspiration
- Retained tracheobronchial secretions
- Chronic upper airway obstruction

---

stoma is mature the tube should be replaced. If the stoma is immature—that is, the stoma is less than a week old—mask ventilation should be employed with the cuff deflated and an orotracheal tube should be inserted. Once the airway is secure the tracheostomy can be revised.[14] The physician should be notified if the tube becomes obstructed and aggressive measures other than routine suctioning are needed to clear the cannula or secretions of debris.

- An initial tracheotomy tube change varies depending on whether the trach was placed via standard surgical procedure or via percutaneous approach. Currently there is no evidence to justify when the initial or subsequent tracheotomy tubes should be changed; it typically occurs by physician preference. The first tube change most commonly occurs around day 5 postoperatively. Some reports state that for a percutaneous tracheotomy the initial change should not occur until postoperative day 10 to allow the stoma to mature. After the initial change, the tracheotomy should be changed approximately every 14 days thereafter. The first change is usually done by the physician.[12,14]

- In all instances, caution should be used to ensure that the tracheostomy tube is not accidentally dislodged or decannulated. The stoma takes approximately 1 week to heal posttracheotomy. Dislodgment of the tube in the first week is considered an emergency; the tissue may collapse, and it may not be possible to replace the tracheal tube. Predisposing factors to tube dislodgement or decannulation include an underinflated cuff, loose ties, neck or airway edema, excessive coughing, agitation or undersedation, morbid obesity, downward traction caused by the weight of the ventilator circuit, and an improperly sized tracheostomy tube. Trach ties should be secure. Weight or traction from the ventilator circuit should be minimized; when transporting or mobilizing the patient the tube should remain in a neutral midline position. Tube position should be noted before and after the patient is moved to ensure safety. Individual institutions usually use protocols to manage new tracheostomy tubes and accidental dislodgment to ensure patient safety.[7,12,14,17,31,33]

- A tracheostomy tube is shorter than but similar in diameter to an endotracheal tube. Some tracheostomy tubes have both outer and inner cannulas. The outer cannula forms the body of the tracheostomy tube with a cuff. The neck flange, attached to the outer cannula, assists in stabilizing the tube in the trachea and provides the small holes necessary for properly securing the tube. Some tracheostomy tubes have an inner cannula inserted into the outer cannula. The inner cannula is removable for easy cleaning without airway compromise and may be disposable. The tracheal tube cuff is an inflatable balloon that surrounds the shaft of the tracheal tube near its distal end. When inflated, the cuff presses against the tracheal wall to prevent air leakage and pressure loss from the lungs during positive pressure ventilation. The tracheal tube cuff is inflated by injecting air through a pilot balloon with a one-way inflation valve. The air in the pilot balloon is used to assess of the amount of pressure in the tracheal tube cuff (Fig. 13-3).

- Tracheostomy tubes are available in various materials, sizes, and styles from several manufacturers. It is important

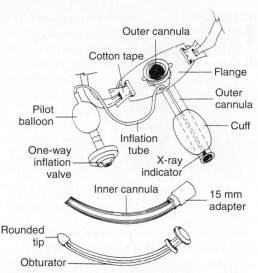

Figure 13-3 Parts of a tracheostomy tube. *(From Eubanks DH, Bone RC: Comprehensive respiratory care, ed 2. St Louis, 1990, Mosby, p. 570.)*

for the clinician to understand the differences between the various tracheostomy tubes to ensure appropriate feature, fit, and size for the patient. The tube should be selected with the goal of minimizing damage to the tracheal wall, allowing adequate ventilation, and when possible promoting translaryngeal airflow for communication to assist with future rehabilitation and therapy. The American Thoracic Society has published guidelines to guide users in selecting the appropriate tube and size.[12,16] Routine patient care and tube maintenance may be affected based on the tube size, style, and construction.

- Tracheostomy tubes can be constructed of metal (silver or stainless steel) or plastic (polyvinyl chloride or silicone). Metal tubes are rarely used due to cost, rigid construction, lack of cuff, the possibility of damage by cleaning with hydrogen peroxide or enzymatic cleaners, and lack of a 15-mm connector needed to attach the tracheostomy tube to a ventilator or bag-valve mask.[8,14] Polyvinyl chloride softens with the patient's body temperature, which helps the tube conform to the patient's anatomy and assists in centering the distal tip in the trachea. Silicone tubes are naturally soft and are not affected by the patient's body temperature.[8]

- Tracheostomy tubes may be angled or curved, and come in standard or extra length, fenestrated, and cuffed or uncuffed. Angled tubes have a straight portion and a curved portion, whereas curved tubes have a uniform angle of curvature. Extra length on the tracheostomy tube may refer to additional length that is proximal (horizontal length) or distal (vertical length). Extra proximal length may facilitate tracheostomy tube placement in patients with large necks (for example, obese patients); extra distal length may facilitate placement in patients with tracheal anomalies or tracheal malacia.[8]

- Fenestrated tracheostomy tubes are similar to standard tracheostomy tubes with an added opening located in the posterior portion of the tube above the cuff. Fenestrated tubes come with an inner cannula and a plastic plug. When the inner cannula is removed, the cuff deflated, and the tracheostomy tube occluded with the plastic plug, the patient can breathe through the fenestration(s) and around the tube, using the normal anatomical airway. When a fenestrated tracheostomy tube is occluded in this manner, the patient can speak, as air is allowed to pass over the vocal cords. Additional oxygen can be provided to the patent via nasal cannula if needed.[8]

- Uncuffed tubes are commonly used in children, in patients with laryngectomies, and during weaning from the tracheostomy. Uncuffed tubes may also be used in long-term mechanically ventilated patients who have adequate pulmonary compliance and sufficient oropharangeal muscle strength for functional swallowing and articulation and laryngeal strength to achieve glottis closure.[8]

- Cuffed tubes are generally used in patients requiring mechanical ventilation. Cuffed tubes allow for airway clearance, and the cuff limits aspiration of oral and gastric secretions in ventilated patients. Cuffed tubes include high-volume, low-pressure cuffs; low-volume, high-pressure cuffs; and foam cuffs (Fig. 13-4). High-volume, low-pressure cuffs are the most desirable. These tubes allow a large surface area to come into contact with the tracheal wall, distributing the pressure over a much greater area. This cuff has a relatively larger inflation volume that requires lower filling pressure to obtain a seal (<25 mm Hg or 34 cm H_2O). The older cuff design (low-volume, high-pressure) may require 40 mm Hg (54.4 cm H_2O) to obtain an effective seal and is undesirable.

- It is generally accepted that cuff pressure should be 20 to 25 mm Hg to minimize the risk of tracheal wall injury and decrease the risk of microaspiration for most tracheostomy tubes.[8,26] The amount of pressure and volume necessary to obtain a seal and prevent mucosal damage depends on tube size and design, cuff configuration, mode of ventilation, and the patient's arterial blood pressure (tracheal capillary perfusion pressure is 25 to 35 mm Hg for normotensive patients). Lower cuff pressures are associated with less mucosal damage but are also associated with silent aspiration, which has been shown when the cuff pressures are less than 20 mm Hg.[8,22,30]

- Appropriate cuff care helps prevent major pulmonary aspirations; prepares for tracheal extubation; decreases the risk of inadvertent decannulation; provides a patent airway for oxygenation, ventilation, and removal of secretions; and decreases the risk of hospital-acquired infections.

- A variety of techniques or devices is available to measure cuff pressures, including bedside pressure manometers. Two techniques, minimal leak technique and minimal occlusion volume (MOV), had historically been listed in the literature as effective methods to assess proper cuff inflation. Both of these methods have fallen out of favor due to the risk of aspiration when the cuff is deflated, increasing the incidence of ventilator-associated pneumonia for some patients. Little research has been conducted regarding the best practices with cuff pressure assessments.[10,15]

  ❖ Measurement of tracheal tube cuff pressures can be achieved through the use of a commercial pressure gauge by assembling equipment to assess pressure via

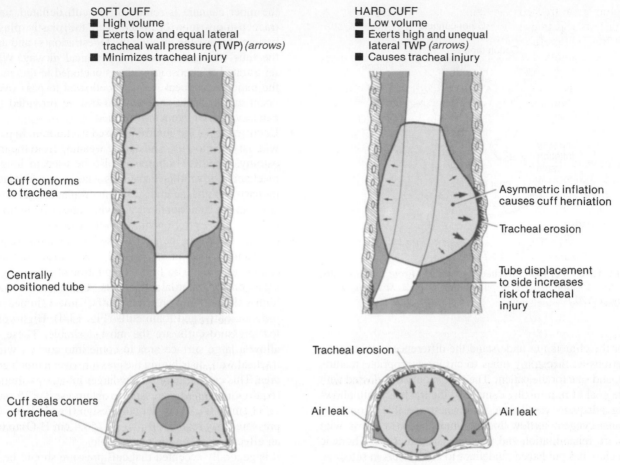

SOFT CUFF
- High volume
- Exerts low and equal lateral tracheal wall pressure (TWP) *(arrows)*
- Minimizes tracheal injury

Cuff conforms to trachea

Centrally positioned tube

Cuff seals corners of trachea

HARD CUFF
- Low volume
- Exerts high and unequal lateral TWP *(arrows)*
- Causes tracheal injury

Asymmetric inflation causes cuff herniation

Tracheal erosion

Tube displacement to side increases risk of tracheal injury

Tracheal erosion

Air leak   Air leak

Figure 13-4 Cross-sectional view in D-shaped trachea. Effects of soft and hard cuff inflation on the tracheal wall. *(From Kersten LD:* Comprehensive respiratory nursing. *Philadelphia 1989, Saunders, p. 648.)*

bedside manometer. An advantage to direct cuff pressure monitoring is that there is no need to deflate then reinflate the cuff, thus decreasing the potential risk for aspiration. Disadvantages are that these devices are designed for high-volume, low-pressure cuffs that are air filled. Saline-filled cuffs would damage the device.[24]

❖ The MOV consists of injection of air into the cuff until no leak is heard, then withdrawal of the air until a small leak is heard on inspiration, and then addition of more air until no leak is heard on inspiration.[1,10,17,25,30] The main advantages of this method are that it is easy to perform and that there is little additional equipment needed to perform the MOV. The main disadvantage is that by withdrawing air from the cuff, a leak is created, thus increasing the patient's potential risk for aspiration.

❖ Although rare since the use of high-volume, low-pressure devices became common, the adverse effects of tracheal tube cuff inflation include tracheal stenosis, necrosis, tracheoesophageal fistulas, and tracheomalacia. These complications may be more likely to occur in conditions that adversely affect tissue response to mucosal injury, such as hypotension. Two major

mechanisms are mainly responsible for airway damage: tube movement and pressure. Duration of intubation also plays a significant role.[16,28]

❖ Routine cuff deflation is unnecessary and is no longer recommended.[17]

• Consideration should be given to obtaining assistance with tracheostomy care, especially when tracheal ties are changed or when the patient is agitated. An assistant can minimize risk for accidental dislodgement.

EQUIPMENT

• Specially designed manometer to measure cuff pressures
• Stethoscope
• Self-inflating manual resuscitation bag-valve device
• Oxygen source and tubing
• Suction supplies (see Procedure 12)
• Personal protective equipment
• Sterile normal saline solution or sterile water
• Two to three sterile containers to place supplies (cotton swabs, normal saline)
• Sterile cotton balls and/or cotton-tipped applicators
• Sterile nylon brush
• Sterile 4 × 4 gauze

- Commercial tracheostomy tube holder
- Sterile precut tracheostomy dressing or dressing used by institutional preference
- If inner cannula is disposable, new sterile disposable inner cannula of the same size
- Extra sterile tracheostomy kit at bedside and obturator

Additional equipment, to have available as needed, includes the following:

- Scissors
- 10-mL syringe
- Three-way stopcock
- Padded hemostats
- Short 18-gauge or 23-gauge blunt needle
- Tongue depressor
- Tape (1 inch wide)
- Reintubation equipment, in case of accidental extubation

PATIENT AND FAMILY EDUCATION

- Explain the procedure and the reason for tracheal tube cuff care, tracheal tube care, and/or tracheostomy dressing change. *Rationale:* This communication identifies patient and family knowledge deficits concerning the patient's condition, procedure, expected benefits, and potential risks, and allows time for questions to clarify information and voice concerns. Explanations decrease patient anxiety and enhance cooperation.
- Explain the patient's role in assisting cuff care. *Rationale:* This information elicits patient cooperation.
- Explain that the procedure may cause the patient to cough. *Rationale:* This explanation prepares the patient for what to expect.

PATIENT ASSESSMENT AND PREPARATION

Patient Assessment

- Assess the presence of bilateral breath sounds. *Rationale:* This assessment provides baseline data.
- Assess signs and symptoms of cuff leakage, including audible or auscultated inspiratory leak over larynx, audible patient vocalizations, inflation (pilot) valve balloon deflation, and loss of inspiratory and expiratory volume on patient with mechanical ventilation. *Rationale:* An adequate seal of the cuff to the tracheal wall does not permit air to flow past the cuff.
- Assess signs and symptoms of inadequate ventilation, including rising arterial carbon dioxide tension, chest-abdominal dyssynchrony, patient-ventilator dyssynchrony, dyspnea, headache, restlessness, confusion, lethargy, increasing (early sign) or decreasing (late sign) arterial blood pressure, and activation of expiratory or inspiratory volume alarms on mechanical ventilator. *Rationale:* This guides needed interventions.
- Assess the amount of air or pressure currently or previously used to inflate the cuff. *Rationale:* The amount of air previously used to inflate the cuff can be used as a guideline to determine changes in volume or pressure or both.
- Assess the size of the tracheal tube and the size of the patient. *Rationale:* The volume and pressure of air needed to seal the airway depends on the relationship between the tracheal tube and the diameter of the trachea.
- Assess the amount of secretions. *Rationale:* This may increase the frequency of suctioning and tube care.
- Assess for the presence of cutaneous tracheal sutures. *Rationale:* After 7 days (when the trach is mature), the sutures may no longer be required. If they remain in place, notify the physician and query for removal. The sutures increase the risk of decanulation due to difficulty with maneuvering to care for the site and dressing. Prolonged suture retention may also promote skin breakdown.

Patient Preparation

- Ensure that the patient and family understand preprocedural teachings. Answer questions as they arise, and reinforce information as needed. *Rationale:* This communication evaluates and reinforces understanding of previously taught information.
- Verify that the patient is the correct patient using two identifiers. *Rationale:* Before performing a procedure, the nurse should ensure the correct identification of the patient for the intended intervention.
- Consider placing the patient in semi-Fowler's position. *Rationale:* This positioning promotes general relaxation, oxygenation, and ventilation. It also reduces stimulation of the gag reflex and risk of aspiration.

Procedure for Tracheostomy Cuff and Tube Care

Steps	Rationale	Special Considerations

Measurement of Cuff Pressure

1. HH
2. PE
3. Hyperoxygenate and suction tracheobronchial tree and pharynx before cuff deflation. Special care should be untaken with subglottic suctioning[16] (see Procedure 12). **(Level D*)** | Clears secretions above the trach cuff and in the lower airway and decreases incidence of aspiration. | If an open suction system is used, a fresh sterile catheter is needed for suctioning the tracheobronchial tree. When suctioning of the tracheobronchial tree is complete, the same catheter may be used to suction the pharynx. If a closed suction system is used in suctioning the tracheobronchial tree, a fresh sterile catheter is needed for suctioning the pharynx.

4. Attach a commercial pressure gauge to the tracheal cuff.[18] | Allows for measurement of the cuff pressure. |

5. Read the measurement. | Intracuff pressure measurement provides an approximation of cuff-to-tracheal wall pressure.[17] | Most cuffs are sufficiently inflated with <10 mL of air.

6. If the cuff pressure is >25 cm H_2O, press the pressure-release button on the pressure gauge until the pressure reaches 20–25 cm H_2O. If the pressure is <20 cm H_2O, add air by squeezing the bulb to increase pressure.[8,28] **(Level D)** | Provides optimal pressure to seal the cuff without causing excessive tracheal pressure. | Hazards of cuff inflation include cuff overinflation, distention, and rupture. The patient who is alert and cooperative may be asked to speak. If the trachea is sealed, vocalization is not possible.

7. If unable to maintain appropriate pressures, notify the physician or advance practice nurse. | Elevated cuff pressures have been associated with tracheal stenosis and necrosis. Inadequate cuff pressures may lead to impaired ability to provide ventilation and increase the risk for aspiration.[28] |

8. Dispose of used supplies and equipment and remove PE.
9. HH

Troubleshooting Tracheal Cuff Problems
Faulty Inflation Valve

1. HH
2. PE
3. Identify the faulty inflation valve by determining that the cuff continually deflates, despite the addition of air to the cuff (Fig. 13-5). | Determines need for repair. | If the inflation valve becomes faulty and reintubation is undesirable, consider instituting an emergency cuff-inflation technique. There are commercial cuff inflation-valve repair kits available. Follow institutional standards regarding who is responsible for repairing a faculty inflation valve.

4. Clamp the inflation tube with the padded hemostat. | Prevents further air loss through the faulty inflation valve. |

5. Insert a three-way stopcock into the inflation valve. | Provides access to the cuff. |

6. Inflate the cuff with the MOV technique. | Allows for cuff inflation; restores tracheal wall and cuff seal. |

---

*Level D: Peer-reviewed professional and organizational standards with the support of clinical study recommendations.

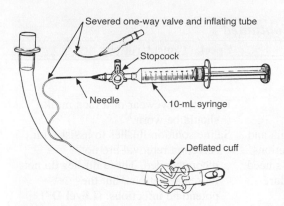

Severed one-way valve and inflating tube

Stopcock

Needle

10-mL syringe

Deflated cuff

Figure 13-5 Attachments for emergency cuff inflation for a faulty inflation line. *(From Sills J: An emergency cuff inflation technique, Respir Care 31:200, 1986.)*

Procedure for Tracheostomy Cuff and Tube Care—*Continued*

Steps	Rationale	Special Considerations
7. Turn the stopcock off to the inflation valve and leave it in place; remove the hemostat.	Temporarily maintains cuff pressure.	
8. Discard used supplies and remove **PE**.		
9. **HH**		
Faulty Inflation Tube		
1. **HH**		
2. **PE**		
3. Identify malfunctioning of the inflation tube by determining that an air leak is present in the tube (see Fig. 13-5).	Determines need for and method of repair.	There are commercial inflation tube repair kits available. Follow institutional standards regarding who is responsible for repairing a faculty inflation tube. Collaborate with respiratory therapy, the advanced practice nurse, and the physician.
4. Clamp the inflation tube, below the leak with the padded hemostat.	Prevents further air loss through the faulty inflation line.	The placement of the padded hemostat should allow adequate inflation tube length to accept the blunt needle.
5. Cut the inflation line above the padded hemostat but below the identified leak.	Allows introduction of the blunt needle for repair.	
6. Insert a short 18 gauge to 23 gauge blunt needle into the inflation tube.	Provides inflation access.	Maintain care to avoid puncture or severing of inflation line or clinician's skin.
7. Attach a three-way stopcock to a blunt needle, "Off" to the inflation tube.	Provides control of airflow in and out of the inflation tube.	
8. With a 10-mL syringe, inflate the cuff with air using the MOV technique.	Allows cuff inflation; restores tracheal wall and cuff seal.	
9. Turn the stopcock off to the inflation tube.	Provides for temporary use of the tracheal tube while maintaining cuff pressure.	
10. Secure the assembled device with tape to a tongue depressor.	Provides for stabilization and protection.	
11. Assemble equipment for tracheal tube replacement.	Prepares for tracheal tube replacement.	Make plans to change the tube as a more permanent solution.
12. Discard used supplies and remove **PE**.	Reduces transmission of microorganisms and body secretions; Standard Precautions.	
13. **HH**		

Procedure continues on following page

Procedure | for Tracheostomy Cuff and Tube Care—*Continued*

Steps	Rationale	Special Considerations
Tracheostomy Tube Care		
1. **HH**		
2. **PE**		Protective eyewear or a face mask should be worn.[22]
3. Hyperoxygenate and suction the trachea and pharynx as needed (see Procedure 12).	Reduces the risk of hypoxemia and arrhythmias; removes secretions and diminishes the patient's need to cough during the procedure.	Saline solution flushes to assist with secretion removal are not recommended. These flushes do not loosen secretions, but they potentiate infections. **(Level D*)**
4. Remove and discard soiled tracheostomy dressing and **PE**.	Provides access and visibility of the tracheostomy site.	
5. **HH**		
6. For disposable inner cannula: A. Open prepackaged inner cannula. B. Apply clean gloves. C. Remove soiled inner cannula. D. Replace with prepackaged cannula.	Replaces the inner cannula.	
7. For nondisposable inner cannula (open prepackaged commercial tracheostomy care kit): A. Prepare sterile saline or sterile water on a sterile field.[22,31,32] B. Apply sterile gloves. C. Remove oxygen source and then inner cannula, placing it in sterile saline or sterile water.	Prepares for cleaning the tracheostomy.	Only sterile normal saline should be used for cleaning tracheostomy tubes. Hydrogen peroxide may cause pitting of metal inner cannula.[25]
8. Place tracheostomy collar, T tube, or ventilator oxygen source over or near the outer cannula.	Maintains oxygen supply.	If the patient cannot tolerate disconnection from a ventilator for the time needed to clean the inner cannula, replace the existing inner cannula with a clean one and reattach the ventilator. Then, clean the cannula just removed from the patient and store it in a sterile container for the next inner cannula change.[29]
9. Clean the inner cannula with a small brush.	Assists in the removal of debris and thick secretions.	
10. Rinse inner cannula by pouring normal saline over the cannula. Remove excess solution by tapping on the inside edge of the sterile container. Do not dry the outside portion of the inner cannula.	Removes any remaining debris from the cannula. Excess solution left on the inside of the inner cannula may lead to aspiration. Solution on the outside portion of the inner cannula may help act as a lubricant for insertion.[29]	
11. Remove the oxygen source from over the outer cannula.	Allows access to the opening of the outer cannula.	
12. Insert the inner cannula and lock it into place.	Secures the inner cannula.	
13. Reapply the oxygen source to the inner cannula hub.	Reestablishes oxygen supply.	

*Level D: Peer-reviewed professional and organizational standards with the support of clinical study recommendations.

Procedure for Tracheostomy Cuff and Tube Care—*Continued*

Steps	Rationale	Special Considerations
14. Moisten 4 × 4 gauze pads with sterile normal saline or sterile water and clean the stoma site, outer cannula, and neck plate surface by wiping with cotton-tipped swabs and 4 × 4 gauze.	Removes debris and secretions from the stoma area.	
15. Dry the skin around the stoma by gently patting it dry.	Decreases the likelihood of microorganism growth and skin breakdown.	
16. If needed, prepare to attach a new tracheostomy tube holder or twill tape tie.	Ties may need to be replaced if they are soiled.	Review individual institutional polices regarding the use of twill tape or commercial trach tie devices. Institutions may prohibit tracheostomy tube holders from being changed for up to 72 hours after tracheostomy tube placement due to the risk of dislodgement. Have an assistant hold the neck plate securely if this procedure is performed.
17. Remove the current tracheostomy tube holder or twill tape.	Prepares for replacement.	Make certain an assistant securely holds the tracheostomy in place.
18. *Tracheostomy tube holder:* Connect one side of the neck plate to the new tracheostomy tube holder, then connect the other side of the neck plate and tighten the tube holder, allowing one finger under the holder to ensure it is secure.	Removes soiled holder or tape.	A variety of commercial tracheostomy tube holders is available. In some instances a newly placed tracheostomy tube may be sutured into place and no holder or ties are used (i.e. for patients with a new laryngectomy and flap). If this occurs, the physician should write clear orders if a tracheostomy holder or twill tape should not be used.
Twill tape: Cut a length long enough to encircle the patient's neck two times. Cut ends diagonally. Insert one end through the faceplate eyelet and pull the ends even. Pass both ends of the tie around the patient's neck and insert one end through the faceplate's second eyelet. Pull snugly to allow space for one finger between tie and the patient's neck and tie the ends securely with a double square knot so that the knot rests on the side of the patient's neck (Fig. 13-6).		
19. Apply a clean, precut tracheostomy dressing under the neck plate.	Provides a dressing between the tracheostomy and the neck plate.	Any precut surgical gauze is sufficient. Never cut a 4 × 4 gauze pad because cut edges fray and provide a potential source for infection.[22,25] **(Level D*)**
20. Provide oral care (see Procedure 4).	Increases patient comfort.	
21. Discard used supplies and remove **PE**.		
22. **HH**		

*Level D: Peer-reviewed professional and organizational standards with the support of clinical study recommendations.

Procedure continues on following page

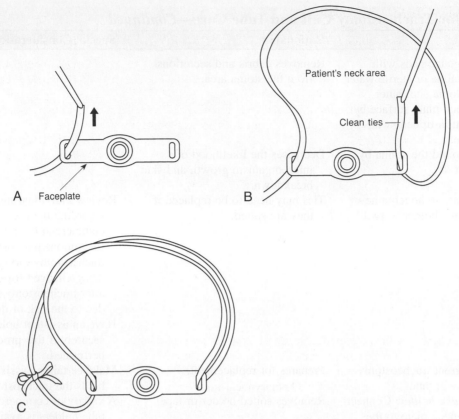

Figure 13-6   Placement of tracheostomy twill tape. **A,** Faceplate with threading of twill tape (for prevention of decannulation, an additional person needs to stabilize faceplate). **B,** Advancing of the twill tape around the back of the neck and looping through the other side of the faceplate. **C,** Doubling of the twill tape and securing it in a knot.

Expected Outcomes

- Tracheal tube remains in correct position
- Cuff pressure is kept at a level to maintain a seal between cuff and tracheal wall (usually between 20 and 25 mm Hg)
- Cuff remains intact
- Airway remains patent
- Stoma site is infection free

Unexpected Outcomes

- Decannulation or tube dislodgment
- Tracheal mucosal ischemia from cuff overinflation
- Faulty inflation valve or tube
- Cuff overinflation and distention over the end of the tube
- Cuff rupture
- Prolonger apnea, increasing hypoxemia, or cardiopulmonary arrest
- Hemorrhage
- Interstitial air: subcutaneous emphysema, pneumothorax, pneumopericardium, pneumomediastinum
- Thyroid gland injury
- Cardiac dysrhythmias
- Tube tip erosion into the innominate artery
- Skin breakdown, pressure areas, stomatitis
- Signs of stoma infection
- Bronchopulmonary infection
- Displacement or dislodgement out of trachea
- Excessive cuff pressure
- Leaking airway cuff
- Airway obstruction from misalignment, cuff overinflation, or dried or excessive secretion
- Tracheal stenosis, malacia, or tracheoesophageal fistula

Patient Monitoring and Care

Steps	Rationale	Reportable Conditions
		These conditions should be reported if they persist despite nursing interventions.
1. Assess respiratory status for optimal ventilation.	Inadequate interface between tracheal cuff and tracheobronchial mucosa decreases inspiratory flow.	• Rising arterial carbon dioxide tension • Chest-abdominal dyssynchrony • Patient-ventilator dyssynchrony • Dyspnea • Headache • Restlessness • Confusion • Lethargy • Increasing (early sign) or decreasing (late sign) arterial blood pressure • Activation of expiratory or inspiratory volume alarms on the mechanical ventilator
2. Measure cuff pressure every 8 hours, or per institutional requirements, maintaining cuff pressure between 20 and 25 mm Hg.[31] **(Level D*)**	Prevents tracheal injury and aspiration. Excessive cuff pressure is cited as the most frequent problem of tracheal intubation and the best predictor of tracheolaryngeal injury.[8,10] If the volume (milliliters) needed to seal the airway increases, evaluate the patient for tracheal dilation with chest radiography of cuff diameter/tracheal diameter ratio. Increasing volumes also may indicate a leak in the cuff, inflation valve, or tube.	• Cuff pressure <20 mm Hg or >25 mm Hg • Inability to maintain cuff pressure
3. Maintain tracheal tube cuff integrity.	Manipulation of the tracheal tube increases the likelihood of cuff disruption. Cuff leak or rupture is evident when the pressure on the manometer continues to decrease.	• Inability to maintain cuff inflation • Audible air through the patient's nose or mouth • Low-pressure or low-volume alarm sounds on the mechanical ventilator • Audible or auscultated inspiratory leak over larynx • Patient able to vocalize audibly • Pilot balloon deflation • Loss of inspiratory and expiratory volume on patients with mechanical ventilation
4. Hyperoxygenate and suction patient based on assessment (see Procedure 12).	Removal of secretions reduces chance for partial or complete airway obstruction.	

---

*Level D: Peer-reviewed professional and organizational standards with the support of clinical study recommendations.

Procedure continues on following page

Patient Monitoring and Care —*Continued*

Steps	Rationale	Reportable Conditions
5. Compare patient's cardiopulmonary status before and after tracheal tube cuff care.	Identifies the effects of tracheal tube cuff care on the cardiovascular system.	• Decreased arterial oxygen saturation • Cardiac dysrhythmias • Bronchospasm • Respiratory distress • Cyanosis • Increased blood pressure or intracranial pressure • Anxiety, agitation, or changes in level of consciousness
6. Reassess cuff pressure and volume when transporting the patient from one altitude to another (i.e., air transport) or during hyperbaric therapy without environmental pressurization.	Changes in altitude may change the volume of gas in the cuff; volume and pressure need to be reevaluated during and after transport.	
7. Provide continuous humidified air or oxygen. Warm or cool as appropriate.[21,25,29] **(Level D*)**	Artificial airways bypass the nose and mouth, preventing normal warming, humidification, and filtering.[4,22]	
8. Maintain the tracheostomy tube in a neutral position, midline with the patient's body.	Traction on the tracheostomy from ventilator circuits, oxygen, or suction tubing may cause the tip of the tracheostomy tube to erode through the trachea and, potentially, into the innominate artery.	• Sutures that prevent adequate stoma care
9. Auscultate lung sounds to check proper placement of tracheostomy tube and ensure tracheostomy tube is securely in place.	Improper placement may lead to inadequate ventilation and complications. An extra sterile tracheostomy kit should be kept at the bedside at all times. Displacement into the subcutaneous tissue can occur. How emergent the situation is depends on whether the upper airway is obstructed. Decannulation inadvertently occurs from lack of tracheotomy securement. If decannulation occurs and if retention sutures are present, pull them apart to lift the trachea up and hold the tracheal stoma open. Do not cross tracheal sutures because this action will close the airway. When help arrives, a second person should reinsert the tracheostomy tube as per individual facility policy.[23] If the patient does not have retention sutures, open a new tracheostomy tube set, remove the inner cannula, insert the obturator into the outer cannula, and slide it into place.[14]	• Decreased chest wall motion • Unilateral breath sounds • Audible expiratory wheeze • Bilateral decreased breath sounds • Oxygen desaturation • Dyspnea and respiratory distress • Stridor • Ventilator alarms
10. Inspect and palpate for air under the skin.	Air may escape into the incision, causing subcutaneous emphysema. Special note: Subcutaneous emphysema does not injure the patient with an artificial airway in place. However, puffiness of the soft tissue may result and, if significant, can change the patient's appearance, alarming the patient and family.	• Subcutaneous emphysema

*Level D: Peer-reviewed professional and organizational standards with the support of clinical study recommendations.

Patient Monitoring and Care —*Continued*

Steps	Rationale	Reportable Conditions
11. Assess for bleeding or a constant ooze of blood.	Surgical procedures increase the risk of potential injury to adjacent tissue or structures. Stoma placement below the second and third cartilaginous rings results in an increased incidence of innominate artery erosion.	• Frank bleeding or constant oozing of blood
12. Gently palpate the tube for pulsation.	Pulsation felt on the tracheal tube is suggestive of potential erosion of major blood vessels.	• Pulsation of the tracheal tube
13. Follow institutional standards for assessing pain and administering analgesia as prescribed.	Identifies pain and need for appropriate interventions.	• Continued pain despite interventions
14. Tracheostomy care should be performed every 4–8 hours and as needed or per institutional policy depending on the type and volume of secretions produced.[13,19,20,23,27] (**Level E***)	Keeps tube free of secretions, mucus, and plugs that may impede airway patency.	• Frequent plugs • Copious drainage • Change in color, odor, or tenacity of secretions
15. Assess stoma for signs of infection, inflammation, or pressure from tension by trach ties or equipment.	Skin irritation or breakdown may occur from the neck plate, tracheostomy tube holder, or sutures, if present.	• Elevated temperature • Swelling • Excoriated or open areas • Redness
16. Monitor secretions for color, consistency, odor, and amount.	Change in secretion characteristic may indicate infection or inadequate hydration.	• Purulent drainage • Excessively thick secretions • Copious or purulent secretions
17. Maintain the head of the bed at 30–45 degrees and during enteral feedings.[24] (**Level D***)	Promotes oropharyngeal and nasopharyngeal drainage and minimizes the risk of aspiration. Prevents ventilator-associated or hospital-acquired pneumonia.[9] Withholding enteral feedings when gastric residuals are high is also important in the prevention if regurgitation and pulmonary aspiration.	
18. Perform oral care every 2–4 hours (see Procedure 4).	Prevents bacterial overgrowth and promotes patient comfort.	
19. Tracheostomy tube care should be completed every 4–8 hours and as needed, or as institutional policy dictates.[21,25,29] (**Level D**)	Prevents bacterial overgrowth and promotes patient comfort.	
20. Promote effective patient-provider communication (paper and pencil, letter or word boards, one-way speaking valves, if appropriate).	The patient cannot talk, which may result in fear and anxiety. Patients need an established communication mechanism. A speaking valve may be used to facilitate speech.	

*Level D: Peer-reviewed professional and organizational standards with the support of clinical study recommendations.
*Level E: Multiple case reports, theory-based evidence from expert opinions, or peer-reviewed professional organizational standards without clinical studies to support recommendations.

Procedure continues on following page

Documentation

Documentation should include the following:

- Patient and family education and comprehension
- Vital signs assessed before and after the procedure
- Date, time, and frequency of tracheostomy care
- Type and size of tracheostomy tube, changing of inner cannula, replacement of tracheostomy tube holder, and general condition of stoma and surrounding skin
- Nursing interventions in response to assessed complications
- Patient and family education
- Cardiopulmonary and vital sign assessment before and after procedure
- Method of cuff inflation
- Cuff inflation volume and cuff pressure
- Patient's tolerance of the procedure.
- Condition of stoma, including inflammation and secretions
- Expected and unexpected outcomes
- Type and amount of secretions, frequency of suctioning
- Performance of oral care
- Pain-assessment interventions, and effectiveness
- Evidence that the securing device is adequate without being excessively tight (2-finger technique)

References and Additional Readings

For a complete list of references and additional readings for this procedure, scan this QR code with any freely available smartphone code reader app, or visit http://booksite.elsevier.com/9780323376624.

14 Continuous End-Tidal Carbon Dioxide Monitoring

Paul Luehrs

PURPOSE: End-tidal carbon dioxide, also referred to as $PetCO_2$, provides a noninvasive continuous measurement of exhaled carbon dioxide (CO_2) concentration commonly referred to as capnometry. A capnograph is a graphic depiction of a waveform tracing of each respiratory cycle. The partial pressure of end-tidal CO_2 is representative of alveolar CO_2 ($PaCO_2$), which under normal ventilation/perfusion matching in the lungs closely parallels arterial levels of CO_2 ($PaCO_2$)

PREREQUISITE NURSING KNOWLEDGE

- There are three broad categories of indications for capnography/capnometry: verification of artificial airway placement; assessment of pulmonary circulation and respiratory status; and optimization of mechanical ventilation.[2,9]
- Capnography provides the clinician with a calculation of airway respiratory rate (RR), and the combination of both $PetCO_2$ and RR can provide clinicians with one of the earliest indications that ventilation is hindered. In fact capnography can detect respiratory depression before changes in pulse oximetry occur. $PetCO_2$ monitoring allows clinicians to actively monitor patients for clinical changes and rapidly correct abnormal ventilatory concerns, such as airway obstruction, congestive heart failure, pulmonary embolism, asthma, and chronic obstructive pulmonary disease (COPD).[6,7,11]
- The principles of arterial blood gas sampling (see Procedure 61) and interpretation should be understood.
- Ventilation is the bulk movement of gases into and out of the lung during the respiratory cycle and is composed of two distinct processes: inspiration and expiration.
  - During inspiration, gas is drawn into the alveoli, at which time it participates in gas exchange. Oxygenation occurs when the oxygen diffuses across the alveolar membrane into the capillary bed. CO_2 exchange occurs during this time as it diffuses across the alveolar membrane into the alveoli. Oxygenated blood is then distributed to and metabolized by the cells of the body. Oxygen saturation can be evaluated with a blood gas machine (oxygen saturation [SaO_2]) or pulse oximetry (SpO_2).
  - During expiration, alveolar gas is exhaled, which results in the elimination of CO_2. Cells produce CO_2 as a byproduct of metabolism; this CO_2 is transported by the vascular system to the lungs, where it is eliminated through exhalation. CO_2 elimination can also be evaluated with a blood gas machine or capnometer.

- In intubated patients, $PetCO_2$ can be monitored through a sensor that is placed directly into the ventilator circuit.
- In nonintubated patients capnography can be performed with a specialized nasal cannula that delivers supplemental oxygen and measures $PetCO_2$ and respiratory rate. Placing the capnography cannula is the same as initiating a nasal cannula for supplemental oxygen. Breath samples are obtained through both nostrils, and oxygen is delivered through the nasal prongs (design depends on manufacturer). For patients who breathe either partially or fully through their mouths, a specially designed nasal cannula can be used that allows for exhaled gas to be captured for analysis.
- The $PetCO_2$ monitor may be a stand-alone system or a module incorporated into the patient's bedside physiological monitor or the mechanical ventilator. An infrared capnometer passes light through an expiratory gas sample and, with a photodetector, measures absorption of that light by the gas. The capnograph determines the amount of CO_2 in the gas sample based on the absorption properties of CO_2. The capnograph provides a display called a capnogram or $PetCO_2$ *waveform*.
- The capnograph samples exhaled CO_2 by one of two methods: aspiration (side stream) or nonaspiration (mainstream) sampling. In the side-stream method, a sample of gas is transported via small-bore tubing to the bedside monitor for analysis. In the mainstream system, analysis occurs directly at the patient-ventilator circuit.
- Normal $PetCO_2$ concentration in a patient with healthy lungs and airway conditions is 30 to 43 mm Hg. As the patient breathes, a characteristic waveform is created that can be divided into two segments: inspiration and expiration.[11] $PaCO_2$ (partial pressure of arterial carbon dioxide)— $PetCO_2$ gradient is the difference between the $PaCO_2$

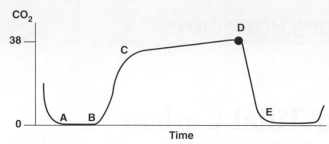

Figure 14-1 Essentials of the normal capnographic waveform. *(Reprinted by permission of Nellcor Puritan Bennett LLC, Boulder, CO, part of Covidien.)*

obtained from an arterial blood gas and the $Petco_2$ measure by the capnometer. A normal gradient is 2 to 5 mm Hg with the $Paco_2$ always higher. A widened gradient can result from increasing dead space ventilation such as is seen in COPD and pulmonary embolism. Additionally a widened gradient can result from low perfusion disease states.

- The normal capnographic waveform has the following characteristics (Fig. 14-1):
  - The zero baseline is seen during inspiration of fresh gas and the beginning of exhalation as CO_2-free gas from anatomical dead space is expelled. This gas comes from the artificial airway (if present) and the large airways, oropharynx, and nasopharynx (see Fig. 14-1*A* and *B*).
  - A rapid sharp upstroke occurs as the gas from the intermediate airways, containing a mixture of fresh gas and CO_2-rich gas, begins to be expelled from the lungs (see Fig. 14-1*B* and *C*).
  - A nearly flat alveolar plateau occurs as exhaled flow velocity slows and mixed gas is displaced by alveolar gas (Fig. 14-1*C* and *D*). Alveolar exhalation of CO_2 is nearing completion.
  - A distinct end-tidal point most closely reflects the maximal concentration of exhaled CO_2 and the end of exhalation (Fig. 14-1*D*).
  - A rapid down stroke occurs as the patient begins the inspiration of fresh gas that is essentially devoid of CO_2 (see Fig. 14-1*D* and *E*).
  - The orientation of the capnogram is commonly confused because the positive aspect of the waveform occurs with exhalation, whereas the negatively deflected limb occurs with inhalation. This is opposite from other respiratory waveforms, including the respirogram, spirogram, and flow-volume loop. The capnogram deviates from normal whenever physiological or mechanical disruption of the breath occurs.

- A ramping waveform is an indication of airway obstruction such as is seen in COPD and asthma.

EQUIPMENT

- Personal protective equipment
- Capnometer
- Airway adapter or $Petco_2$ nasal cannula

PATIENT AND FAMILY EDUCATION

- Discuss the reason for implementation of capnography. *Rationale:* Discussion reduces anxiety for the patient and family associated with an additional monitor, related interventions, and unfamiliar procedures.
- If the patient is alert, explain the procedure to the patient; if the patient is not alert, explain the procedure to the family. *Rationale:* This communication informs the patient and/or the family of the purpose of monitoring, improves cooperation with interventions, and reduces anxiety.

PATIENT ASSESSMENT AND PREPARATION

Patient Assessment

- Assess for indications for $Petco_2$ monitoring, including general anesthesia,[9] monitored anesthesia care, procedural sedation and analgesia,[3] confirmation of endotracheal tube placement,[9–11] adequacy of chest compressions in cardiopulmonary arrest,[8] analysis/monitoring of ventilation in mechanical ventilation,[9] obstructive sleep apnea,[1] and neuromuscular disease. Additional indications (actual or potential) include acute airway obstruction or apnea, dead space ventilation, and incomplete alveolar emptying. *Rationale:* Assessment for initiation of $Petco_2$ monitoring ensures that patients at risk for inadequate ventilation and gas exchange receive monitoring for such occurrences, allowing for early institution of appropriate interventions.

Patient Preparation

- Verify correct patient with two identifiers. *Rationale:* Prior to performing a procedure, the nurse should ensure the correct identification of the patient for the intended intervention.
- Ensure that the patient understands preprocedural teaching. Answer questions as they arise, and reinforce information as needed. *Rationale:* Understanding of previously taught information is evaluated and reinforced.

Procedure   for Continuous End-Tidal Carbon Dioxide Monitoring

Steps	Rationale	Special Considerations
1. **HH**		
2. **PE**		
3. Obtain order or follow institutional protocol for continuous $Petco_2$ monitoring with capnography.	Order provides guideline for duration of monitoring, acceptable parameters for results, and appropriate interventions for abnormal results.	
4. Assess for proper functioning of capnograph, including electronic equipment, self-start, autocalibration, airway adapter, sensor, and display monitor; and secure connections. **(Level M*)**	Ensures reliability of $Petco_2$ values and waveforms obtained.	
5. Connect capnograph into grounded wall outlet, connect the appropriate patient cable into display monitor, and turn on instrument. **(Level M)**	Decreases incidence of electrical interference.	Check capnograph's battery capacity and charging time, if applicable.
6. Perform calibration routine. Calibration procedure should occur daily or more often when instrument is in clinical use.[4] **(Level M)**	Accurate measurement for devices depends on proper calibration. Improper calibration may lead to erroneous $Petco_2$ values.	All monitors have some type of calibration procedure; see operator's manual for exact steps.
7. If the patient is not intubated, apply $Petco_2$ nasal cannula and connect to capnograph.		
8. For intubated patients, assemble airway adapter, sensor, and display monitor; connect to the patient's circuit as close as possible to the patient's ventilation connection.	Decreases incidence of improper gas sampling.	Sampling errors and gas leaks in the system are major causes of inaccurate readings. Placing the sensor or sampling port as close as possible to the patient's airway decreases response time to detect a change in CO_2.
9. Ensure that the light source is on top of the circuit so that condensation and secretions do not pool and obstruct the light transmission in mainstream sensor. **(Level M)**	Decreases condensation and secretion accumulation on CO_2 port where gas is drawn for sampling.	
10. Set appropriate alarms. Alarm limits should include respiratory rate, apnea default, high and low $Petco_2$, and minimal levels of inspiratory CO_2. **(Level M)**	Alerts the nurse to potentially life-threatening problems.	The $Petco_2$ alarm is set 5% above and below acceptable parameter or per institutional standard. If monitor is interfaced with other equipment (electrocardiogram monitor, mechanical ventilator, pulse oximeter), ensure alarms are set consistently among all monitors.
11. Discard supplies		
12. **HH**		

*Level M: Manufacturer's recommendations only.

Procedure continues on following page

Expected Outcomes

- Significant changes in ventilatory status are detected
- Alterations in the alveolar-arterial carbon dioxide gradient are identified

Unexpected Outcomes

- Inaccurate measurements of $Petco_2$ are displayed
- Inaccurate measurements from calibration drift or contamination of optics with moisture or secretions are displayed
- Equipment malfunction occurs
- Inadvertent extubation from weight of sensor

Patient Monitoring and Care

Steps	Rationale	Reportable Conditions
		These conditions should be reported if they persist despite nursing interventions.
1. **HH**		
2. **PE**		
3. Observe artificial airway for patency.[9]	The airway adapter often adds weight to the airway and increases the risk of dislodgment or kinking. If kinking occurs, support the airway with an artificial support or towel.	• Endotracheal or tracheal tube dislodgment
4. If the patient is not intubated, check nasal cannula or mouthpiece for proper placement and ensure that it is clear of secretions.[5]	Poor placement or occlusion of nasal cannula or mouthpiece interferes with accurate $Petco_2$ monitoring.	
5. Observe waveform for quality. **(Level M*)**	If waveform is of poor quality, the numerical $Petco_2$ value should not be accepted. If the $Petco_2$ waveform is acceptable and the $Petco_2$ numerical reading is questionable, obtain arterial blood gas measurement to confirm changes in $Petco_2$.	• Poor-quality waveform • Questionable $Petco_2$ reading
6. Observe waveform for gradually increasing $Petco_2$ (Fig. 14-2).[5,8]	Increasing $Petco_2$ occurs from absorption of CO_2 from exogenous sources and increased CO_2 production. Clinical conditions in which increasing $Petco_2$ is found include increased metabolism, hyperthermia (usually indicated by a rapid rise in $Petco_2$), sepsis, hypoventilation or inadequate minute ventilation, neuromuscular blockade, decreased alveolar ventilation, partial obstruction of the airway, use of respiratory depressant drugs, and conditions that cause metabolic alkalosis.	• $Petco_2$ increase of greater than 10% of baseline

*Level M: Manufacturer's recommendations only.

Patient Monitoring and Care —*Continued*

Steps	Rationale	Reportable Conditions

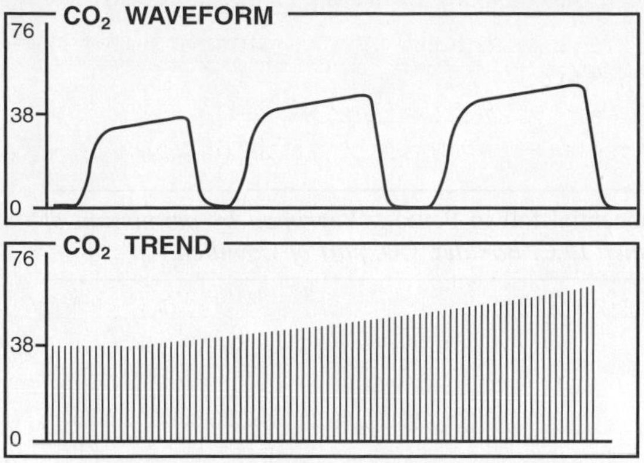

Figure 14-2 Gradually increasing Petco$_2$. *(Reprinted by permission of Nellcor Puritan Bennett LLC, Boulder, CO, part of Covidien.)*

Steps	Rationale	Reportable Conditions
7. Observe for a gradual increase in both baseline CO$_2$ and Petco$_2$ values (Fig. 14-3).[5,8]	Reflects rebreathing of previously exhaled gas. Clinical conditions in which a gradual increase in both baseline CO$_2$ and Petco$_2$ levels is found include defective exhalation valve on mechanical ventilator and excessive mechanical dead space in ventilator circuit.	• Malfunction of the ventilator

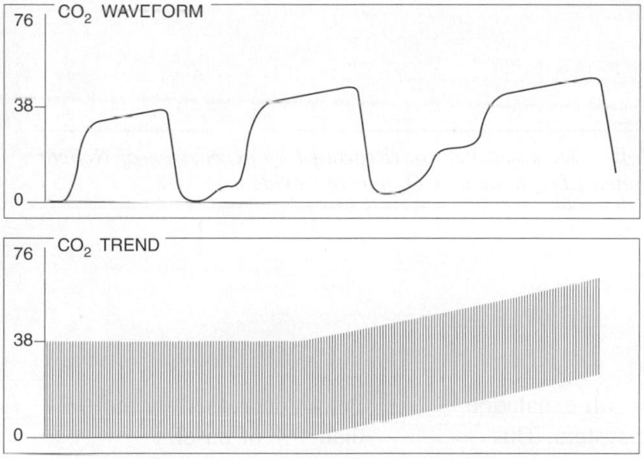

Figure 14-3 Gradual increase in baseline and Petco$_2$. *(Reprinted by permission of Nellcor Puritan Bennett LLC, Boulder, CO, part of Covidien.)*

Steps	Rationale	Reportable Conditions
8. Observe for an exponential fall in Petco$_2$ (Fig. 14-4).[5,8]	Indicates a sudden increase in dead space ventilation seen in clinical conditions such as hypoventilation, cardiopulmonary bypass, pulmonary embolism, and severe pulmonary hypoperfusion.[10]	• Petco$_2$ decreased by more than 10% of baseline

Procedure continues on following page

Patient Monitoring and Care —*Continued*

Steps	Rationale	Reportable Conditions

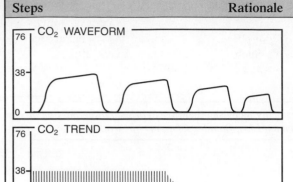

Figure 14-4   Exponential fall in Petco$_2$. *(Reprinted by permission of Nellcor Puritan Bennett LLC, Boulder, CO, part of Covidien.)*

Steps	Rationale	Reportable Conditions
9. Observe for decreased Petco$_2$ (with a normal waveform; Fig. 14-5).[5,8]	Gradual decreases indicate a decrease in perfusion or a decrease in production of CO$_2$ and may be seen in patients with high minute volumes, hypothermia, metabolic acidosis, decreased cardiac output, and hypovolemia.	• Petco$_2$ decreased by more than 10% of baseline

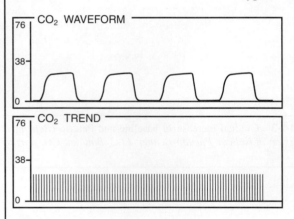

Figure 14-5   Decreased Petco$_2$. *(Reprinted by permission of Nellcor Puritan Bennett LLC, Boulder, CO, part of Covidien.)*

Steps	Rationale	Reportable Conditions
10. Observe for a sudden decrease in Petco$_2$ to low values (Fig. 14-6).[5,8]	Incomplete sampling or full exhalation is not detected in the system. This may be seen in patients with a leak in the airway system, partial airway obstruction, mechanical ventilator malfunction, malpositioning/ dislodgement of the airway, or partial disconnection of a ventilator circuit.	• Petco$_2$ decreased by more than 10% of baseline

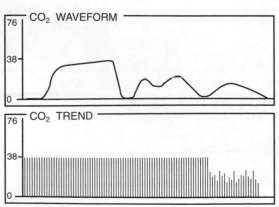

Figure 14-6   Sudden decrease in Petco$_2$ values. *(Reprinted by permission of Nellcor Puritan Bennett LLC, Boulder, CO, part of Covidien.)*

Patient Monitoring and Care —*Continued*

Steps	Rationale	Reportable Conditions
11. Observe for a sudden decrease in Petco$_2$ to near zero (Fig. 14-7).[5,8]	Drop in waveform to baseline or near baseline (baseline equals zero) implies that no respirations are present. Such a drop in waveform may also occur within the case of significant ventilation/perfusion changes such as pulmonary emboli.	• Dislodged endotracheal tube • Complete airway obstruction • Mechanical ventilator malfunction • Airway disconnection • Esophageal intubation • Apnea

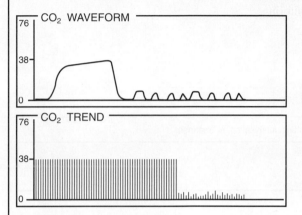

Figure 14-7 Sudden decrease in Petco$_2$ to near zero. *(Reprinted by permission of Nellcor Puritan Bennett LLC, Boulder, CO, part of Covidien.)*

Steps	Rationale	Reportable Conditions
12. Observe for a sustained low Petco$_2$ without alveolar plateau (Fig. 14-8).[5,8]	Sustained low Petco$_2$ values are indicative of incomplete alveolar emptying, such as in partially kinked endotracheal tube, bronchospasm, mucous plugging, improper exhaled gas sampling, or insufficient expiratory time on the ventilator.	• Complete airway obstruction that necessitates reintubation • Petco$_2$ decreased greater than 10% of baseline

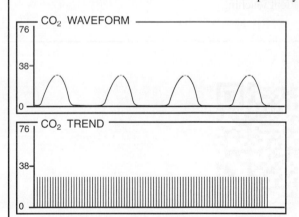

Figure 14-8 Low Petco$_2$, without alveolar plateau. *(Reprinted by permission of Nellcor Puritan Bennett LLC, Boulder, CO, part of Covidien.)*

Steps	Rationale	Reportable Conditions
13. Routinely monitor the airway adapter or sampling port for signs of obstruction.[5,8,9] **(Level M*)**	If the adapter or the port becomes obstructed, the quality of the capnographic waveform is poor and Petco$_2$ is not reliable.	• Obstruction in the airway adapter or sampling port

*Level M: Manufacturer's recommendations only.

Procedure continues on following page

Patient Monitoring and Care —*Continued*

Steps	Rationale	Reportable Conditions
14. Evaluate the patient's response to activities that may positively or negatively affect ventilation (e.g., sedation, analgesia, suctioning, repositioning, change in mechanical support, nutritional supplementation, cardiopulmonary resuscitation, neuromuscular blockade, verification of endotracheal tube placement).[9] **(Level B*)** 15. Discard supplies 16. 🅷🅷	The impact of activities (e.g., suctioning, repositioning, change in mechanical support, nutritional supplementation, cardiopulmonary resuscitation, neuromuscular blockade, verification of endotracheal tube placement) on ventilation can be evaluated with $Petco_2$ monitoring.	• $Petco_2$ values increased or decreased by more than 10% of baseline

*Level B: Well-designed, controlled studies with results that consistently support a specific action, intervention, or treatment.

Documentation

Documentation should include the following:
- Patient and family education
- Mechanical ventilator settings
- $Petco_2$ value and capnogram
- $Paco_2$ (partial pressure of arterial carbon dioxide)—$Petco_2$ gradient (special attention should be given to this gradient as an indication of dead space ventilation)
- Arterial blood gases
- Times of calibration
- Respiratory therapies
- Medications that may affect respiratory system (e.g., neuromuscular blockers, sedatives, or bronchodilators)
- Respiratory assessment (e.g., respiratory rate, breathing patterns, adventitious sounds)
- Unexpected outcomes
- Nursing interventions
- Patient teaching

References and Additional Readings

For a complete list of references and additional readings for this procedure, scan this QR code with any freely available smartphone code reader app, or visit http://booksite.elsevier.com/9780323376624.

15 Continuous Lateral Rotation Therapy

Jamie St. Clair and Jennifer MacDermott

PURPOSE: Continuous lateral rotation therapy (CLRT) or kinetic therapy involves the use of dynamic rotation of a support surface delivered via a specialized overlay or bed to continuously rotate the patient laterally from side to side. Early mobilization is crucial in minimizing the deleterious effects of prolonged immobility but is difficult to achieve in critically ill patients. The purpose of CLRT therapy is to assist in reducing ventilator-associated pneumonia incidence by providing a form of early mobility.[2,3,6,9–13,15,16] There is conflicting evidence as to the effects of CLRT on resolution of atelectasis and reduction in mortality, length of mechanical ventilation, length of intensive care unit and hospital stay, and cost.[2,3,6,10,12,13,15,16]

PREREQUISITE NURSING KNOWLEDGE

- Knowledge is needed regarding the physiological effects of immobility on body systems. Potential complications in the critically ill patient include the following[8]:
  - Pulmonary—pneumonia, atelectasis, pulmonary embolism
  - Cardiovascular—deep vein thrombosis
  - Integumentary—pressure ulcers
  - Gastrointestinal—constipation, fecal impaction
  - Metabolic—glucose intolerance
  - Musculoskeletal—muscle atrophy
- Principles of prevention of ventilator-acquired pneumonia should be understood.[1,4,5,14] CLRT is an adjunct treatment and should not be the sole therapy instituted to prevent ventilator-associated pneumonia.[1,8]
- Indications for CLRT include critically ill patients who are at a higher risk of pulmonary complications, such as the following:
  - Patients at risk for ventilator-associated pneumonia
  - Patients with increasing ventilator support requirements refractory to standard treatment interventions
    - Fraction of inspired oxygen (Fio$_2$) >50% for 1 hour or more[7,18]
    - Positive end-expiratory pressure (PEEP) >8[18]
  - Patients who have clinical indications for acute lung injury or adult respiratory distress syndrome[3]:
    - Partial pressure of arterial oxygen (Pao$_2$/Fio$_2$ ratio <300[7,15,18]
    - Presence of fluffy infiltrates via chest radiograph[8,17]
    - Presence of atelectasis via chest radiograph[8,17]
- Knowledge is needed of contraindications for CLRT, such as
  - Unstable spine or pelvic injury until the injury is stabilized[18]

- Long bone fractures and/or traction[18]
- Unstable intracranial pressure (>20 mm Hg)[18]
- It must be understood when CLRT should be used cautiously, including
  - Extreme agitation and/or motion sickness[18]
  - Immediate postoperative period following open-heart surgery[18]
  - Multiple rib fractures[16,18]
  - Bronchospasm[18]
  - Uncontrollable diarrhea[18]
- Due to the lack of evidence for specific therapy parameters,[8] the degree of rotation and time interval should be set by the clinician or per institution policy. The degree of rotation is set individually on each side; it may be intermittent or constant, or provide unilateral or bilateral rotation, depending on patient condition. For example, if a patient does not tolerate turning to his left side, the surface may be programmed for a shorter time interval or lesser degree of rotation on that side.
- Components necessary for maximal patient benefit include initiation of therapy within 48 hours of intubation and continuous rotation for more than 18 hours per day.[17,20]
- Knowledge of potential physiological changes that occur during CLRT is required. Changes in patient's hemodynamics or oxygen saturation during rotation are often the result of the patient's underlying disease process.[17,20] If hemodynamic and/or oxygenation changes occur, the patient's oxygenation, respiratory rate, ventilator settings, arterial blood gas levels, adequacy of volume resuscitation, cardiac performance, vascular tone, and other appropriate parameters should be assessed and the need for additional intervention should be evaluated.[17,20]
- Knowledge of potential complications associated with CLRT is required. Documented complications include disconnection of intravascular catheters, intolerance to rotation, adverse effects on intracranial pressure, and arrhythmias.[8,17]

- Several support surfaces are available for CLRT. Identify the type of continuous lateral rotational therapy used at the individual institution, whether a framed surface or added overlay, following manufacturer's guidelines. Refer to institutional policy for types of support surfaces that may be used.
- Manufacturer-specific guidelines for implementing CLRT should be reviewed before the patient is placed on the support surface/bed frame.
- Daily evaluation of the patient's response to CLRT and assessment of continued need for CLRT are required.[17,20] Criteria for discontinuation may include resolution of indications for therapy.[17,20]

EQUIPMENT

- Nonsterile gloves
- Sheet, slide board, or other transitioning device to assist with moving a patient onto a surface
- Appropriate CLRT surface

PATIENT AND FAMILY EDUCATION

- Explain to the patient and family the adverse effects of pulmonary complications and complications of immobility. *Rationale:* Explanation encourages understanding when a different bed surface is needed based on the risk assessment of the patient. The patient and family are able to ask questions.
- Explain the purpose of CLRT, properties of the support surface, and possible risks involved with treatment. *Rationale:* Understanding and cooperation are increased when patients and families understand purpose of therapy.

PATIENT ASSESSMENT AND PREPARATION

Patient Assessment

- Assessment of the patient's respiratory status, including breath sounds, respiratory rate, cough, oxygen saturation, arterial blood gas, chest radiograph, and mental status.[17] *Rationale:* Initial and ongoing evaluation of effectiveness of CLRT on body systems.
- Assessment of the patient's skin, including evidence of pressure ulcer formation or other alterations.[11,13,17] *Rationale:* Baseline and ongoing skin status data are provided.
- Assessment of the patient's vascular system, including hemodynamic stability, presence of lower extremity edema, and deep vein thrombosis. *Rationale:* Baseline and ongoing vascular status data are provided.
- Discuss goals for pressure redistribution and CLRT with prescribing provider. *Rationale:* The properties of the CLRT support surface are evaluated to match patient factors.

Patient Preparation

- Ensure the patient and family understand pre-procedural teachings. Answer questions as they arise and reinforce information as needed. *Rationale:* Understanding previously taught clinical information and rationale is evaluated and reinforced.
- Evaluate the properties of the support surface to meet pulmonary needs. *Rationale:* Support surface selection should match clinical indication for patient therapy.
- Verify correct patient with two identifiers. *Rationale:* Prior to performing a procedure, the nurse should ensure the correct identification of the patient for the intended intervention.
- Ensure adequate personnel are available to assist when moving the patient to the new surface. Place the patient in the supine position with the head of the bed elevated to 30 degrees (if not medically contraindicated) in preparation for a move to a specialty surface. *Rationale:* Transfer of the patient from one bed to another is potentiated.

Procedure	Continuous Lateral Rotational Therapy		
Steps	Rationale		Special Considerations
1. **HH**			
2. **PE**			
3. Ensure the bed is locked in the horizontal position and that the drive is disengaged and the brake is on.	Ensures patient and staff safety.		Align both surfaces side by side at a height comfortable for staff to move the patient to new surface, assuring both surfaces are locked and will not move on patient transfer.
4. With use of a draw sheet or other transfer device, move the patient to the center of the surface while maintaining body alignment.	Shearing of patient skin and/or patient or staff injury may be avoided.		Do not leave the patient unattended at any time during the patient transfer.

Procedure   Continuous Lateral Rotational Therapy—*Continued*

Steps	Rationale	Special Considerations
5. Transfer the patient to the center of the bed, aligning the patient using guides on surface or per manufacturer's instructions. (**Level M***)	Assures proper positioning of the patient for rotation.	If using a specialty mattress overlay, it is recommended to place the mattress on the bed frame, then transfer the patient to the new surface.
6. Utilize all securement straps and supports to ensure the patient is held safely in place and prevent shearing over potential areas of friction. (**Level M**)	Prevents unexpected outcomes and promotes patient safety.	
7. Assure all invasive tubing and lines are free from obstruction or risk of dislodgement.[17] (**Level D***)	Assessment leads to early intervention if necessary.[13] (**Level D**)	
8. Initiate therapy per prescriber order or institutional policy.[17] (**Level D**)	Begins therapy.	
9. Monitor the patient through an entire rotational cycle to assess for ventilation or hemodynamic changes. Assure invasive tubing and lines remain free from obstruction or risk of dislodgement.[17] (**Level D**)	Ensures that the patient tolerates, and is safe during, rotation.	Consider longer time intervals, or a decreased angle initially, to allow the patient to increase tolerance to motion.[17] (**Level D**)
10. Discard any used supplies and remove PE.		
11. HH		

*Level D: Peer-reviewed professional and organizational standards with the support of clinical study recommendations.
*Level M: Manufacturer's recommendations only.

Expected Outcomes

- Improved pulmonary function
- Absence of development of ventilator-associated pneumonia
- Intact skin integrity
- Wound healing
- Absence of friction and shearing
- Absence of excessive skin moisture or dryness
- Improved peripheral circulation
- Improved urinary elimination

Unexpected Outcomes

- Desaturation with rotation
- Hemodynamic instability with rotation
- Dislodgement of invasive lines
- Development of worsening pulmonary status
- Development of urinary tract infection
- Friction, shearing, motion sickness, agitation, disorientation, and falls from lateral movement of table if the patient is not strapped in properly
- Pressure ulcer formation or further deterioration of existing pressure ulcers

Patient Monitoring and Care

Steps	Rationale	Reportable Conditions
		These conditions should be reported if they persist despite nursing interventions.
1. Cardiopulmonary resuscitation (CPR): Identify CPR valve or deflate surface to bed frame. If foam base, place backboard under the patient. Begin CPR.	A flat, firm surface is needed for effective CPR.	• Need for CPR

Procedure continues on following page

Patient Monitoring and Care —*Continued*

Steps	Rationale	Reportable Conditions
2. Assess the patient's pulmonary function.[17,19] (**Level D***)	Lateral rotational movement provides continuous postural drainage and mobilization of secretions.[19] (**Level D**)	• Adventitious breath sounds • Decreased respiratory rate and depth • Cough • Cyanosis • Dyspnea • Nasal flaring • Decreased oxygen saturation • Abnormal blood gases • Decreased mental acuity • Restlessness • Abnormal chest radiograph results
3. Assess patient skin for evidence of breakdown, by manually repositioning the patient at least every 2 hours. Closely monitor pressure point areas (occiput, sacrum, and heels) or areas that may rub against support surfaces with rotation (axilla, groin/inner thighs, face/ears, and/or feet) per hospital policy. Consider applying protective dressing to areas prone to shearing.[11,13,19] (**Level D**)	The patient continues to be at risk for skin breakdown and pressure ulcer development. Ensure that routine skin assessments continue throughout rotational therapy.	• Development of pressure ulcers or skin breakdown, or worsening of wounds.
4. Assess the patient's vascular circulation.[17] (**Level D**)	Lateral rotation movement discourages venous stasis.	• Edema, decreased or absent pulses, discoloration, and/or pain
5. Assess the patient for urinary retention.	Lateral rotational movement decreases urinary stasis.	• Decreased urine output • Bladder distention
6. Monitor the patient's tolerance and hemodynamic goals.[17] (**Level D**)	Lateral rotational movement may alter hemodynamics because of the degree of rotation and changes in transducer positioning.[17] (**Level D**)	• Intolerance to device • Vital signs consistently below or above desired goals/parameters
7. Follow institutional standard for assessing pain. Administer analgesia as prescribed.	Identifies need for pain interventions.	• Continued pain despite pain interventions
8. Maintain in motion for 18 out of 24 hours.[17] (**Level D**)	Provides proper rotation and adequate mobility.	• Inability to tolerate rotational therapy angle and time frame
9. Determine when therapy should be discontinued. Reassess need every 24 hours.[17] (**Level D**)	Lateral rotation therapy is no longer required.	

*Level D: Peer-reviewed professional and organizational standards with the support of clinical study recommendations.

Documentation

Documentation should include the following:

- Patient and family education
- Date and time therapy instituted
- Rationale for use of lateral rotation therapy surface
- Number of hours the patient is in rotation mode per 24 hours and the degree of rotation achieved
- Complete a full skin assessment per institutional policy and as needed
- Status of wound healing if applicable
- The patient's response to therapy
- Any unexpected outcomes and interventions taken
- Phone number and name of company representative; keep in easily accessible area of chart, in the event the bed malfunctions
- Pain assessment and management according to institutional policy

References and Additional Readings

For a complete list of references and additional readings for this procedure, scan this QR code with any freely available smartphone code reader app, or visit http://booksite.elsevier.com/9780323376624.

16 Continuous Venous Oxygen Saturation Monitoring

Joni L. Dirks

PURPOSE: Venous oxygen saturation monitoring is performed to measure the oxygen saturation of hemoglobin in the venous blood. The value can be obtained either from the pulmonary artery (PA; mixed venous oxygen saturation—Svo_2) or from the superior vena cava (central venous oxygen saturation—$Scvo_2$). Measurement can be performed intermittently with individual blood samples or continuously with a specialized fiberoptic catheter/probe and an associated computer or module. Assessment of venous oxygen saturation provides an indication of the balance between a patient's oxygen delivery and oxygen consumption.

PREREQUISITE NURSING KNOWLEDGE

- Anatomy and physiology of the cardiopulmonary system should be understood.
- Physiological principles related to invasive hemodynamic monitoring should be understood.
- Technical aspects of central venous catheter (CVC) placement and pressure monitoring (see Procedure 67) should be understood.
- Technical aspects of pulmonary artery catheter (PAC) placement (see Procedures 71 and 72) and pressure monitoring (see Procedure 74) should be understood.
- Physiological concepts of oxygen delivery, oxygen demand, and tissue oxygen consumption should be understood.
- Clinically, venous oxygen saturation provides an index of overall oxygen balance because it is a reflection of the dynamic relationship between the patient's oxygen delivery and oxygen consumption. Early detection of oxygen imbalance can facilitate implementation of goal-directed treatment protocols for sepsis, shock, high-risk surgery, and trauma.[1,11,16]
- Whenever the demand for oxygen exceeds supply, the body's primary compensatory mechanisms are to increase oxygen delivery by increasing cardiac output or to increase oxygen extraction at the tissue level.
- In a critically ill patient with limited cardiac output, increased extraction occurs to meet the demand for oxygen at the tissue level. The result is a decreased level of oxygen returning to the heart and a lower Svo_2 measurement. Many factors can affect the requirements for oxygen and subsequently Svo_2 (Box 16-1).[5,10,12,17]
- Svo_2 does not correlate *directly* with any of the determinants of oxygen delivery (i.e., cardiac output, hemoglobin, and arterial oxygen saturation) or oxygen consumption. Because a critically ill patient is in a dynamic state, Svo_2 must be viewed in the light of these changing determinants and considered an index of oxygen balance.[5,10,12,17]
- A normal Svo_2 generally is considered to be 60% to 80%, and a clinically significant change in Svo_2 (5% to 10%) can be an early indicator of physiological instability.[12,16] Svo_2 values of less than 60% may result from either inadequate oxygen delivery or excessive oxygen consumption. It should be noted that in late stages of sepsis a patient may have a normal or high Svo_2 value, which may indicate impaired cellular function or severe arteriovenous shunting.[13] It is always important to consider the clinical picture along with Svo_2 values.
- The percent of venous oxygen saturation as measured in the PA (Svo_2) is flow weighted and represents a true mixing of all venous blood in the body: inferior vena cava (IVC), superior vena cava (SVC), and coronary sinus.
- PACs are being used less frequently in critically ill patients, so the use of CVCs to measure venous saturation has emerged as an alternative.[12,16] The percent of venous oxygen saturation as measured in the SVC ($Scvo_2$) reflects the mixing of venous blood from the superior half of the body. It does not include blood from the IVC and coronary sinus.
- $Scvo_2$ and Svo_2 do not correlate absolutely, but trend together in a variety of hemodynamic states.[16] In normal conditions, $Scvo_2$ is slightly lower than Svo_2. In periods of hemodynamic instability, $Scvo_2$ is higher than Svo_2, with a difference that ranges from 5% to 7% and up to 18% in severe shock.[17] This difference is in part because of a redistribution of blood flow caused by the various pathophysiologies.[5,10,17] Therefore $Scvo_2$ overestimates Svo_2 in shock conditions; a low $Scvo_2$ likely indicates an even lower Svo_2.[13]
- Continuous venous saturation monitoring is performed with a three-component system (Fig. 16-1):[2–4,7,8]
  - ❖ A fiberoptic central venous or PA *catheter* contains two or three optical filaments that exit at the distal

BOX 16-1	Common Conditions and Activities That Affect Venous Oxygen Saturation Values

DECREASED CENTRAL AND MIXED VENOUS OXYGEN SATURATION

Decreased Oxygen Delivery
- Heart failure
- Hypovolemia
- Anemia
- Hemorrhage
- Hypoxemia

Increased Oxygen Consumption
- Fever
- Pain
- Agitation
- Shivering
- Seizures
- Increased work of breathing
- Infection
- Burns
- Head injury
- Numerous nursing procedures (e.g., dressing changes, suctioning, turning, and chest physiotherapy)

INCREASED CENTRAL AND MIXED VENOUS OXYGEN SATURATION

Increased Oxygen Delivery
- Fluid resuscitation
- Inotropic medications
- Blood transfusion
- Oxygen therapy

Decreased Oxygen Consumption
- Hypothermia
- Analgesia
- Sedation
- Pharmacological paralysis
- Anesthesia
- Cellular dysfunction (shunting, sepsis)
- Mechanical ventilation
- Decreased musculoskeletal activity

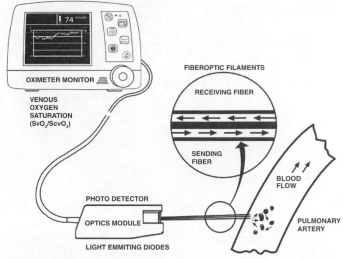

Figure 16-1 Oximetry system with reflectance spectrophotometry. (*From McGee WT, Headley J, Frazier JA, editors:* Quick guide to cardiopulmonary care. *Irvine, CA, 2014, Edwards Lifesciences Corporation.*)

lumen. One filament serves as a sending fiber for the emission of light; the other serves as a receiving fiber for the light reflected back from the blood in the vessel (Fig. 16-2).

❖ The *optic module* houses the light-emitting diodes (LEDs), which transmit various wavelengths of light, and a photodetector, which receives light. The light wavelengths are shone through a blood sample as it travels between the LED and the photodetector. Desaturated hemoglobin, saturated hemoglobin (oxyhemoglobin), and dyshemoglobin (carboxyhemoglobin, methemoglobin) have different light-absorption characteristics. The ratio of hemoglobin to oxyhemoglobin is determined and reported as a percentage value.[2–4,7,8] All patient data, including calibration of saturation values and patient identification information, are stored in this component. This module should not be discon-

nected from the patient's catheter. If the need to disconnect is unavoidable, refer to the manufacturer's instructions for a disconnection procedure that does not result in memory loss.

❖ An oximeter *computer*, either a stand-alone unit or a module for a bedside monitoring system, has a microprocessor that converts the light information from the optic module into an electrical display. This display is updated every few seconds for continuous monitoring. This information may be displayed as a continuous graphic trend, a numeric display, or both, depending on the manufacturer.

- Proper calibration of the monitor and catheter ensures accuracy of venous saturation values. The two types of calibration are in vitro, in which the catheter and optics module are calibrated before insertion; and in vivo, where the venous saturation value from the system is compared with a laboratory cooximeter value from a blood sample drawn from the catheter tip. Follow manufacturer recommendations for performing calibration procedures. Daily in vivo calibrations are recommended by some manufacturers. In addition, proper blood sampling techniques from the distal port of the PAC or CVC catheter are necessary for ensuring accurate values for calibration.[2–4,7,8]

EQUIPMENT

- Fiberoptic PAC for Svo_2 (various sizes, 4 to 8 Fr; various lumens; various lengths, 25 to 110 cm)
- Fiberoptic CVC for $Scvo_2$ (various sizes for pediatric to adult use, 4.5 to 8.5 Fr; various lengths, 5 to 20 cm; single, double, or triple lumen)
- Fiberoptic probe for $Scvo_2$ (2.2 Fr, 37-cm length inserted through a port in an existing CVC)
- Optic module
- Oximeter computer or bedside monitoring system module
- Equipment required for central venous monitoring or PA catheterization and pressure monitoring

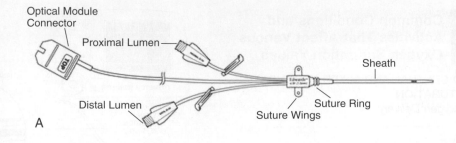

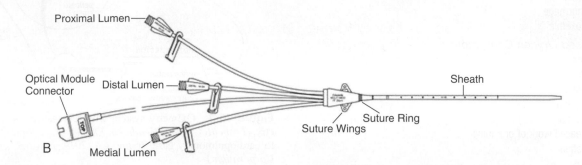

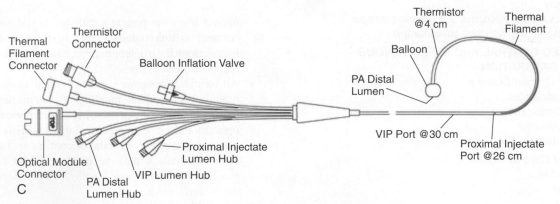

Figure 16-2   Oximetry catheters. **A,** Central venous catheter **B,** Small French size for pediatric applications **C,** Pulmonary artery catheter. *(From McGee WT, Headley J, Frazier JA, editors:* Quick guide to cardiopulmonary care. *Irvine, CA, 2014, Edwards Lifesciences Corporation.)*

Additional equipment, to have available as needed, includes the following:
• Printer (optional)

PATIENT AND FAMILY EDUCATION

• Assess patient and family understanding of the clinical benefits of venous oximetry monitoring. *Rationale:* For information to be the most appropriate, assessment of the level of patient and family understanding of the need for $Scvo_2$ or Svo_2 monitoring is important. By explaining the usefulness of Svo_2 monitoring in language that nonmedical personnel can understand, the patient and family are able to ask appropriate questions, and understand more clearly the clinical presentation of the patient and implications for further treatment therapies.
• Explain the continuous nature of this monitoring system and the significance of the alarms. *Rationale:* Explanation of the procedure to the patient and family helps to allevi-

ate fears and concerns. Additional monitors may produce increased anxiety in the patient and family.

PATIENT ASSESSMENT AND PREPARATION

Patient Assessment

• Indications for use of $Scvo_2$/Svo_2 monitoring include the following:[1,11,15,16,18]
  ❖ High-risk cardiovascular and vascular surgery
  ❖ Heart failure
  ❖ Shock
  ❖ Respiratory failure
  ❖ Severe burns
  ❖ Sepsis (as a component of early goal-directed therapy)
  ❖ Multisystem organ dysfunction
  ❖ Head injury
  ❖ Trauma

* ❖ Acute respiratory distress syndrome
* ❖ Mechanical ventilation (adjustment of settings, weaning)

Patient Preparation

* Verify correct patient with two identifiers. ***Rationale:*** Prior to performing a procedure, the nurse should ensure the correct identification of the patient for the intended intervention.
* Answer patient questions as they arise, and reinforce information as needed. ***Rationale:*** This communication evaluates and reinforces understanding of previously taught information.

Procedure	**for Continuous Mixed Venous Oxygen Saturation Monitoring**	
Steps	**Rationale**	**Special Considerations**
1. **HH**		
2. **PE**		
3. Assemble necessary equipment and supplies for continuous monitoring. (**Level D***)	Ensures equipment is ready and available for the procedure.[9]	
4. Connect power cord to computer, turn on, and observe system check on the computer screen. (**Level M***)	Allows electronics to warm up; confirms component function.[2–4,7,8]	Some monitors allow toggling between Svo_2, $Scvo_2$, or So_2. Ensure the proper label is used.[2–4,7,8]
5. Connect optics module to computer. (**Level M**)	LEDs are housed in optics module. Approximately 5–20 minutes are needed to warm light source sufficiently.[3,4,7,8]	Warm-up times may vary by manufacturer and temperature of location of monitoring.
6. Remove outer wrap of catheter package and aseptically peel back the inner wrap portion that covers the optic connector of the catheter. (**Level M**)	Provides access to inner package; isolates connector from catheter tip to maintain sterility during in vitro calibration.[2–4,7,8]	Catheter packaging may vary according to manufacturer. Follow manufacturer's directions for use to ensure proper handling.
7. Firmly connect the optic connector to the optic module. (**Level M**)	Ensures connections are tight and properly aligned for light transmission.[2–4,7,8]	
8. Perform in vitro calibration or standardization. (**Level M**)	Standardizes or calibrates the light source to the catheter. Calibration is performed before catheter insertion. Catheter tip should be left in the calibration cup or container in the package during in vitro calibration.[2–4,7,8]	Catheter lumens must be dry. Do not flush catheter before performing this step or in vitro calibration is invalid.
9. Pull back remaining wrap covering catheter package with aseptic technique. (**Level M**)	Prepares catheter for insertion.[2–4,7,8]	
10. Carefully remove catheter from tray with sterile technique. Pull catheter tip up and out of the calibration cup. (**Level M**)	Prevents the transmission of microorganisms; prevents damage to the balloon of the PA catheter.[2–4,7,8]	Fiberoptics in the catheter and PA catheter balloon are fragile and may be damaged if not handled properly.
11. Attach pressure tubing, and prime lumens with flush solution (see Procedure 75).	Enables monitoring of chamber pressures during PAC insertion; maintains patency of lumens.	Refer to institutional standards for use of heparinized flush solution.[12]
12. Perform a preprocedure verification and time out if nonemergent.	Ensures patient safety.	

*Level D: Peer-reviewed professional and organizational standards with the support of clinical study recommendations.
*Level M: Manufacturer's recommendations only.

Procedure continues on following page

Procedure	for Continuous Mixed Venous Oxygen Saturation Monitoring—*Continued*

Steps	Rationale	Special Considerations
13. Assist physician or advanced practice nurse with CVC or PAC site preparation and catheter insertion.	Provides assistance to physician or advanced practice nurse while catheter is inserted.	In some cases, a separate fiberoptic probe for Scvo$_2$ monitoring may be inserted through an existing CVC.
14. Observe PA waveforms during insertion.	Central PAC tip placement is necessary for optimal light reflection.[2–4,7–9]	A light intensity or signal indicator verifies adequate reflection of the light signals after the catheter tip is placed correctly.[2–4,7,8]
15. Note amount of air required for inflation of PAC balloon to obtain a wedge tracing. **(Level M*)**	Inflation volume of 1.25–1.5 mL is recommended for proper catheter tip placement.[4,8]	Ensure passive deflation of balloon before proceeding. Less than optimal inflation volume to obtain a wedge tracing may indicate distal catheter migration. A change in the intensity or signal indicator also may alert the clinician to this condition.
16. Set high and low alarm limits and activate alarms. **(Level D*)**	Individualizes alarm settings according to patient baseline. Audible alarms notify the clinician of significant changes in Scvo$_2$/Svo$_2$ values and trends.[9]	
17. Apply a sterile dressing to insertion site. **(Level D)**	Reduces transmission of microorganisms.[14]	Use institutional standard for central venous catheter dressings.
18. Firmly secure the optic module near the patient. **(Level M)**	Excessive tension on catheter or optic module may break the optic fibers.[2–4,7,8]	
19. Input patient height and weight data as per institutional standard.	Allows for calculation of derived hemodynamic parameters.[4,8,9]	This may be done before placement.
20. After calibration and insertion of catheter, obtain baseline set of hemodynamic and oxygenation indices.	Provides baseline information for comparison with patient's response to interventions.	
21. Continuously monitor PA pressure tracings and Svo$_2$/Scvo$_2$ values. **(Level D)**	Spontaneous catheter migration may occur after insertion.	Tip position may influence signal quality if the catheter is positioned against a vessel wall. Signal quality may be compromised by clotting at the tip of the catheter, pulsatility, or hemodilution.[4] If the catheter becomes wedged the readings may reflect postcapillary arterialized blood and the Svo$_2$ value may increase.[9,12]
22. Obtain catheter-placement confirmation per institution standard (i.e., chest radiograph).	Provides confirmation of proper catheter.	

Venous Blood Sampling Skill/In Vivo Calibration

23. **HH** (if independent from catheter placement).		
24. **PE** (if independent from catheter placement).		

*Level D: Peer-reviewed professional and organizational standards with the support of clinical study recommendations.
*Level M: Manufacturer's recommendations only.

Procedure	for Continuous Mixed Venous Oxygen Saturation Monitoring—*Continued*	
Steps	**Rationale**	**Special Considerations**
25. Draw venous blood sample from distal port of catheter for in vivo calibration (see Procedure 63 for mixed venous blood sampling or Procedure 62 for CVC blood sampling).	In vivo calibration may be necessary to verify the accuracy of the computer and value displayed after insertion of the fiberoptic catheter. Ideally, the patient's hemodynamic and oxygenation status should be stable for optimal calibration.[2-4,7,8]	Mixed venous samples should be drawn from the distal port of the PAC.[9] Central venous samples should be drawn from the distal port of the CVC.[6]
26. Perform a verification or in vivo calibration per manufacturer's instructions or institutional standard. **(Level D*)**	In vivo calibration verifies the accuracy of the $Scvo_2$/Svo_2 being displayed.[2-4,7-9] In vivo calibration is required if the catheter was inserted *without* performing preinsertion calibration or if the catheter is disconnected from the optical module. In vivo calibration may also be performed on a routine basis (typically every 24 hours) or whenever the displayed value is in question.	Follow specific recommendations from the manufacturer about the frequency of calibration and specific steps to implement the process.
27. Ensure measurement is performed with a laboratory cooximeter. **(Level D)**	Cooximetry measures direct fractional oxyhemoglobin saturation; blood gas analyzers calculate oxygen saturation from measured partial pressure values. A calculated saturation value from a gas analyzer may not correlate with the actual patient value and, if used for calibration, may produce erroneous results. [2-4,7-9]	
28. Observe bedside monitor display for return of PA/central venous pressure waveform and resume Svo_2/$Scvo_2$ monitoring. **(Level D)**	Reconfirms catheter tip placement in the PA/SVC/right atrium[9,12]	Proper positioning of the catheter is important for accurate measurement of venous oxygen saturation and to prevent possible complications.[12]
29. Dispose of used supplies and equipment.		
30. Remove personal protective equipment. **PE**	Reduces the transmission of microorganisms and body secretions; Standard Precautions.	
31. **HH**		

*Level D: Peer-reviewed professional and organizational standards with the support of clinical study recommendations.

Expected Outcomes

- Svo_2 values and trends within normal range (60%–80%)[9,12,16]
- $Scvo_2$ values and trends greater than 70%[1,17]
- $Scvo_2$/Svo_2 trends not fluctuating greater than 5%–10% of baseline value[12,16]
- Hemodynamic and oxygenation parameters optimal for patient condition

Unexpected Outcomes

- Svo_2 values less than 60% or greater than 80%
- Svo_2 value trends greater than 10% from baseline
- $Scvo_2$ value trends less than 65%–70%[1,17]
- Infection from presence of an indwelling PAC or CVC
- PA occlusion, infarction, or rupture

Procedure continues on following page

Patient Monitoring and Care

Steps	Rationale	Reportable Conditions
		These conditions should be reported if they persist despite nursing interventions.
1. Ensure that no kinks or bends are found in the catheter. **(Level D*)**	Fiberoptics are fragile and can break if not handled carefully. Overtightening of the introducer connector can cause crimping and breakage of the fiberoptics.[4,8] Subclavian or internal jugular approaches for insertion may cause kinking in the vessel if the vessel is tortuous. Sending and receiving wavelengths may show either a change in light signal or values that do not reflect the patient's status.	• Change in PA waveform or Svo_2 value that does not correlate to patient condition • Changes in RA waveforms or $Scvo_2$ value that do not correlate to patient condition
2. Monitor PA waveforms continuously. **(Level D)**	Migration of the catheter tip may reflect postcapillary arterialized blood causing an elevation in the Svo_2 value. Uncorrected catheter migration places the patient at risk for PA infarction or rupture.[9,12]	• Permanent wedge waveform
3. Observe Svo_2 value and trends. **(Level B*)**	Normal Svo_2 values range from 60% to 80%[12,16]; values outside this range may indicate an imbalance between oxygen delivery and consumption. A value change of greater than 5%–10% may signify a clinically significant change.[9,12] A target value of greater than 65% in severe sepsis and septic shock is recommended.[1] If the patient's clinical presentation differs from the observed Svo_2 value or trends, recheck the accuracy of the monitoring system.	• Svo_2 values greater than 80% or less than 60%
4. Observe $Scvo_2$ value and trends. **(Level B)**	$Scvo_2$ values trend with Svo_2. A target value of greater than 70% in severe sepsis and septic shock is recommended.[1]	• $Scvo_2$ values less than 70%

*Level B: Well-designed, controlled studies with results that consistently support a specific action, intervention, or treatment.
*Level D: Peer-reviewed professional and organizational standards with the support of clinical study recommendations.

Documentation

Documentation should include the following:
• Patient and family education
• $Scvo_2$/Svo_2 whenever the hemodynamic profile is recorded
• Additional oxygenation indices as indicated
• Specific nursing activities (e.g., suctioning, turning the patient, or titrating a vasoactive drug) and the

relationship of the event with the continuous trend, especially if the event produces a marked change in the value
• Hard copy printout (as available)
• Unexpected outcomes
• Nursing interventions

References and Additional Readings

For a complete list of references and additional readings for this procedure, scan this QR code with any freely available smartphone code reader app, or visit http://booksite.elsevier.com/9780323376624.

17 Extracorporeal Life Support (ECLS) and Extracorporeal Membrane Oxygenation (ECMO)

Thomas Lawson and Marcia Belcher

PURPOSE: There are multiple indications for extracorporeal life support (ECLS) and extracorporeal membrane oxygenation (ECMO) in adults with acute severe heart and/or lung failure with high mortality risk despite optimal conventional therapy.

PREREQUISITE NURSING KNOWLEDGE

- Advanced cardiac life support knowledge and skills are needed.
- A thorough knowledge of central venous and arterial anatomy, cardiac anatomy and physiology, arterial and venous blood gas interpretation, and ventilator management is important.
- Clinical and technical competence with use of the ECLS/ECMO equipment is essential.
- An understanding of the possible causes of cardiac and/or respiratory failure is needed.
- ECLS/ECMO physiology differs significantly based on cannula location, even though the circuit configuration that delivers oxygenated blood under pressure remains the same. Venous to venous (VV) provides gas exchange and is used exclusively for respiratory failure whereas venous to arterial (VA) also provides mechanical circulatory support by introducing the oxygenated blood under pressure into the arterial system (Fig. 17-1).
- Deoxygenated blood is mechanically pumped out of the vena cava(s) via a drainage cannula placed in the femoral, internal jugular, or subclavian vein into an exchanger where blood is oxygenated and carbon dioxide is removed. The oxygenated blood is then pumped back via the return cannula into either the right atrium (VV) or the aorta (VA). A single dual-lumen bicaval cannula for VV cannulation is also available. An alternative to peripheral cannulation is cannulation of the central vessels via sternotomy during cardiothoracic surgery. Cannula placement includes right atrium to pulmonary artery (VV) or right atrium to aorta (VA).
- Indications:
  - ❖ Respiratory failure, including acute hypoxic respiratory failure of any etiology when the risk of mortality is greater than 50% (Pao_2/Fio_2 <150 on Fio_2 >90%) or when the risk of mortality is greater than 80% (Pao_2/Fio_2 <100 on Fio_2 >90% despite optimal care for >6

hours), hypercarbic respiratory failure refractory to traditional mechanical ventilator support, severe air leak syndromes (such as from a bronchopleural fistula after a pulmonary resection), bridge to lung transplantation, or immediate respiratory collapse (pulmonary emboli, blocked airway)[3]
  - ❖ Cardiogenic shock as a bridge to ventricular assist device or recovery due to inadequate tissue perfusion from low cardiac output despite adequate volume resuscitation, refractory to inotropes, vasopressors, and intraaortic balloon pump counterpulsation. This typically occurs secondary to acute myocardial infarction, myocarditis, peripartum cardiomyopathy, decompensated chronic heart failure, or post cardiotomy shock.[3]
  - ❖ Extracorporeal cardiopulmonary resuscitation; witnessed arrest with refractory pulselessness despite advanced cardiac life support and continuous CPR with an easily reversible etiology[3]
- Absolute Contraindications[3]:
  - ❖ Irreversible central nervous system damage
  - ❖ Multiple organ dysfunction syndrome
  - ❖ Unrecoverable native heart in a patient who is not a candidate for ventricular assist device (VAD), total artificial heart or cardiac transplant
  - ❖ Chronic organ dysfunction (i.e., liver failure, renal failure requiring dialysis)
  - ❖ Prolonged CPR greater than 30 minutes without adequate tissue perfusion
  - ❖ Terminal malignancy
  - ❖ Mechanical ventilation greater than 10 days or with high airway pressures and/or high levels of Fio_2 greater than 7 days[1,3]
- Relative Contraindications[3]:
  - ❖ Contraindication to anticoagulation
  - ❖ Advanced age; there is no specific maximum age, but risk increases with age
  - ❖ Obesity; there is no specific maximum weight or body mass index
  - ❖ Pharmacological immunosuppression

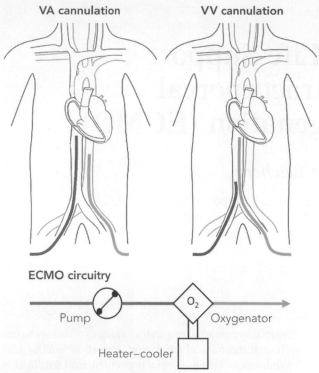

Figure 17-1   Venous to arterial (VA) and venous to venous (VV) cannulation. *(From Lindstrom SJ, Pellegrino, VA, Butt WW: Extracorporeal membrane oxygenation*, Med J Austral *191[3]:178-182, 2009.)*

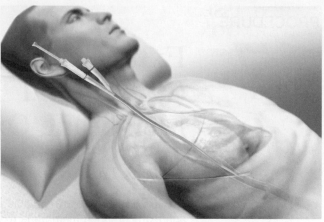

Figure 17-2   Dual lumen cannula. *(From Maquet Getinge Group. Photo of Avalon Elite Bi-Caval Dual Lumen Catheter. Accessed at http://www.maquet.com/int/products/avalon-elite/.)*

- ❖ Recent or expanding central nervous system hemorrhage
- VV cannulation reduces the risk of arterial thrombus and limb ischemia, but the patient must have adequate circulatory function (may be supported with vasoactive medications and inotropes).[1,3]
- In a VV configuration, mixed venous oxygenation saturation measurements are elevated, reflecting that the venous return blood is fully saturated from the exterior oxygenator.[1,3]
- Cannula placement should be assessed upon initial placement with echocardiography, radiographs, or fluoroscopy, and serially by measuring and documenting the length from the skin puncture to the end of the cannula.
- Changes in clinical condition including but not limited to decrease in oxygenation, decrease in pump flow, presence of tube chatter, decreased mentation, or hypotension warrant reevaluating cannula position.

EQUIPMENT

- Nonsterile gloves, masks, and caps
- Sterile gloves, gowns, and drapes
- Central venous catheter insertion supplies (see Procedure 82)
- Arterial catheter insertion supplies (see Procedure 58)
- Normal saline intravenous solutions
- Tape

- Sutures
- Horizontal tube attachment devices
- Cannulas
  - ❖ VV: either large dual lumen cannula (Fig. 17-2) or two large venous cannulas
  - ❖ VA: large venous drainage and arterial return cannulas. Also may need a small catheter for antegrade distal femoral artery perfusion to prevent lower extremity ischemia. The distal perfusion cannula returns a small portion of the oxygenated arterial return blood to the lower extremity, beyond the large arterial cannula.
- Equipment needed:
  - ❖ Pump
  - ❖ Oxygenator
  - ❖ Heat exchanger
  - ❖ Pump controller

Additional equipment, to have available as needed, includes the following:

- Emergency cart (defibrillator, respiratory equipment, cardiac medications)
- Ultrasound equipment
- Fluoroscopy equipment
- Echocardiogram equipment

PATIENT AND FAMILY EDUCATION

- Explain the procedure and the reason for ECLS/ECMO therapy. *Rationale:* Explanation may decrease patient and family anxiety.
- Explain the environment and plan of care to the patient and family on an ongoing basis, including but not limited to the frequency of assessment, sounds and function of equipment, placement of the cannulas, explanation of alarms, dressings, and additional therapies. *Rationale:* This communication provides information to the patient and family, normalizing foreign devices such as an ECLS/ECMO circuit and may alleviate some of the apprehension a patient and family may experience.

PATIENT ASSESSMENT AND PREPARATION

Patient Assessment

- Assess the patient's medical history, including cardiac, pulmonary, renal, and other chronic and acute illnesses. ***Rationale:*** Provides important baseline data.
- If the patient required cardiopulmonary resuscitation, note the length of time CPR was performed and the reported adequacy of compressions. ***Rationale:*** Provides important data that may aid in determining the indication or contraindication to ECLS/ECMO therapy.
- Perform a hemodynamic, cardiovascular, peripheral vascular, pulmonary, and neurological assessment. ***Rationale:*** Provides baseline data that may aid in the determination of which configuration (VV vs. VA) to use.
- Assess the current laboratory profile specifically including complete blood count (CBC), chemistry panel, partial thromboplastin time (PTT), international normalization ratio (INR), liver function panel, arterial blood gas, and central or mixed venous oxygen saturation if access is available. ***Rationale:*** Provides baseline data.
- Assess for active bleeding. ***Rationale:*** The inner surface of the cannulas, the tubing, and the oxygenator are thrombogenic, and the patient will require anticoagulation to prevent thrombus formation. Severe bleeding is a contraindication to anticoagulation and thus is problematic for patients requiring ECLS/ECMO.

Patient Preparation

- Verify that the patient is the correct patient using two identifiers. ***Rationale:*** Before performing a procedure, the physician, advanced practice nurse, or other healthcare professional should ensure the correct identification of the patient for the intended intervention.
- Ensure that the patient and/or family understands preprocedural information. Answer questions as they arise, and reinforce information as needed. ***Rationale:*** Understanding of previously taught information is evaluated and reinforced.
- Obtain informed consent. ***Rationale:*** Informed consent protects the rights of a patient and makes a competent decision possible for the patient.
- Perform a preprocedure verification and time out. ***Rationale:*** Ensures patient safety.
- Administer prescribed sedation or analgesics as needed. ***Rationale:*** Sedation and analgesics minimize anxiety and discomfort.
- Ensure that an echocardiogram has been performed as prescribed. ***Rationale:*** This study documents the nature and severity of heart failure.

Procedure	**for Extracorporeal Life Support and Extracorporeal Membrane Oxygenation**	
Steps	**Rationale**	**Special Considerations**

Assisting With Initial Cannulation (if not already cannulated)

1. Gather equipment; type of equipment will depend on the type of cannulas to be placed (Fig. 17-3).	VV vs. VA configurations require different types of cannulas.	Intraoperatively placed central cannulas may require a subclavian graft.
2. Prime the ECLS/ECMO circuit with sterile saline.	The circuit should be free of air to prevent air embolism.	
3. **HH**		
4. **PE**		

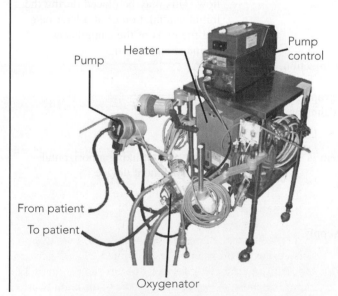

Pump · Heater · Pump control · From patient · To patient · Oxygenator

Figure 17-3 Complete extracorporeal membrane oxygenation (ECMO) circuit. *(From Lindstrom SJ, Pellegrino, VA, Butt WW: Extracorporeal membrane oxygenation, Med J Austral 191[3]:178-182, 2009.)*

Procedure continues on following page

Procedure	for Extracorporeal Life Support and Extracorporeal Membrane Oxygenation—*Continued*	

Steps	Rationale	Special Considerations
5. Assist as needed with preparing the skin with an antiseptic solution (e.g., 2% chlorhexidine-based preparation).	Limits the introduction of potentially infectious skin flora into the vessel during the puncture.	
6. Discard used supplies, perform hand hygiene, and apply sterile gown and gloves.	Reduces the transmission of microorganisms and prepares for the procedure.	Cap and mask are required for everyone in the room once a sterile field is established as in an operating room. Sterile gown and gloves are required for those performing or directly assisting with the cannulation.
7. Assist as needed with placing sterile drapes.	Prepares sterile field.	
8. If ultrasound is to be used, assist as needed with the equipment and ensure the probe is covered with a sterile sheath.	Maintenance of sterile technique is essential to prevent bacteremia and device colonization.	Ultrasound will not provide useable images without adequate conduction gel. Sterile ultrasound gel must be inside and outside the sheath.
9. Assist with cannulation when the physician needs help.	Provides needed assistance.	Ensure that sterility is maintained throughout the procedure.
10. Anticipate the need for large volumes of normal saline solutions when the cannulas are placed.	Normal saline solutions are used to flush air from the cannulas once placed.	
11. When the cannulas are connected to the ECLS/ECMO circuit in: A. VA configuration: Assess for dark venous blood draining from the patient's venous cannula and return of bright red oxygenated blood to the arterial cannula. B. VV configuration: Assess that the oxygenated blood returning to the patient is flowing into the cannula nearest the right atrium.		Note the following terminology: Drainage cannula (deoxygenated blood to the ECMO circuit) Return cannula (oxygenated blood returning to the patient). In a VA configuration, there will be retrograde blood flow to part of the native arterial system. Some VA configurations may require a second, smaller return line to provide distal antegrade perfusion because the large arterial cannula often blocks flow. This may be placed during the initial cannulation or at a later date. Label the ends of the cannulas as drainage and return.
12. Assist as needed with applying sterile dressings.	Decreases the risk of infection.	
13. Assist the insertion team as radiographs, fluoroscopy or bedside echocardiography are obtained.	Aids in determining proper positioning of the cannulas.	
14. Measure the distance from the exterior end of each of the cannulas to the skin, document, and secure tightly with both tape and sutures.	Ensures that the system is secure; maintains safety.	Consider also utilizing a horizontal tube attachment device.
15. Plug the pump controller into electrical outlet.	Provides the power supply.	
16. Remove **PE** and sterile equipment and discard used supplies.		
17. **HH**		

Procedure	for Extracorporeal Life Support and Extracorporeal Membrane Oxygenation—*Continued*	
Steps	**Rationale**	**Special Considerations**

Troubleshooting

1. **HH**
2. **PE**
3. Assess for chatter/chugging of the ECLS/ECMO circuit tubing.
   A. Assess patient's volume status.
      i. Decreasing the flow rate (if hemodynamically appropriate) can temporarily reduce chatter, but the flow setting should be returned to previous settings when possible.
      ii. Flow should be noted before and after decreasing support.
   B. Reassess cannula position by comparing with the baseline cannula position measurement. Radiographic confirmation may also be necessary.

Rationale: Relative or absolute volume depletion will require administration of fluids or blood. Chatter can lead to hemolysis.[3]
A malpositioned cannula may be creating turbulent staccato flow leading to chatter.

Special Considerations: Decreasing the flow rate is a temporary solution; correcting the underlying fluid deficiency needs to be addressed.
When the drainage cannula sucks up against the venous wall turbulent staccato flow through the circuit may cause the tubes to shake.

4. Assess for clots or fibrin deposits within the circuit tubing and oxygenator (clots typically have a dark maroon appearance and fibrin deposits are white) and notify the physician if they are found.

Rationale: Deposits on the oxygenator can decrease its efficiency and lead to decreased gas exchange. Deposits distal to the oxygenator in the return cannula may embolize causing pulmonary embolus, stroke, or organ damage from ischemia. Large deposits may cause hemodynamically significant alterations in flow rate, turbulent flow and hemolysis.

Special Considerations: Turbulent swirling of the blood near clots or fibrin deposits may be seen through the tubing.
Clots may require exchange of the affected part of the circuit. Notify perfusion or ECLS/ECMO specialist if clot is noted.[3]
Ensure anticoagulation is therapeutic (patient-specific PTT goal).
Therapeutic anticoagulation reduces the risk of developing these deposits. Typically heparin but alternatively a direct thrombin inhibitor such as argatroban or bivalirudin may be used if heparin-induced thrombocytopenia is suspected.

5. Assess for high pressure alarms (>300–400 mm Hg) if these alarms are available on the pump controller. If present:
   A. Check the circuit distal to the pump for kinks or occlusions.
   B. Check the patient's blood pressure.
   C. Notify the physician if unable to resolve high pressure alarms.

Rationale: The high pressure alarm indicates increased pressures on the (arterial) return side of the oxygenator.
Small air bubbles caught in the oxygen exchanger may impede blood flow resulting in a high pressure alarm.
In a VA configuration, this alarm may result from an elevated blood pressure.

Procedure continues on following page

Procedure	**for Extracorporeal Life Support and Extracorporeal Membrane Oxygenation**—*Continued*	
Steps	**Rationale**	**Special Considerations**

6. Power outage
  A. Ensure pump switches to battery power.
  B. Switch off the water bath/heater.
  C. If the battery loses power, hand crank the pump:
    i. Remove the pump from its electronic power source.
    ii. Attach the manufacturer-supplied hand crank to the back of the pump and turn.
  D. Notify the physician.
	ECMO machines typically have a short battery life.
	Switching off less essential components such as the heater can conserve power (if both the controller and heater are receiving power from the same source).
	Hand cranking the pump can prevent a low-flow thrombosis and continue to provide some support until power is restored.
		Some pumps may not have a hand cranking backup feature.
		Summon assistance as this will be fatiguing if done for an extended period of time.
		Be aware of the expected battery duration at your institution and take this into consideration when planning to move the patient (e.g., for CT scanning)

7. Assess for hyperthermia. If the patient's temperature is higher than the target:
  A. Use the ice bath.
  B. Use the heater and adjust the temperature knob to the desired temperature.
	Permissive hyperthermia may be indicated in some circumstances, but if allowing a fever is not warranted, it can easily be corrected.	Fevers can be controlled by utilizing an ice bath within the circuit to cool the blood as it passes through.
		If the patient's condition warrants, workup for infection should be completed and empiric antibiotics initiated.

8. Assess for hypothermia.	Due to the large volume of blood circulating outside the body, patients are susceptible to heat loss.	The ECLS/ECMO circuit will have a temperature exchanger with heater and ice bath and desired temperature may be adjusted with a dial and the utilization of an ice bath. The ECLS/ECMO circuit may be utilized to maintain normothermia in hypothermic patients. The ECLS/ECMO circuit may be utilized to induce and maintain hypothermia/targeted temperature management (i.e., post cardiac arrest).

9. Assess for inadequate oxygenation.
  A. If the outlet saturation (determined by drawing a blood gas from the return cannula of the circuit, postoxygenator) is <95%, with a venous saturation (before the oxygenator) of ≥70–75% and the patient's Hgb is ≥12, the oxygenator may need to be exchanged.
  B. Check for water in the gas phase.
  C. Assess hematocrit. It should be >40% for VV ECMO and >30% for VA ECMO.
	Due to the altered cardiopulmonary physiology in ECLS/ECMO patients, oxygenation can provide clues to device malfunction or the need to titrate oxygen delivery. Suggests failure of the oxygenator itself, as opposed to a problem with the patient.
	
	Optimizing the hematocrit improves oxygen-carrying capacity of the blood.
		Increasing oxygen flow to the oxygenator is a quick fix for hypoxia, but further evaluation is typically warranted.
		Address patient conditions contributing to increased oxygen consumption.
		Exchange of components in the ECLS/ECMO circuit is typically performed by a perfusionist or ECLS/ECMO specialist.
		
		Hematocrit targets may vary by center; follow institutional standards.

10. Assess for hypercarbia (P_{CO_2} >70).	Normalized P_{CO_2} contributes to acid-base balance and cerebral perfusion. Elevated P_{CO_2} typically requires adjustment to ECLS settings.	Increasing the airflow through the "sweep" part of the oxygenator removes more CO_2 from the blood. If the initial systemic P_{CO_2} is >70 it may take several hours to normalize, so avoid making adjustments too rapidly.[3]

Procedure	for Extracorporeal Life Support and Extracorporeal Membrane Oxygenation—*Continued*	
Steps	**Rationale**	**Special Considerations**
11. Assess for any air bubbles in circuit. A. If air is found in the circuit, immediately clamp the lines. B. Support the patient by increasing ventilator support and vasoactive support as prescribed. C. Check the circuit proximal to the pump for an open stopcock, leaky connection, tubing compromise, dislodged cannula, or decannulation. Correct the problem identified and notify the physician. D. Check the IV lines for air in line and remove the air if found.	If air is allowed to enter the pulmonary artery or aorta, it may obstruct blood flow causing organ ischemia.	Exercise caution with all venous lines and catheters and central line sites to avoid accidental entrainment of air into the circuit.
12. Assess extremities: A. Check pulses, skin temperature, sensation, movement, and capillary refill. B. Evaluate for compartment syndrome of the extremity (pain, particularly with passive muscle stretch of the affected compartment, tautness of a muscular compartment). Consider consulting the appropriate service to obtain quantitative compartment pressures.	A common complication in the leg ipsilateral to the femoral arterial cannulation is ischemic injury. Ischemia from embolus or mechanical occlusion of the artery at the cannulation site may cause compartment syndrome of the extremity distal to arterial cannulation.	The presence of distal pulses does not rule out compartment syndrome. Consider obtaining an arterial blood gas (ABG) from the right upper extremity and oxygen saturation in either the right upper extremity or the right ear lobe and compare with the left lower extremity or the lower extremities. Regional oxygenation saturation sensors may be helpful in detecting unilateral decreases in oxygenation.
C. Consider placement of a distal perfusion catheter off the return side of the circuit.	A distal perfusion catheter is a second, smaller, return cannula usually placed in the femoral artery distal to the location of the primary return cannula enters the artery.	
D. Evaluate for harlequin syndrome (flow competition in the aorta due to left ventricular recovery with upper body hypoxia).[4]	Harlequin syndrome can occur due to flow competition in the aorta between the native left ventricle output and the ECLS/ECMO return cannula output, leading to poorly oxygenated blood from the left ventricle entering the brachiocephalic and coronary arteries and well-oxygenated blood from the ECLS/ECMO circuit only going to the more distal arteries.	The presence of harlequin syndrome can signal circulatory recovery. Change to VV if lung failure persists as prescribed.

Procedure continues on following page

Procedure	**for Extracorporeal Life Support and Extracorporeal Membrane Oxygenation—*Continued***	
Steps	**Rationale**	**Special Considerations**

13. Assess for hemolysis.
   A. Check plasma-free hemoglobin and lactate dehydrogenase (LD).
   B. Assess urine color.
   C. Check the inlet suction.
   D. Check for clots in the pump chamber.
   E. Notify physician.
14. Remove **PE** and discard used supplies.
15. **HH**
	Hemolysis may be a sign of device malfunction requiring flow adjustment or cannula position adjustment.	Plasma free hemoglobin >10 indicates hemolysis.
		Pink-tinged urine may be due to hemolysis.
		Inlet suction >300 mm Hg can cause hemolysis.
		Turbulent blood flow, from rapidly flowing through a small opening, can cause hemolysis.

Expected Outcomes

- Rapid increase in oxygenation and gas exchange
- Circulatory stabilization but with lower pulse pressure, of ≥15 mm Hg

Unexpected Outcomes

- Related to initial cannulation: Perforation/rupture/tear/dissection of femoral vein/vena cava/femoral artery, aorta. Retroperitoneal hemorrhage. Cannula malposition. Inability to cannulate.
- Secondary: Distal limb ischemia (VA only), coagulopathy, hemorrhage (anticoagulation), organ failure, anoxic brain injury, hemolysis, thromboembolism (VA), increased left ventricular wall tension (VA), maldistribution of oxygenated blood (VA), cannula dislodgement, bleeding, sepsis, air embolism, disseminated intravascular coagulation, skin breakdown, renal failure, heparin-induced thrombocytopenia (HIT)[5]
- Equipment failure
- Hemolysis (membrane failure, turbulence in cannula or pump from hypovolemia)

Patient Monitoring and Care

Steps	Rationale	Reportable Conditions
		These conditions should be reported if they persist despite nursing interventions.
1. Assess level of consciousness.	Monitors for cerebral perfusion. Thrombi may develop and dislodge during ECLS/ECMO therapy. Sudden neurological changes may be an indication of intracerebral hemorrhage.	• Change in level of consciousness • Increased agitation or confusion • Change in saturation levels (per device instructions for use) if utilizing cerebral oxygenation monitors
2. Assess sensory and motor function using a scale (e.g., Glasgow Coma Scale).	Monitors sensory and motor function.	• Change in assessment findings
3. Perform pupil checks every 2–4 hours (more often if administering neuromuscular blockade).[1,3,6]	Assess for adequacy of cerebral perfusion.	• Change in pupil size and reactivity

Patient Monitoring and Care —*Continued*

Steps	Rationale	Reportable Conditions
4. Elevate head of bed.[1,3,6] Prevent pressure on the groin if using femoral cannulation. In order to elevate the head of bed in this paitent population use the reverse Trendelenburg position.	Elevation and maintaining patient's head in midline position encourages venous return.	• Change in venous return as evidence by change in flow rates
5. Provide periods of stimulation and quiet time, provide means of distraction, provide a comforting, restful environment.[1]	Clustering of care, intermittent periods of darkness and promoting prolonged periods of rest can promote neurological recovery.	• Lack of response to therapy
6. Follow institutional standard for assessing pain.[7,9] Administer analgesia as needed.	Identifies need for pain interventions	• Continued pain despite pain interventions
7. Assess agitation and sedation and administer anxiolytics as prescribed.	Identifies need for medications and support	• Continued anxiety despite anxiety interventions
8. Assess vital signs and pulmonary artery pressures every 15–30 minutes to every hour as patient's status dictates. Follow institutional standards.	Demonstrates the effectiveness of ECLS/ECMO therapy.	• Unstable vital signs • Abnormal pulmonary artery pressures
9. Assess circulation to the extremities at least every 2 hours.[1,3,6] Follow institutional standard.	Demonstrates adequate peripheral perfusion. Changes may indicate thrombotic or embolic obstruction of perfusion to extremity	• Capillary refill >3 seconds • Diminished or absent pulses (pulses may be absent on VA support at high flow rates) • Pale color, mottled or cyanotic • Diminished or absent sensation • Pain • Diminished or absent movement • Cold or cool to touch
10. Assess presence or absence of edema (position patient to promote optimal perfusion of extremities and minimize dependent edema).[1,3,6]	Edema of extremities may indicate poor perfusion and may promote lack of skin integrity.	• Change in skin integrity • Presence of edema
11. Measure urine output hourly.	Demonstrates adequate perfusion to the kidneys.	• Urine output <0.5 mL/kg/hr
12. Assess respiratory status by auscultating breath sounds, evaluating respiratory rate and effort, arterial blood gases and peak inspiratory pressure if ventilated.	Demonstrates adequacy of respiratory/ventilator support (gas exchange is controlled primarily by the membrane oxygenator).	• Abnormal ABG results • Abnormal pulse oximetry values • Abnormal breath sounds and pulmonary assessment
13. Monitor platelet count, hematocrit, activated clotting time (ACT), CBC count, prothrombin time (PT), PTT, and INR as prescribed.	Care should be taken to prevent over anticoagulation. Anticoagulation increases risk of intracranial hemorrhage and excessive bleeding.	• Abnormal laboratory values
14. Monitor for systemic evidence of bleeding or coagulation disorders.[1,3,6]	Hematologic and coagulation profiles may be altered as a result of blood loss during ECLS/ECMO insertion, anticoagulation therapy, platelet dysfunction, and hemolysis.	• Bleeding from ECLS/ECMO insertion site • Bleeding from incisions or mucous membranes • Petechiae/ecchymosis • Guaiac-positive nasogastric aspirate or stool • Hematuria • Decreased hemoglobin/hematocrit

Procedure continues on following page

Patient Monitoring and Care —*Continued*

Steps	Rationale	Reportable Conditions
15. Maintain nasogastric/orogastric tube for feeding and/or decompression as prescribed.	Monitors gastrointestinal status.	• Changes in gastric tube drainage • Abnormal bowel sounds • Abdominal distention and tenderness • Changes in bowel activity
16. Obtain daily weights if possible.	Daily weights may assist in assessment of fluid balance.	• Change in weight of more than 2 kg/day
17. Frequent repositioning with close examination of back of head, heels, sacrum (consider utilization of specialty bed with low air loss and continuous lateral rotation, also consider utilizing products to decrease risk of friction injuries such as a turning and positioning glide sheet).[1–3,6,10]	Promotes comfort and skin integrity.	• Skin breakdown • Inability of patient to tolerate movement and repositioning
18. Assess ECLS/ECMO circuit at least every hour. Follow institutional standard.	Demonstrates adequate ECLS/ECMO therapy, such as blood flow, pump speed, FiO_2, sweep gas flow.	• Abnormal ECLS/ECMO circuit findings, such as air in line, clots in oxygenator
19. Maintain sterile dressings on all invasive lines and cannula sites. Change ECMO dressing every 24 hours and as needed.[1]	Decreases incidence of infection and allows for site assessment.	• Signs and symptoms of infection
20. Logroll patient every 2 hours until hemodynamic stability is obtained.[1–3,6,10]	Promotes comfort and skin integrity.	• Disruption of skin integrity
21. When patient is hemodynamically stable and condition allows, ambulate progressively. Use of a multidisciplinary team is essential.[1,8] Follow institutional standards.	Prevents hazards of immobility and begins rehabilitation. Ensures all lines are secure when patient is ambulating.	• Postural hypotension • Decrease in flow with position change • Unrelieved dizziness • Prolonged deconditioning
22. Evaluate family's coping mechanism, strengths, and needs on a continual basis.[1]	Promotes family involvement in care and decision-making.	• Family's inability to cope
23. Consult pastoral care, palliative care, or bereavement specialists.[1]	Team assists with meeting family and patient needs.	• Family's inability to cope
24. Ensure safe transport of patient and equipment to tests and procedures.[1,8]	Ensures entire team, including nurses, physicians, respiratory therapists, and perfusion or ECLS/ECMO specialist, is prepared for transport.	• Patient's inability to be transported such as unstable vital signs or instability of ECLS/ECMO circuit

Documentation

Documentation should include the following:
- Patient and family education
- Plan of care
- Universal protocol requirements, sterile procedure/protocol
- Informed consent
- Patient response to ECLS/ECMO
- Confirmation of placement
- Hemodynamic status
- Pain assessment, interventions and effectiveness
- Activity level
- Additional interventions
- ECLS/ECMO parameters (pump flow, FiO_2, and sweep flow)
- Cannula site and cannula measurements
- Securement of cannulas
- Dressing changes and site assessment
- Skin integrity
- Patient tolerance
- Unexpected outcomes

References and Additional Readings

For a complete list of references and additional readings for this procedure, scan this QR code with any freely available smartphone code reader app, or visit http://booksite.elsevier.com/9780323376624.

18 Oxygen Saturation Monitoring with Pulse Oximetry

Donna Barge Lee

PURPOSE: Pulse oximetry is a noninvasive monitoring technique used to estimate the measurement of arterial oxygen saturation of hemoglobin. Pulse oximetry is indicated in patients at risk for hypoxemia, such as during conscious sedation procedures, transport, and adjustment of fraction of inspired oxygen (Fio_2).

PREREQUISITE NURSING KNOWLEDGE

- Oxygen saturation is an indicator of the percentage of hemoglobin saturated with oxygen at the time of the measurement. The reading, obtained with standard pulse oximetry, uses a light sensor that contains two sources of light (red and infrared) absorbed by hemoglobin and transmitted through tissues to a photodetector. The infrared light is absorbed by the oxyhemoglobin, and the red light is absorbed by the reduced hemoglobin. The amount and type of light transmitted through the tissue is converted to a digital value that represents the percentage of hemoglobin saturated with oxygen (Fig. 18-1).
- Oxygen saturation values obtained with pulse oximetry (Spo_2) represent one part of a complete assessment of a patient's oxygenation status and are not a substitute for measurement of arterial saturation of oxygen (Sao_2) or of ventilation (as measured with arterial partial pressure of carbon dioxide [$Paco_2$]).
- A complete assessment of oxygenation includes evaluation of oxygen content and delivery, which includes the following parameters: arterial partial pressure of oxygen (Pao_2), Sao_2 hemoglobin, cardiac output, and, when available, mixed venous oxygen saturation.
- Normal oxygen saturation values are approximately 97% to 99% in a healthy individual breathing room air. An oxygen saturation value of 95% is clinically accepted in a patient with a normal hemoglobin level. With a normal blood pH and body temperature, an oxygen saturation value of 90% is generally equated with a Pao_2 of 60 mm Hg.
- Tissue oxygenation is not reflected by arterial or oxygen saturation obtained with pulse oximetry.
- The affinity of hemoglobin with oxygen may impair or enhance oxygen release at the tissue level.
  - ❖ Oxygen is more readily released to the tissues when pH is decreased (acidosis), body temperature is increased, $Paco_2$ is increased, and 2,3-diphosphoglycerate levels (a byproduct of glucose metabolism that facilitates the dissociation of oxygen from the hemoglobin molecule to tissue) are increased (decreased oxygen affinity).
  - ❖ When hemoglobin has greater affinity for oxygen, less is available to the tissues (increased oxygen affinity). Conditions such as increased pH (alkalosis), decreased temperature, decreased $Paco_2$, and decreased 2,3-diphosphoglycerate (as found in stored blood products) increase oxygen binding to the hemoglobin and limit its release to the tissue.
- Anemic patients will have normal oxygen saturation levels but may be hypoxic because the total oxygen content of the arterial blood is decreased.
- Oxygen saturation values may vary with the amount of oxygen usage or uptake by the tissues. In some patients, a difference is seen in Spo_2 values at rest compared with values during activity, such as ambulation, motion, or positioning.[19]
- Oxygen saturation does not directly reflect the patient's ability to ventilate. The true measure of ventilation is determination of the $Paco_2$ in arterial blood. Use of Spo_2 in a patient with obstructive pulmonary disease may result in erroneous clinical assessments of a condition. As the degree of lung disease increases, the patient's drive to breathe may shift from an increased carbon dioxide stimulus to a hypoxic stimulus. Enhancing the patient's oxygenation and increasing the Spo_2 may limit the ability to ventilate. The normal baseline Spo_2 for a patient with known severe restrictive disease and more definitive methods of determination of the effectiveness of ventilation must be assessed before consideration of interventions that enhance oxygenation.
- The accuracy of Spo_2 measurements may be influenced by physiological variables, including the following:
  - ❖ Hemoglobin level
  - ❖ Presence of dyshemoglobinemias (i.e., carboxyhemoglobinemia after carbon monoxide exposure)
  - ❖ Arterial blood flow to the vascular bed
  - ❖ Temperature of the digit or the area where the oximetry sensor is located
  - ❖ Vasoconstriction
  - ❖ Venous congestion
  - ❖ Fraction of inspired oxygen (percentage of inspired oxygen)
  - ❖ Degree of ventilation-perfusion mismatch
  - ❖ Venous return at the sensor location

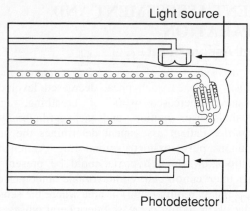

Light source

Photodetector

Figure 18-1 A sensor device that contains a light source and a photodetector is placed around a pulsating arteriolar bed, such as the finger, great toe, nose, or earlobe. Red and infrared wavelengths of light are used to determine arterial saturation. *(Reprinted by permission of Nellcor Puritan Bennett LLC, Boulder, CO, part of Covidien.)*

- The accuracy of SpO_2 measurements may be influenced by environmental variables, including the following:
  - ❖ Nail polish
  - ❖ Pigmentation
  - ❖ Dyes
  - ❖ Ambient light sources
  - ❖ Motion
- Discoloration of the nail bed or obstruction of the nail bed (i.e., blood under the fingernail) can potentially affect the transmission of light through the digit. Dark nail polish, such as blue, green, brown, or black,[4] has been reported to limit the transmission of light and thus affect the SpO_2, although a recent study showed that fingernail polish does not cause a clinically significant change in the pulse oximeter readings in healthy individuals.[17,18] If the nail polish cannot be removed and is believed to be affecting the accuracy of the reading, the sensor can be placed in a lateral side-to-side position on the finger to obtain readings if no other method of sampling the arterial bed is available.[5,18] Bruising under the nail can limit the transmission of light and result in an artificially decreased SpO_2 value. Pulse oximetry has not been shown to be affected by the presence of an elevated bilirubin.[2] The presence of acrylic fingernails may impair the accuracy of the pulse oximetry reading, and removal of the nail covering may be necessary to ensure accurate measurement, although unpolished acrylic nails have been proven not to affect pulse oximetry readings.[16,23]
- Standard pulse oximeters use two wavelengths and are unable to differentiate between oxygen and carbon monoxide bound to hemoglobin and falsely elevated SpO_2 measurements. Standard pulse oximetry equipment should never be used in suspected cases of carbon monoxide exposure. However, recent technology advancements in pulse oximetry have included the introduction of a monitor system that uses up to 12 wavelengths with a digit-based pulse oximeter sensor and that allows for measurement estimates of certain dyshemoglobinemias (i.e., carboxyhemoglobinemia).[12] An arterial blood gas always should be obtained to determine the accurate oxygen saturation and,

if a carbon monoxide (CO) oximeter is available, measurement of carboxyhemoglobin and methemoglobin.[3]
- Dark skin has been suggested to possibly affect the ability of the pulse oximeter to accurately monitor arterial oxygen saturation by interfering with the transmission of light and thus the accuracy of the readings. One study found more frequent differences between the SpO_2 and SaO_2 in dark-skinned patients compared with lighter-skinned patients.[11]
- Certain dyes used intravenously may interfere with the accuracy of measurements, although as a result of rapid clearance the impact is limited. Dyes include methylene blue, indigo carmine, indocyanine green, and fluorescein.[8]
- A pulse oximeter should not be used as a predictive indicator of the actual arterial blood gas saturation; however, the pulse oximetry does provide information about changes in the patient's oxygenation and an early warning sign of hypoxemia. Continuous pulse oximetry monitoring in critical care settings can allow clinicians to recognize early signs of deterioration and provide early interventions that may prevent rescue events such as cardiac arrests or respiratory arrests.[22]
- Low-perfusion states such as hypotension, vasoconstriction, hypothermia, or administration of vasoconstrictive agents limit the ability of the oximeter to distinguish the true pulsatile waveform from background noise.
- The mean oxygen saturation value from the finger of an arm that has been physically restrained has been shown to be significantly different from the finger of an unrestrained arm. Therefore if physical restraints are being used, it is recommended that the pulse oximetry sensor not be placed on the finger of a restrained arm.[2]
- A pulse oximeter should never be used during a cardiac arrest situation because of the extreme limitations of blood flow during cardiopulmonary resuscitation and the pharmacological action of vasoactive agents administered during the resuscitation effort.[9]
- In vasoconstrictive states, oxygen saturation may be measured with a finger probe, but in patients with significant shifts in hemodynamic stability the ear or forehead has been shown to be reasonably resistant to the vasoconstrictive effects of the sympathetic nervous system.[1,15,21]
- Forehead sensors use reflectance and are more accurate in low-flow states but may be affected by venous congestion. Forehead sensors used in patients placed in Trendelenburg's position may require up to 20 mm Hg of external pressure to achieve accurate readings, which may be accomplished with an appropriately applied headband.[1] Disposable pulse oximeters intended for use on fingers should not be used on the forehead, as they are often inaccurate.[20]

EQUIPMENT

- Oxygen saturation monitor
- Oxygen saturation cable and sensor, which may be disposable or nondisposable
- Manufacturer's recommended germicidal agent for cleaning the nondisposable sensor (used for cleaning between patients)

PATIENT AND FAMILY EDUCATION

- Explain the need for determination of oxygen saturation with a pulse oximeter. *Rationale:* This explanation informs the patient of the purpose of monitoring, enhances patient cooperation, and decreases patient anxiety.
- Explain that the values displayed may vary with patient movement, amount of environmental light, patient level of consciousness (awake or asleep), and position of the sensor. *Rationale:* This explanation decreases patient and family anxiety over the constant variability of the values.
- Explain that the use of pulse oximetry is part of a much larger assessment of respiratory status. *Rationale:* This explanation prepares the patient and family for other possible diagnostic tests of oxygenation (e.g., arterial blood gas).
- Explain the equipment to the patient. *Rationale:* This information facilitates patient cooperation in maintaining sensor placement.
- Explain the need for an audible alarm system for alerting clinicians of oxygen saturation values below a set acceptable limit, as determined by the clinician. Demonstrate the alarm system, alerting the patient and family to the possibility of alarms, including causes of false alarms. *Rationale:* Provision of an understanding of the use of an alarm system and its importance in the overall management of the patient's condition and of circumstances in which a false alarm may occur assists in understanding of the SpO$_2$ values seen at the bedside.
- Explain the need to move or remove the sensor on a routine basis to prevent complications related to the type of sensor used and monitoring site (i.e., digit, forehead, ear). *Rationale:* An understanding of the need to move the sensor routinely assists in patient understanding of the frequency of sensor movement.

PATIENT ASSESSMENT AND PREPARATION

Patient Assessment

- Signs and symptoms of decreased oxygenation, including cyanosis, dyspnea, tachypnea, decreased level of consciousness, increased work of breathing, agitation, confusion, disorientation, and tachycardia/bradycardia. *Rationale:* Patient assessment determines the need for continuous pulse oximetry monitoring. Anticipation of conditions in which hypoxia could be present allows earlier intervention before unfavorable outcomes occur.
- Assess the extremity (digit) or area where the sensor will be placed, including decreased peripheral pulses, peripheral cyanosis, decreased body temperature, decreased blood pressure, exposure to excessive environmental light sources (e.g., examination lights), excessive movement or tremor in the digit, presence of dark nail polish or bruising under the nail, presence of artificial nails, clubbing of the digit tips, and blood under the fingernails. *Rationale:* Assessment of factors that may inhibit accuracy of the measurement of oxygenation before attempting to obtain the SpO$_2$ reading enhances the validity of the measurement and allows for correction of factors as is possible.

Patient Preparation

- Verify that the patient is the correct patient using two identifiers. *Rationale:* Before performing a procedure, the nurse should ensure the correct identification of the patient for the intended intervention.
- Ensure that the patient understands preprocedural teachings. Answer questions as they arise, and reinforce information as needed. *Rationale:* This communication evaluates and reinforces understanding of previously taught information.

Procedure	for Oxygen Saturation Monitoring with Pulse Oximetry	
Steps	Rationale	Special Considerations
1. `HH`		
2. `PE`		
3. Select desired sensor site. If digits are chosen, assess for warmth and capillary refill. Confirm the presence of arterial blood flow to the area monitored.	Adequate arterial pulse strength is necessary for obtaining accurate SpO$_2$ measurements.	Avoid sites distal to indwelling arterial catheters, blood pressure cuffs, or venous engorgement (e.g., arteriovenous fistulas, blood transfusions).

Procedure	for Oxygen Saturation Monitoring with Pulse Oximetry—*Continued*	
Steps	**Rationale**	**Special Considerations**
4. Select the appropriate pulse oximeter sensor for the area with the best pulsatile vascular bed to be sampled (Fig. 18-2). The digits are the most common site because of ease of application of the sensor. Consideration of other sites may produce more accurate results in conditions of extreme peripheral vasoconstriction or decreased perfusion.[1,21] **(Level C*)**	The correct sensor optimizes signal capture and minimizes artifact-related difficulties.[5,6,13,14]	Several different types of sensors are available, including disposable and nondisposable sensors, which may be applied over a variety of vascular beds, including the digit, earlobe, nasal bridge or septum, and forehead. The latter requires an appropriately placed headband. Do not use one manufacturer's sensors with another manufacturer's pulse oximeter unless compatibility has been verified.

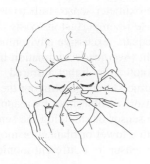
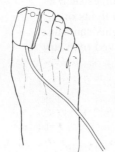
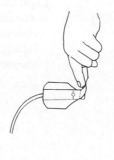

Windows

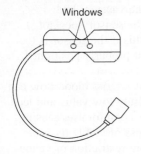
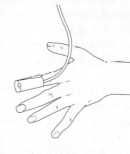
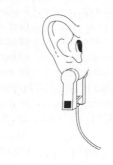

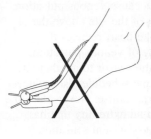
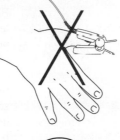
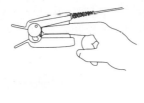

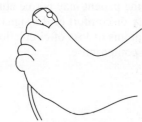
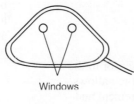

Windows

Figure 18-2 Sensor types and sensor sites for pulse oximetry monitoring. Use "wrap" or "clip" style sensors on the fingers (including thumb), great toe, and nose. The windows for the light source and photodetector must be placed directly opposite each other on each side of the arteriolar bed to ensure accuracy of Spo$_2$ measurements. Choice of the correct size of the sensor helps decrease the incidence of excess ambient light interference and optical shunting. "Clip" style sensors are appropriate for fingers (except the thumb) and the earlobe. Ensuring that the arteriolar bed is well within the clip with the windows directly opposite each other decreases the possibility of excess ambient light interference and optical shunting. *(Reprinted by permission of Nellcor Puritan Bennett LLC, Boulder, CO, part of Covidien.)*

*Level C: Qualitative studies, descriptive or correlational studies, integrative reviews, systematic reviews, or randomized controlled trials with inconsistent results.

Procedure continues on following page

Procedure for Oxygen Saturation Monitoring with Pulse Oximetry—*Continued*

Steps	Rationale	Special Considerations
5. Plug oximeter power cord into grounded wall outlet if the unit is not portable. If the unit is portable, ensure sufficient battery charge by turning it on before use. Plug patient cable into monitor.	With use of electrical outlets, grounded outlets decrease the occurrence of electrical interference.	Portable systems have rechargeable batteries and depend on sufficient time plugged into an electrical outlet to maintain the proper level of battery charge. When system is used in the portable mode, always check battery capacity.
6. Apply the sensor in a manner that allows the light source (LEDs) to be: A. Directly opposite the light detector (photodetector). (**Level C***)	To determine a pulse oximetry value properly, the light sensors must be in opposing positions directly over the area of the sample.[6,7,21]	
B. Shielded from excessive environmental light. (**Level C***)	Light from sources such as examination lights or overhead lights can cause falsely elevated oximetry values.[10,14,21]	If the oximeter sensor fails to detect a pulse when perfusion seems adequate, excessive environmental light (overhead examination lights, phototherapy lights, infrared warmers) may be blinding the light sensor. Troubleshoot by reapplying the sensor or shielding the sensor with a towel or blanket or moving the sensor to a different monitoring site.
C. Positioned so that all sensor-emitted light comes into contact with perfused tissue beds and is not seen by the other side of the sensor or without coming into contact with the area to be read.	If the light from the sensor's LEDs bypasses the tissue bed and is detected at the photodetector, the result is either a falsely high reading or no reading.	Known as *optical shunting,* the light bypasses the vascular bed; shielding the sensor does not eliminate this if the sensor is too large or not properly positioned.
7. Gently position the sensor so that it does not cause restriction to arterial flow or venous return. (**Level C***)	The pulse oximeter is unable to distinguish between true arterial pulsations and fluid waves (e.g., venous engorgement or fluid accumulation).[5,6,13]	Restriction of arterial blood flow can cause a falsely low value and lead to vascular compromise, causing potential loss of viable tissues. Edema from restriction of venous return can cause venous pulsation. Elevation of the site above the level of the heart reduces the possibility of venous pulsation. Moving the sensor to another site on a routine schedule also reduces tissue compromise. Never place the sensor on an extremity that has decreased or absent sensation because the patient may not be able to identify discomfort or the signs and symptoms of loss of circulation or tissue compromise.
8. Plug sensor into oximeter patient cable.	Connects the sensor to the oximeter, which allows SpO_2 measurement and analysis of waveforms.	

*Level C: Qualitative studies, descriptive or correlational studies, integrative reviews, systematic reviews, or randomized controlled trials with inconsistent results.

Procedure for Oxygen Saturation Monitoring with Pulse Oximetry—*Continued*

Steps	Rationale	Special Considerations
9. Turn instrument power switch on.	Applies power to the device.	Allow adequate time for self-testing procedures and for detection and analysis of waveforms before values are displayed. The time required to perform the self-test and adequately warm depends on specific manufacturer.
10. Determine accuracy of detected waveform by comparing the numeric heart rate value with that of a monitored heart rate or an apical heart rate or both. **(Level M*)**	If arterial blood flow through the sensor is insufficient, the heart rate values may vary significantly. If the pulse rate detected with oximeter does not correlate with the patient's heart rate, the oximeter is not detecting sufficient arterial blood flow for accurate values.	This problem occurs particularly with the use of the fingers and the toes in conditions of low blood flow. Consider moving the sensor to another site, such as the earlobe or the forehead (be sure the sensor type is appropriate for the monitoring site).Rotate the site of a reusable sensor every 4 hours; replace an adhesive disposable sensor every 24 hours.[13]
11. Set appropriate alarm limits.	Alarm limits should be set appropriate to the patient's condition.	Oxygen saturation limits should be 5% less than the patient's acceptable baseline. Heart rate alarms should be consistent with the cardiac monitoring limits (if monitored).
13. Cleanse nondisposable sensor, if used, between patients with manufacturer's recommended germicidal agent.	Reduces transmission of microorganisms to other patients.	
12. Discard used supplies and remove PE		
13. HH		

*Level M: Manufacturer's recommendations only.

Expected Outcomes

- All changes in oxygen saturation are detected
- The number of oxygen desaturation events is reduced
- The need for invasive techniques for monitoring oxygenation is reduced
- False-positive pulse oximeter alarms are reduced

Unexpected Outcomes

- Accurate pulse oximetry is not obtainable because of movement artifact
- Low-perfusion states or excessive edema prevents accurate pulse oximetry measurements
- Disagreements occur in Sao_2 and oximeter Spo_2

Procedure continues on following page

Patient Monitoring and Care

Steps	Rationale	Reportable Conditions
		These conditions should be reported if they persist despite nursing interventions.
1. Evaluate laboratory data along with the patient for evidence of reduced arterial oxygen saturation or hypoxemia.	Spo$_2$ values are one segment of a complete evaluation of the patient's oxygenation status and supplemental oxygen therapy. Data should be integrated into a complete assessment to determine the overall status of the patient. If Spo$_2$ is used as an indicator of Sao$_2$, an arterial blood gas with CO oximetry should be done to determine whether the values correlate consistently.	• Inability to maintain oxygen saturation levels as desired
2. Evaluate sensor site every 2–4 hours (if a disposable sensor is used) or every 2 hours (if a reusable or nondisposable sensor is used). Rotate the site of a reusable sensor every 4 hours; replace an adhesive disposable sensor every 24 hours[13] or per manufacturer's recommendations if the securing mechanism is compromised or soiled. Never apply additional adhesive tape to secure a sensor. **(Level M*)**	Assessment of the skin and tissues under the sensor identifies skin breakdown or loss of vascular flow, allowing appropriate interventions to be initiated. Application of additional tape may constrict blood flow at the monitoring site and result in both inaccurate monitor readings and further compromised local skin perfusion.	• Change in skin color • Loss of warmth of tissue unrelated to vasoconstriction • Loss of blood flow to the digit • Evidence of skin breakdown from the sensor • Change in color of the nail bed, which indicates compromised circulation to the nail
3. Monitor the sensor site for excessive movement, which results in motion artifact.	Excessive movement at the monitoring site may result in unreliable saturation values. Moving the sensor to a less physically active site may reduce the risk of motion artifact; use of an adhesive versus reusable sensor may also help as a result of better fit. If the digits are used, ask the patient to rest the hand on a flat or secure surface.	• Inability to obtain pulse oxygen saturation levels
4. Compare and monitor the actual heart rate with the pulse rate value from the pulse oximeter to determine accuracy of values.	The two numeric heart rate values should correlate closely. A difference in pulse rate values reported with pulse oximeter may be from excessive movement, poor peripheral perfusion at the monitoring site, or loss of pulsatile flow detection.	• Inability to correlate actual heart rate and pulse rate from oximeter

Documentation

Documentation should include the following:

Patient and family education
Indications for use of pulse oximetry
Patient's pulse rate with Spo$_2$ measurements
Fio$_2$ delivered (if patient is receiving oxygen)
Patient clinical assessment at the time of the saturation measurement
Sensor site

Simultaneous arterial blood gases (if available)
Recent hemoglobin measurement (if available)
Skin assessment at sensor site
Pulse oximeter monitor alarm settings
Events precipitating acute desaturation
Unexpected outcomes
Nursing interventions

References and Additional Readings

For a complete list of references and additional readings for this procedure, scan this QR code with any freely available smartphone code reader app, or visit http://booksite.elsevier.com/9780323376624.

19

Pronation Therapy

Kathleen Vollman, Sharon Dickinson, and Jan Powers

PURPOSE: The prone position may be indicated in patients diagnosed with acute respiratory distress syndrome demonstrating severe hypoxemia, defined as a partial pressure of arterial oxygen (PaO_2)/fraction of inspired oxygen (FiO_2) ratio of <150 mm Hg with an FiO_2 of at least 60% and positive end-expiratory pressure (PEEP) of at least 5 cm H_2O and a tidal volume close to 6 mL/kg of predicted body weight. The prone position is used in an attempt to improve oxygenation and reduce ventilator-induced lung injury in patients with acute respiratory distress syndrome (ARDS). The position also may be used for mobilization of secretions as a postural drainage technique, posterior wound management that allows excellent visualization and management of the site, relief of pressure in the sacral region, positioning for operative or diagnostic procedures, and therapeutic sleep for critically ill patients who normally sleep on the abdomen at home.

PREREQUISITE NURSING KNOWLEDGE

- Prone positioning is used as an adjunct short-term supportive therapy in an attempt to recruit alveoli to improve gas exchange and reduce ventilator injury in critically ill patients with ARDS with severe hypoxemia.
  - ❖ On the basis of numerous studies and three older and one recent meta-analyses, and the latest prospective randomized controlled trial (RCT), patients with ARDS and severe hypoxemia placed in the prone position significantly increase PaO_2/FiO_2 ratio compared with in the supine position. The greatest effect was seen within the first few days, with continuing benefit up to 8 days.[1–6,10,13,16,17,21,23,29,33,35,37] Guerin and colleagues studied a total of 466 ARDS patients with severe hypoxemia, with 237 in the prone group and 229 in the supine group. Patients were randomly assigned to undergo prone or supine positioning. After eligibility was determined, a stabilization period of 12 to 24 hours took place before randomization. Those in the prone group were turned within 1 hour of randomization and spent at least 16 consecutive hours in the prone position per day. The 28-day mortality was significantly reduced in the prone group. The mortality of the prone group was 16% compared with the supine group at 32.8%. This benefit held out to 90 days.[17] However, the other two of the four meta-analyses showed no improvement in mortality with the use of the prone position.[1,33] The other two meta-analyses showed significant improvement in mortality in patients with severe-hypoxemia ARDS.[3,21] Lee and colleagues also found that >10 hours a day in the prone position was associated with a reduction in mortality.[21]
  - ❖ No significant difference was seen in number of days on mechanical ventilation with the prone position.[1,3,33]

One meta-analysis showed significant reduction in the incidence of ventilator-associated pneumonia (VAP) in the prone position[33]; another showed a trend toward significance in VAP reduction of 23% ($P = 0.09$)[1]; and the third showed no difference in VAP rates between the two positions.[3] The fourth meta-analysis did not evaluate the effect on VAP.[21]

- ❖ Part of the variability in outcomes between the analyses has to do with the inclusion criteria used to choose the studies incorporated in the meta-analysis. The analysis by Alsaghir and Martian[3] resulted in five trials that met inclusion criteria out of 63 with a total of 1316 patients. The meta-analysis performed by Abroung and group[1] included 5 trials out of 72 with a total of 1372 patients, and the analysis by Sud and colleagues[33] included 13 trials out of 1676 studies with analysis being performed on 1559 patients. Lee et al. analyzed 11 trials totaling 2246 patients. They excluded RCTs conducted on pediatric patients and randomized cross over trials that assigned patients to both groups.[21]
- ❖ The last major outcomes to be examined in the meta-analyses were the presence of significant complications when the prone position was compared with the supine position. Three of the four analyses reported on complications. Two analyses showed a statistically significant higher risk for the development of pressure ulcers in the prone position,[21,33] and Abroung and group[1] showed no significant difference in major airway complications in the prone position; however, Lee and colleagues demonstrated that prone positioning was significantly associated with major airway complications.[21] Guerin and colleagues in their recent prospective RCT showed that the incidence of complications did not differ between groups except with cardiac arrests. The supine group had a significantly higher rate of cardiac arrest than the prone group.[17]

- To enhance an understanding of how prone positioning may affect gas exchange, understanding the factors that influence the distribution of ventilation and perfusion within the lung is important.
  - *Distribution of ventilation:* Regional pleural pressures and local lung compliance jointly determine the volume of air distributed regionally throughout the lungs. Three major factors—gravity and weight of the lung, compliance, and heterogeneously diseased lungs—influence regional distribution. In an upright individual, the pleural pressure next to the diaphragm is less negative than at the pleural apices. The weight of the lung and the effect of gravity on the lung and its supporting structures in the upright position create this difference in regional pleural pressures. This relationship results in a higher functional residual capacity (FRC) in the nondependent zone or the apices, redirecting ventilation to the dependent zone.[11,19,41] When body position changes, changes occur in regional pleural pressures, compliance, and volume distribution. In the supine position, distribution becomes more uniform from apex to base. The ventilation of dependent lung units exceeds that of nondependent lung units, however, and a reduction in FRC is seen.[11,41] The two factors that contribute to the reduction in FRC seen in moving from the upright to the supine position include the pressure of the abdominal contents on the diaphragm and the position of the heart and the relationship of the supporting structures to the lung and its influence on pleural pressure gradients.[11,12,22]
  - The first factor to influence pleural pressure, regional volumes, and FRC is the effect of the abdominal contents on the function of the diaphragm. In spontaneously breathing individuals in the supine position, the diaphragm acts as a shield against the pressure exerted by the abdominal contents, preventing the contents from interfering with dependent lung-volume distribution. When patients are mechanically ventilated with positive-pressure breaths, sedated, or paralyzed, the active muscle tension in the diaphragm is lost, which results in a cephalad displacement of the diaphragm and allows abdominal pressures to decrease dependent lung-volume inflation and FRC.[11,19] The only way to modify this influence is to change the posture to a prone position with the abdomen unsupported.[11,29]
  - The second factor to influence pleural pressure, regional volumes, FRC, and compliance is the position of the heart and supporting structures. The heart and the diaphragm extend farther dorsally and rest against a rigid spine in the supine position, squeezing the lungs beneath them. This pressure on the lungs generates more positive pleural pressures, which results in a greater propensity of the alveoli at end expiration to collapse. In the prone position, the heart and upper abdomen rest against the sternum, exerting less weight on the lung tissue. Less effect on pleural pressure occurs, which leaves the pleural pressures more negative, maintaining open alveoli.[22,26,29]
  - A third factor that contributes to the distribution of volume is heterogeneously or unevenly distributed diseased lung. The ARDS lung weight is increased twofold to threefold from normal. The increased weight is from edema and the resulting hydrostatic forces. The result is a progressive squeezing of gas along the vertical-dorsal axis. This decrease of regional inflation along the vertical axis results in dependent or dorsal lung collapse. In the prone position, these densities shift. The pattern almost completely reverts toward normal. The inflation gradient is less steep, and the difference results in a more homogeneous regional inflation. This inflation may be related to a redistribution of gas because of the change in hydrostatic forces caused by differences in pleural pressure, as described previously.[12,14,29]

- *Distribution of perfusion:* Similar to ventilation, regional distribution of perfusion is influenced by three factors: cardiac output, pulmonary vascular resistance, and gravity or body position.
  - In an upright individual, blood flow decreases as it moves from base to apex with virtually no flow at the apex. This decrease is caused by the influence of gravity on pulmonary vascular pressures within the lung
  - In zone 1, near the apex, alveolar pressure exceeds arterial pressure, creating little or no flow.
  - In zone 2, the pulmonary artery pressure exceeds alveolar pressure, which exceeds the venous pressure. Blood flow in this area occurs based on the differences in pressure between the arterial and alveolar bed.
  - In zone 3, the arterial pressure is greater than the venous pressure, which is greater than the alveolar pressure. In this zone, the influence of the alveolar pressure on blood flow is reduced, resulting in freedom of flow in this region.[41,42]
- In supine and lateral positions, apical region blood flow changes. No real change is seen in basilar units, but a greater dependent versus nondependent blood flow occurs. In the prone position, a marked reduction occurs, however, in the gravitational perfusion gradient, which suggests no gravity-dependent benefit to flow in the prone position.[26]
- On the basis of the current available data as outlined here, changes in oxygenation seem to be related to differences in the regional inflation/ventilation of the lung while prone and are not related to a redistribution of blood flow.[7,22,28] In a recent examination of the Guerin et al. trial data, it appears that the improvement in gas exchange did not predict survival. It was suggested that improved survival occurred by reducing ventilator-induced lung injury as it was first discussed in 1997. Prone positioning creates a more uniform distribution of end-expiratory lung volume or FRC and a more uniform tidal volume.[2]
- Suggested criteria for use of the prone position include the following:
  - Consider early use of the prone position for patients with ARDS with severe hypoxemia defined as a Pao_2/Fio_2 ratio <150 mm Hg, with a Fio_2 >60% with at least 5 cm of PEEP.[17]
- Precautions to manual pronation therapy include the following[4,10,28,31,36,37]:
  - Patient unable to tolerate a head-down position
  - Increased intracranial pressure

❖ Unstable spine (unless Stryker Frame [Stryker Medical], Kalamazoo, MI)

❖ Patient with hemodynamically unstable condition (as defined by a systolic blood pressure <90 mm Hg) with fluid and vasoactive support in place

❖ Weight 160 kg or greater (weigh the risk/benefit ratio for the patient and staff)

❖ Extracorporeal membrane oxygenator cannula placement problems

❖ With use of a support frame, patient weight >135 kg (300 lbs)

❖ Open chest or unstable chest wall

❖ Bronchopleural fistula

❖ Unstable pelvis

❖ Facial trauma

❖ Grossly distended abdomen or ischemic bowel

❖ Pregnancy

❖ Bifurcated endotracheal tube (ETT)

• Absolute contraindications for use of Automated Prone Positioning RotoProne Therapy System (Arjohuntleigh, Sweden) include the following:

❖ Unstable cervical, thoracic, lumbar, pelvic, skull, or facial fractures

❖ Cervical or skeletal traction

❖ Uncontrolled intracranial pressure

❖ Patient weight <40 kg (88 lbs)

❖ Patient weight >159 kg (350 lbs)

❖ Patient height >6 ft 6 inches

• The use of the prone position is discontinued when the patient no longer shows a positive response to the position change or mechanical ventilation support has been optimized. In the Guerin et al protocol, prone positioning was stopped when the following criteria were met[17]:

❖ Improvement in oxygenation, defined as PaO_2/FiO_2 ratio <150 mm Hg, with an FiO_2 >60% with ≤10 cm of PEEP (these criteria had to be met in the supine position at least 4 hours after the end of the last prone session)

❖ A PaO_2/FiO_2 ratio of more than 20% relative to the ratio in the supine position before two consecutive prone sessions

❖ Complications occurring during a prone session leading to its immediate interruption, including nonscheduled extubation, main stem bronchus intubation, ETT obstruction, hemoptysis, oxygen saturation <85% for greater than 10 minutes or a PaO_2 of <55 mm Hg for more than 5 minutes. When the FiO_2 was at 100%, cardiac arrest, a heart rate of <30 bpm for more than 1 minute, systolic blood pressure of <60 mm Hg for more than 5 minutes, and any other life-threatening reason

• With use of the RotoProne Therapy System Surface, weaning from the prone position is recommended. Increase supine time while decreasing time in the prone position until the patient is able to tolerate 12 to 24 hours in the supine position with no decrease in oxygenation response. The patient can then be taken off the RotoProne and placed on an appropriate surface to achieve patient goals.

EQUIPMENT

• Pillows, gel or foam blocks, flat sheet

• Four or five staff members

• Resuscitation bag and mask, connected to an oxygen source

• Lift sheets (Figs. 19-1 and 19-2)

or

• RotoProne Therapy System for use in all patient populations (Fig. 19-3): weight limit per manufacturer's recommendations, 88 to 350 lbs (40 to 159 kg); height limit per manufacturer's recommendations, 54 to 78 inches (140 to 200 cm)

or

• Lateral rotation therapy bed with or without prone accessory kit

or

• Vollman Prone Positioner (VPP; Hill-Rom, Inc, Batesville, IN; Fig. 19-4): weight limit per manufacturer's recommendation, 300 lbs (no longer manufactured but may have been purchased in the past)

• Three staff members (with VPP)

• Stryker Frame for use in patients with unstable spines, if available: weight limit per manufacturer's recommendations

Additional equipment, to have available as needed, includes the following:

• Capnography monitor

PATIENT AND FAMILY EDUCATION

• Explain to the patient and family the patient's lung/oxygenation problem and the reason for the use of the prone position. ***Rationale:*** This explanation decreases patient and family anxiety by providing information and clarification.

• Explain the care procedure to the patient and family, including positioning procedure, perceived benefit, frequency of assessments, expected response, and parameters for discontinuation of the positioning technique and equipment (if special bed or frame is initiated). ***Rationale:*** This communication provides an opportunity for the patient and family to verbalize concerns or ask questions about the procedure.

PATIENT ASSESSMENT AND PREPARATION

Patient Assessment

• Assess time interval from initial diagnosis to position change. ***Rationale:*** Prone positioning should be performed within the first 24 hours of the diagnosis of severe-hypoxemia ARDS. Prone positioning should occur for at least 16 hours in a 24-hour period.

• Assess the hemodynamic status of the patient to identify the ability to tolerate a position change.[31,39] Most critically ill patients take 5 to 10 minutes to equilibrate to a position change. Allow for this time period before determining lack of ability to tolerate the prone position.[39] ***Rationale:***

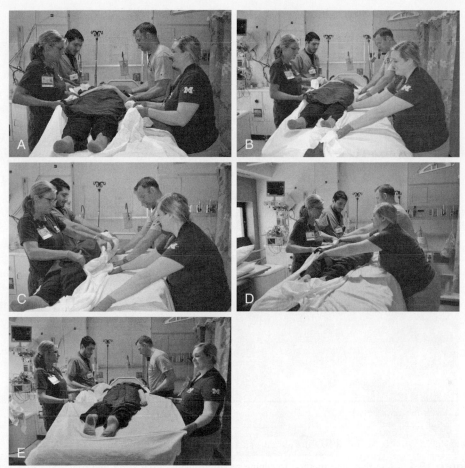

Figure 19-1 The five-step method to prone a patient using a regular bed, flat sheet, and four staff. **A,** Using a flat sheet, pull the patient to one side of the bed using four staff members. **B,** Place the flat sheet around the arm that will pull through (the side you are turning toward). **C,** A second flat sheet is placed on the bed and tucked under the patient. This sheet will pull through as you are turning the patient. **D,** Using the sheet, turn the patient over and position the patient prone. The arm and sheet will pull across the bed. **E,** Pull and center the patient. Discard the sheet that was used to supine the patient. Straighten lines and tubes. *(From University of Michigan Surgical Intensive Care Technique.)*

Imbalances between oxygen supply and demand must be addressed before the pronation procedure to offset any increases in oxygen demand that may be created by the physical turning. The final decision to place a patient with a hemodynamically unstable condition in a prone position rests with the physician or advanced practice nurse who must weigh the risks against the potential benefits of the prone position.

- Assess mental status before use of the prone position. *Rationale:* Agitation, whether caused by delirium, anxiety, or pain, can have a negative effect with the prone position. Nevertheless, agitation is not a contraindication for use of the prone position. The healthcare team should strive to manage the agitation effectively to provide a safe environment for the use of the prone position.
- Assess size and weight load to determine the ability to turn within the narrow critical care bed frame and to weigh the potential risk of injury to the healthcare worker. *Rationale:* When manually turning a patient prone in a hospital bed, with or without a frame, one must determine whether a 180-degree turn can be accomplished within the confines of the space available. Critical care bed frames

are narrow, which makes completion of the turn difficult on patients who weigh more than 160 kg. The team must consider the potential for injury to the healthcare workers when making the decision to turn morbidly obese patients prone. With use of a special bed made specifically for prone positioning, follow the weight and height limitations recommended by the manufacturer.

- Evaluate patient for any history of contraindications for particular arm positions while manually proned. *Rationale:* Identifies patients with arm or shoulder injuries that may preclude proning.

Patient Preparation

- Verify that the patient is the correct patient using two identifiers. *Rationale:* Before performing a procedure, the nurse should ensure the correct identification of the patient for the intended intervention.
- Ensure that the patient and family understand preprocedural teachings. Answer questions as they arise and reinforce information as needed. *Rationale:* This communication evaluates and reinforces understanding of previously taught information.

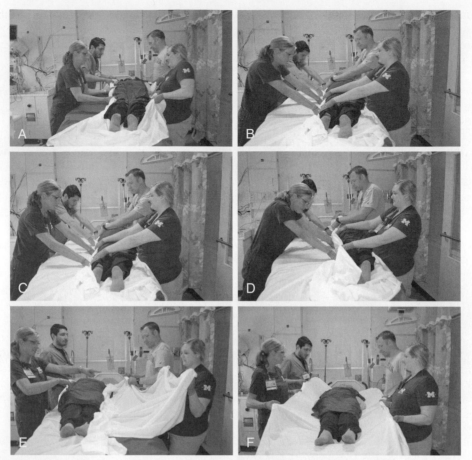

Figure 19-2   The five-step method to supine a patient using a flat sheet and four staff. **A,** Using a flat sheet, pull the patient to one side of the bed. **B,** Place the flat sheet around the arm that will pull through (the side you are turning toward). **C,** A second flat sheet is placed on the bed and tucked under the patient. This sheet will pull through as you are turning the patient. **D,** Using the sheet turn the patient over and position the patient prone. The arm and sheet will pull across the bed. **E,** Discard the sheet that was used to supine patient. **F,** Straighten lines and tubes. *(From University of Michigan Surgical Intensive Care Technique.)*

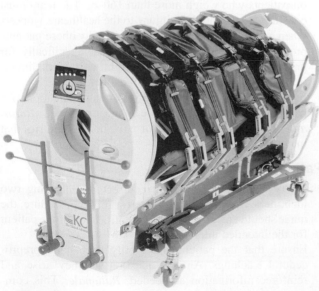

Figure 19-3   The Rotoprone therapy system. *(Courtesy KCI Licensing, Inc, 2008.)*

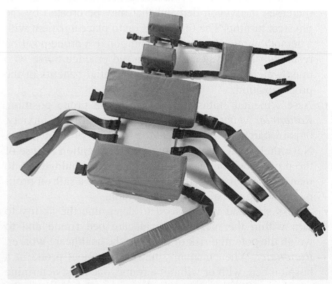

Figure 19-4   Diagram of the Vollman Prone Positioner. *(From Hill-Rom, Inc, San Antonio, TX.)*

- Assess patient's mental condition. *Rationale:* Assessment of pain, anxiety/agitation and delirium using a reliable and valid scale and providing appropriate management before, during, and after the turn are key to accomplishing a safe procedure.
- If using gastric feedings, turn off the tube feeding 1 hour before the prone position turn. *Rationale:* This action assists with gastric emptying and reduces the risk of aspiration during the turning procedure.[38] Enteral feeding can be continued during prone position[34]; use of prokinetic agents or transpyloric feedings is recommended to prevent complications associated with vomiting.[30]
- Before positioning the patient prone, the following care activities should be performed. *Rationale:* These activities prevent areas of pressure and potential skin breakdown; avoid complications related to injury or accidental extubation; and promote the delivery of comprehensive care before, during, and after the pronation therapy.[31,36,37,40]
  - ❖ Order prone positioning.
  - ❖ Remove electrocardiogram (ECG) leads from the anterior chest wall.
  - ❖ Perform eye care, including lubrication and taping of the eyelids closed in a horizontal fashion (or per institutional policy).
  - ❖ Ensure the tongue is inside the patient's mouth. If the tongue is swollen or protruding, insert a dental mouthprop. The dental mouth-prop fits between the teeth (upper and lower) holding the mouth open to prevent the teeth digging into the tongue. Other bite blocks may be used, but do not use bite blocks that fit over the tongue as this will cause undue pressure and increase risk of tongue breakdown.
  - ❖ Ensure the tape or ties of the ETT or tracheotomy tube are secure. Changing of the ties may be necessary on return to the supine position if they are not secure. If adhesive tape is used to secure the ETT, consider double taping or wrapping completely around the head because increased salivary drainage occurs in the prone position and may loosen the adhesive.[31,37] Commercial ETT securement devices are not recommended for use during prone positioning because of the possibility of increased skin breakdown and breakdown of adhesive from increased salivary drainage.[20]
  - ❖ Central and arterial lines should be sutured into place.
  - ❖ If a wound dressing on the anterior body is due to be changed during the prone-position sequence, perform the dressing change before the turn. If saturated on return from the prone position, the dressing needs to be changed.
  - ❖ Empty ileostomy/colostomy bags before positioning. Placement of the drainage bag to gravity drainage and padding around the stoma to prevent pressure directly on stoma are recommended.
  - ❖ Capnography monitoring is suggested to help ensure proper positioning of the ETT during the turning procedure and in the prone position.

Procedure	for Preparation for Manual Prone Therapy	
Steps	**Rationale**	**Special Considerations**
1. **HH**		
2. **PE**		
3. Two staff members are positioned on each side of the bed, with another staff member (often a respiratory therapist [RT]) positioned at the head of the bed. (**Level D***) Ideally, some of the staff should be experienced with proning and moving the patient back to supine in case of an emergency.	Four to five individuals are needed to position a patient safely prone without a frame. Additional stability and position of the personnel may be necessary, based on the size of the patient.[8,9,31,36,37,40]	The RT at the head of the bed is responsible for monitoring the ETT, ventilator tubing. The nurse adjacent to the RT monitors the intravenous (IV) lines located by the patient's head. For increased airway security, the RT or nurse should hold the ETT during the turn.[31,37]
4. Correctly position all tubes and invasive lines. Remove ECG patches from the chest.	All IV tubing and invasive lines are adjusted to prevent kinking, disconnection, or contact with the body during the turning procedure and while the patient remains in the prone position. ECG patches can be a source of pressure when the patient is proned.[8,9]	If the patient is in skeletal traction, one individual needs to apply traction to the leg while the lines and weights are removed for the turn. If a skeletal pin comes into contact with the bed, a pillow needs to be placed in the correct position to alleviate pressure points.

*Level D: Peer-reviewed professional and organizational standards with the support of clinical study recommendations.

Procedure continues on following page

Procedure	for Preparation for Manual Prone Therapy—*Continued*	
Steps	**Rationale**	**Special Considerations**
5. Lines inserted in the upper torso are aligned with either shoulder, and the excess tubing is placed at the head of the bed. The only exception is for the chest tubes or other large-bore tubes (e.g., tubes used for extracorporeal membrane oxygenation). (**Level D***)	Disconnecting IV lines before the turn may help to prevent dislodgement but places the patient at an increased risk for infection.	
6. Chest tubes and lines or tubes placed in the lower torso are aligned with either leg and extend off the end of the bed. (**Level D**)	Consider addition of an extension tube to lines that are too short to be placed at the head of bed or the end of the bed.	
7. If the patient has an open abdomen, cover with a synthetic material or vacuum dressing before positioning. Identify a positioning strategy that allows the abdomen to be free of restriction.	Open abdomens are not a contraindication for use of the prone position. A cover with a synthetic material such as a Wound Vac, or support such as an abdominal binder, may be used effectively to secure the abdomen.[25]	
8. Assess to make sure you have enough bed width to safely turn the patient 180 degrees. If on a low air-loss surface, maximally inflate.[36,40] (**Level E***)	Maximally inflating the air surface firms up the mattress, making the turn easier to perform.	Consider the use of a bariatric bed for patients >300–350 lbs.
9. Preoxygenate the patient with a Fio_2 of 100% for 30 minutes before prone or supine positioning.[8] (**Level E**)	Maximize oxygenation before turning.	
10. Discard used supplies and remove **PE**		
11. **HH**		

Procedure	for Manual Pronation Therapy: The Five-Step Method to Prone the Patient[8,9] (see Fig. 19-1)	
Steps	**Rationale**	**Special Considerations**
1. Start with flat sheet that is under the patient and pull the patient while still supine to the side of the bed away from the ventilator. Turn the patient in the direction of the mechanical ventilator.	The person on the side of the bed closest to the patient maintains body contact with the bed at all times to serve as a side rail and prevent a fall. (**Level C***)	

*Level C: Qualitative studies, descriptive or correlational studies, integrative reviews, systematic reviews, or randomized controlled trials with inconsistent results.

*Level D: Peer-reviewed professional and organizational standards with the support of clinical study recommendations.

*Level E: Multiple case reports, theory-based evidence from expert opinions, or peer-reviewed professional organizational standards without clinical studies to support recommendations.

Procedure	for Manual Pronation Therapy: The Five-Step Method to Prone the Patient[8,9] (see Fig. 19-1)—*Continued*	
Steps	**Rationale**	**Special Considerations**
2. The flat sheet is placed around the arm that is located in the middle of the bed (encircle the arm, that will pull through) side you are turning toward.	This maneuver protects the arm and allows it to be pulled from under the patient after completing the turn.	
3. A second flat sheet is placed on the bed and tucked under the patient and the covered arm. The patient is rolled as far as possible to the side of the bed to allow placement of the second sheet as far under the patient as possible. This sheet will pull through as you are turning the patient.	Both sheets will pull through after turning the patient.	
4. Under direction of the person at the head of the bed, with a count of three, the patient is carefully turned back over by pulling the first sheet from the side of the bed back toward the middle of the bed. The wrapped arm is gently pulled from under the patient using the original sheet while pulling the second sheet under the patient. The original flat sheet is discarded. (**Level E***)	The first flat sheet is pulled through and away from the ventilator, pulling the arm with it. This sheet can be recycled and the second flat sheet pulled through away from the ventilator. Placing the new sheet (second sheet) under the patient allows you to be ready to return the patient to the supine position at any time. It also allows the patient to lay on a clean, absorbent surface.	Chest and/or pelvic support can be done by placing a pillow at the abdomen before completing the turn.
5. The patient is now prone. Pull and center the patient. Straighten and reconnect lines and tubes. Position the head to prevent pressure areas. Place the patient in the reverse Trendelenburg position if not contraindicated. Place feet on pillows. (**Level E**)	Every attempt is made to prevent pressure areas to the face, around lines and tubes, and over bony prominences. The head should lie directly on the bed in a side lying position. Arms are positioned for comfort by either placing them aligned with the body or in a swimmers position, one up and one down.	Patients may have range-of-motion limitations to the shoulder area that may make keeping the arms in a flexed position difficult. The patient should be repositioned every 2 hours, the same as a patient in the supine position. The head should also be rotated every 2 hours from side to side.

Preparation for Returning a Patient to Supine Position

1. Repeat procedure steps 3–9 under Procedure for Preparation for Manual Prone Therapy above.

The Five-Step Method for Returning to the Supine Position From the Prone Position[8,9] (see Fig. 19-2)

1. Start with a flat sheet that is under the patient and pull the patient while still prone to the side of the bed, away from the ventilator. Turn the patient in the direction of the mechanical ventilator.	The person on the side of the bed closest to the patient maintains body contact with the bed at all times to serve as a side rail and prevent a fall. (**Level C***)	The RT at the head of the bed is responsible for monitoring the ETT, ventilator tubing. The nurse adjacent to the RT monitors the intravenous lines located by the patient's head. For increased airway security, the RT or nurse should hold the ETT during the turn.[31,37]

*Level C: Qualitative studies, descriptive or correlational studies, integrative reviews, systematic reviews, or randomized controlled trials with inconsistent results.

^Level E: Multiple case reports, theory-based evidence from expert opinions, or peer-reviewed professional organizational standards without clinical studies to support recommendations.

Procedure continues on following page

Procedure	**for Manual Pronation Therapy: The Five-Step Method to Prone the Patient**[8,9] (see Fig. 19-1)—*Continued*

Steps	Rationale	Special Considerations
2. The flat sheet is placed around the arm that is located in the middle of the bed (encircle the arm that will pull through) while you are turning toward.	This maneuver protects the arm and allows it to be pulled from under the patient after completing the turn.	
3. A second flat sheet is placed on the bed and tucked under the patient and the covered arm. The patient is rolled as far as possible to the side of the bed to allow placement of the second sheet as far under the patient as possible. This sheet will pull through as the patient is turned.	Both sheets will pull through after turning the patient.	
4. Under direction of the person at the head of the bed, with a count of three, the patient is carefully turned back over by pulling the first sheet from the side of the bed back toward the middle of the bed. The wrapped arm is gently pulled from under the patient using the original sheet while pulling the second sheet under the patient. The original flat sheet is discarded. (**Level E***)	The first flat sheet is pulled through and away from the ventilator, pulling the arm with it. This sheet can be recycled and the second flat sheet is pulled through away from the ventilator. Placing the new sheet (second sheet) under the patient allows you to be ready to prone at any time. It also allows the patient to lay on a clean, absorbent surface.	Offloading of bony prominences can be accomplished by placing pillows under the back and buttocks.
5. The patient is now supine. Pull and center the patient. Straighten and reconnect lines and tubes.	Every attempt is made to prevent pressure areas around lines, tubes, and boney prominences.	Position the head to prevent pressure areas. Elevate the head of the bed, 30–45 degrees to prevent a ventilator-associated event, if not contraindicated. Place legs on pillows to free float the heels and reduce edema. Place arms on pillows to reduce edema and prevent pressure. Place head on a pillow, if not contraindicated. Provide range of motion. The patient should be repositioned every 2 hours unless contraindicated.

*Level E: Multiple case reports, theory-based evidence from expert opinions, or peer-reviewed professional organizational standards without clinical studies to support recommendations.

Procedure	**for Automated Pronation Therapy (Using the RotoProne Therapy System; see Fig. 19-3)**	
Steps	**Rationale**	**Special Considerations**
1. **HH**		
2. **PE**		
3. After removing all pieces from the RotoProne Therapy System, move the patient from the intensive care unit bed to the RotoProne Therapy System.	The patient needs to be placed on the RotoProne surface to use this device for proning.	
4. Position the patient in the center of the surface with head positioned in the attached head support.	To appropriately place packs on the patient for the prone procedure, he or she must be centered on the surface with his or her head in the head support.	Ears should be visible through the ear holes on the headpiece.
5. Position all tubes and invasive lines:		
A. Lines inserted in the upper torso are aligned with either shoulder and positioned at the head of the bed in the tube-management system.[8,9] **(Level C*)**	All intravenous tubing and invasive lines are adjusted to prevent kinking, disconnection, or contact with the body during the turning procedure and while the patient remains in the prone position.[8,9]	
B. Chest tubes and lines or tubes placed in the lower torso are aligned with either leg and extend through the center hole at the foot of the surface.	The addition of extension tubing to lines that are too short to be placed at the head of the bed or the end of the bed may be necessary.	
C. If the patient has an open abdomen, it should be supported with some type of supportive dressing. **(Level E*)**	Open abdominal wounds are not a contraindication for use of the prone position. A cover with a synthetic material and a support such as an abdominal binder or vacuum dressing may be used effectively to secure the abdomen.[25]	
6. Follow manufacturer's recommendations for securing patient on therapy surface. **(Level M*)**	For safe operation of the product, manufacturer's recommendations should be followed.	
A. Place leg piece and side packs on surface. Tighten side packs by using the crank at the midpoint of the bed. The packs should fit snugly against the patient's sides.	Ensure the patient is snugly secured within side packs. If the side packs are not secured tightly before the turn, the patient may have shear or friction injuries develop during the turning process. This can also cause the bed to alarm.	
B. Place abdominal support mesh over the patient's abdomen.	Provides abdominal support when patient is in the prone position.	
C. Position additional pads on patient for support if needed. Place chest pad on chest so the top is level with the patient's shoulders.	All packs need to be positioned to prevent undue pressure on the patient's surfaces and to avoid malposition of joints (avoid hyperextension of knees and hips in prone position).	

*Level C: Qualitative studies, descriptive or correlational studies, integrative reviews, systematic reviews, or randomized controlled trials with inconsistent results

*Level E: Multiple case reports, theory-based evidence from expert opinions, or peer-reviewed professional organizational standards without clinical studies to support recommendations.

*Level M: Manufacturer's recommendations only.

Procedure continues on following page

Procedure	**for Automated Pronation Therapy (Using the RotoProne Therapy System; see Fig. 19-3)—*Continued***	
Steps	**Rationale**	**Special Considerations**
D. Tighten the headpiece snugly around the patient's head.	The patient's head needs to be secured during the turning procedure to prevent patient injury and tube dislodgement.	
E. Position all packs snugly over the patient (lower leg below knees, upper leg above knees, pelvic pack over iliac crest, and chest pack over chest/shoulder area) and buckle.	This action prevents direct pressure over bony prominences and provides sufficient distance between the chest and pelvis to allow the abdomen to be free of restriction, and prevents bowing of the back. The chest pack may need to be tightened over the patient last because constriction of the chest may restrict the patient's ventilatory effort and increase peak airway pressures.	
F. Place the face pack on the patient's face and attach to the head piece by inserting black locking straps on both sides. Ensure the top pad is above the eyebrows and the side pieces frame the mouth.	Face pads should be resting on the face; do not tighten because this will create undue pressure.	
7. On the screen at the foot of the bed, set therapy on RotoProne Therapy System to prone toward the direction of the ventilator.	These maneuvers are performed to prevent disconnection of the ventilator tubing or kinking of the ETT during the turning procedure.[31,36,37,40]	
8. Discard used supplies and remove ▣PE.		
9. ▣HH		
Turning Prone With the RotoProne Therapy System		
All steps listed below are performed on the touch screen at the foot of the surface.		Use the touch screen buttons on screen at the foot of the surface, following manufacturer's instructions for turning the patient to the prone position.
1. "Check tubing," "Check airway," "Check head support" (push each button on the screen after checking).	These safety checks are important to prevent complications during the turning procedure.	
2. Push the "Rotate" button.	Must start rotation before turning prone.	
3. Push the "Prone" button.	This will begin instructions for automated prone positioning of the patient.	
4. Push the "Rotate and lower" button. Press and hold button until screen changes.	Surface must be in flat and low position before prone position can be achieved	

Procedure	for Automated Pronation Therapy (Using the RotoProne Therapy System; see Fig. 19-3)—*Continued*	
Steps	**Rationale**	**Special Considerations**
5. "Check tubing," "Check airway," "Check head support," "Check abdominal support," "Check arm slings" (push each button on the screen after checking).	These safety checks are important to prevent complications during the turning procedure.	
6. Reconfirm the face pack and push the button on the touch screen.	Final safety check to assure the face pack is secure before positioning prone to prevent any patient injury.	**Important note:** *The face pack is the only piece without a safety sensor.*
7. Press "Prone." Press and hold the button during the entire turning procedure. (This step can also be accomplished with pushing the "Prone/supine" button on the hand control.) (**Level M***)	This begins the automated prone positioning process.	Release the button if need arises to stop the turning procedure because of kinking or pulling on tubes. It may be helpful to have an additional person present during the actual turning procedure to monitor invasive lines and ventilator tubing to ensure all lines are positioned correctly. In the absence of an additional person, use of the handset at the head of the bed is recommended for turning the patient so all invasive lines and tubes are visible during turning.
8. After the patient is in the prone position, the screen shows additional buttons to "Check tubing," "Check airway," "Check head support" (push each button after checking).	It is important to perform safety checks after the patient is in prone position to assure patient safety.	
9. Press "Rotate."	Patient should rotate 62 degrees to each side while in the prone position as tolerated.	Degree of rotation and pause times on each side can be adjusted based on individual patient response to therapy.
10. Push the "Surface position" button on screen.	This button allows changes in surface height and position.	
11. Place the patient in the reverse Trendelenburg position by pressing the button on screen (push and hold until 11–12 degrees). (**Level M***)	The reverse Trendelenburg position is recommended to keep the head of the bed up to decrease edema and prevent complications associated with feeding or potential aspiration.	
12. Open back hatches in the prone position.	All hatches can be opened to allow for full chest expansion. The foot hatch should be opened and propped open to prevent undue pressure on the heels.	

*Level M: Manufacturer's recommendations only.

Procedure continues on following page

Procedure	for Automated Pronation Therapy (Using the RotoProne Therapy System; see Fig. 19-3)—*Continued*	

Steps	Rationale	Special Considerations
13. Leave patient in the prone position for 3 hours 15 minutes with 62-degree rotation to each side. **(Level C*)**	Recommended time to remain in the prone position is 3 hours 15 minutes, alternating with 45 minutes supine to achieve a total of 19.5 hours prone time in a 24-hour period.[32] After prone time is completed, position the patient supine for 45 minutes as tolerated. The positioning schedule is based on whether the patient is able to sustain improvements in Pao_2 made while in the prone or supine position.	The healthcare team may decide to vary the recommended schedule based on individual patient-care needs. Adjustment of time intervals and rotation times based on the patient's response to therapy may be necessary. Changes to degree of rotation or pause times can be made by pushing the "therapy settings" button. If the need arises to quickly return the patient to the supine position, "CPR buttons" are located on the touch screen and below the screen at the foot of the bed.
14. Discard supplies and remove 〔PE〕.		
15. 〔HH〕		

Turning Supine With the RotoProne Therapy System

1. 〔HH〕		
2. 〔PE〕		
3. Close any open hatches.	All hatches must be closed before moving to the supine position to prevent patient injury. The system will not operate until the hatches are closed.	Make sure all hatches are closed before returning the patient to the supine position.
4. Push the "Supine" button.	Prepares the system to begin the supine function of the surface.	
5. Push the "Rotate and lower" button and hold until screen changes.	Surface must be in the flat and low position before the turning procedure can be achieved	
6. "Check tubing," "Check airway," "Check head support" (push each button after checking).	It is important to perform safety checks to assure patient safety	
7. Press "Supine" and hold the button during the entire turning procedure. (This step can also be accomplished by pushing the "Prone/supine" button on the hand control.) **(Level M*)**	This begins the automated turning process to return the patient to the supine position.	Release the button if need arises to stop the turning procedure because of kinking or pulling on tubes. It may be helpful to have an additional person present during the actual turning procedure to monitor invasive lines and ventilator tubing to ensure all lines are positioned correctly. In the absence of an additional person, use of the handset at the head of the bed is recommended for turning the patient so all invasive lines and tubes are visible during turning.
8. Insert the locking pin after the patient assumes the supine position.	Inserting the locking pin will secure the system in one position and the bed will not alarm when packs are removed from patient.	

*Level C: Qualitative studies, descriptive or correlational studies, integrative reviews, systematic reviews, or randomized controlled trials with inconsistent results.
*Level M: Manufacturer's recommendations only.

Procedure	for Automated Pronation Therapy (Using the RotoProne Therapy System; see Fig. 19-3)—*Continued*	
Steps	**Rationale**	**Special Considerations**
9. Open packs over the patient as needed for patient care.	Allows for easy access to all areas on patient, prevents pressure, and allows for any skin care measures to be provided.	
10. Carefully remove the face pack.	Face pack should be removed in the supine position to prevent undue pressure on the face; this also allows for eye care, oral care, and skin care to be provided as needed.	Care must be taken to prevent dislodging of any tubes positioned within or on the face pack.
11. Rotate the patient supine as tolerated up to 45 minutes or an hour. To rotate patient supine, the bottom pack closest to the foot of the bed, and either the chest or the pelvic pack must be secured over the patient.	Placement of the bottom foot pack and either the chest or the pelvic pack is necessary for supine rotation. Rotation helps provide continued mobilization for oxygenation and reduction of pressure areas	While the patient is supine, complete all assessments and procedures scheduled. After completion, the patient may be rotated in supine position. Placement of the bottom foot pack and either the chest or the pelvic pack is necessary for supine rotation. With automated prone positioning, if the patient is unable to maintain the improvement in gas exchange seen with the prone position when returned to a supine position, the patient can be returned to the prone position. If the patient tolerates the supine position, the patient should optimally remain in the supine/lateral position for only 45 minutes to 1 hour before being repositioned prone.
12. Place in reverse Trendelenburg position to get the head of the bed elevated to maximum 11–12 degrees by pushing the "Surface position" button then "Reverse Trendelenburg." (**Level M***)	The reverse Trendelenburg position is recommended to keep the head of the bed up to decrease edema and prevent complications associated with feeding or potential aspiration.	For increased facial edema, ice packs can also be used. These can be placed over the eyes or lips while in the supine position as needed.
13. Discard used supplies and remove **PE**.		
14. **HH**		

Procedure	for Manual Pronation Therapy With the Vollman Prone Positioner (VPP) (the device is no longer manufactured; see Fig. 19-4)	
Steps	**Rationale**	**Special Considerations**
1. **HH**		
2. **PE**		
3. Bring the VPP to the bedside.	Readies the device for application	With use of the frame, ensure it has been cleaned with an appropriate hospital-approved disinfectant.
4. Ensure that emergency equipment is available.	In the event of an emergency (i.e., accidental extubation or hemodynamic instability), availability of equipment allows for rapid patient stabilization.	

*Level M: Manufacturer's recommendations only.

Procedure continues on following page

Procedure	for Manual Pronation Therapy With the Vollman Prone Positioner (VPP) (the device is no longer manufactured; see Fig. 19-4)—*Continued*	
Steps	**Rationale**	**Special Considerations**
5. Place a lift sheet under the patient to assist with turning.	A lift sheet allows for the use of correct body alignment during the turning procedure.[31,37]	A lift sheet is unnecessary if the patient is on a low air-loss surface and a support frame is used.
6. One staff member is positioned on either side of the bed, with another staff member positioned at the head of the bed.[36,37,40] **(Level C*)**	Three staff members are needed for the turn: two perform the actual lifting and turning, and the third is positioned at the head of the bed.[36,37,40]	The individual at the head of the bed is responsible for monitoring the ETT, ventilator tubing, and monitoring/intravenous lines located by the patient's head.
7. Correctly position all tubes and invasive lines.	All intravenous tubing and invasive lines are adjusted to prevent kinking, disconnection, or contact with the body during the turning procedure and while the patient remains in the prone position.	For increased airway security, the individual at the head of the bed should hold the ETT during the turn.[31,37]
A. Lines inserted in the upper torso are aligned with either shoulder, and the excess tubing is placed at the head of the bed. The only exception to this rule is for chest tubes or other large-bore tubes (e.g., tubes used for extracorporeal membrane oxygenation).	Disconnecting lines before the turn may help to prevent dislodgment but places the patient at an increased risk for infection.	If the patient is in skeletal traction, one individual needs to apply traction to the leg while the lines and weights are removed for the turn. If a skeletal pin comes into contact with the bed, a pillow needs to be placed in the correct position to alleviate pressure points.
B. Chest tubes and lines or tubes placed in the lower torso are aligned with either leg and extend off the end of the bed.	Consider addition of an extension tube to lines that are too short to be placed at the head of the bed or the end of the bed.	
C. If the patient has an open abdomen, cover with a synthetic material or vacuum dressing before positioning and identify a positioning strategy that allows the abdomen to be free of restriction.	Open abdomens are not a contraindication for use of the prone position. A cover with a synthetic material and a support such as an abdominal binder may be used effectively to secure the abdomen.[25]	
8. If on a low air-loss surface, maximally inflate.	Maximally inflating the air surface firms up the mattress, making the turn easier to perform.	

*Level C: Qualitative studies, descriptive or correlational studies, integrative reviews, systematic reviews, or randomized controlled trials with inconsistent results.

Procedure	for Manual Pronation Therapy With the Vollman Prone Positioner (VPP) (the device is no longer manufactured; see Fig. 19-4)—*Continued*	
Steps	**Rationale**	**Special Considerations**
9. Always turn the patient in the direction of the mechanical ventilator.	Helps to maximize the length of the tubing and prevents pulling, which may dislodge the position of the ETT.	
A. Turn the patient's head so that it faces away from the ventilator. Without disconnecting the ventilator tubing from the ETT, place the portion of the tubing that extends out from the ETT on the side of the patient's face that is turned away from the ventilator.	Helps to maximize the length of the tubing and prevents pulling which may dislodge the position of the ETT.	
B. Loop the remaining ventilator tubing above the patient's head.[36,37,40] **(Level C*)**	Helps to maximize the length of the tubing and prevents pulling, which may dislodge the position of the ETT.	
10. The straps that secure the positioner to the body are placed under the patient's head, chest (axillary area), and pelvic region at this time.	Prepares the patient for placement of the VPP to minimize the amount of time during which the device is on top of the patient.	
Placing the Vollman Prone Positioner		
1. Attach the frame to the patient while the patient is in the supine position. Lay the frame gently on top of the patient. Align the chest piece to rest between the clavicle and sixth rib.[36,37,40] **(Level C)**	The chest piece is the only nonmovable part and serves as the marker piece for proper placement and alignment of the device.[36,40]	
2. Adjust the pelvic piece to rest one-half inch above the iliac crest.[36,37,40] **(Level C)**	This placement prevents direct pressure over bony prominences and provides sufficient distance between the chest and pelvis to allow the abdomen to be free of restriction and prevents bowing of the back.[36,40]	
3. Adjust the forehead and chin pieces to provide full facial support in a face-down or a side-lying position without interfering with the ETT.	Allows for correct support without interfering with the clinician's ability to access the ETT.	If the patient has limited neck range of motion or a short neck, the face-down position is optimal. Because readjusting the head to relieve pressure points is difficult, moving both headpieces up to the top of the frame is recommended. Only the head cushion supports the forehead, and the chin is suspended to reduce the risk of skin breakdown from pressure.

*Level C: Qualitative studies, descriptive or correlational studies, integrative reviews, systematic reviews, or randomized controlled trials with inconsistent results.

Procedure continues on following page

Procedure	for Manual Pronation Therapy With the Vollman Prone Positioner (VPP) (the device is no longer manufactured; see Fig. 19-4)—*Continued*

Steps	Rationale	Special Considerations
4. Fasten the positioner to the patient with the soft adjustable straps. As the straps are tightened, the cushions compress. When fastened, lift the positioner to assess whether a secure fit has been obtained. Readjust as necessary. (**Level M***)	If the device is not secured tightly before the turn, the patient may have shear or friction injuries develop on the chest and pelvic area during the turning process.	When the device is secured correctly, it appears uncomfortable and possibly painful. As a result, the practitioner has a tendency not to fasten the device as tightly as is needed to prevent injury. When secured correctly, the device creates a feeling of pressure and a sense of security for the patient during the turning process.

Turning Prone With the Half-Step Technique

Steps	Rationale	Special Considerations
1. With a draw sheet, move the patient to the edge of the bed farthest away from the ventilator in preparation for the prone turn. The individual closest to the patient maintains body contact with the bed at all times, serving as a side rail to ensure a safe environment. (**Level C***)	Provides sufficient room to rotate the body safely 180 degrees within the confines of a narrow critical care bed.[36,37,40]	
2. Turning with the VPP:		
A. Tuck the straps on the bar located between the chest and pelvic piece underneath the patient. (**Level C**)	Helps with forward motion when the turning process begins.[36,37,40]	
B. Tuck the patient's arm and hand that now rest in the center of the bed under the buttocks, after position alignment with the edge of the mattress is achieved. (**Level C**)	Helps with forward motion when the turning process begins.[36,37,40]	
C. Cross the leg closest to the edge of the bed over the opposite leg at the ankle.[36,37,40] (**Level C**)	Helps with forward motion when the turning process begins.[36,37,40]	
3. Turn the patient to a 45-degree angle toward the ventilator.	Use of a wide base of support is extremely important to improve balance and prevent self-injury during the turning procedure.[36,40]	
A. The staff member on the ventilator side of the bed grips the upper steel bar.	Positions staff to be ready for the turn.	
B. The staff member on the opposite side of the bed grasps the straps attached to the lower steel bar.	Positions staff to be ready for the turn.	
C. With a three count, lift the patient by the frame into a prone position.	Count of three provides coordination of effort among the team members.	

*Level C: Qualitative studies, descriptive or correlational studies, integrative reviews, systematic reviews, or randomized controlled trials with inconsistent results.
*Level M: Manufacturer's recommendations only

Procedure	for Manual Pronation Therapy With the Vollman Prone Positioner (VPP) (the device is no longer manufactured; see Fig. 19-4)—*Continued*	
Steps	**Rationale**	**Special Considerations**
D. During the turning procedure, the staff member at the head of the bed ensures that all tubes and lines are secure and patent.[36,37] **(Level C*)**	Provides an extra measure of safety for the ETTs and invasive lines.	
4. Loosen the straps at this time. If the patient is unstable, keeping the straps fastened securely is recommended to facilitate a safe quick return to the supine position in the event of an emergency.	The procedure for returning to the supine position takes less than 1 minute if the straps are fastened and a support frame is used.	
5. Gently rotate the arms parallel to the body, then flex them into a position of comfort so that they are lying adjacent to the head. Minor adjustments of the patient's body may be necessary to obtain correct alignment when in the prone position.	To prevent damage to the brachial plexus.	Many patients have range-of-motion limitations to the shoulder area that may make keeping the arms in a flexed position difficult. Many ways can be used to position the arms for comfort. The arms can be left in a side-lying position, aligned with the body, or positioned one up and one down, similar to a swimmer position.[31]
6. If on a low air-loss surface, release the maximal inflation.	A return to normal pressures on the surface helps to alleviate pressure at various bony prominences in the prone position.	If on a standard hospital mattress, the thigh-knee-calf area must be supported to minimize the risk of pressure injury and prevent discomfort.[31,36,37,40]
7. Place a support or other pillow under the ankle area.	A support in this area allows for correct body alignment and prevents tension on the tendons in the foot and ankle region.	If the patient is tall enough, dangling the feet over the edge of the mattress may be a sufficient alternative to support the ankles and feet in correct alignment.
8. Discard used supplies and remove PE.		
9. HH		
Returning to the Supine Position		
1. HH		
2. PE		
3. Align the patient with the edge of the mattress closest to the ventilator.	Provides sufficient room to rotate the body safely 180 degrees within the confines of a narrow critical care bed.[36,40]	The patient turns toward the center of the mattress, away from the ventilator.
4. Arrange the ventilator tubing to provide sufficient mobility and length to prevent pulling during the turning procedure.	The staff member at the head of the bed is responsible for monitoring placement of the ventilator tubing, monitoring wires, and invasive lines.	
5. Straighten the patient's arms from a flexed position and bring them to rest on either side of the head. Remove leg and ankle pillow supports. If on a low air-loss surface, maximally inflate.	To prevent damage to the brachial plexus area and ready the patient for return to the supine position.	

*Level C: Qualitative studies, descriptive or correlational studies, integrative reviews, systematic reviews, or randomized controlled trials with inconsistent results.

Procedure continues on following page

Procedure	for Manual Pronation Therapy With the Vollman Prone Positioner (VPP) (the device is no longer manufactured; see Fig. 19-4)—*Continued*	
Steps	**Rationale**	**Special Considerations**
6. Cross the leg closest to the edge of the bed over the opposite leg at the ankle.	Prepares the patient for turning.	
7. Stretch the arms parallel to the body and bring them into a downward position.	The process is used to prevent any brachial plexus injury.	
8. With the VPP: fasten the straps tightly before repositioning.	If the device is not secured tightly before the turn, the patient may have shear or friction injuries develop on the chest and pelvic area during the turning process.	
9. Turn the patient to a 45-degree angle with the steel bars, then roll the patient onto his or her back.	The steel bars on the positioning frame allow lifting as the patient is realigned into the center of the bed.	
10. Unfasten the positioner and remove from the patient. The straps may be left under the patient in preparation for the next turn.	The device comes with two sets of straps. The straps were designed to be left underneath the patient to allow for ease of the next prone positioning cycle.	
11. Discard used supplies and remove **PE**.		
12. **HH**		

Expected Outcomes

- Increased oxygenation
- Improved secretion clearance
- Improved compliance of the lungs and alveolar recruitment
- Improved mortality

Unexpected Outcomes

- Agitation
- Disconnection or dislodgment of tubes and lines
- Peripheral arm nerve injury
- Periorbital and conjunctival edema
- Skin injuries or pressure ulcers
- Eye pressure or injury

Patient Monitoring and Care

Steps	**Rationale**	**Reportable Conditions**
		These conditions should be reported if they persist despite nursing interventions.
1. Assess the patient's tolerance to the turning procedure: • Respiratory rate and effort • Heart rate and blood pressure	Oxygen saturation is not used as a measure of intolerance to the turning procedure because patients often have desaturation with a deep lateral turn; however, if the patient responds to the prone position, the condition stabilizes quickly when settled into the prone position. The lateral-turn decrease in oxygen saturation may deter the healthcare team from trying the prone position. If respiratory rate and effort, heart rate, and blood pressure do not return to normal within 10 minutes of the turn, the patient may be displaying initial signs of intolerance.[37,39,43]	• Failure of the respiratory rate, respiratory effort, heart rate, and blood pressure to return to normal 5–10 minutes after the turn[39]

Patient Monitoring and Care —*Continued*

Steps	Rationale	Reportable Conditions
2. Assess the patient's response to the prone position: • Pulse oximetry (SpO_2) • Mixed venous oxygenation saturation (SvO_2) or central mixed venous oxygen saturation ($ScvO_2$) and hemodynamics • Arterial blood gases 30 minutes after position change • PaO_2/FiO_2 ratio	Of all patients with acute lung injury turned prone, more than 70% had improvement in oxygenation.[4,5,10,13,17,23–25,27,28,35,40] A response is defined by a PaO_2/FiO_2 ratio greater than 20% or a PaO_2 greater than 10 mm Hg.[29] The time response varies among patients. Some patients immediately respond, whereas others may take a longer time to show maximal response to the position change. Hemodynamic measurements are accurate in the prone position compared with supine as long as the zero reference point is calibrated at the phlebostatic axis.[38]	• Decrease from baseline in the SpO_2 or failure of the SvO_2 or $ScvO_2$ to return to baseline after 5–10 minutes
3. With manual proning, reposition the patient's head on an hourly basis in the prone position to prevent facial breakdown. While one staff member lifts the patient's head, a second staff member moves the headpieces to provide support for the head in a different position. (**Level D***) Not necessary with automated proning. Arms should be positioned for comfort by either placing them aligned with the body or in a swimmer's position, one up and one down.	The face and ears have minimal structural padding to reduce the risk of skin breakdown. Patients with short necks or limited neck range of motion have difficulty assuming a head side-lying position. These patients are more likely to have facial breakdown develop, making turning the patient more frequently or use of the previous technique necessary to prevent breakdown.[18,31,37]	• Skin breakdown
4. Assess skin frequently for areas of nonblanchable redness or breakdown. Place a hydrocolloid dressing or 5-layer silicone dressing over areas where shearing and friction injuries are likely to occur (i.e., chest, pelvis, elbows, and knees). (**Level M***)	Greater than 2 hours on a standard surface without changing position increases a patient's risk for breakdown. If the patient is on a pressure-reduction surface, the time remaining in a stationary position can be lengthened.[18] The use of a hydrocolloid or a 5-layer silicone dressing may serve as a protective barrier, reducing the risk of pressure, shearing, and friction injuries.[18,31,37] If VPP is used and a skin injury occurs on the chest or pelvis, reassess tightness of the device before the prone position turn. The injury is most often related to a loose-fitting apparatus and is likely a shear injury versus pressure.	• Nonblanchable redness • Shearing and friction injuries

*Level D: Peer-reviewed professional and organizational standards with the support of clinical study recommendations.
*Level M: Manufacturer's recommendations only.

Procedure continues on following page

Patient Monitoring and Care —*Continued*

Steps	Rationale	Reportable Conditions
5. Provide frequent oral care and suctioning of the airway as needed.	The prone position promotes postural drainage through the natural use of gravity. Drainage from the nares may be a clinical sign of an undetected sinus infection.	• Drainage from the nares • Change in amount or character of secretions
6. Maintain eye care to prevent corneal abrasions.	It is important to maintain lubrication via institutional standard protocol to prevent dryness leading to cornel abrasions.	• Changes in the conditions of the eyes
7. Maintain tube feeding as tolerated. **(Level D*)**[33] **(Level C*)**[25]	The risk for aspiration is minimal in the prone position because the patient is already in a head-down, side-lying position that maximizes the use of gravity to move vomited matter safely. A reverse Trendelenburg position changes that relationship. It may reduce the risk of microaspiration and may increase the risk of a large emesis occurring.[38] Use of prokinetic agents or transpyloric feedings is recommended to prevent complications associated with vomiting. Studies have shown increased risk of complications in the prone position in patients receiving gastric feedings. These studies recommend use of promotility agents or postpyloric feedings to reduce the risk of complications such as vomiting and enhance gastric emptying.[30]	• Evidence of tube feeding material when suctioning

8. Scheduling frequency: the positioning schedule is based on the most recent RCT, which suggests at least 16 hours of prone positioning a day.[17]
  A. Time spent in the supine position is based on the length of time the patient is able to sustain or maintain the improvement in gas exchange that occurred while prone. This time may be consecutive or sequential depending on the type of apparatus used and the risk of skin injury and hemodynamic instability experienced.[4,5,13,17,23,27,35,37]
    (Level C)
  B. For automated proning with the RotoProne Therapy System, the suggested time in the prone position is 3 hours 15 minutes prone alternating with 45 minutes as tolerated in the supine position.
	Although the literature demonstrates that longer times in the prone position within a 24-hour period is better, it remains important that the healthcare team weigh other physiological factors when a patient remains in any stationary position for an extended period. Following the principles of pressure relief used when positioning patients laterally or supine can minimize the potential for skin injury and edema formation. Longer time spent in a single position necessitates that the support surface provides greater pressure reduction or relief than a standard hospital mattress.[31,37]
	(Level C)
		• Clinically significant decreases in oxygenation (>10 mm Hg) or oxygen saturation (<88%)

*Level C: Qualitative studies, descriptive or correlational studies, integrative reviews, systematic reviews, or randomized controlled trials with inconsistent results.
*Level D: Peer-reviewed professional and organizational standards with the support of clinical study recommendations.

Patient Monitoring and Care —*Continued*

Steps	Rationale	Reportable Conditions
9. Manual prone positioning should be discontinued if the following criteria have been met: • Improvement in oxygenation defined as PaO_2/FIO_2 ratio <150 mm Hg, with an FIO_2 <60% with ≤10 cm of PEEP (these criteria had to be met in the supine position at least 4 hours after the end of the last prone session). • PaO_2/FIO_2 ratio of more than 20% relative to the ratio in the supine position before two consecutive prone sessions. 10. With automated prone positioning, if the patient is unable to maintain the improvement in gas exchange seen with the prone position when returned to a supine position, the patient can be returned to the prone position. If the patient tolerates supine position, the patient should optimally remain in the supine/lateral position for only 45 minutes to 1 hour before being repositioned prone.	Use of lateral rotation therapy in conjunction with prone positioning is suggested so that when the patient is returned to a supine position, he or she is laterally rotated. The use of continuous lateral rotation therapy has been associated with a reduction in pulmonary complications.[15,24,31,37]	• Complications occurring during a prone session leading to its immediate interruption, including nonscheduled extubation, main-stem bronchus intubation, ETT obstruction, hemoptysis, oxygen saturation of <85% for >10 minutes or a PaO_2 of <55 mm Hg for more than 5 minutes. When the FIO_2 was at 100%, cardiac arrest, a heart rate of <30 bpm for more than 1 minute, systolic blood pressure of less than 60 for more than 5 minutes, and any other life-threatening reason.[17] (**Level B***)

*Level B: Well-designed, controlled studies with results that consistently support a specific action, intervention, or treatment.

Documentation

Documentation should include the following:
- Patient and family education
- Ability to tolerate the turning procedure
- Length of time in the prone position
- Maximal oxygenation response in the prone position
- Oxygenation response when returned to the supine position
- Positioning schedule used
- Complications noted during or after the procedure
- Use of continuous lateral rotation therapy or other devices
- Amount and type of secretions
- Unexpected outcomes
- Nursing interventions

References and Additional Readings

For a complete list of references and additional readings for this procedure, scan this QR code with any freely available smartphone code reader app, or visit http://booksite.elsevier.com/9780323376624.

PROCEDURE

20   Autotransfusion

Kelly McGinty

PURPOSE: Autotransfusion is the collection of the patient's own blood from an active bleeding source within the thoracic cavity, due to trauma or surgery, which is then reinfused to maintain the patient's blood volume.

PREREQUISITE NURSING KNOWLEDGE

- Understanding of infusion therapy and fluid balance is necessary.[8]
- Autotransfusion is commonly used for trauma victims and for patients undergoing cardiothoracic procedures, reducing the need for bank blood transfusions and the associated risks of transfusion reactions and disease transmission.[4,11]
- Indications for autotransfusion include patients that are losing more than 100 mL of blood an hour or collecting more than 300 mL in a collection system.[5,6,11–14]
- A variety of autotransfusion devices are available. Autotransfusion may be a component of a standard water-seal or dry-chest-drainage system (see Fig. 25-1) or a separate system and may be continuous or intermittent.
  - ❖ Continuous systems have an intravenous line connected directly to the patient from the chest-drainage collection unit, via an intravenous pump.
  - ❖ Intermittent systems have an autotransfusion bag that collects the blood either in-line or directly from the chest-drainage collection unit. The autotransfusion bag is disconnected from the chest-drainage collection unit connected to a saline primed blood administration infusion set for delivery to the patient.
- Nurses should be familiar with their institution's autotransfusion system, policies, and procedures.
- Contraindications to autotransfusion include the following:[4,8,10]
  - ❖ Septicemia
  - ❖ Malignant cells in the blood shed
  - ❖ Renal or hepatic insufficiency
  - ❖ Coagulopathies
  - ❖ Blood that has been in the collection system for longer than institutional standards allow
  - ❖ Any of these contraindications may be overruled if the patient is exsanguinating and there is not an adequate supply of banked blood available.[4]

- Patient (or surrogate) consent should always be obtained before any blood infusion in a nonemergent setting. Patients have the right to know risks and benefits of receiving transfusions of any kind. Emergent transfusions will usually include allogeneic blood transfusions and should be administered per institutional protocol.[1,7]
- Patients (or their surrogate) may decline autotransfusions due to religious beliefs. Jehovah's Witnesses may be open to receiving salvaged blood as long as it is not processed and remains attached to their person throughout the collection process. However, consent for transfusion in this population should be strongly considered given their religious views regarding transfusions.[7]

EQUIPMENT

- Personal protection equipment (i.e., gloves, mask, eyeshield)
- Chest-drainage unit
- Autotransfusion collection system
- Blood administration set
- 40-μm microemboli filter
- Normal saline
- Wall suction and regulator

PATIENT AND FAMILY EDUCATION

- If time permits, assess the patient's and family's level of understanding about the condition and rationale for the procedure. **Rationale:** This assessment identifies the patient's and family's knowledge deficits concerning the patient's condition, the procedure, the expected benefits, and the potential risks. It also allows time for questions to clarify information and voice concerns. Explanations decrease patient anxiety and enhance cooperation.
- Explain the procedure and the reason for the procedure, if the clinical situation permits. If not, explain the procedure and reason for the intubation after it is completed. **Rationale:** This explanation enhances patient and family understanding and decreases anxiety.

PATIENT ASSESSMENT AND PREPARATION

Patient Assessment

- Patient should be assessed for signs and symptoms of hypovolemia and shock, which include the following:[4,5,11-14]
  - ❖ Pale, cool, clammy skin
  - ❖ Dyspnea
  - ❖ Tachycardia
  - ❖ Hypotension
  - ❖ Decreased cardiac output or index
  - ❖ Oliguria
  - ❖ Decreased hemoglobin and/or hematocrit
  - ❖ Decreased central venous pressure, pulmonary artery pressure, or pulmonary wedge pressure.

Rationale: Significant blood loss, related systemic hypoperfusion, and the associated decrease in oxygen-carrying capacity, with its effect on hypoxemia, often require the replacement of blood with whole blood or packed red blood cells. In appropriate patient populations (trauma or cardiovascular), autotransfusion should be considered as the need to replace blood becomes apparent.[4,5,11-14]

Patient Preparation

- Ensure the patient (or his or her surrogate) understands the procedural education. Answer questions as they arise, and reinforce information as needed. *Rationale:* This communication evaluates and reinforces understanding of previously provided education.

Procedure	**for Autotransfusion**	
Steps	**Rationale**	**Special Considerations**
1. **HH**		
2. **PE**		
3. Assemble collection system.	Prepares the equipment.	Wall suction will be required to facilitate drainage into chest-drainage system.
4. Addition of anticoagulant into the autotransfusion bag before collecting the blood may be considered, depending on the institution's protocol or manufactures' instructions. **(Level E*)**	There are various anticoagulants that can be used during this transfusion. Citrate phosphate dextrose 2 (CPD2) is commonly used (1 mL per 7 mL blood).[1,3,7,9]	Follow institutional protocol.
5. Connect the patient's drainage system or chest tube to the collection bag directly or via a water-seal system.	Allows for collection of shed blood.	
6. Before disconnecting the filled collection bag for infusion, prepare new collecting bag.	Prevents infection by keeping transfusion system closed and sterile.	
7. Close clamp or clamp tubes on the new collection bag.	Prevents air from entering the system.	
8. Close the clamp on the chest-drainage system.	Stops drainage while changing tubing and adding new collection bag, again decreasing chance for infection and exposure to blood-borne pathogens.	If the collection bag is part of the water-seal system, close the clamps to the water-seal drainage unit. Prepares system for changing of collection bags and prevents infection or air entering system.
9. Disconnect the filled bag from the patient system, maintaining sterility at all times.	Prepares the filled bag for administration of the shed blood to the patient.	
10. Take the previously prepared new collection bag; attach it to the water-seal unit or to the patient's chest tube or drainage tube.	Prepares the chest-drainage system for the collection of further shed blood, if necessary.	

*Level E: Multiple case reports, theory-based evidence from expert opinions, or peer-reviewed professional organizational standards without clinical studies to support recommendations.

Procedure continues on following page

Procedure   for Autotransfusion—*Continued*

Steps	Rationale	Special Considerations
11. Confirm that all connections are secured; open clamps on the autotransfusion bag and patient drainage tubing.	Ensures integrity of the system.	
12. Prime the blood-administration tubing with normal saline.	Prepares the blood-administration set for shed blood infusion.	Do not apply pressure or use with pressure device during transfusion.
13. Add the microfilter to the blood side of the tubing and connect filled collection bag.[1,3,4,9,14] **(Level E*)**	Prevents microembolization from the shed blood.	A 40-mcg filter is always used when transfusing salvaged blood to prevent microembolization.
14. Initiate infusion of the shed blood. **(Level D*)**	Restores blood volume.	Reinfuse blood within 6 hours of collection and ensure it is complete within 4 hours of starting the infusion.[1–3]
15. Repeat this procedure as needed based on reassessment of patient following initial transfusion.	Restores blood volume.	
16. Discard supplies and equipment and remove **PE**.		
17. **HH**		

*Level D: Peer-reviewed professional and organizational standards with the support of clinical study recommendations.
*Level E: Multiple case reports, theory-based evidence from expert opinions, or peer-reviewed professional organizational standards without clinical studies to support recommendations.

Expected Outcomes

- Patient infused with own blood in a timely manner
- Improved hemoglobin and hematocrit
- Improved oxygenation
- Hemodynamic stability

Unexpected Outcomes

- Blood transfusion reaction
- Fluid overload
- Infection; septicemia

Patient Monitoring and Care

Steps	Rationale	Reportable Conditions
		These conditions should be reported if they persist despite nursing interventions.
1. Assess cardiopulmonary status and vital signs every 15 minutes, until 1 hour after transfusion is completed.	Provides baseline and ongoing assessment of the patient's condition.	• Tachycardia • Hypoxia or hypoxemia • Jugular vein distention • Hypotension • Dysrhythmias • Fever
2. Evaluate and maintain chest tube patency every 2 hours.	Obstruction of the drainage interferes with drainage of blood from the chest.	• Inability to establish patency

Patient Monitoring and Care —*Continued*

Steps	Rationale	Reportable Conditions
3. Monitor the amount of blood accumulation in the chest-drainage unit and mark the drainage on the outside of the unit in hourly or shift increments, as necessary.	Volume loss can cause patients to become hypovolemic.	• Blood accumulation of >200 mL/hr • New onset of clots • Sudden decrease or absence of drainage
4. Monitor for blood-transfusion reaction.	A patient receiving autotransfusion is unlikely to experience a blood-transfusion reaction.	• Fever >101°F (38.5°C) • Chills • Tachycardia • Abdominal or back pain • Hypotension • Hematuria

Documentation

Documentation should include the following:

- Patient and surrogate education
- Amount of drainage
- Amount of transfusion volume
- Date and start time of collection and when it was infused

- Patient response, including vital signs
- Nursing interventions
- Unexpected outcomes

References and Additional Readings

For a complete list of references and additional readings for this procedure, scan this QR code with any freely available smartphone code reader app, or visit http://booksite.elsevier.com/9780323376624.

21 Chest Tube Placement (Perform)

Julie Waters

PURPOSE: Chest tubes are placed for the removal or drainage of air, blood, or fluid from the intrapleural space. They also are used to introduce sclerosing agents into the pleural space to prevent a reaccumulation of fluid.

PREREQUISITE NURSING KNOWLEDGE

- The thoracic cavity is a closed airspace in normal conditions. Any disruption results in the loss of negative pressure within the intrapleural space. Air or fluid that enters the space competes with the lung, resulting in collapse of the lung. Associated conditions are the result of disease, injury, surgery, or iatrogenic causes.
- Chest tubes are sterile flexible polyvinyl chloride (PVC) or silicone nonthrombogenic catheters approximately 20 inches (51 cm) long, varying in size from 8 to 40 Fr. The size of the tube placed is determined by the indication and viscosity of the drainage.[6] The side of the chest tube usually has a radiopaque strip down the side to assist in visualization on chest radiographs.
- Indications for chest tube insertion include the following:
  - Pneumothorax (collection of air in the pleural space)
  - Hemothorax (collection of blood)
  - Hemopneumothorax (accumulation of air and blood in the pleural space)
  - Thoracotomy (e.g., open heart surgery, pneumonectomy)
  - Pyothorax or empyema (collection of pus)
  - Chylothorax (collection of chyle from the thoracic duct)
  - Cholothorax (collection of fluid containing bile)
  - Hydrothorax (collection of noninflammatory serous fluid)
  - Pleural effusion
  - Pleurodesis (instillation of anesthetic solutions and sclerosing agents)
- Chest tubes inserted for traumatic hemopneumothorax or hemothorax (blood) should be large (36 to 40 Fr). Medium tubes (24 to 36 Fr) should be used for fluid accumulation (pleural effusions). Tubes inserted for pneumothorax (air) should be small (≤24 Fr).[2,6]

- A pneumothorax may be classified as an open, closed, or tension pneumothorax.
  - *Open pneumothorax:* The chest wall and the pleural space are penetrated, which allows air to enter the pleural space, as in a penetrating injury or trauma; a surgical incision in the thoracic cavity (i.e., thoracotomy); or a complication of surgical treatment (e.g., unintentional puncture during invasive procedures, such as thoracentesis or central venous catheter insertion).
  - *Closed pneumothorax:* The pleural space is penetrated, but the chest wall is intact, which allows air to enter the pleural space from within the lung, as in spontaneous pneumothorax. A closed pneumothorax occurs without apparent injury and often is seen in individuals with chronic lung disorders (e.g., emphysema, cystic fibrosis, tuberculosis, necrotizing pneumonia) and in young, tall men who have a greater than normal height-to-width chest ratio; after blunt traumatic injury; or iatrogenically, occurring as a complication of medical treatment (e.g., intermittent positive-pressure breathing, mechanical ventilation with positive end-expiratory pressure).
  - *Tension pneumothorax:* Air leaks into the pleural space through a tear in the lung and has no means to escape from the pleural cavity, creating a one-way valve effect. With each breath the patient takes, air accumulates and pressure within the pleural space increases, and the lung collapses. This condition causes the mediastinal structures (i.e., heart, great vessels, and trachea) to be compressed and shift to the opposite or unaffected side of the chest. Venous return and cardiac output are impeded, and collapse of the unaffected lung is possible. This life-threatening emergency requires prompt recognition and intervention.
- *Absolute Contraindications:* A lung that is densely adherent to the chest wall throughout the hemithorax is an absolute contraindication to chest tube therapy.[5]
- *Relative Contraindications:* Use of chest tubes in patients with multiple adhesions, giant blebs, or coagulopathies should be carefully considered; however, these relative contraindications are superseded by the need to reexpand the lung. When possible, any coagulopathy or platelet defect should be corrected before chest tube insertion. The differential diagnosis between a pneumothorax

---

AP This procedure should be performed only by physicians, advanced practice nurses, and other healthcare professionals (including critical care nurses) with additional knowledge, skills, and demonstrated competence per professional licensure or institutional standard.

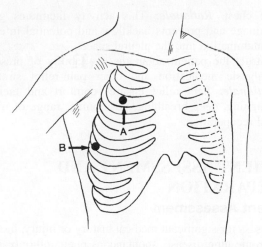

Figure 21-1 Standard sites for tube thoracostomy. **A,** The second intercostal space, midclavicular line. **B,** The fourth or fifth intercostal space, midaxillary line. Most clinicians prefer midaxillary line placement for all chest tubes, regardless of pathology. Placement of the tube too far posteriorly does not allow the patient to lie down comfortably. *(From Roberts JR, Hedges JR, editors: Clinicals in emergency medicine, ed 4, Philadelphia, 2004, Saunders.)*

and bullous disease necessitates careful radiological assessment.[5]

- Ultrasound guidance for chest tube placement is strongly recommended because it can localize fluid accumulation and decrease the risk of complications.[3]
- Chest tubes should be inserted into the "triangle of safety." This is an area bordered inferiorly by a horizontal line at the level of the fifth intercostal space, anteriorly by the lateral border of the pectoralis major, and posteriorly by the lateral border of the latissimus dorsi.[3]
- The tube size and insertion site selected for the chest tube are determined by the indication.[5,6] If draining air, the tube is placed near the apex of the lung (second intercostal space); if draining fluid, the tube is placed near the base of the lung (fourth or fifth intercostal space; Fig. 21-1).
  - ❖ Once the tube is in place, it should be sutured to the skin to prevent displacement, and an occlusive dressing applied (Fig. 21-2). The chest tube also is connected to a chest drainage system (see Procedure 25) to remove air and fluid from the pleural space, which facilitates reexpansion of the collapsed lung. All connection points are secured with tape or zip ties (Parham Martin bands) to ensure that the system remains airtight (Fig. 21-3).
  - ❖ The water-seal chamber should bubble gently immediately on insertion of the chest tube during expiration and with coughing. Continuous bubbling in this chamber indicates a leak within the patient or in the chest-drainage system. Fluctuations in the water level in the water-seal chamber of 5 to 10 cm, rising during inhalation and falling during expiration, should be observed with spontaneous respirations. If the patient is on mechanical ventilation, the pattern of fluctuation is just the opposite. Any suction applied must be disconnected temporarily to assess correctly for fluctuations in the water-seal chamber.

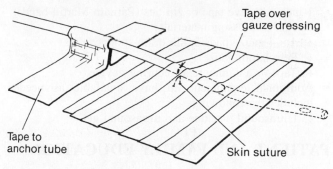

Figure 21-2 Occlusive chest tube dressing. *(From Kersten LD: Comprehensive respiratory nursing, Philadelphia, 1989, Saunders.)*

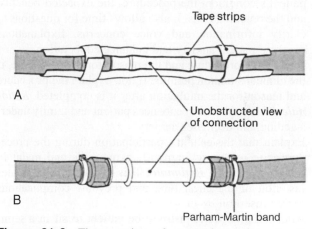

Figure 21-3 The securing of connection points. **A,** Tape. **B,** Parham-Martin bands. *(From Kersten LD: Comprehensive respiratory nursing, Philadelphia, 1989, Saunders.)*

EQUIPMENT

- Caps, masks, sterile gloves, gowns, drapes
- Protective eyewear (goggles)
- Antiseptic solution: 2% chlorhexidine or povidone-iodine
- Local anesthetic: 1% or 2% lidocaine solution (with or without epinephrine)
- 10-mL syringe with 20-gauge 1½-inch needle
- 5-mL syringe with 25-gauge 1-inch needle
- Tube thoracostomy insertion tray
  - ❖ Sterile towels, 4 × 4 sterile gauze
  - ❖ Scalpel with No. 10 or 11 blade
  - ❖ Two Kelly clamps
  - ❖ Needle holder
  - ❖ Monofilament or silk suture material (No. 0 or 1-0)
  - ❖ Sterile basin or medicine cup
  - ❖ Suture scissors
  - ❖ Two hemostats
- Thoracostomy tubes (8 to 40 Fr, as appropriate)
- Closed chest-drainage system
- Suction source
- Suction connector and connecting tubing (usually 6 feet for each tube)

- 1-inch adhesive tape or zip ties (Parham-Martin bands)
- Occlusive dressing materials:
  - ❖ 4 × 4 gauze pads or slit drain sponges
  - ❖ Petrolatum gauze
  - ❖ Tape or a commercial securing device
- Additional equipment, to have available as needed, includes the following:
  - ❖ Ultrasound machine and ultrasound gel

PATIENT AND FAMILY EDUCATION

- If time permits, assess the patient's and family's level of understanding about the condition and rationale for the procedure. *Rationale:* This assessment identifies the patient's and family's knowledge deficits concerning the patient's condition, the procedure, the expected benefits, and the potential risks. It also allows time for questions to clarify information and voice concerns. Explanations decrease patient anxiety and enhance cooperation.
- Explain the procedure and the reason for the procedure, if the clinical situation permits. If not, explain the procedure and reason for the intubation after it is completed. *Rationale:* This explanation enhances patient and family understanding and decreases anxiety.
- Explain that the patient's participation during the procedure is to remain as immobile as possible and maintain relaxed breathing. *Rationale:* This explanation facilitates insertion of the chest tube and prevents complications during insertion.
- After the procedure, instruct the patient to sit in a semi-Fowler's position (unless contraindicated). *Rationale:* This position facilitates drainage, if present, from the pleural space by allowing air to rise and fluid to settle to be removed via the chest tube. This position also makes breathing easier.
- Instruct the patient to turn and change position every 2 hours. The patient may lie on the side with the chest tube but should keep the tubing free of kinks. *Rationale:* Turning and changing position may prevent complications related to immobility and retained pulmonary secretions. Keeping the tube free of kinks maintains patency of the tube, facilitates drainage, and prevents the accumulation of pressure within the pleural space that interferes with lung reexpansion.
- Instruct the patient to cough and deep breathe, with splinting of the affected side. *Rationale:* Coughing and deep breathing increase pressure within the pleural space, facilitating drainage, promoting lung reexpansion, and preventing respiratory complications associated with retained secretions. The application of firm pressure over the chest tube insertion site (i.e., splinting) may decrease pain and discomfort.
- Encourage active or passive range-of-motion exercises of the arm on the affected side. *Rationale:* The patient may limit movement of the arm on the affected side to decrease the discomfort at the insertion site, which may result in joint discomfort and potential joint contractures.
- Instruct the patient and family about activity as prescribed while maintaining the drainage system below the level of

the chest. *Rationale:* This activity facilitates gravity drainage and prevents backflow and potential infectious contamination into the pleural space.
- Instruct the patient about the availability of prescribed analgesic medication and other pain-relief strategies. *Rationale:* Pain relief ensures comfort and facilitates coughing, deep breathing, positioning, range of motion, and recuperation.

PATIENT ASSESSMENT AND PREPARATION

Patient Assessment

- Assess for significant medical history or injury, including chronic lung disease, spontaneous pneumothorax, hemothorax, pulmonary disease, therapeutic procedures, and mechanism of injury. *Rationale:* Medical history or injury may provide the etiological basis for the occurrence of pneumothorax, empyema, pleural effusion, or chylothorax.
- Evaluate diagnostic test results (if patient's condition does not necessitate immediate intervention), including chest radiograph and arterial blood gases. *Rationale:* Diagnostic testing confirms the presence of air or fluid in the pleural space, a collapsed lung, hypoxemia, and respiratory compromise.
- Assess baseline cardiopulmonary status for signs and symptoms that necessitate chest tube insertion.[4] *Rationale:* Accurate assessment of signs and symptoms allows for prompt recognition and treatment. Baseline assessment provides comparison data for evaluation of changes and outcomes of treatment.
  - ❖ Tachypnea
  - ❖ Decreased or absent breath sounds on affected side
  - ❖ Crackles adjacent to the affected area
  - ❖ Shortness of breath, dyspnea
  - ❖ Asymmetrical chest excursion with respirations
  - ❖ Cyanosis
  - ❖ Decreased oxygen saturation
  - ❖ Hyperresonance in the affected side (pneumothorax)
  - ❖ Subcutaneous emphysema (pneumothorax)
  - ❖ Dullness or flatness in the affected side (hemothorax, pleural effusion, empyema, chylothorax)
  - ❖ Sudden, sharp chest pain
  - ❖ Anxiety, restlessness, apprehension
  - ❖ Tachycardia
  - ❖ Hypotension
  - ❖ Dysrhythmias
  - ❖ Tracheal deviation to the unaffected side (tension pneumothorax)
  - ❖ Neck vein distention (tension pneumothorax)
  - ❖ Muffled heart sounds (tension pneumothorax)

Patient Preparation

- Verify that the patient is the correct patient using two identifiers. *Rationale:* Before performing a procedure, the nurse should ensure the correct identification of the patient for the intended intervention.

- Ensure that the patient understands preprocedural teachings. Answer questions as they arise, and reinforce information as needed. **Rationale:** This communication evaluates and reinforces understanding of previously taught information.
- Obtain informed consent if circumstances allow. **Rationale:** Invasive procedures, unless performed with implied consent in a life-threatening situation, require written consent of the patient or significant other.
- Ensure patient has a patent intravenous access. **Rationale:** This access provides a route for analgesic, sedation, and emergency medications.
- Determine the insertion site and mark the skin with an indelible marker. **Rationale:** The insertion site is determined by the indication for the chest tube and diagnostic images. For a pneumothorax, the tube may be directed anterior and apical. For fluid drainage, it may be aimed posterior and basilar.[6]

- Determine the size of chest tube needed. **Rationale:** Evacuation of air necessitates a smaller tube; evacuation of fluid necessitates a larger tube.
- Assist the patient to a supine position with the ipsilateral arm abducted and flex the elbow so that the patient's hand is comfortably positioned above his or her head.[2,8] **Rationale:** This positioning enhances accessibility to the insertion site for positioning of the chest tube.
- Administer prescribed analgesics or sedatives as needed; follow institutional policy for moderate or procedural sedation. **Rationale:** Analgesics and sedatives reduce the discomfort and anxiety experienced and facilitate patient cooperation.
- Administer supplemental oxygen as needed. Monitor pulse oximeter and/or end-tidal carbon dioxide level. **Rationale:** Real-time assessment of patient's respiratory status during the procedure is provided.

Procedure for Performing Pleural Chest Tube Placement		
Steps	**Rationale**	**Special Considerations**
1. HH		
2. PE		
3. Don sterile gloves, sterile gown, mask, eye protection, and head covering.	*Chest tube insertion is a sterile procedure and requires full surgical attire, unless performed in a life-threatening situation.*	
4. Have an assistant open the outer wrapper of the tube thoracotomy insertion tray, remove the tray from wrapper, and open it with sterile technique.	Reduces transmission of microorganisms.	
5. Prepare equipment.	Facilitates insertion of the tube.	
A. Check that all equipment is present.		
B. Have an assistant pour antiseptic solution into the sterile cup or basin with aseptic technique (or open the swab packet and stand by).		
C. Have an assistant open the chest tube package and empty it onto the open tray.		
D. Grasp suture needle with needle holder.		
E. Remove the trocar from the chest tube and grasp the proximal end of the chest tube with a large Kelly clamp (Fig. 21-4).		
F. Prepare the syringe with lidocaine solution.		

Procedure continues on following page

Procedure | for Performing Pleural Chest Tube Placement—*Continued*

Steps	Rationale	Special Considerations

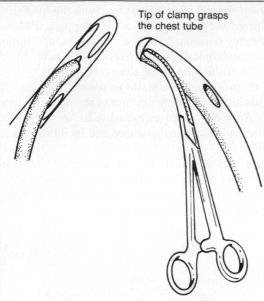

Tip of clamp grasps the chest tube

Figure 21-4   The tube is grasped with the curved clamp, with the tube tip protruding from the jaws. *(From Roberts JR, Hedges JR, editors: Clinicals in emergency medicine, ed 4, Philadelphia, 2004, Saunders.)*

Steps	Rationale	Special Considerations
6. Identify the insertion site and have an assistant position the patient. **(Level E*)**	Assists in preparation of area for insertion and proper placement of tube.[8]	Insertion site for air removal is right or left second intercostal space. Insertion site for fluid removal is right or left fifth or sixth intercostal space, midaxillary line. Incision site is one rib below insertion site.
7. Perform a preprocedure verification and time out, if nonemergent.	Ensures patient safety.	
8. Surgically prepare the skin with antiseptic solution, and drape the area surrounding the insertion site. **(Level E)**	Inhibits growth of bacteria at insertion site; maintains sterility.[2,8]	Prepare the area from the clavicle to the umbilicus, midchest to anterior axillary line.
9. Anesthetize the skin, subcutaneous tissue, muscle, and periosteum one intercostal space below the intercostal space that will be used to place the tube with lidocaine solution.	Results in loss of sensation and decreased pain during insertion.[2,8]	When infiltrating with lidocaine, aspirate repeatedly as the needle is inserted to identify the presence of air or fluid; 30–40 mL of lidocaine may be needed for anesthesia.
A. With a 5-mL syringe (25-gauge needle), inject a subcutaneous wheal of lidocaine at the insertion site.		
B. With a 10-mL syringe (20-gauge, 1½-inch needle), advance the needle/syringe, aspirating as you go, until air or pleural fluid is confirmed.		
C. Inject the lidocaine deeper, and slowly withdraw the syringe, generously anesthetizing rib periosteum, subcutaneous tissue, and pleura (Fig. 21-5). **(Level E)**		

*Level E: Multiple case reports, theory-based evidence from expert opinions, or peer-reviewed professional organizational standards without clinical studies to support recommendations.

Procedure	**for Performing Pleural Chest Tube Placement—*Continued***	
Steps	**Rationale**	**Special Considerations**

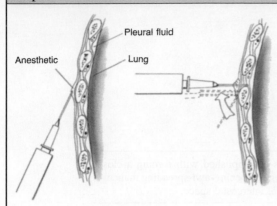

Pleural fluid

Anesthetic

Lung

Figure 21-5 Insertion of a chest tube can be relatively painless with proper infiltration of the skin and pleura with local anesthetic. The liberal use of buffered 1% lidocaine without epinephrine (maximal lidocaine dose, 5 mg/kg) is recommended. *(From Roberts JR, editor: Roberts and Hedges' clinical procedures in emergency medicine, ed 6, Philadelphia, 2014, Saunders.)*

---

10. An incision should be made, similar to the diameter of the tube being inserted, directly over the inferior aspect of the anesthetized rib below the insertion site (Fig. 21-6). **(Level E*)**

Allows for the diameter of the chest tube.[2,8]

When making the incision, incise down through the subcutaneous tissue; the space should be large enough to admit a finger.

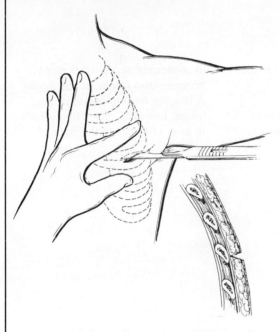

Figure 21-6 Transverse skin incision is made directly over the inferior aspect of the anesthetized rib down to the subcutaneous tissue. *(From Dumire SM, Paris PM: Atlas of emergency procedures, Philadelphia, 1994, Saunders.)*

---

11. Introduce the Kelly clamp through the incision, with the tips down, creating a tunnel through the subcutaneous tissue and muscle; use an opening and spreading maneuver; aim toward the superior aspect of the rib until the pleural space is reached (Fig. 21-7). **(Level E)**

Facilitates insertion of the tube. Blunt dissection minimizes trauma to the neurovascular bundle.[2,8]

Additional lidocaine is infiltrated as needed. The direction of the tunnel created through the subcutaneous tissue and muscle determines the direction the chest tube takes after insertion. Be sure the clamp stays close to the ribs to avoid injury to the neurovascular bundle.

---

*Level E: Multiple case reports, theory-based evidence from expert opinions, or peer-reviewed professional organizational standards without clinical studies to support recommendations.

Procedure continues on following page

Procedure for Performing Pleural Chest Tube Placement—*Continued*

Steps	Rationale	Special Considerations

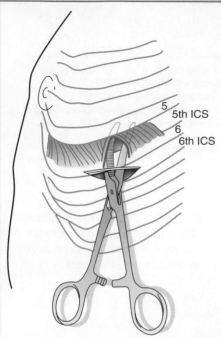

Figure 21-7 Blunt dissection is accomplished with forcing a closed clamp through the incision and using an opening-and-spreading maneuver to create a tunnel to the pleura. *ICS,* intercostal space.

Steps	Rationale	Special Considerations
12. When the clamp is just over the superior portion of the rib, close the clamp and push it with steady pressure through the parietal pleura and into the pleural space, then widen the hole in the pleural space by spreading the clamp (Fig. 21-8). **(Level E*)**	Ensures opening is large enough for the chest tube. Steady, even, controlled pressure provides control of the clamp once the pleura is perforated.[2,8]	This maneuver necessitates more pressure than might be anticipated. A lunging motion or use of the trocar, however, may cause a hole in lung or injury to the liver or spleen.

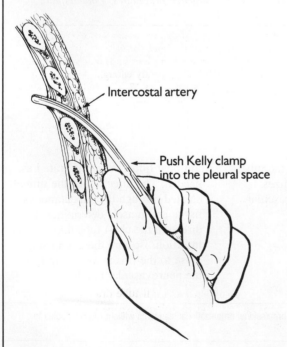

Intercostal artery

Push Kelly clamp into the pleural space

Figure 21-8 Just over the superior portion of the rib, close the clamp and push with steady pressure into the pleura. *(From Dumire SM, Paris PM: Atlas of emergency procedures, Philadelphia, 1994, Saunders.)*

*Level E: Multiple case reports, theory-based evidence from expert opinions, or peer-reviewed professional organizational standards without clinical studies to support recommendations.

Procedure	for Performing Pleural Chest Tube Placement—*Continued*	
Steps	**Rationale**	**Special Considerations**
13. Insert the index finger to dilate the tract and hole in the pleura.	Relieves air or fluid when penetration of the space is made and ensures entry into the pleural space and not into a space inadvertently created between the parietal pleura and chest wall.[8]	Feel for lung tissue (lung should expand and meet finger on inspiration), diaphragm, or adhesions. Manually break up any clot, if found. If significant adhesions are unexpectedly encountered, abandon that site and select another one.
14. Insert the chest tube into the chest cavity with a curved Kelly clamp, holding the proximal end to guide the tip into the pleural space. Remove the clamp and guide the tube, in a rotating motion, through the tract and into the space. The tube is advanced until the last hole is in the pleural space. Condensation of air or fluid in the tube should be noted.	The Kelly clamp provides stiffness to the chest tube, allowing for more control as it is inserted into the pleural space.	To drain air, aim the tube posteriorly and superiorly toward the apex of the lung; to drain fluid, aim the tube inferiorly and posteriorly. Do not allow any side holes of the tube to remain outside the thoracic cavity.
15. Connect the chest tube to the closed chest-drainage system (see Procedure 25) and check for rise and fall (tidaling) of the H_2O column. Assistant applies ordered amount of suction.	Ensures the tube is properly positioned.	
16. Suture the tube to the chest wall. Wrap the free ends of the suture around the tube (similar to lacing a shoe). Tie the ends of the suture snugly around the top of the tube (Fig. 21-9).	Secures the position of the tube.[4] Sutures should be snug to prevent free air from passing into the subcutaneous tissue.	Type of stitch used depends on the preference of the physician; the goal is to prevent displacement of the chest tube.

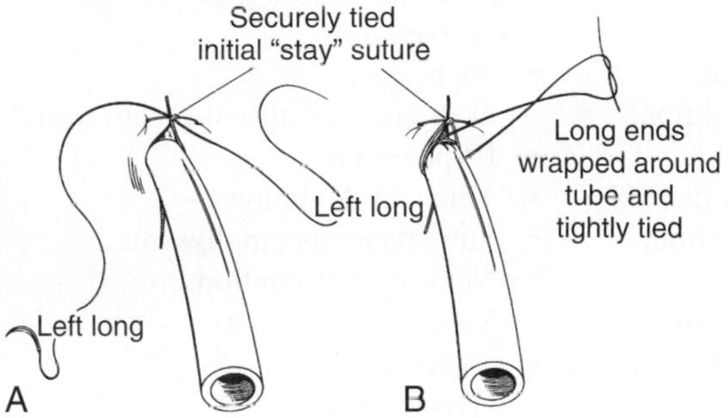

Securely tied
initial "stay" suture

Long ends
wrapped around
tube and
tightly tied

Left long

Left long

A　B

Figure 21-9　A "stay" suture is placed first next to the tube to close the skin incision. **A,** The knot is tied securely, and the ends, which subsequently are wrapped around the chest tube, are left long. **B,** The ends of the suture are wound twice about the tube, tightly enough to indent the tube slightly, and are tied securely. *(From Roberts JR, editor: Roberts and Hedges' clinical procedures in emergency medicine, ed 6, Philadelphia, 2014, Saunders.)*

17. Apply occlusive dressing. 　A. Slit drain sponges or 4 × 4 gauze are applied under and over top of the chest tube insertion site. Petrolatum gauze is used around the chest tube, or follow institutional standards.[7] 　B. Secure with a tape dressing.	Provides cover for the wound, secures the dressing to the wound, and creates an airtight dressing.	
18. Tape all connection points to the drainage system or secure with zip ties (Parham-Martin bands). **(Level E*)**	Creates an airtight system. Airtight connections prevent air leaks into the pleural space.[1,4]	Check that all tube drainage holes are in the pleural space.

*Level E: Multiple case reports, theory-based evidence from expert opinions, or peer-reviewed professional organizational standards without clinical studies to support recommendations.

Procedure continues on following page

Procedure   for Performing Pleural Chest Tube Placement—*Continued*

Steps	Rationale	Special Considerations
19. Secure the tube below the dressing to the patient's skin with a commercial securing device or tape.	Functions as a strain relief to prevent tube and dressing dislodgment.	
20. Obtain a chest radiograph. (**Level E***)	Chest radiograph confirms placement of tube, expansion of lung, and removal of fluid.[8]	Ensure that the distal drainage hole is within the pleural space. Document result of chest radiograph in the patient's record.
21. Dispose of equipment and remove **PE**.		
22. **HH**		

Expected Outcomes

- Removal of air, fluid, or blood from the pleural space
- Relief of respiratory distress
- Reexpansion of the lung (validated with chest radiograph)
- Restoration of negative pressure within the pleural space

Unexpected Outcomes

- Hemorrhage or shock
- Increasing respiratory distress
- Infection
- Damage to intercostal nerve that results in neuropathy or neuritis
- Incorrect tube placement
- Chest tube kinking, clogging, or dislodgment from chest wall
- Subcutaneous emphysema
- Reexpansion pulmonary edema

Patient Monitoring and Care

Steps	Rationale	Reportable Conditions
		These conditions should be reported if they persist despite nursing interventions.
1. Assess cardiopulmonary and vital signs every 1–4 hours and as needed.	Provides baseline and ongoing assessment of patient's condition. Abnormalities can indicate recurrence of the condition that necessitated chest tube insertion. On the basis of the patient's clinical condition or physician orders, vital signs may need to be checked more frequently.	• Tachypnea • Decreased or absent breath sounds • Hypoxemia • Tracheal deviation • Subcutaneous emphysema • Neck vein distention • Muffled heart tones • Tachycardia • Hypotension • Dysrhythmias • Fever
2. Monitor chest tube output every 1–4 hours, and record amount and color.	Provides data for diagnosis. Higher drainage amounts require more frequent assessment. On the basis of the patient's clinical condition or physician orders, output may need to be checked more frequently.	• Bloody drainage greater than or equal to 200 mL/hr • Sudden cessation of drainage • Change in character of drainage
3. Assess for pain at the insertion site or for chest discomfort.	Pain interferes with adequate deep breathing. Pain at insertion site, particularly with inspiration, may indicate improper tube placement.	• Continued pain despite pain interventions

*Level E: Multiple case reports, theory-based evidence from expert opinions, or peer-reviewed professional organizational standards without clinical studies to support recommendations.

Patient Monitoring and Care —*Continued*

Steps	Rationale	Reportable Conditions
4. Evaluate the chest drainage system for rise and fall (tidaling) in water-seal chamber. Check connections.[4] **(Level E*)**	Water level normally rises and falls with respiration until lung is expanded. Bubbling immediately after insertion signifies that air is being removed from the pleural space; bubbling with exhalation and coughing is normal. Persistent bubbling indicates an air leak either in the patient's lung or in the chest drainage system.	• Absence of tidaling in water-seal chamber • Persistent bubbling
5. Assess insertion site and surrounding skin with daily dressing change for presence of subcutaneous emphysema and signs of infection or inflammation.	Skin integrity is altered during insertion, which can lead to infection.	• Fever • Redness around insertion site • Purulent drainage • Subcutaneous emphysema

*Level E: Multiple case reports, theory-based evidence from expert opinions, or peer-reviewed professional organizational standards without clinical studies to support recommendations.

Documentation

Documentation should include the following:
- Patient and family education
- Reason for chest tube insertion
- Respiratory and vital sign assessment before and after insertion
- Description of procedure, including tube size, date and time of insertion, insertion site, and any complications associated with procedure
- Type and amount of drainage

- Presence of fluctuation and bubbling
- Amount of suction
- Patient's tolerance to procedure
- Postinsertion chest radiograph results
- Unexpected outcomes
- Nursing interventions
- Pain assessment, interventions, and effectiveness

References and Additional Readings

For a complete list of references and additional readings for this procedure, scan this QR code with any freely available smartphone code reader app, or visit http://booksite.elsevier.com/9780323376624.

22 Chest Tube Placement (Assist)

Julie Waters

PURPOSE: Chest tubes are placed for the removal or drainage of air, blood, or fluid from the intrapleural space. They also are used to introduce sclerosing agents into the pleural space to prevent a reaccumulation of fluid.

PREREQUISITE NURSING KNOWLEDGE

- The thoracic cavity is a closed airspace in normal conditions. Any disruption results in the loss of negative pressure within the intrapleural space. Air or fluid that enters the space competes with the lung, resulting in collapse of the lung. Associated conditions are the result of disease, injury, surgery, or iatrogenic causes.
- Chest tubes are sterile flexible polyvinyl chloride (PVC) or silicone nonthrombogenic catheters approximately 20 inches (51 cm) long, varying in size from 8F to 40F. The size of the tube placed is determined by the indication and viscosity of the drainage.[6] The side of the chest tube usually has a radiopaque strip down the side to assist in visualization on chest radiographs.
- Indications for chest tube insertion include the following:
  - ❖ Pneumothorax (collection of air in the pleural space)
  - ❖ Hemothorax (collection of blood)
  - ❖ Hemopneumothorax (accumulation of air and blood in the pleural space)
  - ❖ Thoracotomy (e.g., open heart surgery, pneumonectomy)
  - ❖ Pyothorax or empyema (collection of pus)
  - ❖ Chylothorax (collection of chyle from the thoracic duct)
  - ❖ Cholothorax (collection of fluid containing bile)
  - ❖ Hydrothorax (collection of noninflammatory serous fluid)
  - ❖ Pleural effusion
  - ❖ Pleurodesis (instillation of anesthetic solutions and sclerosing agents)
- Chest tubes inserted for traumatic hemopneumothorax or hemothorax (blood) should be large (36F to 40F). Medium tubes (24F to 36F) should be used for fluid accumulation (pleural effusions). Tubes inserted for pneumothorax (air) should be small (12F to 24F).[2,6]
- A pneumothorax may be classified as an open, closed, or tension pneumothorax.
  - ❖ *Open pneumothorax:* The chest wall and the pleural space are penetrated, which allows air to enter the pleural space, as in a penetrating injury or trauma; a surgical incision in the thoracic cavity (i.e., thoracotomy); or a complication of surgical treatment (e.g.,

unintentional puncture during invasive procedures, such as thoracentesis or central venous catheter insertion).
  - ❖ *Closed pneumothorax:* The pleural space is penetrated but the chest wall is intact, which allows air to enter the pleural space from within the lung, as in spontaneous pneumothorax. A closed pneumothorax occurs without apparent injury and often is seen in individuals with chronic lung disorders (e.g., emphysema, cystic fibrosis, tuberculosis, necrotizing pneumonia) and in young tall men who have a greater than normal height-to-width chest ratio; after blunt traumatic injury; or iatrogenically, occurring as a complication of medical treatment (e.g., intermittent positive-pressure breathing, mechanical ventilation with positive end-expiratory pressure).
  - ❖ *Tension pneumothorax:* Air leaks into the pleural space through a tear in the lung and has no means to escape from the pleural cavity, creating a one-way valve effect. With each breath the patient takes, air accumulates and pressure within the pleural space increases, and the lung collapses. This condition causes the mediastinal structures (i.e., heart, great vessels, and trachea) to be compressed and shift to the opposite or unaffected side of the chest. Venous return and cardiac output are impeded, and collapse of the unaffected lung is possible. This life-threatening emergency requires prompt recognition and intervention.
- *Absolute contraindications:* Lung that is densely adherent to the chest wall throughout the hemithorax is an absolute contraindication to chest tube therapy.[5]
- *Relative contraindications:* Use of chest tubes in patients with multiple adhesions, giant blebs, or coagulopathies should be carefully considered; however, these relative contraindications are superseded by the need to reexpand the lung. When possible, any coagulopathy or platelet defect should be corrected before chest tube insertion. The differential diagnosis between a pneumothorax and bullous disease necessitates careful radiological assessment.[5]
- The tube size and insertion site selected for the chest tube are determined by the indication.[5,6] If draining air, the tube is placed near the apex of the lung (second intercostal space); if draining fluid, the tube is placed near the base of the lung (fifth or sixth intercostal space; see Fig. 21-1).

- Once the tube is in place, it should be sutured to the skin to prevent displacement and an occlusive dressing should be applied (see Fig. 21-2). The chest tube also is connected to a chest-drainage system (see Procedure 25) to remove air and fluid from the pleural space, which facilitates reexpansion of the collapsed lung. All connection points are secured with tape or zip ties (Parham-Martin bands) to ensure that the system remains airtight (see Fig. 21-3).
- The water-seal chamber should bubble gently immediately on insertion of the chest tube and during expiration and with coughing. Continuous bubbling in this chamber indicates a leak within the patient or in the chest-drainage system. Fluctuations in the water level in the water-seal chamber of 5 to 10 cm, rising during inhalation and falling during expiration, should be observed with spontaneous respirations. If the patient is on mechanical ventilation, the pattern of fluctuation is just the opposite. Any suction applied must be disconnected temporarily to assess correctly for fluctuations in the water-seal chamber.

EQUIPMENT

- Caps, masks, sterile gloves, gowns, drapes
- Protective eyewear (goggles)
- Antiseptic solution: 2% chlorhexidine or povidone-iodine
- Local anesthetic: 1% or 2% lidocaine solution (with or without epinephrine)
  - ❖ 10-mL syringe with 20-gauge, 1½-inch needle
  - ❖ 5-mL syringe with 25-gauge, 1-inch needle
- Tube thoracostomy tray
  - ❖ Sterile towels, 4 × 4 sterile gauze
  - ❖ Scalpel with No. 10 or 11 blade
  - ❖ Two Kelly clamps
  - ❖ Needle holder
  - ❖ Monofilament or silk suture material (No. 0 or 1-0)
  - ❖ Sterile basin or medicine cup
  - ❖ Suture scissors
  - ❖ Two hemostats
- Thoracotomy tubes (8 to 40Fr, as appropriate)
- Closed chest-drainage system
- Suction source
- Suction connector and connecting tubing (usually 6 feet for each tube)
- 1-inch adhesive tape or zip ties (Parham-Martin bands)
- Occlusive dressing materials
  - ❖ 4 × 4 gauze pads or slit drain sponges
  - ❖ Petrolatum gauze
  - ❖ Tape or a commercial securing device

Additional equipment, to have available as needed, includes the following:

- Ultrasound machine and ultrasound gel

PATIENT AND FAMILY EDUCATION

- If time permits, assess the patient's and family's level of understanding about the condition and rationale for the procedure. *Rationale:* This assessment identifies the patient's and family's knowledge deficits concerning the patient's condition, the procedure, the expected benefits, and the potential risks. It also allows time for questions to clarify information and voice concerns. Explanations decrease patient anxiety and enhance cooperation.
- Explain the procedure and the reason for the procedure, if the clinical situation permits. If not, explain the procedure and reason for the intubation after it is completed. *Rationale:* This explanation enhances patient and family understanding and decreases anxiety.
- Explain that the patient's participation during the procedure is to remain as immobile as possible and to do relaxed breathing. *Rationale:* This explanation facilitates insertion of the chest tube and prevents complications during insertion.
- After the procedure, instruct the patient to sit in a semi-Fowler's position (unless contraindicated). *Rationale:* This position facilitates drainage, if present, from the pleural space by allowing air to rise and fluid to settle to be removed via the chest tube. This position also makes breathing easier.
- Instruct the patient to turn and change position every 2 hours. The patient may lie on the side with the chest tube but should keep the tubing free of kinks. *Rationale:* Turning and changing position prevent complications related to immobility and retained pulmonary secretions. Keeping the tube free of kinks maintains patency of the tube, facilitates drainage, and prevents the accumulation of pressure within the pleural space that interferes with lung reexpansion.
- Instruct the patient to cough and deep breathe, with splinting of the affected side. *Rationale:* Coughing and deep breathing increase pressure within the pleural space, facilitating drainage, promoting lung reexpansion, and preventing respiratory complications associated with retained secretions. The application of firm pressure over the chest tube insertion site (i.e., splinting) may decrease pain and discomfort.
- Encourage active or passive range-of-motion exercises of the arm on the affected side. *Rationale:* The patient may limit movement of the arm on the affected side to decrease the discomfort at the insertion site, which may result in joint discomfort and potential joint contractures.
- Instruct the patient and family about activity as prescribed while maintaining the drainage system below the level of the chest. *Rationale:* This activity facilitates gravity drainage and prevents backflow and potential infectious contamination into the pleural space.
- Instruct the patient about the availability of prescribed analgesic medication and other pain-relief strategies. *Rationale:* Pain relief ensures comfort and facilitates coughing, deep breathing, positioning, range of motion, and recuperation.

PATIENT ASSESSMENT AND PREPARATION

Patient Assessment

- Assess significant medical history or injury, including chronic lung disease, spontaneous pneumothorax, hemothorax, pulmonary disease, therapeutic procedures, and mechanism of injury. *Rationale:* Medical history or injury may provide the etiological basis for the occurrence of pneumothorax, empyema, pleural effusion, or chylothorax.

- Evaluate diagnostic test results (if patient's condition does not necessitate immediate intervention), including chest radiograph and arterial blood gases. *Rationale:* Diagnostic testing confirms the presence of air or fluid in the pleural space, a collapsed lung, hypoxemia, and respiratory compromise.
- Assess baseline cardiopulmonary status for the following signs and symptoms that necessitate chest tube insertion.[4] *Rationale:* Accurate assessment of signs and symptoms allows for prompt recognition and treatment. Baseline assessment provides comparison data for evaluation of changes and outcomes of treatment.
  - ❖ Tachypnea
  - ❖ Decreased or absent breath sounds on affected side
  - ❖ Crackles adjacent to the affected area
  - ❖ Shortness of breath, dyspnea
  - ❖ Asymmetrical chest excursion with respirations
  - ❖ Cyanosis
  - ❖ Decreased oxygen saturation
  - ❖ Hyperresonance in the affected side (pneumothorax)
  - ❖ Subcutaneous emphysema (pneumothorax)
  - ❖ Dullness or flatness in the affected side (hemothorax, pleural effusion, empyema, chylothorax)
  - ❖ Sudden, sharp chest pain
  - ❖ Anxiety, restlessness, apprehension
  - ❖ Tachycardia
  - ❖ Hypotension
  - ❖ Dysrhythmias
  - ❖ Tracheal deviation to the unaffected side (tension pneumothorax)
  - ❖ Neck vein distention (tension pneumothorax)
  - ❖ Muffled heart sounds (tension pneumothorax)

Patient Preparation

- Verify correct patient with two identifiers. *Rationale:* Prior to performing a procedure, the nurse should ensure the correct identification of the patient for the intended intervention.
- Ensure that the patient understands preprocedural teachings. Answer questions as they arise, and reinforce information as needed. *Rationale:* This communication evaluates and reinforces understanding of previously taught information.
- Obtain consent if circumstances allow. *Rationale:* Invasive procedures, unless performed with implied consent in a life-threatening situation, require written consent of the patient or significant other.
- Ensure patient has a patent intravenous access. *Rationale:* This access provides a route for analgesics, sedation, and emergency medications.
- Consult with the practitioner for the appropriate-size chest tube to be inserted. *Rationale:* Evacuation of air necessitates a smaller tube; evacuation of fluid necessitates a larger tube.
- Assist the patient to a supine position with the ipsilateral arm abducted and flex the elbow so that the patient's hand is comfortably positioned above his or her head.[2,8] *Rationale:* This positioning enhances accessibility to the insertion site for positioning of the chest tube.
- Administer prescribed analgesics or sedatives as needed; follow institutional policy for moderate or procedural sedation. *Rationale:* Analgesics and sedatives reduce the discomfort and anxiety experienced and facilitate patient cooperation.
- Administer supplemental oxygen as needed. Monitor pulse oximeter or end-tidal carbon dioxide level. *Rationale:* Real-time assessment of patient's respiratory status during the procedure is provided.

Procedure	**for Assisting with Pleural Chest Tube Placement**	
Steps	Rationale	Special Considerations
1. ▣▣		
2. ▣▣		
3. Open the chest tube insertion tray using sterile technique.	Reduces transmission of microorganisms.	
4. Assist with preparation of the equipment.	Facilitates insertion of the tube.	
A. Check that all equipment is present.		
B. Pour antiseptic solution into basin or medicine cup with aseptic technique or open antiseptic swab packet and stand by.		
C. Open the chest tube package and empty it onto the open sterile tray.		
D. Assist to prepare a syringe with lidocaine.		

Procedure for Assisting with Pleural Chest Tube Placement—*Continued*		
Steps	**Rationale**	**Special Considerations**
5. Assist the physician or advanced practice nurse with preparation of the insertion site.	Assists in preparation of area for insertion and proper placement of tube.[8]	Insertion site for air removal is right or left second intercostal space. Insertion site for fluid removal is right or left fifth or sixth intercostal space, midaxillary line. Incision site is one rib below insertion site (see Fig. 21-1).
6. Perform a preprocedure verification and time out, if nonemergent.	Ensures patient safety.	
7. After tube insertion, connect the chest tube to the closed chest-drainage system and check for rise and fall (tidaling) of the H_2O column. Apply ordered amount of suction.	Ensures the tube is properly positioned.[3]	
8. Assist with suturing of the tube to the chest wall.	Secures the position of the tube.[4] Sutures should be snug to prevent free air from passing into the subcutaneous tissue.	Type of stitch used depends on the individual; the goal is to prevent displacement of the chest tube.
9. Apply occlusive dressing (see Fig. 21-2). A. May use slit drain sponge or 4×4 gauze under and over top of the chest tube insertion site. Petrolatum gauze is used around the chest tube, or follow institutional standards.[7] B. Secure with tape dressing.	Provides cover for the wound with the least damage to the surrounding skin.	
10. Tape all connection points to the drainage system or secure with zip ties (Parham-Martin bands). **(Level E*)**	Creates an airtight system. Airtight connections prevent air leaks into the pleural space.[1,4]	Check that all tube drainage holes are in the pleural space.
11. Secure the tube below the dressing to the patient's skin with a commercial securing device or tape.	Functions as a strain relief to prevent tube and dressing dislodgement.	
12. Confirm tube placement with chest radiography. **(Level E)**	Chest radiograph confirms placement of tube, expansion of lung, and removal of fluid.[8]	Ensure that the distal drainage hole is within the pleural space. Document result of chest radiograph in the patient's record.
13. Dispose of used supplies and remove **PE**.		
14. **HH**		

*Level E: Multiple case reports, theory-based evidence from expert opinions, or peer-reviewed professional organizational standards without clinical studies to support recommendations.

Procedure continues on following page

Expected Outcomes

- Removal of air, fluid, or blood from the pleural space
- Relief of respiratory distress
- Reexpansion of the lung (validated with chest radiograph)
- Restoration of negative pressure within the pleural space

Unexpected Outcomes

- Hemorrhage or shock
- Increasing respiratory distress
- Infection
- Damage to intercostal nerve that results in neuropathy or neuritis
- Incorrect tube placement
- Chest tube kinking, clogging, or dislodgment from chest wall
- Subcutaneous emphysema
- Reexpansion pulmonary edema

Patient Monitoring and Care

Steps	Rationale	Reportable Conditions
		These conditions should be reported if they persist despite nursing interventions.
1. Assess cardiopulmonary and vital signs every 1–4 hours and as needed.	Provides baseline and ongoing assessment of patient's condition. Abnormalities can indicate reoccurrence of the condition that necessitated chest tube insertion. On the basis of the patient's clinical condition or physician orders, vital signs may need to be checked more frequently.	• Tachypnea • Decreased or absent breath sounds • Hypoxemia • Tracheal deviation • Subcutaneous emphysema • Neck vein distention • Muffled heart tones • Tachycardia • Hypotension • Dysrhythmias • Fever
2. Monitor chest tube output every 1–4 hours and record amount and color.	Provides data for diagnosis. Higher drainage amounts require more frequent assessment. On the basis of the patient's clinical condition or physician orders, output may need to be checked more frequently.	• Bloody drainage greater than or equal to 200 mL/hr • Sudden cessation of drainage • Change in character of drainage
3. Assess for pain at the insertion site or for chest discomfort.	Pain interferes with adequate deep breathing. Pain at insertion site, particularly with inspiration, may indicate improper tube placement.	• Continued pain despite pain interventions
4. Evaluate the chest-drainage system for rise and fall (tidaling) or bubbling in water-seal chamber. Check connections.	Water level normally rises and falls with respiration until lung is expanded. Bubbling immediately after insertion signifies that air is being removed from the pleural space; bubbling with exhalation and coughing is normal. Persistent bubbling indicates an air leak either in the patient's lung or in the chest-drainage system.[3]	• Absence of tidaling in water-seal chamber • Persistent bubbling
5. Assess insertion site and surrounding skin with daily dressing change for presence of subcutaneous emphysema and signs of infection or inflammation.	Skin integrity is altered during insertion, which can lead to infection.[3]	• Fever • Redness around insertion site • Purulent drainage • Subcutaneous emphysema

Documentation

Documentation should include the following:
- Patient and family education
- Reason for chest tube insertion
- Respiratory and vital sign assessment before and after insertion
- Description of procedure, including tube size, date and time of insertion, insertion site, and any complications associated with the procedure
- Type and amount of drainage
- Presence of tidaling and bubbling
- Amount of suction
- Patient's tolerance of procedure
- Postinsertion chest radiograph results
- Unexpected outcomes
- Nursing interventions
- Pain assessment, interventions, and effectiveness

References and Additional Readings

For a complete list of references and additional readings for this procedure, scan this QR code with any freely available smartphone code reader app, or visit http://booksite.elsevier.com/9780323376624.

23 Chest Tube Removal (Perform) AP

Peggy Kirkwood

PURPOSE: Chest tube removal is performed to discontinue a chest tube when it is no longer needed for the removal or drainage of air, blood, or fluid from the intrapleural or mediastinal space.

PREREQUISITE NURSING KNOWLEDGE

- Chest tubes are placed in the pleural or mediastinal space to evacuate an abnormal collection of air or fluid or both.
- For interpleural chest tubes, the air leak detector should bubble gently immediately on insertion of the chest tube during expiration and with coughing. Continuous bubbling in the air leak detector indicates a leak in the patient or the chest-drainage system. Fluctuations in the water level (also known as tidaling) in the water-seal chamber of 5 to 10 cm, rising during inhalation and falling during expiration, should be observed with spontaneous respirations. If the patient is on mechanical ventilation, the pattern of fluctuation is just the opposite. Any suction applied must be disconnected temporarily to assess correctly for fluctuations in the water-seal chamber.
- Flexible Silastic (Blake; Ethicon, Inc., Somerville, NJ) drains may be used in place of large-bore chest tubes in the mediastinal and pleural spaces after cardiac surgery. These tubes provide more efficient drainage and improved patient mobility with minimized tissue trauma and pain with removal.[3,16]
- Chest radiographs are done periodically to determine whether the lung has reexpanded. Daily chest radiographs have been found not to be necessary while the tube is in place.[5,7,16,19,21] Reexpanded lungs, along with respiratory assessments that show improvement in the patient's respiratory status, are the basis for the decision to remove the chest tube.
- While the tubes are in place, patients may have related discomfort. Prompt removal of chest tubes encourages patients to increase ambulation and respiratory measures to improve lung expansion after surgery (e.g., coughing, deep breathing). However, removal of the chest tube may also be a painful procedure for the patient.[4,9,12–14]
- The types of sutures used to secure chest tubes vary according to the preference of the physician, the physician assistant, or the advanced practice nurse. One common type is the horizontal mattress or purse-string suture, which is threaded around and through the wound edges in a U shape with the ends left unknotted until the chest tube is removed. Usually one or two anchor stitches accompany the purse-string suture (Fig. 23-1).
- A primary goal of chest tube removal is removal of tubes without introduction of air or contaminants into the pleural space.
- Available data indicate there is no consensus as to the rate of drainage that should be used as a threshold for tube removal and no evidence to suggest that it is unsafe to remove tubes that still have a relatively high rate of fluid drainage.[5,20] Research has shown that, depending on the reason for the chest tube, volumes of 200 to 450 mL/day do not adversely affect length of stay or overall costs compared with lower threshold volumes, nor does the risk of pleural fluid reaccumulation increase.[5,22] However, some suggested guidelines include the following:
  - Drainage has decreased to 50 to 200 mL in the prior 24 hours if tube was placed for hemothorax, empyema, or pleural effusion.
  - If tube was placed after cardiac surgery, drainage has changed from bloody to serosanguineous, no air leak is present, and amount is less than 100 mL in the past 8 hours.[1,10]
  - Pleural tubes are placed after cardiac surgery if the pleural cavity has been entered. They typically are removed within 24 to 48 hours after surgery.[1,10]
  - Mediastinal chest tubes most often are removed 24 to 36 hours after cardiac surgery.[1]
  - Lungs are reexpanded (as shown on chest radiographic results).
  - Respiratory status has improved (i.e., nonlabored respirations, equal bilateral breath sounds, absence of shortness of breath, decreased use of accessory muscles, symmetrical respiratory excursion, and respiratory rate less than 24 breaths/min).
  - Fluctuations are minimal or absent in the water-seal chamber of the collection device, and the level of solution rises in the chamber.
  - For interpleural chest tubes, air leaks have resolved for at least 24 hours (the absence of continuous bubbling in the water-seal chamber or absence of air bubbles from right to left in the air leak detector), and lung is fully reinflated on chest radiographic results.

AP This procedure should be performed only by physicians, advanced practice nurses, and other healthcare professionals (including critical care nurses) with additional knowledge, skills, and demonstrated competence per professional licensure or institutional standard.

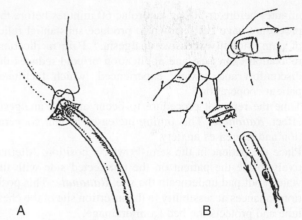

Figure 23-1 Purse-string suture. Removing the chest tube. **A,** First throw of a knot in the mattress suture. **B,** Removal of the chest tube and tying of purse-string suture. (*From Leonar S, Nikaidoh H: Thoracentesis and chest tube insertion. In Levin D, Morriss F, editors. Essentials of pediatric intensive care, St Louis, 1990, Quality Medical Publishing.*)

EQUIPMENT

- Suture-removal set
- Antiseptic swabs (povidone-iodine, chlorhexidine gluconate with alcohol, etc.)
- Petrolatum gauze, as per hospital protocol
- Rubber-tipped Kelly clamps or disposable umbilical clamps
- Wide occlusive tape (2 inches)
- Elastic closure device, such as Steri-Strips (3M, St. Paul, MN)
- Dry 4 × 4 gauze sponges (two to four)
- Waterproof pad
- Personal protective equipment (goggles, sterile and non-sterile gloves, mask, gown)

Additional equipment, to have available as needed, includes the following:

- Specimen collection cup (if catheter tip is to be sent to the laboratory for analysis)
- Scissors

PATIENT AND FAMILY EDUCATION

- Assess the patient's and family's level of understanding about the condition and rationale for the procedure. *Rationale:* This assessment identifies the patient's and family's knowledge deficits concerning the patient's condition, the procedure, the expected benefits, and the potential risks. It also allows time for questions to clarify information and voice concerns. Explanations decrease patient anxiety and enhance cooperation.
- Explain the procedure, reason for removal, and sensations to be expected.[15,19] The most commonly reported sensations are pulling, pain or hurting, and burning.[14] *Rationale:* This explanation decreases patient anxiety and enhances cooperation.
- Explain the patient's role in assisting with removal. Explain that the patient should perform the Valsalva

maneuver on the count of three. Have the patient practice the maneuver before the procedure. *Rationale:* This explanation elicits patient cooperation and facilitates removal.

- Instruct the patient to turn and reposition every 2 hours after the chest tube has been removed. *Rationale:* This action prevents complications related to immobility and retained secretions.
- Instruct the patient to cough and breathe deeply after the chest tube has been removed, with splinting of the affected side or sternum (with mediastinal tubes). *Rationale:* This action prevents respiratory complications associated with retained secretions. The application of firm pressure over the insertion site (i.e., splinting) decreases pain and discomfort.
- Instruct the patient about the availability of prescribed analgesic medication after the chest tube is removed. *Rationale:* Analgesics alleviate pain and facilitate coughing, deep breathing, and repositioning.[9,13,19]
- Instruct the patient and family to report signs and symptoms of respiratory distress or infection immediately. *Rationale:* Immediate reporting facilitates prompt intervention to relieve a recurrent pneumothorax or to treat an infection.

PATIENT ASSESSMENT AND PREPARATION

Patient Assessment

- Assess respiratory status. *Rationale:* Assessment of respiratory status verifies the patient's readiness for chest tube removal.
  - ❖ Oxygen saturation within normal limits
  - ❖ Nonlabored respirations
  - ❖ Absence of shortness of breath
  - ❖ Decreased use of accessory muscles
  - ❖ Respiratory rate of less than 24 breaths/min
  - ❖ Equal bilateral breath sounds
- Assess chest tube drainage (less than 200 mL in 24 hours or less than 100 mL in 8 hours after cardiac surgery).[1,5,10] *Rationale:* Assessment of drainage verifies patient readiness for chest tube removal.
- For interpleural chest tubes, assess for minimal or no air leak in the air leak detector zone or indicator with pleural tubes. *Rationale:* This assessment indicates whether the lung is reexpanded and whether air leak is present.
- Evaluate chest radiographic results. *Rationale:* Lung reexpansion indicates that need for chest tube is resolved.
- Assess vital signs and (optional) arterial blood gases. *Rationale:* Vital sign assessment indicates whether the patient can tolerate chest tube removal.
- Assess laboratory results for clotting capability and medications that may affect clotting. *Rationale:* Low platelet levels or thrombolytic medications may precipitate excessive bleeding.[17]

Patient Preparation

- Verify correct patient with two identifiers. *Rationale:* Prior to performing a procedure, the nurse should ensure the correct identification of the patient for the intended intervention.

- Ensure that the patient understands preprocedural teachings. Answer questions as they arise, and reinforce information as needed. *Rationale:* This communication evaluates and reinforces understanding of previously taught information. Anticipatory preparation may prepare patients for a better experience.[12,18]
- Administer premedication of adequate analgesics at least 20 minutes before the procedure. Alternatively, subfascial lidocaine may be injected into the chest tube tract. In addition to opioids, adjunct methods shown to decrease pain during chest tube removal include slow deep-breathing relaxation exercises and application of cold packs.[8,9] *Rationale:* Intravenous 4-mg morphine 20 minutes before or 30-mg ketorolac 60 minutes before the procedure have been shown to produce substantial relief of pain without excessive analgesia.[13] Pain medication, relaxation exercises, and application of cold reduces the discomfort and anxiety experienced, which facilitates patient cooperation.[8,9,12,13]

- Time the removal procedure to occur at peak analgesic effect. *Rationale:* This timing increases patient cooperation and decreases anxiety.[13]
- Place the patient in the semi-Fowler's position. Alternatively, place the patient on the unaffected side with the waterproof pad underneath the site. *Rationale:* This position enhances accessibility to the insertion site of the chest tube and protects the bed from drainage.

Procedure for Performing Chest Tube Removal

Steps	Rationale	Special Considerations
1. **HH**		
2. **PE**		
3. Open the sterile suture removal set and prepare petrolatum gauze dressing and two to four 4 × 4 gauze sponges, as per hospital protocol.	Aseptic technique is maintained to prevent contamination of the wound.	
4. Perform a preprocedure verification and time out, if nonemergent.	Ensures patient safety.	
5. Discontinue suction from chest-drainage system and check for air leakage in air leak detector zone or indicator. Observe the air leak detector zone or indicator while the patient coughs.	Bubbling in the air leak detector is associated with an air leak. When an air leak is present, removal of the chest tube may cause development of a pneumothorax. Ensures a recurrent pneumothorax has not occurred.	If an air leak is present, the tube should not be removed. Consult with the physician, physician assistant, or advanced practice nurse to determine appropriate action.
6. Remove existing tape, and clean area around tubes with antiseptic solution or swab. Determine type of suture that secures each chest tube. Clip appropriately. If a purse-string suture is present, leave the long suture ends intact. **(Level D*)**	Allows access to the chest tube at the skin level and prepares the sutures for removal.	Antiseptic swabs remove a broad spectrum of microbes quickly and provide high-level antimicrobial action for up to 6 hours after use.[6]
7. Confirm that the tube is free from the suture and the tape.	Allows ease of removal and avoids tearing the skin.	
8. Cover pleural insertion sites with petrolatum gauze dressing and mediastinal insertion site with 4 × 4 gauze pads, as per hospital protocol.	Avoids the influx of air.	

*Level D: Peer-reviewed professional and organizational standards with the support of clinical study recommendations.

Procedure	for Performing Chest Tube Removal—*Continued*	
Steps	**Rationale**	**Special Considerations**
9. Clamp each tube to be removed with two Kelly clamps or umbilical clamps.[11] **(Level E*)**	Possibly prevents air from being introduced into the pleural space, although controversy is found in the literature.[11]	
10. Instruct the patient to perform a Valsalva maneuver at either end inspiration or end expiration.[2] **(Level E)**	Valsalva maneuver is needed to provide positive pressure in the pleural cavity and decrease the incidence of an involuntary gasp by the patient when the tube is removed.[2]	
A. End inspiration: Instruct patient to take a deep breath and hold it while performing the Valsalva maneuver for each tube removed. If the patient is receiving ventilator support and is unable to follow instructions, remove the tube during peak inspiration.		
B. End expiration: Instruct patient to forcibly exhale and perform the Valsalva maneuver at end expiration.		
C. If possible, patients may need to hold their breath until sutures are tied.		
11. Remove chest tubes rapidly, smoothly, and individually while patient is performing Valsalva maneuver or during peak inspiration if the patient is on a mechanical ventilator.	Prevents accidental entrance of air into the pleural space. Removal of pleural chest tubes should be accomplished rapidly with the simultaneous application of an occlusive dressing or closure with purse-string sutures to decrease possibility of air from entering the pleural space.	*Some resistance is expected; however, if strong resistance is encountered and rapid removal of the tube is not possible, stop the procedure and consult with the physician, physician's assistant, or advanced practice nurse immediately.* Resistance may indicate that the tube was inadvertently sutured during surgery or sternal closure.
A. Hold sutures in hand closer to head of patient, and apply mild pressure over exit site with folded 4 × 4 gauze pad.		
B. If tube was "Y" connected to another tube, cut the removed tube below the clamp to allow for easier manipulation when removing the remaining chest tubes.		
12. If a purse-string suture is present, tie it off with a square knot (see Fig. 23-1). If no purse-string was used, the site may be closed with adhesive skin closure strips.	Creates a firm closure of the chest tube site.	*Avoid pulling the suture too tight to prevent tissue necrosis at the site and to facilitate easier removal later.*

*Level E: Multiple case reports, theory-based evidence from expert opinions, or peer-reviewed professional organizational standards without clinical studies to support recommendations.

Procedure continues on following page

Procedure   for Performing Chest Tube Removal—*Continued*

Steps	Rationale	Special Considerations
13. Secure dressing with tape.	Creates a firm closure of the chest tube site.	This action is easier with a second person to place the tape while holding pressure over the site.
14. Examine each chest tube to verify that the entire tube has been removed.	If portion of tube is not removed, surgical removal is necessary to remove it.	Consult with physician, physician assistant, or advanced practice nurse immediately if a portion of the tube remains in the patient.
15. Assess the patient's condition after the procedure and compare the results with the preprocedure assessment, as described previously.	Ensures stable respiratory status after the procedure.	Increased work of breathing, decreased oxygen saturation, increased restlessness, symptoms of chest discomfort, and diminished breath sounds on the affected side are warning signs to be observed.
16. Obtain a chest radiograph (generally 1–4 hours after removal) only as clinically indicated.[7,16,19,21] **(Level B*)**	Assesses that the lung has remained expanded.	Low incidence of complication. Recommended to perform chest radiograph only if patient is clinically deteriorating.[7,16,19,21]
17. Dispose of used supplies and equipment and remove PE.		
18. HH		

*Level B: Well-designed, controlled studies with results that consistently support a specific action, intervention, or treatment.

Expected Outcomes

- Patient is comfortable and has no respiratory distress
- Lung remains expanded after chest tube removal
- Site remains free of infection

Unexpected Outcomes

- Pneumothorax
- Bleeding
- Skin necrosis
- Retained chest tube
- Infected chest tube insertion site

Patient Monitoring and Care

Steps	Rationale	Reportable Conditions
		These conditions should be reported if they persist despite nursing interventions.
1. Assess respiratory status, including oxygen saturation, work of breathing, breath sounds, and symptoms of chest discomfort. Obtain chest radiograph if significant changes are found.	Diminished respiratory status could indicate a pneumothorax. Pneumothorax could be from removal of the chest tube before all the air, fluid, or blood in the pleural space had been drained, or it may recur after removal of the chest tube if air is introduced accidentally into the pleural space through the chest tube tract.	• Decreased oxygen saturation on pulse oximetry • Increased work of breathing • Diminished breath sounds on affected side • Increased restlessness and symptoms of chest discomfort
2. Monitor insertion site for bleeding. If bleeding is found, apply pressure and place a tight occlusive dressing over site, which may be removed after 48 hours.	Persistent bleeding from insertion site could mean chest tube was against a vein or artery of chest wall before removal.	• Persistent bleeding

Patient Monitoring and Care —*Continued*

Steps	Rationale	Reportable Conditions
3. Monitor purse-string suture site for signs of skin necrosis.	If purse-string suture was pulled too tightly closed when chest tube was removed, skin necrosis may be seen.	• Dark or inflamed skin with necrotic areas visible
4. Monitor site for signs of infection.	Prolonged insertion of a chest tube increases the risk that the tract created by the chest tube may become infected, or infection may occur after removal of the chest tube if the opening created by the removal becomes contaminated.	• Purulent drainage • Increased body temperature • Inflammation • Tenderness • Warmth at site
5. Monitor insertion area for development of subcutaneous emphysema.	Air may leak into the surrounding tissues and cause crepitus.	• Crepitus
6. Monitor for signs and symptoms of pericardial effusion or cardiac tamponade.	Removal of chest tubes may cause increased bleeding into pericardium. Pericardial bleeding may continue after chest tubes are removed.	• Distant heart tones • Decreased blood pressure, tachycardia • Pulsus paradoxus • Narrowed pulse pressure • Equalized pulmonary artery pressures
7. Follow institution standard for assessing pain. Administer analgesia as prescribed.	Identifies need for pain interventions.	• Continued pain despite pain interventions

Documentation

Documentation should include the following:
- Patient and family education
- Respiratory and vital signs assessments before and after procedure
- Date and time of procedure and who performed the procedure
- Amount, color, and consistency of any drainage
- Application of a sterile occlusive dressing
- Type of suture in place and what was done to it (cut and removed or tied)

- Patient's tolerance of the procedure
- Completion and results of chest radiograph
- Specimens sent to laboratory (if applicable)
- Unexpected outcomes
- Nursing interventions
- Pain assessment, interventions, and effectiveness

References and Additional Readings

For a complete list of references and additional readings for this procedure, scan this QR code with any freely available smartphone code reader app, or visit http://booksite.elsevier.com/9780323376624.

24 Chest Tube Removal (Assist)

Peggy Kirkwood

PURPOSE: Chest tube removal is performed to discontinue a chest tube when it is no longer needed for the removal or drainage of air, blood, or fluid from the intrapleural or mediastinal space.

PREREQUISITE NURSING KNOWLEDGE

- Chest tubes are placed in the pleural or mediastinal space to evacuate an abnormal collection of air or fluid or both.
- For interpleural chest tubes, the air leak detector should bubble gently immediately on insertion of the chest tube during expiration and with coughing. Continuous bubbling in the air leak detector indicates a leak in the patient or the chest-drainage system. Fluctuations in the water level (also known as tidaling) in the water-seal chamber of 5 to 10 cm, rising during inhalation and falling during expiration, should be observed with spontaneous respirations. If the patient is on mechanical ventilation, the pattern of fluctuation is just the opposite. Any suction applied must be disconnected temporarily to assess correctly for fluctuations in the water-seal chamber.
- Flexible Silastic (Blake; Ethicon, Inc, Somerville, NJ) drains may be used in place of large-bore chest tubes in the mediastinal and pleural spaces after cardiac surgery. These tubes provide more efficient drainage and improved patient mobility with minimized tissue trauma and pain with removal.[3,16]
- Chest radiographs are done periodically to determine whether the lung has reexpanded. Daily chest radiographs have been found to be unnecessary while the tube is in place.[5,7,16,19,21] Reexpanded lungs, along with respiratory assessments that show improvement in the patient's respiratory status, are the basis for the decision to remove the chest tube.
- While the tubes are in place, patients may have related discomfort. Prompt removal of chest tubes encourages patients to increase ambulation and respiratory measures to improve lung expansion after surgery (e.g., coughing, deep breathing). However, removal of the chest tube may also be a painful procedure for the patient.[4,9,12–14]
- The types of sutures used to secure chest tubes vary according to the preference of the physician, the physician assistant, or the advanced practice nurse. One common type is the horizontal mattress or purse-string suture, which is threaded around and through the wound edges in a U shape with the ends left unknotted until the chest tube is removed. Usually, one or two anchor stitches accompany the purse-string suture (Fig. 23-1).
- A primary goal of chest tube removal is removal of tubes without introduction of air or contaminants into the pleural space.
- Available data indicate there is no consensus as to the rate of drainage that should be used as a threshold for tube removal and no evidence to suggest that it is unsafe to remove tubes that still have a relatively high rate of fluid drainage.[5,20] Research has shown that, depending on the reason for the chest tube, volumes of 200 to 450 mL/day do not adversely affect length of stay or overall costs compared with lower threshold volumes, nor does the risk of pleural fluid reaccumulation increase.[5,22] However, some suggested guidelines include the following:
  - ❖ Drainage has decreased to 50 to 200 mL in the prior 24 hours if tube was placed for hemothorax, empyema, or pleural effusion.
  - ❖ If tube was placed after cardiac surgery, drainage has changed from bloody to serosanguineous, no air leak is present, and amount is less than 100 mL in the past 8 hours.[1,10]
  - ❖ Pleural tubes are placed after cardiac surgery if the pleural cavity has been entered. They typically are removed within 24 to 48 hours after surgery.[1,10]
  - ❖ Mediastinal chest tubes most often are removed 24 to 36 hours after cardiac surgery.[1]
  - ❖ Lungs are reexpanded (as shown on chest radiographic results).
  - ❖ Respiratory status has improved (i.e., nonlabored respirations, equal bilateral breath sounds, absence of shortness of breath, decreased use of accessory muscles, symmetrical respiratory excursion, and respiratory rate less than 24 breaths/min).
  - ❖ Fluctuations are minimal or absent in the water-seal chamber of the collection device, and the level of solution rises in the chamber.
  - ❖ For interpleural chest tubes, air leaks have resolved for at least 24 hours (the absence of continuous bubbling in the water-seal chamber or absence of air bubbles

from right to left in the air leak detector), and the lung is fully reinflated on chest radiographic results.

EQUIPMENT

- Suture-removal set
- Antiseptic swabs (povidone-iodine, chlorhexidine gluconate with alcohol, etc.)
- Petrolatum gauze, as per hospital protocol
- Rubber-tipped Kelly clamps or disposable umbilical clamps
- Wide occlusive tape (2 inches)
- Elastic closure device, such as Steri-Strips (3M, St. Paul, MN)
- Dry 4×4 gauze sponges (two to four)
- Waterproof pad
- Personal protective equipment (goggles, sterile and non-sterile gloves, mask, gown)

Additional equipment, to have available as needed, includes the following:

- Specimen collection cup (if catheter tip is to be sent to the laboratory for analysis)
- Scissors

PATIENT AND FAMILY EDUCATION

- Assess the patient's and family's level of understanding about the condition and rationale for the procedure. **Rationale:** This assessment identifies the patient's and family's knowledge deficits concerning the patient's condition, the procedure, the expected benefits, and the potential risks. It also allows time for questions to clarify information and voice concerns. Explanations decrease patient anxiety and enhance cooperation.
- Explain the procedure, reason for removal, and sensations to be expected.[15,19] The most commonly reported sensations are pulling, pain or hurting, and burning.[14] **Rationale:** This explanation prepares the patient and enhances cooperation.
- Explain the patient's role in assisting with removal. Explain that the patient should perform the Valsalva maneuver on the count of three. Have the patient practice the maneuver before the procedure. **Rationale:** This explanation elicits patient cooperation and facilitates removal.
- Instruct the patient to turn and reposition every 2 hours after the chest tube has been removed. **Rationale:** This action prevents complications related to immobility and retained secretions.
- Instruct the patient to cough and breathe deeply after the chest tube has been removed, with splinting of the affected side or sternum (with mediastinal tubes). **Rationale:** This action prevents respiratory complications associated with retained secretions. The application of firm pressure over the insertion site (i.e., splinting) decreases pain and discomfort.
- Instruct the patient about the availability of prescribed analgesic medication after the chest tube is removed. **Rationale:** Analgesics alleviate pain and facilitate coughing, deep breathing, and repositioning.[9,13,19]

- Instruct the patient and family to report signs and symptoms of respiratory distress or infection immediately. **Rationale:** Immediate reporting facilitates prompt intervention to relieve a recurrent pneumothorax or to treat an infection.

PATIENT ASSESSMENT AND PREPARATION

Patient Assessment

- Assess respiratory status. **Rationale:** Assessment of respiratory status verifies the patient's readiness for chest tube removal.
  - ❖ Oxygen saturation within normal limits
  - ❖ Nonlabored respirations
  - ❖ Absence of shortness of breath
  - ❖ Decreased use of accessory muscles
  - ❖ Respiratory rate of less than 24 breaths/min
  - ❖ Equal bilateral breath sounds
- Assess chest tube drainage (less than 200 mL in 24 hours or less than 100 mL in 8 hours after cardiac surgery).[1,5,10] **Rationale:** Assessment of drainage verifies patient readiness for chest tube removal.
- For interpleural chest tubes, assess for minimal or no air leak in the air leak detector zone or indicator. **Rationale:** This assessment indicates whether the lung is reexpanded and whether or not air leak is present.
- Obtain chest radiographic results. **Rationale:** Lung reexpansion indicates that need for chest tube is resolved.
- Assess vital signs. **Rationale:** Vital sign assessment indicates whether the patient can tolerate chest tube removal.
- Assess laboratory results for clotting capability and medications that may affect clotting. **Rationale:** Low platelet levels or thrombolytic medications may precipitate excessive bleeding.[17]

Patient Preparation

- Verify correct patient with two identifiers. **Rationale:** Prior to performing a procedure, the nurse should ensure the correct identification of the patient for the intended intervention.
- Ensure that the patient understands preprocedural teachings. Answer questions as they arise, and reinforce information as needed. **Rationale:** This communication evaluates and reinforces understanding of previously taught information. Anticipatory preparation may prepare patients for a better experience.[12,18]
- Administer premedication of adequate analgesics at least 20 minutes before the procedure. Alternatively, subfascial lidocaine may be injected into the chest tube tract. In addition to opioids, adjunct methods shown to decrease pain during chest tube removal include slow deep-breathing relaxation exercises and application of cold packs.[8,9] **Rationale:** Intravenous 4-mg morphine 20 minutes before or 30-mg ketorolac 60 minutes before the procedure have been shown to have substantial relief of pain without excessive analgesia.[12] Pain medication, relaxation exercises, and application of cold reduces the

discomfort and anxiety experienced, which facilitates patient cooperation.[8,9,12,13]

- Time the removal procedure to occur at peak analgesic effect. ***Rationale:*** This timing increases patient cooperation and decreases anxiety.[13]

- Place the patient in the semi-Fowler's position. Alternatively, place the patient on the unaffected side with the waterproof pad underneath the site. ***Rationale:*** This position enhances accessibility to the insertion site of the chest tube and protects the bed from drainage.

Procedure	for Assisting with Chest Tube Removal		
Steps	**Rationale**	**Special Considerations**	
1. HH			
2. PE			
3. Assist with opening the sterile suture removal set and preparing petrolatum gauze dressing and two to four 4×4 gauze sponges, as per hospital protocol.	Aseptic technique is maintained to prevent contamination of the wound.		
4. Perform a preprocedure verification and time out, if nonemergent.	Ensures patient safety.		
5. Assist with discontinuing suction from chest-drainage system and check for air leakage in air leak detector zone or indicator. Observe the air leak detector zone or indicator while the patient coughs.	Bubbling in the air leak detector is associated with an air leak. When an air leak is present, removal of the chest tube may cause development of a pneumothorax. Ensures a recurrent pneumothorax has not occurred.	If an air leak is present, the tube should not be removed. Consult with the physician, physician assistant, or advanced practice nurse to determine appropriate action.	
6. Assist with removing existing tape, and clean area around tubes with antiseptic swab. **(Level D*)**	Allows access to the chest tube at the skin level and prepares the sutures for removal.	Antiseptic swabs remove a broad spectrum of microbes quickly and provide high-level antimicrobial action for up to 6 hours after use.[6]	
7. Assist with covering the pleural insertion sites with petrolatum gauze dressing and mediastinal insertion site with 4×4 gauze pads, as per hospital protocol.	Avoids the influx of air.		
8. Assist with clamping each tube to be removed with two Kelly clamps or umbilical clamps.[11] **(Level E*)**	Possibly prevents air from being introduced into the pleural space, although controversy is found in the literature.[11]		
9. The tube is removed while the patient is performing a Valsalva maneuver at either end inspiration or end expiration.[2] **(Level E)**	Valsalva maneuver is needed to provide positive pressure in the pleural cavity and decrease the incidence of an involuntary gasp by the patient when the tube is removed.[2]		
A. End inspiration: Instruct patient to take a deep breath and hold it while performing the Valsalva maneuver for each tube removed. If the patient is receiving ventilator support and is unable to follow instructions, remove the tube during peak inspiration.	Removal of pleural chest tubes should be accomplished rapidly with the simultaneous application of an occlusive dressing or closure with purse-string sutures to decrease possibility of air from entering the pleural space.		

*Level D: Peer-reviewed professional and organizational standards with the support of clinical study recommendations.
*Level E: Multiple case reports, theory-based evidence from expert opinions, or peer-reviewed professional organizational standards without clinical studies to support recommendations.

Procedure for Assisting with Chest Tube Removal—*Continued*

Steps	Rationale	Special Considerations
B. End expiration: Instruct patient to forcibly exhale and perform the Valsalva maneuver at end expiration.		
C. If possible, patients may need to hold their breath until sutures are tied.		
10. Assist with securing the dressing with tape.	Creates a firm closure of the chest tube site.	This action is easier with a second person to place the tape while holding pressure over the site.
11. Assess the patient's condition after the procedure, and compare the results with preprocedure assessment as noted previously.	Ensures stable respiratory status after the procedure.	Increased work of breathing, decreased oxygen saturation, increased restlessness, symptoms of chest discomfort, and diminished breath sounds on the affected side are warning signs to be observed.
12. Ensure a chest radiograph is obtained, if ordered (generally 1–24 hours after removal) only as clinically indicated.[7,16,19,21] **(Level B*)**	Assesses that the lung has remained expanded.	Low incidence of complication. Recommended to perform chest radiograph only if patient is clinically deteriorating.[7,16,19,21]
13. Dispose of used supplies and equipment and remove PE.		
14. HH		

*Level B: Well-designed, controlled studies with results that consistently support a specific action, intervention, or treatment.

Expected Outcomes

- Patient is comfortable and has no respiratory distress
- Lung remains expanded after chest tube removal
- Site remains free of infection

Unexpected Outcomes

- Pneumothorax
- Bleeding
- Skin necrosis
- Retained chest tube
- Infected chest tube insertion site

Patient Monitoring and Care

Steps	Rationale	Reportable Conditions
		These conditions should be reported if they persist despite nursing interventions.
1. Assess respiratory status, including oxygen saturation, work of breathing, breath sounds, and symptoms of chest discomfort. Obtain chest radiograph if significant changes are found.	Diminished respiratory status could indicate a pneumothorax. Pneumothorax could be from removal of the chest tube before all the air, fluid, or blood in the pleural space had been drained, or it may recur after removal of the chest tube if air is introduced accidentally into the pleural space through the chest tube tract.	• Decreased oxygen saturation on pulse oximetry • Increased work of breathing • Diminished breath sounds on affected side • Increased restlessness and symptoms of chest discomfort

Procedure continues on following page

Patient Monitoring and Care —*Continued*

Steps	Rationale	Reportable Conditions
2. Monitor insertion site for bleeding. If bleeding is found, apply pressure and place a tight occlusive dressing over site, which may be removed after 48 hours.	Persistent bleeding from insertion site could mean chest tube was against a vein or artery of chest wall before removal.	• Persistent bleeding
3. Monitor purse-string suture site for signs of skin necrosis.	If purse-string suture was pulled too tightly closed when chest tube was removed, skin necrosis may be seen.	• Dark or inflamed skin with necrotic areas visible
4. Monitor site for signs of infection.	Prolonged insertion of a chest tube increases the risk that the tract created by the chest tube may become infected, or infection may occur after removal of the chest tube if the opening created by the removal becomes contaminated.	• Purulent drainage • Increased body temperature • Inflammation • Tenderness • Warmth at site
5. Monitor insertion area for development of subcutaneous emphysema.	Air may leak into the surrounding tissues and cause crepitus.	• Crepitus
6. Monitor for signs and symptoms of pericardial effusion or cardiac tamponade.	Removal of chest tubes may cause increased bleeding into pericardium. Pericardial bleeding may continue after chest tubes are removed.	• Distant heart tones • Decreased blood pressure, tachycardia • Pulsus paradoxus • Narrowed pulse pressure • Equalized pulmonary artery pressures
7. Follow institution standard for assessing pain. Administer analgesia as prescribed.	Identifies need for pain interventions.	• Continued pain despite pain interventions

Documentation

Documentation should include the following:
- Patient and family education
- Respiratory and vital signs assessments before and after procedure
- Date and time of procedure and who performed the procedure
- Amount, color, and consistency of any drainage
- Application of a sterile occlusive dressing
- Patient's tolerance of the procedure
- Completion and results of chest radiograph
- Specimens sent to laboratory (if applicable)
- Unexpected outcomes
- Nursing interventions
- Pain assessment, interventions, and effectiveness

References and Additional Readings

For a complete list of references and additional readings for this procedure, scan this QR code with any freely available smartphone code reader app, or visit http://booksite.elsevier.com/9780323376624.

25 Closed Chest-Drainage System

Joya D. Pickett

PURPOSE: Closed chest-drainage systems are used to facilitate the evacuation of fluid, blood, and air from the pleural space, the mediastinum, or both; to restore negative pressure to the pleural space; and to promote reexpansion of a collapsed lung.

PREREQUISITE NURSING KNOWLEDGE

- The clinical need for chest drainage arises whenever the negative pressure in the pleural cavity is disrupted by the presence of air and/or fluid, resulting in pulmonary compromise. The purpose of a chest-drainage system (CDS) is to evacuate the air and/or fluid from the chest cavity to reestablish normal intrathoracic pressure.
- Closed CDSs are integrated disposable systems (also known as chest-drainage units) that are modeled after the classic three-bottle CDS.
- Normal anatomy and physiology of the thorax:
  - Under usual conditions, normal intrapleural pressures measure approximately -4 cm H_2O during expiration, whereas at end inspiration, pressure decreases to -8 cm H_2O.[15]
  - The mediastinum is within the musculoskeletal cage of the thorax and contains three subdivisions. The two lateral subdivisions hold the lungs. Between the lungs is the mediastinum, which contains the heart, the great vessels, parts of the trachea and esophagus, and other structures.
  - The lungs consist of the trachea and the bronchi, which divide into smaller branches until they reach the alveoli, known as the air sacs.
- Thoracic pathophysiology requiring a chest tube and CDS, which may occur spontaneously or as the result of trauma and/or surgery:
  - Pneumothoraces (e.g., open, closed, and tension)
  - Hemothorax
  - Pleural effusions
  - Chylothorax
  - Empyema
  - Pericardial effusions, including cardiac tamponade
- CDSs include the following types:
  - Dry suction with a traditional water-seal, dry suction with a one-way valve, and wet suction with a traditional water-seal
  - Those that implement the use of gravity, suction, or both to restore negative pressure and remove air, fluid, and blood from the pleural space or the mediastinum
- Some CDSs use dry suction with a traditional water-seal and either a regulator or a restricted orifice mechanism.

Although water is added to the water-seal chamber, water does not need to be added to the suction chamber. Instead, the suction source (usually a wall regulator) is increased until an indicator appears.
- Some CDSs are waterless, referred to as dry-dry drains, and have a one-way valve, which eliminates the need to fill any chambers (except an air-leak indicator zone, as needed). A valve opens on expiration and allows patient air to exit, then closes to prevent atmospheric air from entering during inspiration. This one-way valve feature allows the system to be used in the vertical or horizontal position without loss of the seal. These systems are safe if accidentally tipped. The amount of suction delivered is regulated with an adjustable dial.
  - Advantages of dry suction are ease of setup; ease of application if higher, more precise levels of suction are needed; and a quiet system.
- CDSs may have some of the following components:
  - Tubing, which may or may not be latex free. See manufacturer guidelines for specific information
  - Collection chambers, which may be replaceable, allowing them to be removed when filled and replaced with a new collection chamber without changing the entire unit
  - Fluid-collection ports, which may be self-sealing ports or collection tubes for aspiration of drainage samples and removal of excess chamber fluid levels
  - A one-way mechanism created by a water-seal that permits air and fluid to be removed and prevents backflow into the chest[20]
  - Accessories that may be used to convert systems to autotransfusion units
- Examples of CDSs include the Pleur-Evac, Thora-Klex, Argyle, and Atrium systems.
- CDSs contain the following chambers (Fig. 25-1):
  - The collection chamber, the largest of the three chambers, generally on the far-right side of the CDS, is the drainage reservoir. This is where drainage from the pleural space accumulates. A window with calibrated markings is located on the exterior of the drainage collection for observation of the color, amount, and consistency of fluid.
  - The suction-control chamber, generally on the far-left side of the CDS, is the suction chamber that regulates the amount of negative pressure applied to the system.

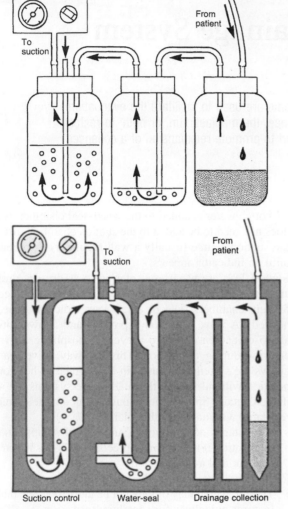

Figure 25-1 Disposable system correlates with three-bottle system. *(From Luce JM, Tyler ML, Pierson DJ: Intensive respiratory care, Philadelphia, 1984, Saunders.)*

TABLE 25-1	**Pressure Conversion Chart***
cm H$_2$O	mm Hg
20	15
25	18
30	22
35	26
40	30
45	33
50	37
60	44

*Approximate values.
Reprinted with permission of Atrium Medical Corporation, Hudson, NH.

- ❖ The water-seal chamber, in traditional water-seal CDSs (wet systems), is usually the middle chamber and provides a one-way relief valve between the atmospheric pressure and the patient's negative intrapleural pressure.
- ❖ Positive-pressure relief valves are used to prevent a tension pneumothorax if the suction tubing becomes accidentally occluded or if the suction source fails. In addition, automatic and manual pressure relief valves vent excessive negative pressure, such as may occur during deep inspiration or with milking of the chest tube.
- Suction guidelines include the following:
  - ❖ When clinically indicted, the addition of a suction source can enhance drainage when large volumes of air or fluid must be evacuated.
  - ❖ Currently guidelines recommend that a water-seal alone is safe for most patients with a pneumothorax or small air leak.[2-5,8,9,21] However, if the pneumothorax or air leak is large, expanding, or persistent, suction is recommended.[5,8,9]

- ❖ The most common amount of suction pressure ranges from −10 to −20 cm H$_2$O.[1,3,8,14] High suction levels may cause persistent pleural air leaks, air stealing, lung tissue entrapment, and reexpansion pulmonary edema.[14,17]
- ❖ There are differences in flow rates and in accuracy of delivered negative pressures noted in CDSs; however, they are not likely to be clinically important.[6,7]
- ❖ Some systems contain an exit vent from the water-seal chamber that ensures the drainage unit remains vented when the suction device is off. Do not close or occlude the exit vent.[21,29] When using CDSs without an exit vent, the drainage systems should be disconnected from suction before they are turned off.[21,29]
- ❖ Some wall-mounted suction devices need control and pressure gauges to regulate and monitor for potential surges in suction levels.[15,22,25]
- ❖ If clinically appropriate, some wet suction with traditional water-seal drainage systems can provide suction levels greater than −25 cm H$_2$O. The suction-chamber vent holes can be occluded with nonporous tape or by replacing them with the manufacturer's special pronged vent plug and connecting directly to wall regulator suction. Suction levels must be converted from prescribed levels of cm H$_2$O suction to mm Hg of wall suction (Table 25-1).
- General guidelines in the proper care of the CDC include the following:
  - ❖ Greater pressure within the chest than within the system is needed to maintain proper functioning of the closed system; this requirement is accomplished by keeping the drainage unit at least 1 foot below the chest tube insertion site and the tubing free of dependent loops and obstructions,[1,11,13,25,27] which prevents siphoning of the contents back into the pleural cavity.[25]
  - ❖ Except for the exit vent, an airtight system is required to assist in maintaining negative pressure in the pleura and to prevent air entrapment in the pleural space.
  - ❖ Tidaling, fluctuations that occur with inspiration and expiration, provides a continuous manometer of the pressure changes in the pleural space and indicates overall respiratory effort. Absence of fluctuations suggests obstruction of the drainage system from clots, contact with lung tissue, kinks, loss of subatmospheric

pressure from fluid-filled dependent loops, or complete reexpansion of the lung.[1,10,19]

* In general, clamping of chest tubes is contraindicated. ***Clamping a chest tube in a patient with a pleural air leak may cause a tension pneumothorax.*** The few situations in which chest tubes may be clamped briefly (i.e., less than a minute) include locating the source of an air leak, replacing the CDS, determining whether a patient is ready to have the chest tube removed, and during chest tube removal.[1,14,15,21,29]

EQUIPMENT
Disposable Setup (Wet and Dry Systems)

* Disposable chest-drainage unit
* Gloves
* Suction source and regulator
* Connecting tubing
* 1-L bottle of sterile water or normal saline (for systems that use water)
* 50-mL irrigation syringe (if not supplied with unit) for systems that use water
* Tape (1 inch), one roll, or zip ties (e.g., Parham-Martin bands)

PATIENT AND FAMILY EDUCATION

* Explain the procedure, the indication for the chest tube insertion, and how the closed CDS works. ***Rationale:*** This communication identifies patient and family knowledge deficits about the patient's condition, procedure, expected benefits, and potential risks and allows time for questions to clarify information and to voice concerns. Explanations decrease patient anxiety and enhance cooperation.
* After chest tube insertion, instruct the patient to sit in a semi-Fowler's position (unless contraindicated). ***Rationale:*** Proper positioning facilitates drainage from the lung by allowing air to rise and fluid to settle, enhancing removal via the chest tube. This position also makes breathing easier.
* Instruct the patient to turn and reposition every 2 hours to facilitate drainage. The patient may lie on the side with the chest tube but should keep the tubing free of kinks. ***Rationale:*** Turning and positioning prevents complications related to immobility and retained secretions. Keeping the tubing free of kinks maintains patency of the tube, facilitates drainage, and prevents the accumulation of pressure within the pleural space, which interferes with lung reexpansion.
* Instruct the patient to cough and deep breathe, with splinting of the affected side or sternum (if mediastinal tube is in place). ***Rationale:*** Coughing and deep breathing increase pressure within the pleural space, facilitating drainage, promoting lung reexpansion, and preventing respiratory complications associated with retained secretions. The application of firm pressure over the chest tube insertion site (e.g., splinting) may decrease pain and discomfort.
* Encourage active or passive range-of-motion exercises of the arm on the affected side. ***Rationale:*** The patient may limit the movement of the arm on the affected side to decrease the discomfort at the insertion site, which may result in joint discomfort and potential joint complications.
* Instruct the patient and family about activity as prescribed while maintaining the drainage system below the level of the chest. ***Rationale:*** The drainage system is maintained below the level of the chest to facilitate gravity drainage and to prevent backflow into the pleural space and potential infectious contamination into the pleural space.
* Instruct the patient and family about the availability of prescribed analgesic medication and other pain-relief strategies. ***Rationale:*** Pain relief ensures comfort and facilitates coughing, deep breathing, positioning, and range-of-motion exercises, and promotes healing.

PATIENT ASSESSMENT AND PREPARATION
Patient Assessment

* Assess significant medical history or injury, including chronic lung disease, spontaneous pneumothorax, pulmonary disease, therapeutic procedures, and mechanism of injury. ***Rationale:*** Medical history or injury may provide the etiological basis for the occurrence of pneumothorax, hemothorax, empyema, pleural effusion, or chylothorax.
* Assess patient's baseline cardiopulmonary status (if patient's condition does not necessitate immediate intervention). ***Rationale:*** Provides reference points for future assessments upon completion of the procedure.
* Assess baseline cardiopulmonary status, as follows:
  * Vital signs (blood pressure, heart rate, respiratory rate)
  * Shortness of breath or dyspnea
  * Anxiety, restlessness, or apprehension
  * Cyanosis
  * Decreased oxygen saturation (e.g., pulse oximetry [Spo_2])
  * Decreased or absent breath sounds on the affected side
  * Crackles adjacent to the affected area
  * Asymmetrical chest excursion with respirations
  * Hyperresonance with percussion on the affected side (pneumothorax)
  * Dullness or flatness with percussion on the affected side (hemothorax, pleural effusion, empyema, or chylothorax)
  * Subcutaneous emphysema or crepitus (pneumothorax)
  * Sudden sharp focal chest pain
  * Tracheal deviation to the unaffected side (tension pneumothorax)
  * Neck vein distention (tension pneumothorax, cardiac tamponade)
  * Muffled heart sounds (cardiac tamponade)
  Rationale: Provides reference points for future tests upon completion of the procedure.
* Assess diagnostic tests (if patient's condition does not necessitate immediate intervention):
  * Chest radiograph
  * Arterial blood gases

Patient Preparation

- Ensure the patient understands preprocedural teachings. Answer questions as they arise, and reinforce information as needed. *Rationale:* This communication evaluates and reinforces understanding of previously presented information.
- Verify that the patient is the correct patient using two identifiers. *Rationale:* Before performing a procedure, the nurse should ensure the correct identification of the patient for the intended intervention.
- Administer prescribed analgesics or sedatives as needed. *Rationale:* Analgesics and sedatives reduce the discomfort and anxiety experienced, facilitating patient cooperation and improving outcomes.

Procedure **for Dry Suction Closed Chest-Drainage Systems**		
Steps	Rationale	Special Considerations
1. HH		
2. PE		
3. Open sterile packages.	Maintains aseptic technique whenever changes are made to the system.	
4. Stabilize the unit. Some systems have a floor stand. For systems with an in-line connector, move the patient tube clamp down next to the in-line connector.	Keeping the clamp visible helps prevent inadvertent clamping.	Clamping of chest tubes can cause air trapped in the pleural space to accumulate and may cause tension pneumothorax.
5. *Dry suction with a traditional water-seal:* Remove the connector cap from the short tubing of the water-seal chamber and use the funnel provided or a 50-mL syringe to add sterile water or normal saline to the 2-cm level. Some systems provide prefilled sterile water containers. *Dry suction with a one-way valve:* Fill air-leak monitor zone.	Depth of solution required to establish a water-seal; the water-seal permits air and fluid to be removed from the patient and prevents the backflow of air into the chest.[1,19]	Water-seal levels greater than 2 cm increase the work of breathing; levels less than 2 cm can expose the water-seal to air and increase the risk for pneumothorax.[19]
6. Hang drainage unit from bed frame or set it on a floor stand. **(Level E*)**	Drainage unit must be kept below the level of the chest to promote gravity drainage and to prevent backflow of drainage into the pleural space, which interferes with lung expansion.[1,25]	Avoid hanging drainage unit from bed rails or other movable structures.
7. Connect the long tubing from the drainage collection chamber to the chest tube. **(Level C*)**	Creates the closed CDS; avoid dependent or fluid-filled loops.[13,24]	Avoid dependent or fluid-filled loops, which may create back pressure and decrease the effectiveness of suction.[13,24]
8. For gravity drainage, leave the suction-control chamber open to air. **(Level M*)**	Creates the exit vent for the escape of air.	*Clamping of chest tubes can cause air trapped in the pleural space to accumulate and may cause tension pneumothorax.*

*Level C: Qualitative studies, descriptive or correlational studies, integrative reviews, systematic reviews, or randomized controlled trials with inconsistent results.

*Level E: Multiple case reports, theory-based evidence from expert opinions, or peer-reviewed professional organizational standards without clinical studies to support recommendations.

*Level M: Manufacturer's recommendations only.

Procedure	**for Dry Suction Closed Chest-Drainage Systems—*Continued***	
Steps	Rationale	Special Considerations
9. To initiate suction, connect the CDS to the suction source and dial in the prescribed amount of suction (usually −10 to −20 cm H_2O), and then increase suction source until indicator mark appears according to manufacturer's guidelines.	Activates suction.	Apply suction as per manufacturer's guidelines. For example, to apply −20 cm H_2O suction, use a minimum vacuum pressure of −80 mm Hg. Suction source vacuum should be >−80 mm Hg when multiple chest drains are used. For a suction level <−20 cm H_2O, any observed bellows expansion across the monitor window confirms adequate suction operation. To decrease suction, set the dial, confirm patient on suction, then depress the high-negativity vent, venting to the newer lower amount.
10. Tape all connection points in the CDS (see Fig. 21-2). A. One-inch tape is placed horizontally, extending over the connections (a portion of the connector may be left unobstructed by the tape). B. Reinforce the horizontal tape with tape placed vertically so that it encircles both ends of the connector.	Except for the exit vent, a secure and airtight system is required to avoid inadvertent disconnection that could cause air entrapment in the pleural space and decreased pleural negative pressure. This technique secures the connections but allows visualization of drainage in the connector.	Zip ties (Parham-Martin bands) may be used to secure connections instead of tape.
11. Dispose of soiled equipment and supplies and remove **PE**.		
12. **HH**		

Procedure	**for Wet Suction Closed Chest-Drainage Systems**	
1. **HH**		
2. **PE**		
3. Open sterile packages.	Maintains aseptic technique whenever changes are made to the system.	
4. Stabilize the unit. Some systems have a floor stand. For systems with an in-line connector, move the patient tube clamp down next to the in-line connector.	Keeping the clamp visible helps prevent inadvertent clamping.	Clamping of chest tubes can cause air trapped in the pleural space to accumulate and may cause tension pneumothorax.
5. Remove the connector cap from the short tubing of the water-seal chamber and use the funnel provided or a 50-mL syringe to add sterile water or normal saline to the 2-cm level.	Depth of solution required to establish a water-seal; the water-seal permits air and fluid to be removed from the chest and prevents backflow of air.[1,19]	Water-seal levels >2 cm increase the work of breathing; levels <2 cm can expose the water-seal to air and increase the risk for pneumothorax.[19]
6. For gravity drainage, leave the short tubing from the suction control chamber open to air by turning stopcock to "open" or "on" position.	Creates the exit vent for the escape of air.	Clamping or occlusion of the exit vent can cause air to remain trapped in the pleural space, which may cause tension pneumothorax.

Procedure continues on following page

Procedure	**for Wet Suction Closed Chest-Drainage Systems—*Continued***	
7. For suction drainage, fill the suction-control chamber with sterile water or normal saline to the prescribed level (usually −10 to −20 cm H$_2$O suction). Connect the short tubing from the suction-control chamber to the suction source.	Suction is regulated by the height of the solution level in this chamber.	Refill the solution level as necessary to the prescribed amount to replace solution lost through evaporation. Remove excess fluid as necessary via self-sealing grommet.
8. Hang chest-drainage unit from bed frame, or set it on a floor stand. **(Level E*)**	Drainage unit must be kept below the level of the chest to promote gravity drainage and to prevent backflow of drainage into the pleural space, which interferes with lung expansion.[1,25]	Avoid hanging drainage unit from bed rails or other movable structure.
9. Connect the long tubing from the drainage collection chamber to the chest tube. **(Level C*)**	Creates the drainage-collection system; avoid dependent or fluid-filled loops.[13,24]	Dependent or fluid-filled loops may create back pressure and decrease the effectiveness of suction.[13,24]
10. Turn on the suction source, if prescribed, to elicit gentle constant bubbling. Leave stopcock between CDS and suction source fully open and adjust force of bubbling at suction source to decrease risk for pneumothorax.	Activates suction.	Some systems have a suction-control feature to maintain the desired suction level automatically despite fluctuations in the suction source. The stopcock should be kept fully in "open" or "on" position and force of bubbling should be adjusted at suction source.
11. Tape all connection points in the CDS (see Fig. 21-2).[15] A. One inch tape is placed horizontally extending over the connections (a portion of the connector may be left unobstructed by the tape). B. Reinforce the horizontal tape with tape placed vertically so that it encircles both ends of the connector.	Except for the exit vent, a secure and airtight system is required to avoid inadvertent disconnection that could cause air entrapment in the pleural space and decreased pleural negative pressure. This technique secures the connections but allows visualization of drainage in the connector.	Zip ties (Parham-Martin bands) may be used to secure connections instead of tape.
12. Dispose of soiled equipment and supplies and remove **PE**.		
13. **HH**		

---

*Level C: Qualitative studies, descriptive or correlational studies, integrative reviews, systematic reviews, or randomized controlled trials with inconsistent results.
*Level E: Multiple case reports, theory-based evidence from expert opinions, or peer-reviewed professional organizational standards without clinical studies to support recommendations.

Expected Outcomes	**Unexpected Outcomes**
• Removal of air, fluid, or blood from the thoracic cavity • Fluctuation or tidaling noted in the water-seal chamber (until lung reexpanded) • Relief of respiratory distress • Reexpansion of the collapsed lung as validated with chest radiograph	• Tension pneumothorax • Hemorrhagic shock • Absence of drainage and fluctuation or tidaling, or continuous bubbling in the water-seal chamber with continued respiratory distress • No evidence of reexpansion of lung • Fever, purulent drainage, and redness around the insertion site or purulent drainage in the chest tube

Patient Monitoring and Care

Steps	Rationale	Reportable Conditions
		These conditions should be reported if they persist despite nursing interventions.
1. Assess every 1–2 hours and with any change in patient condition or according to institution protocol.	Provides baseline and ongoing assessment of patient's condition.	• Tachypnea • Decreased or absent breath sounds • Hypoxemia • Tachycardia • Dysrhythmias • Hypotension • Muffled heart tones • Subcutaneous emphysema (crepitus) • Neck vein distention • Tracheal deviation • Fever • Absence of fluctuations in water-seal chamber with respiratory distress
2. Monitor the amount and type of drainage by marking the drainage level on the outside of the drainage-collection chamber in hourly or shift increments (depending on the amount of drainage) or in time increments established by institution policy or per practitioner orders. Monitor amount and type of drainage.	Marking container provides reference point for future measurements. Volume loss can cause patients to become hypovolemic or can signal intrapulmonary bleeding. Drainage should decrease gradually and change from bloody to pink to straw colored. Sudden flow of dark bloody drainage that occurs with position change is often old blood. Decreased or absent drainage associated with respiratory distress may indicate obstruction; decreased or absent drainage without respiratory distress may indicate lung reexpansion. Autotransfusion: if chest-drainage transfusion (autotransfusion) is being considered, please see Autotransfusion (Procedure 20).	• Drainage >100 mL/hr[1] or according to practitioner order • Sudden decrease or absence of drainage • Change in characteristics of drainage, such as unexpectedly bloody, cloudy, or milky • New onset of clots

Procedure continues on following page

Patient Monitoring and Care —*Continued*

Steps	Rationale	Reportable Conditions
3. Assess patient and CDS for an air leak. If a suction source has been added, momentarily turn suction off or pinch suction tubing to accurately assess.[1] An air leak is present if air bubbles are observed in the water-seal chamber or going from right-to-left in the leak detector zone. When assessing the air-leak chamber, ask the patient to take deep breaths in and out. If you do not note an air leak, ask the patient to cough.[8] When the patient's pleural space is leaking air, intermittent bubbling is seen corresponding to respirations. If bubbling is continuous, suspect an air leak in the system. To locate the source, intermittently pinch the chest tube or drainage tubing for a moment (i.e., less than a minute), beginning at the insertion site and progressing to the chest-drainage unit.[1]	Assessing for an air leak is one way to determine whether the patient is experiencing a pneumothorax. Bubbling when suction is initially turned on occurs with air displaced by fluid drainage in the collection chamber, loose connections in the system, or an air leak in the pleural space.[10] With a minor air leak, bubbling may occur only with coughing when airway pressures reach their peak.[8,29] An airtight system is required to help reestablish negative pressure in the pleural space. If bubbling in the water-seal chamber stops when the chest tube is occluded at the dressing site, the air leak is inside the patient's chest or under the dressing. If a new-onset air leak, reinforce the dressing and notify the physician. If the bubbling stops when the drainage tubing is occluded along its length, the air leak is between the occlusion and the patient's chest; check to ensure all connections are airtight.[1,8] If bubbling does not stop with occlusion, replace the CDS.	• New or increasing air leaks in the chest or around the chest tube insertion site • Chest tube drainage from a mediastinal tube does not normally cause bubbling in the water-seal chamber; if noted, it may indicate communication with the pleural space; notify physician • Notify physician of system knock over and changing of the CDS (e.g., chest radiograph may be ordered).[29]

4. Assess chest tube and CDS patency on insertion, every 1–2 hours, and with a change in patient condition. Routine chest tube stripping or milking is not recommended. Upon identification of a visible clot or other obstructing drainage, gently milk (manual squeezing and releasing of small segments of tubing, or fan-folding and compressing small segments of tubing[13]) between the fingers.[10–12,16,18,22,23,26, 28-30]
(Level C*)
Ensure there are no clamps on the chest tubes during milking.
	Obstruction of drainage from the chest tube interferes with lung reexpansion or may cause cardiac tamponade.
	Stripping the entire length of the chest tube is contraindicated because it results in transient high negative pressures in the pleural space that could lead to lung entrapment.[11]
	No significant differences are reported in the amount of drainage when the tubing is milked as opposed to stripped.[12] Milking can cause excessive negativity. Use the high negativity relief value to restore negativity to prescribed levels (see Step 8). Milking with a clamp on can result in the build-up of excessive thoracic pressure.
		• Inability to establish patency
		• Excessive drainage
		• Signs and/or symptoms of increasing:
		  • Pneumothorax
		  • Cardiac tamponade
		  • Hemothorax

5. Maintain drainage tubing free of dependent loops (i.e., place the tube horizontally on the bed and down into the collection chamber, coiling the tubing on the bed). If a dependent loop cannot be avoided, lift and drain the tubing every 15 minutes.[13,14,24] **(Level C)**	Drainage that accumulates in dependent loops obstructs chest drainage into the collecting system and increases pressure within the lung.[10,12,13,15,22,24] Allow enough length for patient movement.	• Loops or kinks that cannot be removed

---

*Level C: Qualitative studies, descriptive or correlational studies, integrative reviews, systematic reviews, or randomized controlled trials with inconsistent results.

Patient Monitoring and Care —*Continued*

Steps	Rationale	Reportable Conditions
6. Monitor fluid levels in the CDS chambers by briefly turning off the suction and refill (usually every 8 hours for suction chamber and every 24 hours for water-seal) or remove solution levels as necessary to the prescribed amount.	To maintain prescribed water-seal and suction levels and to prevent complications. Water-seal levels >2 cm increase the work of breathing; levels <2 cm expose the water-seal to air and increase the risk for pneumothorax.[1,19]	• Inability to maintain a water-seal or to keep suction at prescribed level
7. Assess for CDS patency: note fluctuations or tidaling of fluid level in the water-seal chamber (disposable CDS) or the long straw of the water-seal bottle (bottle CDS) with respirations.[1,19] If a suction source has been added, momentarily turn suction off or pinch suction tubing to accurately assess for fluctuations or tidaling.	Tidaling, fluid fluctuation up and down or back and forth, indicates effective communication between the pleural space and drainage system and provides an indication of lung expansion. Fluctuations or tidaling stops when the lung is reexpanded or when the tubing is obstructed by a kink, a fluid-filled loop, the patient lying on the tubing, or a clot or tissue at the distal end.[1,10,19] Suction must be turned off to accurately assess for tidaling.	• Absence of fluctuations or tidaling
8. Assess CDS equipped with a float valve for increases in the patient's negative intrathoracic pressure. Inspect water-seal chamber for increased levels (e.g., after milking of chest tube or when decreasing the amount of suction). Ensure the CDS is operating on suction. Second, temporarily depress the filtered manual vent until the float valve releases and the water column lowers.	Changes in the patient's intrathoracic pressure are reflected by the height of the water in the water-seal column. Do not lower water-seal column when suction is not operating or when patient is on gravity drainage. Resume suction while performing this operation. If suction is not operative, or operating on gravity drainage, depressing the high-negative relief valve can reduce negative pressure within the collection chamber to zero (atmosphere), possibly resulting in a pneumothorax.	• Sustained increases in negative pressures
9. Assess insertion site and surrounding skin for the presence of subcutaneous emphysema (crepitus) and signs of infection or inflammation daily and with each dressing change. Dressings should be changed when soiled, per institution protocol, or when ordered by practitioner. Routine petroleum dressings are not recommended.[15] **(Level E*)**	Crepitus may indicate chest tube obstruction or improper tube position. Skin integrity is altered during insertion and can lead to infection. Petroleum gauze dressing has been noted to cause skin maceration, potentiating the risk of infection.[15]	• New or increasing subcutaneous emphysema (crepitus) • Fever • Redness around insertion site • Purulent drainage

*Level E: Multiple case reports, theory-based evidence from expert opinions, or peer-reviewed professional organizational standards without clinical studies to support recommendations.

Procedure continues on following page

Patient Monitoring and Care —*Continued*

Steps	Rationale	Reportable Conditions
10. Monitor collection chamber for total amount of fluid. Change CDS when approaching full or if system integrity is interrupted (i.e., cracked). Assess cardiopulmonary status and vital signs (including SpO$_2$) before and after procedure. Prepare new CDS according to manufacturer's instructions. Then, briefly (i.e., for less than a minute) cross clamp the chest tube close to the patient's chest. Attach the new system, unclamp the chest tube, check connections, and assess function of drainage system.	When the patient has an air leak or pneumothorax, clamping of the chest tube may precipitate a tension pneumothorax because the air has no escape route and may accumulate in the pleural space.[1,15,17] Clamping of the chest tube should be as brief as possible.	• Respiratory distress noted during or after procedure • Changes in breath sounds after procedure • Nonfunctioning CDS
11. During gravity drainage, ambulation, or transport with gravity drainage, ensure CDS is upright, below the chest tube insertion site, and maintain the suction control stopcock in the "on" or "open" position. Do not clamp chest tube during transport.[1,25] **(Level E*)**	The suction control stopcock should always remain in the "on" or "open" position. Do not clamp or cap the suction line. Leaving the port open allows air to exit and minimizes the possibility of tension pneumothorax.	• Notify physician of inadvertent clamping or capping of the suction line
12. Follow institution standard for assessing pain. Administer analgesia as prescribed.	Identifies need for pain interventions.	• Continued pain despite pain interventions.
13. Obtain a drainage specimen from some disposable CDSs. Cleanse the site with antiseptic solution and use a syringe with a smaller (e.g., 20-gauge) needle to withdraw the specimen from the self-sealing diaphragm, or self-sealing drainage tubing, as available. Momentarily forming a dependent loop in the fluid collection tubing may be necessary to obtain a specimen.	Provides a specimen for analysis.	• Inability to obtain specimen

*Level E: Multiple case reports, theory-based evidence from expert opinions, or peer-reviewed professional organizational standards without clinical studies to support recommendations.

Documentation

Documentation should include the following:
• Patient and family education
• Pain assessment, interventions, and effectiveness
• Cardiopulmonary and vital sign assessment
• Type of drainage system used
• Amount of suction, fluctuation or tidaling, type and amount of drainage
• Air leak: absence, presence, severity, and resolution

• Respiratory, thoracic, and vital sign assessment at baseline and with changes in therapy
• Completion and results of the postinsertion chest radiograph and any other ordered diagnostic tests
• Unexpected outcomes
• Nursing interventions
• Patient's tolerance of the therapy

References and Additional Readings

For a complete list of references and additional readings for this procedure, scan this QR code with any freely available smartphone code reader app, or visit http://booksite.elsevier.com/9780323376624.

26 Needle Thoracostomy (Perform) AP

Cindy Goodrich

PURPOSE: Needle thoracostomy is performed to reduce a tension pneumothorax to a simple pneumothorax in a patient with a rapidly deteriorating condition. This temporary measure is followed quickly by the insertion of a chest tube for more definitive management.

PREREQUISITE NURSING KNOWLEDGE

- Anatomy and physiology of the pulmonary system should be understood.
- The thoracic cavity, in normal conditions, is a closed air space. Any disruption results in the loss of negative pressure within the intrapleural space. Air or fluid that enters the space competes with the lung, which results in collapse of the lung. Associated conditions are the result of disease, injury, surgery, or iatrogenic causes.
- A pneumothorax is classified as an open, closed, or tension pneumothorax. In patients with tension pneumothorax, air leaks into the pleural space through a tear in the lung and, with no means to escape from the pleural cavity, creates a one-way valve effect. With each breath the patient takes, air accumulates, pressure within the pleural space increases, and the lung collapses. As a result, the mediastinal structures (i.e., heart, great vessels, and trachea) shift to the opposite or unaffected side of the chest. Venous return and cardiac output are impeded, and the possibility of collapse of the unaffected lung exists.[1]
- Tension pneumothorax is a medical emergency that necessitates *immediate* intervention. Accurate assessment of the following signs and symptoms allows for prompt recognition and treatment:
  - ❖ Tracheal deviation to the unaffected side
  - ❖ Jugular vein distention
  - ❖ Sudden, sharp chest pain
  - ❖ Decreased or absent breath sounds on the affected side
  - ❖ Asymmetrical chest excursion with respirations
  - ❖ Tachypnea, shortness of breath, dyspnea, increased work of breathing
  - ❖ Decreased oxygen saturation
  - ❖ Subcutaneous emphysema
  - ❖ Anxiety, restlessness, apprehension
  - ❖ Tachycardia
  - ❖ Hypotension
  - ❖ Dysrhythmias
  - ❖ Cyanosis
  - ❖ Decreased pulse oximetry readings
  - ❖ Pulseless electrical activity
- Needle thoracostomy is performed by placing a needle into the pleural space to remove air and reestablish negative pressure in patients who are rapidly deteriorating from a life-threatening tension pneumothorax (Fig. 26-1). Definitive treatment requires the insertion of a chest tube as soon as possible after this temporary measure.[1]
- Needle decompression success is influenced by the chest wall thickness. Current evidence suggests that an 8-cm needle will reach the pleural space more than 90% of the time, whereas a 5-cm length needle will only reach the pleural space more than 50% of the time.[1]

EQUIPMENT

- Personal protective equipment including eye protection
- 14- to 16-gauge hollow needle or catheter at least 5 cm in length
- Antiseptic solution
- 4 × 4 gauze dressing
- Tape
- Oxygen
- Self-inflating manual resuscitation bag-valve-mask device
- Oxygen source and tubing
- Commercially available (Heimlich) flutter valve to attach to the needle or catheter, or, as an emergency alternative, a one-way valve may be created by using the following:
  - ❖ Scissors
  - ❖ Sterile glove (powder-free)
  - ❖ Small rubber band
  - ❖ Cut a finger off the glove, cut the very tip of the glove finger off, and attach it to the needle with the rubber band.[1]

PATIENT AND FAMILY EDUCATION

- If time permits, assess the patient's and family's level of understanding about the condition and rationale for the procedure. ***Rationale:*** This assessment identifies the patient's and family's knowledge deficits concerning the

---

AP   This procedure should be performed only by physicians, advanced practice nurses, and other healthcare professionals (including critical care nurses) with additional knowledge, skills, and demonstrated competence per professional licensure or institutional standard.

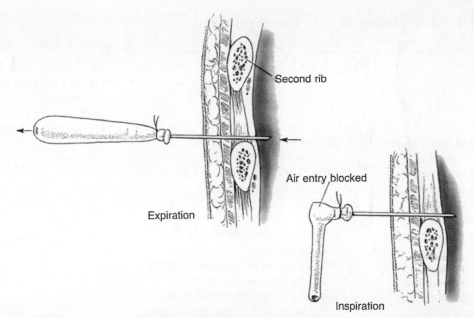

Figure 26-1 Use of a needle and a sterile finger cot or a finger from a sterile glove to fashion a one-way (flutter) valve for emergency evacuation of a tension pneumothorax. A small opening is made in the free end of the glove finger to allow air to escape during expiration. *(From Cosrniff JH: An atlas of diagnostic and therapeutic procedures for emergency personnel, Philadelphia, 1978, J.B. Lippincott.)*

patient's condition, the procedure, the expected benefits, and the potential risks. It also allows time for questions to clarify information and voice concerns. Explanations decrease patient anxiety and enhance cooperation.
- Explain the procedure and the reason for the procedure, if the clinical situation permits. If not, explain the procedure and reason for its implementation after it is completed. *Rationale:* This explanation enhances patient and family understanding and decreases anxiety.
- If indicated, explain the patient's role in assisting with needle thoracostomy. *Rationale:* Eliciting the patient's cooperation assists with insertion of a needle and flutter valve.

PATIENT ASSESSMENT AND PREPARATION

Patient Assessment
- Assess whether signs and symptoms are consistent with tension pneumothorax, as noted previously. *Rationale:* Accurate assessment of signs and symptoms allows for prompt recognition and treatment. Baseline assessment provides comparison data for evaluation of changes and outcomes of treatment. Tension pneumothorax is a medical emergency that necessitates immediate intervention.
- If the situation allows, assess vital signs, including pulse oximetry. *Rationale:* Baseline assessment data provide information about the patient's condition and allows for comparison during and after the procedure.

Patient Preparation
- Verify correct patient with two identifiers. *Rationale:* Prior to performing a procedure, the nurse should ensure the correct identification of the patient for the intended intervention.
- Ensure that the patient and family understand the emergency nature of the procedure and preprocedural teachings, if appropriate. Answer questions as they arise, and reinforce information as needed. *Rationale:* This communication evaluates and reinforces understanding of previously taught information.
- Position the patient in supine position with the head of the bed flat. *Rationale:* This positioning allows for identification of landmarks for proper placement of needle and flutter valve.
- Perform a preprocedure verification and time out, if nonemergent. *Rationale:* Ensures patient safety.

Procedure   for Performing Needle Thoracostomy

Steps	Rationale	Special Considerations
1. **HH**		
2. **PE**		Protective eyewear prevents exposure to secretions that may be expelled as the needle penetrates the pressurized pleural space.
3. Administer high-flow oxygen and ventilate as needed.	Allows for oxygenation and ventilation before needle insertion.	
4. Locate the second intercostal space at the midclavicular line on the side of the suspected tension pneumothorax.	Identification of landmarks for needle thoracostomy.	
5. Prepare the skin with antiseptic solution using a circular motion.	Cleanses area before needle insertion.	
6. Locate the upper margin of the third rib with several fingers. Insert needle into the second intercostal space at the midclavicular line, pointing the needle posterior but slightly upward and sliding it over the top of the third rib.[1-4] **(Level D*)**	Allows the proper placement of the needle into the pleural space. Inserting the needle above third rib avoids damaging the nerve, artery, and vein that lie just beneath each rib.	
7. Puncture the parietal pleural space. Listen for an audible escape of air as the needle enters the pleural space. If a catheter over needle device is used, remove the needle.[1-4] **(Level D)**	Although an audible rush of air indicates that needle decompression has been successful, a dramatic improvement in the patient's clinical condition is the best indicator of successful intervention.	This procedure may not be successful due to chest wall thickness, anatomical complications, or kinking of the catheter.[1] May need to repeat procedure with a longer catheter to puncture the parietal pleura in patients with large, thick chests. Verify catheter is not kinked and that it is has been inserted into the proper anatomical location.
8. Attach a flutter valve to the needle or catheter, if not already attached.[1-4] **(Level D)**	Allows air to escape the pleural space and prevents air from entering.	Needle and flutter valve act as a one-way valve, preventing reentry of air into pleural space but allowing for escape of air during expiration (see Fig. 26-1).
9. Apply a small dressing around the needle or catheter and secure, or suture, it in place.	Allows for temporary stabilization of needle or catheter until a chest tube can be inserted.	
10. Prepare for immediate chest tube insertion (see Procedures 21 and 22).	Definitive treatment of tension pneumothorax.	
11. Discard used supplies and remove **PE**.		
12. **HH**		

*Level D: Peer-reviewed professional and organizational standards with the support of clinical study recommendations.

Expected Outcomes

- Removal of air from pleural space
- Reestablishment of negative intrapleural pressure
- Tension pneumothorax conversion to simple pneumothorax
- Improved oxygenation and ventilation

Unexpected Outcomes

- Resultant pneumothorax in patient without tension pneumothorax
- Damage to nerves, veins, or arteries because of improper flutter-valve placement
- Local hematoma or cellulitis
- Pleural infection
- Unsuccessful placement of needle due to chest wall thickness, anatomical complications, or kinking of catheter

Patient Monitoring and Care

Steps	Rationale	Reportable Conditions
		These conditions should be reported if they persist despite nursing interventions.
1. Assess vital signs.	Provides information regarding the patient's condition.	• Significant changes in the patient's vital signs
2. Stabilize the needle or catheter with dressing until chest tube is inserted.	Prevents movement and dislodgment of needle or catheter. A chest tube should be inserted as soon as practical.	• Dislodged needle or catheter
3. Continuously monitor for signs and symptoms of tension pneumothorax.[1-4] **(Level D*)**	Determines whether chest decompression has been successful and allows for early identification of new pneumothorax until chest tube has been placed.	• Tracheal deviation to the unaffected side • Jugular vein distention • Sudden, sharp chest pain • Decreased or absent breath sounds on the affected side • Asymmetrical chest excursion with respirations • Tachypnea, shortness of breath, dyspnea, increased work of breathing • Decreased oxygen saturation • Subcutaneous emphysema • Anxiety, restlessness, apprehension • Tachycardia • Hypotension • Dysrhythmias • Cyanosis
4. Continuously monitor for catheter/needle occlusion due to clot formation at the catheter/needle tip.	Determines need for repeated needle decompression and rapid insertion of a chest tube.	• Return of signs and symptoms of tension pneumothorax as listed previously
5. Follow institution standard for assessing pain. Administer analgesia as prescribed.	Identifies need for pain interventions.	• Continued pain despite pain interventions

*Level D: Peer-reviewed professional and organizational standards with the support of clinical study recommendations.

Procedure continues on following page

Documentation

Documentation should include the following:

- Vital signs before and after insertion of needle or catheter, including pain, as appropriate
- Location of needle or catheter
- Size and length of needle or catheter used
- Response after needle or catheter placement

- Occurrence of unexpected outcomes
- Nursing interventions
- Patient and family education
- Pain assessment, interventions, and effectiveness

References and Additional Readings

For a complete list of references and additional readings for this procedure, scan this QR code with any freely available smartphone code reader app, or visit http://booksite.elsevier.com/9780323376624.

27 Thoracentesis (Perform) AP

Susan Yeager

PURPOSE: Thoracentesis is performed to assist in the diagnosis and therapeutic management of patients with pleural effusions.

PREREQUISITE NURSING KNOWLEDGE

- Thoracentesis is performed with insertion of a needle or a catheter into the pleural space, which allows for removal of pleural fluid.
- Pleural effusions are defined as the accumulation of fluid in the pleural space that exceeds 10 mL and results from the overproduction of fluid or disruption in fluid reabsorption.[1]
- Thoracentesis is not used to verify the presence of pleural effusion. Diagnosis of pleural effusion is made via clinical examination, patient symptoms, and diagnostic techniques. A number of techniques can demonstrate pleural effusion with varying levels of sensitivity. Percussion requires a minimum of 300 to 400 mL for identification of a pleural effusion, whereas a standard chest radiography requires 200 to 300 mL. Lateral decubitus radiographs can be used to recognize smaller fluid amounts and highlight whether present fluid is free flowing. Ultrasound scan, computed tomography (CT) scan, and magnetic resonance imaging (MRI) technology can detect 100 mL of fluid with 100% sensitivity.[1] Therefore, initial diagnosis of pleural effusion may be optimized via imaging techniques such as chest radiographs, ultrasound scans, CT scans, or MRI combined with patient symptoms and clinical examination findings.
- Diagnostic thoracentesis is indicated for differential diagnosis for patients with pleural effusion of unknown etiology. A diagnostic thoracentesis may be repeated if initial results fail to yield a diagnosis.
- Therapeutic thoracentesis is indicated to relieve the symptoms (e.g., dyspnea, cough, hypoxemia, or chest pain) caused by a pleural effusion.
- Pleural effusions are classified as either transudative or exudative effusions.
- Samples of pleural fluid are analyzed and assist in distinguishing between exudative and transudative etiologies of effusion. Results of laboratory tests on pleural fluid alone

do not establish a diagnosis; instead the laboratory results must be correlated with the clinical findings and serum laboratory results.
- Light's criteria should be used to distinguish between a pleural fluid exudate and transudate. In order to apply Light's criteria, the total protein and lactate dehydrogenase (LDH) should be measured in both blood and pleural fluid (Box 27-1).[2,3]
- Exudative effusions indicate a local etiology (e.g., pulmonary embolus, infection), whereas transudative effusions usually are associated with systemic etiologies (e.g., heart failure).[3]
- Exudative pleural effusions meet one of the following criteria:
  - Pleural fluid LDH/serum LDH ratio is greater than 0.6 international units/mL.
  - Pleural fluid LDH is more than two thirds of the upper limit of normal for serum LDH.
  - Pleural fluid protein/serum protein ratio is greater than 0.5 g/dL.[3]
- Relative contraindications for thoracentesis include the following:
  - Patient anatomy that hinders the practitioner from clearly identifying the appropriate landmarks
  - Patients actively undergoing anticoagulation therapy or with an uncorrectable coagulation disorder
  - Patients receiving positive end-expiratory pressure therapy
  - Patients with splenomegaly, elevated left hemidiaphragm, or left-sided pleural effusion
  - Patients with only one lung as a result of a previous pneumonectomy
  - Patients with known lung disease
  - Patients with active skin infection at the point of needle insertion[4]
- Ultrasound scan guided thoracentesis is thought to reduce complications.
- Complications commonly associated with thoracentesis include pneumothorax, hemopneumothorax, hemorrhage, hypotension, cough, pain, visceral injury, and reexpansion pulmonary edema.[4–6]
- The most common complications from pleural aspiration are pneumothorax, pain, hemorrhage, and procedure failure. The most serious complication is visceral injury.[5]
- Hypotension can occur as part of the vasovagal reaction, causing bradycardia, during or hours after the procedure.

AP   This procedure should be performed only by physicians, advanced practice nurses, and other healthcare professionals (including critical care nurses) with additional knowledge, skills, and demonstrated competence per professional licensure or institutional standard.

BOX 27-1   Light's Criteria for Exudative Pleural Effusions (Applies If One or More Criteria Are Met)

EXUDATIVE CRITERIA

Ratio of pleural fluid protein to serum protein is >0.5

Ratio of pleural fluid lactate dehydrogenase (LDH) to serum LDH is >0.6

Pleural fluid LDH level is >⅔ of the upper limit of normal for serum LDH

Modified from Porcel J, Light R: Diagnostic approach to pleural effusion in adults, Am Fam Physician 73(7):1211–1220, 2006.

If it occurs during the procedure, cessation of the procedure and intravenous (IV) atropine may be necessary. If hypotension occurs after the procedure, it is likely the result of fluid shifting from pleural effusion reaccumulation. In this situation, the patient is likely to respond to fluid resuscitation.[7]

- Development of cough generally initiates toward the end of the procedure and should result in procedure cessation.
- Reexpansion pulmonary edema is thought to occur from overdraining of fluid too quickly. The incidence is less than 1% but asymptomatic radiologically apparent reperfusion pulmonary edema may be slightly more frequent.[5] The maximum volume of fluid that can be safely removed is uncertain because the volume removed does not clearly correlate with the onset of symptoms. Traditionally, to avoid this complication, discontinuation of fluid removal occurs with the onset of symptoms or when the total fluid removed reaches 1000 to 1500 mL.[5,6]
- If using continuous positive airway pressure, caution should be taken to avoid potential pneumothorax following aspiration if there is no pleural drain in place.[5] Patients receiving positive airway pressure can undergo thoracentesis with an ultrasound-guided incidence of less than 7% pneumothorax noted.[4,8]
- Baseline diagnostic study results (i.e., lateral decubitus chest radiograph, ultrasound imaging, CT scan, or MRI) should be reviewed before the procedure to identify the location and extent of pleural fluid accumulation.

EQUIPMENT

- Indelible marker
- Sterile gloves
- Sterile drapes
- Sterile towels
- Adhesive bandage or adhesive strip
- Antiseptic solution
- Sterile 4 × 4 gauze pads
- Intervention medications (opioid, sedative, or hypnotic agents, local anesthetic 1% or 2% lidocaine)
- One small needle (25-gauge, ⅝-inch long)
- 5-mL syringe for local anesthetic
- Three large needles (20- to 22-gauge, 1½ to 2 inches long)

- Three-way stopcock
- Sterile 20-mL syringe
- Sterile 50-mL syringe
- Two chemistry blood tubes
- Hemostat or Kelly clamp
- Pulse oximetry equipment
- Side table
- Pillow or blanket to be placed on side table
- 14-gauge needle
- 16-gauge catheter
- Vacutainers or evacuated bottles (1 to 2 L) with pressure tubing

Additional equipment, to have available as needed, includes the following:

- Atropine, oxygen, thoracostomy supplies, advanced cardiac life-support equipment
- Ultrasound-scan equipment as available and with a credentialed provider
- Two complete blood count tubes
- One anaerobic and one aerobic media bottle for culture and sensitivity
- Sterile tubes for fungal and tuberculosis cultures specimen tubes
- Commercially prepackaged thoracentesis kits, which are available in some institutions

PATIENT AND FAMILY EDUCATION

- Assess patient's and family's level of understanding about the condition and rationale for the procedure. ***Rationale:*** This assessment identifies the patient's and family's knowledge deficits concerning the patient's condition, the procedure, the expected benefits, and the potential risks. It also allows time for questions to clarify information and voice concerns. Explanations decrease patient anxiety and enhance cooperation.
- Explain the procedure and the reason for the procedure, if the clinical situation permits. If not, explain the procedure and reason for the intubation after it is completed. ***Rationale:*** This explanation enhances patient and family understanding and decreases anxiety.
- Explain the patient's role in thoracentesis. ***Rationale:*** This explanation increases patient compliance, facilitates needle and catheter insertion, and enhances fluid removal.

PATIENT ASSESSMENT AND PREPARATION
Patient Assessment

- Assess medical history of symptoms, occupational exposure, pleuritic chest pain, malignancy disease, heart failure, and medication usage. ***Rationale:*** Medical history may provide valuable clues to the cause of a patient's pleural effusion or presence of hypercoagulable states as a result of medications. Knowledge of medication usage can indicate the need for anticoagulation reversal. In addition, an increasing number of medications are noted to contribute to exudative effusions. See http://www.pneumotox.com.[9]

- Assess for signs and symptoms of pleural effusion. *Rationale:* Physical findings may suggest a pleural effusion.
  - ❖ Trachea deviated away from the affected side
  - ❖ Affected side dull to flat with percussion
  - ❖ Absent or decreased breath sounds
  - ❖ Tactile fremitus
  - ❖ Pleuritic chest pain
  - ❖ Hypoxemia
  - ❖ Tachypnea
  - ❖ Dyspnea
  - ❖ Cough, weight loss, night sweats, anorexia, and malaise may also occur with pleural infection or malignancy disease
- Assess chest radiograph or other imaging findings. Posterior-anterior chest radiographs should be performed in the assessment of all suspected pleural effusions.[2] *Rationale:* If at least half the hemidiaphragm is obliterated on erect anterior-posterior radiograph results, sufficient fluid is in the pleural space for a thoracentesis. Greater than 200 mL of fluid is considered abnormal in erect chest radiograph results.
- If a small amount of loculated fluid is noted, a lateral decubitus radiograph should be obtained. *Rationale:* Lateral decubitus radiographs assist with distinguishing between free-moving fluid and pleural thickening. Lateral radiographs show blunting of the costophrenic angle with 50 mL. If the pleural effusion is measured to be greater than 10 mm deep on a lateral decubitus radiograph, a diagnostic thoracentesis can be performed.[10]
- Anterior-posterior chest radiographs completed in the intensive-care setting are typically completed in the supine position and are less sensitive in the identification of pleural effusions. In this setting, hazy opacification of one lung field or minor fissure thickening may be the only clues to the presence of a pleural effusion.[10] *Rationale:* In the supine position, pleural effusions tend to spread out across the posterior thoracic surface and are less evident on supine radiographs.
- Thoracic ultrasound guidance is strongly recommended for all pleural procedures for pleural fluid acquisition.[5] Marking of the site using thoracic ultrasound for subsequent remote aspiration is not recommended except for large pleural effusions.[5] *Rationale:* Ultrasound-guided pleural aspiration has been shown to increase the yield and reduce the risks of complications, particularly pneumothoraces and inadvertent organ puncture. Ultrasound detects pleural fluid septations with greater sensitivity than computed tomography.[2] However, it should be noted that ultrasound may not impact the incidence of intercostal vessel laceration as vessels are not visualized on ultrasound.[5]
- CT scans with contrast should be performed for pleural enhancement before complete drainage of the fluid. *Rationale:* CT scans are useful in distinguishing malignant from benign pleural thickening. CT scan results may also be helpful when complicated pleural infection is present

or if initial tube drainage is unsuccessful and surgery is to be considered.[2]

- Assess baseline vital signs, including pulse oximetry. *Rationale:* Baseline assessment data provide information about patient status and allow for comparison during and after the procedure.
- Assess recent serum laboratory results, including the following. *Rationale:* These studies help determine whether the patient is at risk for bleeding. Although thoracentesis is considered to have a low risk of bleeding, an international normalized ratio of 1.5 or less is acceptable for invasive procedures.[5,11] Platelet transfusion is recommended for counts less than 50,000. No consensus/recommendations exist for partial thromboplastin time and hematocrit thresholds. There is no evidence to support the use of bleeding times before minimally invasive procedures.[11]
  - ❖ Hematocrit
  - ❖ Platelet count
  - ❖ Prothrombin time/international normalized ratio
  - ❖ Partial thromboplastin time
- Assess timing of day that the procedure is to occur. Unless it is a patient emergency, pleural procedures should not take place out of hours.[5] *Rationale:* Avoiding out-of-hour procedures when possible increases the likelihood of having additional staff and resources available to support potential untoward sequelae.

Patient Preparation

- Verify that the patient is the correct patient using two identifiers. *Rationale:* Before performing a procedure, the nurse should ensure the correct identification of the patient for the intended intervention.
- Ensure that the patient understands preprocedural teachings. Answer questions as they arise and reinforce information. *Rationale:* This communication evaluates and reinforces understanding of previously taught information.
- Obtain written informed consent for the procedure. *Rationale:* Invasive procedures, unless performed with implied consent in a life-threatening situation, require written consent of the patient or significant other.
- Consider medications for pain, sedation, or chemical paralysis, as indicated by the patient's condition. *Rationale:* Pain and sedation medications or chemical paralysis may be necessary to maximize positioning. If utilizing sedation or paralysis, ensure that airway adjuncts or definitive airways are secured before induction.
- Have atropine available. *Rationale:* Bradycardia, from a vasovagal reflex, can occur during thoracentesis.
- Initiate pulse oximetry monitoring. *Rationale:* Pulse oximetry provides a noninvasive means for monitoring oxygenation and heart rate at the bedside, which allows for prompt recognition and intervention should problems develop.
- Ensure patent intravenous access. *Rationale:* Provides IV access for both procedural and emergency medications, as necessary

Procedure for Diagnostic and Therapeutic Thoracentesis

Steps	Rationale	Special Considerations

Diagnostic Thoracentesis
1. **HH**
2. **PE**
3. Assemble equipment and review of available imaging.

Ensures proper equipment is readily available throughout procedure and in emergency situations. Review of imaging ensures the proper side has been selected and provides anatomical guidance to the practitioner.[6]

Ultrasound guidance reduces complications associated with pleural procedures in the critical care setting and its routine use is recommended.[5] **(Level C*)**

4. Position patient for procedure with assistant standing in front of patient.

If the patient is alert and able, position the patient on the edge of the bed with feet supported on a stool and arms resting on a pillow on an elevated bedside table (Fig. 27-1A). The patient may sit on a chair backward and rest arms on a pillow on the back of the chair. If the patient is unable to sit, position the patient in the lateral recumbent position on the unaffected side, with the back near the edge of the bed and the arm on the affected side above the head. Elevate the head of the bed to 30 or 45 degrees, as tolerated.

Positioning enhances ease of withdrawal of pleural fluid. Assuring patient is comfortable increases the chance that the procedure will be successfully completed. Having the assistant in front of the patient ensures visualization of facial cues and enables the cessation of inadvertent patient movements that might interfere with the procedure.

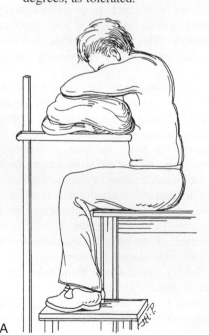

Figure 27-1   Thoracentesis. **A,** Ideal patient position for thoracentesis.

A

*Level C: Qualitative studies, descriptive or correlational studies, integrative reviews, systematic reviews, or randomized controlled trials with inconsistent results.

Procedure	for Diagnostic and Therapeutic Thoracentesis—*Continued*	
Steps	**Rationale**	**Special Considerations**
5. If not utilizing ultrasound, the following physical examination utilizing landmarks should be completed. Percuss the affected side posteriorly to determine the highest point of the pleural effusion. Effusion is generally noted using the following: one to two interspaces below the level at which breath sounds disappear on auscultation or become decreased, percussion becomes dull, or fremitus disappears. Identify the intercostal space below this point but above the ninth rib. Once the level is noted, a mark should be made 9–10 cm lateral to the spine moving toward the posterior axillary line.	Identifies the superior border of the pleural effusion and identifies and validates the planned site for thoracentesis. Palpation midway between the spine and posterior axillary line is a location where the ribs can generally be palpated. Accessing above the ninth rib minimizes potential injury to solid organs. Accessing 9–10 cm lateral to the spine below the eighth rib was noted to be associated with decreased canulation of tortuous vessels and has been deemed the "safe zone."[2,4,5]	Use the posterior axillary line as the insertion point to avoid the spinal cord. If the space identified for insertion is below the eighth intercostal space (area is approximated at the posterior edge of scapula), ultrasound scan should be done to mark the fluid level and its relationship to the diaphragm, which helps identify a safe point of entry to avoid solid-organ damage. When able, ultrasound guidance should be utilized to identify effusion location.[2,5] **(Level D*)**
6. Apply sterile personal protective equipment, while an assistant opens the necessary equipment onto a sterile field or opens the appropriate sterile tray with the equipment.	Reduces the transmission of microorganisms and body secretions during an invasive procedure.	
7. Have an assistant provide preprocedural medications.	Premedication with opioid, antianxiolytic, sedative, or hypnotic assures patient comfort throughout procedure.	
8. Perform a preprocedure verification and time out, if nonemergent.	Ensures patient safety.	
9. Sterilize a wide area surrounding the insertion site using 0.05% chlorhexidine or 10% povidone-iodine solution. Use concentric circles from insertion site mark outward, and drape area with sterile drape.	Although the pleural space is efficient in clearing bacteria, aseptic technique minimizes skin contaminants, which reduces the risk of infection.[4]	
10. Anesthetize the skin with 1%–2% lidocaine (25-gauge, ⅝-inch needle) in the typical wheal fashion around the insertion site.	Increases comfort for patient by anesthetizing the skin.	

*Level D: Peer-reviewed professional and organizational standards with the support of clinical study recommendations.

Procedure continues on following page

Procedure for Diagnostic and Therapeutic Thoracentesis—*Continued*

Steps	Rationale	Special Considerations
11. With lidocaine, insert a 20–22-gauge, $1\frac{1}{2}$–2-inch needle through the wheal. Advance the needle toward the rib, injecting the lidocaine into the deep tissue. "Walk" the needle over the superior edge of the rib and periosteum of the underlying rib superiorly and laterally. The exact puncture site should be immediately above the superior aspect of a rib and, when possible, 8–10 cm lateral from the spine.[6]	Anesthetizes the work area for optimal patient comfort. Insertion above the rib minimizes manipulation or laceration of the vascular bundle located beneath the rib and the intercostal arteries (Fig. 27-1*B*).[4,6] **(Level C*)**	Always aspirate before injecting to prevent lidocaine from entering a blood vessel or the pleural space. A longer needle may be needed in extremely obese patients.

Figure 27-1, cont'd   **B,** Ideal placement of needle insertion.

B

12. After anesthetizing the periosteum of the underlying rib, gently advance the needle and alternately aspirate and inject lidocaine until pleural fluid is obtained in the syringe.	In addition to anesthetizing the parietal pleura, utilizing this technique the pleural space is identified by pleural fluid aspirate in the syringe.[4,12] If air bubbles are noted, the lung tissue may have been violated or air may have been introduced by the thoracentesis system. Withdraw syringe to tissue and redirect. Withdrawal of needle minimizes manipulation of lung tissue.	
13. When pleural fluid is obtained, place a sterile gloved finger on the needle at the point where the needle exits the skin. Withdraw the needle and syringe. For therapeutic thoracentesis, **proceed to step 21**.	Approximates the length of insertion for the thoracentesis needle or catheter.	
14. Attach a three-way stopcock and 50-mL syringe to a 20–22-gauge, $1\frac{1}{2}$- or 2-inch needle. Open the stopcock valve between the syringe and the needle.	The open stopcock valve allows for aspiration of pleural fluid during needle insertion and minimizes atmospheric air introduction.	Longer needles may be necessary in the obese patient.

*Level C: Qualitative studies, descriptive or correlational studies, integrative reviews, systematic reviews, or randomized controlled trials with inconsistent results.

Procedure	for Diagnostic and Therapeutic Thoracentesis—*Continued*	
Steps	Rationale	Special Considerations
15. Insert the selected needle via the anesthetized tract, superior to the rib, and continually aspirate until pleural fluid is obtained, filling the 50-mL syringe. Fluid should be separated into three sterile containers for microbiology, biochemistry, and cytology analysis.	Inserting the needle superior to the rib avoids disruption of the vascular and lymph systems (Fig. 27-1B). The pleural fluid is used for laboratory testing for the differential diagnosis. A sample of 35–50 mL is needed for a diagnostic analysis of fluid. A change in patient position can be attempted to facilitate fluid drainage.	It is possible that no fluid is accessed (dry tap). If a dry tap occurs, the needle may be withdrawn and reinserted in a slightly different angle if the patient tolerated the initial "dry tap." A second tap warrants reevaluation with an ultrasound if not initially employed.[4] A larger gauge needle may be needed for thick or loculated fluid, or the needle may have been inserted above or below the pleural fluid. When pleural fluid is aspirated, the needle may be stabilized with placing a hemostat or clamp on the needle at the skin site to keep the needle from advancing farther into the pleural space, preventing lung puncture. Note the appearance of the aspirated fluid because this may provide clues to the underlying etiology of effusion. Straw-colored fluid is common and typical of transudates. Blood-stained fluid is suggestive of hemothorax, malignancy disease, pulmonary infarction, trauma, or postcoronary artery bypass surgery. Fluid turbidity suggests empyema or chylothorax, and food particles indicates esophageal rupture.
16. Fill the specimen tubes from the pleural fluid–filled syringe by turning the stopcock "off" to the patient and allowing the tubes to fill passively by vacuum or by depressing the syringe plunger (Fig. 27-1C). Send the specimen tubes to the laboratory for appropriate analysis.	Analysis may aid in determining an etiology of the pleural effusion.	To interpret pleural fluid laboratory values utilizing Light's criteria, serum and pleural fluid chemistry laboratory values must be obtained (e.g., total protein and LDH). Initial laboratory testing may also include cytology, gram stain, culture, amylase, and glucose.[4]

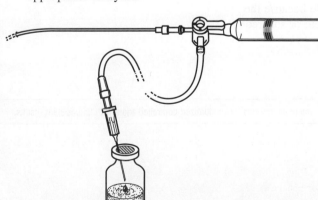

Figure 27-1, cont'd   C, Attach catheter to three-way stopcock syringe and vacutainer. *Barton ED: Thoracentesis. In Rosen P, Chan TC, Vilke M, Sternbach G, editors: Atlas of emergency procedures, St. Louis, Mosby, 2001. pp. 36–37.*

C

Procedure continues on following page

Procedure for Diagnostic and Therapeutic Thoracentesis—*Continued*		
Steps	Rationale	Special Considerations
17. Evaluate patient response throughout procedure.	Monitoring patient heart rate, pulse oximetry, and clinical response throughout the procedure enables prompt intervention or cessation of procedure should complications arise.	
18. On completion of diagnostic thoracentesis, withdraw the needle. Apply pressure to the puncture site for a few minutes, then apply an adhesive strip or adhesive bandage over the puncture site. Without concrete clinical indications, (i.e., withdraw of air, multiple needle passes, or clinical changes), a chest radiograph is not necessary after a routine thoracentesis.[2,4,6] **(Level C*)**	If the patient is nonventilated and asymptomatic, only 1% of patients were noted to have a pneumothorax on a postthoracentesis chest radiograph.[4]	If air is aspirated during the procedure, multiple needle passes are required, or the patient develops signs of a pneumothorax, imaging should be ordered. Postthoracentesis chest radiograph in mechanically ventilated patients remains controversial.[4]
19. Discard used supplies and remove **PE**.		
20. **HH**		
Therapeutic Thoracentesis		
21. Insert a 14-gauge needle attached to a 20-mL syringe, bevel down, into the anesthetized tract until pleural fluid is returned.	The 14-gauge needle is selected because it allows for insertion and passage of a 16-gauge catheter; a smaller-sized catheter may be unstable and fold or kink on itself.	
22. When pleural fluid is obtained, remove the syringe from the needle, occluding the needle with an index finger.	Occluding the needle helps prevent the possible occurrence of a pneumothorax.	
23. Insert the 16-gauge catheter through the 14-gauge needle. Advance the catheter slowly through the needle, angling the catheter in a downward fashion toward the costodiaphragm until the catheter moves freely in the pleural space.	Advancing the catheter toward the costodiaphragm allows for optimal drainage of pleural fluid.	In therapeutic thoracentesis, a catheter is preferred over a needle because the lung is expected to reexpand. A needle could puncture the lung during reexpansion and cause a pneumothorax.
24. While advancing the catheter beyond the needle tip, remove the needle and leave the catheter in the pleural space. Attach a three-way stopcock with a 50-mL syringe to the end of the catheter.	Never pull the catheter back through the needle because the catheter may be cut or sheared by the needle tip.	

*Level C: Qualitative studies, descriptive or correlational studies, integrative reviews, systematic reviews, or randomized controlled trials with inconsistent results.

Procedure | for Diagnostic and Therapeutic Thoracentesis—*Continued*

Steps	Rationale	Special Considerations
25. Fill the 50-mL syringe with pleural fluid. Fill the specimen tubes from the pleural fluid–filled syringe by turning the stopcock "Off" to the patient and allowing the tubes to fill passively by vacuum or by depressing the syringe plunger (Fig. 27-1*C*). Send the specimen tubes to the laboratory for appropriate analysis.	When changing syringes, be certain the stopcock is positioned such that air does not enter the pleural space. Analysis may aid in determining an etiology of the pleural effusion.	To interpret pleural fluid chemistry laboratory values, serum chemistry laboratory values also must be obtained (see Diagnostic Thoracentesis section). Local anesthetics (i.e., lidocaine) are acidic; therefore, care should be taken during pleural sampling to avoid contamination of sample.[4]
26. Attach the vacutainer or evacuated bottles with tubing to the three-way stopcock. Open the valve to the vacutainer and fill the vacutainer.	The vacutainer or evacuated bottles use negative pressure to withdraw pleural fluid from the pleural space, providing therapeutic relief. Reposition catheter or patient, or both, if drainage stops to determine whether fluid is still present.	The maximum volume of fluid that can be safely reviewed is uncertain because the volume removed does not clearly correlate with the onset of symptoms. Traditionally, to avoid this complication, discontinuation of fluid removal occurs with the onset of symptoms or when the total fluid removed reaches 1000–1500 mL.[5,6] **(Level E*)** The patient may feel the need to cough as the lung reexpands.
27. On completion of thoracentesis, remove the catheter. Apply pressure to the puncture site for a few minutes, then apply an adhesive strip or adhesive bandage over the puncture site. **(Level C*)**	If the patient is nonventilated and asymptomatic, only 1% of patients were noted to have a pneumothorax on a postthoracentesis chest radiograph.[4]	If air is aspirated during the procedure, multiple needle passes are required, or if the patient develops signs of a pneumothorax, imaging should be ordered. Postthoracentesis chest radiograph in mechanically ventilated patients remains controversial.[4]
28. Reposition the patient to optimize comfort.	Patient may desire to lie down after procedure. Head of bed placement may vary if dyspnea, hypotension, or other symptoms re-present during procedure.	
29. Dispose of equipment and remove **PE**.		
30. **HH**		

*Level C: Qualitative studies, descriptive or correlational studies, integrative reviews, systematic reviews, or randomized controlled trials with inconsistent results.
*Level E: Multiple case reports, theory-based evidence from expert opinions, or peer-reviewed professional organizational standards without clinical studies to support recommendations.

Expected Outcomes

- Patient is comfortable and has decreased respiratory distress
- Lung reexpansion occurs
- Site remains infection free
- Procedure aids in diagnosis of etiology of pleural effusion

Unexpected Outcomes

- Pneumothorax
- Vasovagal response
- Dyspnea
- Hypovolemia
- Hematoma
- Hemothorax
- Liver or splenic laceration
- Reexpansion pulmonary edema

Procedure continues on following page

Patient Monitoring and Care

Steps	Rationale	Reportable Conditions
		These conditions should be reported if they persist despite nursing interventions.
1. Monitor vital signs and cardiopulmonary status before and after thoracentesis and as needed.	Any change in vital signs may alert the practitioner of possible unexpected outcomes. Use of supplemental oxygen may be necessary.	• Tachypnea • Decreased or absent breath sounds on the affected side • Shortness of breath, dyspnea • Asymmetrical chest excursion with respirations • Decreased oxygen saturation • Subcutaneous emphysema • Sudden sharp chest pain • Anxiety, restlessness, apprehension • Tachycardia • Hypotension • Dysrhythmias • Tracheal deviation to the unaffected side • Neck vein distention • Muffled heart sounds • Pneumothorax • Expanding pleural effusion • Catheter migration
2. If indicated, obtain a postthoracentesis expiratory chest radiograph.[10] **(Level D*)**	A chest radiograph is used to evaluate for lung reexpansion and evidence of a possible pneumothorax or hemothorax. If a pneumothorax or hemothorax is present, a chest tube may be necessary. Without concrete clinical indications, chest radiograph is not necessary after a routine thoracentesis	
3. Follow institution standard for assessing pain. Administer analgesia as prescribed.	Identifies need for pain interventions.	• Continued pain despite pain interventions

*Level D: Peer-reviewed professional and organizational standards with the support of clinical study recommendations.

Documentation

Documentation should include the following:

- Patient and family teaching
- Consent for procedure
- Adherence to Universal Protocol
- Patient positioning and monitoring devices
- Medication administration and patient response
- Patient tolerance, including procedural pain and instillation and response to pain medications
- Insertion of catheter or needle
- Catheter or needle size used
- Any difficulties in insertion
- Pleural fluid aspirate characteristics

- Total amount of pleural fluid aspirated
- Site assessment
- Intact catheter on withdrawal
- Occurrence of unexpected outcomes
- Postthoracentesis radiograph acquisition and results, as needed/available
- Laboratory test ordered and results as available
- Interpretation of laboratory results
- Nursing interventions
- Pain assessment, interventions, and effectiveness

References and Additional Readings

For a complete list of references and additional readings for this procedure, scan this QR code with any freely available smartphone code reader app, or visit http://booksite.elsevier.com/9780323376624.

28 Thoracentesis (Assist)

Susan Yeager

PURPOSE: Thoracentesis is performed to assist in the diagnosis and therapeutic management of patients with pleural effusions.

PREREQUISITE NURSING KNOWLEDGE

- Thoracentesis is performed with insertion of a needle or a catheter into the pleural space, which allows for removal of pleural fluid.
- Pleural effusions are defined as the accumulation of fluid in the pleural space that exceeds 10 mL and results from the overproduction of fluid or disruption in fluid reabsorption.[1]
- Diagnostic thoracentesis is indicated for differential diagnosis for patients with pleural effusion of unknown etiology. A diagnostic thoracentesis may be repeated if initial results fail to yield a diagnosis.
- Therapeutic thoracentesis is indicated to relieve the symptoms (e.g., dyspnea, cough, hypoxemia, or chest pain) caused by a pleural effusion.
- Samples of pleural fluid are analyzed and assist in distinguishing between exudative and transudative etiologies of effusion. Results of laboratory tests on pleural fluid alone do not establish a diagnosis; instead the laboratory results must be correlated with the clinical findings and serum laboratory results.
- Exudative effusions indicate a local etiology (e.g., pulmonary embolus, infection), whereas transudative effusions usually are associated with systemic etiologies (e.g., heart failure).
- Relative contraindications for thoracentesis include the following:
  - ❖ Patient anatomy that hinders the practitioner from clearly identifying the appropriate landmarks
  - ❖ Patients actively undergoing anticoagulation therapy or with an uncorrectable coagulation disorder
  - ❖ Patients receiving positive end-expiratory pressure therapy
  - ❖ Patients with splenomegaly, elevated left hemidiaphragm, or left-sided pleural effusion
  - ❖ Patients with only one lung as a result of a previous pneumonectomy
  - ❖ Patients with known lung disease
  - ❖ Patients with active skin infection at the point of needle insertion[4]
- Ultrasound scan–guided thoracentesis is thought to reduce complications.
- Complications commonly associated with thoracentesis include: pneumothorax, hemopneumothorax, hemorrhage, hypotension, cough, pain, visceral injury, and reexpansion pulmonary edema.[4-6]
- The most common complications from pleural aspiration are pneumothorax, pain, hemorrhage, and procedure failure. The most serious complication is visceral injury.[5]
- Hypotension can occur as part of the vasovagal reaction, causing bradycardia, during or hours after the procedure. If it occurs during the procedure, cessation of the procedure and intravenous (IV) atropine may be necessary. If hypotension occurs after the procedure, it is likely the result of fluid shifting from pleural effusion reaccumulation. In this situation, the patient is likely to respond to fluid resuscitation.[7]
- Development of cough generally initiates toward the end of the procedure and should result in procedure cessation.
- Reexpansion pulmonary edema is thought to occur from overdraining of fluid too quickly. The incidence is less than 1%, but asymptomatic radiological pulmonary edema may be slightly more frequent.[5] The maximum volume of fluid that can be safely removed is uncertain because the volume removed does not clearly correlate with the onset of symptoms. Traditionally, to avoid this complication, discontinuation of fluid removal occurs with the onset of symptoms or when the total fluid removed reaches 1000 to 1500 mL.[5,6]
- If using continuous positive airway pressure, caution should be taken to avoid potential pneumothorax following aspiration if there is no pleural drain in place.[5] Patients receiving positive airway pressure can undergo thoracentesis with an ultrasound-guided incidence of less than 7% pneumothorax noted.[4,8]

EQUIPMENT

- Indelible marker
- Sterile gloves
- Sterile drapes
- Sterile towels
- Adhesive bandage or adhesive strip
- Antiseptic solution
- Sterile 4 × 4 gauze pads
- Intervention medications (opioid, sedative, or hypnotic agents, local anesthetic 1% or 2% lidocaine)
- One small needle (25-gauge, ⅝-inch long)
- 5-mL syringe for local anesthetic

- Three large needles (20- to 22-gauge, 1½ to 2 inches long)
- Three-way stopcock
- Sterile 20-mL syringe
- Sterile 50-mL syringe
- Two chemistry blood tubes
- Hemostat or Kelly clamp
- Pulse oximetry equipment
- Side table
- Pillow or blanket to be placed on side table
- 14-gauge needle
- 16-gauge catheter
- Vacutainers or evacuated bottles (1 to 2 L) with pressure tubing

Additional equipment, to have available as needed, includes the following:

- Atropine, oxygen, thoracostomy supplies, advanced cardiac life-support equipment
- Ultrasound-scan equipment as available and with a credentialed provider
- Two complete blood count tubes
- One anaerobic and one aerobic media bottle for culture and sensitivity
- Sterile tubes for fungal and tuberculosis cultures specimen tubes
- Commercially prepackaged thoracentesis kits which are available in some institutions

PATIENT AND FAMILY EDUCATION

- Assess patient's and family's level of understanding about the condition and rationale for the procedure. ***Rationale:*** This assessment identifies the patient's and family's knowledge deficits concerning the patient's condition, the procedure, the expected benefits, and the potential risks. It also allows time for questions to clarify information and voice concerns. Explanations decrease patient anxiety and enhance cooperation.
- Explain the procedure and the reason for the procedure, if the clinical situation permits. If not, explain the procedure and reason for the intubation after it is completed. ***Rationale:*** This explanation enhances patient and family understanding and decreases anxiety.
- Explain the patient's role in thoracentesis. ***Rationale:*** This explanation increases patient compliance, facilitates needle and catheter insertion, and enhances fluid removal.

PATIENT ASSESSMENT AND PREPARATION

Patient Assessment

- Assess medical history of symptoms, occupational exposure, pleuritic chest pain, malignancy disease, heart failure, and medication usage. ***Rationale:*** Medical history may provide valuable clues to the cause of a patient's pleural effusion or presence of hypercoagulable states as a result of medications. Knowledge of medication usage can indicate the need for anticoagulation reversal. In addition, an increasing number of medications are noted to contribute to exudative effusions. See http://www.pneumotox.com.[9]

- Assess for signs and symptoms of pleural effusion. ***Rationale:*** Physical findings may suggest a pleural effusion.
  - ❖ Trachea deviated away from the affected side
  - ❖ Affected side dull to flat with percussion
  - ❖ Absent or decreased breath sounds
  - ❖ Tactile fremitus
  - ❖ Pleuritic chest pain
  - ❖ Hypoxemia
  - ❖ Tachypnea
  - ❖ Dyspnea
  - ❖ Cough, weight loss, night sweats, anorexia, and malaise may also occur with pleural infection or malignancy disease
- Anterior-posterior chest radiographs completed in the intensive-care setting are typically completed in the supine position and are less sensitive in the identification of pleural effusions. In this setting, hazy opacification of one lung field or minor fissure thickening may be the only clues to the presence of a pleural effusion.[10] ***Rationale:*** In the supine position, pleural effusions tend to spread out across the posterior thoracic surface and are less evident on supine radiographs.
- Assess baseline vital signs, including pulse oximetry. ***Rationale:*** Baseline assessment data provide information about patient status and allow for comparison during and after the procedure.
- Assess recent serum laboratory results, including the following. ***Rationale:*** These studies help determine whether the patient is at risk for bleeding. Although thoracentesis is considered to have a low risk of bleeding, an international normalized ratio of 1.5 or less is acceptable for invasive procedures.[5,11] Platelet transfusion is recommended for counts < 50,000. No consensus/recommendations exist for partial thromboplastin time and hematocrit thresholds. There is no evidence to support the use of bleeding times before minimally invasive procedures.[11]
  - ❖ Hematocrit
  - ❖ Platelet count
  - ❖ Prothrombin time/international normalized ratio
  - ❖ Partial thromboplastin time

Patient Preparation

- Verify that the patient is the correct patient using two identifiers. ***Rationale:*** Before performing a procedure, the nurse should ensure a timeout was completed to verify the correct identification of the patient for the intended intervention.
- Ensure that the patient understands preprocedural teachings. Answer questions as they arise and reinforce information. ***Rationale:*** This communication evaluates and reinforces understanding of previously taught information.
- Ensure written informed consent for the procedure has been completed. ***Rationale:*** Invasive procedures, unless performed with implied consent in a life-threatening situation, require written consent of the patient or significant other.
- Assist with patient positioning. Several alternative positions may be used, as follows. ***Rationale:*** Positioning enhances patient comfort and ease of pleural fluid withdraw.

- ❖ On the edge of the bed with legs supported and arms resting on a pillow on the elevated bedside table (see Fig. 27-1).
- ❖ Backwards on a chair with arms resting on a pillow over the chair back.
- If the patient is unable to sit, position the patient on the unaffected side, with his or her back near the edge of the bed and the arm on the affected side above the head. Elevate the head of the bed to 30 or 45 degrees, as tolerated. Position yourself or another member of the healthcare team in front of the patient. *Rationale:* This positioning enables visualization of facial cues and a close proximity to reassure or comfort the patient.

- Inquire about the need for sedation or paralysis. *Rationale:* Sedation or paralysis may be necessary to maximize positioning.
- Have atropine available. *Rationale:* Bradycardia, from a vasovagal reflex, is not uncommon during thoracentesis.
- Initiate pulse oximetry monitoring. *Rationale:* Pulse oximetry provides a noninvasive means for monitoring oxygenation and heart rate at the bedside, which allows for prompt recognition and intervention should problems develop.
- Ensure patent IV access. *Rationale:* Provides IV access for both procedural and emergency medications, as necessary

Procedure for Assisting with Diagnostic and Therapeutic Thoracentesis		
Steps	Rationale	Special Considerations
1. **HH**		
2. **PE**		
3. Assemble equipment and procedure tray.	Ensures proper equipment is readily available throughout procedure and in emergency situations.	
4. Assist with patient positioning.	Positioning that optimizes patient comfort aids in patient cooperation and completion of the procedure.	
5. Assume a position in front of the patient and provide physical support for positioning, as necessary.	Positioning in front of the patient ensures visualization of facial cues and enables the cessation of inadvertent patient movements that might interfere with the procedure.	
6. As directed by physician or advanced practice provider, administer procedural medications.	Premedication with opioid, antianxiolytic, sedative, or hypnotic ensures patient comfort throughout procedure.	
7. Throughout procedure, assist with providing continuous monitoring of patient vital signs and response to the procedure and interventions.	The physician or advanced practice provider is focused on the technique required to obtain the fluid and may be delayed in noticing patient changes.	
8. As directed by physician or advanced practice provider, assist with filling of the specimen tubes from the pleural fluid–filled syringe. Label appropriately and send the specimen tubes to the laboratory for appropriate analysis.	Analysis may aid in determining an etiology of the pleural effusion.	To interpret pleural fluid laboratory values, serum chemistry laboratory values must be obtained (e.g., pH, total protein, glucose, and lactate dehydrogenase).
9. As directed by physician or advanced practice provider, assist with attaching the vacutainer or evacuated bottles with tubing to the three-way stopcock.	The vacutainer or evacuated bottles use negative pressure to withdraw pleural fluid from the pleural space, providing therapeutic relief. Assist in repositioning the patient if drainage stops, as directed.	Evacuating more than 1000–1500 mL of pleural fluid at one time may cause hypovolemia, hypoxemia, or reexpansion pulmonary edema. The patient may feel the need to cough as the lung reexpands.

Procedure for Assisting with Diagnostic and Therapeutic Thoracentesis—*Continued*

Steps	Rationale	Special Considerations
10. On completion of thoracentesis, the physician or advanced practice provider may apply pressure to the puncture site for a few minutes. After pressure application has been completed, apply an adhesive bandage over the puncture site.		Without concrete clinical indications, chest radiograph is not necessary after a routine thoracentesis.
11. Reposition patient to optimize comfort.	Patient may desire to lie down after procedure completion. Head-of-bed placement may vary if dyspnea, hypotension, or other symptoms are present during procedure.	
12. Dispose of soiled supplies and remove personal **PE**.		
13. **HH**		

Expected Outcomes

- Patient is comfortable and has decreased respiratory distress
- Lung reexpansion occurs
- Site remains infection free
- Procedure aids in diagnosing of etiology of pleural effusion

Unexpected Outcomes

- Pneumothorax
- Vasovagal response
- Dyspnea
- Hypovolemia
- Hematoma
- Hemothorax
- Liver or splenic laceration
- Reexpansion pulmonary edema

Patient Monitoring and Care

Steps	Rationale	Reportable Conditions
1. Monitor vital signs and cardiopulmonary status before, during, and after thoracentesis.	Any change in vital signs may alert the practitioner of possible unexpected outcomes. Use of supplemental oxygen may be necessary.	*These conditions should be reported if they persist despite nursing interventions.* • Tachypnea • Decreased or absent breath sounds on the affected side • Shortness of breath, dyspnea • Asymmetrical chest excursion with respirations • Decreased oxygen saturation • Subcutaneous emphysema • Sudden sharp chest pain • Anxiety, restlessness, apprehension • Tachycardia • Hypotension • Dysrhythmias • Tracheal deviation to the unaffected side • Neck vein distention • Muffled heart sounds

Procedure continues on following page

Patient Monitoring and Care —*Continued*

Steps	Rationale	Reportable Conditions
2. If indicated, obtain a postthoracentesis expiratory chest radiograph. **(Level C*)**	A chest radiograph is used to evaluate for lung reexpansion and evidence of a possible pneumothorax or hemothorax. If a pneumothorax or hemothorax is present, a chest tube may be necessary. Without concrete clinical indications, chest radiograph is not necessary after a routine thoracentesis.[2,3,5]	• Pneumothorax • Catheter migration • Expanding pleural effusion
3. Follow institution standard for assessing pain. Administer analgesia as prescribed.	Identifies need for pain interventions.	• Continued pain despite pain interventions

*Level C: Qualitative studies, descriptive or correlational studies, integrative reviews, systematic reviews, or randomized controlled trials with inconsistent results.

Documentation

Documentation should include the following:
- Patient and family teaching
- Presence of completed consent for procedure
- Adherence to Universal Protocol
- Patient positioning and monitoring devices
- Medication administration and patient response
- Patient tolerance, including procedural pain and instillation and response to pain medications
- Pleural fluid aspirate characteristics

- Total amount of pleural fluid aspirated
- Site assessment
- Occurrence of unexpected outcomes
- Postthoracentesis radiograph acquisition and results, as needed/available
- Laboratory test ordered and results, as available
- Nursing interventions
- Pain assessment, interventions, and effectiveness

References and Additional Readings

For a complete list of references and additional readings for this procedure, scan this QR code with any freely available smartphone code reader app, or visit http://booksite.elsevier.com/9780323376624.

PROCEDURE

29 Invasive Mechanical Ventilation (Through an Artificial Airway): Volume and Pressure Modes

John Gallagher

PURPOSE: Initiation and maintenance of positive-pressure ventilation through an artificial airway are accomplished to maintain or improve oxygenation and ventilation and to provide respiratory muscle rest. Selection of volume or pressure modes is dependent on the available evidence, clinical goals, availability of modes, and practitioner preference.

PREREQUISITE NURSING KNOWLEDGE

- Indications for the initiation of mechanical ventilation include the following:
  - Apnea (e.g., neuromuscular or cardiopulmonary collapse)
  - Acute ventilatory failure, which is generally defined as a pH of less than or equal to 7.25 with an arterial partial pressure of carbon dioxide ($Paco_2$) greater than or equal to 50 mm Hg
  - Impending ventilatory failure (serial decrement of arterial blood gas values or progressive increase in signs and symptoms of increased work of breathing)
  - Severe hypoxemia: an arterial partial pressure of oxygen (Pao_2) of less than or equal to 50 mm Hg on room air indicates a critical level of oxygen in the blood. Although oxygen-delivery devices may be used before intubation, the refractory nature of shunt (perfusion without ventilation) may necessitate that positive pressure be applied to reexpand closed alveoli. Restoration of functional residual capacity (FRC; lung volume that remains at the end of a passive exhalation) is the goal.
  - Respiratory muscle fatigue: the muscles of respiration can become fatigued if they are made to contract repetitively at high workloads.[86] Fatigue occurs when muscle-energy stores become depleted. Weakness, hypermetabolic states, and chronic lung disease are examples of conditions in which patients are especially prone to fatigue. When fatigue occurs, the muscles no longer contract optimally and hypercarbia results.[8,24] Twelve to 24 hours of rest are typically needed to rest the muscles. Respiratory muscle rest requires that the workload of the muscles (or muscle loading) be offset

so that mitochondrial energy stores can be repleted.[8,24] Respiratory work and rest vary with different modes and the application of the same. In general, when hypercarbia is present, mechanical ventilation is necessary to relieve the work of breathing. Muscle unloading is accomplished differently and depends on patient-ventilator interaction and the mode.[13,14,63,67]

- Ventilators are categorized as either negative or positive pressure. Although negative-pressure ventilation (i.e., the iron lung) was used extensively in the 1940s, introduction of the cuffed endotracheal tube resulted in the dominance of positive-pressure ventilation (PPV) in clinical practice during the second half of the 20th century. Although sporadic interest in negative-pressure ventilation continues, the cumbersome nature of the ventilators and the lack of airway protection associated with this form of ventilation preclude a serious resurgence of this mode of ventilation.[11,21]
  - Positive-pressure ventilation: positive-pressure modes of ventilation have traditionally been categorized into volume and pressure. However, with the advent of microprocessor technology, sophisticated iterations of traditional volume and pressure modes of ventilation have evolved.[11,25] Many of the modes have names that are different from traditional volume and pressure modes, but they are similar in many characteristics. Little data exist to show that the newer modes improve outcomes.[11,17,25,57] A wide variety of modes described in this procedure are actually a combination of volume and pressure but for ease of learning are classified into specific categories.
  - Volume ventilation has traditionally been the most popular form of PPV, largely because tidal volume (Vt) and minute ventilation (MV) are ensured, which is an essential goal in the patient with acute illness. With

volume ventilation, a predetermined Vt is delivered with each breath regardless of resistance and compliance. Vt is stable from breath to breath, but airway pressure may vary. The gas flow-rate pattern of volume ventilation is generally constant from the beginning to the end of the breath (square wave). In modern ventilators, this can be changed to accelerating, decelerating, or even sine patterns. To rest the respiratory muscles with volume ventilation, the ventilator rate must be increased until spontaneous respiratory effort ceases. When spontaneous effort is present, such as with initiation of an assist/control (A/C) breath, respiratory muscle work continues throughout the breath.[67,96]

❖ With traditional *pressure ventilation,* the practitioner selects the desired pressure level and the Vt is determined by the selected pressure level, airway resistance, and lung compliance. This characteristic is important to note in caring for a patient with an unstable condition on a pressure mode of ventilation. Careful attention to Vt is necessary to prevent inadvertent hyperventilation or hypoventilation. To ensure respiratory muscle rest on pressure-support ventilation (PSV), workload must be offset with the appropriate adjustment of the pressure-support level. To accomplish this adjustment, the pressure-support level is increased to lower the spontaneous respiratory rate to less than or equal to 20 breaths/min and to attain a Vt of 6 to 10 mL/kg of predicted body weight (PBW).[13,14,17,61]

❖ Pressure ventilation provides for an augmented inspiration (pressure is maintained throughout inspiration). The flow pattern (speed of the gas) is described as decelerating; that is, gas-flow delivery is high at the beginning of the breath and tapers off toward the end of the breath. This pattern is in contrast to volume ventilation, in which the flow rate is typically more consistent during inspiration (i.e., the same at the beginning of the breath as at the end of the breath). The decelerating flow pattern associated with pressure ventilation is thought to provide better gas distribution and more efficient ventilation.[61,63,87]

❖ Increasingly, sophisticated ventilator technology has resulted in the development of volume-assured pressure modes of ventilation. Ventilator manufacturers have responded rapidly to the request of practitioners that pressure modes of ventilation be designed in such a way that the minimum desired tidal volume be can be achieved on a breath-to-breath basis. These are called *adaptive pressure control* or *dual control pressure modes.* The potential value of such modes is obvious. The more desirable decelerating flow pattern may be provided and plateau pressures controlled, with more consistent Vt and MV.

❖ Additional modes of ventilation have been promoted for use in patients with acute respiratory distress syndrome (ARDS), including high-frequency oscillation, airway pressure-release ventilation (APRV), and other ventilator-specific modes, such as biphasic, adaptive support, and proportional assist ventilation. Although some data exist that suggest the modes may be beneficial in patients with ARDS, to date no change in

mortality rate has been noted, although positive trends have been demonstrated in some variables of interest such as oxygenation.[17,28,31,39,46,47,69,83,84]

• Summary descriptions of modes, mode parameters, and ventilator alarms are provided within this procedure and in Boxes 29-1 and 29-2, and Table 29-1.

BOX 29-1 **Traditional Modes of Mechanical Ventilation (On All Ventilators)**

VOLUME MODES

Control Ventilation (CV) or Controlled Mandatory Ventilation (CMV)
Description: With this mode, the ventilator provides all of the patient's minute ventilation. The clinician sets the rate, Vt, inspiratory time, and PEEP. Generally, this term is used to describe situations in which the patient is chemically relaxed or is paralyzed from a spinal cord or neuromuscular disease and is unable to initiate spontaneous breaths. This mode does not exist as a standard mode on modern ventilators. Patients on assist/control (A/C) mode who are unable to trigger the machine are essentially in CMV.

Assist/Control (A/C) Ventilation
Description: This option requires that a rate, Vt, inspiratory time, and PEEP be set for the patient. The ventilator sensitivity also is set, and when the patient initiates a spontaneous breath, a full-volume breath is delivered.

Synchronized Intermittent Mandatory Ventilation (SIMV)
Description: This mode requires that rate, Vt, inspiratory time, sensitivity, and PEEP are set by the clinician. In between mandatory breaths, patients can spontaneously breathe at their own rates and Vt. With SIMV, the ventilator synchronizes the mandatory breaths with the patient's own breaths.

PRESSURE MODES

Pressure Support Ventilation (PSV)
Description: This mode provides augmented inspiration to a patient who is spontaneously breathing. With pressure support (PS), the clinician selects an inspiratory pressure level, PEEP, and sensitivity. When the patient initiates a breath, a high flow of gas is delivered to the preselected pressure level, and pressure is maintained throughout inspiration. The patient determines the parameters of Vt, rate, and inspiratory time.

Pressure-Controlled (PC) and Pressure-Controlled Inverse Ratio Ventilation (PC/IRV)
Description: This mode may provide pressure-limited ventilation (PC) alone, or combined with an inverse ratio of inspiration to expiration (PC/IRV). The clinician selects the pressure level, rate, inspiratory time (1:1, 2:1, 3:1, 4:1), and PEEP level. With prolonged inspiratory times, auto-PEEP may result. The auto-PEEP may be a desirable outcome of the inverse ratios. In PC without IRV, conventional inspiratory times are used, and rate, pressure level, and PEEP are selected.

Positive End-Expiratory Pressure (PEEP) and Continuous Positive Airway Pressure (CPAP)
Description: This ventilatory option creates positive pressure at end exhalation. PEEP restores functional residual capacity. The term PEEP is used when end-expiratory pressure is provided during ventilator positive pressure breaths.

| BOX 29-2 | Ventilator Alarms |

DISCONNECT ALARMS (LOW-PRESSURE OR LOW-VOLUME ALARMS)

When disconnection occurs, the clinician must be immediately notified. Generally, this alarm is a continuous one and is triggered when a preselected inspiratory pressure level or minute ventilation is not sensed. With circuit leaks, this same alarm may be activated even though the patient may still be receiving a portion of the preset breath. Physical assessment, digital displays, and manometers are helpful in troubleshooting the cause of the alarms.

PRESSURE ALARMS

High-pressure alarms are set to ensure notification of pressures that exceed the selected threshold. These alarms are usually set 10–15 cm H_2O above the usual peak inspiratory pressure (PIP). Some causes for alarm activation (generally an intermittent alarm) include secretions, condensate in the tubing, biting on the endotracheal tubing, increased resistance (i.e., bronchospasm), decreased compliance (e.g., pulmonary edema, pneumothorax), and tubing compression. When this alarm is triggered, the breath delivery is halted and the remaining tidal volume to be delivered by the machine is not delivered. This will then often result in the occurrence of a low-volume alarm.

Low-pressure alarms are used to sense disconnection, circuit leaks, and changing compliance and resistance. They are generally set 5–10 cm H_2O below the usual PIP or 1–2 cm H_2O below the PEEP level or both.

Minute ventilation alarms may be used to sense disconnection or changes in breathing pattern (rate and volume). Generally, low-minute ventilation and high-minute ventilation alarms are set (usually 5–10 L/min above and below usual minute ventilation). When stand-alone pressure support ventilation (PSV) is in use, this alarm may be the only audible alarm available on some ventilators.

FiO_2 alarms are provided on most new ventilators and are set 5–10 mm Hg above and below the selected FiO_2 level.

Alarm silence or pause options are built in by ventilator manufacturers so that clinicians can temporarily silence alarms for short periods (i.e., 20 seconds) because alarms must stay activated at all times. The ventilators reset the alarms automatically.

Alarms provide important protection for patients on ventilation. However, inappropriate threshold settings decrease usefulness. When threshold gradients are set too narrowly, alarms occur needlessly and frequently. Conversely, alarms that are set too loosely (wide gradients) do not allow for accurate and timely assessments.

From Burns SM: Mechanical ventilation and weaning. In Kinney MR, et al, editors: AACN clinical reference for critical care nursing, ed 4. St Louis, 1998, Mosby.

- Complications of PPV include volume-pressure trauma, hemodynamic changes, and pulmonary barotrauma.
  - ❖ Volume-pressure trauma, in contrast to barotrauma (or air-leak disease), was first described in animals with stiff noncompliant lungs who were ventilated with traditional lung volumes (range, 10 to 12 mL/kg PBW). The investigators noted that the large volumes translated into high plateau pressures (also known as static, distending, or alveolar pressure) and subsequent acute lung injury. The lung injury was described as a loss of alveolar integrity (i.e., alveolar fractures) and movement of fluids and proteins into the alveolar space (sometimes called non-ARDS-ARDS).[33,34,43,52] Plateau pressures of 30 cm H_2O or more for greater than 48 to 72 hours were associated with the injury.[34,49,52]
  - ❖ Studies in humans followed the recognition that large Vts may be associated with lung injury.[1] The ARDS Network conducted a randomized controlled trial of adult patients with ARDS that compared low lung-volume ventilation (6 mL/kg) with more traditional volumes (i.e., 12 mL/kg). The results showed that the lower-volume ventilation resulted in a lower mortality rate.[1] As a result, current recommendations are to limit volumes (and lower pressures) in patients with stiff lungs. With pressure ventilation, pressure is limited by definition; however, until additional evidence emerges on the efficacy of controlling pressures versus volumes in ARDS, a goal should be to ensure a Vt in the 6 mL/kg range. Another lung-protective strategy is that of "recruitment" and the prevention of "derecruitment." Investigators showed that stiff noncompliant lungs were at risk of trauma from the repetitive opening associated with tidal breaths. The application of higher levels of positive end-expiratory pressure (PEEP) was associated with better recruitment and resulted in improved mortality rates.[3,4,18,44,85]
  - ❖ The extent of hemodynamic changes associated with PPV depends on the level of applied positive pressure, the duration of positive pressure during different phases of the breathing cycle, the amount of pressure transmitted to the vascular structures, the patient's intravascular volume, and the adequacy of hemodynamic compensatory mechanisms. PPV can reduce venous return, shift the intraventricular septum to the left, and increase right-ventricular afterload as a result of increased pulmonary vascular resistance.[22,38,53,54] The hemodynamic effects of PPV may be prevented or corrected by optimizing filling pressures to accommodate the PPV-induced changes in intrathoracic pressures; by minimizing the peak pressure, plateau pressure, and PEEP; and by optimizing the inspiratory-to-expiratory (I : E) ratio.
  - ❖ Pulmonary barotrauma (i.e., air-leak disease) is damage to the lung from extrapulmonary air that may result from changes in intrathoracic pressures during PPV. Barotrauma is manifested by pneumothorax, pneumomediastinum, pneumopericardium, pneumoperitoneum, and subcutaneous emphysema. The risk of barotrauma in a patient receiving PPV is increased with preexisting lung lesions (e.g., localized infections, blebs), high inflation pressures (i.e., large Vt, PEEP, main-stem bronchus intubation, patient-ventilator asynchrony), and invasive thoracic procedures (e.g., subclavian catheter insertion, bronchoscopy, thoracentesis). Barotrauma from PPV may be prevented by controlling peak and plateau pressures, optimizing PEEP, preventing auto-PEEP, ensuring patient-ventilator synchrony, and ensuring proper artificial airway position.

TABLE 29-1   Volume and Pressure Modes and Corresponding Ventilator Parameters

Mode Name and Description	Main Parameters	Comments
Assist Control (A/C)	Vt Rate Inspiratory time (Ti) Sensitivity Fio$_2$ PEEP	Generally considered a support mode. Must switch to another mode or method for weaning.
Synchronized Mandatory Ventilation (SIMV)	Vt Rate Ti Sensitivity Fio$_2$ PEEP	Originally used as a weaning mode; however, work of breathing is high at low SIMV rates. Often used in conjunction with PSV.
Pressure Support Ventilation (PSV)	PS level Sensitivity Fio$_2$ PEEP	Often pressure is arbitrarily selected (e.g., 10–20 cm H$_2$O) then adjusted up or down to attain the desired tidal volume. Some use the plateau pressure if transitioning from volume ventilation as a starting point.
Pressure-Controlled Ventilation (PCV)	Inspiratory pressure limit (IPL) Rate Ti Sensitivity Fio$_2$ PEEP	Variants of PCV include Volume-Assured Pressure Options and some other modes such as Airway Pressure Release Ventilation and Bilevel Ventilation.
Pressure Controlled–Inverse Ratio Ventilation	As for PCV, but an inverse inspiratory : expiratory (I : E) ratio is attained by lengthening the Ti. Inverse ratios include 1:1, 2:1, 3:1, and 4:1.	Some ventilators allow for the I : E ratio to be selected.
Bilevel Positive Airway Pressure (Bilevel or BiPAP)	Pressure$_{HIGH}$ (P$_{HIGH}$) Pressure$_{LOW}$ (P$_{LOW}$) T$_{HIGH}$ (Similar to I Time in PC) T$_{LOW}$ (Similar to E time in PC) Or set ratio T$_{HIGH}$/T$_{LOW}$ ratio Rate Fio$_2$	Similar in many ways to PC in that an inspiratory pressure (Pressure$_{HIGH}$) and PEEP (Pressure$_{LOW}$) are set. However, unlike PC, the patient may take spontaneous breaths as well. If additional support is desired for patient-initiated breathing, pressure support in bilevel mode (Psupp) may be selected as well. Attention to Vt is important because the patient can augment Vt significantly with supported spontaneous breaths.
Airway Pressure Release Ventilation (APRV)	Pressure high (P$_{HIGH}$): high CPAP level. Pressure low (P$_{LOW}$) is generally 0–5 cm H$_2$O. Time high (T$_{HIGH}$). Time low (T$_{LOW}$). Fio$_2$	APRV is a form of biphasic ventilation with a very short expiratory time. Generally, the CPAP level is adjusted to ensure adequate oxygenation while the rate of the releases are increased or decreased to meet ventilation goals. Vt is variably dependent on the CPAP level, compliance and resistance of the patient, and patient spontaneous effort.
Dual Control or Volume-Assured Pressure Modes (1–5 listed here)	These modes provide pressure breaths with a minimum tidal volume assurance.	These modes are ventilator specific. Although the similarities are greater than the differences, they are called different names. Often the names suggest that the mode is a volume mode, yet a decelerating flow pattern (associated with pressure ventilation) is always provided.
1. Volume Support (VS)	Vt Sensitivity Fio$_2$ PEEP	The pressure level is automatically adjusted to attain the desired Vt. If control of pressure is desired, it must be carefully monitored.
2. Pressure-Regulated Control (PRVC)	Rate and Ti set in addition to those set for VS.	As with VS. The difference is that this is a control mode. Spontaneous breaths, however, may also occur.

TABLE 29-1	Volume and Pressure Modes and Corresponding Ventilator Parameters—cont'd	
Mode Name and Description	**Main Parameters**	**Comments**
3. Volume Control Plus (VC+)	Rate and Ti are set in addition to those set for VS.	This is a mode option listed in the category called Volume Ventilation Plus. To access this mode, the user selects the SIMV or A/C (both control modes) then selects VC+. For some clinicians, this is confusing because it appears that the patient is on two different modes versus VC+.
4. Adaptive Support Ventilation (ASV)	Body weight %MinVol (minute volume), high pressure limit	Once basic settings are selected, ASV is started and %MinVol is adjusted if indicated. Spontaneous breathing is automatically encouraged, and when the inspiratory pressure (Pinsp) is consistently 0 and rate is 0, extubation may be considered.
5. Proportional Assist Ventilation (PAV)	Proportional Pressure Support (PPS): PEEP, FiO_2, percent volume assist and flow assist Proportional Assist Plus: PAV+: PEEP, FiO_2, percent support	Depending on the ventilator, the amount of assist that is provided is determined by the clinician and different parameters are selected to do so. Default percent support numbers are recommended, but the clinician must determine the timing of reductions of same.
6. Automatic Tube Compensation (ATC)	Endotracheal tube internal diameter Percent compensation	This is not a mode but rather a pressure option to offset the work associated with tube resistance. It can be combined with other modes or used alone as in a CPAP weaning trial.

Adapted with permission from Burns S: *Pressure modes of mechanical ventilation: The good, bad and the ugly,* AACN Adv Crit Care *19:399–411, 2008.*

- ❖ Auto-PEEP is a common complication of mechanical ventilation and can result in hemodynamic compromise and even death. Because increased intrathoracic pressures are transmitted to the adjacent capillaries, venous return is decreased and the effect can be profound. Auto-PEEP and dynamic hyperinflation should be assumed in the patient on ventilation with acute severe asthma whose condition is hemodynamically compromised, and a brief cessation of mechanical ventilation or decrease in rate and shortening of inspiratory time should be accomplished.[16,59,65,79] Auto-PEEP is caused by inadequate expiratory time relative to the patient's lung condition. Auto-PEEP is often seen in patients with prolonged inspiratory times, short expiratory times, high minute ventilation requirements, bronchospasm, low elastic recoil, mucus hypersecretion, increased wall thickness, airway closure or collapse, and mechanical factors (e.g., water in the ventilator circuit, pinched ventilator tubing).[16,59,65,79] Correcting these factors reduces auto-PEEP. In some cases where auto-PEEP cannot be eliminated, adding set PEEP to the level of auto-PEEP results in reduction of the inspiratory trigger threshold and thus improvement of patient triggering.[16,59,62,79]
- Complications of PPV include ventilator-associated pneumonia (VAP).
  - ❖ VAP occurs after 3 to 5 days of mechanical ventilation and accounts for one third of all healthcare-associated infections and between 50% and 83% of infections in the patient with MV.[23,74,75,82]
  - ❖ Modifiable risk factors to the aspiration of colonized organisms in the patient on ventilation include interventions such as proper endotracheal tube cuff inflation (secretions that collect above the cuff of the endotracheal or tracheostomy tube and leak past the cuff into the lungs), use of continuous-aspiration subglottic suctioning (CASS) tubes, decreased ventilator tubing changes, use of heat and moisture exchangers (HMEs), stringent hand washing, backrest elevation (BRE) of greater than 30 degrees, and when possible the use of noninvasive ventilation (especially in patients with immunocompromise).[23,74,75,82]
  - ❖ Other interventions with a lower level of evidence supporting their use include oral care techniques such as mouth care and oral decontamination with agents such as chlorhexidine or oral antibiotics.[45] Of interest, gastric residual volumes have not been found to be consistently associated with VAP.[73] Box 29-3 lists the top recommendations of authoritative professional organizations for the prevention of VAP.

EQUIPMENT

- Endotracheal or tracheostomy tube
- Electrocardiogram and pulse oximetry
- Supplemental oxygen source
- Manual self-inflating resuscitation bag-valve device (with PEEP adjusted to patient baseline level or with a PEEP valve)
- Appropriately sized resuscitation face mask
- Ventilator
- Suction equipment

PATIENT AND FAMILY EDUCATION

- Explain the procedure and the reasons for PPV to the patient and family. *Rationale:* Communication and explanations for therapy are important needs of patients and families.
- Discuss the potential sensations the patient will experience, such as relief of dyspnea, lung inflations, noise of

BOX 29-3 | **Top Modifiable VAP Prevention Interventions: Guidelines by Authoritative Professional Organizations***

- Back rest elevation (>30–45 degrees)
- Continuous aspiration of subglottic secretions tubes
- Limit/interrupt sedation (spontaneous awakening trial)
- Spontaneous breathing trial/assess readiness to extubate daily.
- Noninvasive ventilation when possible
- Early Mobility
- No routine ventilator circuit change
- Hand washing and aseptic technique

*Professional Associations:
- AHRQ, Prevention of Ventilator Associated Pneumonia (2011). http://www.guideline.gov/content.aspx?id=36063. Accessed January 27, 2016.
- Association for Professionals in Infection Control (APIC) (2009). Guideline to Eliminating Ventilator Associated Pneumonia. http://www.apic.org/Resource_/EliminationGuideForm/18e326ad-b484-471c-9c35-6822a53ee4a2/File/VAP_09.pdf: Accessed: January 27, 2016.
- Institute for Clinical Systems Improvement (2011). https://www.icsi.org/_asset/y24ruh/VAP.pdf. Accessed: January 27 2016.
- Society for Healthcare Epidemiology in America (SHEA) (2014). Strategies to Prevent Ventilator Associated Pneumonia in Acute Care Hospitals.

ventilator operation, and alarm sounds. *Rationale:* Knowledge of anticipated sensory experiences reduces anxiety and distress.
- Encourage the patient to relax. *Rationale:* This encouragement promotes general relaxation, oxygenation, and ventilation.
- Explain that the patient will be unable to speak. Establish a method of communication in conjunction with the patient and family before initiating mechanical ventilation, if necessary. *Rationale:* Ensuring the patient's ability to communicate is important to alleviate anxiety.
- Teach the family how to perform desired and appropriate activities of direct patient care, such as pharyngeal suction with the tonsil-tip suction device, range-of-motion exercises, and reconnection to ventilator if inadvertent disconnection occurs. Demonstrate use of the call bell. *Rationale:* Family members have identified the need and desire to help in the patient's care.
- Explain to the patient and family the importance of not touching the ventilator controls, including silencing and resetting alarms. *Rationale:* Families may become familiar with the ventilator over time and, in a desire to help, reset or silence an alarm without an understanding of the cause/underlying problem.
- Provide the patient and family with information on the critical nature of the patient's dependence on PPV. *Rationale:* Knowledge of the prognosis, probable outcome, or chance for recovery is cited as an important need of patients and families.
- Offer the opportunity for the patient and family to ask questions about PPV. *Rationale:* Asking questions and having questions answered honestly are cited consistently as the most important need of patients and families.

PATIENT ASSESSMENT AND PREPARATION
Patient Assessment

- Assess for signs and symptoms of acute ventilatory failure and fatigue. *Rationale:* Ventilatory failure indicates the need for initiation of PPV. While PPV is being considered and assembled, support ventilation via a self-inflating manual resuscitation bag-valve-mask (BVM), if necessary.
  - ❖ Rising arterial carbon dioxide tension
  - ❖ Chest-abdominal dyssynchrony
  - ❖ Shallow or irregular respirations
  - ❖ Tachypnea, bradypnea, or dyspnea
  - ❖ Decreased mental status
  - ❖ Restlessness, confusion, or lethargy
  - ❖ Increasing or decreasing arterial blood pressure
  - ❖ Tachycardia
  - ❖ Atrial or ventricular dysrhythmias
- Determine arterial pH and carbon dioxide tension. *Rationale:* Acute ventilatory failure is confirmed by an uncompensated respiratory acidosis. Ventilatory failure is an indication for PPV.
- Assess for signs and symptoms of inadequate oxygenation. *Rationale:* Hypoxemia may indicate the need for PPV. While PPV is being considered and assembled, provide 100% oxygen via manual resuscitation bag and mask or via an oxygen delivery device, such as a nonrebreather mask.
  - ❖ Decreasing arterial oxygen tension
  - ❖ Tachypnea
  - ❖ Dyspnea
  - ❖ Central cyanosis
  - ❖ Alterations in level of consciousness
  - ❖ Restlessness
  - ❖ Confusion
  - ❖ Agitation
  - ❖ Tachycardia
  - ❖ Bradycardia
  - ❖ Dysrhythmias
  - ❖ Intercostal and suprasternal retractions
  - ❖ Increasing or decreasing arterial blood pressure
  - ❖ Adventitious breath sounds
  - ❖ Decreasing urine output
  - ❖ Metabolic acidosis
- Determine PaO_2 or arterial oxygen saturation (SaO_2). *Rationale:* Hypoxemia is confirmed by PaO_2 of <60 mm Hg or SaO_2 of less than 90% on supplemental oxygen. Hypoxemia may indicate the need for PPV.
- Assess for signs and symptoms of inadequate breathing patterns. *Rationale:* Respiratory distress is an indication for PPV.
  - ❖ Dyspnea
  - ❖ Chest-abdominal dyssynchrony
  - ❖ Rapid-shallow breathing pattern
  - ❖ Irregular respirations
  - ❖ Intercostal or suprasternal retractions
  - ❖ Inability to say a whole sentence

Patient Preparation

- Verify that the patient is the correct patient using two identifiers. *Rationale:* Before performing a procedure, the nurse should ensure the correct identification of the patient for the intended intervention.
- Perform a preprocedure verification and time out, if non-emergent. *Rationale:* Ensures patient safety.
- If patient is not in distress ensure that the patient understands preprocedural teachings. Answer questions as they arise, and reinforce information as needed. *Rationale:* This communication evaluates and reinforces understanding of previously taught information.
- Premedicate as needed. *Rationale:* Administration of sedatives, narcotics, or muscle relaxants may be necessary to provide adequate oxygenation and ventilation in some patients.
- Ensure patient is positioned properly for optimum ventilation. *Rationale:* Placement of the patient in a head-of-bed elevation of at least 30 degrees enhances diaphragmatic excursion, decreases intrathoracic pressure, and helps prevent aspiration and VAP.

Procedure	for Invasive Mechanical Ventilation (Through an Artificial Airway): Volume and Pressure Modes	
Steps	**Rationale**	**Special Considerations**

1. **HH**
2. **PE**

Volume-Control Modes

3. Select mode (see Box 29-1 and Table 29-1). The three traditional volume modes and mode settings are control mechanical ventilation (CMV), assist/control (A/C), and synchronized intermittent mandatory ventilation (SIMV).

   A. CMV: The intent of control ventilation is to have volume and rate ensured. As with all modes of ventilation, the patient is never completely "locked out" and can breathe between the control breaths, which is ensured by setting the sensitivity or flow triggers **(see Step 8)**. However, should control over ventilation be desired, sedation and often paralytic agents are provided to ensure the goal.

   B. A/C: Ventilation ensures that a control rate and volume are set. Patient-initiated breaths are delivered at the predetermined volume selected for the control breaths.

   C. SIMV: With this mode, a rate (fx) and Vt are set and are delivered in synchrony with the patient's respiratory effort. Between mandatory breaths, the patient may initiate breaths at a patient-determined volume and rate.

Mode selection varies depending on the clinical goal and clinician preference.

Traditional volume modes that may provide total ventilatory support include control, SIMV, and A/C. With SIMV and A/C the ventilator rate must be high enough or the patient sedated so that spontaneous effort is not present. Other modes may also provide complete support depending on the settings. Remember that the goal is to offset the patient's work of breathing. See subsequent description of other modes and their application.

SIMV is often used in conjunction with PSV (to overcome circuit resistance and to decrease the work of breathing associated with spontaneous effort).

The use of SIMV plus PSV has been associated with prolonged weaning times. If respiratory muscle rest is the goal with SIMV plus PSV, the level of PSV should be high enough to provide a Vt of 6–12 mL/kg and to maintain a total rate (IMV plus PSV breaths) of ≤20 breaths/min.[13,14,36,37,41,67,68,86]

Procedure continues on following page

Procedure	for Invasive Mechanical Ventilation (Through an Artificial Airway): Volume and Pressure Modes—*Continued*	

Steps	Rationale	Special Considerations
4. Set Vt <10 mL/kg PBW. In patients with ARDS, Vt should be set at 4–6 mL/kg PBW. **(Level B*)**	Vt is selected in conjunction with fx to attain an MV 5–10 L/min with a $Paco_2$ 35–45 mm Hg. Large Vt values (12 mL/kg) have been associated with lung injury in patients with ARDS.[3,4,18,44,85]	When lower Vt values are used in an attempt to reduce lung injury, patients may need sedation and potentially muscle relaxants if they are dyssynchronous with the ventilator. Hypercarbia is an expected outcome of low Vt values.[7,26,27,78] Permissive hypercarbia is generally well tolerated in patients if the pH is reduced gradually (over 24–48 hours); pH around 7.2 is cited as an end point if tolerated.[77] Occasionally, bicarbonate infusions are used to keep the pH within an acceptable range. However, this temporizing maneuver may result in a higher $Paco_2$ because bicarbonate is metabolized into CO_2 and H_2O. Permissive hypercarbia should not be attempted in patients with elevated intracranial pressure or patients with myocardial ischemia, myocardial injury, or dysrhythmias. Patients who are allowed to become hypercarbic may need sedation and often muscle relaxants (paralytic agents) to control ventilation.
5. Select respiratory rate (frequency) between 10 and 20 breaths/min.	Vt and rate are selected to maintain an acceptable $Paco_2$ with an MV between 5 and 10 L/min. Generally, once Vt is selected, rate is the parameter adjusted to attain a desired $Paco_2$; the rate selected depends on whether or not the clinical goal is to rest or work the respiratory muscles.	When low Vts are used, as in ARDS, a higher rate may be necessary to maintain pH and $Paco_2$ at acceptable levels because smaller Vt provides less-efficient ventilation; the result is higher CO_2 and lower pH.[27,33,34,78]

*Level B: Well-designed, controlled studies with results that consistently support a specific action, intervention, or treatment.

Procedure	**for Invasive Mechanical Ventilation (Through an Artificial Airway): Volume and Pressure Modes—*Continued***	
Steps	**Rationale**	**Special Considerations**
6. For I:E times, select inspiratory time (this parameter name is different, depending on the ventilator). Examples of parameter names include percent inspiratory time, inspiratory time, flow rate, and peak flow. I:E ratios are usually 1:2 or 1:3. A typical inspiratory time for an adult is in the range of 0.75–1.2 second.	Inspiratory flow refers to the speed with which Vt is delivered during inspiration. Increasing the flow rate shortens the inspiratory time. Conversely, slowing the flow rate lengthens the inspiratory time.	Generally, flow rates of approximately 50 L/min are used initially and adjusted to provide an inspiratory time that synchronizes with patient effort. Short inspiratory times and long expiratory times are necessary in patients with obstructive lung diseases (e.g., emphysema, asthma). In contrast, patients with restrictive diseases, such as ARDS, have noncompliant lungs. Longer inspiratory times enhance recruitment and prevent derecruitment.[1,3,16,59,65,79]
7. Adjust flow as necessary to attain patient ventilator synchrony.	Achieves the desired I:E ratio and comfortable breathing patterns.	
8. Set the sensitivity (trigger sensitivity). Most ventilators have pressure-sensing sensitivity mechanisms that trigger flow, which means that the patient must generate a decrease in the system pressure with an inspiratory effort. When the ventilator senses the drop in pressure, flow (or a breath) is delivered. If a pressure trigger is used, sensitivity is set between −1 and −2 cm H_2O pressure.	The more negative the number, the less sensitive the ventilator is to patient effort, which increases the patient respiratory workload and may lead to dyssynchrony.	When auto-PEEP is present, the patient has to generate a negative pressure equal to the set sensitivity plus the level of auto-PEEP. Auto-PEEP is common in patients with asthma, chronic obstructive pulmonary disease, and high respiratory rates and minute ventilation. This additional work may fatigue the patient. Patient ventilator dyssynchrony is likely.[6,62,65]
9. If the ventilator has a flow-triggering option, select the flow trigger in L/min. The smaller the number, the more sensitive the ventilator. Flow triggering is set in conjunction with a base flow (flow in L/min that is provided between ventilator breaths). Flow rate is monitored in the expiratory limb of the ventilator. When flow is disrupted during a spontaneous breath, a decrease in flow downstream is sensed; additional flow or a breath is delivered.	Flow triggering has been associated with faster ventilator response times and less work of breathing than pressure sensing.[6]	
10. Set Fio_2 to 0.60–1.0 (60%–100%), if Pao_2 is unknown. A. Adjust Fio_2 downward as tolerated by monitoring Sao_2 and arterial blood gas values.	Initiation of PPV with maximal oxygen concentration avoids hypoxemia while optimal ventilator settings are being determined and evaluated. In addition, it permits measurement of the percentage of venous admixture (shunt), which provides an estimate of the severity of the gas-exchange abnormality.	The goal is an Fio_2 ≤0.5; high levels of Fio_2 result in increased risk of oxygen toxicity, absorption atelectasis, and reduction of surfactant synthesis.[30,42,48]

Procedure continues on following page

Procedure	for Invasive Mechanical Ventilation (Through an Artificial Airway): Volume and Pressure Modes—*Continued*		
Steps	**Rationale**		**Special Considerations**
11. Select PEEP or continuous positive airway pressure (CPAP) level. Initial setting is often 5 cm H_2O. A. PEEP may be adjusted as needed after evaluation of tolerance (e.g., SaO_2, PaO_2, physical assessment). PEEP levels are increased to restore FRC and allow for reduction of FiO_2 to safe levels (i.e., ≤0.5) to decrease the risk of oxygen toxicity.	A PEEP level of 5 cm H_2O is considered physiological (essentially the amount of pressure at end exhalation normally provided by the glottis). Higher levels of PEEP may be used to prevent alveolar collapse during the expiratory phase of the ventilator breath in atelectasis or ARDS.		High levels of PEEP ≥10 cm H_2O rarely should be interrupted because reestablishment of FRC (and PaO_2) may take hours. Prevention of this derecruitment in the patient with ARDS is especially important. Super-PEEP levels (i.e., ≥20 cm H_2O) may be necessary in patients with noncompliant lungs (e.g., patients with ARDS) to prevent lung injury. The repetitive opening and closing of stiff alveoli is thought to result in alveolar damage; to that end, the use of high PEEP levels to maintain alveolar distention and to prevent injury during PPV is considered a protective lung strategy.[3–5,12,33,34,44] In general, when high PEEP levels are used, Vt values are lower than normal and subsequent hypercarbia may be anticipated. Use of muscle relaxants, sedatives, and narcotics is often necessary to prevent patient spontaneous breathing.
B. CPAP is often referred to as PEEP without the positive pressure breaths. CPAP is a spontaneous breathing mode that provides continuous pressure throughout the ventilator cycle. It is commonly used as a mode for spontaneous-breathing weaning trials.	Patients who are spontaneously breathing may not require delivery of ventilator breaths, but positive pressure applied to the airways and alveoli to prevent collapse or obstruction during exhalation.		Generally, the pressure levels of CPAP are relatively low but vary with individual patient conditions. A traditional application of CPAP is for obstructive sleep apnea (OSA) through a noninvasive mask or prongs. When used for OSA, the mode provides a pneumatic splint to the airways to prevent obstruction during sleep.
Pressure Modes (Invasive) 1. Select mode: PSV, pressure-controlled/inverse ratio ventilation (PC/IRV), volume-assured pressure support option, APRV, adaptive support ventilation, proportional assist ventilation (PAV), automatic tube compensation (ATC), or high-frequency oscillation (HFO).	Mode selection depends on clinical goals, mode availability (these vary widely with different ventilators), and clinician preference. To date, no mode has emerged as superior.[17,81,89] Modes include those designed for spontaneous breathing and those for control or partial control of ventilation.		Many new modes that use microprocessor technology are available on specific ventilators. Although many are similar to traditional modes, others are not. Parameter names also vary. Refer to specific ventilator operating manuals and websites for details not contained in this procedure.

Procedure	**for Invasive Mechanical Ventilation (Through an Artificial Airway): Volume and Pressure Modes—*Continued***	
Steps	**Rationale**	**Special Considerations**
2. PSV augments spontaneous respirations with a clinician-selected pressure level. Adjust the PSV level to attain a Vt <10 mL/kg PBW with a spontaneous respiratory rate (RR) ≤20 breaths/min (if respiratory muscle rest is desired; this is called PSVmax). Decrease PSV level during weaning trials as tolerated by patient. Tolerance criteria for trials may be predetermined by protocols or on an individual basis. Often during trials, Vt values are allowed to be lower (i.e., 5–8 mL/kg) and RR higher (i.e., 25–30 breaths/min) than when rest is the goal. However, these parameters are always evaluated in conjunction with other signs and symptoms of fatigue and intolerance.[13,14,41,61,63,95] **(Level B*)**	Pressure level in conjunction with compliance and resistance determines delivered Vt.	PSV sometimes is used between IMV breaths to offset the work of breathing associated with artificial airways and circuits during spontaneous breathing. PSV generally is considered a weaning mode of ventilation, which necessitates stability of patient condition. PSV may be used in patients with less stable conditions provided that close attention is given to changes in Vt and RR. High levels of PSV may provide respiratory muscle unloading.
A. Set sensitivity (as with volume ventilation).	The more negative the number, the less sensitive the ventilator is to patient effort, which increases the patient respiratory workload and may lead to dyssynchrony.	
B. Set Fio₂ (as with volume ventilation).	Initiation of PPV with maximal oxygen concentration avoids hypoxemia while optimal ventilator settings are being determined and evaluated. In addition, it permits measurement of the percentage of venous admixture (shunt), which provides an estimate of the severity of the gas-exchange abnormality.	
C. Set PEEP (as with volume ventilation).	A PEEP level of 5 cm H₂O is considered physiological (essentially the amount of pressure at end exhalation normally provided by the glottis). Higher levels of PEEP may be used to prevent alveolar collapse during the expiratory phase of the ventilator breath in atelectasis or ARDS.	

*Level B: Well-designed, controlled studies with results that consistently support a specific action, intervention, or treatment.

Procedure continues on following page

Procedure	**for Invasive Mechanical Ventilation (Through an Artificial Airway): Volume and Pressure Modes—*Continued***		
Steps	**Rationale**	**Special Considerations**	

Steps	Rationale	Special Considerations
3. PC/IRV are both control modes of ventilation. With these modes, a pressure level is selected; the rate and inspiratory time are selected as well. They were originally used to manage patients with ARDS in whom the goal was to limit the pressure level. In addition, the decelerating flow pattern of the modes was considered desirable. PC/IRV was used to enhance lung recruitment by prolonging inspiration. Expiration was shortened, thereby decreasing the potential for derecruitment.	Absolute pressure level is the sum of the inspiratory pressure level (IPL) and PEEP.	If the clinical goal is to ensure a plateau pressure of ≤30 cm H_2O, the pressure level may be lowered gradually over 24–48 hours to prevent sudden changes in $Paco_2$ and pH.[50,76,78]
A. Select IPL. With this pressure mode, the level of pressure support is often identified as IPL versus PSV.	Rate and IPL determine MV.	
B. Select rate.	Vt and rate are selected to maintain an acceptable $Paco_2$ with an MV between 5 and 10 L/min. Generally, once Vt is selected, rate is the parameter adjusted to attain a desired $Paco_2$; the rate selected depends on whether or not the clinical goal is to rest or work the respiratory muscles.	When low Vts are used, as in ARDS, a higher rate may be necessary to maintain pH and $Paco_2$ at acceptable levels because smaller Vts provide less-efficient ventilation; the result is higher CO_2 and lower pH.[27,33,34,79]
C. Select inspiratory time or inverse I:E ratio (ventilators vary).	I:E ratios are set at 1:1, 2:1, 3:1, or 4:1 by selecting the appropriate inspiratory time. Ratios are adjusted upward to improve shunt and oxygenation. Blood pressure may be adversely affected. Rate is usually relatively high (e.g., 20–25 breaths/min).	Generally, clinicians start with 1:1 ratios and increase as necessary to improve oxygenation. A limiting factor related to prolonged inspiratory times is hemodynamic compromise and hypotension, which is generally why the use of ratios >2:1 rarely is seen clinically. Auto-PEEP is common and may be a desired outcome of PC/IRV.[66,76]
D. Select PEEP level. When transitioning from volume ventilation to PC/IRV, the PEEP initially is maintained at the level used previously until the effect of the IRV is assessed. **(Level C*)**	Because IRV may result in auto-PEEP, evaluation of the total amount of PEEP present is important. This can be measured through the performance of an expiratory hold maneuver on the ventilator.	Auto-PEEP generated by IRV is expected and helpful in expanding collapsed alveoli.

*Level C: Qualitative studies, descriptive or correlational studies, integrative reviews, systematic reviews, or randomized controlled trials with inconsistent results.

Procedure	for Invasive Mechanical Ventilation (Through an Artificial Airway): Volume and Pressure Modes—*Continued*	
Steps	**Rationale**	**Special Considerations**
E. Set Fio$_2$ to 0.60–1.0 (60%–100%) if Pao$_2$ is unknown. Adjust Fio$_2$ downward as tolerated by monitoring Sao$_2$ and arterial blood gas values.	Initiation of PPV with maximal oxygen concentration avoids hypoxemia while optimal ventilator settings are being determined and evaluated. In addition, it permits measurement of the percentage of venous admixture (shunt), which provides an estimate of the severity of the gas-exchange abnormality.	The goal is an Fio$_2$ ≤0.5; high levels of Fio$_2$ result in increased risk of oxygen toxicity, absorption atelectasis, and reduction of surfactant synthesis.[30,42,48]
F. Set sensitivity (as with volume ventilation). **(Level B*)**	The goal of PC/IRV is to improve oxygenation and allow for reduction of Fio$_2$ to ≤0.5.[17,50,76,87] This is done in conjunction with the addition of PEEP. Always set sensitivity so that the patient can get a breath if needed.	If controlled ventilation is the goal, chemical relaxation may be necessary in conjunction with sedatives and narcotics. Patient tolerance of IRV (i.e., the prolonged inspiratory times) is unlikely without such interventions. Remember that IRV may result in auto-PEEP (which may be a desirable outcome of the mode). Regardless, auto-PEEP should be anticipated and measured regularly.
4. Dual-control pressure mode options are pressure modes that assure a minimum set tidal volume. The breath delivery varies with the specific mode. For dual control pressure support options, parameter selection (i.e., pressure, volume, rate) is specific to the ventilator; however, selection of desired (or guaranteed) Vt is required. Some ventilators also require selection of the pressure level. Spontaneous breathing modes and controlled modes are available.[2,11,15,17, 58,87,90] **(Level C*)** A. For volume-guaranteed pressure options, please see specific ventilator manual for parameter setting. **(Level M*)** B. PEEP, Fio$_2$ and sensitivity are set as per volume ventilation, as are rate and inspiratory time if the mode is a control mode. However, the desired Vt must be selected as well.[17]	Specific names vary depending on ventilator manufacturer. Examples include Pressure Augmentation (Carefusion, San Diego, CA) and Volume Support and Pressure Regulated Volume Control (Maquet, Wayne, NJ); similar modes are available on other manufacturers' ventilators.	Few studies have been accomplished that show the superiority of these modes. In addition, many modes are available only on specific ventilators. These modes are complex; concurrent use of pressure, flow, and volume waveform displays may be necessary to assess the modes accurately. Refer to specific ventilator operating manuals or websites for additional information. See Table 29-1 parameters for volume-guaranteed pressure options.

*Level B: Well-designed, controlled studies with results that consistently support a specific action, intervention, or treatment.

*Level C: Qualitative studies, descriptive or correlational studies, integrative reviews, systematic reviews, or randomized controlled trials with inconsistent results.

*Level M: Manufacturer's recommendations only.

Procedure continues on following page

| Procedure | for Invasive Mechanical Ventilation (Through an Artificial Airway): Volume and Pressure Modes—*Continued* |

Steps	Rationale	Special Considerations
5. Biphasic and APRV ventilation are relatively new modes that appear on selected ventilators. Used most commonly for patients with ARDS, the modes use relatively high levels of pressure to recruit the lung (restore FRC). APRV is a type of biphasic ventilation with a very short expiratory (release) time.[56,69,71,80,81,88, 89,97] **(Level C*)**	Although the modes appear to be safe and effective, randomized controlled trials are not available. Regardless, one big advantage to these modes is that they do not require that the patient be heavily sedated or paralyzed. Spontaneous breathing is expected. Generally, the patient's breathing pattern is rapid.	Few studies have been accomplished that show the superiority of these modes. In addition, many modes are available on specific ventilators. These ventilatory modes require a steep learning curve on the part of physician, advanced practice nurse, and other healthcare professionals who care for the patients; as with most new forms of ventilation, education of staff should occur before the mode is used. Although the appeal of APRV and biphasic ventilation is in part because the patient may breath spontaneously, it is unclear whether the associated workload is advantageous.[72]
A. With APRV, a high level of CPAP is selected, and brief expiratory "releases" are provided at set intervals (similar to setting a RR); the releases are very brief (≤1.5 seconds).	The high level of CPAP helps "recruit" the lung. Alveolar filling and emptying time constants in the ARDS lung vary; the brief expiratory releases provided with APRV allow for more uniform emptying throughout the lung and ultimately improved gas distribution. An additional benefit of periodic airway pressure releases is that they may decrease the potential negative effect of the high CPAP level on venous return. At the high CPAP level, the patient may take spontaneous breaths at the rate that they require.[47,56,70,84]	On some machines, the formal mode name APRV may not be used. It may be incorporated under biphasic ventilation.
B. With the biphasic mode, two different levels of PEEP are selected and are called high-PEEP and low-PEEP. This is really an interaction of traditional PC ventilation. A rate is set, and the cycles look similar to PC or PC/IRV ventilation (depending on the I:E ratio). The major difference is that flow is available to the patient for spontaneous breathing at both pressure levels. In addition, Pressure Support (PS) may be added to assist in decreasing the work associated with spontaneous breathing.[17,56,81] **(Level E*)**	The theoretical advantage of this mode over traditional PC/IRV is that the mode may fully support lung recruitment while still allowing for spontaneous breathing at the two pressure levels.[17,56,81] In contrast to traditional PC/IRV, the patient receives additional flow adequate to meet inspiratory demands throughout the ventilatory cycle. Deterioration with spontaneous effort is less likely; as a result, heavy sedation and paralytics may be avoided.	APRV mode as described previously may be achieved in ventilators with biphasic modes. Biphasic modes have many trade names (BiVent, BiLevel, BiPAP, DuoPap). The APRV settings are achieved on each type of ventilator in a slightly different manner. Refer to the specific ventilator manual for parameter settings.

*Level C: Qualitative studies, descriptive or correlational studies, integrative reviews, systematic reviews, or randomized controlled trials with inconsistent results.
*Level E: Multiple case reports, theory-based evidence from expert opinions, or peer-reviewed professional organizational standards without clinical studies to support recommendations.

Procedure	for Invasive Mechanical Ventilation (Through an Artificial Airway): Volume and Pressure Modes—*Continued*	
Steps	**Rationale**	**Special Considerations**
C. For APRV and biphasic mode options, please see specific ventilator manual for parameter settings. (**Level M***)	Manufacturers have different names for parameters settings. Although there are similarities among the ventilator models, it is important to be familiar with the ventilators used in your practice area.	
D. Specific APRV settings: i. Pressure high (P_{HIGH}), which is the high-PEEP level. May be set at the measured plateau pressure to start. ii. Pressure low (P_{LOW}), which is the low-PEEP level, is generally set at 0 cm H_2O. iii. Time high (T_{HIGH}): 4–6 seconds. iv. Time low (T_{LOW}): 0.4–0.8 seconds (keep <1.5 seconds). Rate is determined by the combined inspiratory (T_{HIGH}) expiratory time (T_{LOW}).	The combination of the inspiratory pressure (P^{HIGH}) and inspiratory time (T^{HIGH}) determine the machine-delivered tidal volume. The expiratory time (T_{Low}) determines the duration of exhalation. In APRV, the expiratory time is very short (usually <1.0 second). Therefore, the P_{Low} is set at 0 cm H_2O, because there is insufficient time for the alveoli to collapse before the next breath.	Patients on APRV should be transported on the ventilator to avoid alveolar derecruitment associated with disconnection from the ventilator circuit. This can occur when the patient is transitioned to a bag-valve mask for transport. If the patient must be disconnect from the ventilator, the endotracheal tube may be clamped during the inspiratory phase before circuit disconnection to reduce the chance of alveolar derecruitment.
E. Specific biphasic settings: i. Pressure high (P_{HIGH}) Set to achieve the desired tidal volume for the patient ii. Pressure low (P_{LOW}). Set to attain best PEEP iii. Rate: 8–10 iv. Inspiratory time (T_{HIGH}): 1.5 seconds or set T_{HIGH}/T_{LOW} ratio (I:E ratio) v. Fio_2.	The combination of the inspiratory pressure (P^{HIGH}) and inspiratory time (T^{HIGH}) determines the machine-delivered tidal volume. The expiratory time (T_{Low}) determines the duration of exhalation. In biphasic (non-APRV), the I:E ratio is usually set at conventional ratios (1:2 or 1:3).	
F. Fio_2 and sensitivity are set as outlined in **Steps 8 and 9** above under Volume Control Modes.	See Steps 8 and 9.	

*Level M: Manufacturer's recommendations only.

Procedure continues on following page

| **Procedure** | **for Invasive Mechanical Ventilation (Through an Artificial Airway): Volume and Pressure Modes—*Continued*** | |

Steps	Rationale	Special Considerations
6. Adaptive support ventilation: The mode is referred to by the ventilator manufacturer as "intelligent ventilation" and is designed to assess lung mechanics on a breath-to-breath basis (controlled loop ventilation) for spontaneous and control settings. It achieves an optimal Vt by automatically adjusting mandatory respiratory fx and inspiratory pressure. Built into the mode are algorithms that are "lung protective." The protective strategies are designed to minimize auto-PEEP and prevent apnea, tachypnea, excessive dead space, and excessively large breaths.[2,15,19,25,58,90] **(Level C*)**	The working concept with this mode is that the patient will breathe at fx and Vt that minimize elastic and resistive loads. In all modes, the opportunity for spontaneous breathing is promoted (the user does not have to switch back and forth from one mode to another to encourage spontaneous breathing because this is automatically done). Thus the interactions required by the clinician are few.	The higher the %MinVol, the higher the level of support provided to the patient.
Parameters to set include predicted body weight, minute volume (%MinVol), and high pressure limit in addition to Fio$_2$. **(Level M*)**		
7. PAV: The concept with this pressure mode is to prevent fatiguing workloads although still allowing the patient to breathe spontaneously. Current PAV modes take measurements throughout the inspiratory cycle and automatically adjust the pressure, flow, and volume proportionally to offset the resistance and elastance of the system with each inspiration (patient and circuit). Different names for the modes are provided by specific manufacturers, and parameters that require adjustment vary somewhat between the ventilators. **(Level M)**	PAV may provide a more physiological breathing pattern.[10,17,25,45,60,94] The modes recognize that patient effort reflects work and demand, and base the adjustments accordingly. The percent of assist is adjusted to a higher percent if less work is desired and a lower percent if more work is necessary.	Few studies have been accomplished that show the superiority of this mode. In addition, many modes are available on specific ventilators.
Parameter settings include PEEP, Fio$_2$, percent volume assist, and percent flow assist.		
8. ATC is a ventilatory adjunct rather than a mode and is available on many current ventilators. It is designed to overcome the work of breathing imposed by the artificial airway. Parameters include internal diameter size of the endotracheal tube and the desired percent of compensation.[17, 35,93] **(Level C)**	ATC adjusts the pressure (proportional to tube resistance) needed to provide a variable fast inspiratory flow during spontaneous breathing.	ATC is increased during inspiration and lowered during expiration, thus decreasing the work of breathing as a result of tube resistance. In some patients, the use of ATC has resulted in auto-PEEP.[35,93]

*Level C: Qualitative studies, descriptive or correlational studies, integrative reviews, systematic reviews, or randomized controlled trials with inconsistent results.
*Level M: Manufacturer's recommendations only.

Procedure	for Invasive Mechanical Ventilation (Through an Artificial Airway): Volume and Pressure Modes—*Continued*	
Steps	**Rationale**	**Special Considerations**
9. High-frequency oscillation ventilation (HFOV) differs significantly from conventional ventilator modes or mode options. HFOV does not require bulk movement of volume in and out of the lungs; rather, a bias flow of gases is provided, and an oscillator disperses the gases throughout the lung in what has been called augmented dispersion at high frequencies.[31,32,39,83] **(Level C*)**	The method achieves oscillation of the lung around a constant airway pressure (essentially opening the lung and keeping it open).[31,32,39,83]	Studies to date have not shown the superiority of this mode over traditional modes in adults with ARDS. The mode is safe if appropriately applied by those with experience in its use; however, it is not easily understood by clinicians. Especially of concern is the fact that patients on the mode often need sedation and neuromuscular blockade.
The parameters for HFOV are different from conventional ventilation and are outlined in the following.		
A. Bias flow: flow in L/min (usual range, 40–50 L/min).	The bias flow combined with the oscillatory activity (extremely rapid pulses in a back and forth motion) results in the constant infusion of fresh gases and evacuation of old gases.	
B. Oscillatory frequency (fx): In Hz (usual range, 3–6 Hz).[20,39,40]	Increases in frequency in HFOV actually reduces CO_2 elimination because there is less time for CO_2 to be removed from the lungs between the oscillatory breaths. This is different from conventional ventilation, with which an increase in rate may reduce CO_2.[20,39,40]	1 Hz is equivalent to 60 breaths.
C. Mean airway pressure: generally slightly greater than conventional ventilation initially.		
D. ΔP: The change in pressure or pressure amplitude (generally adjusted to achieve chest wall vibration).	ΔP and fx are adjusted to achieve $Paco_2$ within a target range.	
E. Fio_2 level and PEEP level: as in conventional ventilation (generally PEEP is >10).		
F. Percent inspiratory time: controls the percentage of time the oscillator spends in the inspiratory phase. A starting place is 33%.		
10. Discard used supplies and remove PE.		
11. HH		
Humidity		
1. Humidity is essential to prevent the drying effect of the gases provided by the ventilator.	Inspired gases may be humidified with the use of standard cascade or high-volume humidifiers. Many institutions use disposable HMEs in place of conventional humidifiers.	HMEs are popular because they decrease the risk of infection and are inexpensive.

*Level C: Qualitative studies, descriptive or correlational studies, integrative reviews, systematic reviews, or randomized controlled trials with inconsistent results.

Procedure continues on following page

Procedure	for Invasive Mechanical Ventilation (Through an Artificial Airway): Volume and Pressure Modes—*Continued*		
Steps	**Rationale**	**Special Considerations**	
2. For conventional humidifiers, ensure that the humidifier has adequate fluid (sterile distilled water) and that the thermostat setting is adjusted according to manufacturer's recommendations. **(Level M*)**	Gases generally are humidified before entering the artificial airway. Temperature is measured at the patient's airway; temperatures between 35°C and 37°C (95°F and 98°F) are considered optimal.[72]	Cool circuits may be tolerated well in patients without secretions. In patients with thick or tenacious secretions, attention to inspired temperature is important to prevent mucus plugging; circuit temperatures may need to be closer to body temperature (37°C versus 35°C) in these cases.	
3. HMEs are placed between the airway and the ventilator circuit.	The moisture in warmed exhaled gases passes through the vast surface area of the HME and condenses. With inspiration, dry gases pass through the HME and become humidified. The use of HMEs has been associated with decreased incidence of ventilator-associated pneumonias in patients on ventilation.[9,29,51,91,92] **(Level B*)**		
A. Change HMEs per manufacturer's instructions. **(Level M*)**	The longer the HME is in line, the more efficient the humidification; however, inspiratory resistance increases over time. HMEs are often changed every 2–3 days (refer to manufacturer's instructions).	In patients undergoing weaning, the additional resistive load added by these humidifiers may preclude their use.[51,55,64,77]	
B. Do not use if secretions are copious or bloody.	Obstruction is possible, and HMEs are not indicated in these conditions.		
4. Discard used supplies and remove **PE**.			
5. **HH**			

*Level B: Well-designed, controlled studies with results that consistently support a specific action, intervention, or treatment.
*Level M: Manufacturer's recommendations only.

Expected Outcomes

- Maintenance of adequate pH and $PaCO_2$
- Maintenance of adequate PaO_2
- Maintenance of adequate breathing pattern
- Respiratory muscle rest

Unexpected Outcomes

- Abnormal pH, $PaCO_2$, and PaO_2
- Hemodynamic instability
- Pulmonary barotrauma
- Inadvertent extubation
- Malpositioned endotracheal tube
- Nosocomial lung infection
- Acid-base disturbance
- Respiratory muscle fatigue

Patient Monitoring and Care

Steps	Rationale	Reportable Conditions
		These conditions should be reported if they persist despite nursing interventions.
1. Ensure activation of all alarms each shift (see Box 29-2).	Ensures patient safety.	• Continued activation of alarms
2. Check for secure stabilization and maintenance of endotracheal or tracheostomy tube.	Reduces risk of inadvertent extubation or decannulation.	• Unplanned extubation or decannulation,
		• Dislodgment of airway
3. Monitor in-line thermometer to maintain inspired gas temperature (in the range 35–37°C [95–98°F]).	Reduces risk of thermal injury from overheated inspired gas and risk of poor humidity from underheated inspired gas.	• Temperature <35°C or >37°C
4. Keep ventilator tubing clear of condensation. Drain any condensation in the ventilator tubing toward condensation-collection reservoirs on the expiratory limb of the circuit (clean to dirty). Avoid draining condensation back toward the patient. (dirty to clean).	Reduces risk of respiratory infection by decreasing inhalation of contaminated water droplets.	• Continued condensation
5. Ensure availability of self-inflating manual resuscitation bag-valve device attached to supplemental oxygen at the head of the bed. Attach or adjust PEEP valve if the patient is on >5 cm H_2O.	Provides capability for immediate delivering of ventilation and oxygenation to relieve acute respiratory distress caused by hypoxemia or acidosis.	• Inability to oxygenate or ventilate
6. Check ventilator for baseline Fio_2, peak inspiratory pressure (PIP), Vt, fx, and alarm activation with initial assessment and after removal of ventilator from patient for suctioning, bagging, or draining ventilator tubing.	Ensures that prescribed ventilator parameters are used (e.g., 100% oxygen used for suctioning is not inadvertently delivered after suctioning procedure), provides diagnostic data to evaluate interventions (e.g., PIP is reduced after suctioning or bagging), and ensures that the monitoring and warning functions of the ventilator are functional (i.e., alarms).	• Fio_2, PIP, Vt, or fx settings different from prescribed
7. Explore any changes in peak inspiratory pressure >4 cm H_2O or decreased (sustained) Vt on PSV. Immediately explore the cause of high-pressure alarms.	Acute changes in PIP or Vt may indicate mechanical malfunction, such as tubing disconnection, cuff or connector leaks, tubing or airway kinks, or changes in resistance and compliance. Always consider possibility of tension pneumothorax.	• Unexplained high-pressure alarms
8. Place bite-block between the teeth if the patient is biting on the oral endotracheal tube.	An oral airway serves the same purpose but may not be tolerated as well as the bite-block because it may induce gagging.	• Biting on tube

Procedure continues on following page

Patient Monitoring and Care —*Continued*

Steps	Rationale	Reportable Conditions
9. Evaluate patient-ventilator dyssynchrony by manually ventilating the patient with a self-inflating manual resuscitation bag-valve device.	By taking the patient off the ventilator for manual ventilation, synchrony may be accomplished more quickly than on the ventilator. This intervention may reduce risk of barotrauma and cardiovascular depression. If patient breathes in synchrony with bagging, consider changes in ventilatory parameters. If patient does not breathe synchronously with bagging, explore differential diagnoses of problems distal to the airway. Respiratory care practitioner, nurse practitioner, or physician consultation may be necessary.	• Patient-ventilator dyssynchrony
10. Assess for signs of atelectasis.	May occur as a result of hypoventilation as well as mucous plugging of bronchioles. Early detection of atelectasis indicates the need for alteration to promote resolution (tidal volume adjustment, recruitment maneuver, PEEP adjustment).	• Localized changes in auscultation (increased or bronchial breath sounds) • Localized dullness to percussion • Increased breathing effort • Tracheal deviation toward the side of abnormal findings • Increased peak and plateau pressures • Decreased compliance • Decreased Pao_2 or Sao_2 (with constant ventilator parameters) • Localized consolidation ("whiteout," opacity) on chest radiograph
11. Assess for signs and symptoms of pulmonary barotrauma (i.e., pneumothorax).	Early detection of pneumothorax is essential to minimize progression to cardiac tamponade and death. Tension pneumothorax requires immediate emergency decompression with a large-bore needle (i.e., 14-gauge) into the second or third intercostal space, midclavicular line on the affected side, followed by immediate chest tube placement.	• Acute, increasing, or severe dyspnea • Restlessness • Agitation • Localized changes in auscultation (decreased or absent breath sounds) on the affected side • Localized hyperresonance or tympany to percussion on the affected side • Elevated chest on the affected side • Increased breathing effort • Tracheal deviation away from the side of abnormal findings • Increased peak and plateau pressures • Decreased compliance • Decreased Pao_2 or Sao_2 • Subcutaneous emphysema • Localized increased lucency with absent lung markings on chest radiograph. • Hypotension

Patient Monitoring and Care —*Continued*

Steps	Rationale	Reportable Conditions
12. Assess for signs of volume-pressure trauma that are consistent with ARDS.	Volume-pressure trauma is assumed if the patient has the last three criteria noted. Ventilatory management should focus on ensuring that lung-protective strategies are in place so that additional injury does not ensue. Some examples include Vt of 6 mL/kg and lung recruitment with PEEP. In general, these strategies result in hypercarbia because ventilation is not efficient.	• Acute, increasing, or severe dyspnea • Restlessness • Agitation • Generalized crackles, especially in the dependent portions of the lung • Refractory hypoxemia • Increased peak and plateau pressures • Decreased compliance • Decreased Pao_2 or Sao_2 • Bilateral diffuse lung opacity on chest radiograph or computer axial tomography (CAT) scan of the chest • $Pao_2:Fio_2$ of <200 • A noncardiac etiology for the "wet" lung
13. Monitor for signs and symptoms of acute respiratory distress, hypoxemia, hypercarbia, and fatigue.	Respiratory distress indicates the need for changes in PPV. While troubleshooting the difficulties, support ventilation via a manual self-inflating resuscitation bag if necessary.	• Chest-abdominal dyssynchrony • Shallow or irregular respirations • Tachypnea, bradypnea, or dyspnea • Decreased mental status • Restlessness, confusion, lethargy • Increasing or decreasing arterial blood pressure • Tachycardia • Atrial or ventricular dysrhythmias • Significant changes in arterial pH, Pao_2, $Paco_2$, or Sao_2
14. Assess for signs and symptoms of a malpositioned endotracheal tube.	Early detection and correction of a malpositioned endotracheal tube can prevent inadvertent extubation, atelectasis, barotrauma, and problems with gas exchange.	• Dyspnea • Restlessness or agitation • Unilateral decreased or absent breath sounds • Unilateral dullness to percussion • Increased breathing effort • Asymmetrical chest expansion • Increased PIP • Changes in endotracheal tube depth • Radiographic evidence of malposition. • Decreased Sao_2
15. Assess for signs and symptoms of inadvertent extubation.	Inadvertent extubation is sometimes obvious (e.g., the endotracheal tube is in the patient's hand). Often, the tip of the endotracheal tube is in the hypopharynx or in the esophagus; however, an inadvertent extubation may not be immediately apparent. Reintubation may be necessary, although some patients may not need reintubation. If reintubation is necessary, ventilation and oxygenation are assisted with a manual self-inflating resuscitation bag-valve device and face mask.	• Vocalization • Activated ventilator alarms • Low pressure • Low minute ventilation • Inability to deliver preset pressure • Decreased or absent breath sounds • Gastric distention • Changes in endotracheal tube depth • Signs and symptoms of inadequate ventilation, oxygenation, and breathing pattern

Procedure continues on following page

Patient Monitoring and Care —*Continued*

Steps	Rationale	Reportable Conditions
16. Evaluate the patient's need for long-term mechanical ventilation.	This evaluation allows the nurse to anticipate patient and family needs for the patient's discharge to an extended-care facility, rehabilitation center, or home on PPV.	• Spontaneous breathing trial failure • Inability to wean from the ventilator
17. Observe for hemodynamic changes associated with increased Vt, PEEP/CPAP, or recruitment maneuver.	PPV can cause decreased venous return and afterload because of the increase in intrathoracic pressure. This mechanism often manifests immediately after initiation of mechanical ventilation and with large Vt, increases in PEEP or CPAP levels and manual hyperinflation techniques. Cardiovascular depression associated with manual or periodic ventilator hyperinflation is immediately reversible with cessation of hyperinflation. Decreases in blood pressure with PPV also may be seen with hypovolemia. Always consider potential for pneumothorax with acute changes.	• Decreased blood pressure • Change in heart rate (increase or decrease of >10% of baseline) • Weak peripheral pulses, pulsus paradoxus, or decreased pulse pressure • Decreased cardiac output • Decreased mixed venous oxygen tension • Increased arterial-venous oxygen difference

Documentation

Documentation should include the following:

- Patient and family education
- Date and time ventilatory assistance was instituted
- Ventilator settings, including the following: Fio_2, mode of ventilation, Vt, respiratory frequency (total and mandatory), PEEP level, I:E ratio or inspiratory time, PIP, dynamic compliance, and static compliance
- Arterial blood gas results
- Sao_2 readings
- Reason for initiation of PPV
- Assessment of pain, interventions and response to intervention
- Patient responses to PPV (including the patient's indication of level of comfort and respiratory symptoms)
- Depth of endotracheal tube at the teeth or gum
- Hemodynamic values
- Vital signs
- Respiratory assessment findings
- Unexpected outcomes
- Nursing interventions
- Degree of backrest elevation
- Humidifier change maintenance

References and Additional Readings

For a complete list of references and additional readings for this procedure, scan this QR code with any freely available smartphone code reader app, or visit http://booksite.elsevier.com/9780323376624.

30 Noninvasive Positive Pressure Ventilation: Continuous Positive Airway Pressure (CPAP) and Bilevel Positive Airway Pressure (BiPAP)

Susan K. Frazier

PURPOSE: Noninvasive positive pressure ventilation is delivery of ventilatory support without the placement of an artificial airway (an oral or nasal endotracheal tube or tracheostomy); ventilatory support is provided through a nasal mask, nasal pillows, full face mask, or helmet mask. Noninvasive positive pressure ventilation is used to prevent airway obstruction during sleep, to maintain or improve ventilation and/or oxygenation, and to provide respiratory muscle rest in patients in whom invasive mechanical ventilation is not possible, acceptable, or desired. Continuous positive airway pressure (CPAP) is the provision of continuous positive airway pressure throughout inspiration and expiration; bilevel positive airway pressure is the administration of two levels of airway pressure, one during inspiration and another during expiration. Bilevel positive airway pressure (BiPAP) is a proprietary name of Respironics Inc., but for the purposes of this procedure, the acronym BiPAP indicates bilevel positive airway pressure.

PREREQUISITE NURSING KNOWLEDGE

- Although invasive mechanical ventilation delivered through an artificial airway has been the principal support strategy for patients with impaired ventilation and oxygenation in critical care since the early 1970s, Sullivan and colleagues[39] introduced the use of CPAP delivered through a nasal mask to patients with obstructive sleep apnea in 1981, and in 1987 to patients with acquired muscle weakness and muscular dystrophy.[12]
- The use of noninvasive positive pressure ventilation has become common, and often a first-line support. Recently Ugurlu and colleagues[40] determined that nearly 40% of patients who required ventilator support initially received noninvasive ventilation; most common diagnoses managed with noninvasive ventilation were acute exacerbation of chronic obstructive pulmonary disease (COPD) and cardiogenic pulmonary edema. Nearly three quarters of these patients were successful users of noninvasive ventilation, and the mortality rate of those who received noninvasive ventilation was nearly half that of patients ventilated invasively.
- Lin and colleagues[21] demonstrated that noninvasive ventilation was effective in the prevention of postextubation respiratory failure in a meta-analysis of 10 clinical trials; they identified a 25% reduction in the likelihood of postextubation respiratory failure, a 35% decrease in the likelihood of reintubation, and a reduction in the likelihood of intensive care unit (ICU) and hospital mortality by 41% and 59% respectively, compared with standard therapy. Chandra and colleagues[10] reported a 400% increase in the use of noninvasive ventilation for patients with an acute exacerbation of COPD over the decade from 1998 to 2008, and a subsequent reduction in invasive ventilation of 42%.
- The use of noninvasive ventilation maintains upper-airway protective reflexes and the ability to speak and swallow and avoids complications associated with intubation and invasive ventilation such as airway trauma, barotrauma, ventilation-induced acute lung injury, and hospital-acquired ventilator-associated pneumonia.[26] Carron and colleagues[8] reviewed the prevalence of complications associated with noninvasive ventilation from a meta-analysis. Airway dryness was reported in 10% to 20% of patients, nasal congestion in 20% to 50%, gastric insufflation in 10% to 50%, facial erythema in 20% to 32%, nasal/sinus/ear pain in 10% to 30%, minor air leaks in 80% to 100%, major air leaks in 18% to 68%, claustrophobia in 5% to 20%, carbon dioxide (CO_2) rebreathing in 50% to 100%, nasal skin in lesions in 10% to 50%, and general discomfort in 30% to 50% of patients.
- Patient predictors of potential failure of noninvasive ventilation before application of noninvasive ventilation

include established severe acute respiratory distress syndrome, reduced level of consciousness, shock of any etiology, Glasgow coma score less than 11, Acute Physiology and Chronic Health Evaluation (APACHE) II severity of illness score higher than 29, profuse secretions, tachypnea (>35 breaths/minute), pH less than 7.25, hypotension (systolic blood pressure <90 mm Hg), age over 40 years, edentulism, severe agitation, and asynchronous breathing.[17,26] Predictors observed after initiation of noninvasive ventilation include major air leaks, poor tolerance, and ventilatory asynchrony. After 1 hour of ventilation, continued tachypnea, lack of improvement in oxygenation, hypercarbia, acidosis, and evident fatigue predict failure of noninvasive ventilation.[17]

Indications for Noninvasive Positive Pressure Ventilation

- *Obstructive sleep apnea.* Obstructive sleep apnea (OSA) is characterized by repeated episodes of upper-airway collapse during sleep with subsequent oxyhemoglobin desaturation, hypoxemia, and recurrent sleep arousal. OSA produces fragmented sleep; daytime sleepiness; exaggerated fluctuation in intrathoracic pressure, blood pressure, and cardiac rhythm; systemic inflammation; sympathetic activation; and endothelial dysfunction.[3] Long-term consequences of OSA include hypertension,[47] atherosclerosis and cardiovascular disease,[7] cognitive dysfunction, decreased quality of life, depression,[1] and premature all-cause mortality.[25,28] Additionally, individuals with OSA are two and a half times more likely to have a motor vehicle accident, particularly those who are 65 years of age and older.[19] Recently, investigators estimated the prevalence of moderate to severe OSA at 10% for 30- to 49-year-old men, 3% for 30- to 49-year-old women, 17% for 50- to 70-year-old men, and 9% for 50- to 70-year-old women; these findings represented a 14% to 55% increase in prevalence of OSA over the past 2 decades.[34] Although CPAP is highly effective as a pneumatic split to the upper airway, investigators have reported poor adherence, with nonadherence rates of 46% to 83%.[31,43] Predictors of adherence include the initial 1-month experience and adverse effects attributed to CPAP therapy[9] and variability of more than 75 minutes in bedtime.[37] A systematic evaluation of interventions to improve adherence to nocturnal CPAP found that ongoing supportive interventions, educational interventions, and behavioral therapy increased CPAP use by 50, 35, and 90 minutes/night, respectively; however, these studies were generally of low quality.[46]
- *Acute exacerbation of COPD.* The use of noninvasive ventilation to manage patients with acute exacerbation of COPD has been associated with a 36% reduction in mortality, a 35% reduction in hospital-acquired pneumonia, an 18% reduction in hospital length of stay, a 30% reduction in costs, and 78%, 55%, and 29% reductions in mortality in patients with low, moderate, and high comorbidity burdens compared with patients managed with invasive ventilation.[24] Noninvasive ventilation is the established standard of care for acute exacerbations of COPD with concomitant administration of appropriate antibiotics, corticosteroids, and bronchodilators.[36] Predictors of those patients who failed noninvasive ventilation included weak

cough, high severity of illness (APACHE II >19), and malnutrition as indicated by total protein less than 5.8 mg; those with one, two, or three of these risk factors increased their risk of failure by 4.7, 13.6, and 21.6 times, respectively.[14]
- *Acute cardiogenic pulmonary edema.* CPAP was demonstrated to reduce the need for intubation by 56% and mortality by 36% in patients with acute cardiogenic pulmonary edema, particularly those with edema subsequent to myocardial ischemia or infarction. Bilevel noninvasive ventilation reduced the risk for intubation by 46% but had no effect on mortality in a meta-analysis.[44] The use of noninvasive ventilation in this patient population before arrival in the emergency department has also been studied, but trials have been small with methodological issues. A systematic review of these trials provided minimal evidence that the need for intubation was reduced, but mortality was unchanged with prehospital initiation of noninvasive ventilation in acute cardiogenic pulmonary edema.[4] In a recent well-designed trial, investigators compared CPAP and bilevel noninvasive ventilation in patients with cardiogenic pulmonary edema; bilevel ventilation use was associated with more rapid improvement in oxygenation, reduction in dyspnea, and a significantly lower need for intensive care admission compared with CPAP.[23] There were no differences in need for intubation, mortality, or acute myocardial infarction between these two strategies.
- *Asthma.* There is theoretical support for the use of noninvasive positive pressure ventilation in the management of acute asthma; however, there currently are few data to support its use. Small trials have described improvements in dyspnea, respiratory rate, and airflow, which were attributed to the use of positive airway pressure and improved dispersal of inhaled bronchodilators.[33]
- *Pneumonia.* The use of noninvasive ventilation in the management of community-acquired pneumonia was associated with significantly shorter length of ventilation, shorter length of intensive care stay, fewer hospital days, and lower mortality compared with intubated patients in a large trial of more than 500 patients.[27] In a large cohort of elderly, immunocompromised patients with pneumonia, noninvasive ventilation was associated with a 34% reduction in mortality.[18] However, in a recent trial the failure rate for noninvasive ventilation was 76%; mortality was not different from patients ventilated invasively.[30] Thus there are equivocal data to support the effective use of noninvasive ventilation for community-acquired pneumonia.
- *Postextubation respiratory failure.* The use of noninvasive positive pressure ventilation after planned tracheal extubation reduced reintubation rate by 35%, ICU mortality by 59%, and hospital mortality by 41%.[21] However, when respiratory failure after tracheal extubation was established, there was no improvement in outcomes, and some evidence suggested that mortality was increased because of delayed reintubation.[13] The efficacy of noninvasive ventilation after extubation is dependent on patient risk for failure and the reason for invasive ventilation, the timing of application, patient motivation, and the skill and experience of clinicians.[15] Those patients at high risk of

extubation failure, postoperative patients, immediate application of noninvasive ventilation after extubation, and an experienced and skilled cohort of clinicians may reduce morbidity and mortality, particularly in carefully selected postoperative patients.[2]

- *Thoracic trauma.* There is evidence to support the effective use of noninvasive ventilation in the thoracic trauma population. Pooled data from 10 studies demonstrated a 74% reduced risk of mortality; as well as a 68% reduced risk for intubation, a reduction of intensive care stay by nearly 2.5 days, improved oxygenation, and reduced respiratory rate.[11] However, the optimal type of noninvasive ventilation has not been determined.

- *Palliative care and neuromuscular disorders.* The use of noninvasive ventilation with neuromuscular disorders such as Duchenne muscular dystrophy and amyotrophic lateral sclerosis increased minute ventilation, reduced respiratory rate, reduced hypoxemia time, decreased energy expenditure, and prolonged survival.[29,42] There was also a demonstrated reduction in dyspnea and need for morphine, with subsequent improvement in quality of life for end-stage patients with COPD, cancer, and neuromuscular disorders.[16,31] Thus noninvasive ventilation may be a useful strategy for symptom palliation at end of life.

Contraindications for Use of Noninvasive Positive Pressure Ventilation

Absolute Contraindications
- Respiratory arrest, apnea
- Uncontrolled vomiting
- Absence of upper-airway reflexes
- Pneumothorax (untreated)
- Acute, copious upper-gastrointestinal bleeding
- Recent gastric, laryngeal, or esophageal surgery
- Facial and/or airway trauma
- Total airway obstruction

Relative Contraindications
- Medically unstable—hypotension, cardiac dysrhythmias, need for vasopressors
- Agitated or uncooperative
- Excessive secretions
- Impaired swallow reflex
- Cardiac ischemia
- Cardiac dysrhythmias

Noninvasive Positive Pressure Ventilation Interfaces

An interface is the device that connects the positive pressure source (ventilator) to the patient airway. Interfaces can be categorized as nasal, face, or helmet (Fig. 30-1).[17,26]

- *Nasal interfaces* are the most commonly used in patients with chronic conditions such as OSA.[26] Nasal interfaces include nasal pillows and nasal masks. Nasal interfaces permit speech and feeding; unfortunately, these interfaces are also associated with greater resistance to gas flow and the potential for considerable leak of gas from the mouth.[45] Thus nasal interfaces are of minimal use during critical illness.

- *Facial interfaces* are the most common in critical care clinical practice and include oronasal masks, face masks, and full face masks.[26] These interfaces vary in size and the area of the face covered and are particularly useful for patients who are mouth breathers. An oronasal and traditional face mask covers the mouth and nose, whereas a total face mask covers the mouth, nose, and eyes. These interfaces are associated with nasal congestion, skin breakdown, nasal and mouth dryness, and claustrophobia and are less useful in patients who are vomiting.[26] Total face masks may be better tolerated and induce fewer adverse effects, but their superiority for outcomes such as mortality has not been demonstrated.[22]

- The *helmet interface* is the least frequently used; this interface covers the entire head and part of the neck. The helmet allows maximal interaction with the surrounding environment and is not associated with skin breakdown; however, it cannot be used with traditional ventilator as a high gas flow is required to prevent rebreathing, and the associated noise with a helmet use may reduce tolerance.[32,41]

Modes of Noninvasive Positive Pressure Ventilation

- *CPAP* does not provide inspiratory support but maintains positive airway pressure at end-expiration. Thus collapsed alveoli are recruited, functional residual capacity is increased, ventilation perfusion match is improved, lung compliance is optimized, and the work of breathing is lessened.[26]

- *Noninvasive bilevel positive pressure* provides two levels of pressure, an inspiratory positive airway pressure (IPAP), which may also be referred to as pressure support, and an expiratory positive airway pressure (EPAP). The use of regular intensive-care ventilators permits the addition of intermittent mandatory ventilation.[48] Bilevel ventilation is commonly used in acute-care patients.[26]

- *Other modes of noninvasive ventilation* include assist-control, where a preset rate is used; proportional assist, where the degree of inspiratory support is determined by the patient effort; neurally adjusted, where ventilatory support is triggered by electrical activity in the diaphragm;[5,35,38] and adaptive pressure control or volume-assured pressure support, where the ventilator titrates the degree of pressure based on inspiratory effort and tidal volume.[26] These modes are typically used in complex patient situations, and none have been demonstrated to be superior.

EQUIPMENT

- Noninvasive interface (see Fig. 30-1)
- CPAP or BiPAP ventilator
- Electrocardiographic monitor
- Pulse oximeter—stand alone or monitor module
- Self-inflating manual resuscitation bag-valve-mask device
- Oxygen source and tubing
- Suction equipment
- Intubation equipment and endotracheal tubes
- Equipment for needle thoracostomy or tube thoracostomy

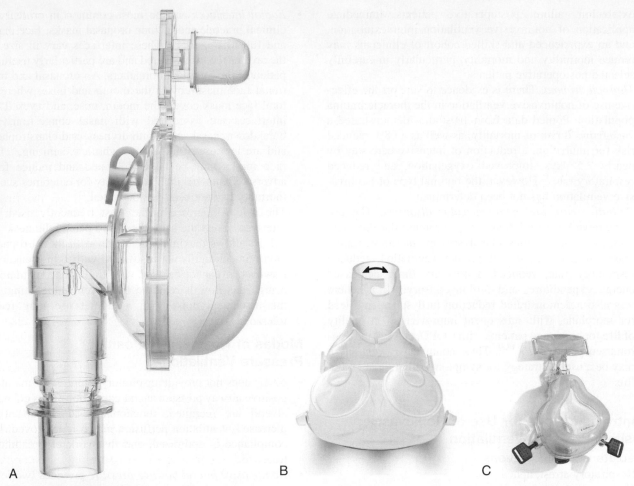

Figure 30-1 Noninvasive patient interfaces. **A,** Nasal mask. **B,** Nasal pillow. **C,** Full face mask. *(Images used with permission of Philips Respironics, Inc, Murrysville, PA.)*

- Personal protective equipment (gloves, mask, goggles, gown, as appropriate)
- Humidification equipment as required

Additional equipment (to have available depending on patient need) includes the following:

- Medications, as indicated

PATIENT AND FAMILY EDUCATION

- If time permits, assess patient and family level of understanding about the condition and rationale for the procedure. *Rationale:* This assessment identifies knowledge deficits about the patient's condition, the procedure, the expected benefits, and the potential risks. The nurse should provide sufficient time for questions to clarify information and for patient and family to voice concerns. Explanations decrease patient anxiety and enhance cooperation.
- Explain the procedure and the reason for the procedure before and during the institution of noninvasive ventilation. Reinforce the information as required by the patient's condition. *Rationale:* This explanation enhances patient and family understanding, decreases anxiety, and increases cooperation.
- Provide details about the potential sensations associated with noninvasive ventilation (dyspnea, claustrophobia, lung inflation, noise, alarms). *Rationale:* Clear, complete

explanations will reduce anxiety, fear, and distress and may improve patient tolerance.

- Promote relaxation in the patient. Techniques such as distraction may be useful. *Rationale:* Relaxation and cooperation promote optimal delivery of positive pressure gas flow, improve ventilation and oxygenation, and reduce the work of breathing.
- Establish a method of communication in conjunction with patient and family before initiation of ventilation. Explain that the patient will be able to speak, but this should be minimized to optimize the therapy. *Rationale:* The ability to communicate needs, symptoms, and feelings is vital to effective patient care and will reduce anxiety and fear.
- Instruct the patient and family about how to use the call system to obtain assistance and how to perform selected activities to improve patient comfort. This includes how to remove the mask if nausea and vomiting occur. *Rationale:* This supports autonomy of patient and family; includes family in caregiving, which is an identified need; and reduces anxiety of patient and family members. Air insufflation may produce gastric distension, nausea, and vomiting with potential for pulmonary aspiration.
- Explain that the patient will not be permitted oral intake during noninvasive ventilation. *Rationale:* Reduces the risk for pulmonary aspiration.

- Offer information about the goals of noninvasive ventilation for the patient and frequent reports about progress. *Rationale:* Information about care, goals, and probable outcome is a stated need of patients and family members.
- Provide the opportunity for questions during noninvasive ventilation. *Rationale:* Family members state that the ability to ask questions and receive honest understandable answers is their most important need.

PATIENT ASSESSMENT AND PREPARATION

Patient Assessment

- Evaluate for the signs and symptoms of respiratory muscle fatigue and impending acute ventilatory failure. These include rising arterial partial pressure of carbon dioxide ($PaCO_2$) and end-tidal CO_2, chest wall-abdominal dyssynchrony, shallow or irregular respirations, tachypnea, bradypnea, dyspnea, reduced level of consciousness, confusion, lethargy, restlessness, change in arterial blood pressure (increase or decrease), tachycardia, and cardiac dysrhythmias. *Rationale:* Early detection of inadequate ventilation permits the clinician to intervene and improve ventilation with the noninvasive method or rapidly institute intubation and invasive mechanical ventilation.
- Evaluate patient for signs and symptoms of inadequate oxygenation. These include decreased oxygen saturation by pulse oximetry (SpO_2), PaO_2 ≤60 mm Hg, tachypnea, dyspnea, central cyanosis, restlessness, confusion, decreased level of consciousness, agitation, tachycardia, bradycardia, cardiac dysrhythmias, intercostal and suprasternal retractions, alteration in arterial blood pressure (increased or decreased), adventitious breath sounds, reduced urine output, and acidosis. *Rationale:* Early detection of hypoxemia permits the clinician to intervene and institute additional supports to maintain adequate tissue oxygenation.
- Evaluate ventilation with measurement of $PaCO_2$ and pH. Hypercarbia and respiratory acidosis indicate inadequate ventilation. *Rationale:* $PaCO_2$ is the best indicator of adequacy of ventilation. Early detection of inadequate ventilation permits the clinician to intervene and improve ventilation with the noninvasive method or rapidly institute intubation and invasive mechanical ventilation.

Patient Preparation

- Verify that the patient is the correct patient by two independent clinicians. *Rationale:* Ensures correct identification of the appropriate patient for the procedure.
- Evaluate patient understanding of the information provided. Answer questions and reinforce information as needed. *Rationale:* Determines patient understanding, reinforces information, and reduces anxiety of patient and family.
- Premedicate the patient as needed. *Rationale:* Cautious use of low-dose narcotics, sedatives, or anxiolytics may be required to improve patient tolerance, reduce anxiety, and promote optimal ventilation. Medication should not reduce level of consciousness or central ventilatory drive.

Procedure	**for Noninvasive Ventilation (CPAP and Bilevel Ventilation)**	
Steps	**Rationale**	**Special Considerations**
1. **HH**		
2. **PE**		
3. Assemble and prepare equipment.	Readies equipment for the procedure.	
4. Select noninvasive interface for use with noninvasive ventilation (see Fig. 30-1).[20,21,41,45] **(Level C*)**	Interface device fit is essential to efficacy. The interface should be carefully selected with attention to patient preference, face and nose size, facial deformities, skin integrity, presence of nasal or oral gastric tubes, and availability.	Not all interfaces may be available. The presence of a nasal or oral gastric tube does not preclude noninvasive ventilation. Most of the ventilators have leak compensation built into the system. However, a large leak may make patient-initiated cycling more difficult. Obtunded patients and patients with excessive secretions are not good choices.[26] **(Level E*)** Helmet and full face mask ventilation should be used cautiously. The patient should be able to remove the interface quickly if nausea and vomiting are imminent; otherwise the potential for aspiration is high.

*Level C: Qualitative studies, descriptive or correlational studies, integrative reviews, systematic reviews, or randomized controlled trials with inconsistent results.
*Level E: Multiple case reports, theory-based evidence from expert opinions, or peer-reviewed professional organizational standards without clinical studies to support recommendations.

Procedure continues on following page

References and Additional Readings

For a complete list of references and additional readings for this procedure, scan this QR code with any freely available smartphone code reader app, or visit http://booksite.elsevier.com/9780323376624.

31 Manual Self-Inflating Resuscitation Bag-Valve Device

Thomas Levins

PURPOSE: The use of a manual self-inflating resuscitation bag, otherwise known as "bagging," is an essential skill for all levels of providers. It is also one of the most difficult to perform. It is used to provide ventilation when spontaneous respirations are inadequate or absent.

PREREQUISITE NURSING KNOWLEDGE

- Bagging is an essential skill utilized in many emergency situations:
  - ❖ Cardiac arrest
  - ❖ General anesthesia/neuromuscular blockade
  - ❖ Altered level of consciousness
  - ❖ To assess the patency of airway devices such as an endotracheal tube
  - ❖ To assist patients in respiratory distress
  - ❖ To provide oxygenation and ventilation before and after airway suctioning
  - ❖ To provide oxygenation and ventilation during patient transport
  - ❖ To evaluate the interaction of the patient and ventilator
- Bagging should result in chest movement and auscultatory evidence of bilateral air entry.
- In patients without an artificial airway in place, effective bagging requires an unobstructed airway, slight head and neck extension (i.e., the same technique used for mouth-to-mouth ventilation), and firm placement of the face mask over the nose and mouth (Fig. 31-1). An exception to this technique is with known or suspected cervical spine injury, in which the patient's airway is opened with the jaw thrust (without neck hyperextension). Effective bagging is best accomplished with two people: one to secure the mask and ensure head and neck placement and one to bag.[1] In patients with artificial airways, such as endotracheal or nasotracheal tubes or tracheostomies, the nurse must understand the components of artificial airways and their relationship to the upper-airway anatomy.
- When signs and symptoms of respiratory distress are noted in a patient on mechanical ventilation and troubleshooting the ventilator does not immediately resolve the issue, the patient should be bagged on 100% oxygen.
- Monitor the rate and depth of bagged breaths.
  - ❖ Large bagged breaths or rapid rates during bagging may result in dynamic hyperinflation and resultant hypotension.[2]
  - ❖ Dynamic hyperinflation may also occur in ventilated patients who "breath stack," which is initiating an additional ventilator breath *before* completion of the preceding ventilator-delivered breath. Hyperinflation occurs when exhalation time is inadequate, which results in auto–positive end-expiratory pressure (PEEP).
  - ❖ Dynamic hyperinflation is most commonly associated with bronchospasm and chronic obstructive pulmonary disease.[2] A high index of suspicion is necessary for the presence of dynamic hyperinflation if hemodynamic instability or worsening respiratory distress occurs with bagging.
  - ❖ Auto-PEEP increases intrathoracic pressures and may decrease venous return, which may result in hypotension. It may also result in significant barotrauma and the possibility of pneumothorax or tension pneumothorax. A rapid solution to auto-PEEP with hemodynamic or respiratory compromise is a brief disconnection from the bag to allow passive deflation and a decrease in intrathoracic pressures. This should result in improved hemodynamics. With resumption of bagging, providing a longer exhalation time (smaller tidal volumes with a lower respiratory rate) will help to minimize auto-PEEP.

EQUIPMENT

- Manual self-inflating resuscitation bag and mask of appropriate size (Fig. 31-2)
- Appropriately sized airway adjuncts in the nonintubated patient
  - ❖ Oral pharyngeal airway
  - ❖ Nasopharyngeal airway
- Oxygen source and regulator
- Large-bore suction
- McGill forceps of various sizes
- Personal protective equipment
  - ❖ Eye protection
  - ❖ Face mask/shield
  - ❖ Gloves
  - ❖ Gown

Additional equipment, to have available as needed, includes the following:
- PEEP valve, if required

PATIENT AND FAMILY EDUCATION

- If time permits, assess the patient's and family's level of understanding about the condition and rationale for the procedure. ***Rationale:*** This assessment identifies the patient's and family's knowledge deficits concerning the patient's condition, the procedure, the expected benefits, and the potential risks. It also allows time for questions to clarify information and voice concerns. Explanations decrease patient anxiety and enhance cooperation.
- Explain the procedure and the reason for the procedure, if the clinical situation permits. If not, explain the procedure and reason for the intubation after it is completed. ***Rationale:*** This explanation enhances patient and family understanding and decreases anxiety.
- If the patient is currently on a ventilator, inform the patient if possible and the family if present that the patient will be disconnected from the ventilator and bagging will be performed. Describe the reason (e.g., ventilator malfunction, suctioning, patient comfort, the need for patient transport) for bagging. Explain that if the patient is in respiratory distress, bagging must be done immediately. ***Rationale:*** Information about the patient's therapy is an important need of the patient and family members. Dyspnea is uncomfortable and frightening. It leads to anxiety, fear, and distrust. Failure to diagnose promptly and alleviate the cause of respiratory distress puts the patient at risk for further decompensation.
- Discuss the sensory experience associated with bagging. ***Rationale:*** Knowledge of anticipated sensory experiences decreases anxiety and distress.
- Instruct the patient to communicate discomfort with breathing during bagging, if possible. ***Rationale:*** The bagging technique can be altered to produce a more comfortable breathing pattern by working with the patient's spontaneous respiratory efforts.
- Offer the opportunity for the patient if possible and the family to ask questions about bagging. ***Rationale:*** The ability to ask questions and have questions answered honestly is cited consistently as the most important need of patients and families.

PATIENT ASSESSMENT AND PREPARATION

Patient Assessment

- Verify that the patient is the correct patient using two identifiers if possible. ***Rationale:*** Before performing a procedure, the nurse should ensure the correct identification of the patient for the intended intervention, though completing this in patients in severe distress should *not* delay intervention.
- Assess for signs of respiratory distress, including mental status changes; respiratory rate, rhythm, and quality; breath sounds; heart rhythm and rate; hypoxemia or hypoxia; hypertension or hypotension; or diaphoresis. ***Rationale:*** Any acute change in patient status may indicate that bagging is necessary.
- If present, assess for sudden increase or decrease in end-tidal carbon dioxide ($Etco_2$) readings. ***Rationale:*** Any acute change in patient status may indicate that bagging is necessary.
- Assess the patency of the patient's airway. ***Rationale:*** Establishes if there are any obstructions of the patient's airway and the patency of the patient's ability to maintain an open airway. Suction as necessary with a large-bore suction device or utilize McGill forceps to remove larger foreign bodies. If *no* protective airway reflexes are present, consider inserting an oropharyngeal airway or nasopharyngeal airway.

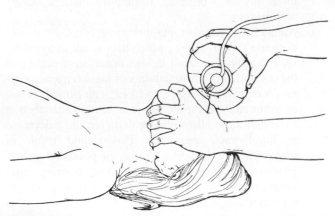

Figure 31-1 Proper technique of ventilation with manual self-inflating resuscitation bag-valve device and face mask. *(From Wilkins RL, Stoller JK, Kacmarek RM: Egan's fundamentals of respiratory care, ed 8, St Louis, 2008, Mosby.)*

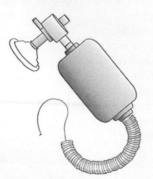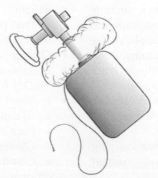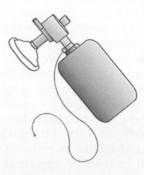

Bag-valve assembly with rear bag reservoir   Bag-valve assembly with collar reservoir   Bag-valve assembly without reservoir

Figure 31-2 Manual self-inflating bags: bag-valve assembly with and without reservoir.

- Use ventilator alarms if patient is receiving mechanical ventilation, including low- or high-pressure or apnea alarms. *Rationale:* Any acute change in patient status may indicate that bagging is necessary. Rapid response with 100% fraction of inspired oxygen (Fio_2) protects the patient and allows for rapid evaluation of airway resistance, placement, and function of the artificial airway if one is in place.
- If present, ensure proper placement and function of any artificial airway. *Rationale:* The positioning and patency of the airway must be ensured.

Patient Preparation

- Ensure that the patient understands preprocedural teachings if possible. Answer questions as they arise and reinforce information as needed. *Rationale:* This communication evaluates and reinforces understanding of previously taught information.

Procedure   for Manual Self-Inflating Resuscitation Bag

Steps	Rationale	Special Considerations
Using the Manual Self-Inflating Bag Device without an Advanced Airway		
1. HH		
2. PE		
3. Attach the bag to an oxygen source and open the oxygen source to a minimum of 15 L/min.	A minimum amount of oxygen is required to provide a high Fio_2, usually >15 L/min flow.	If a reservoir bag is present, it must be fully inflated to provide a high concentration of oxygen.
4. If the patient is spontaneously breathing, place mask over the patient's face and attempt to assist spontaneous respirations	Working with the patient's spontaneous respirations will minimize patient discomfort.	Use thumb and index fingers to provide downward pressure on mask while using the 3rd, 4th, and 5th fingers to lift mandible toward mask (see Fig. 31-1). Avoid placing the 3rd, 4th, and 5th fingers beneath the mandible on the soft tissue because this may worsen airway obstruction. Fingers/pressure should be placed on the mandible itself.
5. If the patient is *not* breathing spontaneously, open the airway using either the head tilt/chin lift or jaw thrust maneuvers.	Opening the airway allows the patient either to attempt self-ventilation or to be bagged.	Jaw thrust if cervical spine trauma is suspected. If the patient is unable to maintain his or her own airway, consider inserting an oropharyngeal airway or nasopharyngeal airway.
6. After obtaining an adequate seal with mask, slowly compress the bag over 1 second, at approximately 10–12 breaths/min (1 breath every 5–6 seconds).[3]	Compressing the bag too fast may result in gastric insufflation, emesis, and the possibility of breath stacking (dynamic hyperinflation).	If adequate mask seal cannot be obtained and ventilations are inadequate with a single provider, utilize a two-person technique with one provider maintaining a mask seal while the other ventilates the patient by compressing the bag-valve mask.[4]
		Obtaining an adequate mask seal with a single provider is frequently difficult. If bagging the patient is difficult, look for causes of high airway resistance (e.g., obstructed airway) or low lung compliance (e.g., bronchospasm, mucus plugging, pulmonary edema, pneumonia, acute lung injury, or pneumothorax).

Procedure continues on following page

Procedure	**for Manual Self-Inflating Resuscitation Bag—*Continued***	
Steps	**Rationale**	**Special Considerations**
7. Assess chest rise and fall and bilateral breath sounds with each bag compression. Is the chest rising? Do you still have an adequate seal with the mask?	Confirm the effectiveness of the bagging.	If ventilations are not effective, be prepared to intervene by assessing the mask size and seal and/or adjusting hand placement to obtain a better seal. Call for assistance and prepare for intubation or other rescue airway-device placement.
8. When assistance arrives, discard used supplies and **PE**.		
9. **HH**		

Using the Manual Self-Inflating Bag-Valve Device in a Patient with an Advanced Airway (i.e., Endotracheal Tube, Tracheostomy, Laryngeal Mask Airway, or King Airway)

Steps	Rationale	Special Considerations
1. **HH**		
2. **PE**		
3. Attach the bag to an oxygen source and open the oxygen source to a minimum of 15 L/min.	A minimum amount of oxygen is required to provide a high Fio_2, usually >15 L/min flow.	Attach a PEEP valve, if the patient is on a ventilator with a PEEP of 5 cm H_2O or more, and adjust the bag's PEEP level to that of the ventilator settings.
4. Silence the ventilator alarms.	Eliminates the ventilator alarms when the circuit is disconnected.	
5. Disconnect patient from the ventilator.	Allows for attachment of the bag-valve device.	
6. Connect bag to artificial airway.	Allows for manual ventilation.	
7. Slowly compress the bag over 1 second, at approximately 10–12 breaths/min (1 breath every 5–6 seconds).[3]	Compressing the bag too fast may result in breath stacking (dynamic hyperinflation).	If bagging the patient is difficult, look for causes of high airway resistance (e.g., obstructed airway, misplaced artificial airway) or low lung compliance (e.g., bronchospasm, mucus plugging, pulmonary edema, pneumonia, acute lung injury, or pneumothorax).
8. Observe patient's breathing pattern and rate and attempt to synchronize manual breaths with the patient's spontaneous effort. **(Level C*)**	Helps patient gain control over breathing by ensuring ventilation and adequate oxygenation.[1]	A higher manual rate may be required initially because larger breaths are more difficult to provide with manual ventilation compared with breaths provided by the ventilator.
9. If the patient is awake and alert, encourage the patient to relax and breathe with the manual breaths that are provided.	Provides synchrony between patient breaths and manual breaths.	
10. Gradually adjust the rate of manual breaths to a rate that meets the patient's demand.	Reestablishes synchrony.	A return to higher ventilator support settings may be necessary after bagging.
11. Ascertain whether the patient is comfortable with the manual breaths.	Promotes comfort.	
12. Assess the ease or difficulty with which the bag is compressed.	Difficulty in bag compression may identify presence of a pneumothorax or pulmonary emboli.	
13. If signs and symptoms of distress are resolved, reconnect the patient to the ventilator.	Indicates that respiratory distress is relieved.	Reassess the patient once placed back on ventilator.

*Level C: Qualitative studies, descriptive or correlational studies, integrative reviews, systematic reviews, or randomized controlled trials with inconsistent results.

Procedure for Manual Self-Inflating Resuscitation Bag—*Continued*

Steps	Rationale	Special Considerations

14. If the patient's distress is not eliminated with bagging, consider the following steps:
  A. Hyperoxygenate and suction.
  B. Assess for the presence of bilateral breath sounds and symmetrical chest expansion.
  C. Assess the ease (or difficulty) with which the bag can be compressed.
  D. Assess anxiety and discomfort as potential causes of dyspnea.
	Indicates respiratory distress cannot be relieved with bagging. Further assessment is needed.
	Suctioning provides information related to the presence of secretions or airway obstruction.
	By auscultating the lungs during bagging, essential information related to tube placement (e.g., migration to right mainstem or displaced) or patient status (e.g., bronchospasm, pulmonary edema) may be obtained. Asymmetrical chest expansion may be the result of a displaced artificial airway, pneumothorax, or obstruction.
	A change in ease of bag compression provides gross data about increasing (improved) or decreasing (deteriorating) lung compliance.
	Although psychological reasons for respiratory distress are possible, rule out physiological causes first.
		In some situations, such as pulmonary embolus, no distinct physical assessment findings may be immediately evident.
		Support the patient until appropriate interventions are accomplished.
		The use of anxiolytics or analgesics or both may be appropriate to decrease anxiety and pain. However, a thorough evaluation of the cause of distress must be undertaken both before and after administration.

15. Return patient to ventilator when respiratory distress is relieved.	Returns the patient to his or her baseline.	
16. Reactivate and check ventilator alarms and settings.	Safety precautions. Ensures the nurse is alerted to actual or potential life-threatening problems.	
17. Observe breathing pattern, patient ventilator synchrony, peak inspiratory pressure (volume ventilation), and tidal volume and respiratory frequency (patient initiated).		
18. Check that call system is within patient's reach, if appropriate.		
19. Discard used supplies and remove **PE**.		
20. **HH**		

Maintenance Ventilation, with an Advanced Airway, during Patient Transport

Portable ventilators are highly recommended for use during transport instead of manual bagging. If a transport ventilator is not available, bagging may be required. Procedures may vary depending on institutional standards.

1. **HH**		
2. **PE**		
3. Obtain an appropriate-sized bag and mask.	Ensures that appropriate equipment is available during the transport.	An appropriately sized mask must accompany the patient in the event of inadvertent removal of the invasive airway.

Procedure continues on following page

Procedure   for Manual Self-Inflating Resuscitation Bag—*Continued*

Steps	Rationale	Special Considerations
4. Attach the bag to an oxygen source and open the oxygen source to a minimum of 15 L/min.	A minimum amount of oxygen is required to provide a high Fio_2, usually >15 L/min flow.	Attach a PEEP valve if the patient is on a ventilator with a PEEP of 5 cm H_2O or more and adjust the bag's PEEP level to that of the ventilator settings.
5. Confirm airway placement and the patient's tolerance to ventilator and settings.	Establishes patency of the airway and ventilator's settings.	
6. Silence the ventilator alarms.	Eliminates the ventilator alarm when the circuit is disconnected.	
7. Disconnect patient from ventilator.	Allows for attachment of the spirometer and bag-valve device.	
8. Connect the bag-valve device and bag patient with Fio_2 of 1.0, at an approximate rate depth and pattern as ventilator breaths.	Maintains ventilation pattern similar to that being provided by the ventilator.	1.0 Fio_2 is typically used during patient transports. Adjust liter flow of oxygen to maintain the patient's arterial blood oxygen saturation (Sao_2) at the desired level. If bagging the patient is difficult, look for causes of high airway resistance (e.g., obstructed airway, misplaced artificial airway) or low lung compliance (e.g., bronchospasm, mucus plugging, pulmonary edema, pneumonia, acute lung injury, or pneumothorax).
9. Attach continuous $Etco_2$ monitor.	$Etco_2$ monitoring continuously monitors airway placement and the adequacy of ventilations.	$Etco_2$ monitoring is a vital part of monitoring during patient transport to ensure continued airway patency and adequate ventilations.[5] **(Level E*)**
10. Frequently reassess the patient to ensure that the patient is comfortable with the bagging technique.	Promotes patient comfort.	Frequent reassessment is vital to patient comfort and safety. Adjustments may be needed to maintain patient comfort with manual ventilation.
11. Reattach the patient's advanced airway to the ventilator when the transport is completed.	Reestablishes mechanical ventilation.	
12. Discard used supplies and remove **PE**.		
13. **HH**		

*Level E: Multiple case reports, theory-based evidence from expert opinions, or peer-reviewed professional organizational standards without clinical studies to support recommendations.

Expected Outcomes

- Maintenance of adequate oxygenation and ventilation
- Resolution of respiratory distress if present

Unexpected Outcomes

- Hemodynamic instability from dynamic hyperinflation
- Pulmonary barotrauma (e.g., pneumothorax)
- Inability to restore adequate ventilation and oxygenation with bagging
- Inadvertent extubation during bagging
- Equipment failure and inability to bag

Patient Monitoring and Care

Steps	Rationale	Reportable Conditions
		These conditions should be reported if they persist despite nursing interventions.
1. Evaluate trends or sudden changes in lung compliance, airway resistance, or the patient's condition.	Impairment of the patient's lung function or airway may be identified by changes in the patient's condition or the ability to bag the patient.	• Difficulty bagging (stiff) • No observable chest wall movement • Agitation • Diaphoresis • Hyper- or hypotension • Tachy- or bradycardia
2. Observe for signs and symptoms of synchrony with the bagging, including adequate chest rise and fall.	Proper technique results in a comfortable synchronous breathing pattern.	• Dyssynchronous breathing
3. Monitor SpO_2 and $EtcO_2$ values and trends.	SpO_2 and $EtcO_2$ provide information regarding the adequacy of oxygenation and ventilation.	• Decrease in SpO_2 >10% • Increase in $EtcO_2$ >10%

Documentation

Documentation should include the following:
- Patient and family education
- Reason for bagging (e.g., to transport, suction, etc.)
- Frequency
- Patient's response to the procedure
- Unexpected outcomes
- Nursing interventions

References and Additional Readings

For a complete list of references and additional readings for this procedure, scan this QR code with any freely available smartphone code reader app, or visit http://booksite.elsevier.com/9780323376624.

32 Peripheral Nerve Stimulators

Nathan W. Howard

PURPOSE: Peripheral nerve stimulators (PNSs) are used in association with the administration of neuromuscular-blocking medication agents to assess nerve-impulse transmission at the neuromuscular junction of select skeletal muscles.

PREREQUISITE NURSING KNOWLEDGE

- PNSs are used in association with the administration of neuromuscular-blocking drugs (NMBDs) to block skeletal muscle activity.
- NMBDs are given in the intensive care unit, along with sedatives and opioids, most commonly to coordinate contemporary modes of mechanical ventilation with breathing in patients with severe lung injury. Neuromuscular-blocking agents are also used to assist with the management of increased intracranial pressure after a head injury; for severe muscle spasms associated with seizures, tetanus, and drug overdose; to reduce intraabdominal hypertension[1]; in hypothermia protocols for cardiac arrest[6]; and for preservation of delicate reconstructive surgery.
- NMBDs do not affect sensation or level of consciousness. Because NMBDs lack amnesic, sedative, and analgesic properties, sedatives and analgesics should *always* be given concurrently to minimize the patient's awareness of blocked muscle activity and discomfort. Sedatives and analgesics should be initiated *before* NMBDs because neuromuscular blockade hinders the assessment of anxiety and pain.[5]
- Numerous medications, such as aminoglycosides and other antibiotics, beta blockers, calcium channel blockers, corticosteroids, and anesthetics, and conditions, such as acidosis and various electrolyte imbalances, potentiate the effects of neuromuscular-blocking agents. Thus the level of blockade is subject to variation, which necessitates vigilant monitoring with a PNS and titration of the NMBD.[6]
- The muscle twitch response to a small electrical stimulus delivered by the PNS corresponds to an estimated number of nerve receptors blocked by the NMBDs and assists the clinician in the assessment and titration of the medication dosage. The level of blockade is estimated by observing the muscle twitch after stimulating the appropriate nerve with a small electrical current delivered by the PNS.
- The train-of-four (TOF) method of stimulation is most commonly used for ongoing monitoring of NMBD use. After delivery of four successive stimulating currents to a select peripheral nerve with the PNS, in the absence of significant neuromuscular blockade, four muscle twitches follow. The four twitches signify that 70% or fewer of the receptors are blocked. Three twitches correspond to approximately 75% blockade, and two to one twitches in response to four stimulating currents correlate with approximately 80% to 90% blockade of the neuromuscular junction receptors.[9] One to two twitches is the recommended level of block, although the appropriate level has not yet been determined through research in the critically ill population.[5] Absence of twitches may indicate that 100% of receptors are blocked, which exceeds the desired level of blockade (Table 32-1).
- The stimulating current is measured in milliamperes (mA). The usual range of milliamperes required to stimulate a peripheral nerve and elicit a muscle twitch is 20 to 50 mA, although increasing the current to 70 or 80 mA may be necessary, especially in the obese patient.[9]
- Some stimulators do not indicate the milliamperes. Instead, digital or dialed numbers ranging from 1 to 10 represent the range of milliamperes from 20 to 80 mA. With use of these instruments, the usual setting is 2 to 5, although a setting of 10 is sometimes necessary. Other stimulators (with and without digital displays) automatically adjust the voltage output relative to resistance and deliver the current accordingly.[10]
- The ulnar nerve in the wrist is recommended for testing, although the facial and the posterior tibial nerves may also be used.
- Peripheral nerve monitoring is used in conjunction with the assessment of clinical goals, and *clinical decisions should never be made solely on the basis of the twitch response.*
- Titration of the drugs according to clinical assessment and muscle twitch response may help provide a sufficient level of blockade without overshooting the goal. Overshooting the level of blockade with use of excessive doses of NMBDs is of special concern in the critically ill patient because it may predispose the patient to prolonged paralysis and muscle weakness, reported in the literature.[6] Monitoring with a PNS during the administration of NMBDs results in the use of less medication, hastens recovery of spontaneous ventilation, and accelerates restoration of neuromuscular transmission (NMT),[2] which is necessary for resumption of muscle activity. Although some patients have severe muscle weakness after neuromuscular blockade, peripheral nerve monitoring during NMBD therapy facilitates prompt recovery of NMT when therapy is terminated.[2]

TABLE 32-1	Train-of-Four (TOF) Stimulation as a Correlation of Blocked Nerve Receptors

TOF (No. of Twitches)	Percent of Receptors Blocked (Approximately)[7]
0/4	100
1/4	90
2/4	80
3/4	75
4/4	<70

Adapted from Figure 4, p. e5, Train-of-four suppression in Wilson J, Collins AS, Rowan BO: Residual neuromuscular blockade in critical care, Crit Care Nurse 32(3):e1–e10, 2012.

EQUIPMENT

- Peripheral nerve stimulator
- Two pregelled electrode pads (the same as is used for electrocardiography monitoring)
- Two lead wires packaged with the peripheral nerve stimulator
- Alcohol pads for skin degreasing and cleansing

Additional equipment, to have available as needed, includes the following:

- A bipolar touch stimulator probe may be substituted for the pregelled electrodes and lead wires
- Scissors or clippers if hair removal is necessary

PATIENT AND FAMILY EDUCATION

- If time permits, assess the patient's and family's level of understanding about the condition and rationale for the procedure. *Rationale:* This assessment identifies the patient's and family's knowledge deficits concerning the patient's condition, the procedure, the expected benefits, and the potential risks. It also allows time for questions to clarify information and voice concerns. Explanations decrease patient anxiety and enhance cooperation.
- Explain the procedure and the reason for the procedure, if the clinical situation permits. If not, explain the procedure and reason for the intubation after it is completed. *Rationale:* This explanation enhances patient and family understanding and decreases anxiety.
- Describe the equipment to be used. *Rationale:* This description may decrease anxiety.
- Reassure the patient and family that medications for sedation and analgesia are provided throughout this therapy so the patient is comfortable while paralyzed. *Rationale:* Reassurance that the patient's pain and anxiety will be treated during therapy is provided.
- Describe the experience of the stimuli as a slight prickly sensation. *Rationale:* The use of sensation descriptors may reduce anxiety.
- Explain that the electrodes require periodic changing, which feels like removing an adhesive-backed bandage. *Rationale:* This explanation may elicit decreased anxiety.

PATIENT ASSESSMENT AND PREPARATION

Patient Assessment

- Verify that the patient is the correct patient using two identifiers. *Rationale:* Before performing a procedure, the nurse should ensure the correct identification of the patient for the intended intervention.
- Assess the patient for the best location for electrode placement. Consider criteria such as edema, fat, hair, diaphoresis, wounds, dressings, and arterial and venous catheters. *Rationale:* This assessment improves conduction of stimulating current through dermal tissue.
- Assess the patient for history or presence of hemiplegia, hemiparesis, or peripheral neuropathy. *Rationale:* Motor response to nerve stimulation of the affected limb may be diminished; receptors may be resistant to NMBDs and lead to excess doses.[9]
- Assess whether burns are present or whether topical ointments are being used. *Rationale:* In patients with burns or topical ointments, for whom electrode adherence is difficult, a bipolar touch probe may be more effective than the electrode pads and lead wires. Poor electrode adherence interferes with the conduction of the stimulating current.

Patient Preparation

- Ensure that the patient and family understand preprocedural teachings. Answer questions as they arise and reinforce information as needed. *Rationale:* Evaluates and reinforces understanding of previously taught information.
- Clip hair at the electrode placement sites if necessary. *Rationale:* This action improves electrode contact, which facilitates current flow to the nerve.
- Cleanse skin and degrease with alcohol. *Rationale:* Cleansing improves electrode contact, which facilitates current flow to the nerve.
- Apply the electrodes and test the TOF response to determine the adequacy of the location before initiating administration of an NMBD. In an emergent situation, testing the TOF response before the administration of an NMBD may not be possible. *Rationale:* Testing improves the reliability of the interpretation of the TOF response.
- Whenever possible, determine the supramaximal stimulation (SMS) level before initiating NMBDs. The SMS is the level at which additional stimulating current elicits no further increase in the intensity of the four twitches. In an emergent situation, determination of the SMS level before the administration of an NMBD may not be possible. *Rationale:* This determination helps establish adequate stimulating current and improves reliability of testing.

Procedures for Peripheral Nerve Stimulators

Steps	Rationale	Special Considerations

Testing the Ulnar Nerve

1. **HH**
2. **PE**
3. Extend the arm, palm up, in a relaxed position; cleanse with alcohol pad (Fig. 32-1).

The ulnar nerve is superficial and easy to locate; degreasing increases conduction.

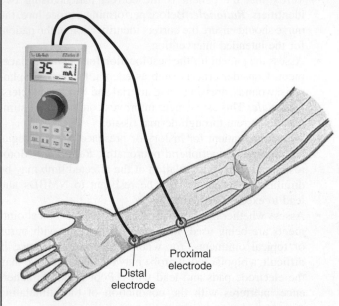

Figure 32-1 Placement of electrodes along the ulnar nerve.

4. Apply two pregelled electrodes over the path of the ulnar nerve (see Fig. 32-1). Place the distal electrode on the skin at the flexor crease on the ulnar surface of the wrist, as close to the nerve as possible. Place the second electrode approximately 1–2 cm proximal to the first, parallel to the flexor carpi ulnaris tendon. **(Level E*)**

Enables stimulation of the ulnar nerve. Skin resistance causes the greatest impediment to current flow, which can be reduced through clean dry skin and secure electrodes. The electrode gel enhances conduction. Maintaining the electrodes as close as possible in alignment with the nerve minimizes artifact from direct muscle stimulation.[9]

Ensure that the patient's wrist is clean and dry.

5. Use caution in selecting the site of the electrode placement to avoid direct stimulation of the muscle rather than the nerve. **(Level E*)**

Direct muscle stimulation elicits a response similar to the TOF, which makes evaluation of blocked nerve-impulse transmission difficult.

In patients with hemiplegia, place the electrodes on the unaffected limb because resistance to NMBDs on the affected side may lead to excess doses.[9] In patients with limbs immobilized from orthopedic casts, use the unaffected limb because possible resistance to some NMBDs on the affected limb may lead to excess doses.[4]

---

*Level E: Multiple case reports, theory-based evidence from expert opinions, or peer-reviewed professional organizational standards without clinical studies to support recommendations.

Procedures | for Peripheral Nerve Stimulators—*Continued*

Steps	Rationale	Special Considerations
6. Plug the lead wires into the nerve stimulator, matching the negative (black) and positive (red) leads to the black and red connection sites.	Necessary for the conduction of electrical current.	
7. Attach the lead wires to the electrodes. Connect the negative (black) lead to the distal electrode over the crease in the palmar aspect of the wrist. Connect the positive (red) lead to the proximal electrode.	Prepares the equipment.	
8. Turn on the PNS and select the current determined by the SMS or, if not performed, a low current (10–20 mA is typical).	Excessive current results in overstimulation and can cause repetitive nerve firing.	Patients with diabetes mellitus may need higher stimulating current than patients without diabetes because of impaired motor nerve fibers and nerve endings.[8]
9. Depress the TOF key; through tactile assessment, determine twitching of the thumb and count the number of twitches. Do not count finger movements, only the thumb.	Finger movements result from direct muscle stimulation. The quality of the twitches may be subtle and decrease in amplitude with increasing edema; detection with tactile methods increases sensitivity and accuracy.	Placing the operator's hand over the fingers helps reduce interpretation of artifactual movement. Use the dominant hand for tactile assessment because it may more accurately detect the TOF response.
10. Maintain a consistent current with each stimulation.	Increases reliability and validity in the quality of the twitch response.	
11. Discard used supplies and remove **PE**.		
12. **HH**		
Testing the Facial Nerve		
1. **HH**		
2. **PE**		
3. Place one electrode on the face at the outer canthus of the eye and the second electrode approximately 2 cm below, parallel with the tragus of the ear (Fig. 32-2).	Stimulates the facial nerve. Maintaining the electrodes as close as possible in alignment with the nerve minimizes artifact from direct muscle stimulation.[9]	Ensure that the patient's face is clean and dry. When wounds, edema, invasive lines, and other factors interfere with ulnar nerve testing, the facial or posterior tibial nerves may be substituted. The risk for direct muscle stimulation is greater, however, with resulting underestimation of blockade. Also, the alternate nerves correlate less well with blockade of the diaphragm.[7] (**Level C***)

*Level C: Qualitative studies, descriptive or correlational studies, integrative reviews, systematic reviews, or randomized controlled trials with inconsistent results.

Procedure continues on following page

Procedures for Peripheral Nerve Stimulators—*Continued*

Steps	Rationale	Special Considerations

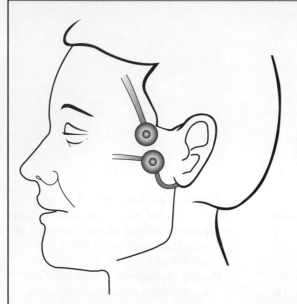

Figure 32-2 Placement of electrodes along the facial nerve.

4. Plug the lead wires into the nerve stimulator, matching the black and red leads to the black and red connection sites.

Necessary for conduction of the electrical current.

5. Attach the lead wires to the electrodes. Connect the negative (black) lead to the distal electrode at the tragus of the ear. Connect the positive (red) lead to the proximal electrode at the outer canthus of the eye.

Prepares the equipment.

6. Turn on the PNS and select the current determined by the SMS or, if not performed, a low current (10–20 mA is typical).

Excessive current results in overstimulation and can cause repetitive nerve firing.

7. Depress the TOF key; through tactile assessment, determine twitching of the muscle above the eyebrow and count the number of twitches.

Determines the neuromuscular blockade at the junction between a branch of the facial nerve and orbicularis muscle.

8. Discard used supplies and remove PE.

9. HH

Testing the Posterior Tibial Nerve

1. HH

2. PE

3. Place one electrode approximately 2 cm posterior to the medial malleolus (Fig. 32-3). **(Level E*)**

Stimulates the posterior tibial nerve. Maintaining the electrodes as close as possible in alignment with the nerve minimizes artifact from direct muscle stimulation.[9]

Ensure that the patient's skin is clean and dry.

---

*Level E: Multiple case reports, theory-based evidence from expert opinions, or peer-reviewed professional organizational standards without clinical studies to support recommendations.

Procedures for Peripheral Nerve Stimulators—*Continued*

Steps	Rationale	Special Considerations

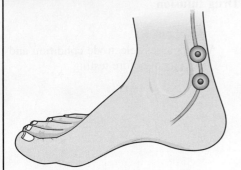

Figure 32-3 Placement of electrodes along the posterior tibial nerve.

4. Place the second electrode approximately 2 cm above the first (see Fig. 32-3).

   Maintaining the electrodes as close as possible in alignment with the nerve minimizes artifact from direct muscle stimulation.[9]

5. Plug the lead wires into the nerve stimulator, matching the black and red leads to the black and red connection sites.

   Necessary for conduction of the electrical current.

6. Attach the lead wires to the electrodes. Connect the negative (black) lead to the distal electrode 2 cm posterior to the medial malleolus. Connect the positive (red) lead to the proximal electrode 2 cm above the medial malleolus.

   Prepares the equipment.

7. Turn on the PNS and select the current determined by the SMS or, if not performed, a low current (10–20 mA is typical).

   Excessive current results in overstimulation and can cause repetitive nerve firing.

8. Depress the TOF key; through tactile assessment of plantar flexion of the great toe, count the number of twitches.

   Determines the neuromuscular blockade at the junction between the posterior tibial nerve and the flexor hallucis brevis muscle.

9. Discard used supplies and remove **PE**.

10. **HH**

Determining the Supramaximal Stimulation

1. **HH**
2. **PE**
3. Beginning at 5 mA, increase the milliamperes in increments of 5 mA until four twitches are observed.

   Uses the lowest level necessary to elicit the twitches.

4. Note the amount of current (in milliamperes) that corresponds to four vigorous twitches. Administer one to two more TOF stimuli to confirm the response. This current level is then used in TOF testing for that site.

   If no increase in intensity of the muscle twitch is found when the milliamperes are increased, the SMS is the level at which four vigorous twitches were observed.

   For example, if a strong response is observed at 30 mA, raise the current to 35 mA. If no increase is seen in intensity of the twitch, the SMS is 30 mA. If an increase is seen, raise the milliamperes to 40 mA. If an additional increase is seen in twitch intensity, raise it to 45 mA. If the intensity shows no further increase, the SMS is 40 mA.

Procedure continues on following page

Procedures for Peripheral Nerve Stimulators—*Continued*

Steps	Rationale	Special Considerations

Determining the Train-of-Four Response during Neuromuscular-Blocking Drug Infusion

Steps	Rationale	Special Considerations
1. HH		
2. PE		
3. Retest the TOF 10–15 minutes after a bolus dose or when continuous infusion of NMBD is given/initiated/changed.	Evaluates the level of blockade provided.	Always assess electrode condition and placement before testing.
4. If more than one or two twitches occur and neuromuscular blockade is unsatisfactory for clinical goals, increase the infusion rate as prescribed or according to hospital protocol and retest in 10–15 minutes.	Signifies that less than 85–90% of receptors are blocked.	
5. Retest every 4–8 hours after a clinically stable and satisfactory level of blockade is achieved.	Evaluates the level of blockade and avoids underestimation and overestimation of blockade.	
6. Discard supplies and remove PE.		
7. HH		

Troubleshooting with Zero Twitches

Steps	Rationale	Special Considerations
1. HH		
2. PE		
3. Change the electrodes and ensure that the patient's skin is clean and dry. (**Level E***)	Drying of the gel or poor contact from moisture or soiling compromises conduction.[10]	
4. Check the lead connections and the PNS for mechanical failure and change the battery if needed. (**Level E***)	One of the most common causes of PNS malfunction is low battery voltage.[9]	
5. Increase the stimulating current. (**Level E***)	The current may be inadequate to stimulate the nerve, especially for increasingly edematous patients.[9]	
6. Retest another nerve (the other ulnar nerve or facial or posterior tibial nerves).	Avoids overestimating the level of blockade with false zero twitch responses.	
7. If no other explanations are found for a zero response, check the NMBD infusion for the rate, dose, and concentration. Reduce the infusion rate of the NMBD as prescribed or according to hospital protocol. (**Level E**)	Excessive neuromuscular blockade produces absence of a twitch response and, if allowed to persist, may contribute to prolonged paralysis or severe weakness.[6] Peripheral hypothermia causes a decrease in twitch response and may require a decrease in NMBD by 80%.[9]	
8. Discard supplies and remove PE.		
9. HH		

*Level E: Multiple case reports, theory-based evidence from expert opinions, or peer-reviewed professional organizational standards without clinical studies to support recommendations.

Expected Outcomes

- Slight discomfort during the TOF test
- The muscles of the thumb twitch, rather than the fingers, when the ulnar nerve is stimulated
- The twitch response approximates the number of blocked peripheral nerve receptors; for example, four twitches before initiating the NMBD infusion and one to two twitches when a desired level of blockade is achieved
- The NMBD dosage is titrated according to the TOF test and clinical goals
- Resumption of four twitches occurs within 2 hours when the NMBD is discontinued[7]

Unexpected Outcomes

- Moderate to severe discomfort from the TOF test
- Impaired skin integrity when the electrodes are removed
- The fingers twitch when the ulnar nerve is stimulated as a result of artifact; if the thumb does not twitch, this signifies direct muscle rather than ulnar nerve stimulation
- Resumption of four twitches does not occur within 2 hours of discontinuation of NMBD[7]

Patient Monitoring and Care

Steps	Rationale	Reportable Conditions
		These conditions should be reported if they persist despite nursing interventions.
1. Cleanse and thoroughly dry the skin before applying electrodes.	Improves the electrode adherence.	
2. Change the electrodes every 24 hours or whenever they are loose or when the gel becomes dry.	Optimizes conduction of the stimulating current. This action also assists with decreasing the risk for skin breakdown from the adhesive on the electrodes. Use caution when removing the old electrodes so as not to disrupt skin integrity.	• Skin breakdown
3. Select the most accessible site with the smallest degree of edema and hair and with no wounds, catheters, or dressings that impede accurate electrode placement over the selected nerve.	Facilitates ease in testing, electrode adherence, and the conduction of current.	
4. Never use the Single Twitch, Tetany, or Double Burst settings, if available on the PNS. (**Level E***)	These methods are designed for profound neuromuscular blockade and may cause extreme discomfort.[10]	
5. Assess the patient's oxygenation and ventilation, neurological function, and tissue perfusion before increasing the rate of the NMBD infusion.	The patient may have subtle movement of the extremities with an acceptable TOF response. Clinical decisions should never be made solely on the TOF test results.	• Excessive patient movement despite acceptable TOF • Change in vital signs • Decreased oxygenation (e.g., measured via arterial blood gas or pulse oximetry) • Change in neurological function • Cardiac dysrhythmias or change in patient condition
6. Extreme caution must be exercised to prevent the PNS lead wires from contacting an external pacing catheter or pacing lead wires.	Direct electrical current can be conducted from the PNS through the pacing wires to the heart.	

*Level E: Multiple case reports, theory-based evidence from expert opinions, or peer-reviewed professional organizational standards without clinical studies to support recommendations.

Procedure continues on following page

Patient Monitoring and Care —*Continued*

Steps	Rationale	Reportable Conditions
7. Perform the TOF testing every 4–8 hours during NMBD infusion after the patient's condition is clinically stable and a satisfactory level of neuromuscular blockade is achieved, or per institution policy.	Determines an effective dose of NMBD.	• Abnormal TOF results
8. Consider objective methods of sedation monitoring, such as bispectral index monitoring (see Procedure 88) or evoked potentials, during NMBD therapy.[3] **(Level E*)**	Muscle paralysis during therapy with NMBDs hinders sedation assessment with subjective instruments.	
9. Remove the electrodes, lead wires, and PNS from the patient for magnetic resonance imaging or exposure to any magnetic field.	Metal objects are attracted to the magnetic field.	
10. Follow institution standard for assessing pain. Administer analgesia as prescribed.	Identifies need for pain interventions.	• Continued pain despite pain interventions

*Level E: Multiple case reports, theory-based evidence from expert opinions, or peer-reviewed professional organizational standards without clinical studies to support recommendations.

Documentation

Documentation should include the following:
- Patient and family education
- The time, baseline SMS milliamperes, most recent milliamperes, TOF twitch response, and nerve site tested
- The TOF response as $\frac{0}{4}$, $\frac{1}{4}$, $\frac{2}{4}$, $\frac{3}{4}$, or $\frac{4}{4}$
- Dosage of NMBD

- Assessment data (e.g., neurological, pulmonary, cardiovascular)
- Unexpected outcomes
- Troubleshooting attempts
- Additional interventions
- Pain assessment, interventions, and effectiveness

References and Additional Readings

For a complete list of references and additional readings for this procedure, scan this QR code with any freely available smartphone code reader app, or visit http://booksite.elsevier.com/9780323376624.

33 Weaning Mechanical Ventilation

Susan K. Frazier

PURPOSE: Weaning from mechanical ventilation is a process whereby the work of breathing is transferred from the mechanical ventilator to the individual, who is liberated from mechanical support; satisfactory spontaneous ventilation is indicated by optimal oxygenation and carbon dioxide removal for 30 to 120 minutes.

PREREQUISITE NURSING KNOWLEDGE

- Scientists classify successful weaning as adequate oxygenation and carbon dioxide removal for 24 to 48 hours after cessation of mechanical ventilation support, regardless of when extubation occurs.[41,47,48]

- Positive pressure mechanical ventilation use is associated with the need for sedation and the possibility for excess sedation, potential exposure to high airway pressures with subsequent barotrauma, disruption of upper-airway protective mechanisms, and increased risk for lower respiratory infection or ventilator-associated pneumonia.[48]

- To date, none of the predictors of readiness to wean are sufficiently sensitive and specific in all populations; thus the use of mechanical ventilation may continue even when the patient has the ability to ventilate independently.[59] After the requirement for ventilatory support is adequately addressed, ventilator discontinuation should be initiated. However, premature ventilator removal is also linked with potential for airway obstruction, hypoxemia, pulmonary aspiration, respiratory muscle failure, respiratory arrest, and mortality.[48] Thus clinicians seek the ideal point in the clinical course to initiate ventilator discontinuation. The transition from mechanical to spontaneous ventilation, known as weaning, is a process that requires as much as 40% of total ventilator time in adults who require ventilatory support.[6,19]

- Annually in the United States, approximately 300,000 patients require invasive ventilation for more than 4 days; scientists estimate that by 2020, 600,000 individuals annually will require mechanical ventilation.[73,74] These patients may be classified as those who require simple, difficult, or prolonged ventilator weaning.[48,57] Patients who require simple weaning are those who are successful on the initial attempt; difficult weaning requires at least three spontaneous breathing trials and as long as 7 days to achieve a successful transition. Those who require prolonged weaning need more than three spontaneous breathing trials and longer than 7 days to achieve successful independent ventilation.

- Trials of spontaneous ventilation consist of cessation of mechanical ventilation and administration of supplemental humidified oxygen, most often accompanied by varied levels of continuous positive airway pressure (CPAP), pressure support (PS), or automatic tube compensation (ATC), a strategy whereby the degree of pressure needed to overcome the resistance imposed by the endotracheal tube for the measured flow is applied in patients capable of spontaneous ventilation.[22] These supports are intended to reduce work of breathing imposed by the endotracheal tube; however, work of breathing is highly variable due to the nonlinear, flow-dependent nature of the pressure decrease across the airway.[56] PS adequate to overcome the work produced by the endotracheal tube can range from 5 to 22 cm H_2O pressure.[24] ATC uses a continuous measurement of flow to calculate the inspiratory pressure needed to compensate for the flow-dependent work. ATC assumes a constant lumen and normal shaped endotracheal tube; however, Oto and colleagues[56] found that deformations in the tube and secretion buildup in the lumen after 48 hours of placement increased the imposed resistance and reduced the efficacy of ATC. A superior technique for spontaneous breathing trials has not been identified.[44]

- Typically, a majority of patients (55% to 81%) required simple ventilator weaning; difficult weaning was required by 16% to 39% and prolonged weaning by less than 1% to 6%.[26,29] Difficult and prolonged weaning were associated with a greater comorbid burden, higher severity of illness, longer intensive care and hospital stay, and higher mortality.[29] Clinical factors associated with weaning success included normal respiratory rate, optimal cardiovascular function, adequate nutrition, sufficient hemoglobin, electrolyte homeostasis, adequate respiratory muscle strength, psychological and neurological stability, adequate oxygenation, normal bowel function, fluid homeostasis, and normal blood pH.[8,28,30,41]

- The use of weaning protocols directed by registered nurses,[14,61] respiratory therapists,[29,62] or computer-driven protocols[49] has demonstrated significant reductions in ventilator hours,[29,61] intensive care days, and hospital length of stay compared with usual care.[5,14,29,62]

- Well-established evidence-based guidelines support the use of a daily spontaneous breathing trial for 30 to 120 minutes to evaluate individual ability to sustain independent spontaneous ventilation.[25,49] Respiratory pattern, arterial blood gas concentrations for adequacy of ventilation

TABLE 33-1	Weaning Criteria Identified as Potential Predictors by McMaster Review		
Variable	Threshold Values	Criterion Evaluated	Likelihood Ratios*
V_E in L/min	10–15	Respiratory muscle endurance	0.8–2.37
NIF in cm H_2O	−20 to −30	Effort-independent inspiratory respiratory muscle strength	0.23–3.01
Pi_{max} in cm H_2O	−15 to −30	Respiratory muscle function	0.98–3.01
$P0.1/Pi_{max}$	0.30	Respiratory drive and inspiratory muscle strength	2.14–25.3
CROP index	13	Compliance, ventilatory drive, oxygenation, respiratory muscle function	1.05–19.74
Respiratory rate in breaths/min	30–38	Ventilatory drive and pattern	1.00–3.89
Vt in mL	325–408 or 4–6 mL/kg ideal body weight	Respiratory muscle endurance	0.71–3.83
f/Vt	60–105	Ventilatory pattern and drive	0.84–4.67

*A likelihood ratio of <1 indicates a reduced likelihood of successful weaning; a ratio of 0.5 to 2.0 indicates a small, clinically unimportant likelihood; ratios of <0.1 or >10 indicate a high likelihood of failure or success; V_E = minute ventilation; NIF = negative inspiratory force; Pi_{max} = maximal inspiratory pressure; $P0.1/Pi_{max}$ = ratio of inspiratory pressure at 0.1 second and maximal inspiratory pressure; CROP index = index of compliance, respiratory rate, oxygenation, and airway pressures; Vt = tidal volume; f/Vt = rapid shallow breathing index.

From Cook D, Meade M, Guyatt G, et al: Evidence report on criteria for weaning from mechanical ventilation. Rockville, MD: Agency for Health Care Policy and Research, 1999, (classic reference); MacIntyre NR, Cook DJ, Ely EW, et al: Evidence-based guidelines for weaning and discontinuing ventilatory support: A collective task force facilitated by the American College of Chest Physicians, the American Association for Respiratory Care, and the American College of Critical Care Medicine, Chest 120(6 suppl):375S–395S, 2001.

and oxygenation, hemodynamic stability, and patient comfort are used as indicators of tolerance. Failure of the spontaneous breathing trial is identified by tachypnea, a rapid shallow breathing pattern, partial pressure of O_2 in arterial blood (PaO_2) <60 mm Hg with a fraction of inspired oxygen (FiO_2) of 0.40, oxygen saturation values (SpO_2) obtained with pulse oximetry, heart rate and/or blood pressure increase or decrease of >20% of baseline values, increase in work of breathing as indicated by respiratory accessory muscle effort, intercostal retractions, nasal flaring, and/or asynchronous thoracic cavity-abdominal movement, diaphoresis, agitation, and alteration in level of consciousness.[58]

• In 1999 the Agency for Health Care Policy Research funded a comprehensive review of published studies intended to identify predictors of the likelihood of successful ventilator weaning.[13] Sixty six potential predictors were identified; the investigators calculated the odds that each measure would accurately predict successful weaning. Only eight of these measures demonstrated statistically significant predictive ability; however, the likelihood of accurate prediction by these was generally poor and highly variable. These measures included minute ventilation (V_E), negative inspiratory force (NIF), maximal inspiratory pressure (Pi_{max}), and the ratio of pressure at 0.1 second to maximal inspiratory pressure ($P0.1/Pi_{max}$) all measured during mechanical ventilation; measures made during a 1- to 2-minute spontaneous breathing trial included an index score that was comprised of compliance, respiratory rate, oxygenation, pressure (CROP index), respiratory rate, tidal volume (Vt), and the respiratory frequency to tidal volume ratio (f/Vt) or the rapid shallow breathing index. Although these criteria are included in evidence-based guidelines[49] and were evaluated in as many as 24 studies, there have been no consistently robust predictors of weaning success in all patient populations.[48,49] Over the past decade, investigators have failed to identify effective predictors of ventilator weaning success; thus, success predictors are not consistently used in clinical practice (Table 33-1).[32,48]

Other Criteria That May Be Used for Evaluation of Weaning Readiness

• *Vital capacity (VC) or forced vital capacity (FVC)* is the maximal volume exhaled after a maximal inspiration or the volume forcibly exhaled during a forced expiratory volume maneuver. The normal VC is double to triple the tidal volume, or 10 to 15 mL/kg ideal body weight in a normal adult. VC is the sum of the inspiratory and expiratory reserve volumes and the tidal volume. VC and FVC are used as indicators of ventilatory and respiratory muscle reserve, adequacy, and function. These measures may be particularly useful in evaluation of patients with neuromuscular disorders who require mechanical ventilation, but are more often used to determine the need for ventilation in that patient population.[11,36,55,60]

• *B-type natriuretic peptide (BNP)* is a hormone produced and secreted by cardiac myocytes in response to stretching, which occurs with increased preload associated with fluid overload. BNP concentration is an independent predictor of ventilator weaning failure due to cardiac dysfunction.[72] BNP-guided fluid management that consisted of furosemide administration and fluid restriction when BNP concentration was ≥200 pg/mL was associated with an average reduction of 26 hours in time to successful extubation and an increase of nearly 3 ventilator-free days compared with usual care during ventilator weaning.[51]

- *Diaphragm thickening fraction/diaphragm electromyography derived indices* are recently evaluated predictors of ventilator weaning ability.[16,17,21,53] The diaphragm is the primary ventilatory muscle. During ultrasound measurement of diaphragm thickening with spontaneous ventilation, diaphragm thickness was calculated as thickness at end-inspiration minus thickness at end-expiration divided by thickness at end-expiration. A value greater than 36% predicted successful weaning with sensitivity 0.82, specificity 0.88, positive predictive value 0.92, and negative predictive value 0.75.[21] Diaphragm electrical activity has also been evaluated using a neurally adjusted ventilatory assist catheter (NAVA), a nasogastric catheter with multiple electrodes placed in the distal esophagus, that captured real-time electrical activity of the diaphragm.[17] When diaphragm electrically derived values were compared between those patients who were successfully weaned and those who failed weaning, patients who failed had significantly higher derived values compared with the successful patients; these values occurred early in a spontaneous breathing trial and persisted throughout the trial. Investigators have proposed that these derived values provided an evaluation of the balance between ventilatory drive and the sustainability of the demand for ventilation.[53]

- *Heart rate variability (HRV)* is an indicator of the balance between sympathetic and parasympathetic stimulation to the heart; measurement of the interval between successive cardiac electrical stimulations producing contraction is used to calculate measures of HRV. Time domain measures use statistical analysis of these time intervals. Frequency domain measures are determined by separating electrical activity into different frequency ranges and calculating the total power within a given time period.[66] There are four primary frequency bands produced in this analysis, high frequency, low frequency, very low frequency, and ultralow frequency bands. The high frequency band (0.15 to 0.4 Hz) is a reflection of parasympathetic activity; this band may be referred to as the respiratory band because of its association with heart rate variation produced with respiration. The low frequency band (0.04 to 0.15 Hz) reflects baroreceptor activity during rest and during 24-hour recordings has been demonstrated to respond to increased sympathetic innervation. The very low frequency (0.0033 to 0.04 Hz) is generated by sensory neurons in the heart and is an intrinsic cardiac rhythm that is essential to health; reductions in very low frequency power are associated with all-cause mortality, sudden cardiac death, and systemic inflammation. The ultralow frequency (<0.0033 Hz) reflects 24-hour cardiac oscillations associated with circadian rhythm, as well as temperature regulation, metabolic rate, and the renin-angiotensin-aldosterone system. Investigators have identified significantly reduced total power in those patients who failed the transition to spontaneous ventilation; those who were successfully weaned increased low frequency and total power in response to a spontaneous breathing trial.[31] Other investigators developed nonlinear analysis techniques of heart rate variability during weaning to identify differences between patients who were successfully weaned and those who failed.[1]

- *Other clinical indicators* of weaning readiness that have been tested included hemoglobin concentration,[41] ineffective cough,[32] heart rate less than 105 beats/minute, and $Paco_2$ <54 mm Hg at the end of a 30-minute spontaneous breathing trial,[65] presence of depressive disorder,[35] maintenance of central venous oxygen saturation during a spontaneous breathing trial,[70] and knee tissue oxygen saturation (Sto_2) and skin mottling score change during a spontaneous breathing trial.[50] Burns and colleagues developed the Burns Weaning Assessment Program (BWAP), an instrument that contained 26 clinical factors for evaluation before ventilator weaning. In a recent evaluation of the BWAP, 20 of these factors were significantly associated with weaning success in a variety of specialty intensive care unit patients.[8] Another investigative group found that a modified BWAP using a cut-off point of 60 provided a sensitivity of 81% and a specificity of 82%, which was superior to traditional measures like the rapid shallow breathing index and Pi_{max}.[34] Although numerous investigators have identified multiple independent predictors of weaning success and failure, the lack of consistent predictive power in heterogeneous patient populations limits their clinical utility and significantly reduces their utility in clinical care.

Methods of Ventilator Weaning

- *Standardized weaning protocol use* is associated with significantly increased weaning success and reduced ventilator days, along with reduced ICU and hospital lengths of stay.[5,38,39] For example, implementation of a standardized protocol for ventilator weaning was demonstrated to increase the use of spontaneous breathing trials by 26% and subsequently reduce the occurrence of ventilator-associated conditions by 37%, infection-related ventilator-associated conditions by 65%, and probable pneumonia by 49%.[39] In addition, these investigators found that standardized weaning reduced ventilator time by 2.4 days, ICU length of stay by 3 days, and hospital length of stay by 6.3 days. However, investigators also reported difficulty with protocol adherence and lack of any change in ventilator time after protocol implementation, probably due to nonadherence to the specific protocol components.[37] To date, the use of a standardized protocol for ventilator weaning has been demonstrated to be superior to usual care, regardless of the specific method used for weaning.

- *T-piece spontaneous breathing trial* with administration of supplemental oxygen by T-piece is recommended for discontinuation of mechanical ventilation.[49,59] Spontaneous breathing trials with T-piece were associated with superior arterial and central venous oxygenation compared with CPAP with PS and CPAP with automatic tube compensation during spontaneous breathing trials.[45] However, other investigators found no difference in weaning success, hemodynamic values, and arterial blood gas values between T-piece and CPAP weaning.[10] Currently, spontaneous breathing trials are widely recommended because they are safe, effective, and efficient strategies to evaluate tolerance of independent ventilation, and they may be accompanied by supplemental oxygen via T-piece, PS, CPAP, or automatic tube compensation.

However, none of these methods has demonstrated superiority in all patient populations.

- *Pressure support (PS)* permits the patient to trigger inspiration and control respiratory rate, depth, length, and flow during each spontaneous breath. Inspiration is supported by a preset inspiratory pressure; the tidal volume achieved with each breath is determined by individual effort, pulmonary compliance, airway and endotracheal tube resistance, and the set level of PS. Several investigators have concluded that PS weaning was associated with greater weaning success compared with T-piece weaning, particularly in patients who required simple weaning.[20,40] However, with conventional PS, the level of support is constant and ventilatory variability is reduced; breathing variability reductions have been previously associated with weaning failure.[71] The use of variable PS, also known as noisy PS, improved tidal volume variability and was significantly associated with improved patient ventilator synchrony.[68] In an experimental model of acute lung injury, variable PS was superior to conventional PS in improvement of gas exchange, reduction of work of breathing, alveolar edema, and inflammatory infiltrates.[67] Variable pressure support for ventilator weaning is currently in clinical trials to evaluate its efficacy as a weaning mode for adult patients.

- *Continuous positive airway pressure (CPAP)* consists of adding positive airway pressure throughout the ventilatory cycle during spontaneous breathing. Positive pressure at end-expiration in particular increases functional residual capacity and redistributes extravascular lung water to the interstitial space, which improves pulmonary compliance, oxygenation, and ventilation-perfusion match.[27,46] Comparison of ventilator weaning with CPAP to T-piece provided evidence that CPAP was superior, because 16% more patients in the CPAP group were weaned;[52] however, other investigators have found no significant difference in weaning outcome when CPAP was compared with the application of automatic tube compensation[23] and worse outcomes when CPAP combined with PS was compared with T-piece.[45] Thus there is equivocal evidence to support the superiority of CPAP to other methods of ventilator weaning.

- *Automated weaning systems* with the use of computer-driven automated systems to support earlier removal of mechanical ventilation have been tested over the past decade. An automated ventilator system monitors and interprets clinical data that include end-tidal CO_2 concentration, respiratory rate, and tidal volume and adapts the level of PS in 2- to 4-cm H_2O increments based on these values. A minimal level of PS is the goal, and the system can automatically initiate a spontaneous breathing trial with automatic tube compensation or PS. Early investigators reported significant reductions in weaning time, ventilator days, and intensive care length of stay,[42] and more recent studies supported these findings.[43] However, recently investigators found no improvement in weaning outcomes of surgical patients with the computer-automated strategy,[64] and scientists in two recent systematic reviews concluded that evidence to date did not provide definitive support for comprehensive superior outcomes with this weaning strategy.[7,62]

EQUIPMENT

- Standardized weaning protocol approved for your facility
- Personal protective equipment (i.e., gloves, mask, goggles, gown)
- Force meter/aneroid pressure manometer—typically a component of the mechanical ventilator
- Spirometer to measure volumes—typically a component of the mechanical ventilator
- Equipment for endotracheal suctioning

Additional equipment, to have available as needed, includes the following:

- Self-inflating manual resuscitation bag-valve device connected to oxygen source as needed
- Oxygen flow meter connected to oxygen source with heated aerosol humidifier with in-line thermometer and water trap for T-piece weaning or tracheostomy collar as appropriate for those using this method of weaning

PATIENT AND FAMILY EDUCATION

- Assess patient and family level of understanding about the condition and rationale for the procedure. *Rationale:* Assessment identifies the patient and family knowledge deficits about the patient's condition, the procedure, the expected benefits, and the potential risks. The clinician should permit time for questions to clarify information and voice concerns. Explanations decrease patient anxiety and enhance cooperation.
- Explain the procedure and the reason for the procedure before and during the procedure. Reinforce information frequently. *Rationale:* Explanation enhances patient and family understanding and decreases anxiety.
- Maintain the clear and frequent transmission of information about patient progress, change in status, and prognosis with the patient and family members. *Rationale:* Establishes an open trusting relationship and encourages realistic perception of the situation and patient prognosis.
- Describe the potential sensations (dyspnea, increased airway resistance, increased ventilatory effort, palpitations) that the patient may experience during evaluation and spontaneous breathing trials, and explain the importance of cooperation and maximal effort. Explain that prolonged ventilation may require muscle conditioning and produce more sensations associated with distress. *Rationale:* A clear understanding of expected sensations reduces anxiety and improves understanding and cooperation.
- Provide reassurance during the procedure; ensure continuous presence of qualified, experienced clinician(s). *Rationale:* May reduce anxiety, promote patient cooperation, and improve and enhance effort.
- Explain how the patient will be monitored and evaluated for tolerance of spontaneous breathing and ensure patient and family that mechanical ventilation will be reinstituted should the patient demonstrate intolerance. *Rationale:*

Provides assurance to the patient and family that clinicians will protect the patient from harm during the procedure.

PATIENT ASSESSMENT AND PREPARATION

Patient Assessment

- Evaluate the patient for objective and subjective measures of adequacy of ventilation and oxygenation. Objective measures include oxygenation (Pao_2, Spo_2), carbon dioxide removal ($Paco_2$, end-tidal CO_2), arterial pH, respiratory rate (tachypnea, bradypnea, apnea), synchrony of chest and abdominal movements, level of consciousness, agitation, arterial blood pressure and heart rate within normal limits or less than 20% change from values normal for the individual, new cardiac dysrhythmias, and volume and characteristics of secretions. Subjective indicators include self-reported dyspnea, sensation of excessive work of breathing, anxiety, and fatigue. *Rationale:* Early detection of inadequate ventilation and oxygenation permits the clinician to quickly intervene and return the patient to the prior ventilator settings.

- Evaluate the level of patient responsiveness and degree of sedation for those patients receiving intermittent or continuous sedation infusion using a reliable and valid instrument like the Richmond Agitation-Sedation Scale.[4,63] Assess the patient for delirium with a reliable and valid instrument like the Confusion Assessment Method for the Intensive Care Unit (CAM-ICU)[4,18] because the presence of delirium has previously been hypothesized to be associated with the use of sedation and mechanical ventilation, and this combination may trigger weaning failure.[3,12] *Rationale:* Adequate cognitive function supports the ability of the patient to cooperate and participate in the procedure and increases the likelihood of success.

- Evaluate the patient for factors that induced the need for mechanical ventilation in the individual, particularly those that are reversible, and address those before weaning trials. These factors include correction of the underlying cause of the respiratory failure, neurological function and adequate ventilatory drive in particular, cardiovascular stability demonstrated by heart rate and blood pressure within normal limits without the use of vasoactive medications, absence of evidence of myocardial ischemia, adequacy of hemoglobin concentration for oxygen transport, electrolyte and acid-base homeostasis, adequate nutritional status, fluid volume state, lack of localized or systemic infection, and adequacy of respiratory muscle function (muscle fatigue or lack of endurance). These factors should be effectively managed before the initiation of weaning. *Rationale:* Adequate attention to all factors that influence ability to ventilate spontaneously improves the likelihood of successful weaning from ventilation.

Patient Preparation

- Verify patient identity for the prescribed procedure to ensure the correct patient will receive the appropriate treatment. *Rationale:* Ensures correct identification of the appropriate patient for the procedure.

- Review the procedure and expected sensations with the patient and family; answer questions as they arise. Reinforce the importance of patient relaxation, cooperation, and maximal effort. *Rationale:* Determines patient understanding, reinforces information, and reduces anxiety of patient and family.

- Position the patient for comfort and physiological support of ventilation; consider the use of a position elevated 45 degrees, as this supported optimal respiratory muscle function.[15] *Rationale:* Investigators found that a 45-degree elevation reduced work of breathing and intrinsic positive end-expiratory pressure level, compared with supine and sitting positions.[15]

- Initiate titration/reduction or cessation of sedation (sedation interruption, sedation vacation) following hospital protocol. Some prior investigations have demonstrated that sedation interruption is safe and reduced length of ventilation.[2,33] However, recently other investigators found no difference in ventilator time, length of stay, medication use, or mortality with this strategy, but unplanned extubation rate was increased with daily sedation interruption.[9,54,69] However, the patient should be relaxed, able to cooperate, and free from pain/discomfort during this experience. *Rationale:* Minimal sedation optimizes the ability of the patient to understand the procedure, the sensations detected during weaning, and to cooperate, thereby increasing the likelihood of success.

Procedure　for Ventilator Weaning

Steps	Rationale	Special Considerations
Evaluation of Readiness		
1. HH		
2. PE		
3. Assemble and prepare equipment and supplies.	Prepares equipment for procedure.	
4. Use the spirometer as indicated in the facility protocol to evaluate specific indicators if they are to be measured before weaning trial.	Spirometer in the ventilator may be used to measure spontaneous Vt and V_E and VC.	Ensure that there is minimal leak around the endotracheal tube cuff because this will give inaccurate measures of volumes measured through the tube. Provide patient with rest periods on the ventilator between measurements.
5. Request the patient breathe normally for 1 minute; the spirometer in the ventilator may be used to determine values required by your facility protocol.	Ventilator may measure the V_E, the total volume exhaled in 1 minute. Spontaneous Vt is also measured breath to breath or determined by dividing the 1-minute total exhaled volume by the measured respiratory rate.	Evaluate patient status and discontinue evaluation if intolerance detected ($SpO_2 < 90\%$, tachypnea, bradypnea, agitation, diaphoresis, tachycardia, etc.)
6. Measure the rapid shallow breathing index (f/Vt), divide the measured spontaneous Vt by the respiratory rate if required in your facility protocol.	Threshold values for weaning are 60–105.	
7. Measure the VC and/or FVC if these are a component of your facility protocol. For a VC measure, instruct the patient to exhale then inhale as deeply as possible (maximal inspiration), followed by an exhalation of all the gas possible (maximal expiration). For the FVC measure, the patient is instructed to maximally inhale and then forcibly exhale the maximal amount as quickly as possible.	VC and FVC measures require patient cooperation and effort. These measures are typically repeated at least three times and the average value used.	Most often used with patients who have a neuromuscular disorder.
8. When indicated by your facility protocol, measure the negative inspiratory force. Instruct the patient to maximally inhale. Determine the maximal pressure generated during the inspiratory effort over a 20-sec period.	This measure is typically repeated at least three times and either the best effort achieved or the average value used. This measure can be effort independent in patients who are unable to cooperate. Threshold −20 to −30 cm H_2O pressure (a greater negative value is desirable).	There are ventilators that will permit this measure to be made while the patient is connected to the ventilator. The patient will be unable to ventilate normally during this measure and may become anxious. Prior explanation should reduce this anxiety. Abort the measure with signs of excessive anxiety and intolerance.
9. Evaluate patient condition; return to mechanical ventilation using previous settings or initiate spontaneous breathing trial based on facility weaning protocol.	Patient measures that indicate adequate ventilatory drive, respiratory muscle strength, and endurance lead to initiating a spontaneous breathing trial in most protocols.	Spontaneous breathing trial in those deemed ready to wean may be supported with PS, CPAP, ATC to reduce the effect of the endotracheal tube on flow.

Procedure for Ventilator Weaning—*Continued*

Steps	Rationale	Special Considerations
10. Discard used supplies and remove **PE**.		
11. **HH**		
Spontaneous Breathing Trial with T-Piece or Tracheostomy Collar		
1. **HH**		
2. **PE**		
3. Position patient for optimal respiratory muscle function and comfort.	Head of the bed elevated 45 degrees provides optimal support of respiratory muscle function.[15]	
4. Remove patient from the ventilator and connect the endotracheal tube or tracheostomy to a humidified, heated oxygen source with the same Fio_2 as patient received via the ventilator unless otherwise prescribed. Recommended time for spontaneous breathing trials is 30–120 minutes, driven by patient tolerance.[25,49] **(Level B*)**	Endotracheal tube or tracheostomy removes the upper-airway mechanisms that warm and humidify inhaled gas.	Monitor respiratory frequency, breathing pattern, heart rate, cardiac rhythm, Sao_2, and general appearance of patient continuously during the trial. General appearance includes skin color and temperature, presence of mottling or cyanosis, perceived anxiety, degree of subjective work of breathing, and patient report of tolerance.
5. Stay with the patient during the trial. Provide coaching, encouragement, and information to the patient and family during the trial. Celebrate successes, and provide encouragement for those who are not tolerant of the trial.	Patient and family require frequent accurate information about status and care. Frequent encouragement and reminders that spontaneous breathing will have different sensation from mechanical ventilation may increase tolerance of the trial.	Abort the trial if patient intolerance develops. This type of weaning may require repeated conditioning of respiratory muscles with subsequently longer trial periods, as muscles become trained.[59]
6. At the end of the trial time, return patient to the mechanical ventilator at the prior settings.	Report the measures obtained before the trial, the length and tolerance of the trial to the care team.	As many as 80–90% of patients require simple weaning most commonly with spontaneous breathing trials, and can be extubated after the initial weaning trial. For those who require difficult or prolonged weaning, gradual reduction of support strategies like PS or CPAP are more common.[58]
7. Discard used supplies and remove **PE**.		
8. **HH**		
Spontaneous Breathing Trial and Gradual Reduction of Support with CPAP or PS		
1. **HH**		
2. **PE**		
3. Position patient for optimal respiratory muscle function and comfort.	Head of the bed elevated 45 degrees provides optimal support of respiratory muscle function.[15]	

*Level B: Well-designed, controlled studies with results that consistently support a specific action, intervention, or treatment.

Procedure continues on following page

Procedure for Ventilator Weaning—*Continued*

Steps	Rationale	Special Considerations
4. Set the ventilator to the prescribed level of CPAP or PS and spontaneous ventilation. Typical levels of CPAP are 5–8 cm H_2O; PS may begin with higher levels of support and be titrated downward according to patient tolerance.	Patient will remain connected to the ventilator, but all ventilation will be patient-initiated/spontaneous. CPAP will maintain a positive pressure throughout the ventilatory cycle; PS will provide inspiratory gas with the set level of inspiratory support. The initial PS level should be that which attains a spontaneous respiratory rate of ≤20 breaths/min with the absence of accessory muscle use, and a Vt of 6–10 mL/kg ideal body weight.	Monitor respiratory frequency, breathing pattern, heart rate, cardiac rhythm, Sao_2, and general appearance of patient during the trial. Use caution with high levels of PS, because patients who have obstructive lung disease may develop alveolar overdistension and air trapping.
5. Stay with the patient during the trial. Provide coaching, encouragement, and information to the patient and family during the trial. Celebrate successes and provide encouragement for those who do not tolerate the trial.	Patient and family require frequent accurate information about status and care. Frequent encouragement and reminders that spontaneous breathing with these modes will have different sensations from mechanical ventilation may increase tolerance of the trial.	Abort the trial if patient intolerance develops. This type of weaning increases endurance of respiratory muscles as levels of support are decreased. Full ventilatory support should be provided at night to promote rest, especially early in the weaning process. If the endotracheal or tracheostomy cuff is insufficiently inflated, the PS cycle-off mechanism may not activate (i.e., the ventilator cycles off when it senses that flow is one fourth the original flow). If this decrement of flow is not recognized, the result is an inappropriately long inspiratory time.
6. Depending on the facility protocol, CPAP or PS level may be titrated downward until a lower limit is reached and tolerated by the patient. In patients who have difficult or require prolonged weaning, gradual reduction in support may be performed with an automatic ventilator system or with use of a nurse, physician, or respiratory therapist-driven protocol. (**Level A***)[5]	Report the measures obtained before the trial, the length and tolerance of the trial, and the titration of CPAP or PS to the care team.	As many as 80–90% of patients require simple weaning, most commonly with spontaneous breathing trials, and can be extubated after the initial weaning trial (see Procedures 5 and 6). For those who have difficult or require prolonged weaning, gradual reduction of support strategies like pressure support or CPAP are more common.[58]
7. Discard used supplies and remove **PE**.		
8. **HH**		

*Level A: Meta-analysis of quantitative studies or metasynthesis of qualitative studies with results that consistently support a specific action, intervention, or treatment (including systematic review of randomized controlled trials).

Expected Outcomes

- Identification of the appropriate time for ventilator weaning
- Effective transition from mechanical to spontaneous independent ventilation without complication
- Ability to sustain adequate independent ventilation for more than 48 hours

Unexpected Outcomes

- Cardiac or respiratory distress or arrest during trial
- Cardiac dysrhythmias that influence hemodynamic state during weaning
- Pulmonary aspiration
- Ventilator-associated pneumonia
- Respiratory muscle fatigue/failure
- Hypoxemia and/or hypercapnia with acidosis
- Dyspnea, anxiety and agitation
- Unsuccessful, demoralizing weaning trials

Patient Monitoring and Care

Steps	Rationale	Reportable Conditions
		These conditions should be reported if they persist despite nursing interventions.
1. Evaluate patient responses to ventilation and weaning systematically. Be vigilant for deviations from a homeostatic condition.	Premature spontaneous breathing trials are associated with worse patient outcomes.[48]	Abort trial with signs of intolerance to prevent complications and subsequently worse outcomes. These signs and symptoms include development of anxiety, agitation, tachypnea or bradypnea, thoracic abdominal asynchrony, worsening dyspnea, altered level of consciousness, reduction in Pao_2, Spo_2, and Sao_2, increase in end-tidal CO_2 or $Paco_2$, tachycardia or bradycardia, cardiac dysrhythmias, and/or change in blood pressure or heart rate more than 20% from baseline.

Documentation

Documentation should include the following:
- Patient and family education provided before and during ventilator weaning
- Individualized goals set by multidisciplinary team and patient for weaning
- Method and procedures used for weaning
- Preweaning measures of readiness for spontaneous breathing trial per facility protocol
- Patient physiological and psychological responses to weaning trial

- Duration of trial and measured criteria per protocol at the end of trial time
- Titration of support level, decreases in support level timing, and tolerance of titration
- Complications and unexpected outcomes
- Notification of multidisciplinary team
- Extubation and subsequent status

References and Additional Readings

For a complete list of references and additional readings for this procedure, scan this QR code with any freely available smartphone code reader app, or visit http://booksite.elsevier.com/9780323376624.

PROCEDURE

34

Automated External Defibrillation

Kiersten Henry

PURPOSE: An automated external defibrillator (AED) is a defibrillator that, by using a computerized detection system, analyzes cardiac rhythms, distinguishes between rhythms that require defibrillation and rhythms that do not, and delivers a series of preprogrammed electrical shocks. The automated external defibrillator is designed to allow early defibrillation by physicians, advanced practice nurses, and other healthcare professionals who have minimal or no training in rhythm recognition or manual defibrillation.

PREREQUISITE NURSING KNOWLEDGE

- Defibrillation is the therapeutic use of an electrical shock that temporarily stops or stuns an irregularly beating heart and allows the spontaneously repolarizing pacemaking cells within the heart to recover and resume more normal electrical activity. Ventricular fibrillation (VF) and ventricular tachycardia (VT) are the only two rhythms recognized as shockable by an automated external defibrillator (AED; Fig. 34-1).
- Time is the major determining factor in the success rates of defibrillation. In out-of-hospital cardiac arrests, for every minute defibrillation is delayed the chance of success decreases by 7% to 10%. When used in conjunction with effective CPR, the decrease in the likelihood of success is more gradual and averages 3% to 4% per minute. Effective CPR increases the amount of time in which defibrillation may be effective.[1,10]
- Although defibrillation is the definitive treatment for VF and pulseless VT, the use of the AED is not a stand-alone skill; it is used in conjunction with CPR. CPR should be started as soon as the patient is found to be pulseless and not stopped until the AED has been turned on, the pads have been attached, and the machine is prompting the provider to "stand clear" or "don't touch the patient."[1,2] Immediate postshock CPR starting with compressions has been documented to lead to increased return of spontaneous circulation and increased cerebral survival,[1,9] which is why time is not taken to check for a rhythm or pulse after defibrillation.
- Ventricular fibrillation depletes the cardiac energy stores of adenosine triphosphate (ATP) more rapidly than a normal rhythm. The longer the heart goes without circulation, the more depleted its energy stores. In a heart with depleted energy stores, defibrillation is more likely to result in asystole because no fuel remains to support spontaneous depolarization or myocardial contraction. Effective CPR can supply the needed oxygen and energy substrates to the heart cells and allow them to return to a perfusing rhythm.[1,6]
- Three stages of VF are seen in cardiac arrest. The first phase is the electrical phase. During this phase, which is considered the first 4 to 5 minutes of VF, defibrillation is most likely to be effective, and the sooner the shock can be delivered the more likely it is to work. During the next 5 to 10 minutes after VF occurs, the hemodynamic or circulatory phase, a brief period of CPR may "prime the pump" and provide oxygen to the myocardial cells, improving the effectiveness of the defibrillation. The metabolic phase starts 10 minutes after VF. During this phase, the cardiac cells have experienced global ischemia and energy depletion if no CPR has been initiated. CPR before defibrillation is more likely to be successful and needs to be used in conjunction with advanced cardiac life support (ACLS) therapies.[1,6]
- The AED is attached to the patient with adhesive electrode pads. Through these pads, the rhythm is analyzed and a shock delivered, if indicated. If the AED recognizes VF or VT, visual and/or verbal prompts guide the operator to deliver a shock to the patient. The AED, not the operator, makes the decision about whether the rhythm is appropriate for defibrillation.
- The chance of the AED shocking inappropriately is minimal. There is a higher incidence of inappropriate shocks with manual defibrillation than AED.[8] The AED

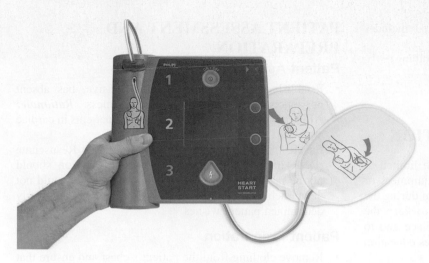

Figure 34-1 Automated external defibrillator device. (*Courtesy Philips Medical Systems.*)

should be applied only to unresponsive, nonbreathing, pulseless patients. To keep artifact interference to a minimum, the patient should not be touched or moved during the analysis time.

- The mnemonic "PAAD" makes it easy for the rescuer to remember the steps of operation of the AED: "P" for Power on, "A" for Attach the pads, "A" for clear to Analyze, and "D" for clear to Defibrillate.

- Although AEDs are simple to use, healthcare personnel should be familiar with and technically competent in use of AEDs.

- The AED is recommended for use in children ages 1 through 8 years if the child shows no signs of circulation. Approximately 15% of children in arrest have initial VT or VF.[5] Primary VF in children rapidly changes to asystole; rhythm detection and rapid defibrillation in children is most effective. It is best if the defibrillator has a pediatric switch or pediatric pads, which have an attenuator in the cord that decreases the amount of energy delivered. If pediatric pads are not available, adult pads should be used.[3-5] With use of adult pads, ensure that they do not touch each other because this may cause electrical arcing and skin burns and divert defibrillation energy. The pads should be at least 1 inch apart. If the pads cannot be fit on the child's chest in a lead-II position, an anterior-posterior pad placement should be used.[3] Never use pediatric pads on an adult or large child because the reduced energy levels delivered by these electrodes may not be effective for treatment of VF.

- The use of AEDs in prehospital settings has increased the success of defibrillation. The goal in the hospital should be to have the ability to defibrillate any person in cardiac arrest within 3 minutes or less of discovery. Placement of AED units in nonmonitored patient units and in public use areas of a hospital decreases the time to defibrillation. The largest study of in-hospital cardiac arrest found overall survival to discharge to be 15%.[2,10] AEDs are also needed in freestanding or ambulatory care settings. The majority of in-hospital cardiac arrests do not involve VT/VF and therefore are not indications for defibrillation.[5,10] High

quality CPR and rapid initiation of ACLS should remain a focus for in-hospital cardiac arrest.

- Many manual defibrillators have analysis capability that allows a tiered response (i.e., individuals with different skill levels can use the same defibrillator).

- Most AEDs in use in emergency response systems (EMS) or in the hospital have a method of recording the event in the form of rhythm strip printouts, audio and event recording devices, data cards, or computer chips that can print an event summary.

- AEDs may or may not have monitor screens. AEDs with screens may allow the provider with rhythm recognition skills to override the AED's analysis and recommendations.

- An important safety issue an AED operator must address is the possibility of inadvertently shocking a bystander or other provider at the scene. The operator must clear the patient verbally and visibly by looking at the patient from head to toe before and during the discharge of the energy to the patient.

- All defibrillation programs need to include training for the potential operators. Training should include psychomotor skills, troubleshooting, equipment maintenance, and interfacing with ACLS providers. Physicians, advanced practice nurses, and other healthcare professionals have the responsibility to be familiar with the machine they will use.

- When a resuscitation team (e.g., 911 responders, code team, ACLS providers) arrives, the team assumes responsibility for monitoring and treating the patient.

EQUIPMENT

- AED
- Nonsterile gloves
- Barrier device or airway management equipment (bag-valve device with mask and oxygen)
- Hand towel
- At least two sets of adult defibrillation pads and potentially one set of child defibrillation pads

Additional equipment, to have available as needed, includes the following:
- Trauma shears (with ability to cut through clothing)
- Clippers or scissors
- Extra electrocardiographic (ECG) paper
- Cardiac board

PATIENT AND FAMILY EDUCATION

- AEDs are used in emergency situations with limited or no time to educate the family about the equipment or the procedure. If family is present in the room during the arrest, a staff member should be assigned to keep the family informed of the procedures taking place and to offer support. *Rationale:* Information provides education and support.
- After a sudden cardiac event, a patient may be discharged from an institution with an implanted cardioverter defibrillator or a wearable cardioverter defibrillator. In these situations, patient and family education is essential and should include information regarding performing CPR. *Rationale:* Education prepares the family for potential future procedures and emergencies.

PATIENT ASSESSMENT AND PREPARATION

Patient Assessment

- Establish that the patient is unresponsive, has absent or abnormal breathing, and is pulseless. *Rationale:* AEDs are indicated for the treatment of patients in cardiac arrest.
- Ensure that patient does not have a Do Not Resuscitate (DNR) order indicating CPR and defibrillation should not be performed. Gathering this information should not delay delivery of care. *Rationale:* Honors previously determined patient wishes.

Patient Preparation

- Remove clothing from the patient's chest and ensure that the skin is dry where the AED electrodes will be placed. *Rationale:* This action prepares the patient for placement of the AED electrodes and minimizes the risk of electrical burns.
- Call for or obtain the AED; activate emergency response procedures for your setting. *Rationale:* Ensures the availability of the AED and additional emergency personnel.

Procedure | for Automated External Defibrillation

Steps	Rationale	Special Considerations
1. HH		
2. PE		
3. Assess patient. Perform CPR until the AED is available, turned on, attached to the patient, and prompts you to clear the patient. (If another provider is not nearby, it is reasonable for the healthcare provider to leave the patient and quickly obtain the AED.)	CPR helps keep the patient in a shockable rhythm longer, increasing the chance that defibrillation will be effective.	Place a backboard under the patient who is in bed.
4. The person in charge of the AED should: A. Open the AED. B. Press the "on" button. C. Proceed with the next steps as instructed by the AED.	When the AED is on, the prompts tell you what to do.	Some AEDs automatically turn on when they are opened. CPR should continue during the next few steps.
5. Attach the electrode pads to the patient's bare, dry chest:	Moisture under the pads can decrease the effectiveness of the contact of the electrode pads. Ensure the appropriate-sized pads are used.	Patients ages 1–8 may use pediatric or adult pads, adult patients must use adult-sized pads.[2]

Procedure for Automated External Defibrillation—*Continued*		
Steps	**Rationale**	**Special Considerations**
A. Place one pad below the right clavicle to the right of the sternum and the other to the left of the left nipple or slightly lower than the nipple line with the center of the electrode pad on the midaxillary line. The electrode pads have pictures that indicate where to place them (see Fig. 34–1).	This placement ensures that the heart is between the two electrode pads, maximizing the current flow through the heart.	Placing an electrode pad on the sternum decreases effectiveness. Bone blocks some of the energy. Even with proper placement, only 4–25% of the delivered current actually passes through the heart, so proper pad placement is crucial.[1] Polarity of the electrode pads is interchangeable for defibrillation purposes. However, if ECG monitoring is being done, the QRS complex is inverted if the positive and negative pads are reversed.
B. An alternative electrode pad position is anterior-posterior placement, where one pad is anterior over the left apex and the other is posterior behind the heart in the infrascapular location.	This placement also ensures that the heart is between the two electrode pads.	Ensure that the electrode pads are directly above and below each other.
6. Connect the cables from the electrode pads to the AED.	Prepares equipment.	
7. Place the electrode pads firmly to eliminate air pockets and to form a complete seal.	The AED uses the electrode pads to monitor and to shock. Good contact must be ensured to defibrillate most effectively; air pockets under the electrode can cause electrical sparks and skin burns.	
A. Do not place the electrode pads over any medication or monitoring patches. Remove any medication pads from the chest and wipe the chest clean.	Defibrillating over medication patches can cause burns and block the transfer of energy from the electrode pad to the heart.	
B. For the patient with an implantable cardioverter defibrillator (ICD) or pacemaker, keep the electrode pads 3 inches from the device generator. When possible for these patients, anterior-posterior placement is preferred. Other acceptable placement options are on the lateral chest wall on the right and left sides (biaxillary) or placement of the left pad in the standard apical position and the other pad on the right or left upper back.	Placement of electrode pads directly over an implanted device can divert energy away from the heart and can damage the device.	Some manufacturers recommend placing electrode pads 6 inches away from the device generators if possible. The ICD or pacemaker should be checked for possible damage to the device after defibrillation. Try to place the pads without interrupting CPR. Pad placement should not delay defibrillation.[1,2]

Procedure continues on following page

Procedure   for Automated External Defibrillation—*Continued*

Steps	Rationale	Special Considerations
8. Once the electrode pads are in place and plugged in, most AEDs sense an electrical pattern and tell the operator to make sure no one is touching the patient ("stand clear" or "don't touch the patient").	The machine needs to analyze the rhythm to determine whether defibrillation is needed, and touching the patient or doing CPR may give the machine a false message or delay the ability of the AED to analyze the rhythm.	CPR must be stopped at this point. No one should be touching the patient when the AED is analyzing.
9. Wait for the AED to analyze the patient's rhythm:		
A. If a shock is advised, clear the patient visually and verbally.	The AED has determined that the rhythm is either VF or VT; defibrillation is needed. Maintain safety for everyone around the patient. Anyone touching the patient or any conductive apparatus that is in contact with the patient (e.g., stretcher frame, intubation stylet) when the energy is discharged receives some of that shock.	Use a mnemonic such as "I'm clear, you're clear, we're all clear," and look at the patient while talking to ensure that no one is touching the patient. Another mnemonic is "Shocking on three. One, I am clear. Two, you are clear. Three, we are all clear. Shocking now."
B. If no shock is advised, restart CPR.	If the patient is not in a shockable rhythm and was pulseless, the only treatment is CPR until the ACLS team arrives.	
10. Push the shock button or buttons, as prompted while looking at the patient.	Delivering the shock quickly is the best way to convert the fatal rhythm. Most AEDs discharge the energy into the machine if the shock button is not pushed within a preset time frame, usually about 10–15 seconds.	The energy levels for AEDs are preset to an energy level recommended by the manufacturer. Some AEDs are fully automatic and deliver a shock if needed without user interaction. In this case the AED warns the user to stand clear before delivering the shock.
11. Immediately restart CPR, beginning with compressions. Continue CPR for 2 minutes, approximately five cycles of 30 compressions to two breaths. If an advanced airway has been achieved, an asynchronous breath should be delivered 10 times/min.[9] **(Level D*)**	Providing immediate postshock compressions increases the probability of return of spontaneous circulation.[1,2,9]	Change compressors every 2 minutes to ensure effectiveness of CPR. Performing chest compressions is tiring, and effectiveness decreases after 2 minutes.[1]
12. After 2 minutes, the AED prompts the physicians, advanced practice nurses, and other healthcare professionals "stand clear" or "don't touch the patient" to allow it to analyze the rhythm, determining whether the rhythm remains shockable.	Checks to see whether the initial shock was effective or whether the patient needs to be defibrillated again.	Ensure that no one touches the patient during the analysis. A good time to change compressors is during the analysis pause.
13. **Repeat steps 8-11** if prompted to shock again.	If the patient remains in a shockable rhythm, CPR and defibrillation are most likely to be effective in return of spontaneous circulation.	Be sure to clear the patient for analysis and shocking.

*Level D: Peer-reviewed professional and organizational standards with the support of clinical study recommendations.

Procedure for Automated External Defibrillation—*Continued*

Steps	Rationale	Special Considerations
14. If you receive a "no shock advised" message, resume CPR until the ACLS team arrives and the rhythm can be checked, or the patient begins to move.[7]	Continues emergency intervention.	If a change occurs in the patient's condition, check a pulse. If a pulse is found, check for adequate breathing. If adequate breathing is not found and the patient has a pulse, provide rescue breaths at a rate of one every 5–6 seconds with a bag-valve device with mask and oxygen if available.
15. Once the patient has a pulse, obtain vital signs and assess level of consciousness.	Determines the patient's response to CPR and use of the AED.	
16. Transfer the patient to a critical care unit.	Continues assessment and medical intervention.	
17. Ensure that AED is cleaned and electrodes are replaced.	Prepares emergency equipment for future use.	
18. Discard **PE** and used supplies in appropriate receptacle.	Reduces the transmission of microorganisms; Standard Precautions.	
19. **HH**		

Expected Outcomes°

- Restoration of perfusing rhythm
- Restoration of spontaneous respirations
- Transfer to a critical care unit for postresuscitation care

Unexpected Outcomes

- Operator or bystander shocked
- Skin burns
- Pain
- Unsuccessful resuscitation; death

Patient Monitoring and Care

Steps	Rationale	Reportable Conditions
		These conditions should be reported if they persist despite nursing interventions.
1. Monitor vital signs at least every 15 minutes until stable.	Determines hemodynamic stability.	• Abnormal vital signs
		• Dysrhythmias
2. Monitor ECG rate and rhythm.	A patient with VF or VT is at risk for additional dysrhythmias.	• Dysrhythmias
3. Administer antidysrhythmic and vasopressor medications as prescribed.	Antidysrhythmic medications may prevent the risk of additional dysrhythmias. Vasopressors may be required to maintain adequate blood pressure in patients who are hypotensive postarrest.	• Dysrhythmias • Hypotension
4. Follow institution standard for assessing pain. Administer analgesia as prescribed.	Identifies need for pain interventions.	• Continued pain despite pain interventions
5. Initiate induced hypothermia postarrest if prescribed.	Reduces the incidence of hypoxic brain injury after cardiac arrest.	

Procedure continues on following page

Documentation

Documentation should include the following:

- Type of arrest (witnessed or not witnessed)
- Time from patient collapse to first shock (only if witnessed)
- CPR information (including start and stop times)
- CPR performed before AED application: yes/no
- Time of application of AED
- Time of first shock
- Number of times patient was defibrillated

- Preshock and postshock rhythms
- Any complications
- Assessment after resuscitation (if applicable)
- Pain assessment, interventions, and effectiveness
- Unexpected outcomes
- Nursing interventions
- Patient and family education

References and Additional Readings

For a complete list of references and additional readings for this procedure, scan this QR code with any freely available smartphone code reader app, or visit http://booksite.elsevier.com/9780323376624.

35 Cardioversion

Cynthia Hambach

PURPOSE: Cardioversion is the therapy of choice for terminating hemodynamically unstable tachydysrhythmias. It also may be used to convert hemodynamically stable atrial fibrillation or atrial flutter into normal sinus rhythm.

PREREQUISITE NURSING KNOWLEDGE

- Understanding the anatomy and physiology of the cardiovascular system, principles of cardiac conduction, basic dysrhythmia interpretation, and electrical safety is needed.
- Basic and advanced cardiac life support knowledge and skills are essential.
- Clinical and technical competence in the use of the defibrillator is important.
- Synchronized cardioversion is recommended for termination of those dysrhythmias that result from a reentrant circuit, which include unstable supraventricular tachycardia, atrial fibrillation, atrial flutter, and unstable monomorphic ventricular tachycardia with a pulse.[3,4,8]
- The electrical current delivered with cardioversion depolarizes the myocardial tissue involved in the reentrant circuit. This depolarization renders the tissue refractory; thus, it is no longer able to initiate or sustain reentry. A countershock synchronized to the QRS complex allows for the electrical current to be delivered outside the heart's vulnerable period in which a shock can precipitate ventricular fibrillation. This synchronization occurs a few milliseconds after the highest part of the R wave but before the vulnerable period associated with the T wave.[3,4,8]
- Cardioversion may be implemented in the patient with an emergent condition. The aforementioned dysrhythmias are converted with synchronized cardioversion when the patient develops symptoms from the rapid ventricular response. Symptoms may include hypotension, acutely altered mental status, signs of shock, ischemic chest pressure, and acute heart failure.[4,8]
- Elective cardioversion may be used to convert hemodynamically stable atrial fibrillation or atrial flutter into normal sinus rhythm. When used to convert atrial fibrillation or atrial flutter, anticoagulation therapy is considered for 3 weeks before cardioversion to decrease the risk of thromboembolism. Anticoagulation therapy may not be necessary if atrial fibrillation or atrial flutter has been present for less than 48 hours, depending on thromboembolic risk. A physician, advanced practice nurse, or other healthcare professional may choose to perform a transesophageal echocardiogram to exclude the possibility of an atrial thrombus before cardioversion for patients at high risk for thromboembolism. The patient is immediately placed on an anticoagulant, and the cardioversion is performed once anticoagulation is achieved. Anticoagulation therapy should be continued for 4 weeks after cardioversion because of the possibility of delayed embolism.[2]

- Elective cardioversion also may be used in patients with hemodynamically stable ventricular or supraventricular tachydysrhythmias unresponsive to medication therapy.[3]
- If time and clinical condition permit, the patient should be given a combination of analgesia and sedation to minimize discomfort.[4,8,9]
- Defibrillators deliver energy or current in waveform patterns. Delivered energy levels may differ among the various defibrillators and waveforms. Various types of monophasic waveforms are used in older defibrillators. Biphasic waveforms have been designed more recently and are used currently in implantable cardioverter defibrillators (ICDs), automated external defibrillators, and manual defibrillators sold at the present time.
  - ❖ Monophasic waveforms deliver energy in one direction. The energy travels through the heart from one pad or paddle to the other.[3]
  - ❖ Biphasic waveforms deliver energy in two directions. The energy travels through the heart in a positive direction and then reverses itself and flows back through the heart in a negative direction.[3]
  - ❖ Due to their increased success in terminating dysrhythmias, defibrillators with biphasic waveforms are preferred for the treatment of atrial and ventricular dysrhythmias.[6]
- When performing synchronized cardioversion, use energy recommendations as specified by the American Heart Association (Table 35-1).[3,8]

EQUIPMENT

- Defibrillator/monitor with electrocardiogram (ECG) oscilloscope/recorder capable of delivering a synchronized shock
- ECG cable
- Self-adhesive defibrillation pads connected directly to the defibrillator or conductive gel, paste, or prepackaged gelled conduction pads to be used with defibrillator paddles
- Intravenous sedative and/or analgesic pharmacological agents as prescribed

TABLE 35-1	American Heart Association Energy Level Recommendations for Treatment of Tachydysrhythmias
Tachydysrhythmia	**Initial Dose**
Unstable atrial fibrillation	200 J (monophasic) 120–200 J (biphasic)
Unstable monomorphic ventricular tachycardia	100 J (monophasic or biphasic)
Other unstable supraventricular tachycardia or atrial flutter	50–100 J (monophasic or biphasic)
Unstable polymorphic ventricular tachycardia (irregular form and rate)	Treat as ventricular fibrillation with high-energy shock (defibrillation doses)

Note: Escalate subsequent doses as needed.
(From Sinz, E. et al, editors: Advanced cardiac life support provider manual. Dallas, 2011, American Heart Association.)

- Bag-valve device with mask and oxygen delivery
- Flow meter for oxygen administration, oxygen source
- Emergency suction and intubation equipment
- Blood pressure monitoring equipment
- Pulse oximeter
- Intravenous infusion pumps

Additional equipment, to have available as needed, includes the following:
- Cardiac board
- Emergency medications
- Emergency transcutaneous pacing equipment

PATIENT AND FAMILY EDUCATION

- Assess patient and family understanding of the etiology of the dysrhythmia. *Rationale:* This assessment determines the patient and family understanding of the condition and additional educational needs.
- Explain the procedure to the patient and family. *Rationale:* This explanation decreases anxiety and promotes patient cooperation.
- Discuss the use of sedative and analgesic pharmacology agents. *Rationale:* This discussion will help alleviate the patient's fear and anxiety about receiving an electrical shock.
- Explain the signs and symptoms of hemodynamic compromise associated with the preexisting cardiac dysrhythmias to the patient and family. *Rationale:* This explanation enables the patient and family to recognize when the patient needs to notify the nurse or physician.
- Evaluate and discuss with the patient the need for long-term pharmacological support. *Rationale:* This discussion allows the nurse to anticipate educational needs of the patient and family regarding specific discharge medications.
- Assess and discuss with the patient the need for lifestyle changes. *Rationale:* The underlying pathophysiology may necessitate alterations in the patient's current lifestyle and require a plan for behavioral changes.

PATIENT ASSESSMENT AND PREPARATION

Patient Assessment

- Assess the patient's ECG results for tachydysrhythmias, including paroxysmal supraventricular tachycardia, atrial fibrillation, atrial flutter, and monomorphic ventricular tachycardia with a pulse, which could require synchronized cardioversion. *Rationale:* Tachydysrhythmias may precipitate deterioration of hemodynamic stability.[4,8]
- Assess the patient's vital signs and any associated symptoms of hemodynamic compromise with each significant change in ECG rate and rhythm. *Rationale:* Deterioration of vital signs or the presence of associated symptoms indicates hemodynamic compromise that could become life threatening.[4,8]
- Assess for the presence or absence of peripheral pulses and the patient's level of consciousness. *Rationale:* This baseline determination assists in the detection of cardioversion-induced peripheral embolization.[1]
- Obtain the patient's serum potassium, magnesium, digitalis levels (if taking this medication), and arterial blood gas results. *Rationale:* Electrolyte imbalances, acid-base disturbances, and digitalis toxicity contribute significantly to electrical instability and may potentiate postconversion dysrhythmias.[1] Hypokalemia should be corrected to prevent postconversion dysrhythmias. Although cardioversion is considered a safe practice in patients taking digitalis glycosides, the medication is generally discontinued on the day of cardioversion.

Patient Preparation

- Verify correct patient with two identifiers. *Rationale:* Before performing a procedure, the nurse should ensure the correct identification of the patient for the intended intervention.
- Ensure that the patient and family understand preprocedural teaching. Answer questions as they arise, and reinforce information as needed. *Rationale:* This communication evaluates and reinforces understanding of previously taught information.
- Ensure that informed consent is obtained. *Rationale:* Informed consent protects the rights of the patient and makes competent decision making possible for the patient; however, in emergency circumstances, time may not allow the consent form to be signed.
- Perform a preprocedure verification and time out if nonemergent. *Rationale:* Ensures patient safety.
- Obtain 12-lead ECG. *Rationale:* Provides baseline data.
- Give the patient nothing by mouth per institution policy. *Rationale:* Decreases the risk of aspiration.
- Establish a patent intravenous access. *Rationale:* Medication administration may be necessary.[3,4,8]
- Assist the patient to a supine position. *Rationale:* Supine positioning provides the best access for procedure initiation, intervention, and management of possible adverse effects.
- Remove all metallic objects from the patient. *Rationale:* Metallic objects are excellent conductors of electrical current and could result in burns.

- Remove transdermal medication patches from the patient's chest and wipe area clean or ensure the defibrillator pad or paddle does not touch the patch. *Rationale:* Transdermal medication patches may block the transfer of energy from the pad or paddle to the patient and produce a chest burn when the pad or paddle is placed over it.[3,8]
- Ensure that the patient is in a dry environment and dry the patient's chest if it is wet. *Rationale:* Water is a conductor of electricity. If the patient and rescuer are in contact with water, the rescuer may receive a shock or the patient may receive a skin burn. Also, if the patient's chest is wet, the current may travel from one paddle across the water to the other, resulting in a decreased amount of energy to the myocardium.[8]
- If the patient has a hairy chest, self-adhesive defibrillation pads may stick to the patient's hair instead of the skin. Apply pressure to pads to ensure contact. If this is not working and it is an emergency, remove pads briskly to remove hair. Hair may also be clipped if time is available. *Rationale:* This action allows the electrodes to adhere to the chest.[3,8]
- Remove loose-fitting dentures, partial plates, or other mouth prostheses. *Rationale:* Removal decreases the risk of airway obstruction during the procedure. Evaluate each individual situation (e.g., dentures may facilitate a tighter seal for airway management).
- Preoxygenate the patient as prescribed and appropriate to the condition. *Rationale:* This will optimize oxygen delivery until the patient is stabilized.[4,8]
- If time allows, consider administration of sedation and analgesia as prescribed. *Rationale:* These medications provide amnesia and decrease anxiety and pain during the procedure.[4,8,9]
- Maintain a patent airway with oxygenation throughout the procedure. *Rationale:* Respiratory depression and hypoventilation can occur after administration of sedatives and analgesics.[9]

Procedure for Cardioversion		
Steps	**Rationale**	**Special Considerations**
1. HH		
2. PE		
3. Connect the patient to the monitoring lead wires on the defibrillator.	The R wave must be sensed by the defibrillator to achieve synchronization for cardioversion.[3,4,8]	
4. Select a monitor lead that displays an R wave of sufficient amplitude to activate the synchronization mode of the defibrillator. In most models, synchronization is achieved when the monitoring lead produces a tall R wave. **(Level M*)**	Synchronized cardioversion must sense the R wave to deliver the current outside the heart's vulnerable period.[3,4,8] Lead II generally produces a large R wave.	If a combination defibrillator/monitor is not being used, a converter cable must connect the monitor to the defibrillator to achieve synchronization.
5. Place the defibrillator in the synchronization mode. Ensure that the patient's QRS complexes appear with a marker to signify correct synchronization of the defibrillator with the patient's ECG rhythm (Fig. 35-1). To confirm that the synchronization has been achieved, observe for visual flashing on the screen or listen for auditory beeps. If necessary, adjust the R wave gain until the synchronization marker appears on each R wave. **(Level D*)**	Synchronization prevents the random delivery of an electrical charge, which may cause ventricular fibrillation.[3,4,8]	

*Level D: Peer-reviewed professional and organizational standards with the support of clinical study recommendations.
*Level M: Manufacturer's recommendations only.

Procedure continues on following page

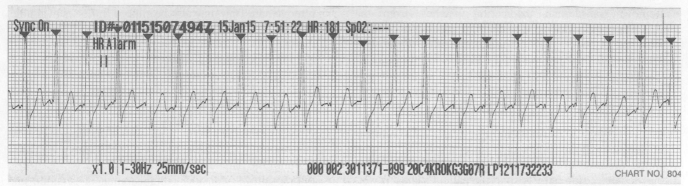

Figure 35-1 R-wave synchronization. Note the synchronization marker above each R wave. *(Courtesy Drexel University Center for Interdisciplinary Clinical Simulation and Practice.)*

Procedure	**for Cardioversion—*Continued***	
Steps	**Rationale**	**Special Considerations**
6. If the defibrillator is unable to distinguish between the peak of the QRS complex and the peak of the T wave, as in polymorphic ventricular tachycardia, proceed with unsynchronized defibrillation (see Procedure 36).	Avoids a delay or failure of shock delivery in the synchronized mode.[3,4,8]	
7. Apply self-adhesive defibrillation pads or prepare defibrillation paddles with proper conductive agent. (**Level D***)	Reduces transthoracic resistance, enhancing electrical conduction through subcutaneous tissue.[3,8] Minimizes erythema from the electrical current.	Self-adhesive defibrillation pads connected directly to the defibrillator have been found to be as effective as paddles.[8] Advantages of hands-free cardioversion are safety and convenience of use. These devices can be used for monitoring, and they allow for rapid delivery of a shock if necessary. For that reason, they are recommended for routine use instead of standard paddles.[8] Prepackaged gelled conductive pads are available for placement in the area of each paddle.[3,8] Gel pads should be replaced if they appear to be drying out or as per manufacturer recommendations. Conductive gel should be evenly dispersed on the defibrillator paddles and should adequately cover the surface. Be careful not to smear gel between paddles because current may follow an alternate pathway over the chest wall and avoid the heart. It may also cause a potential for a spark, causing a fire hazard. For that reason, gel pads are preferred.[3]

*Level D: Peer-reviewed professional and organizational standards with the support of clinical study recommendations.

Procedure for Cardioversion—*Continued*

Steps	Rationale	Special Considerations
8. Follow these steps for pad or paddle placement: A. Place one pad or paddle at the heart's apex, just to the left of the nipple at the midaxillary line. Place the other pad or paddle just below the right clavicle to the right of the sternum (Fig. 35-2).	Cardioversion is achieved by passing an electrical current through the cardiac muscle mass to restore a single source of impulse generation; this pathway maximizes current flow through the myocardium.[3,8]	Most pads or paddles are 8–12 cm in diameter.[3] Avoid placing pads or paddles over lead wires or implanted devices (ports, pacemakers, ICD).[3,8]

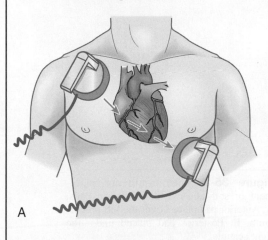

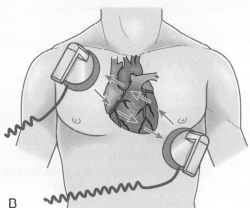

Figure 35-2 Paddle placement and current flow in **A,** monophasic defibrillation and **B,** biphasic defibrillation. *(From Lewis SL, et al: Medical-surgical nursing: Assessment and management of clinical problems, ed 9, St Louis, 2014, Mosby.)*

Steps	Rationale	Special Considerations
B. In women, the apex pad or paddle is placed at the fifth to sixth intercostal space with the center of the pad or paddle at the midaxillary line.	Placement over a woman's breast should be avoided to reduce transthoracic resistance.	

Procedure continues on following page

Procedure **for Cardioversion—*Continued***

Steps	Rationale	Special Considerations

C. Anterior-posterior placement also may be used.
  i. Self-adhesive defibrillation pads are used for this approach.
  ii. The anterior pad is placed in the anterior left precordial area, and the posterior pad is placed posteriorly behind the heart in the right or left infrascapular area (Fig. 35-3).
  iii. An alternative approach is to place the anterior pad in the right infraclavicular area and the posterior pad in the left infrascapular position.
	All methods of pad or paddle placement are effective.[3,8]	

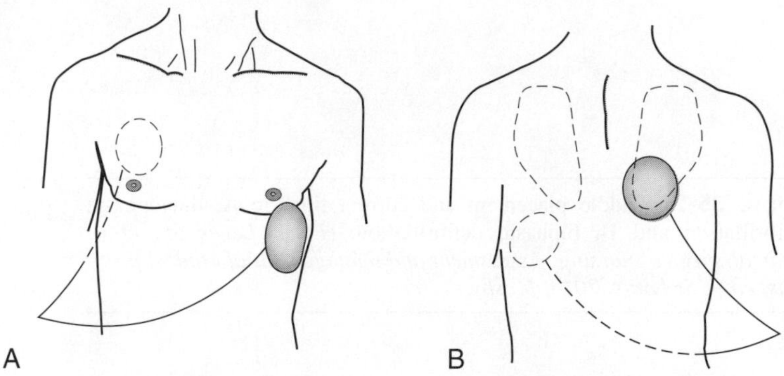

Figure 35-3 Anterior-posterior placement of self-adhesive defibrillation pads. **A,** Anterior pad placed over the left precordium. **B,** Posterior pad placed under the right scapula.

Steps	Rationale	Special Considerations
D. In a patient with a permanent pacemaker, do not place pads or paddles directly over the pulse generator.	Cardioversion over an implanted pacemaker may impair passage of current to the patient and may cause the device to malfunction or become damaged.[3,8]	Do not place the pad or paddle over the pulse generator and lead wire.[3,8] Anterior-posterior placement is also suggested.[3] The pacemaker should be assessed after any electrical countershock. Standby emergency pacing equipment should be available should pacemaker failure occur.
E. Pad or paddle placement in the patient with an ICD is the same as standard paddle placement for cardioversion (see Fig. 35-2). Pads or paddles should not be placed over the device. **(Level D*)**	Cardioversion over an ICD may impair passage of current to the patient and cause the device to malfunction or become damaged.[3,8]	Do not place the pad or paddle over the pulse generator and lead wire.[3,8] Anterior-posterior placement is also suggested.[3] The ICD should be checked after external countershock. If the ICD is delivering shocks to the patient, wait 30–60 seconds before defibrillating the patient with the manual defibrillator.[3,8]
9. Ensure that the defibrillator cables are positioned to allow for adequate access to the patient.	Allows cardioversion to occur without excessive tension on the cables.	

*Level D: Peer-reviewed professional and organizational standards with the support of clinical study recommendations.

Procedure	**for Cardioversion—*Continued***	
Steps	**Rationale**	**Special Considerations**
10. Turn on the ECG recorder for a continuous printout.	Establishes a visual recording of the patient's current ECG status and response to intervention. Provides a permanent record of the patient's response to intervention.	
11. Charge the defibrillator as prescribed or in accordance with the recommendations of the American Heart Association (see Table 35-1). **(Level D*)**	The defibrillator is charged with the lowest energy level necessary to convert the tachydysrhythmia.[3,8]	
12. Disconnect the oxygen source during actual cardioversion.	Decreases the risk of combustion in the presence of electrical current.[3]	Arcing of electrical current in the presence of oxygen could precipitate an explosion and subsequent fire hazard.[3]
13. State "all clear" or similar wording three times, and visually verify that everyone is clear of contact with the patient, bed, and equipment.	Maintains safety to caregivers because electrical current can be conducted from the patient to another individual if contact occurs.	Use a mnemonic such as "I'm clear, you're clear, we're all clear" and look at the patient while talking to ensure that no one is touching or is in contact with the patient. When using hands-free cardioversion, take special care to clear other personnel from patient contact because they do not have the visual cue of the paddles being placed on the patient's chest.
14. Verify that the defibrillator is in the synchronization mode and that the patient's QRS complexes appear with a marker to signify correct synchronization of the defibrillator with the patient's ECG rhythm (see Fig. 35-1). **(Level D*)**	Synchronization prevents the random delivery of an electrical charge, which may potentiate ventricular fibrillation.[3,8]	
15. When using self-adhesive hands-free defibrillation pads, depress the discharge button on the defibrillator to deliver the charge. In the synchronized mode, a delay occurs before the charge is released, which allows the sensing mechanism to detect the QRS complex.	Depolarizes the cardiac muscle.[8]	
16. If using handheld paddles, apply pressure to each paddle against the chest wall and depress both buttons on the paddles simultaneously and hold until the defibrillator fires.	Firm paddle pressure decreases transthoracic resistance, thus improving the flow of electrical current across the axis of the heart.[3]	This application of pressure is not necessary for defibrillator models with hands-free and automatic transthoracic impedance sensing/correction options built in.

*Level D: Peer-reviewed professional and organizational standards with the support of clinical study recommendations.

Procedure continues on following page

Procedure   for Cardioversion—*Continued*

Steps	Rationale	Special Considerations
17. Observe the monitor for conversion of the tachydysrhythmia, and assess the patient's carotid pulse. If a pulse is palpated, assess the patient's vital signs and level of consciousness.	Simultaneous depolarization of the myocardial muscle cells should reestablish a single source of impulse generation.[8]	If unsuccessful in converting the rhythm, proceed with repeated energy recommendations (see Table 35-1). Ensure that the defibrillator is still in the synchronization mode; many defibrillators revert back to the unsynchronized mode after cardioversion. Ventricular fibrillation may develop after cardioversion. If so, deactivate the synchronizer and follow the procedure for defibrillation (see Procedure 36).[3,8]
18. Clean the defibrillator, and remove any gel from the paddles.	Conductive gel accumulated on the defibrillator paddles impedes surface contact and increases transthoracic resistance.	
19. If self-adhesive defibrillation pads were used, evaluate the placement and integrity of pads.	Self-adhesive defibrillation pads may crimp, crack, or fold with loss of adhesiveness.	Loss of adhesive integrity in self-adhesive defibrillation pads may occur in restless or diaphoretic patients.
20. Remove PE and discard used supplies in appropriate receptacle.	Reduces the transmission of microorganisms; standard precautions.	
21. HH		

Expected Outcomes

- Reestablishment of a single source of impulse generation for the cardiac muscle
- Hemodynamic stability

Unexpected Outcomes

- Continued tachydysrhythmias
- Ventricular fibrillation that progresses to cardiopulmonary arrest
- Bradycardia
- Asystole
- Pulmonary edema
- Systemic embolization
- Respiratory complications
- Hypotension
- Pacemaker or ICD dysfunction
- Skin burns
- Pain

Patient Monitoring and Care

Steps	Rationale	Reportable Conditions
		These conditions should be reported if they persist despite nursing interventions.
1. Evaluate neurological status before and after cardioversion. Reorient as needed to person, place, and time.	An altered level of consciousness may occur after hemodynamically unstable dysrhythmias.[5,8] Cerebral emboli may develop as a postprocedural complication.[1,2]	• Change in level of consciousness • Sensory or motor changes
2. Monitor pulmonary status before and after cardioversion.	Hemodynamically unstable tachydysrhythmias may cause respiratory complications.[4,8] Respiratory depression and hypoventilation can occur after administration of sedatives and analgesics.[9]	• Dyspnea • Crackles • Rhonchi • Slow shallow respirations • Decrease in oxygen saturation as measured with pulse oximetry
3. Monitor cardiovascular status (blood pressure, heart rate, and rhythm) before and after cardioversion.	Dysrhythmias may develop after cardioversion.[5,7,8]	• Hypotension • Supraventricular dysrhythmias • Ventricular dysrhythmias • Bradycardia • Asystole
4. Prepare for administration of intravenous antidysrhythmic medications as prescribed.	Dysrhythmias may develop after cardioversion.[5,7,8]	• Supraventricular dysrhythmias • Ventricular dysrhythmias • Bradycardia • Asystole
5. Assess for burns.	Erythema at electrode sites may be seen from local hyperemia in the current pathway. Skin burns may be minimized with use of gel pads or placement of appropriate paste or gel on the paddles. Local cold application to electrode site after cardioversion may decrease the incidence and severity of burns and pain at site.[10]	• Skin burns
6. Follow institution standard for assessing pain. Administer analgesia as prescribed.	Identifies need for pain interventions.	• Continued pain despite pain interventions

Documentation

Documentation should include the following:

- Patient and family education
- Signed informed consent
- Universal Protocol requirements, if nonemergent
- Neurological, pulmonary, and cardiovascular assessment before and after cardioversion
- Interventions to prepare the patient for cardioversion
- The joules used and the number of cardioversion attempts made

- Pain assessment, interventions, and effectiveness
- Printout of the ECG tracing depicting the cardiac rhythm before and after cardioversion (before and after each attempt if more than one attempt is used)
- Condition of the skin of the chest wall
- Unexpected outcomes and nursing interventions
- Serum electrolytes, digoxin level, and coagulation laboratory results

References and Additional Readings

For a complete list of references and additional readings for this procedure, scan this QR code with any freely available smartphone code reader app, or visit http://booksite.elsevier.com/9780323376624.

36 Defibrillation (External)

Cynthia Hambach

PURPOSE: External defibrillation is performed to eradicate life-threatening ventricular fibrillation or pulseless ventricular tachycardia. The goal for defibrillation is to restore coordinated cardiac electrical and mechanical pumping action, resulting in restored cardiac output, tissue perfusion, and oxygenation.

PREREQUISITE NURSING KNOWLEDGE

- Understanding the anatomy and physiology of the cardiovascular system, principles of cardiac conduction, basic dysrhythmia interpretation, and electrical safety is needed.
- Basic and advanced cardiac life support (ACLS) knowledge and skills are necessary.
- Clinical and technical competence in the use of the defibrillator is needed.
- Ventricular fibrillation and pulseless ventricular tachycardia (VT) are lethal dysrhythmias. Early emergent defibrillation is the treatment of choice to restore normal electrical activity and coordinated contractile activity within the heart.[1,7]
- The electrical current delivered with defibrillation depolarizes the myocardium, terminating all electrical activity and allowing the heart's normal pacemaker to resume electrical activity within the heart.[7] Defibrillator pads or paddles placed over the patient's chest wall surface in the anterior-apex or anterior-posterior position maximize the current flow through the myocardium.[1,7]
- Defibrillators deliver energy or current in waveform patterns. Delivered energy levels may differ among different defibrillators and waveforms. Various types of monophasic waveforms are used in older defibrillators. Biphasic waveforms have been designed more recently and are used currently in implantable cardioverter defibrillators (ICDs), automated external defibrillators, and manual defibrillators sold at the present time.
- Monophasic waveforms deliver energy in one direction. The energy travels through the heart from one pad or paddle to the other.[1]
- Biphasic waveforms deliver energy in two directions. The energy travels through the heart in a positive direction and then reverses itself and flows back through the heart in a negative direction. Investigators in both in-hospital and out-of-hospital studies concluded that lower energy biphasic waveform shocks had equal or higher success rates for eradicating ventricular fibrillation than monophasic defibrillators.[1] Due to their increased success in terminating dysrhythmias, defibrillators with biphasic waveforms are preferred for the treatment of atrial and ventricular dysrhythmias.[4] More research is needed to determine a specific recommendation for the optimal energy level for biphasic waveform defibrillation. Biphasic energy recommendations are device specific, using a variety of waveforms that are effective in terminating fatal dysrhythmias. When using biphasic defibrillators, the American Heart Association (AHA) recommends using the amount of energy specified by the manufacturer (120–200 J). If operators are unaware of the effective biphasic dose, they should use the maximal amount specified on the defibrillator for the first shock, followed by escalating doses for subsequent shocks.[4]

- A wearable cardioverter defibrillator (WCD) has been developed for patients at high risk for sudden cardiac arrest. Patient populations may include those who do not meet the current guidelines for an immediate ICD implantation but who are at risk, those who may need protection when ICD therapy is interrupted because of infection or lead malfunction, patients with nonischemic cardiomyopathy, and those patients at high risk who are in need of a ventricular assist device or cardiac transplant. It may also be used to protect patients with syncope until a definitive diagnosis is found. The WCD has the ability to detect and treat life-threatening tachydysrhythmias without bystander support and allows the patient to ambulate freely. Results have shown that the WCD is a safe and effective method to terminate life-threatening dysrhythmias in this high-risk patient population.[6] (See Procedure 41.)

EQUIPMENT

- Defibrillator with electrocardiogram (ECG) oscilloscope/recorder
- ECG cable
- Self-adhesive defibrillation pads connected directly to the defibrillator or conductive gel, paste, or prepackaged gelled conduction pads to be used with defibrillator paddles
- Bag-valve device with mask and oxygen delivery
- Flow meter for oxygen administration, oxygen source
- Emergency suction and intubation equipment
- Blood pressure monitoring equipment
- Pulse oximeter
- End-tidal carbon dioxide ($ETco_2$) monitoring equipment
- Intravenous infusion pumps

Additional equipment, to have available as needed, includes the following:

*   Cardiac board
*   Emergency medications
*   Emergency transcutaneous pacing equipment

PATIENT AND FAMILY EDUCATION

*   Teaching may need to be performed after the procedure. *Rationale:* If emergent defibrillation is performed in the face of hemodynamic collapse, education may be impossible until after the procedure has been performed.
*   Assess patient and family understanding of the etiology of the dysrhythmia. *Rationale:* This assessment determines the patient and family understanding of the condition and guides additional educational needs.
*   Explain the procedure to the patient and the family. *Rationale:* This explanation decreases anxiety and promotes understanding.
*   Explain to the patient and the family the signs and symptoms of hemodynamic compromise associated with pre-existing cardiac dysrhythmias. *Rationale:* This explanation enables the patient and the family to recognize when to contact the nurse or physician.
*   Evaluate and discuss with the patient the need for long-term pharmacological support. *Rationale:* This evaluation and discussion allows the nurse to anticipate educational needs of the patient and family regarding specific discharge medications.
*   Assess and discuss with the patient the need for lifestyle changes. *Rationale:* Underlying pathophysiology may necessitate alterations in the patient's current lifestyle and require a plan for behavioral changes.
*   Assess and discuss with the patient the need as applicable for an ICD. *Rationale:* Life-threatening dysrhythmias may persist after initial defibrillation and pharmacological interventions.[2]
*   Assess and discuss with the patient the need as applicable for an emergency communication system. *Rationale:* People with recurrent life-threatening dysrhythmias are at risk for cardiac arrest.[2]

PATIENT ASSESSMENT AND PREPARATION

Patient Assessment

*   Assess the ECG monitor for tachydysrhythmias, including paroxysmal supraventricular tachycardia, atrial fibrillation, atrial flutter, atrial tachycardia, and ventricular tachycardia. *Rationale:* Tachydysrhythmias often precede ventricular fibrillation, can be life-threatening, and can precipitate deterioration of hemodynamic stability.[7]
*   Assess the ECG monitor for ventricular fibrillation. *Rationale:* Ventricular fibrillation is life-threatening; if not terminated immediately, death ensues.[7]

*   Assess vital signs. *Rationale:* Blood pressure and pulse are absent in the presence of ventricular fibrillation because of the loss of cardiac output.[7]

Patient Preparation

*   Verify correct patient with two identifiers. *Rationale:* Before performing a procedure, the nurse should ensure the correct identification of the patient for the intended intervention.
*   If family is present during the procedure, a staff member should be assigned, if possible, to provide support and keep family informed. *Rationale:* By relaying information and answering questions, a staff member may provide support to ease family members' anxiety during the procedure.
*   If possible, ask a member of pastoral care or another designated healthcare provider to provide support for family members during the procedure. *Rationale:* Pastoral care team members or other members of the healthcare team should be available to provide family support.
*   Remove all metallic objects from the patient. *Rationale:* Metallic objects are excellent conductors of electrical current and could result in burns.
*   Remove transdermal medication patches from the patient's chest and wipe area clean or ensure the defibrillator pad or paddle does not touch the patch. *Rationale:* Transdermal medication patches may block the transfer of energy from the pad or paddle to the patient and produce a chest burn when the pad or paddle is placed over it.[1,7]
*   Ensure that the patient is in a dry environment and dry the patient's chest if it is wet. *Rationale:* Water is a conductor of electricity. If the patient and rescuer are in contact with water, the rescuer may receive a shock or the patient may receive a skin burn. Also, if the patient's chest is wet, the current may travel from one paddle across the water to the other, resulting in a decreased amount of energy to the myocardium.[7]
*   If the patient has a hairy chest, self-adhesive defibrillation pads may stick to the patient's hair instead of the skin. Apply pressure to pads to ensure contact. If this is not working, remove pads briskly to remove hair. *Rationale:* This action allows the electrodes to adhere to the chest.[1,7]
*   Initiate basic life support (BLS) if immediate defibrillation is not available. *Rationale:* Basic life support maintains cardiac output to diminish irreversible organ and tissue damage.[2,7]
*   Oxygenate the patient with a bag-valve device with mask and 100% oxygen. *Rationale:* This will optimize oxygen delivery until the patient is stabilized.[2,4,7] Use of bag-mask ventilation is more effective with two rescuers.[2]
*   Place the defibrillator in the defibrillation mode. *Rationale:* The defibrillation mode must be set to disperse the electrical charge randomly because the synchronization mode does not fire in the absence of a QRS complex.[1,7]

Procedure   for Defibrillation (External)

Steps	Rationale	Special Considerations
1. HH		
2. PE		
3. Apply self-adhesive defibrillation pads or prepare defibrillation paddles with proper conductive agent. **(Level D*)**	Reduces transthoracic resistance, thus enhancing electrical conduction through subcutaneous tissue.[1,7] Minimizes erythema from the electrical current.	Self-adhesive defibrillation pads connected directly to the defibrillator have been found to be as effective as paddles. Advantages of hands-free defibrillation are safety and convenience of use.[7] Self-adhesive defibrillation pads decrease the risk of arcing, they can be used for monitoring, and they allow for fast delivery of a shock if necessary. For that reason, the pads are recommended for routine use instead of standard paddles.[7] Prepackaged gelled conductive pads are available for placement in the area of the defibrillation paddles.[1,7] Gel pads should be replaced if they appear to be drying out or as per manufacturer recommendations. Conductive gel should be evenly dispersed on the defibrillator paddles and should adequately cover the surface. Be careful not to smear gel between paddles because current may follow an alternate pathway over the chest wall and avoid the heart. It may also cause a potential for a spark, causing a fire hazard. For that reason, gel pads are preferred.[1]
4. Ensure that the defibrillator cables are positioned to allow for adequate access to the patient.	Allows defibrillation to occur without excessive tension on cables.	
5. Turn on the ECG recorder for continuous printout.	Establishes a visual recording of the patient's current ECG, verifies response to intervention, and provides a permanent record of the response to defibrillation.	
6. Follow these steps for pad or paddle placement: A. Place one pad or paddle at the heart's apex, just to the left of the nipple at the midaxillary line. Place the other pad or paddle below the right clavicle to the right of the sternum (see Fig. 35-2).	Defibrillation is achieved by passing an electrical current through the cardiac muscle mass to restore a single source of impulse generation. This pathway maximizes current flow through the myocardium.[1,7]	Most pads or paddles range from 8–12 cm in diameter and are effective.[1] Avoid placing pads or paddles over lead wires or implanted devices (ports, pacemakers, ICD).[1,7]

*Level D: Peer-reviewed professional and organizational standards with the support of clinical study recommendations.

Procedure	for Defibrillation (External)—*Continued*	
Steps	**Rationale**	**Special Considerations**
B. In women, the apex pad or paddle is placed at the fifth to sixth intercostal space with the center of the pad or paddle at the midaxillary line.	Placement over a woman's breast should be avoided to reduce transthoracic resistance.	

C. Anterior-posterior placement may also be used.
  i. Self-adhesive defibrillation pads are used for this approach.
  ii. The anterior pad is placed in the anterior left precordial area, and the posterior pad is placed posteriorly behind the heart in the right or left infrascapular area (see Fig. 35-3).
  iii. An alternative approach is to place the anterior pad in the right infraclavicular area and the posterior pad in the left infrascapular position.
	All methods of pad placement are effective.[1,7]	

D. If the patient has a permanent pacemaker, do not place pads or paddles directly over the pulse generator.	Defibrillation over an implanted pacemaker may impair passage of current to the patient and may cause the device to malfunction or become damaged.[1,7]	Do not place the pad or paddle over the pulse generator and lead wire.[1,7] Anterior-posterior placement is also suggested.[1] The pacemaker should be assessed after any electrical countershock. Standby emergency pacing equipment should be available in case the patient's permanent pacemaker does not function appropriately.
E. Pad or paddle placement in the patient with an ICD is the same as standard placement for defibrillation (see Fig. 35-2). Pads or paddles should not be placed over the device. **(Level D*)**	Defibrillation over an implanted ICD may impair passage of current to the patient and cause the device to malfunction or become damaged.[1,7]	Do not place the pad or paddle over the pulse generator and lead wire.[1,7] Anterior-posterior placement is also suggested.[1] The ICD should be checked after external countershock. If the ICD is delivering shocks to the patient, wait 30–60 seconds before defibrillating the patient with the manual defibrillator.[1,7]
7. Charge the defibrillator as prescribed or in accordance with AHA recommendations. **(Level D*)**	The defibrillator is charged with the lowest energy level needed to convert ventricular fibrillation or pulseless ventricular tachycardia.[1,7]	AHA monophasic energy recommendations for adults are for a 360-J shock.[1,7] When using biphasic defibrillators, AHA recommends using the amount of energy specified by the manufacturer (120–200 J). If operators are unaware of the effective biphasic dose, they should use the maximal amount specified on the defibrillator for the first shock, followed by escalating doses for subsequent shocks.[4]

*Level D: Peer-reviewed professional and organizational standards with the support of clinical study recommendations.

Procedure continues on following page

Procedure   for Defibrillation (External)—*Continued*

Steps	Rationale	Special Considerations
8. Disconnect the oxygen source during actual defibrillation.	Decreases the risk of combustion in the presence of electrical current.[1]	Arcing of electrical current in the presence of oxygen could precipitate an explosion and subsequent fire hazard.[1]
9. State "all clear" or similar wording three times and visually verify that all personnel are clear of contact with the patient, bed, and equipment.	Maximizes safety to self and caregivers because electrical current can be conducted from the patient to another person if contact occurs.	Use a mnemonic such as "I'm clear, you're clear, we're all clear," and look at the patient while talking to ensure that no one is touching or is in contact with the patient. With use of a hands-free defibrillation, take special care to clear other personnel from patient contact because they do not have the visual cue of the paddles being placed on the patient's chest.
10. Verify that the patient is still in ventricular fibrillation or pulseless ventricular tachycardia.	Ensures that defibrillation is necessary.	
11. When using self-adhesive hands-free defibrillation pads, depress the discharge button on the defibrillator to deliver the charge. In the defibrillation mode, an immediate release of the electrical charge occurs.	Depolarizes the cardiac muscle.[7]	
12. If using handheld paddles, apply pressure to each paddle against the chest wall and depress both buttons on the paddles simultaneously and hold until the defibrillator fires.	Firm paddle pressure decreases transthoracic resistance, thus improving the flow of electrical current across the axis of the heart.[1]	This application of pressure is not necessary for defibrillator models with hands-free and automatic transthoracic impedance sensing/correction options built in.
13. Administer 2 minutes (approximately five cycles) of CPR. **(Level D*)**	CPR is needed for 2 minutes to provide some coronary and cerebral perfusion until adequate heart function resumes.[1,7]	
14. Observe the monitor for conversion of the dysrhythmia. If a stable rhythm is noted, assess for the presence of a carotid pulse. If a pulse is palpated, assess vital signs and level of consciousness.	Simultaneous depolarization of the myocardial muscle cells should reestablish a single source of impulse generation.[7]	If using $ETCO_2$ monitoring, observe for capnography waveform that indicates return of spontaneous circulation (ROSC).[2]
15. If the patient is still in ventricular fibrillation or pulseless VT, continue CPR and immediately charge the paddles to 360 J (monophasic) or device-specific value (escalating; biphasic) and **repeat Steps 8–14. (Level D*)**	Immediate action increases the chance of successful subsequent depolarization of cardiac muscle.[1,7]	A vasopressive medication such as epinephrine may be given during CPR to improve cardiac output and blood pressure.[4] It has been proven to assist with initial resuscitation although there is no evidence that it improves the rate of survival to hospital discharge.[2,7]

*Level D: Peer-reviewed professional and organizational standards with the support of clinical study recommendations.

Procedure   for Defibrillation (External)—*Continued*

Steps	Rationale	Special Considerations
16. If the second attempt is unsuccessful, continue CPR and immediately charge the paddles to 360 J (monophasic) or device-specific value (escalating; biphasic) and repeat Steps 8–14. **(Level D*)**	Immediate action increases the chance of successful subsequent depolarization of cardiac muscle.[1,7]	An antidysrhythmic medication such as amiodarone or lidocaine may be given during CPR to assist in terminating the dysrhythmia. There is no evidence that the use of an antidysrhythmic medication will increase long-term survival or survival with a positive neurologic outcome after cardiac arrest.[4]
17. If the third attempt is unsuccessful, continue with ACLS. **(Level D*)**	Actions necessary to maintain the delivery of oxygenated blood to vital organs.[2,7]	BLS must be continued throughout resuscitation.[2,7]
18. Obtain vital signs and assess level of consciousness.	Determines patient response to defibrillation.	
19. Transfer patient to a critical care unit (if not there already).	Continues assessment and medical intervention.[7]	
20. After the emergency has ended, clean the defibrillator and remove the gel.	Prepares emergency equipment for future use.	
21. If the self-adhesive defibrillation pads were used, evaluate the placement and integrity of the pads.	Self-adhesive defibrillation pads may crimp, crack, or fold with loss of adhesiveness.	Loss of adhesive integrity in self-adhesive defibrillator pads can occur in restless or diaphoretic patients.
22. Remove **PE** and discard used supplies in appropriate receptacle.	Reduces transmission of microorganisms; standard precautions.	
23. **HH**		

*Level D: Peer-reviewed professional and organizational standards with the support of clinical study recommendations.

Expected Outcomes

- Reestablishment of a single source of impulse generation for the cardiac muscle
- Hemodynamic stability

Unexpected Outcomes

- Continued ventricular fibrillation
- Continued cardiopulmonary arrest
- Asystole
- Myocardial infarction (MI)
- Respiratory complications
- Cerebral anoxia and brain death
- Systemic embolization
- Hypotension
- Pacemaker or ICD dysfunction
- Skin burns
- Pain

Procedure continues on following page

Patient Monitoring and Care

Steps	Rationale	Reportable Conditions
		These conditions should be reported if they persist despite nursing interventions.
1. Evaluate neurological status before and after defibrillation. Reorient as necessary to person, place, and time.	Altered level of consciousness may occur after cardiac arrest.[3,7]	• Change in level of consciousness
2. If patient's neurological status is decreased (unable to follow verbal commands), prepare for procedures to achieve targeted temperature management. Maintain patient's temperature between 32°C to 36°C for 24 hours. Follow institution standards.	Therapeutic hypothermia has been shown to improve neurological recovery for patients post cardiac arrest.[3,5,7]	• Core temperature >32–36°C during treatment protocol
3. Monitor the patient's airway and pulmonary status after defibrillation.	Goal is to support cardiac and pulmonary function to optimize tissue perfusion to vital organs, especially the brain.[3,7]	• Change in respirations • Change in breath sounds • Decreased oxygen saturation as measured with pulse oximetry • Abnormal arterial blood gas results • Abnormal $Paco_2$ results • Abnormal $ETco_2$ results
4. Prepare for insertion of an advanced airway if patient remains unconscious or unresponsive and administer 10–12 breaths/min to achieve a $Paco_2$ of 35–45 mm Hg or an $ETco_2$ of 30–40 mm Hg. Mechanical ventilatory support may be necessary.	Hyperventilation of the patient should be avoided as it may cause adverse hemodynamic effects secondary to increased thoracic pressure. It may also decrease $Paco_2$ leading to decreased cerebral blood flow.[3,7]	
5. Administer sedation and analgesia in mechanically ventilated patients as prescribed.	Intubation and mechanical ventilation can cause the patient pain and anxiety.[3]	• Continued pain or anxiety despite interventions
6. Administer oxygen therapy as prescribed.	Goal is to administer enough oxygen to maintain oxygen saturation (Sao_2) ≥94% and to avoid oxygen toxicity.[3,7]	• Sao_2 <94%
7. Monitor vital signs immediately after defibrillation and at least every 15 minutes until stable.	Vital signs should stabilize after achieving a normal heart rate and rhythm.	• Hypotension • Hypertension • Tachycardia • Bradycardia
8. Administer intravenous fluids or vasopressive medications to support cardiac output and maintain normal blood pressure as prescribed.	Goal is a systolic blood pressure ≥90 mm Hg or mean arterial pressure ≥65 mm Hg.[3,5,7]	• Hypotension • Hypertension
9. Continue to monitor the ECG after defibrillation.	Postdefibrillation dysrhythmias may occur. Administration of antidysrhythmic medications may be prescribed.[2,4,7]	• Dysrhythmias
10. Monitor electrolyte levels.	Abnormal electrolyte levels may have contributed to the development of ventricular dysrhythmias.	• Abnormal electrolyte results
11. Obtain a 12-lead ECG and prepare for emergent coronary angiography if warranted.	Cardiac arrest may be caused by acute coronary syndrome.[3,5]	• ECG changes

Patient Monitoring and Care —*Continued*

Steps	Rationale	Reportable Conditions
12. Assess for burns.	Erythema at electrode sites may be seen from local hyperemia in the current pathway. Skin burns may be minimized with use of gel pads or placement of appropriate paste or gel on the paddles. Local cold application to electrode site after defibrillation may decrease the incidence and severity of burns and pain at the site.[8]	• Skin burns
13. Consider other possible causes for ventricular fibrillation or pulseless ventricular tachycardia.	Interventions may be aimed at correcting underlying pathophysiology and preventing the recurrence of lethal dysrhythmias.[3,7]	
14. Closely monitor neurological status.	The goal is to return patients to their precardiac arrest neurological function.[3,7]	• Changes in level of consciousness • Changes in neurological examination

Documentation

Documentation should include the following:

- Neurological, pulmonary, and cardiovascular assessments before and after defibrillation
- Interventions to prepare the patient for defibrillation
- The joules (J) used and the number of defibrillation attempts made
- Printout of ECG tracings that depict the cardiac rhythm before and after defibrillation
- Pain assessment, interventions, and effectiveness
- Patient response to defibrillation
- Condition of skin of the chest wall
- Unexpected outcomes and nursing interventions
- Patient and family education

References and Additional Readings

For a complete list of references and additional readings for this procedure, scan this QR code with any freely available smartphone code reader app, or visit http://booksite.elsevier.com/9780323376624.

37 Defibrillation (Internal) Perform

Marion E. McRae

PURPOSE: The purpose of internal defibrillation is to deliver electrical current directly to the epicardial surface of the heart via sterile internal defibrillation paddles when a shockable rhythm is present.

PREREQUISITE NURSING KNOWLEDGE

- Cardiac arrest after cardiac surgery, which occurs in about 0.7% to 2.9% of patients, is the most common scenario in which internal defibrillation is needed.[3,11]
- Understanding is needed of cardiovascular anatomy and physiology, principles of cardiac conduction, dysrhythmia interpretation, and electrical safety.
- Advanced cardiac life support knowledge and skills are needed.
- If open-chest resuscitation with internal defibrillation is attempted in cardiac arrest, it should be performed within the first 5 minutes after cardiac arrest for the best outcomes.[11]
- Clinical and technical competence in the use of the defibrillator is needed.
- Knowledge of aseptic and sterile technique is necessary.
- Emergent sternotomy or thoracotomy precedes internal defibrillation (see Procedure 39).
- Knowledge of internal paddle placement and energy requirements for internal defibrillation is needed.
- Internal paddle placement should ensure that the axis of the heart is situated between the sources of current.
- Energy requirements for internal defibrillation usually range from 5 to 20 J for biphasic shocks and 10 to 40 J for monophasic shocks.[11] It has been suggested that biphasic shocks for ventricular fibrillation and pulseless ventricular tachycardia should start at 10 to 20 J[10] or at 20 J.[1] Biphasic shocks are more effective than monophasic shocks at the same energy level in internal defibrillation.[10,12] The amount of myocardial damage from internal defibrillation does not differ between monophasic and biphasic shocks.[12]

EQUIPMENT

- Surgical head covers, masks, eye protection, sterile gowns, sterile gloves, large sterile drape
- Open sternotomy or thoracotomy tray

- Large sterile suction catheter (Yankauer), sterile tubing, suction canisters, suction regulator, and suction source
- Sterile internal paddles (ensure compatibility with the defibrillator). Adult internal paddles are usually 5 to 7.5 cm in diameter.
- Defibrillator

Additional equipment, to have available as needed, includes the following:
- Intubation equipment
- Flow meter for oxygen administration
- Bag-valve device with mask capable of delivering 100% oxygen and at least 500-mL volumes
- Intravenous (IV) fluids (e.g., 500 mL of normal saline)
- Emergency medications
- Temporary pacemaker equipment
- Antiseptic skin prep solution (e.g., 2% chlorhexidene-based preparation)

PATIENT AND FAMILY EDUCATION

- Teaching may need to be performed after the procedure. *Rationale:* Internal defibrillation usually is performed in the face of sudden hemodynamic collapse.
- Explain to the family the need for internal defibrillation. *Rationale:* This information keeps the family informed.

PATIENT ASSESSMENT AND PREPARATION

Patient Assessment

- Assess for dysrhythmias, especially ventricular ectopy. *Rationale:* Ventricular dysrhythmias may precede ventricular tachycardia and ventricular fibrillation.
- Assess vital signs when dysrhythmias occur. *Rationale:* This assessment provides data about the patient's response to dysrhythmias.
- Assess for pulseless ventricular tachycardia or ventricular fibrillation. *Rationale:* Assessment determines the need for resuscitation, which includes internal cardiac defibrillation. If immediate intervention is not initiated, return of circulation may not be possible.

Patient Preparation

- Verify correct patient with two identifiers. *Rationale:* Before performing a procedure, the nurse should ensure

AP   This procedure should be performed only by physicians, advanced practice nurses, and other healthcare professionals (including critical care nurses) with additional knowledge, skills, and demonstrated competence per professional licensure or institutional standard.

310

the correct identification of the patient for the intended intervention.

- Ensure the patient has a patent airway and ventilation before the initiation of the procedure. Assign responsibility to this task to another qualified provider. ***Rationale:*** The patient's airway is protected and maintained, and a means for adequate ventilation and oxygenation is provided.
- Place the patient in a flat supine position. ***Rationale:*** This position provides the best access during the procedure and during intervention for management of adverse effects.

- Prepare for this procedure by opening the chest and draping the patient in a sterile fashion (refer to Procedure 39). ***Rationale:*** Allows the internal paddles to be inserted into the patient's chest.
- Remove all metallic objects from the patient's skin. ***Rationale:*** Metallic objects are conductors of electrical current and may cause burns.
- Order sedation and analgesia as needed. ***Rationale:*** Promotes patient comfort.

Procedure	for Internal Defibrillation	
Steps	**Rationale**	**Special Considerations**
1. HH		
2. PE		
3. Confirm that the patient is in ventricular fibrillation *or* pulseless ventricular tachycardia.	Reconfirms that defibrillation is needed.	External defibrillation should be attempted first whenever possible (see Procedure 36) unless the chest is already open and there is rapid access for internal defibrillation. Follow institution's standard.
4. Initiate basic and advanced cardiac life support.[11] **(Level D*)**	Life-saving interventions are necessary.	It is controversial whether external cardiac compressions (because of potential damage to the postoperative cardiac patient) should be started if rapid defibrillation can be accomplished.[2,8] External cardiac compressions should be delivered while awaiting a defibrillator.[6] The American Heart Association's 2010 advanced cardiovascular life support guidelines recommend external chest compressions if emergency resternotomy is not immediately available.[11] Deformation of transcatheter aortic valves with external chest compressions has been reported.[5,9] Left hemithorax compressions may be safer with transcatheter than compressions over the sternum.[9] Follow institution's standards regarding initiation of external cardiac compressions.

*Level D: Peer-reviewed professional and organizational standards with the support of clinical study recommendations.

Procedure continues on following page

Procedure for Internal Defibrillation—*Continued*

Steps	Rationale	Special Considerations
5. Don sterile equipment.	Prepares for sterile procedure.	The physician, advanced practice nurse, or other healthcare professional(s) performing the procedure should perform hand antisepsis and hand scrub if possible.[1,4] However, if a closed sleeve technique for gowning and gloving technique is used, handwashing is not necessary in cardiac arrest as it delays resuscitation. Increased time to defibrillation decreases the likelihood of successful resuscitation.[1]
6. If there is blood/fluid in the mediastinum, connect a sterile Yankauer suction to a sterile suction tubing and suction the mediastinum before defibrillation.	Fluid/blood may need to be evacuated from the mediastinum before defibrillation.	
7. Ask for internal paddles (Fig. 37-1) to be opened and placed on the sterile field and hand off the connection cable for the defibrillator to an unsterile assistant to connect to the defibrillator.	Prepares the equipment.	

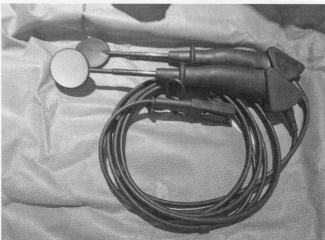

Figure 37-1   Internal paddles. *(Courtesy Marion E. McRae.)*

Steps	Rationale	Special Considerations
8. If the internal paddles are two-part paddles, connect the defibrillation paddles to the handles (usually via screw mechanism).	Prepares the equipment.	
9. Identify the number of joules the defibrillator is to be charged to (usually 5–20 J for biphasic shocks, 10–40 J for monophasic shocks).[11,12] **(Level D*)**	The lowest energy level that will convert the rhythm and minimize damage to the myocardium is used.	Biphasic shocks of 5–20 J usually are sufficient to convert pulseless rhythms.[10–12] Refer to the defibrillator manufacturer's operation guidelines for specific recommendations and follow institution guidelines.

*Level D: Peer-reviewed professional and organizational standards with the support of clinical study recommendations.

Procedure	for Internal Defibrillation—*Continued*	
Steps	**Rationale**	**Special Considerations**

Steps	Rationale	Special Considerations
10. Position one paddle over the right atrium or right ventricle; the other paddle is placed over the apex of the heart (Fig. 37-2).	This will aid in depolarizing the entire myocardium.	

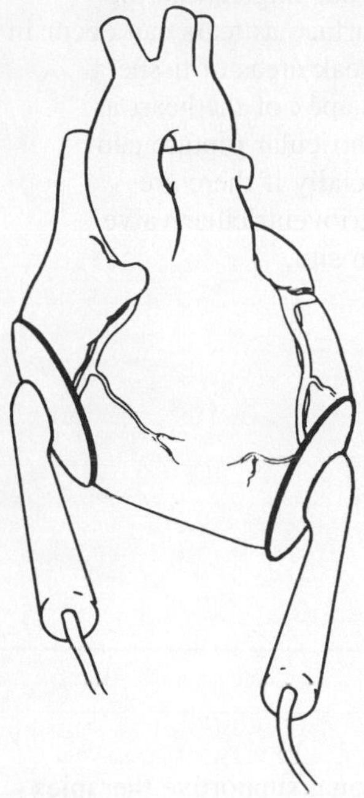

Figure 37-2 Paddle placement for internal defibrillation. *(From Kinkade S, Lohrman JE: Critical care nursing procedures: a team approach, Philadelphia, 1990, BC Decker.)*

Steps	Rationale	Special Considerations
11. State "all clear" three times and visually verify that all personnel are clear of contact with the patient, bed, and equipment.	Electrical current can be conducted from the patient to another person if contact occurs.	Use a mnemonic such as "I'm clear, you're clear, we're all clear," and look at the patient while talking to ensure that no one is touching or is in contact with the patient.
12. Simultaneously depress and hold the buttons on each paddle until the defibrillator discharges if the paddles are equipped with defibrillation buttons. If the paddles are not equipped with defibrillation buttons, ask for the defibrillation button on the defibrillator to be activated. **(Level M*)**	In the defibrillation mode, an immediate release of the electrical charge depolarizes cardiac muscle. Simultaneous depolarization of the myocardial muscle cells may result in simultaneous repolarization of enough myocardial cells to reestablish a single cardiac impulse.	Follow manufacturer's recommendations.
13. Assess the patient's response to defibrillation (heart rate and rhythm, blood pressure, level of consciousness).	Determines whether additional interventions may be needed.	

*Level M: Manufacturer's recommendations only

Procedure continues on following page

Procedure for Internal Defibrillation—*Continued*

Steps	Rationale	Special Considerations
A. If the first defibrillation is not successful, perform additional defibrillations as needed.[11] **(Level D*)**	Continues emergency treatment.	
B. Open chest cardiac compressions may be initiated if needed: i. Place one hand around the surface of the apex of the heart toward the posterior aspect of the heart with the palm up and fingers straight. ii. Avoid lifting the apex of the heart. iii. Avoid any grafts or other structures on the heart such as epicardial pacemaker leads. iv. Place the palm of the other hand on the anterior surface of the heart keeping the fingers straight. v. Squeeze the heart between your two hands at 100/min.[4] **(Level E*)**	Open-chest cardiac compression may be initiated if internal defibrillation is not successful. Internal cardiac massage is superior to external cardiac massage.[4]	Do not press your fingers into the epicardial surface as tears can occur in thinner or weak areas of tissue. Do not lift the apex of the heart as posterior ventricular rupture can occur,[4] especially if there are prosthetic atrioventricular valve prostheses in situ.
C. If defibrillation is successful, obtain vital signs and assess the patient.	Aids in determining whether additional interventions are needed.	Provide additional supportive therapies as needed. Epicardial pacing and vasoactive agents may be needed.
14. Prepare the patient for transfer to the operating room to close the chest; cover the patient's chest with a sterile drape or sterile occlusive dressing before transporting the patient to the operating room.	Prepares for chest closure.	Follow institution standard for closing the chest in the unit or in the operating room. The chest may be left open with a sterile occlusive dressing in place particularly if the patient remains unstable.
15. Remove sharps from the open chest tray and discard in a sharp container.	Reduces risk for injury.	
16. Place the internal paddles in the appropriate bag or container and ensure that it is sent for decontamination, disinfection, and sterilization.	Prepares for sterilization of equipment.	Follow manufacturer and institutional guidelines for cleansing the defibrillator and internal paddles. Discard disposable internal paddles if used.
17. Remove PE and sterile equipment and discard used supplies in appropriate receptacles.	Reduces the transmission of microorganisms; Standard Precautions.	
18. HH		
19. Request that sterile internal paddles and an open chest tray are immediately restocked.	Prepares for another emergency.	

*Level D: Peer-reviewed professional and organizational standards with the support of clinical study recommendations.
*Level E: Multiple case reports, theory-based evidence from expert opinions, or peer-reviewed professional organizational standards without clinical studies to support recommendations.

Expected Outcomes

- Reestablishment of a single origin of the cardiac impulse
- Hemodynamic stability

Unexpected Outcomes

- Inability to resuscitate; death
- Cerebral anoxia, brain impairment
- Infection
- Myocardial injury (e.g., from hypoxia, defibrillation, sternotomy/thoracotomy, internal compressions)
- Pain

Patient Monitoring and Care

Steps	Rationale	Reportable Conditions
		These conditions should be reported if they persist despite nursing interventions.
1. Continue to monitor the patient's cardiac rate and rhythm after defibrillation.	Dysrhythmias may develop.	• Dysrhythmias
2. Assess the patient's neurological status after defibrillation. Order the frequency of neurological assessments. If resuscitation is successful but the patient remains unresponsive after the resuscitation, consideration should be given to therapeutic hypothermia at 32–34°C for at least 12–24 hours.[7] (**Level E* in this population**)	Determines patient's neurological status after arrest and defibrillation. The benefit of therapeutic hypothermia in cardiac arrest after cardiac surgery is unknown. However, due to the strength of evidence in other populations it should be considered. Hypothermia can impair coagulation which is a concern if a patient is bleeding.	• Change in level of consciousness
3. Order arterial blood gases and ventilator settings for ongoing patient care.	Determines oxygenation and acid-base balance after arrest and defibrillation and provides for ongoing respiratory support.	• Abnormal respirations • Abnormal oxygen saturation • Abnormal arterial blood gas results
4. Order vital sign monitoring immediately after defibrillation and at least every 15 minutes until stable.	Determines the patient's hemodynamic stability.	• Abnormal vital signs
5. Prescribe intravenous antidysrhythmic medications as needed.	Antidysrhythmic medications may be prescribed to prevent or control dysrhythmias.	• Dysrhythmias
6. Order hemoglobin/hematocrit levels if blood loss occurred during the procedure.	Ensures sufficient hemoglobin for oxygen transport.	• Abnormal hemoglobin and hematocrit results
7. Order blood replacement products if needed.	Replaces blood loss that occurred during the procedure.	
8. Order electrolyte levels and replace electrolytes if low.	Abnormal electrolyte levels may contribute to the development of ventricular dysrhythmias.	• Abnormal electrolyte results
9. Order and interpret a 12-lead electrocardiogram (ECG).	Assesses for myocardial ischemia.	• ECG abnormalities
10. Order analgesia and sedation as needed.	Ensures patient comfort.	• Continued pain or agitation despite pain and sedation interventions

---

*Level E: Multiple case reports, theory-based evidence from expert opinions, or peer-reviewed professional organizational standards without clinical studies to support recommendations

Procedure continues on following page

Documentation

Documentation should include the following:

- Orders given during the resuscitation
- A procedure note describing the procedure performed, the sequential events occurring, patient assessment before and after defibrillation, and complications of the procedure
- Printout of ECG tracings with cardiac events before, during, and after each defibrillation
- Patient response to defibrillation
- Pain assessment, interventions, and effectiveness
- Medications and IV fluids given during the resuscitation

- Any unexpected outcomes and interventions taken
- Amount of chest drainage/blood loss
- Time chest was covered with a sterile occlusive dressing or when the chest was closed.
- Laboratory values obtained immediately before and after defibrillation.
- Family notification of the event.
- Patient (if applicable) and family education about the event

References and Additional Readings

For a complete list of references and additional readings for this procedure, scan this QR code with any freely available smartphone code reader app, or visit http://booksite.elsevier.com/9780323376624.

38

Defibrillation (Internal) Assist

Marion E. McRae

PURPOSE: The purpose of internal defibrillation is to deliver electrical current directly to the epicardial surface of the heart when a shockable rhythm is present.

PREREQUISITE NURSING KNOWLEDGE

- Cardiac arrest after cardiac surgery, which occurs in about 0.7% to 2.9% of patients, is the most common scenario in which internal defibrillation is needed.[6] About 25% to 50% of cardiac arrest after cardiac surgery results from ventricular fibrillation.[1]
- Understanding is needed of cardiovascular anatomy and physiology, principles of cardiac conduction, dysrhythmia interpretation, and electrical safety.
- Advanced cardiac life support knowledge and skills are needed.
- If open-chest resuscitation with internal defibrillation is attempted in cardiac arrest, it should be performed within the first 5 minutes after cardiac arrest for the best outcome.[2,6]
- Clinical competence in the use of the defibrillator is needed.
- Knowledge of aseptic and sterile technique is necessary.
- Emergent open sternotomy or thoracotomy precedes internal defibrillation (see Procedures 39 and 40).
- Energy requirements for internal defibrillation usually range from 5 to 20 J for biphasic (electrical current goes from one paddle to the other and then back to the first paddle) shocks and 10 to 40 J for monophasic (electrical current travels from one paddle to the other) shocks.[6] It has been suggested that biphasic shocks for ventricular fibrillation or pulseless ventricular tachycardia should start at 10 to 20 J[3] or 20 J.[1] Biphasic shocks are more effective than monophasic shocks at the same energy level in internal defibrillation.[5,7] The amount of myocardial damage from internal defibrillation does not differ between monophasic and biphasic shocks.[7]

EQUIPMENT

- Surgical head covers, masks, eye protection, sterile gowns, sterile gloves, large sterile drape
- Open sternotomy or thoracotomy tray
- Large sterile suction catheter (Yankauer), sterile tubing, suction canisters, suction regulator, and suction source
- Sterile internal paddles (ensure compatibility with the defibrillator). Adult internal paddles are usually 5 to 7.5 cm in diameter.
- Defibrillator

Additional equipment, to have available as needed, includes the following:

- Intubation equipment
- Flow meter for oxygen administration
- Bag-valve device with mask capable of delivering 100% oxygen and at least 500-mL volumes
- Intravenous (IV) fluids (e.g., 500 mL of normal saline)
- Emergency medications
- Temporary pacemaker equipment
- Antiseptic skin prep solution (e.g., 2% chlorhexidine-based preparation)

PATIENT AND FAMILY EDUCATION

- Teaching may need to be performed after the procedure. *Rationale:* Internal defibrillation usually is performed in the face of sudden hemodynamic collapse.
- Explain to the family the need for internal defibrillation. *Rationale:* This information keeps the family informed.

PATIENT ASSESSMENT AND PREPARATION

Patient Assessment

- Assess for dysrhythmias, especially ventricular ectopy. *Rationale:* Ventricular dysrhythmias may precede ventricular tachycardia and ventricular fibrillation.
- Assess vital signs when dysrhythmias occur. *Rationale:* This assessment provides data about the patient's response to dysrhythmias.
- Assess for pulseless ventricular tachycardia or ventricular fibrillation. *Rationale:* Assessment determines the need for resuscitation, which may include internal cardiac defibrillation. If immediate intervention is not initiated, return of circulation may not be possible.

Patient Preparation

- Verify correct patient with two identifiers. *Rationale:* Before performing a procedure, the nurse should ensure the correct identification of the patient for the intended intervention.
- Ensure the patient has a patent airway and ventilation before the initiation of the procedure. *Rationale:* The patient's airway is protected and maintained, and a means for adequate ventilation and oxygenation is provided.

- Place the patient in a flat supine position. *Rationale:* This position provides the best access during the procedure and during intervention for management of adverse effects.
- Remove all metallic objects from the patient's skin. *Rationale:* Metallic objects are conductors of electrical current and may cause burns.

- Establish or ensure patency of IV access. *Rationale:* Medication administration may be necessary.
- Administer sedation and analgesia as prescribed. *Rationale:* Promotes patient comfort.

Procedure for Defibrillation Internal

Steps	Rationale	Special Considerations
1. **HH**		
2. **PE**		
3. Confirm that the patient is in ventricular fibrillation or pulseless ventricular tachycardia.	Reconfirms that defibrillation is needed.	External defibrillation should be attempted first whenever possible (see Procedure 36) unless the chest is already open and there is rapid access for internal defibrillation.
4. Initiate basic and advanced cardiac life support.[3,6] **(Level D*)**	Life-saving interventions are necessary.	Follow institution standards regarding initiating external cardiac compressions.
5. Assist the physician, advanced practice nurse, or other healthcare provider performing the procedure with applying personal protective and sterile equipment.	Prepares for sterile procedure.	The provider performing the procedure should perform hand antisepsis and hand scrub if possible.[1,3] However, if a closed sleeve technique for gowning and gloving is used, handwashing is not necessary in cardiac arrest as it delays resuscitation. Increased time to defibrillation decreases the likelihood of successful resuscitation.[1]
6. As needed, place a sterile Yankauer and suction tubing onto the sterile field.	Fluid/blood may need to be evacuated from the mediastinum before defibrillation.	
7. As needed, have the provider performing the procedure hand one end of the suction tubing back to you to connect to the suction source.	Prepares equipment.	
8. Ensure that the defibrillator is positioned within reach of the defibrillator cables with the screen facing toward the provider performing the procedure if possible.	Facilitates access to the defibrillator.	The defibrillator cannot touch the patient, field, or healthcare providers but must be close enough to treat the patient.
9. When requested open the package with the internal paddles and place them on the sterile field.	Prepares equipment.	
10. Connect the internal paddle cable to the defibrillator when the healthcare provider performing the procedure hands the cable off the sterile field to you.	Prepares the equipment.	Maintain asepsis by not touching the healthcare provider handing off the paddle cable. Use caution when pulling the connector to the defibrillator so that objects on the sterile field are not dislodged or entangled.

*Level D: Peer-reviewed professional and organizational standards with the support of clinical study recommendations.

Procedure	for Defibrillation Internal—*Continued*	
Steps	**Rationale**	**Special Considerations**
11. Charge the defibrillator when requested to the prescribed energy level (usually 5–20 J for biphasic shocks, 10–40 J for monophasic shocks).[6,7] **(Level D*)**	The defibrillator is charged with the lowest energy level necessary to convert the rhythm and minimize damage to the myocardium.	Biphasic shocks of 5–20 J usually are sufficient to convert ventricular tachycardia or ventricular fibrillation.[5-7] Refer to the defibrillator manufacturer's operation guidelines for specific recommendations and to your institutional policy.
12. Ensure that the healthcare provider delivering the shock states "all clear" three times and visually verifies that all personnel are clear of contact with the patient, bed, and equipment.	Electrical current can be conducted from the patient to another person if contact occurs.	
13. If the internal paddles being used can only be discharged by depressing the defibrillation button on the defibrillator, press the button when all personnel are clear. (Some internal paddles are equipped with a defibrillation button that the provider can activate on the paddles). **(Level M*)**	In the defibrillation mode, an immediate release of the electrical charge depolarizes cardiac muscle. Simultaneous depolarization of the myocardial muscle cells may result in simultaneous repolarization of enough myocardial cells to reestablish a single cardiac impulse.	Follow manufacturer's recommendations.
14. Assess the patient's response to defibrillation (heart rate and rhythm, blood pressure, level of consciousness):	Determines whether additional interventions may be needed.	
A. If the first defibrillation is not successful, assist the team with additional defibrillations as needed.	Continues emergency treatment.	
B. If defibrillation is successful, obtain vital signs and assess the patient.	Aids in determining whether additional interventions are needed.	Provide additional supportive therapies as needed. Epicardial pacing and vasoactive agents may be prescribed.
15. Assist with transferring the patient to the operating room.	Prepares for chest closure.	Follow institution standard for closing the chest in the unit or in the operating room. The chest may be left open with a sterile occlusive dressing in place particularly if the patient remains unstable.
16. Assist as needed with placing the internal paddles in the appropriate bag or container and ensure that it is sent for decontamination, disinfection, and sterilization.	Prepares for sterilization of equipment.	

*Level D: Peer-reviewed professional and organizational standards with the support of clinical study recommendations.
*Level M: Manufacturer's recommendations only.

Procedure continues on following page

Procedure for Defibrillation Internal—*Continued*

Steps	Rationale	Special Considerations
17. Remove **PE** and discard used supplies in appropriate receptacles.	Reduces the transmission of microorganisms; Standard Precautions.	
18. **HH**		
19. Obtain sterile internal paddles to restock emergency supplies.	Prepares for another emergency.	

Expected Outcomes

- Reestablishment of a single origin of the cardiac impulse
- Hemodynamic stability

Unexpected Outcomes

- Inability to resuscitate; death
- Cerebral anoxia, brain impairment
- Infection
- Myocardial injury (e.g., from hypoxia, defibrillation, sternotomy/thoracotomy, internal compressions)
- Pain

Patient Monitoring and Care

Steps	Rationale	Reportable Conditions
		These conditions should be reported if they persist despite nursing interventions.
1. Continue to monitor the patient's cardiac rate and rhythm after defibrillation.	Dysrhythmias may develop.	• Dysrhythmias
2. Assess the patient's neurological status after defibrillation. Initiate therapeutic hypothermia if prescribed. (**Level E* in this population**)[1,3,4]	Determines patient's neurological status after arrest and defibrillation.	• Change in level of consciousness
3. Monitor the patient's vital signs immediately after defibrillation and at least every 15 minutes until stable.	Determines the patient's hemodynamic stability.	• Abnormal vital signs
4. Initiate intravenous antidysrhythmic medications as prescribed.	Antidysrhythmic medications may be prescribed to prevent or control dysrhythmias.	• Dysrhythmias
5. Obtain blood samples for laboratory analysis as prescribed (e.g., electrolyte levels).	Abnormal electrolyte levels may contribute to the development of ventricular dysrhythmias (specifically low potassium and magnesium levels).	• Abnormal electrolyte results
6. After successful internal defibrillation obtain a 12-lead electrocardiogram (ECG) if prescribed.	Assesses for myocardial ischemia.	• ECG abnormalities
7. Administer analgesia and sedation as prescribed.	Ensures patient comfort.	• Continued pain or agitation despite pain and sedation interventions

*Level E: Multiple case reports, theory-based evidence from expert opinions, or peer-reviewed professional organizational standards without clinical studies to support recommendations.

Documentation

Documentation should include the following:

- Cardiovascular, respiratory, and neurological assessments before and after defibrillation
- Each defibrillation and joules used
- Printout of ECG tracings with cardiac events before, during, and after each defibrillation
- Patient response to defibrillation
- Pain assessment, interventions and effectiveness
- Medications and IV fluids given during the resuscitation

- Any unexpected outcomes and interventions taken
- Amount of chest drainage
- Any unexpected outcomes and interventions taken
- Laboratory values obtained immediately before, during, and after defibrillation
- Family notification of the event
- Patient (if applicable) and family education about the event

References and Additional Readings

For a complete list of references and additional readings for this procedure, scan this QR code with any freely available smartphone code reader app, or visit http://booksite.elsevier.com/9780323376624.

39 Emergent Open Sternotomy AP (Perform)

Alice Chan

PURPOSE: Emergent open sternotomy for a patient after cardiac surgery is performed to identify and eliminate areas of persistent hemorrhage, relieve pericardial tamponade, and provide access for open cardiac massage and internal defibrillation.

PREREQUISITE NURSING KNOWLEDGE

- Knowledge of anatomy and physiology of the cardiovascular system is necessary.
- Advanced cardiac life support knowledge and skills are needed.
- Understanding of the signs and symptoms of cardiac tamponade is necessary.
- Emergent open sternotomy is performed for patients who have undergone a median sternotomy.
- Emergent open sternotomy is indicated for exsanguinating hemorrhage or cardiac tamponade with imminent cardiac arrest.[4,7]
  - The goal of mediastinal exploration for persistent hemorrhage is to stop the bleeding and retain circulating blood volume. The requirement for homologous blood transfusion and incidence of wound infection associated with an undrained mediastinal hematoma may be decreased.[2]
  - The goal of mediastinal exploration for cardiac tamponade is to relieve the pressure on the ventricles during diastole. The decreased pressure allows the ventricles to fill during diastole, which should increase contractility, stroke volume, and cardiac output to improve systemic perfusion.
- Knowledge and skills related to aseptic and sterile technique, surgical instrumentation, sternal opening, sternal exploration, sternal closure, and suturing are needed.[1,4-6]
- Paralytic agents may be a necessary adjunct to sedation and analgesia to improve oxygenation, diminish muscle activity, and enhance visualization.
- Internal defibrillation may be necessary if life-threatening dysrhythmias occur (see Procedure 37).

EQUIPMENT

- Antiseptic solution (e.g., 2% chlorhexidine gluconate skin preparation)
- Head cover, masks, eye protection, sterile gown, sterile gloves, sterile drapes
- Sterile thoracic pack and sternotomy tray
  - Wire cutter
  - Rib spreader
  - Kelly clamps and skin snaps
  - Knife handle
  - Scissors
- Electrocautery equipment: generator, cautery, electrical dispersing pad (e.g., grounding pad)
- Large sterile suction catheter (e.g., Yankauer)
- Suction containers, tubing, regulator, and suction source
- Radiopaque gauze or other surgical sponge materials
- Polypropylene (Prolene) suture (cutting needle) and other suture material according to preference
- Clip applicator and clips
- Syringes: 3 mL, 5 mL, 10 mL, and 20 mL
- Knife blades: Nos. 10, 11, 15
- Sternal wires or bands
- Sterile stapler or sutures
- Sterile dressing supplies
- Emergency medication and resuscitation equipment, including internal defibrillation paddles and external defibrillation pads or paddles
- Prescribed analgesia or sedation

Additional equipment, to have available as needed, includes the following:

- Prescribed blood products and intravenous solutions
- Warm saline solution with or without an antibiotic, as prescribed
- Chest tubes and chest tube drainage system
- Epicardial wires
- Intraaortic balloon catheter and pump console or other mechanical assist device
- Peripheral nerve stimulator (used if paralytic agents are administered)
- Sterile staple remover

AP   This procedure should be performed only by physicians, advanced practice nurses, and other healthcare professionals (including critical care nurses) with additional knowledge, skills, and demonstrated competence per professional licensure or institutional standard.

PATIENT AND FAMILY EDUCATION

- Teaching may not be provided until after the procedure. *Rationale:* When an emergent sternotomy is performed for rapid hemodynamic collapse, education of the patient and family may not be possible before the procedure.
- Explain the reason that the open sternotomy procedure was performed and its outcome or anticipated outcome. *Rationale:* This explanation provides information and encourages the patient and family to ask questions and clarify details about the patient and procedure.

PATIENT ASSESSMENT AND PREPARATION

Patient Assessment

- Assess hemodynamic and neurological status. *Rationale:* This assessment identifies baseline data that may indicate the need for emergent open sternotomy and provides comparison data.
- Assess the patient's medical history, specifically for coagulation disorders, renal disease with coexistent uremia, and functional status of the right and left ventricle. *Rationale:* Baseline data are obtained.
- Assess current laboratory data, specifically complete blood cell count, platelet count, international normalized ratio, activated partial thromboplastin time, and fibrinogen. *Rationale:* Near-normal baseline coagulation study results decrease the likelihood of coagulopathy as a possible cause for ongoing hemorrhage.
- Assess for signs and symptoms of cardiac tamponade. *Rationale:* The presence of some or all of these signs and symptoms help the physician, advanced practice nurse, or other healthcare professional determine whether the emergent open sternotomy is indicated:
  - ❖ Sudden decrease or cessation in chest tube drainage
  - ❖ Hypotension (mean arterial blood pressure, <60 mm Hg)
  - ❖ Altered mental status
  - ❖ Apical heart rate greater than 110 beats/min
  - ❖ Narrowing of pulse pressure

  - ❖ Distended neck veins
  - ❖ Distant heart sounds
  - ❖ Equalization of intracardiac pressures, including right atrial, pulmonary artery diastolic, and pulmonary artery occlusion pressures
  - ❖ Decreased cardiac output and cardiac index
- Pulsus paradoxus
- Assess for excessive chest tube drainage. *Rationale:* Severity of bleeding assists with the determination of the need for emergent mediastinal exploration. Follow the institution's guidelines regarding determination of the timing of mediastinal exploration. One recommendation for timing the procedure is when chest tube drainage continues at equal to or greater than 3 mL/kg/hr for at least 3 hours.[3]

Patient Preparation

- Verify that the patient is the correct patient using two identifiers. *Rationale:* Before performing a procedure, the nurse should ensure the correct identification of the patient for the intended intervention.
- Ensure that the patient and family understand procedural teaching (if time is available). Answer questions as they arise and reinforce information as needed. *Rationale:* Understanding of the information provided is evaluated and reinforced.
- Obtain informed consent (may not be possible if the procedure is an emergency). *Rationale:* Informed consent protects the rights of the patient and ensures a competent decision for the patient and the family.
- Perform a preprocedure verification and time out, if nonemergent. *Rationale:* Ensures patient safety.
- Ensure the patient's airway is protected and that supplemental oxygen is delivered. *Rationale:* The probability that the patient's ventilatory needs will be met is enhanced.
- Position the patient in the supine position with the head of the bed flat. *Rationale:* This position ensures visualization of the chest and enhances hemodynamic stability.
- Prescribe and ensure that an analgesic and/or sedative are administered. *Rationale:* Promotes patient comfort.

Procedure   for Performing Emergent Open Sternotomy

Steps	Rationale	Special Considerations
1. Call the physician and operative team.	The physician can assess the need for further surgical intervention. The operative team may be needed to assist at the bedside or to prepare the operating room if further exploration is needed.	Follow the institution's standard.
2. **HH**		
3. **PE**		
4. Prepare the electrocautery device for possible use: Apply the electrical dispersing pad (i.e., grounding pad) to the patient's dry skin over a large well perfused muscle mass and attach the grounding cable to the device.[1] **(Level D*)**	Electrocautery is used to terminate capillary oozing or bleeding.	Grounding is essential to avoid burning the patient and possible electrical shock to the healthcare providers. Electrocautery may not be immediately available in the critical care setting; follow institution standard.
5. Ensure that a new sterile suction system is set up.	Suction within the mediastinum is necessary during the procedure.	
6. Remove the sternal dressing and cleanse the chest with an antiseptic solution (e.g., 2% chlorhexidine gluconate solution). Remove gloves when cleansing is completed and wash hands.	Inhibits microorganism transmission.	Prepare the skin beginning at the incision line, extending outward to include the area from the chin to the midabdomen (caudal to the umbilicus) and to include the area outward to one anterior axillary line and then outward to the opposite anterior axillary line. Minimize solution from running off the surgical site, dripping, pooling, and soaking fabric and the patient's hair. Ensure alcohol-based preparation agents have not wet the patient's hair or bedding nor pooled in skin-folds or the umbilicus because the risk of fire is increased (nonflammable preparations eliminate the risk of fire).[1]

7. Don personal protective equipment and sterile equipment:
  A. Surgical head cover, mask, and eye protection.
  B. Perform hand antisepsis/hand scrub.
  C. Sterile gown and sterile gloves.
	Removes debris and transient microorganisms.[1]
	Inhibits rebound microorganism growth.[1]
		All personnel in the room must don caps and masks.

8. Ask the critical care nurse or person assisting to open the sternotomy tray and to hand it to the person performing the procedure.	Prepares equipment.	The critical care nurse or person assisting with the procedure can help by opening sterile packs and the instrument tray.

*Level D: Peer-reviewed professional and organizational standards with the support of clinical study recommendations.

Procedure	for Performing Emergent Open Sternotomy—*Continued*	
Steps	**Rationale**	**Special Considerations**
9. Fully drape the patient with exposure of only the surgical site.[1,3,5] **(Level D*)**	A large sterile field minimizes the risk of infection and provides space to maintain asepsis of instruments and supplies during the procedure.	Allows good view of the incision.
10. Hand off the distal end of the electrocautery cable (active electrode) to the critical care nurse or assisting healthcare provider.	Cautery is used to stop bleeding from small vessels.	The cautery control is not sterile. The connection must be handed off of the sterile field without the healthcare provider performing the procedure and the assisting personnel touching each other.
11. Open the incision down to the sternum with the staple remover or scalpel, exposing the sternal wires or bands.	Ensures visualization of the sternal wires or bands.	Remove staples with a staple remover; cut sutures and tissue with a scalpel.
12. Cut the sternal wires (or bands) from the top to the bottom with the wire cutter or untwist the wires with the heavy needle holder.	Provides access to the mediastinum. The sternal wires fatigue and break when untwisted with the heavy needle holders.	Use care when removing the sternal wires to minimize damage to the heart, underlying equipment (e.g., epicardial pacing wires, chest tubes), and coronary artery bypass grafts and injury to the healthcare provider.
13. With your hands, gently separate the sternum.	Caution must be taken to separate the sternum gently because the heart, bypass grafts, and pacing wires rest just under the sternal bone.	
14. Place the sternal retractor under the sternal bone. Slowly crank it open while feeling along the edge of the retractor blades and observing the mediastinal cavity and heart for anything caught in the retractor.	Exposes the heart and mediastinum.	Sternal retractor blades can trap and tear bypass grafts and pacing wires if caught and pulled apart when the retractor is cranked open.
15. For bleeding, apply pressure with a finger over any bleeding site and suction the remainder of the chest, evacuating any clots.	Pressure on the bleeding site may minimize blood loss.	Resuscitate with intravenous fluids, inotropic medications, and blood products as necessary.
16. Control and ligate bleeding sites, enhance the sternal retraction, and provide suctioning and electrocautery as needed.	May eliminate the need for further exploration and assists with better visualization of the surgical field.	The physician determines whether the patient needs to be transferred to the operating room for further surgical intervention.
17. If pulseless ventricular tachycardia or ventricular fibrillation occurs, internal defibrillation is needed (see Procedure 37).	Emergency intervention is needed.	The critical care nurse or additional assistive personal can help to obtain the defibrillator and the internal defibrillation paddles.
18. Insert or assist with insertion of chest tubes or epicardial pacing wires as needed.	Chest tubes and epicardial pacing wires can be displaced during sternal retraction or mediastinal exploration.	
19. Warm saline solution with or without an antibiotic may be used to flush the chest cavity before closing the incision.	May decrease the incidence of infection.	Determine whether additional antibiotic coverage is needed.

*Level D: Peer-reviewed professional and organizational standards with the support of clinical study recommendations.

Procedure continues on following page

Procedure	for Performing Emergent Open Sternotomy—*Continued*	
Steps	**Rationale**	**Special Considerations**
20. Assist with the placement of mechanical assist devices if needed.	Cardiac tamponade may conceal right or left ventricular dysfunction; mechanical assistance may be necessary to improve cardiac output.	
21. Assist with patient transport to the operating room if necessary.	The patient may need further exploration; surgical repair of coronary artery bypass grafts, cardiac valves, or the myocardium; or insertion of an assist device (e.g., intraaortic balloon pump, ventricular assist device).	Ensure that the patient's chest is covered with sterile drapes or with a dressing during transportation.

22. If the patient does not need to return to the operating room, assist the physician with reinsertion of sternal wires as follows:
  A. Grasp the sternal wire with the needle holder.
  B. From under the sternum, push one end of the wire up between two ribs at the sternal border.
  C. Repeat step B with the other end of the wire on the opposite side of the sternum (same intercostal space).
  D. Pull the sternum together with the wire and twist the edges of the wires together with the needle holder.
  E. Cut off the excess wire and bend the twisted edges flat against the sternum.
  F. Repeat with additional wires every two to three ribs until the sternum is closed.
	Ensures sternal closure.	Caution must be taken not to penetrate the heart, pericostal vessels, lungs, or bypass grafts with the sternal wires.
		Multiple wiring techniques can be used for sternal wound closure; the advanced practice nurse or physician performing the procedure may use an alternate method or use sternal bands to close the sternum.

23. Assist the physician with tissue and skin closure according to preference (staples or sutures).	Promotes wound healing.	The patient's chest may be left open and covered with a sterile occlusive dressing if severe tissue swelling or ventricular dysfunction exists.
24. Apply an occlusive dressing to the sternal incision, epicardial pacing wires, and chest tube sites.	Dressings provide a physical barrier to external sources of contamination and cushion from physical contact and trauma; they absorb drainage, maintain a moist environment at body temperature to enhance wound healing, and are used for aesthetics.	
25. Dispose of sharps per facility standard.[1,5]	Minimizes risk of sharps injury.	A chest radiograph may be prescribed to rule out the presence of any retained surgical sponges, needles, or instruments.

Patient Monitoring and Care —*Continued*

Steps	Rationale	Special Considerations
26. Discard used supplies in appropriate receptacles, and remove and discard **PE**.	Reduces the transmission of microorganisms and body secretions; Standard Precautions.	
27. **HH**		
28. Remove and package instruments for sterilization.	Prepares for another emergency.	

Expected Outcomes

- Resolution of the condition that necessitated the emergent open sternotomy
- Increased cardiac output
- Increased tissue perfusion, including cerebral, renal, and peripheral perfusion
- Minimal chest tube drainage
- Decreased need for blood transfusions

Unexpected Outcomes

- Severe right or left ventricular dysfunction
- Continued dysrhythmias, bleeding, or coagulation disorders
- Myocardial, aortic, coronary artery, or coronary artery bypass graft perforation
- Cardiac arrest
- Pneumothorax
- Intracardiac infarction
- Atrial and ventricular dysrhythmias
- Pain
- Surgical infection
- Death

Patient Monitoring and Care

Steps	Rationale	Reportable Conditions
		These conditions should be reported if they persist despite nursing interventions.
1. Perform cardiovascular, hemodynamic, and peripheral vascular assessments every 15–30 minutes as patient status requires (including vital signs, pulmonary artery pressures, cardiac index, level of consciousness, and urine output).	Determines hemodynamic stability and volume status; recurrent tamponade or dysrhythmias may develop during and after sternotomy. Determines the adequacy of cerebral perfusion; hemodynamic instability can lead to cerebral anoxia. Determines adequate perfusion to the kidneys.	• Mean arterial blood pressure <60 mm Hg • Abnormal changes in heart rate • Decrease in cardiac index • Abnormal pulmonary artery pressures • Urine output <0.5 mL/kg/hr • Equalizing pulmonary artery pressures • Change in level of consciousness
2. Assess heart and lung sounds every 2 hours and as needed.	Abnormal heart and lung sounds may indicate the need for additional treatment.	• Distant heart sounds • Abnormal lung sounds
3. Monitor coagulation, hematologic, and electrolyte laboratory blood study results.	Coagulation and hematologic profiles provide data that indicate the risk of bleeding and indicate the need for additional treatment. Electrolyte studies provide data regarding the risk for dysrhythmias and decreased contractility.	• Abnormal hemoglobin and hematocrit, activated partial thromboplastin time, international normalized ratio, platelets, fibrinogen, calcium, magnesium, or potassium
4. Closely monitor chest tube drainage.	Determines functioning of the chest tube drainage system and the amount of chest drainage.	• Cessation of chest tube drainage • Increased chest tube drainage • Clots in the chest tube drainage system
5. Assess pain and prescribe analgesia as needed.	Identifies need for pain interventions.	• Continued pain despite pain interventions

Procedure continues on following page

Documentation

Documentation should include the following:
- Patient and family education
- Signed informed consent, if nonemergent
- Universal Protocol requirement, if nonemergent
- Pain assessment, interventions and effectiveness
- Indications for the procedure and the procedure performed
- Amount of blood collected from chest suctioning; estimated blood loss

- Patient therapies and response, including hemodynamic parameters, inotropic or vasopressor agents, analgesia, sedation, ventilation, and neurological status
- Additional interventions
- Unexpected outcomes

References and Additional Readings

For a complete list of references and additional readings for this procedure, scan this QR code with any freely available smartphone code reader app, or visit http://booksite.elsevier.com/9780323376624.

Emergent Open Sternotomy (Assist)

Alice Chan

PURPOSE: Emergent open sternotomy for a patient after cardiac surgery is performed to identify and eliminate areas of persistent hemorrhage, relieve pericardial tamponade, and provide access for open cardiac massage and internal defibrillation.

PREREQUISITE NURSING KNOWLEDGE

- Knowledge of the anatomy and physiology of the cardiovascular system is necessary.
- Advanced cardiac life support knowledge and skills are needed.
- Understanding of signs and symptoms of cardiac tamponade is necessary.
- Emergency open sternotomy is performed for patients who have undergone a median sternotomy.
- Emergent open sternotomy is indicated for exsanguinating hemorrhage or cardiac tamponade with imminent cardiac arrest.[3,6]
  - ❖ The goal of mediastinal exploration for persistent hemorrhage is to stop the bleeding and retain circulating blood volume. The requirement for homologous blood transfusion and incidence of wound infection associated with an undrained mediastinal hematoma may be decreased.[3]
  - ❖ The goal of mediastinal exploration for cardiac tamponade is to relieve the pressure on the ventricles during diastole. The decreased pressure allows the ventricles to fill during diastole, which should increase contractility, stroke volume, and cardiac output to improve systemic perfusion.
- Knowledge and skills related to aseptic and sterile technique are needed.
- Paralytic agents may be a necessary adjunct to sedation and analgesia to improve oxygenation, diminish muscle activity, and enhance visualization.
- Internal defibrillation may be necessary if life-threatening dysrhythmias occur (see Procedures 37 and 38).

EQUIPMENT

- Antiseptic solution (e.g., 2% chlorhexidine gluconate skin preparation)
- Head cover, masks, eye protection, sterile gown, sterile gloves, sterile drapes
- Sterile thoracic pack and sternotomy tray
  - ❖ Wire cutter
  - ❖ Rib spreader

- ❖ Kelly clamps and skin snaps
- ❖ Knife handle
- ❖ Scissors
- Electrocautery equipment: generator, cautery, electrical dispersing pad (e.g., grounding pad)
- Large sterile suction catheter (e.g., Yankauer)
- Suction containers, tubing, regulator, and suction source
- Radiopaque gauze or other surgical sponge materials
- Polypropylene (Prolene) suture (cutting needle), other suture material as requested
- Clip applicator and clips
- Syringes: 3 mL, 5 mL, 10 mL, and 20 mL
- Knife blades: Nos. 10, 11, 15
- Sternal wires or bands
- Sterile stapler or sutures
- Sterile dressing supplies
- Emergency medication and resuscitation equipment

Additional equipment, to have available as needed, includes the following:

- Prescribed analgesia and sedation
- Blood products and intravenous solutions as prescribed
- Warm saline solution with or without an antibiotic, as prescribed
- Chest tubes and chest tube drainage system
- Epicardial wires
- Intraaortic balloon catheter and pump console or other mechanical assist device
- Peripheral nerve stimulator (used if paralytic agents are administered)
- Sterile staple remover

PATIENT AND FAMILY EDUCATION

- Teaching may not be provided until after the procedure. *Rationale:* When an emergent sternotomy is performed for rapid hemodynamic collapse, education of the patient and family may not be possible before the procedure.
- Explain the reason that the open sternotomy procedure was performed. *Rationale:* This explanation provides information and encourages the patient and family to ask questions and clarify details about the patient and procedure.

PATIENT ASSESSMENT AND PREPARATION

Patient Assessment

- Assess hemodynamic and neurological status. ***Rationale:*** This assessment identifies baseline data that may indicate the need for emergent open sternotomy and provides comparison data.
- Assess current laboratory data, specifically complete blood cell count, platelet count, international normalized ratio, activated partial thromboplastin time, and fibrinogen. ***Rationale:*** Near-normal baseline coagulation study results decrease the likelihood of coagulopathy as a possible cause for ongoing hemorrhage.
- Assess for signs and symptoms of cardiac tamponade. ***Rationale:*** The presence of some or all of these signs and symptoms assists the healthcare team to decide whether an emergent open sternotomy is necessary:
  - ❖ Sudden decrease or cessation in chest tube drainage
  - ❖ Hypotension (mean arterial blood pressure, <60 mm Hg)
  - ❖ Altered mental status
  - ❖ Apical heart rate greater than 110 beats/min
  - ❖ Narrowing of pulse pressure
  - ❖ Distended neck veins
  - ❖ Distant heart sounds
  - ❖ Equalization of intracardiac pressures, including right atrial, pulmonary artery diastolic, and pulmonary artery occlusion pressures
  - ❖ Decreased cardiac output and cardiac index
  - ❖ Pulsus paradoxus
- Assess for excessive chest tube drainage. ***Rationale:*** Presence of bleeding assists with the determination of the need for mediastinal exploration. Follow the institution's guidelines regarding determination of the timing of mediastinal exploration. One recommendation for timing the procedure is when chest tube drainage continues at equal to or greater than 3 mL/kg/hr for at least 3 hours.[2]

Patient Preparation

- Verify that the patient is the correct patient using two identifiers. ***Rationale:*** Before performing a procedure, the nurse should ensure the correct identification of the patient for the intended intervention.
- Ensure that the patient and family understand procedural teachings (if time available). Answer questions as they arise, and reinforce information as needed. ***Rationale:*** Understanding of the information provided is evaluated and reinforced.
- Ensure that informed consent was obtained (may not be possible if the procedure is an emergency). ***Rationale:*** Informed consent protects the rights of the patient and ensures a competent decision for the patient and the family.
- Perform a preprocedure verification and time out, if nonemergent. ***Rationale:*** Ensures patient safety.
- Ensure the patient's airway is protected and that supplemental oxygen is delivered. ***Rationale:*** Ensures adequate ventilation and oxygenation.
- Position the patient in the supine position with the head of the bed flat. ***Rationale:*** This position ensures visualization of the chest and enhances hemodynamic stability.
- Administer analgesia and sedation as prescribed. ***Rationale:*** Promotes patient comfort.

Procedure	for Assisting with Emergent Open Sternotomy	
Steps	**Rationale**	**Special Considerations**
1. Assist as needed with calling the patient's physician and operative team.	The physician can reassess the need for further surgical intervention. The operative team may be needed to assist at the bedside or to prepare the operating room if further exploration is needed.	Follow the institution's standard.
2. **HH**		
3. **PE**		
4. Assist with preparation of the electrocautery device for possible use: A. Apply the electrical dispersing pad (i.e., grounding pad) to the patient's dry skin over a large well perfused muscle. B. Attach the grounding cable to the electrocautery device.[1] **(Level D*)**	Electrocautery may be used to terminate capillary oozing or bleeding.	Grounding is essential to avoid burning the patient and possible electrical shock to the healthcare providers. Electrocautery may not be immediately available in the critical care setting; follow institution standard.

*Level D: Peer-reviewed professional and organizational standards with the support of clinical study recommendations

Procedure for Assisting with Emergent Open Sternotomy—*Continued*

Steps	Rationale	Special Considerations
5. Set up a new sterile suction system.	Suction within the mediastinum is necessary during the procedure.	
6. Assist if needed with removing the sternal dressing.	Prepares for the procedure.	
7. Assist if needed with cleansing the patient's chest with an antiseptic solution (e.g., 2% chlorhexidine gluconate solution).	Inhibits microorganism transmission.	The skin is cleansed beginning at the incision line, extending outward to include the area from the chin to the midabdomen (caudal to the umbilicus) and to include the area outward to one anterior axillary line and then outward to the opposite anterior axillary line. Minimize solution from running off of the surgical site, dripping, pooling, and soaking fabric and the patient's hair. Ensure alcohol-based preparation agents have not wet the patient's hair or bedding nor pooled in skin-folds or the umbilicus because the risk of fire is increased (nonflammable preparations eliminate the risk of fire).[1]
8. If needed, assist the physician, advanced practice nurse, or other healthcare provider performing the procedure with: A. Donning surgical head cover, mask, and eye protection. B. Donning sterile gown and sterile gloves.	Inhibits rebound microorganism growth.[1]	All personnel in the room must don head covers and masks.
9. Assist as needed, with opening the sternotomy tray on a clean dry surface.	Prepares equipment.	
10. Assist as needed with fully draping the patient with exposure of only the surgical site.[1,4,5] **(Level D*)**	A large sterile field minimizes the risk of infection and provides space to maintain asepsis of instruments and supplies during the procedure.	Allows good view of the incision.
11. Assist as needed with setting up the electrocautery system (e.g., adjusting the controls).	Cautery is used to stop bleeding from small vessels.	The cautery control is not sterile. The connection must be handed off of the sterile field without the healthcare provider performing the procedure and the assisting personnel touching each other.
12. Assist as needed with providing supplies and with removing sharp objects (e.g., cut wires) from the surgical field.	Assists with procedure and ensures that removed wires are safely discarded.	
13. Assist with suctioning as needed.	Clears blood from the field.	

*Level D: Peer-reviewed professional and organizational standards with the support of clinical study recommendations.

Procedure continues on following page

Procedure for Assisting with Emergent Open Sternotomy—*Continued*

Steps	Rationale	Special Considerations
14. If pulseless ventricular tachycardia or ventricular fibrillation occurs, assist with obtaining equipment for internal defibrillation (see Procedures 37 and 38).	Provides emergent intervention.	
15. Prepare chest drainage system and pacemaker to be connected after placement of chest tubes or epicardial pacing wires.	Epicardial pacing wires and chest tubes can be displaced during sternal retraction.	
16. Assist as needed with obtaining or preparing warm saline solution with or without an antibiotic for flushing chest cavity.	May decrease the incidence of infection.	
17. Prepare equipment for placement of mechanical assist devices if needed.	Cardiac tamponade can conceal right or left ventricular dysfunction; mechanical assistance may be necessary to improve cardiac output.	
18. Assist with transporting the patient to the operating room if necessary.	The patient may need further exploration or surgical repair of coronary artery bypass grafts, cardiac valves, the myocardium, or placement of an assist device (e.g., intraaortic balloon pump, ventricular assist device).	Ensure that the patient's chest is covered with sterile drapes or with a dressing during transportation.
19. If the patient does not return to the operating room, assist the healthcare provider performing the procedure by providing supplies for reinsertion of the sternal wires.	Ensures sternal closure.	
20. Provide supplies for tissue and skin closure.	Ensures closure of the sternal incision.	
21. Assist or apply an occlusive dressing to the sternal incision, epicardial pacing wires, and chest tube sites after the procedure is completed.	Dressings provide a physical barrier to external sources of contamination and cushion from physical contact and trauma; they absorb drainage, maintain a moist environment at body temperature to enhance wound healing, and are used for aesthetics.	The patient's chest may be left open and covered with a sterile occlusive surgical dressing if severe ventricular dysfunction exists.
22. Discard used supplies, and remove and discard **PE**.	Reduces the transmission of microorganisms and body secretions; Standard Precautions.	A chest radiograph may be ordered to rule out the presence of any retained surgical sponges, needles, or instruments.
23. Assist if needed with packaging used instruments for sterilization.	Prepares equipment for future use.	
24. **HH**		

Expected Outcomes

- Resolution of the condition that necessitated the emergent open sternotomy
- Increased cardiac output
- Increased tissue perfusion, including cerebral, renal, and peripheral perfusion
- Minimal chest tube drainage
- Decreased need for blood transfusions

Unexpected Outcomes

- Severe right or left ventricular dysfunction
- Continued dysrhythmias, bleeding, or coagulation disorders
- Myocardial, aortic, coronary artery, or coronary artery bypass graft perforation
- Cardiac arrest
- Pneumothorax
- Intracardiac infarction
- Atrial and ventricular dysrhythmias
- Pain
- Surgical site infection
- Death

Patient Monitoring and Care

Steps	Rationale	Reportable Conditions
		These conditions should be reported if they persist despite nursing interventions.
1. Perform cardiovascular, hemodynamic, and peripheral vascular assessments every 15–30 minutes as patient status requires (including vital signs, pulmonary artery pressures, cardiac index, level of consciousness, and urine output).	Determines hemodynamic stability and volume status; recurrent tamponade or dysrhythmias may develop during and after sternotomy. Determines the adequacy of cerebral perfusion; hemodynamic instability can lead to cerebral anoxia. Determines perfusion to the kidneys.	- Mean arterial blood pressures <60 mm Hg - Abnormal changes in heart rate - Decrease in cardiac index - Abnormal pulmonary artery pressures - Urine output <0.5 mL/kg/hr - Equalizing pulmonary artery pressures - Change in levels of consciousness - Distant heart sounds - Abnormal lung sounds
2. Assess heart and lung sounds every 2 hours and as needed.	Abnormal heart and lung sounds may indicate the need for additional treatment.	
3. Monitor coagulation, hematologic, and electrolyte laboratory blood study results as prescribed.	Coagulation and hematologic profiles provide data that indicate the risk of bleeding and indicate the need for additional treatment. Electrolyte studies provide data regarding the risk for dysrhythmias and decreased contractility.	- Abnormal hemoglobin and hematocrit, activated partial thromboplastin time, international normalized ratio, platelets, fibrinogen, calcium, magnesium, or potassium levels
4. Monitor chest tube drainage.	Determines functioning of the chest tube drainage system and the amount of chest drainage.	- Cessation of chest tube drainage - Increased chest tube drainage - Clots in chest tube drainage system
5. Follow institution standard for assessing pain. Administer analgesia as prescribed.	Identifies need for pain interventions.	- Continued pain despite pain interventions

Documentation

Documentation should include the following:
- Patient and family education
- Signed informed consent, if nonemergent
- Universal Protocol requirement, if nonemergent
- Indications for procedure and the procedure performed
- Amount of blood collected from chest suctioning; estimated blood loss
- Patient therapies and response, including hemodynamic values, inotropic or vasopressor agents, ventilation, and neurological status
- Additional interventions
- Unexpected outcomes
- Pain assessment, interventions and effectiveness

References and Additional Readings

For a complete list of references and additional readings for
this procedure, scan this QR code with any freely available
smartphone code reader app, or visit
http://booksite.elsevier.com/9780323376624.

41

External Wearable Cardioverter-Defibrillator

Kiersten Henry

PURPOSE: The external wearable cardioverter-defibrillator (WCD) is a temporary device that is used to prevent sudden cardiac death from malignant ventricular dysrhythmias. The WCD continuously monitors a patient's heart rate and rhythm and attempts to convert ventricular tachycardia or ventricular fibrillation via defibrillation.

PREREQUISITE NURSING KNOWLEDGE

- Knowledge of the anatomy and physiology of the cardiovascular system, principles of cardiac conduction, and basic dysrhythmia interpretation is needed.
- Knowledge of basic functioning of the WCDs and patient response to WCD therapy is needed.
- Knowledge of principles of defibrillation threshold, antidysrhythmia medications, alteration in electrolytes, and effect on the defibrillation threshold is necessary.
- Basic life support (BLS) and advanced cardiac life support (ACLS) knowledge and skills are needed.
- The WCD may be utilized as a bridge therapy to the implantable cardioverter-defibrillator (ICD).
- The WCD is different from an automated external defibrillator because it requires no bystander assistance.
- The WCD currently commercially available in the United States is the Zoll LifeVest. The LifeVest is worn by the patient underneath his or her clothes. The purpose of the vest is to sense malignant ventricular arrhythmias and defibrillate as appropriate.[1]
- The vest contains four nonadhesive electrodes that continuously monitor the cardiac rhythm. Three defibrillator pads release gel just before defibrillation to protect the skin from burns.[1]
- The WCD monitor and batteries are worn in a holster around the waist (Fig. 41-1).
- Patients are advised to change the rechargeable battery daily. Batteries need approximately 1 to 2 hours to recharge on the charging unit.
- If the WCD senses ventricular fibrillation or ventricular tachycardia, it can deliver a series of up to five defibrillations. The energy delivered is selected by the provider when the device is ordered. The LifeVest can deliver up to 150 joules per defibrillation. The heart rate threshold for defibrillation is also determined by the ordering provider.[2,3]
- When a shockable ventricular rhythm is detected, the vest begins a series of audible warnings and physical vibrations to alert the patient and bystanders. The warnings

continue for at least 25 seconds, allowing the patient to deactivate the device if the detected arrhythmia is actually interference due to electronic devices or motion artifact. The patient can deactivate the WCD by pushing a button located on the battery pack. If defibrillation is indicated, the device will audibly warn bystanders to stand clear.[2,3]
- Audible alerts with the Zoll LifeVest[8]:
  - Gong followed by "Contact your physician" or "Treatment has been given, call your doctor." This indicates that therapy has been given and the patient is being monitored.
  - Two-tone alarm followed by "If patient is not responsive, call for help, perform CPR," or "Device disabled, call ambulance." These mean that the Zoll LifeVest is not sensing a shockable rhythm, has delivered the maximum number of therapies, or cannot detect the electrocardiogram (ECG).
  - Two-tone alarm accompanied by "Electrical shock possible, do not touch patient. Bystanders do not interfere." A shock will be delivered within 25 to 60 seconds unless the patient deactivates the device. Bystanders should stand clear until defibrillation is completed, as they can be shocked if the patient is touched during defibrillation.
  - The presence of blue gel on the patient's chest indicates that a defibrillation has likely been delivered.
- The WCD monitors patient rhythm and stores data about vest utilization. This information is transmitted electronically to the manufacturing company, which provides clinical information to the prescribing provider.
- Indications for the WCD include any situation in which a patient is at risk for sudden cardiac death but is not eligible for an ICD. Delays in ICD eligibility are related to the fact that a patient may regain left ventricular function with optimal medical therapy, reducing the patient's risk of sudden cardiac death.[7]
- Explanation of an ICD due to infection:[8]
  - Patients who may require ICD implantation but are within the mandated waiting period:[4,6]
    - Patients within 40 days of a myocardial infarction who did not undergo coronary intervention

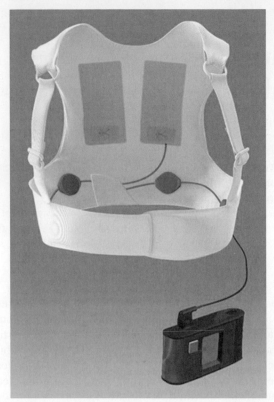

Figure 41-1   LifeVest wearable cardioverter-defibrillator. *(From ZOLL, Pittsburgh, PA.)*

○ Patients within 90 days of a myocardial infarction who underwent percutaneous coronary intervention or coronary artery bypass grafting
○ Patients with cardiomyopathy who have not been on optimal medical therapy for at least 90 days
○ Patients awaiting cardiac transplantation
○ Patients with ICD indications when the patient's condition prohibits ICD implantation
• A clinical trial of the WCD in patients after myocardial infarction who were not eligible for ICD implantation due to mandatory waiting periods found a survival rate of 91% in patients wearing the WCD who had ventricular tachycardia or ventricular fibrillation arrest. The greatest benefit was seen in the first 30 days after hospital discharge.[4]
• Studies of WCD patients show that 24.5% of sudden cardiac deaths were due to respiratory arrest, asystole, or sudden cardiac death. In patients with ventricular tachycardia or ventricular fibrillation arrest while wearing the WCD, survival was 90%. This trial also showed a 90% compliance rate in the majority of patients utilizing the LifeVest WCD.[2]
• If a patient meets eligibility criteria for an ICD, the ICD is preferable to the WCD.[2]
• Research on use of the WCD in children is limited.[5]
• For patients presenting to the hospital wearing a WCD, refer to facility-specific protocols regarding management of the device, including communication to all team members regarding safety precautions with WCD use. Some facilities require the device be removed during hospitalization, whereas others encourage patients to wear it at all times.

EQUIPMENT

• LifeVest garment
• Sensing electrodes
• Defibrillator pads
• Battery pack with waist holster
• Extra battery pack
• Charging/transmission station
• Cardiac monitor
• Nonsterile gloves

Additional equipment, to have available as needed, includes the following:

• Emergency medications
• Cardiac board
• Resuscitation equipment

PATIENT AND FAMILY EDUCATION

• Assess learning needs, readiness to learn, and factors that influence learning. *Rationale:* This assessment allows the nurse to individualize teaching in a meaningful manner.
• Assess patient and family understanding of WCD therapy and the reason for its use. *Rationale:* This assessment provides information regarding knowledge level and necessity of additional teaching.
• Provide information about the normal conduction system, such as the structure of the conduction system, the source of the heartbeat, the normal and abnormal heart rhythms, the symptoms of abnormal heart rhythms, and the potentially life-threatening nature of VT and VF. *Rationale:* Understanding the conduction system and dangerous dysrhythmias assists the patient and family in recognizing the seriousness of the patient's condition and the need for WCD therapy.
• Provide information about WCD therapy, including the reason for the WCD, device operation, location of the device, types of therapy given by the device, risks and benefits of the device, and follow-up. This will occur in conjunction with the provider who ordered the device and the WCD company representative, who provides fitting of the device and patient education. *Rationale:* Understanding WCD functioning assists the patient and family in developing realistic perceptions of WCD therapy.
• Reinforce with the patient and family members the importance of wearing the vest at all times (including during sleep), except when showering or bathing. Another responsible adult should be present during showering or bathing to obtain help in the event of a life-threatening dysrhythmia. The device is not waterproof, but should be worn at all other times. *Rationale:* Understanding the importance of compliance with wearing the vest will help decrease the risk of death from sudden cardiac death.
• Reinforce with the patient and family members that only the patient should press the button to cancel defibrillation if the device begins alert. If the patient is not coherent to abort the defibrillation, it is likely indicated. Family members should be educated to stand clear of the patient if defibrillation occurs, and immediately call 911. *Rationale:* Understanding that the device is likely functioning

appropriately if defibrillating an unconscious patient will help limit the likelihood of inappropriate deactivation by bystanders or risk of the bystander injury due to an electrical shock.

PATIENT ASSESSMENT AND PREPARATION

Patient Assessment

- In conjunction with the physician, advanced practice nurse, and other healthcare professionals, assess the patient for orientation and mental capacity to manage the WCD. *Rationale:* Patients who cannot exercise compliance with the WCD, or deactivate the device before inappropriate defibrillation, are not candidates for WCD therapy.[1]
- Monitor and document the cardiac rhythm per unit protocol during hospitalization. *Rationale:* This will allow real-time assessment of any arrhythmias that occur in the WCD patient and early diagnosis of lethal arrhythmias during hospitalization.

Patient Preparation

- Verify that the patient is the correct patient using two identifiers. *Rationale:* Before performing a procedure, the nurse should ensure the correct identification of the patient for the intended intervention.
- Ensure that the patient and family understand preprocedural teaching. Answer questions as they arise, and reinforce information as needed. *Rationale:* Understanding of previously taught information is evaluated and reinforced.
- Consent for monitoring and using the device is obtained from the patient by the WCD product representative. *Rationale:* Placement of the WCD is not an invasive procedure. The patient is consenting to the company monitoring vest utilization and therapy.

Procedure	for External Wearable Cardioverter-Defibrillator	
Steps	**Rationale**	**Special Considerations**
1. HH		
2. PE		
3. Assist the WCD product representative as needed in determining the appropriate vest size for the patient.	There are different vest sizes. Utilization of the appropriate-size vest will increase compliance as well as increase cardiac monitoring accuracy.	
4. Assist if needed with placing the WCD on the patient.	Provides assistance and begins therapy.	
5. The patient should wear the device as prescribed.	This provides an opportunity for the patient to get comfortable with the fit of the device and how it operates.	The patient should demonstrate an understanding of WCD placement, the rationale for wearing the device, and appropriate utilization of the device.
6. Continue cardiac monitoring even though the patient is wearing the WCD.	Monitors for changes in heart rate and rhythm.	The WCD does not protect against arrest from pulseless electrical activity/asystole.
7. If the device indicates that defibrillation is indicated:[9]		
A. Assess and stay with the patient. Do not touch the patient.	A bystander can be shocked during defibrillation with the WCD.	
B. Wait for the device to function. The device may deliver up to 5 shocks. **(Level M*)**	The audible alerts will indicate which phase of the process the WCD is in, monitoring or preparing to defibrillate.	Observe the heart rate and rhythm on the cardiac monitor.
C. If the device successfully converts a life-threatening dysrhythmia:	Determines the patient's response to the therapy.	
i. Assess the patient's level of consciousness.		
ii. Assess the patient's vital signs and heart rhythm.		

*Level M: Manufacturer's recommendations only.

Procedure continues on following page

Procedure   for External Wearable Cardioverter-Defibrillator—*Continued*

Steps	Rationale	Special Considerations
D. If the device is not successful in converting a life-threatening dysrhythmia:		CPR can be interpreted by the device as ventricular arrhythmia.
i. Remove the WCD battery and/or vest after defibrillation attempts are complete.	Disconnecting the battery will deactivate the defibrillator. If anterior/posterior placement of defibrillator pads is required, the vest should be removed.	The battery should be removed or disconnected before initiation of CPR to avoid inappropriate defibrillation. When removing the WCD, if cutting the cloth vest off is required, make every attempt to avoid cutting through the ECG leads. This allows the device to be utilized by the patient at a later time.
ii. Initiate BLS and ACLS.	Provides emergency interventions.	Patients may progress to pulseless electrical activity/asystole, which the device will not treat.
8. After successful or unsuccessful treatment, contact the WCD product representative to download the device information.	The device download can be helpful in determining rhythm type (if not captured on a hospital-based monitor).	The device will store pre- and posttherapy ECG strips. This information can also be obtained from the cardiac monitoring system.
9. Discard used supplies and personal protective equipment in appropriate receptacles.	Reduces the transmission of microorganisms and body secretions; Standard Precautions.	
10. 🅗🅗		
11. Obtain an additional WCD vest and defibrillator pads from the company representative.	Provides equipment needed for ongoing therapy.	

Expected Outcomes

- WCD detects life-threatening VT or VF
- WCD delivers appropriate defibrillation
- Patient deactivates the WCD if audible/physical warnings begin and the patient is conscious
- Emergency treatment is provided

Unexpected Outcomes

- WCD delivers inappropriate defibrillation
- Failure of the WCD to detect VF/VT
- Patient is noncompliant with wearing of the WCD
- Staff/bystander injury

Patient Monitoring and Care

Steps	Rationale	Reportable Conditions
		These conditions should be reported if they persist despite nursing interventions.
1. Continuous cardiac monitoring.	Detects dysrhythmias.	• Abnormal heart rate • Dysrhythmias
2. Assess the patient's response to WCD defibrillation, including anxiety, cardiac rate and rhythm, level of consciousness, and vital signs.	Determines patient status after defibrillation.	• Anxiety • Abnormal heart rate • Dysrhythmias • Hypotension • WCD therapy • Defibrillation • WCD malfunction • Hemodynamic instability • Neurological changes
3. Follow institution standard for assessing pain. Administer analgesia as prescribed.	Identifies need for pain interventions.	• Continued pain despite pain interventions

Documentation

Documentation should include the following:

- WCD settings
- Patient and family education
- Patient's return demonstration of device placement and utilization
- All rhythm-strip recordings

- Pain
- Patient response to WCD therapy
- Anxiety assessment, interventions, and effectiveness
- Occurrence of any unexpected outcomes
- Additional interventions

References and Additional Readings

For a complete list of references and additional readings for this procedure, scan this QR code with any freely available smartphone code reader app, or visit http://booksite.elsevier.com/9780323376624.

42   Pericardiocentesis (Perform) **AP**

Kathleen M. Cox

PURPOSE: Pericardiocentesis is the removal of excess fluid from the pericardial sac for identification of the etiology of pericardial effusion by fluid analysis (diagnostic pericardiocentesis) and/or prevention or treatment of cardiac tamponade (therapeutic pericardiocentesis).

PREREQUISITE NURSING KNOWLEDGE

- Advanced cardiac life support (ACLS) knowledge and skills are required.
- Knowledge and skills related to sterile technique are needed.
- Clinical and technical competence in the performance of pericardiocentesis is required.
- Knowledge of cardiovascular anatomy and physiology is needed.
- The pericardial space normally contains 20–50 mL of fluid.
- Pericardial fluid has electrolyte and protein profiles similar to plasma.
- Pericardial effusion is generally defined as the accumulation of fluid within the pericardial sac that exceeds the stretch capacity of the pericardium, generally more than 50 to 100 mL.[7]
- The space within the pericardial sac is finite; however, initially large increases in intrapericardial volume result in relatively small changes in intrapericardial pressure. If fluid continues to accumulate and increases intrapericardial pressures above the filling pressures of the right heart, right–ventricular diastolic filling is compromised, resulting in cardiac tamponade.[5]
- Intrapericardial fluid accumulation can be acute or chronic and therefore varies in presentation of symptoms. Acute effusions are usually a rapid collection of fluid occurring over minutes to hours and may result in hemodynamic compromise with volumes of less than 250 mL.[6] Chronically developing effusions occurring over days to weeks allow for hypertrophy and distention of the fibrous pericardial membrane. Patients with chronic effusions may accumulate greater than or equal to 2000 mL of fluid before exhibiting symptoms of hemodynamic compromise.[6]
- Symptoms of cardiac tamponade are nonspecific so the diagnosis relies on clinical suspicion and associated signs and symptoms. Acute pericardial effusions are usually a result of trauma, myocardial infarction, or iatrogenic injury, whereas chronic effusions can result from conditions such as bacterial or viral pericarditis, cancer, autoimmune disorders, uremia, etc.[2] With a decrease in cardiac output, the patient often develops chest pain, dyspnea, tachycardia, tachypnea, pallor, cyanosis, impaired cerebral and renal function, diaphoresis, hypotension, neck vein distention, distant or faint heart sounds, and pulsus paradoxus.[4]
- The amount of fluid in the pericardium is evaluated through chest radiograph, two-dimensional echocardiogram, electrocardiography (ECG), and clinical findings. Chest x-rays may not be diagnostically significant in patients with acute traumatic tamponade.[6]
- Pericardiocentesis to remove fluid from the pericardial sac is performed therapeutically to relieve tamponade or to diagnose the etiology of the effusion. An acute tamponade resulting in hemodynamic instability necessitates an emergency procedure. Blind pericardiocentesis should be performed only in extreme emergency situations.[7]
- Pericardiocentesis is usually performed via a subxiphoid approach.
- Two-dimensional echocardiography or ultrasound to assist in guiding the needle during pericardiocentesis is strongly recommended.[2,6,7]
- This procedure may also be performed with fluoroscopy in a cardiac catheterization or interventional radiology suite.
- Urgent or emergent chest exploration is necessary in the face of cardiac injury, rapid reaccumulation of pericardial fluid, or ineffective drainage of the pericardium.
- There are no absolute contraindications to pericardiocentesis in the setting of life-threatening hemodynamic instability. Relative contraindications include coagulopathy, prior thoracic surgery or pacemaker placement, artificial heart valves or other cardiac devices, or inability to directly visualize the effusion using ultrasound during procedure.[6]
- Cardiac output is generally improved after pericardiocentesis.

EQUIPMENT

- Pericardiocentesis tray (or thoracentesis tray)
- 16-gauge or 18-gauge, 3-inch cardiac needle or catheter over the needle

---

AP   This procedure should be performed only by physicians, advanced practice nurses, and other healthcare professionals (including critical care nurses) with additional knowledge, skills, and demonstrated competence per professional licensure or institutional standard.

- Antiseptic skin preparation solution (e.g., 2% chlorhexidine-based preparation)
- Two packs of 4 × 4 gauze sponges
- No. 11 knife blade with handle (scalpel)
- Sterile 50-mL to 60-mL, 10-mL, 5-mL, and 3-mL syringes
- Sterile drapes and towels
- Masks, goggles or face shields, surgical head covers, sterile gowns, and gloves
- Two three-way stopcocks
- 1% lidocaine (injectable)
- 10 mL syringe with 25-gauge needle
- Culture bottles and specimen tubes for fluid analysis
- 2-inch and 3-inch tape

Additional equipment, to have available as needed, includes the following:

- Emergency cart (defibrillator, emergency respiratory equipment, emergency cardiac medications, and temporary pacemaker)
- Two-dimensional echocardiography equipment
- 12-lead ECG machine
- Sterile marker
- Echocardiogram contrast medium
- Suture supplies
- Scissors
- If continuous drainage is necessary:
  - ❖ J guidewire, 0.035 diameter
  - ❖ Vessel dilator, 7 Fr
  - ❖ Pigtail catheter, 7 Fr
  - ❖ Tubing and drainage bag or bottle
  - ❖ Three-way stopcock and nonvented caps

PATIENT AND FAMILY EDUCATION

- Explain to the patient and family the reason necessitating the pericardiocentesis (e.g., relief of pressure on the heart); describe the procedure in detail, to include risks, benefits, alternatives, expected outcomes, and potential complications. **Rationale:** Communication of pertinent information helps the patient and family to understand the procedure and the potential risks and benefits, subsequently reducing anxiety and apprehension.[1]
- Teach the patient and family about the signs and symptoms of pericardial effusion (e.g., dyspnea, dull ache or pressure within the chest, dysphagia, cough, tachypnea, hoarseness, hiccups, or nausea).[4,5] **Rationale:** Early recognition of signs and symptoms of recurrent pericardial effusion may prompt detection of a potentially life-threatening problem.

PATIENT ASSESSMENT AND PREPARATION

Patient Assessment

- Elicit the patient's history of the present illness and mechanism of injury (if applicable), past medical history, and current medications and/or medical therapies from the patient or reliable source. **Rationale:** A thorough history is necessary to determine the patient's baseline health status and to identify potential risk factors. The nurse-patient interaction provides an opportunity for the nurse to establish a therapeutic relationship focused on the patient.[2]

- Assess the patient's neurological status, heart rate, cardiac rhythm, heart sounds (S_1, S_2, rubs, murmurs), pulmonary artery pressures, central venous pressure (noninvasive or invasive), blood pressure, mean arterial pressure (MAP), oxygen saturation via pulse oximetry (SpO_2), and respiratory status. **Rationale:** Provides baseline data.

- Evaluate current laboratory values to include a complete blood cell count, electrolytes, and coagulation profile. **Rationale:** Review of these data is essential to identify the potential risk of cardiac dysrhythmias or abnormal bleeding. If the international normalized ratio or partial thromboplastin time or both are elevated, reversing the level of anticoagulation therapy should be considered before performing the procedure. It may be prudent to defer the procedure until the blood levels indicate a reduction in bleeding risk.[6]

Patient Preparation

- Confirm that the patient and family understand preprocedural teaching by having them verbalize understanding. Clarify key points by reinforcing important information and answer all questions. **Rationale:** Preprocedure communication provides a framework of patient expectations, enhances cooperation, and reduces anxiety.[2]
- Verify that the patient is the correct patient using two identifiers. **Rationale:** The nurse should always ensure the correct identification of the patient for the intended intervention for patient safety.
- Obtain informed consent by providing specific and relevant information about the procedure. Implied consent may be assumed if emergent life-saving intervention is necessary. **Rationale:** Informed consent is based on the autonomous right of the patient and facilitates a competent decision for the patient and the family.[2]
- Perform a preprocedure verification and time out, if nonemergent. **Rationale:** Ensures patient safety.
- Coordinate the procedure with the echocardiogram technician or ultrasonographer to assist with the two-dimensional echocardiogram or ultrasound if this approach is being used. **Rationale:** Echocardiogram- or ultrasound-directed pericardiocentesis allows for more precise localization of the effusion and is associated with higher success rates and lower complication rates.[5–7]
- If nonemergent, prescribe and ensure that an analgesic and/or sedative is administered. **Rationale:** Analgesia and sedation reduce anxiety and promote comfort and cooperation.
- Apply the limb leads and connect the leads to the cardiac bedside monitoring system or to the 12-lead ECG machine. **Rationale:** The ECG is monitored during and after the procedure for changes that may indicate cardiac injury.

Procedure for Performing Pericardiocentesis

Steps	Rationale	Special Considerations
1. **HH**		
2. **PE**		Consider putting a mask on the patient during the actual procedure if the patient is not intubated (in a contained system), especially if the patient has methicillin-resistant *Staphylococcus aureus* (MRSA)–positive results on nasal swab or known colonization.
3. Prepare the pericardiocentesis tray and supplies with aseptic technique.	Reduces the potential for infection.	
4. Position patient in the supine position with the head of the bed elevated 30–45 degrees as the patient's condition allows.	Facilitates patient comfort, decreases work of breathing, and aids adequate aspiration of fluid.	
5. Cleanse the skin with antiseptic solution (e.g., 2% chlorhexidine-based preparation) and perform HH.	Minimizes the potential for infection.	Clipping the hair may be necessary before applying antiseptic solution.
6. If two-dimensional echocardiogram or ultrasound is being used, **skip to step 14.**		
7. Using maximal barrier precautions, fully drape the patient with exposure of only the surgical site and apply mask, goggles or face shield, surgical cap, sterile gown, and sterile gloves.[2]	Minimizes the risk of infection; maintains aseptic and sterile precautions.	
8. Attach a three-way stopcock to a 3-inch cardiac needle, and attach to a 50-mL or 60-mL syringe.	Provides the mechanism to aspirate fluid.	
9. If time and patient condition permit, inject access site with 2–3 mL 1% lidocaine using a 10-mL syringe and a 25-gauge needle, raising a wheal. If unable to perform this step, attach a syringe with 1% lidocaine to one side of the stopcock to inject analgesia during the access procedure.	Reduces patient discomfort.	Local infiltration of analgesia reduces patient discomfort. Alternatively, as the needle is introduced, the physician, advanced practice nurse, or other healthcare professional may insert a small amount of 1% lidocaine to add analgesic effect.
10. Continuously monitor the bedside ECG, vital signs, SpO2, and venous pressure during needle aspiration and fluid withdrawal.[2,4,5]	Determines patient response during the procedure.	A 12-lead ECG machine can also be used for cardiac monitoring.

Procedure for Performing Pericardiocentesis—*Continued*

Steps	Rationale	Special Considerations
11. Subxiphoid approach to pericardiocentesis (Fig. 42-1): A. A 16- or 18-gauge needle is slowly inserted into the left xiphocostal angle perpendicular to the skin 3–4 mm below the left costal margin. Slowly advance the needle under the xiphoid toward the left shoulder while maintaining negative pressure on the syringe (aspirating). B. After the needle is advanced to the inner aspect of the rib cage, the needle's hub is depressed while the needle points toward the patient's left shoulder. The needle is slowly advanced 5–10 mm until fluid is aspirated. You may feel a distinct "give" when the needle penetrates the pericardium. Successful removal of fluid confirms needle position.	Minimizes the risk of cardiac injury; angles >45 degrees may lacerate the liver or stomach.	The movement of the heart usually defibrinates blood in the pericardial space so that it cannot clot.[8] Clotting usually indicates penetration of the heart chamber and blood obtained from within a ventricle or atrium.[5] If clotting occurs with the fluid obtained, withdraw the needle. If no fluid is aspirated, withdraw the needle completely and redirect it working from the patient's left to right.
12. When the needle position is confirmed, obtain the fluid samples and remove the needle. No more than 50–150 mL of pericardial fluid should be removed at one time.[5,6] (Level E*) **If continuous drainage is needed, go to step 19.**	Removes the pericardial fluid for analysis.	Usual tests include body fluid cytology, cell count, electrolytes, routine aerobic and anaerobic cultures, acid-fast bacilli cultures, and other tests as indicated.
13. Label the specimen and send the specimen to the laboratory.	Prepares the sample for analysis.	

When Two-Dimensional Echocardiogram or Ultrasound Is Used

Steps	Rationale	Special Considerations
14. Perform a two-dimensional echocardiogram or ultrasound to determine the location and size of the effusion.	Two-dimensional echocardiogram or ultrasound can help to identify the location and size of the pericardial effusion.	
15. Determine the ideal entry site and needle trajectory for the pericardiocentesis.	The ideal entry site is the point where the effusion is closest to the transducer and fluid accumulation is maximal.[4,6,7]	A straight trajectory that best avoids vital structures, including the liver, myocardium, and lung, should be chosen. The internal mammary artery also should be avoided.[6–8]
16. Mark the skin with a sterile marker.	May aid with the procedure.	
17. **Return to Step 7** and follow the procedural steps.		

*Level E: Multiple case reports, theory-based evidence from expert opinions, or peer-reviewed professional organizational standards without clinical studies to support recommendations.

Procedure continues on following page

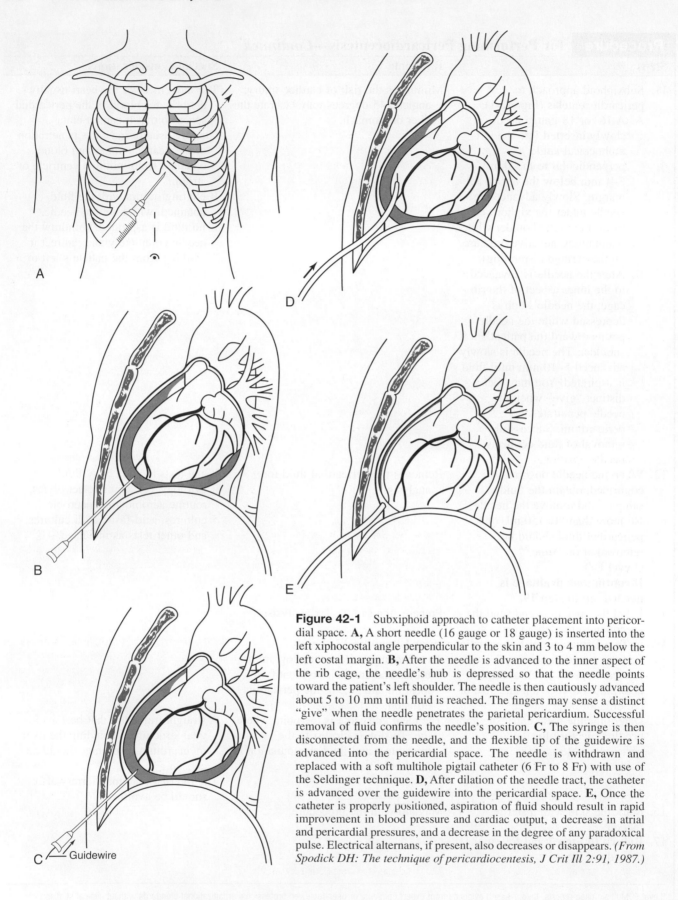

Figure 42-1   Subxiphoid approach to catheter placement into pericordial space. **A,** A short needle (16 gauge or 18 gauge) is inserted into the left xiphocostal angle perpendicular to the skin and 3 to 4 mm below the left costal margin. **B,** After the needle is advanced to the inner aspect of the rib cage, the needle's hub is depressed so that the needle points toward the patient's left shoulder. The needle is then cautiously advanced about 5 to 10 mm until fluid is reached. The fingers may sense a distinct "give" when the needle penetrates the parietal pericardium. Successful removal of fluid confirms the needle's position. **C,** The syringe is then disconnected from the needle, and the flexible tip of the guidewire is advanced into the pericardial space. The needle is withdrawn and replaced with a soft multihole pigtail catheter (6 Fr to 8 Fr) with use of the Seldinger technique. **D,** After dilation of the needle tract, the catheter is advanced over the guidewire into the pericardial space. **E,** Once the catheter is properly positioned, aspiration of fluid should result in rapid improvement in blood pressure and cardiac output, a decrease in atrial and pericardial pressures, and a decrease in the degree of any paradoxical pulse. Electrical alternans, if present, also decreases or disappears. *(From Spodick DH: The technique of pericardiocentesis, J Crit Ill 2:91, 1987.)*

Procedure   for Performing Pericardiocentesis—*Continued*

Steps	Rationale	Special Considerations
18. If bloody fluid is aspirated, a few milliliters of echo contrast medium can be infused to confirm position.[6,7] A. Echocardiogenic saline can be prepared by using two 5-mL syringes attached to a three-way stopcock, one filled with sterile normal saline and one with air. B. Agitate the saline between the two syringes and inject into the sheath. The agitated saline should appear as an echogenic stream.[7] C. When the fluid is determined to be pericardial, **return to Step 12.**	If the contrast material appears in the pericardial space, the procedure can be continued. If the contrast material disappears, the needle may be in one of the heart chambers and must be withdrawn and repositioned.	Two-dimensional echocardiogram or ultrasound assists in determining the position of the needle. Echo contrast is agitated saline solution that is injected via the side port of the stopcock.[6]
When Continuous Drainage Is Desired		
19. When the needle tip position is confirmed to be within the pericardial space, insert the flexible tip of the guidewire through the needle into the pericardial space and then remove the needle, leaving the guidewire in place. The guidewire is passed so that it wraps around the heart within the pericardial space.[6,7]	A soft guidewire minimizes the risk of cardiac injury and allows for the passage of the guidewire and placement within the pericardial space.	
20. A multiholed pigtail or straight soft catheter is passed over the guidewire using the Seldinger technique[5] (see Fig. 42-1).	A flexible-tipped soft catheter with multiple holes in the tip is used to facilitate drainage of the effusion. Use of a soft-tipped catheter reduces the chances of causing myocardial injury and dysrhythmias during the procedure.[1]	Either a pigtail catheter or a straight catheter with multiple holes can be used for better drainage.
21. Remove the guidewire and connect the end of the catheter to the three-way stopcock and the drainage collection bag.[5–7]	Maintains asepsis; allows for continual drainage of the effusion.	If the effusion is small, when fluid is drained remove the catheter.
22. If an indwelling catheter is placed to continuously drain a large pericardial effusion, attach the catheter to the sterile bag or bottle using aseptic technique (see Procedure 78).	Facilitates fluid drainage; minimizes the potential for infection.	
23. If an indwelling catheter is to remain in place, secure the catheter by suturing the catheter securely to the patient's chest wall.	Prevents dislodging or accidental removal.	
24. Cleanse the area around the catheter with an antiseptic solution and apply an occlusive sterile dressing.[3]	May reduce the risk of infection.	

Procedure continues on following page

Procedure for Performing Pericardiocentesis—*Continued*

Steps	Rationale	Special Considerations
25. Continue bedside ECG monitoring, and discontinue 12-lead ECG if used.	Allows monitoring of cardiac rate and rhythm.	
26. Dispose of **PE**, sharps, and used supplies in appropriate receptacles.		
27. **HH**		
28. If an indwelling catheter is placed, consider prescribing antibiotics.	May reduce the risk of infection.	

Expected Outcomes

- Fluid removed from the pericardial sac
- Relief of pain, discomfort, or other symptoms that indicated the need for the procedure
- Improved cardiac output
- Patient's blood pressure, venous pressure, heart sounds, pulse pressure, and cardiac rhythm within normal limits

Unexpected Outcomes

- Decrease in blood pressure, increase in venous pressure, cardiac dysrhythmias, or excessive bleeding
- Hemodynamic instability
- ST-segment depression
- PR-segment elevation
- Cardiac tamponade
- Pain

Patient Monitoring and Care

Steps	Rationale	Reportable Conditions
		These conditions should be reported if they persist despite nursing interventions.
1. Continuously monitor ECG; assess pulmonary artery (PA) pressures, venous pressure, blood pressure, SpO₂, and neurological status during and every 15 minutes after the procedure until stable (if available, continuously monitor cardiac index and systemic vascular resistance).	A change in these signs may indicate cardiac tamponade, cardiac injury, or hemodynamic instability.	- Increasing venous pressure - Decreasing arterial pressure - Change in level of consciousness - Pulsus paradoxus - Equalizing PA pressures - Decreased cardiac index - Abnormal systemic vascular resistance
2. Treat dysrhythmias if they occur.	Dysrhythmias may lead to cardiac decompensation.	- Persistent dysrhythmias despite appropriate intervention
3. Auscultate heart and lung sounds immediately after the procedure.	Evaluates potential pericardial fluid reaccumulation or puncture of the lung.	- Asymmetrical breath sounds - Dyspnea - Tachypnea - Decreased SpO₂ - Distant or faint heart sounds
4. Obtain a portable chest radiograph immediately after the procedure.	Assesses for pneumothorax and hemothorax.	- Pneumothorax - Hemothorax
5. Obtain a two-dimensional echocardiogram within several hours after the procedure.	Determines the effectiveness of the pericardial drainage.	- Pericardial effusion

Patient Monitoring and Care —*Continued*

Steps	Rationale	Reportable Conditions
6. Monitor the pericardiocentesis site for bleeding every 15 minutes after the procedure is completed until the patient's condition is stable, then every 4 hours for 24 hours. If an indwelling catheter is present, continue to monitor the site every 4 hours until the catheter is removed.	Assesses for post-procedural hemostasis and possible drainage.	• Bleeding or hematoma at site
7. Monitor hemoglobin, hematocrit, and coagulation studies every 8 hours after the procedure for 24 hours or as indicated.	Assesses for potential of effusion recurrence or bleeding at the site.	• Bleeding or hematoma at site • Decrease in hemoglobin or hematocrit values • Changes in coagulation study results
8. Assess pericardiocentesis site every day.	Determines the presence of infection.	• Erythema • Edema • Purulent drainage • Foul odor • Temperature >100.5°F (>38°C)

9. Prescribe site care:
  A. Cleanse the area surrounding the pericardial catheter with an antiseptic solution (e.g., 2% chlorhexidine-based preparation).
  B. Apply a dry sterile gauze or transparent dressing with the date and time of the dressing change.
	May reduce infection. The Centers for Disease Control and Prevention (CDC) do not have a specific recommendation for care of pericardial catheters or site care. The CDC recommends replacing intravascular catheter dressings when the dressing becomes damp, loosened, or soiled or when inspection of the site is necessary.[3]	

10. Evaluate the size of the effusion within 24 hours of the indwelling catheter placement with the use of a two-dimensional echocardiogram.	Records how effective drainage was and whether the need for the indwelling catheter continues to exist.	• Increased size of the effusion
11. Remove the indwelling catheter using aseptic technique when no longer needed.	Minimizes the potential for infection.	
12. Be prepared for emergent chest exploration if sudden deterioration in the patient's condition occurs.	Deterioration may indicate reaccumulation of cardiac tamponade or cardiac damage.	• Decreased blood pressure • Presence of dysrhythmias • Increased venous pressure • Change in mental or respiratory status • Diaphoresis • Distant heart sounds
13. Provide emotional support to the patient throughout the procedure.	Minimizes apprehension and anxiety.	
14. Keep the patient and family informed about the patient's condition. Be available to answer patient's and family's questions and facilitate meeting their needs as appropriate.	The unknown increases the anxiety and apprehension of the patient and family.	
15. Assess pain and prescribe analgesia as needed.	Identifies need for pain interventions.	• Continued pain despite pain interventions

Procedure continues on following page

Documentation

Documentation should include the following:

- Specific preprocedure instruction and patient's and family's satisfactory understanding
- Universal Protocol requirement, if nonemergent
- Legally signed consent form
- Pre- and postprocedure level of consciousness; blood pressure; venous pressures; pulmonary arterial pressures; cardiac index, cardiac output, systemic vascular resistance, if available; heart sounds and cardiac rhythm; respiratory status and pulse oximetry reading
- Pre- and postprocedure hemoglobin, hematocrit, and coagulation results, if performed
- Medications administered with dosage and times noted
- Placement of indwelling catheter (if used) to include total length, diameter, and length from skin to hub
- Removal of indwelling catheter, if used
- Assessment of pericardiocentesis fluid
- Amount and consistency of postprocedure drainage
- Occurrence of unexpected outcomes
- Pain assessment, interventions and effectiveness
- Pre- and postprocedural evaluation and location of effusion with two-dimensional echocardiogram, if used
- ECG rhythm strips
- Emergency interventions performed if necessary
- Specimens sent to the laboratory

References and Additional Readings

For a complete list of references and additional readings for this procedure, scan this QR code with any freely available smartphone code reader app, or visit http://booksite.elsevier.com/9780323376624.

43 Pericardiocentesis (Assist)

Kathleen M. Cox

PURPOSE: Pericardiocentesis is the removal of excess fluid from the pericardial sac for identification of the etiology of pericardial effusion by fluid analysis (diagnostic pericardiocentesis) and/or prevention or treatment of cardiac tamponade (therapeutic pericardiocentesis).

PREREQUISITE NURSING KNOWLEDGE

- Advanced cardiac life support (ACLS) knowledge and skills are required.
- Knowledge and skills related to aseptic technique are necessary.
- Knowledge of cardiovascular anatomy and physiology is needed.
- The pericardial space normally contains 20–50 mL of fluid.
- Pericardial fluid has electrolyte and protein profiles similar to plasma.
- Pericardial effusion is generally defined as the accumulation of fluid within the pericardial sac that exceeds the stretch capacity of the pericardium, generally more than 50 to 100 mL.[7]
- The space within the pericardial sac is finite; however, initially large increases in intrapericardial volume result in relatively small changes in intrapericardial pressure. If fluid continues to accumulate and increases intrapericardial pressures above the filling pressures of the right heart, right-ventricular diastolic filling is compromised, resulting in cardiac tamponade.[5]
- Intrapericardial fluid accumulation can be acute or chronic and therefore varies in presentation of symptoms. Acute effusions are usually a rapid collection of fluid occurring over minutes to hours and may result in hemodynamic compromise with volumes of less than 250 mL.[6] Chronically developing effusions occurring over days to weeks allow for hypertrophy and distention of the fibrous pericardial membrane. Patients with chronic effusions may accumulate greater than or equal to 2000 mL of fluid before exhibiting symptoms of hemodynamic compromise.[6]
- Symptoms of cardiac tamponade are nonspecific so the diagnosis relies on clinical suspicion and associated signs and symptoms. Acute pericardial effusions are usually a result of trauma, myocardial infarction, or iatrogenic injury, whereas chronic effusions can result from conditions such as bacterial or viral pericarditis, cancer, autoimmune disorders, uremia, etc.[2] With a decrease in cardiac output, the patient often develops chest pain, dyspnea, tachycardia, tachypnea, pallor, cyanosis, impaired cerebral and renal function, diaphoresis, hypotension, neck vein distention, distant or faint heart sounds, and pulsus paradoxus.[4]
- The amount of fluid in the pericardium is evaluated through chest radiograph, two-dimensional echocardiogram, electrocardiography (ECG), and clinical findings. Chest x-rays may not be diagnostically significant in patients with acute traumatic tamponade.[6]
- Pericardiocentesis to remove fluid from the pericardial sac is performed therapeutically to relieve tamponade or to diagnose the etiology of the effusion. An acute tamponade resulting in hemodynamic instability necessitates an emergency procedure. Blind pericardiocentesis should be performed in emergency situations.[7]
- Pericardiocentesis is usually performed via a subxiphoid approach.
- Two-dimensional echocardiography or ultrasound to assist in guiding the needle during pericardiocentesis is strongly recommended.[2,6,8]
- This procedure may also be performed with fluoroscopy in a cardiac catheterization or interventional radiology suite.
- Urgent or emergent chest exploration is necessary in the face of cardiac injury, rapid reaccumulation of pericardial fluid, or ineffective drainage of the pericardium.
- There are no absolute contraindications to pericardiocentesis in the setting of life-threatening hemodynamic instability. Relative contraindications include coagulopathy, prior thoracic surgery or pacemaker placement, artificial heart valves or other cardiac devices, or inability to directly visualize the effusion using ultrasound during the procedure.[6]
- Cardiac output is generally improved after pericardiocentesis.

EQUIPMENT

- Pericardiocentesis tray (or thoracentesis tray)
- 16-gauge or 18-gauge, 3-inch cardiac needle or catheter over the needle
- Antiseptic skin preparation solution (e.g., 2% chlorhexidine-based preparation)
- Two packs of 4 × 4 gauze sponges
- No. 11 knife blade with handle (scalpel)
- Sterile 50-mL to 60-mL, 10-mL, 5-mL, and 3-mL syringes
- Sterile drapes and towels

- Masks, goggles or face shields, surgical head covers, sterile gowns, and gloves
- Two three-way stopcocks
- 1% lidocaine (injectable)
- 10-mL syringe with 25-gauge needle
- Culture bottles and specimen tubes for fluid analysis
- 2-inch and 3-inch tape

Additional equipment, to have available as needed, includes the following:

- Emergency cart (defibrillator, emergency respiratory equipment, emergency cardiac medications, and temporary pacemaker)
- Two-dimensional echocardiography equipment
- 12-lead ECG machine
- Sterile marker
- Echocardiogram contrast medium
- Suture supplies
- Scissors
- If continuous drainage is necessary:
  - J guidewire, 0.035 diameter
  - Vessel dilator, 7 Fr
  - Pigtail catheter, 7 Fr
  - Tubing and drainage bag or bottle
  - Three-way stopcock and nonvented caps

PATIENT AND FAMILY EDUCATION

- Explain to the patient and family the reason necessitating the pericardiocentesis (e.g., relief of pressure on the heart). *Rationale:* Communication of pertinent information helps the patient and family to understand the procedure and may reduce anxiety and apprehension.[1]
- Teach the patient and family about the signs and symptoms of pericardial effusion (e.g., dyspnea, dull ache or pressure within the chest, dysphagia, cough, tachypnea, hoarseness, hiccups, or nausea).[4,5] *Rationale:* Early recognition of signs and symptoms of recurrent pericardial effusion may prompt detection of a potentially life-threatening problem.

PATIENT ASSESSMENT AND PREPARATION

Patient Assessment

- Elicit complete history of present illness and mechanism of injury (if applicable), past medical history, and current medications and/or medical therapies from the patient or reliable source. *Rationale:* A thorough history is necessary to determine the patient's baseline health status and to identify potential risk factors. The nurse-patient interaction provides an opportunity for the nurse to establish a therapeutic relationship focused on the patient.[2]
- Assess the patient's neurological status, heart rate, cardiac rhythm, heart sounds (S_1, S_2, rubs, murmurs), pulmonary artery pressures, central venous pressure (noninvasive or invasive), blood pressure, mean arterial pressure, oxygen saturation via pulse oximetry (SpO_2), and respiratory status. *Rationale:* Provides baseline data.
- Evaluate current laboratory values to include a complete blood cell count, electrolytes, and coagulation profile. *Rationale:* Review of these data is essential to identify the potential risk of cardiac dysrhythmias or abnormal bleeding. If the international normalized ratio or partial thromboplastin time or both are elevated, reversing the level of anticoagulation therapy should be considered before performing the procedure. It may be prudent to defer the procedure until the blood levels indicate a reduction in bleeding risk.[6]

Patient Preparation

- Confirm that the patient and family understand preprocedural teaching by having them verbalize understanding. Clarify key points by reinforcing important information and answer all questions. *Rationale:* Preprocedure communication provides a framework of patient expectations, enhances cooperation, and reduces anxiety.[2]
- Verify that the patient is the correct patient using two identifiers. *Rationale:* The nurse should always ensure the correct identification of the patient for the intended intervention for patient safety.
- Ensure that informed consent is obtained. Implied consent may be assumed if emergent life-saving intervention is necessary. *Rationale:* Informed consent is based on the autonomous right of the patient and facilitates a competent decision for the patient and the family.[2]
- Assist as needed with a preprocedure verification and time out, if nonemergent. *Rationale:* Ensures patient safety.
- Assist with coordinating the procedure with the echocardiogram technician or ultrasonographer to assist with the two-dimensional echocardiogram or ultrasound if this approach is being used. *Rationale:* Echocardiogram- or ultrasound-directed pericardiocentesis allows for more precise localization of the effusion and is associated with higher success rates and lower complication rates.[5-7]
- Administer analgesics or sedatives as prescribed. *Rationale:* Analgesia and sedation reduce anxiety and promote comfort and cooperation.
- Continue cardiac monitoring or initiate bedside cardiac monitoring. *Rationale:* The ECG is monitored during and after the procedure for changes that may indicate cardiac injury.

Procedure	for Assisting With Pericardiocentesis	
Steps	**Rationale**	**Special Considerations**
1. ▣HH		
2. ▣PE		Consider putting a mask on the patient during the actual procedure if the patient is not intubated (in a contained system), especially if the patient has methicillin-resistant *Staphylococcus aureus* (MRSA)–positive results on nasal swab or known colonization.
3. Using aseptic technique, assist as needed with opening the pericardiocentesis tray and supplies.	Prepares for procedure.	
4. If tolerated, ensure that the patient is positioned in the supine position with the head of the bed elevated 30–45 degrees.	Facilitates patient comfort, decreases work of breathing, and aids adequate aspiration of fluid.	
5. Assist the physician, advance practice nurse, or healthcare provider performing the procedure with cleansing the patient's skin with antiseptic solution (e.g., 2% chlorhexidine-based preparation) and perform ▣HH.	Minimizes the potential for infection.	Clipping hair from the area may be necessary before applying the antiseptic solution.
6. If two-dimensional echocardiogram or ultrasound is being used, **skip to Step 14.**		
7. Assist as needed with applying personal protective, and sterile equipment (e.g., masks, head covers, sterile gowns, and sterile gloves) and if needed assist with fully draping the patient with exposure of only the surgical site.	Protects provider and maintains aseptic and sterile technique.	
8. Assist if needed with providing a three-way stopcock, 3-inch cardiac needle, and 50-mL or 60-mL syringe.	Provides needed supplies.	
9. Assist if needed with preparing for a local injection (e.g., 10-mL syringe with 1% lidocaine and a 25-guge needle).	Reduces patient's discomfort.	As the needle is introduced, the physician, advanced practice nurse, or other healthcare professional may insert a small amount of 1% lidocaine to add analgesic effect.
10. Continuously monitor the bedside ECG, vital signs, Spo$_2$, pulmonary artery pressures, and venous pressure during needle aspiration and fluid withdrawal.[2,4,5]	Determines the patient's response during the procedure.	
11. Continuously monitor the patient as the physician, advanced practice nurse, or other healthcare professional slowly inserts the needle.	Continues to determine patient response during the procedure.	The movement of the heart usually defibrinates blood in the pericardial space so that it cannot clot. Clotting usually indicates penetration of the heart chamber and blood obtained from within a ventricle or atrium.[1,3]

Procedure continues on following page

Procedure for Assisting With Pericardiocentesis—*Continued*		
Steps	Rationale	Special Considerations
12. Assist if needed with obtaining pericardial fluid samples. If continuous drainage is used, **go to step 17.**	Provides diagnosis of the organism involved in pericardial effusion.	Usual tests include body fluid cytology, cell count, electrolytes, routine aerobic and anaerobic cultures, acid-fast bacilli cultures, and other tests as indicated.
13. Assist if needed with labeling the specimens and send the specimens to the laboratory.	Prepares the samples for analysis.	
When Two-Dimensional Echocardiogram or Ultrasound Is Used		
14. Assist the physician, advanced practice nurse, or other healthcare professional and the echocardiogram/ultrasound technician as needed.	Provides assistance.	Assist if needed with marking the skin with a sterile marker.
15. **Return to Step 7** and proceed.		
16. If bloody fluid is aspirated, be prepared to assist the physician, advanced practice nurse, or other healthcare professional in infusing a few milliliters of echo contrast medium into the space where the needle is to confirm position.[6,7] If requested, prepare echocardiogenic saline with aseptic technique by: A. Attaching two 5-mL syringes to a three-way stopcock, one filled with air and one with 5 mL sterile normal saline. B. Hand the syringes attached to the stopcock using aseptic technique to the physician, advanced practice nurse, or other healthcare professional performing the procedure. When this is determined to be pericardial fluid, **return to step 12.**	Provides assistance.	
When Continuous Drainage Is Desired		
17. Assist the physician, advanced practice nurse, or other healthcare professional if needed as he or she removes the steel needle and inserts a soft floppy-tipped guidewire through the needle. The guidewire is passed so that it wraps around the heart within the pericardial space.[6,7]	Provides assistance.	
18. Assist the physician, advanced practice nurse, or other healthcare professional with removing the guidewire and connecting the end of the catheter to the three-way stopcock and the drainage collection bag.[5–7]	Maintains asepsis; allows for continual drainage of the effusion.[1]	
19. If an indwelling catheter is placed to continuously drain a large pericardial effusion, assist the physician, advanced practice nurse, or other healthcare professional with attaching the sterile bag or bottle with aseptic technique (see Procedure 78).	Facilitates fluid drainage; minimizes the potential for infection.	

Procedure   for Assisting With Pericardiocentesis—*Continued*

Steps	Rationale	Special Considerations
20. If an indwelling catheter is in place, assist the physician, advanced practice nurse, or other healthcare professional if needed by providing suture supplies.	Prevents dislodging or accidental discontinuation of the drainage.	
21. Assist if needed with cleansing the area around the catheter with antiseptic solution and apply an occlusive sterile dressing.[3]	May reduce the risk of infection.	
22. Continue bedside ECG monitoring and discontinue the 12-lead ECG if used.	Allows monitoring of cardiac rate and rhythm.	
23. Dispose of **PE** and used supplies in appropriate receptacles.	Reduces the transmission of microorganisms; Standard Precautions.	
24. **HH**		
25. Administer antibiotics as prescribed.	May reduce the risk of infection.	

Expected Outcomes

- Fluid removed from the pericardial sac
- Relief of pain, discomfort, or other symptoms that indicated the need for the procedure
- Improved cardiac output
- Patient's blood pressure, venous pressure, heart sounds, pulse artery pressures, and cardiac rhythm within normal limits

Unexpected Outcomes

- Decrease in blood pressure, rise in pulmonary artery pressures, venous pressure, cardiac dysrhythmias, or excessive bleeding
- Hemodynamic instability
- ST-segment depression
- PR-segment elevation
- Cardiac tamponade
- Pain

Patient Monitoring and Care

Steps	Rationale	Reportable Conditions
		These conditions should be reported if they persist despite nursing interventions.
1. Continuously monitor the patient's ECG; assess pulmonary artery (PA) pressures, venous pressure, blood pressure, SpO$_2$, and neurological status during and every 15 minutes after the procedure until stable (if available, continuously monitor cardiac index and systemic vascular resistance).	A change in these signs may indicate cardiac tamponade, cardiac injury, or hemodynamic instability.	• Increasing venous pressure • Decreasing arterial pressure • Decrease in intensity of heart sounds • Change in level of consciousness • Pulsus paradoxus • Equalizing PA pressures • Decreased cardiac index • Decreased systemic vascular resistance
2. Treat dysrhythmias as prescribed.	Dysrhythmias may lead to cardiac decompensation.	• Persistent dysrhythmias despite appropriate intervention
3. Auscultate heart and lung sounds immediately before and after the procedure.	Evaluates potential fluid reaccumulation or puncture of the lung.	• Asymmetrical breath sounds • Dyspnea • Tachypnea • Decreased SpO$_2$ • Distant or faint heart sounds
4. Ensure a portable chest radiograph is obtained immediately after the procedure as prescribed.	Assesses for pneumothorax and hemothorax.	• Pneumothorax • Hemothorax

Procedure continues on following page

Patient Monitoring and Care —*Continued*

Steps	Rationale	Reportable Conditions
5. Ensure a two-dimensional echocardiogram is obtained within several hours after the procedure as prescribed.	Shows the effectiveness of the pericardial drainage.	• Pericardial effusion
6. Monitor the pericardiocentesis site for bleeding every 15 minutes after the procedure is completed until the patient's condition is stable, then every 4 hours for 24 hours. If an indwelling catheter is present, continue to monitor the site every 4 hours until the catheter has been removed.	Assesses for postprocedural hemostasis and possible drainage.	• Bleeding or hematoma at the site • Drainage at the insertion site
7. Monitor hemoglobin, hematocrit, and coagulation levels as prescribed (e.g., every 8 hours after the procedure for 24 hours and then as indicated).	Assesses for the potential of effusion recurrence or bleeding at the site.	• Bleeding or hematoma at site • Decrease in hemoglobin or hematocrit • Changes in coagulation study results
8. Assess the pericardiocentesis site every day.	Determines the presence of infection.	• Erythema • Edema • Purulent drainage • Foul odor • Temperature >100.5°F (>38°C) • Signs and symptoms of infection
9. Perform site care as prescribed or according to institutional standards: A. Cleanse the area surrounding the pericardial catheter with an antiseptic solution (e.g., 2% chlorhexidine-based preparation).	Reduces infection. The Centers for Disease Control and Prevention (CDC) do not have a specific recommendation for care of pericardial catheters or site care.	
B. Apply a dry sterile gauze or transparent dressing with the date and time of the dressing change. Follow institutional standards. (**Level E***)	The CDC recommends replacing intravascular catheter dressings when the dressing becomes damp, loosened, or soiled or when inspection of the site is necessary.[3]	
10. Be prepared for chest exploration if the patient's status deteriorates.	Deterioration in the patient's hemodynamic status may indicate an increasing effusion and the need for immediate surgical intervention.	• Decreased blood pressure • Dysrhythmias • Increased venous pressure • Change in mental or respiratory status • Diaphoresis • Distant or faint heart sounds
11. Provide emotional support to the patient throughout and after the procedure.	Minimizes apprehension and anxiety.	
12. Keep the patient and family informed about the patient's condition. Be available to answer patient's and family's questions and facilitate meeting their needs as appropriate.	The unknown increases the anxiety and apprehension of the patient and family.	
13. Follow institutional standards for assessing pain. Administer analgesia as prescribed.	Identifies need for pain interventions.	• Continued pain despite pain interventions

* Level E: Multiple case reports, theory-based evidence from expert opinions, or peer-reviewed professional organizational standards without clinical studies to support recommendations.

Documentation

Documentation should include the following:

- Specific preprocedure instruction and patient's and family's satisfactory understanding
- Legally signed informed consent
- Universal Protocol requirement, if nonemergent
- Pre- and postprocedure level of consciousness; blood pressure; venous pressures; pulmonary arterial pressures; cardiac index, cardiac output, and systemic vascular resistance, if available; heart sounds and cardiac rhythm; respiratory status and pulse oximetry reading.

- Preprocedure and postprocedure hemoglobin, hematocrit, and coagulation results, if performed
- Medications administered
- Assessment of pericardiocentesis fluid
- Amount and consistency of postprocedure drainage
- Occurrence of unexpected outcomes
- Pain assessment, interventions, and effectiveness
- ECG rhythm strips
- Emergency interventions necessary
- Specimens sent to the laboratory

References and Additional Readings

For a complete list of references and additional readings for this procedure, scan this QR code with any freely available smartphone code reader app, or visit http://booksite.elsevier.com/9780323376624.

PROCEDURE

44   Atrial Electrogram

Marion E. McRae

PURPOSE: An atrial electrogram (AEG) is obtained to determine the presence of atrial activity in a dysrhythmia or to identify the relationship between atrial and ventricular depolarizations.

PREREQUISITE NURSING KNOWLEDGE

- Understanding of the anatomy and physiology of the cardiovascular system, principles of cardiac conduction, and basic dysrhythmia interpretation is necessary.
- Principles of general electrical safety apply with use of epicardial pacing wires. Gloves should always be worn when handling pacing electrodes to prevent microshock because even small amounts of electrical current can cause serious dysrhythmias if transmitted to the heart.[1,9–11]
- Advanced cardiac life support knowledge and skills are needed.
- AEG is a method of recording electrical activity that originates from the atria with use of temporary atrial epicardial wires placed during cardiac surgery. Standard electrocardiogram (ECG) monitoring records electrical events from the heart with electrodes located on the surface of the patient's body, which is a considerable distance from the myocardium. One limitation of ECG monitoring may be its inability to detect P waves effectively.[3]
- AEGs detect electrical events directly from the atria, which provides a greatly enhanced tracing of atrial activity. This enhanced tracing allows for determination of the presence of atrial activity, comparison of atrial events with ventricular events and determination of the relationship between the two.
- The American Heart Association Practice Standards for Electrocardiographic Monitoring in Hospital Settings recommend recording an AEG whenever tachycardia of unknown origin develops in a patient after cardiac surgery.[2]
- Indications for AEG are as follows:[2]
  - ⋄ When atrial activity is not clearly detected on ECG monitoring
  - ⋄ For determining the relationship between atrial and ventricular activity
  - ⋄ For differentiating wide-complex rhythms (i.e., ventricular tachycardia and supraventricular tachycardia with aberrant ventricular conduction)
  - ⋄ For differentiating narrow-complex supraventricular tachycardias (i.e., sinus tachycardia, atrial tachycardia, paroxysmal supraventricular tachycardia, atrial flutter, atrial fibrillation with relatively regular ventricular rate intervals, or junctional tachycardia)
- AEGs can be performed with multichannel telemetry or a bedside ECG monitor that allows for simultaneous display of the AEG along with the surface ECG.[4–6] A 12-lead ECG machine also can be used to obtain an AEG.
- Accurate identification of the epicardial atrial pacing wire or wires is important.
- The two types of AEGs that can be obtained from epicardial pacing wires are unipolar and bipolar.
  - ⋄ A unipolar electrogram measures electrical activity between one atrial epicardial wire and a surface ECG electrode. The unipolar AEG detects atrial and ventricular activity.
  - ⋄ A bipolar electrogram detects electrical activity between the two atrial epicardial wires. The bipolar AEG predominantly detects atrial activity because both electrodes are attached to the atria.
- Atrial electrograms increase the accuracy of nurses' diagnoses of cardiac arrhythmias.[5,8] However, they remain underused in clinical practice.[6,10]
- An AEG cannot be performed if the patient is dependent on atrial pacing for hemodynamic stability since at least one atrial pacing wire must be disconnected from the pacemaker to perform the AEG, resulting in a loss of atrial pacing.

EQUIPMENT

- Nonsterile gloves
- Temporary atrial epicardial pacing wires placed during cardiac surgery
- Multichannel ECG monitor and recorder or 12-lead ECG machine (ensure that biomedical safety standards are met and the machine is safe for use with epicardial wires)
- Sterile dressings and materials needed for site care including antiseptic solution

Additional equipment, to have available as needed, includes the following:
- ECG electrodes
- Lead wire with alligator clips

- Insulating material for epicardial pacing wires (e.g., finger cots, needle caps, glove, ear plug)

PATIENT AND FAMILY EDUCATION

- Provide information about the normal conduction system, normal and abnormal heart rhythms, and symptoms of abnormal heart rhythms. *Rationale:* This information helps the patient and family to understand the patient's condition and encourages the patient and family to ask questions.
- Provide information about the AEG and the reason for the AEG and explanation of the equipment. *Rationale:* This communication may decrease patient anxiety and help the patient and family to understand the procedure, why it is needed, and how it will help the patient.
- Explain the patient's expected participation during the procedure. *Rationale:* This explanation encourages patient assistance.

PATIENT ASSESSMENT AND PREPARATION

Patient Assessment

- Assess the patient's cardiac rhythm for the presence of atrial activity in more than one lead from the multichannel ECG monitor or 12-lead ECG. *Rationale:* This assessment determines the presence or absence of P waves and the potential need for an AEG.
- Assess the patient's cardiac rhythm for the relationship between atrial and ventricular activity. *Rationale:* This assessment determines the relationship between P waves and QRS complexes and the potential need for an AEG.
- Assess for dysrhythmias. *Rationale:* This assessment determines the patient's baseline cardiac rhythm.
- Assess the patient's hemodynamic status (e.g., systolic, diastolic, and mean arterial pressure; level of consciousness; dizziness; dyspnea; nausea; vomiting; cool or clammy skin; and chest pain). *Rationale:* The patient's hemodynamic status and need for immediate intervention are determined.

Patient Preparation

- Verify that the patient is the correct patient using two identifiers. *Rationale:* Before performing a procedure, the nurse should ensure the correct identification of the patient for the intended intervention.
- Ensure that the patient understands preprocedure teaching. Answer questions as they arise, and reinforce information as needed. *Rationale:* This communication evaluates and reinforces understanding of previously taught information.
- Expose the patient's chest and identify the epicardial pacing wires. *Rationale:* This action provides access to the atrial pacing wires.

Procedure	for Atrial Electrogram	
Steps	**Rationale**	**Special Considerations**
1. HH		
2. PE		Epicardial wires are a direct source of electrical conduction to the myocardium. Use of gloves prevents microshocks with handling of epicardial wires that could cause arrhythmias.[2,9-11]
3. Touch a large metal object such as the patient's bed before touching the wires.[9] (**Level E***)	This prevents microshock that can cause arrythmias.[8]	Any static electricity is discharged before touching the pacing wires.
4. Expose and identify the atrial epicardial pacing wires.	Differentiation of the atrial from the ventricular wires is important to ensure that the appropriate epicardial wires are used.	Typically the atrial wires exit the chest to the right of the patient's sternum and the ventricular wires exit to the left of the patient's sternum (Fig. 44-1).
5. Ensure that you are not using a ground wire (only one sutured to the chest wall).[5]	Using a ground wire will record only a surface ECG not an AEG.	

*Level E: Multiple case reports, theory-based evidence from expert opinions, or peer-reviewed professional organizational standards without clinical studies to support recommendations.

Procedure continues on following page

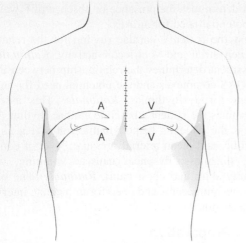

Figure 44-1 Atrial wires exit the chest to the right of the patient's sternum. Ventricular wires exit the chest to the left of the patient's sternum. *(Drawing by Todd Sargood.)*

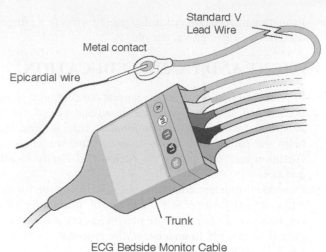

Figure 44-2 Tip of atrial epicardial wire in direct contact with the metal on the end of the V lead wire. *(Drawing by Paul W. Schiffmacher, Thomas Jefferson University, Philadelphia.)*

Procedure	for Atrial Electrogram—*Continued*	
Steps	**Rationale**	**Special Considerations**
Obtaining a Unipolar AEG with Multichannel Telemetry or Bedside ECG Monitor: Lead V		
1. Detach the V lead wire from the electrode on the patient's chest.	Prepares equipment.	Determine that the ECG monitoring system meets all safety requirements.
2. Place the tip of one of the atrial epicardial wires in direct contact with: A. The metal on the end of the V lead wire (Fig. 44-2).[2] **(Level D*)**	Electrical activity is transmitted from the epicardial wire to the ECG monitoring system.	A lead wire with alligator clips at both ends also can be used to connect the epicardial pacing wire to the monitor.
or		
B. The conductive gel on the adhesive side of the electrode attached to the V lead wire (Fig. 44-3).[4-6]	Electrical activity is transmitted from the epicardial wire to the ECG monitoring system.	The electrode can be wrapped around the atrial wire if continuous monitoring of the AEG is indicated to diagnose an unknown intermittent rhythm (Fig. 44-4).[4]
3. Select lead V on the ECG monitor and a surface ECG lead (I, II, III, augmented vector foot, augmented vector right, or augmented vector left).	Use of the precordial lead allows for detection of atrial electrical activity between the lead V and an indifferent limb lead in a unipolar configuration.	
4. Record a dual-channel strip.	Displays the AEG simultaneously with a surface ECG lead.	Label lead V on the ECG strip as the AEG.

*Level D: Peer-reviewed professional and organizational standards with the support of clinical study recommendations.

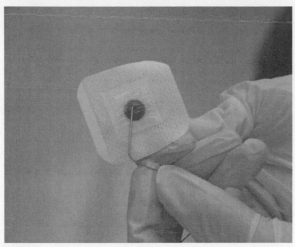

Figure 44-3 The tip of the atrial epicardial wire in direct contact with the conductive gel on the adhesive side of the electrode. *(Kern LS, McRae ME, Funk M: ECG monitoring after cardiac surgery: Postoperative atrial fibrillation and the atrial electrogram, AACN Adv Crit Care 18[3]:298, 2007.)*

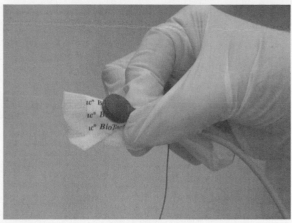

Figure 44-4 An electrode wrapped around the tip of the atrial epicardial wires. *(Kern LS, McRae ME, Funk M: ECG monitoring after cardiac surgery: Postoperative atrial fibrillation and the atrial electrogram, AACN Adv Crit Care 18[3]:299, 2007.)*

Procedure for Atrial Electrogram—*Continued*

Steps	Rationale	Special Considerations
5. Analyze the AEG strip and compare the surface ECG with the AEG: A. Vertically line up the QRS complexes on the ECG strip with the ventricular deflections on the AEG. B. All other spikes should be atrial activity either being initiated in the atrium or being conducted retrograde to the atrium (Fig. 44-5).	Identifies P waves and QRS complexes and determines the relationship between the P waves and the QRS complexes.	Multiple atrial spikes will exist between ventricular spikes if the atrial rate is greater than the ventricular rate (e.g., atrial flutter, atrial fibrillation, second or third degree atrioventricular block).

Obtaining a Unipolar AEG with Multichannel Telemetry or Bedside ECG Monitor: Lead I

Steps	Rationale	Special Considerations
1. Detach the right arm (RA) lead wire from the electrode on the patient's chest.	Prepares equipment.	Determine that the ECG bedside monitoring system meets all safety requirements.
2. Place the tip of one of the atrial epicardial wires in direct contact with: A. The metal on the end of the RA lead wire.[2] **(Level D*)**	Electrical activity is transmitted from the epicardial wire to the ECG monitoring system.	A lead wire with alligator clips at both ends also can be used to connect the epicardial pacing wire to the monitor.
or		
B. The conductive gel on the adhesive side of the electrode attached to the RA lead wire (see Fig. 44-3).[4]	Electrical activity is transmitted from the epicardial wire to the ECG monitoring system.	The electrode can be wrapped around the atrial wire if continued monitoring is indicated to diagnose an unknown intermittent rhythm (see Fig. 44-4).[4]

*Level D: Peer-reviewed professional and organizational standards with the support of clinical study recommendations.

Procedure continues on following page

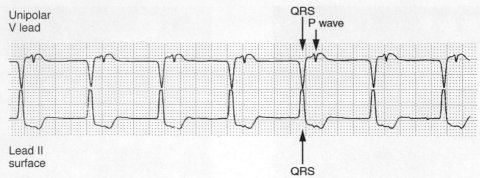

Figure 44-5   Unipolar AEG strip from lead V. The surface ECG was obtained in lead II. On the basis of the surface ECG, the rhythm appears to be junctional with no evidence of P waves or atrial activity. The unipolar AEG shows retrograde P waves that follow the QRS complex, confirming the junctional rhythm interpretation.

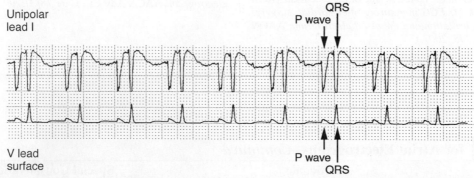

Figure 44-6   Unipolar AEG strip from lead I. The surface ECG was obtained in lead V. The unipolar AEG was obtained in lead I. The atrial activity is magnified in lead I.

Procedure	**for Atrial Electrogram—*Continued***	
Steps	**Rationale**	**Special Considerations**
3. Select lead I and a surface ECG lead on the ECG monitor.	Lead I detects electrical activity between the RA limb lead and the left arm (LA) limb lead. Because the atrial pacing wire is in contact with the RA lead, lead I detects the electrical activity between the atrial wire and the surface LA limb lead.	Label lead I on the ECG strip as the AEG.
4. Record a dual-channel strip.	Displays the AEG simultaneously with a surface ECG lead.	A dual-channel recorder permits the comparison of the surface ECG with the AEG.
5. Analyze the AEG strip and compare the surface ECG with the AEG (Fig. 44-6). A. Vertically line up the QRS complexes on the ECG strip with the ventricular deflections on the AEG. B. All other spikes should be atrial activity either being initiated in the atrium or being conducted retrograde to the atrium (see Fig. 44-6).	Identifies P waves and QRS complexes and determines the relationship between the P waves and the QRS complexes.	

Procedure	for Atrial Electrogram—*Continued*		
Steps	**Rationale**	**Special Considerations**

Obtaining a Unipolar AEG with a 12-Lead ECG Machine

1. Connect the patient to the 12-lead ECG machine (see Procedure 57).	Provides another method of obtaining an AEG.	Determine that the 12-lead ECG machine meets all safety requirements.
2. Attach one atrial epicardial pacing wire to the clip of the RA lead wire of the 12-lead ECG machine (Fig. 44-7).	Prepares for the AEG.	
3. Run a 12-lead ECG.	Lead I measures the electrical activity between the RA and LA. Because the atrial pacing wire is connected to the RA lead, lead I detects the electrical activity between the atrial wire and surface LA limb lead. Lead II measures the electrical activity between the RA and left leg (LL) leads. Because the atrial pacing wire is connected to the RA lead, lead II detects the electrical activity between the atrial wire and the surface LL lead.	
4. Analyze leads I and II.	Identifies P waves and QRS complexes and determines the relationship between the P waves and the QRS complexes.	

Obtaining a Bipolar AEG with Multichannel Telemetry or Bedside ECG Monitor

1. Detach the RA and LA lead wires from the electrodes on the patient's chest.	Two atrial pacing wires are used when obtaining a bipolar AEG.	Determine that the ECG monitoring system meets all safety requirements.

Procedure continues on following page

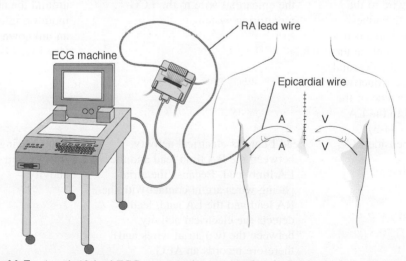

Figure 44-7 Attach 12-lead ECG per procedure except that the RA lead wire connects to one of the atrial epicardial pacing wires. *(Drawing by Todd Sargood.)*

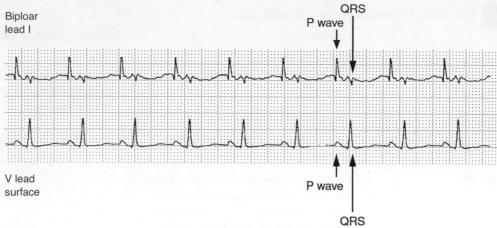

Figure 44-8   Bipolar AEG strip from lead I. The surface ECG was obtained in lead V. The bipolar AEG was obtained in lead I. The atrial activity is magnified in lead I. Also note how small the ventricular activity is in lead I.

Procedure	for Atrial Electrogram—*Continued*	
Steps	**Rationale**	**Special Considerations**
2. Atrial pacing wires: A. Place the tip of one atrial epicardial pacing wire to the metal on the end of the RA lead wire and limb lead and place the tip of the other atrial epicardial pacing wire to the metal on the end of the LA lead wire and limb lead.	Connection to the limb leads of the ECG monitor allows for the detection and recording of atrial electrical activity.	A lead wire with alligator clips at both ends also can be used to connect the epicardial pacing wires to the monitor leads.
or B. Place the tip of one atrial epicardial pacing wire to the conductive gel on the adhesive side of the electrode attached to the RA lead wire and place the tip of the other atrial epicardial pacing wire to the conductive gel on the adhesive side of the electrode attached to the LA lead wire (see Fig. 44-3).	Electrical activity is transmitted from the epicardial wire to the ECG monitoring system.	The electrodes can be wrapped around the atrial wires if continued monitoring is indicated to diagnose an unknown intermittent rhythm (see Fig. 44-4).[4]
3. Select lead I on the bedside ECG monitor.	Lead I detects electrical activity between the RA limb lead and the LA limb lead. Because the atrial pacing wires are in contact with the RA lead and the LA lead, lead I detects the electrical activity between the two atrial wires and therefore records an AEG.	Bipolar tracings magnify atrial activity and minimize ventricular activity.
4. Record a dual-channel strip of lead I and another surface lead.	Displays the AEG simultaneously with a surface ECG.	Label lead I on the ECG strip as the bipolar AEG.
5. Analyze the AEG strip (Fig. 44-8).	Identifies P waves and QRS complexes; determines the relationship between the P waves and the QRS complexes.	

Procedure for Atrial Electrogram—*Continued*

Steps	Rationale	Special Considerations
Obtaining a Bipolar AEG with a 12-Lead ECG Machine		
1. Connect the patient to the 12-lead ECG machine (see Procedure 57).	Provides another method of obtaining an AEG.	Determine that the ECG monitoring system meets all safety requirements.
2. Attach one atrial epicardial pacing wire to the RA limb lead and the other atrial epicardial pacing wire to the LA limb lead of the 12-lead ECG machine.	Connection to the limb leads of the ECG machine allows for the detection and recording of atrial electrical activity.	
3. Run a 12-lead ECG.	Lead I measures the electrical activity between the RA and LA limb leads, which sense atrial activity from both epicardial wires, to provide a bipolar AEG tracing.	
4. Analyze lead I (Fig. 44-9).	Displays the bipolar AEG for analysis. Identifies P waves and QRS complexes and determines the relationship between the P waves and the QRS complexes.	Bipolar tracings magnify atrial activity and minimize ventricular activity. With this method, unipolar AEGs also are obtained in lead II and lead III.

Procedure continues on following page

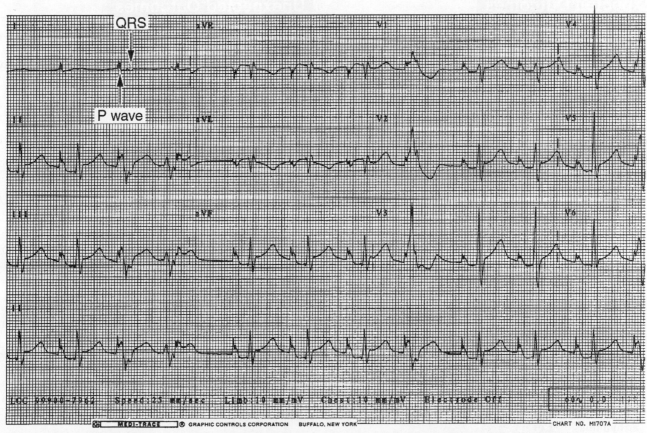

Figure 44-9 A 12-lead ECG obtained with two atrial pacing wires connected to the RA and LA lead wires. Lead I shows a bipolar AEG. The P swave is greater in size than the QRS complex. Leads II and III show unipolar AEGs. In leads II and III, atrial activity is enhanced. Atrial activity is enhanced throughout the 12-lead ECG.

Procedure for Atrial Electrogram—*Continued*

Steps	Rationale	Special Considerations
After AEG Is Obtained		
1. Disconnect the atrial epicardial wires.	Disconnects the wires from the bedside monitoring system or the 12-lead ECG machine.	
2. Reconnect or ensure that the ECG lead wire(s) are connected to the electrode(s) on the patient's chest.	Establishes continuous ECG monitoring.	
3. Apply a dry sterile dressing to the epicardial wire exit sites if this was removed to access the atrial epicardial wires.	Reduces the transmission of microorganisms; Standard Precautions.	Follow institution's guidelines for site care.
4. Place the uninsulated portion of the epicardial wires in an insulated material (e.g., finger cot, needle cap, needle barrel, glove, ear plug).[9–11] **(Level E*)**	Prevents microshock.	
5. Remove gloves and discard used supplies in appropriate receptacle.	Reduces the transmission of microorganisms; Standard Precautions.	
6. 🅷🅷		

Expected Outcomes

- Atrial activity is identified
- The relationship between atrial and ventricular activity is determined

Unexpected Outcomes

- Hemodynamically significant dysrhythmias
- Dysrhythmias in which atrial activity is unclear or the relationship between atrial and ventricular activity is unclear
- Microshocks that cause dysrhythmias

Patient Monitoring and Care

Steps	Rationale	Reportable Conditions
		These conditions should be reported if they persist despite nursing interventions.
1. Evaluate the AEG for the presence of atrial activity and its relationship to ventricular activity. Compare with the surface ECG for interpretation.	AEG determines the presence or absence of atrial activity.	• Inability to identify atrial activity • Inability to determine the relationship between the atrial and ventricular activity
2. Monitor the ECG rhythm for changes.	The underlying dysrhythmia may change during the AEG.	• Altered hemodynamic status caused by change in ECG rhythm
3. Monitor vital signs and level of consciousness during the AEG and as needed.	Ensures adequate tissue perfusion.	• Hemodynamic instability • Change in level of consciousness
4. Assess and treat dysrhythmias identified by the AEG and ECG. AEG can increase diagnostic accuracy of arrhythmias.[5,8] **(Level C*)**	Identifies dysrhythmias that need intervention.	• Return of rhythm stability • Change in cardiac rate or rhythm

*Level C: Qualitative studies, descriptive or correlational studies, integrative reviews, systematic reviews, or randomized controlled trials with inconsistent results.

*Level E: Multiple case reports, theory-based evidence from expert opinions, or peer-reviewed professional organizational standards without clinical studies to support recommendations.

Patient Monitoring and Care —*Continued*

Steps	Rationale	Reportable Conditions
5. Site care should be as follows:		
A. Cleanse the area surrounding the epicardial pacing wires with an antiseptic solution (e.g., 2% chlorhexidine-based preparation). **(Level D*)**	May reduce infection. There are no specific recommendations for epicardial pacing wire site care.[7]	• Any signs or symptoms of infection
B. Apply a dry sterile dressing with the date and time of the dressing change. Institutional standard should be followed for frequency and type of dressing. **(Level D*)**	There are no specific recommendations for epicardial pacing wire dressing care. The Centers for Disease Control and Prevention recommends replacing gauze dressings every 2 days and transparent dressings at least every 7 days.[7] Dressings should be replaced when they become damp, loosened, or soiled or when inspection of the site is necessary.[7] Wet materials increase the likelihood of microshock as electrical current travels more effectively through fluid.	
C. Protect the exposed uninsulated portion of the epicardial pacing wires in an insulated environment according to institutional standards (e.g., finger cot, glove, plastic needle cap, needle barrel, ear plug).[9–11] **(Level E*)**	Prevents microshocks and potentially lethal dysrhythmias.	• Dysrhythmias • Hemodynamic instability • Microshocks

*Level D: Peer-reviewed professional and organizational standards with the support of clinical study recommendations.
*Level E: Multiple case reports, theory-based evidence from expert opinions, or peer-reviewed professional organizational standards without clinical studies to support recommendations.

Documentation

Documentation should include the following:
- Patient and family education
- AEG tracing with interpretation
- Treatment undertaken for arrhythmias present
- Hemodynamic status and level of consciousness
- Patient tolerance of the procedure
- Occurrence of unexpected outcome

References and Additional Readings

For a complete list of references and additional readings for this procedure, scan this QR code with any freely available smartphone code reader app, or visit http://booksite.elsevier.com/9780323376624.

45 Atrial Overdrive Pacing AP (Perform)

Jillian Hamel

PURPOSE: The purpose of atrial overdrive pacing is to attempt to restore sinus rhythm in the setting of reentrant atrial dysrhythmias, especially atrial flutter, by intermittently pacing at a rate faster than the tachycardia. Sinus rhythm enhances cardiac output by allowing atrial contraction to contribute to ventricular filling.

PREREQUISITE NURSING KNOWLEDGE

- Knowledge of the anatomy and physiology of the cardiovascular system, principles of cardiac conduction, and basic and advanced dysrhythmia interpretation is necessary.
- Supraventricular dysrhythmias (e.g., atrial flutter, reentrant atrial tachycardia, atrioventricular [AV] nodal reentry tachycardia, reentrant tachycardias that use an accessory pathway, such as Wolff-Parkinson-White [WPW] syndrome) sometimes can be terminated by overdrive atrial pacing.[1,2]
- Atrial fibrillation occasionally terminates with overdrive atrial pacing, but this is not a reliable therapy for atrial fibrillation. Many contemporary permanent pacemakers have arrhythmia response algorithms that include antitachycardia pacing, but research has not yet shown that continuous atrial overdrive pacing prevents the progression to permanent atrial fibrillation or reduces other major adverse cardiac events.[3,4]
- Knowledge of pacemaker function and patient response to pacemaker therapy is needed.
- Principles of general electrical safety need to be applied with use of temporary invasive pacing.
- Gloves always should be worn when handling pacemaker electrodes to prevent microshock because even small amounts of electrical current can cause serious dysrhythmias if they are transmitted to the heart.[5,9–12]
- Clinical and technical competence related to the use of a temporary atrial pacemaker pulse generator and the rapid atrial pacing feature is needed (Fig. 45-1).
- Advanced cardiac life support knowledge and skills are necessary.
- In the acute care setting, overdrive atrial pacing is performed most commonly with epicardial atrial pacing wires placed during cardiac surgery. A transvenous atrial pacing lead with an active fixation tip to help keep the lead in the atrium also can be used.
- Overdrive atrial pacing involves the delivery of short bursts of rapid pacing stimuli through an epicardial atrial pacing wire or a transvenous lead in the atrium. The physician or advanced practice nurse determines the duration and rate of the burst.
  - ❖ One approach to overdrive pacing is to atrial pace the heart with 20 milliampere (mA) at a rate 20% to 30% faster than the intrinsic atrial rate for 30 seconds, then abruptly stop pacing. An alternate approach is to initiate atrial pacing at a rate 20 beats/min faster than the intrinsic atrial rate; if 1:1 capture does not occur after 30 seconds, the paced rate can be increased by 20 beats/min; repeat every 30 seconds until 1:1 capture is achieved. Continue pacing until the heart rate decreases from AV block (e.g., 2:1, 3:1) or 1 to 2 minutes of 1:1 pacing have occurred, then stop pacing.[6]
  - ❖ Successive bursts usually are performed at gradually increasing rates (maximal capability of the pulse generator for overdrive atrial pacing is 800 pulses/min) and may be delivered for up to 2 minutes.[7]
- The atrial pacing wire or atrial pacing lead needs to be accurately identified with initiation of overdrive pacing because pacing the ventricle at rapid rates may induce ventricular tachycardia or ventricular fibrillation.
- Rapid atrial pacing may result in degeneration of the atrial rhythm to atrial fibrillation with a rapid ventricular response. This pacemaker-induced atrial fibrillation usually does not sustain itself for more than a few minutes before it converts to normal sinus rhythm.[6]
- If an accessory pathway is present, rapid atrial pacing can result in conduction to the ventricles over the accessory pathway, leading to ventricular fibrillation.
- Overdrive suppression of the sinus node may result in periods of bradycardia, asystole, junctional or ventricular escape rhythms, or polymorphic ventricular tachycardia.
- Conversion of an atrial tachydysrhythmia can result in dislodgment of atrial thrombus and embolization of clots to the pulmonary or systemic circulation.

AP   This procedure should be performed only by physicians, advanced practice nurses, and other healthcare professionals (including critical care nurses) with additional knowledge, skills, and demonstrated competence per professional licensure or institutional standard.

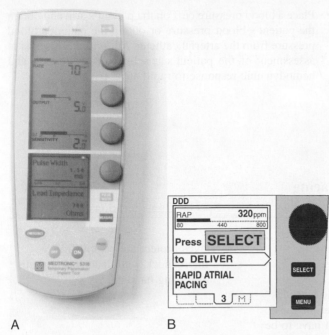

Figure 45-1 **A,** Temporary dual-chamber pulse generator with overdrive atrial pacing capability. **B,** Enlargement of lower screen on the pacemaker showing rapid atrial pacing controls. *(Courtesy Medtronic, Inc.)*

EQUIPMENT

- Nonsterile gloves
- External pulse generator capable of rapid atrial pacing
- Connecting cable (between the pulse generator and the patient's pacemaker leads)
- Cardiac monitor and recorder
- Electrocardiogram (ECG) electrodes
- Double alligator clip or wire with connector pins (if needed to create a ground wire)
- Materials for epicardial pacing wire site care:
  - ❖ Antiseptic pads or swab sticks (e.g., 2% chlorhexidine-based preparation)
  - ❖ Gauze pads
  - ❖ Tape
- Insulating material for epicardial pacing wires or transvenous pacing electrode connector pins (e.g., finger cot, needle cap, needle barrel, glove, ear plug)
- Blood pressure monitoring system

Additional equipment, to have available as needed, includes the following:
- Defibrillator
- Emergency medications
- Airway management equipment
- Standard pulse generator or transcutaneous pacemaker and equipment
- Subcutaneous needle for a ground wire

PATIENT AND FAMILY EDUCATION

- Explain the procedure and its purpose to the patient and family. *Rationale:* This explanation may decrease patient and family anxiety and promote cooperation with the procedure.
- Reassure the patient that atrial pacing usually cannot be felt and that any sensation most likely will be a "fluttering" feeling in the chest. *Rationale:* This reassurance prepares the patient and may decrease the patient's anxiety.

PATIENT ASSESSMENT AND PREPARATION

Patient Assessment

- Assess the patient's ECG rhythm and intervals, verifying atrial and ventricular rates. *Rationale:* This assessment determines baseline cardiac conduction.
- Assess the patient's vital signs and hemodynamic parameters. *Rationale:* This assessment determines baseline cardiovascular function.
- Assess for signs and symptoms that might be caused by the dysrhythmia (e.g., shortness of breath, dizziness, nausea, chest pain, signs of poor peripheral perfusion). *Rationale:* The patient's response to the dysrhythmia is determined.
- Assess the patency of the intravenous access. *Rationale:* Intravenous access is needed for possible administration of fluids and medications.
- Note any medications that might have an effect on the patient's cardiac rhythm or hemodynamic parameters (e.g., beta blockers, calcium channel blockers, antidysrhythmics, and digoxin). *Rationale:* Knowledge of medication therapy can alert the healthcare providers to potential cardiac rhythms (e.g., bradycardia or atrioventricular block) after termination of the atrial dysrhythmia.
- Verify the patient's coagulation study results. *Rationale:* Therapeutic coagulation levels may decrease the risk of embolization.[2,6–8]

Patient Preparation

- Verify that the patient is the correct patient using two identifiers. *Rationale:* Before performing a procedure, the nurse should ensure the correct identification of the patient for the intended intervention.
- Obtain informed consent (may not be possible in an emergency). *Rationale:* Informed consent protects the rights of the patient and makes a competent decision possible for the patient.
- Ensure that the patient and family understand preprocedural teaching. Answer questions as they arise and reinforce information as needed. *Rationale:* This communication evaluates and reinforces understanding of previously taught information.
- Perform a preprocedure verification and time out, if nonemergent. *Rationale:* Ensures patient safety.
- Initiate continuous bedside cardiac monitoring (if not already in place). *Rationale:* The patient's cardiac rate and rhythm must be visible at the bedside during the procedure to determine atrial capture during pacing and to evaluate the response of the patient's cardiac rate and rhythm after pacing.

- Obtain a 12-lead ECG as needed. ***Rationale:*** The ECG may aid in determining the patient's baseline cardiac rhythm.
- Assist the patient to a supine position. ***Rationale:*** This position facilitates access to the epicardial pacemaker wires or the transvenous atrial pacing lead wire.

- Place a blood pressure cuff on the patient's arm and obtain the patient's blood pressure or obtain the patient's blood pressure from the arterial catheter. ***Rationale:*** This aids in assessment of the patient's baseline blood pressure and hemodynamic response to rapid atrial pacing.

Procedure	**for Performing Atrial Overdrive Pacing**	
Steps	Rationale	Special Considerations
1. **HH**		
2. **PE**		Gloves protect the patient from microshock while pacemaker wires are being handled.[5,9-12]
3. Attach the connecting cable to the external pulse generator, making sure that the positive (+) pole of the cable is connected to the (+) terminal of the pulse generator and the negative (−) pole of the cable is connected to the (−) terminal.	The connecting cable provides extra length so that the pulse generator does not have to be placed on the patient's chest or abdomen.	
4. For epicardial atrial pacing:		
A. Expose the atrial epicardial pacing wires.	The atrial epicardial wires usually exit the chest to the right of the patient's sternum (see Fig. 44-1).	The atrial epicardial pacing wires can be verified by performing an atrial electrogram (see Procedure 44).
B. Connect an atrial epicardial pacing wire to the negative terminal of the connecting cable.	The pacing current is delivered through the negative terminal of the pulse generator; an epicardial pacing wire on the atrium must be connected to the negative terminal for the atrium to receive pacing impulses.	
C. Connect a second epicardial pacing wire or a ground wire to the positive terminal of the connecting cable.	The pacing circuit is completed as energy reaches the positive electrode.	If only one atrial pacing wire is present, additional options for a ground wire include an ECG monitoring electrode on the chest near the epicardial pacing wire exit site or a subcutaneous needle in the tissue on the chest. The positive terminal of the connecting cable is connected to the metal snap of the monitoring electrode or the subcutaneous needle hub with a double alligator clip.
5. For transvenous atrial pacing:		
A. Identify the proximal and the distal electrode connector pins on the external portion of the atrial pacing lead.	The pacing stimulus travels from the pulse generator to the negative terminal and energy returns to the pulse generator via the positive terminal.	
B. Connect the distal (negative) electrode connector pin to the negative terminal of the connecting cable.	Energy from the pulse generator is directed to the distal electrode in contact with the atrium.	

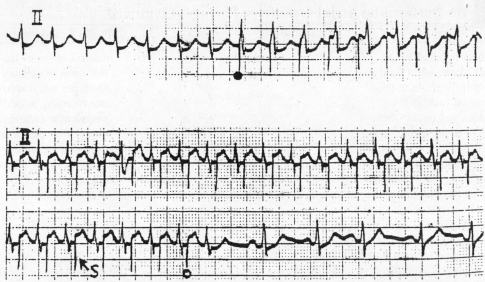

Figure 45-2 The *top trace* shows ECG lead II recorded during an episode of paroxysmal atrial tachycardia at a rate of 150 beats/min. Beginning with the eighth beat in this trace *(black dot)*, rapid atrial pacing at a rate of 165 beats/min was initiated. In the *middle trace*, which begins 12 seconds after the top trace, atrial capture is shown clearly. In the *bottom trace*, which is continuous with the middle trace, sinus rhythm appears when atrial pacing is terminated abruptly *(open circle)*. Paper recording speed was 25 mm/sec. *S*, Stimulus artifact. *(From Cooper TB, MacLean WAH, Waldo AL: Overdrive pacing for supraventricular tachycardia: A review of theoretical implications and therapeutic techniques, Pacing Clin Electrophysiol 1:200, 1978.)*

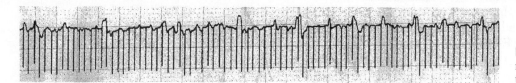

Figure 45-3 Rhythm strip shows rapid atrial pacing in an attempt to terminate atrial flutter.

Procedure for Performing Atrial Overdrive Pacing —*Continued*

Steps	Rationale	Special Considerations
C. Connect the proximal (positive) electrode connecting pin to the positive terminal of the connecting cable.	The pacing circuit is completed as energy reaches the positive electrode.	
6. Set the rate and the milliampere (mA/output) controls on the pulse generator.	The settings are based on the characteristics of the patient's dysrhythmia and the threshold needed for atrial capture.	
7. Initiate atrial overdrive pacing. Pace the atrium for a brief period of 30 seconds to 2 minutes, then abruptly terminate pacing (Figs. 45-2 and 45-3).	Short bursts of pacing stimuli at a rapid rate are intended to create refractory tissue in the atrium and interrupt the reentry circuit responsible for the tachydysrhythmia.	Bursts can be repeated at faster rates and for longer intervals until the dysrhythmia terminates or changes.
A. Pace the heart with 20 mA at a rate 20–30% faster than the intrinsic atrial rate for 30 seconds, then stop pacing.		Refer to the pulse generator's technical manual for instructions on how to initiate rapid atrial pacing.

Procedure continues on following page

Procedure for Performing Atrial Overdrive Pacing—*Continued*

Steps	Rationale	Special Considerations
B. An alternate approach is to initiate atrial pacing at a rate 20 beats/min faster than the intrinsic atrial rate; if 1:1 capture does not occur after 30 seconds, increase the paced rate by 20 beats/min; repeat every 30 seconds until 1:1 capture is achieved. Continue pacing until the heart rate decreases from AV block (e.g., 2:1, 3:1) or 1–2 minutes of 1:1 pacing have occurred, then stop pacing.[6] **(Level E*)**		On termination of the dysrhythmia, the sinus node may be suppressed for a period, resulting in bradycardia, asystole, junctional or ventricular escape rhythms, or ventricular tachycardia. Initiation of temporary atrial, ventricular, or transcutaneous pacing may be necessary until normal sinus function returns.
8. When atrial pacing is completed, disconnect the connecting cable from the epicardial pacing wires or from the transvenous pacing electrode connector pins.	Removes the rapid atrial pacemaker.	Standard pacemaker therapy can be initiated if necessary.
9. Apply a sterile occlusive dressing to the pacemaker site if not already in place.	May reduce the incidence of infection.	
10. Protect the exposed pacemaker electrode connector pins or epicardial pacemaker wires with an insulating material (e.g., finger cot, needle cap, needle barrel, glove, ear plug).[9–12] **(Level E)**	Prevents microshock, which can result in symptomatic dysrhythmias.	
11. Secure the pacing wires or connector pins.	Prevents accidental dislodgment.	
12. Label each epicardial pacemaker wire or dressing to identify atrial and ventricular pacing wires.	Aids identification of the epicardial pacemaker wires.	
13. Remove gloves and discard used supplies in appropriate receptacles.	Reduces the transmission of microorganisms; Standard Precautions.	
14. 🅗🅗		

*Level E: Multiple case reports, theory-based evidence from expert opinions, or peer-reviewed professional organizational standards without clinical studies to support recommendations.

Expected Outcomes

- Return to normal sinus rhythm
- Stable or improved hemodynamic status

Unexpected Outcomes

- Continuation of the tachydysrhythmia
- Conversion to atrial fibrillation
- Prolonged period of bradycardia or asystole after termination of the tachydysrhythmia
- Rapid conduction of atrial paced impulses to the ventricle through an accessory pathway, resulting in ventricular tachycardia or ventricular fibrillation
- Emergence of a slow junctional or ventricular escape rhythm or ventricular tachycardia after termination of the tachydysrhythmia
- Microshock that results in ventricular tachycardia or fibrillation
- Pain

Patient Monitoring and Care

Steps	Rationale	Reportable Conditions
		These conditions should be reported if they persist despite nursing interventions.
1. Monitor the patient's cardiac rhythm continuously at the bedside during the procedure and after the procedure.	Allows for immediate recognition of rhythm changes or return of the initial tachydysrhythmia.	• Heart rate or rhythm changes • Return of initial tachydysrhythmia • Any significant or hemodynamically unstable dysrhythmia • Need for additional temporary pacing to maintain adequate heart rate after conversion of the tachydysrhythmia
2. Monitor the patient's vital signs before initiating overdrive pacing, every 5–10 minutes during attempts to overdrive pace, with any significant heart rate or rhythm change during the procedure, and on termination of the procedure. If the patient's condition is not hemodynamically stable after the procedure, monitor vital signs every 5–10 minutes until stable. Monitor vital signs per unit standard if the patient's condition is stable after the procedure.	Changes in vital signs may indicate significant change in the patient's condition. Blood pressure often improves with cessation of the tachydysrhythmia or restoration of normal sinus rhythm; blood pressure may deteriorate if the ventricular rate accelerates because of overdrive pacing. If the patient is receiving antidysrhythmic medications, changes in vital signs may indicate an adverse medication reaction.	• Abnormal heart rate or rhythm • Hypotension
3. Replace gauze dressings every 2 days and transparent dressings at least every 7 days.[13] Cleanse the site with an antiseptic solution (e.g., 2% chlorhexidine-based solution). Follow institution standard. **(Level D*)**	Although guidelines specific to epicardial wires and transvenous pacemaker sites do not exist, the Centers for Disease Control and Prevention (CDC) recommend replacing dressings on intravascular catheters when the dressing becomes damp, loosened, or soiled or when inspection of the site is necessary.[13]	• Redness or exudate around site • Increased white blood cell count, increased band neutrophil values • Elevated temperature
4. Monitor the patient's response to antidysrhythmic medications.	Antidysrhythmic medications may be necessary to prevent recurrence of the initial tachydysrhythmia or to control the ventricular rate.	• Prolongation of QT interval • Rhythm changes
5. Follow institution standard for assessing pain. Administer analgesia as prescribed.	Identifies need for pain interventions.	• Continued pain despite pain interventions

*Level D: Peer-reviewed professional and organizational standards with the support of clinical study recommendations.

Procedure continues on following page

Documentation

Documentation should include the following:
- Signed informed consent, if nonemergent
- Universal Protocol requirements, if nonemergent
- Patient and family education provided and an evaluation of their understanding of the procedure
- Rhythm strip documenting initial cardiac rate and rhythm
- Initial vital signs
- Pacemaker settings for each attempt of overdrive pacing: rate, mA, duration
- Rhythm strip documenting each overdrive pacing burst

- Number of pacing attempts
- Patient's response to the procedure (e.g., anxiety, pain)
- Pain assessment, interventions and effectiveness
- Post procedure rhythm strip
- Post procedure vital signs
- Any medications given during procedure
- Any unexpected outcomes
- Additional interventions

References and Additional Readings

For a complete list of references and additional readings for this procedure, scan this QR code with any freely available smartphone code reader app, or visit http://booksite.elsevier.com/9780323376624.

46

Epicardial Pacing Wire Removal AP

Marion E. McRae

PURPOSE: Temporary epicardial pacing wires are inserted into the epicardium during cardiac surgery and are removed when pacing therapy is no longer needed.

PREREQUISITE NURSING KNOWLEDGE

- Knowledge of the cardiovascular anatomy and physiology is necessary.
- Knowledge of placement and function of epicardial pacing wires is necessary.
- Advanced cardiac life support knowledge and skills are needed.
- Knowledge of where atrial, ventricular, and ground wires are placed on the chest is necessary.
- Principles of general electrical safety need to be applied with use of temporary epicardial pacemaker wires.[10]
- Gloves always should be worn when handling epicardial pacemaker electrodes to prevent microshock because even small amounts of electrical current can cause serious dysrhythmias if they are transmitted to the heart.[1,13]
- Knowledge of cardiac dysrhythmias and treatment of life-threatening dysrhythmias is necessary.
- Relative contraindications to epicardial pacing wire removal include, abnormal coagulation study results (elevated international normalized ratio [INR], partial thromboplastin time [PTT], heparin level, or heparin anti-Xa level), very low platelet counts, presence of dysrhythmias that necessitate pacing, and compromised hemodynamic status.[4,10] Acceptable levels for INR, PTT, heparin level, or anti-Xa level are determined by institutional policy.
- Knowledge of signs and symptoms of cardiac tamponade is needed (e.g., hemodynamic instability, dyspnea, muffled heart sounds, diaphoresis, equalizing pulmonary artery pressures, jugular venous distention, pulsus paradoxus, narrowed pulse pressure, orthopnea, altered level of consciousness).[2,9,15]
- Epicardial pacing wires should not be cut but should be removed. Retained epicardial pacing wires can cause long-term problems. The wires can eventually protrude through the skin, cause local infection or infective endocarditis, and they can migrate, causing serious tissue and organ injury.[16,18]
- Although it is not recommended, if cut epicardial pacemaker wires are left in situ, the patient must be educated

about this, what warning signs to look for, and to identify that the wires are in situ before magnetic resonance image (MRI) scanning, although MRI scanning with retained epicardial wires is considered safe at 1.5 Tesla.[6,7,12,18]

EQUIPMENT

- Nonsterile gloves
- Antiseptic solution (e.g., 2% chlorhexidine-based solution)
- Suture removal kit
- Sterile gauze
- Tape

Additional equipment, to have available as needed, includes the following:
- Emergency equipment including resuscitation cart and sternotomy tray
- Temporary transcutaneous or transvenous pacing equipment

PATIENT AND FAMILY EDUCATION

- Assess patient and family readiness to learn, and identify factors that affect learning. *Rationale:* This assessment allows the nurse to individualize teaching.
- Provide information about the epicardial pacing wires, the reason for their removal, and an explanation of the procedure. *Rationale:* This information helps the patient and family to understand the procedure and why it is needed and may decrease anxiety.
- Explain the patient's expected participation during and after the procedure. *Rationale:* Encourages patient participation in the treatment plan and may decrease anxiety.
- Explain that the patient may feel mild pain and a burning or pulling sensation during the procedure.[11,14] *Rationale:* This explanation prepares the patient for the procedure.

PATIENT ASSESSMENT AND PREPARATION
Patient Assessment

- Assess the patient's baseline cardiovascular, hemodynamic, and peripheral vascular status. *Rationale:* This assessment provides data that can be used for comparison with postremoval assessment data and hemodynamic values.

AP   This procedure should be performed only by physicians, advanced practice nurses, and other healthcare professionals (including critical care nurses) with additional knowledge, skills, and demonstrated competence per professional licensure or institutional standard.

- Assess the patient's current laboratory data, including electrolyte and coagulation study results. ***Rationale:*** This assessment identifies laboratory abnormalities. Baseline coagulation studies (INR [if on warfarin], PTT or heparin levels [if on heparin], anti-Xa levels [if on low molecular weight heparin]) and platelet counts are helpful in determining the patient's risk for bleeding.[4] Electrolyte abnormalities such as hypokalemia, hyperkalemia, or hypomagnesemia may increase cardiac irritability.
- Ensure that the patient is not fully anticoagulated and/or that the platelet count is not very low. Based on the half-life of heparin,[8] stop a heparin infusion 2 hours before pacemaker wire removal and start the heparin infusion 1 hour after pacemaker removal.[4,8] Remove pacemaker wires at the nadir of low molecular weight heparin doses or hold for several hours when the next dose is due. Ensure that the INR is less than 1.5 to 2 before removing pacemaker wires if the patient is on warfarin.[4,10] Ensure the platelet count is greater than 50,000. ***Rationale:*** Bleeding is more likely to occur if the patient is anticoagulated or the platelet count is low.

Patient Preparation

- Verify that the patient is the correct patient using two identifiers. ***Rationale:*** Before performing a procedure, the nurse should ensure the correct identification of the patient for the intended intervention.
- Ensure that the patient and family understand preprocedural teaching. Answer questions as they arise, and reinforce information as needed. ***Rationale:*** Evaluates and reinforces understanding of previously taught information.
- Remove epicardial pacing wires at least the day before discharge (approximately 24 hours or longer).[10] ***Rationale:*** Removal at this time provides time for observation for potential complications.
- Administer prescribed analgesic medication before removing the epicardial pacing wires.[11,14] ***Rationale:*** Analgesics may minimize discomfort during epicardial pacing wire removal. Patients report mild pain and a burning or pulling sensation during the procedure.[11,14]
- Determine the patency of an intravenous (IV) catheter. ***Rationale:*** A patent IV is necessary should emergency fluids or medications be needed.
- Ensure that patient has electrocardiographic (ECG) monitoring. ***Rationale:*** ECG monitoring provides assessment for the presence of potential dysrhythmias during epicardial wire removal.[2]

Procedure   for Epicardial Pacing Wire Removal

Steps	Rationale	Special Considerations
1. **HH**		
2. **PE**		Gloves minimize the possibility of microshock when in contact with the epicardial pacing wires.[1,13]
3. Assist the patient into the supine position with head of bed (HOB) up 30 degrees.	This position provides the best access during the procedure.	Epicardial pacing wires are removed with the patient lying in bed.
4. Touch a large metal object such as the patient bed before touching the wires to ensure any static electricity is discharged.[13] **(Level E*)**	Static electricity could be conducted to the pacemaker wires resulting in microshock.	
5. Remove the dressing and tape over the epicardial wires.	Exposes the epicardial wire exit sites.	
6. Cleanse each of the epicardial pacing wire exit sites with an antiseptic solution (e.g., 2% chlorhexidine solution).	May reduce the risk of infection.	Cleanse at least a 3-inch area around each of the exit sites.
7. Untie or cut the suture knot of each of the epicardial pacing wires at the skin.	Prepares for epicardial pacing wire removal.	
8. Obtain an ECG strip and observe the patient's ECG monitor while removing epicardial wires.	Dysrhythmias may occur during epicardial wire removal, particularly ventricular ectopy.[2]	

*Level E: Multiple case reports, theory-based evidence from expert opinions, or peer-reviewed professional organizational standards without clinical studies to support recommendations.

Procedure for Epicardial Pacing Wire Removal—*Continued*

Steps	Rationale	Special Considerations
9. Remove each epicardial atrial pacing wire and then right ventricular epicardial pacing wires by pulling with a steady, slow, gentle tension. There may also be epicardial wires on the left ventricle for right atrial-left ventricular or biventricular pacing that require removal.[5] Ground pacing wires are anchored only in the skin and are removed similar to skin sutures.	Steady, slow, gentle tension uncoils the pacing lead from the epicardial surface of the heart. Removing the atrial wires first allows ventricular pacing if hemodynamic instability occurs.	Follow institution standard. If slow, steady, gentle tension does not remove the wires, stop the procedure and notify the surgeon. Wires can become trapped in adhesions.
10. Inspect each epicardial pacing wire to ensure that each wire is intact and to assess for the presence of tissue.[3,19] **(Level E*)**	Ensures that each epicardial wire extracted is completely intact.	If bleeding occurs at the epicardial pacing wire site, apply direct pressure until bleeding stops. If tissue is noted on the epicardial wire(s) observe the patient for hemodynamic instability. Notify the physician if tissue is noted on the epicardial wire(s) and if bleeding or oozing continues.
11. Apply a sterile dressing over the epicardial exit sites.	Decreases the risk of infection until the exit sites heal. Contains drainage from the site.	
12. Remove **PE** and discard used supplies in appropriate receptacle.	Reduces the transmission of microorganisms and body secretions; Standard Precautions.	
13. **HH**		

Expected Outcomes

- Removal of the epicardial pacing wires
- Stable cardiac rate and rhythm
- Stable vital signs

Unexpected Outcomes

- Dysrhythmias
- Hemodynamic instability
- Pain
- Hemorrhage
- Cardiac tamponade
- Hematoma
- Infection

Patient Monitoring and Care

Steps	Rationale	Reportable Conditions
		These conditions should be reported if they persist despite nursing interventions.
1. Ask the patient to let you know if any pain, changes in breathing, sweating, or lightheadedness occur. **(Level C*)**	These signs and symptoms have been found to correlate with cardiac tamponade after pacemaker wire removal.[9] Dyspnea has a sensitivity of 87–89% for cardiac tamponade.[15]	• Dyspnea • Bleeding • Palpitations • Diaphoresis • Chest pressure • Presyncope

*Level C: Qualitative studies, descriptive or correlational studies, integrative reviews, systematic reviews, or randomized controlled trials with inconsistent results.
*Level E: Multiple case reports, theory-based evidence from expert opinions, or peer-reviewed professional organizational standards without clinical studies to support recommendations.

Procedure continues on following page

Patient Monitoring and Care —*Continued*

Steps	Rationale	Reportable Conditions
2. After the epicardial wires are removed, monitor vital signs frequently for at least 2 hours. Follow institution standard. **(Level C*)**	Determines the patient's hemodynamic status. Abrupt hypotension can occur within 2 hours of pacemaker wire removal.[9]	• Abnormal vital signs
3. Continue ECG monitoring for at least 24 hours after removal of epicardial pacing wires.[10] **(Level E*)**	Provides assessment of possible dysrhythmias.	• Dysrhythmias • ECG changes
4. Follow institution standard regarding activity limitations after epicardial pacing wire removal.	There is little evidence that activity limitation after removal of pacemaker wires prevents complications.[17]	
5. When obtaining vital signs, assess for signs and symptoms of cardiac tamponade.	Early detection is important because cardiac tamponade is a potentially fatal complication.	• Hypotension and tachycardia • Pulsus paradoxus • Beck's triad (jugular venous distention, hypotension, and muffled heart sounds) • Presyncope • Altered level of consciousness • Orthopnea
6. Follow the institution's standard for assessing pain. Administer analgesia as prescribed.	Identifies need for pain interventions.	• Continued pain despite pain interventions

*Level C: Qualitative studies, descriptive or correlational studies, integrative reviews, systematic reviews, or randomized controlled trials with inconsistent results.
*Level E: Multiple case reports, theory-based evidence from expert opinions, or peer-reviewed professional organizational standards without clinical studies to support recommendations.

Documentation

Documentation should include the following:
- Patient and family education
- Removal of epicardial pacing wires
- Patient tolerance of the procedure
- Pain assessment, interventions, and effectiveness
- Site assessment
- Vital signs and ECG strip
- Occurrence of unexpected outcomes and interventions

References and Additional Readings

For a complete list of references and additional readings for this procedure, scan this QR code with any freely available smartphone code reader app, or visit http://booksite.elsevier.com/9780323376624.

47 Implantable Cardioverter-Defibrillator

Kiersten Henry

PURPOSE: The implantable cardioverter-defibrillator (ICD) is a device that is used to prevent sudden cardiac death from malignant ventricular dysrhythmias. The ICD continuously monitors a patient's rhythm and attempts to convert ventricular tachycardia or ventricular fibrillation via antitachycardia pacing, cardioversion, defibrillation, or some combination of these. The ICD has the capability for backup bradycardia pacing.

PREREQUISITE NURSING KNOWLEDGE

- Knowledge of the anatomy and physiology of the cardiovascular system, principles of cardiac conduction, and basic dysrhythmia interpretation is needed.
- Knowledge of basic functioning of ICDs and patient response to ICD therapy is needed.
- Knowledge of principles of defibrillation threshold, antidysrhythmia medications, alteration in electrolytes, and effect on the defibrillation threshold is necessary.
- Advanced cardiac life support (ACLS) knowledge and skills are needed.
- Clinical and technical competence related to use of the external defibrillator is necessary.
- Indications for ICD implantation, based on the 2012 Update of the American College of Cardiology (ACC)/American Heart Association (AHA)/Heart Rhythm Society (HRS) guidelines[8]:
  - ❖ Class I: Indicated in:
    - ○ Survivors of cardiac arrest as a result of ventricular fibrillation (VF) or sustained unstable ventricular tachycardia (VT)
    - ○ Patients with structural heart disease and sustained VT (hemodynamically stable or unstable)
    - ○ Patients with syncope of undetermined origin with hemodynamically significant VT or VF at electrophysiology study (EPS)
    - ○ Patients with nonischemic dilated cardiomyopathy (DCM) with left ventricular ejection fraction (LVEF) less than or equal to 35%, New York Heart Association (NYHA) functional class II or III
    - ○ Patients with LVEF less than 35% as a result of prior myocardial infarction (MI; more than 40 days after MI), NYHA class II or III; or LVEF less than 30%, NYHA functional class I
    - ○ Patients with nonsustained VT as a result of prior MI, LVEF less than 40%, with inducible VF or sustained VT at EPS

- ❖ Class IIa: Reasonable for:
  - ○ Patients with unexplained syncope, significant left ventricular (LV) dysfunction, nonischemic dilated cardiomyopathy
  - ○ Patients with sustained VT with normal or near-normal ventricular function
  - ○ Patients with hypertrophic cardiomyopathy (HCM) or arrhythmogenic right ventricular dysplasia (ARVD) and with one or more major risk factors for sudden cardiac death (SCD)
  - ○ Patients with long QT syndrome who are having syncope or VT while receiving beta blockers
  - ○ Patients who are not hospitalized and are waiting transplantation
  - ○ Patients with Brugada syndrome, with either syncope or with documented VT that has not resulted in cardiac arrest
  - ○ Patients with catecholaminergic polymorphic VT with syncope or documented sustained VT on beta blocker therapy
  - ○ Patients with cardiac sarcoidosis, giant cell myocarditis, or Chagas' disease
- ❖ Class IIb: May be considered in:
  - ○ Patients with nonischemic cardiomyopathy with LVEF less than or equal to 35%, NYHA functional class I
  - ○ Patients with long QT syndrome and risk factors for SCD
  - ○ Patients with syncope and advanced structural heart disease in whom thorough invasive and noninvasive investigations have failed to define a cause
  - ○ Patients with familial cardiomyopathy associated with SCD
  - ○ Patients with LV noncompaction
- ❖ Class III: Not indicated in:
  - ○ Patients without a clinical expectation of survival for at least 1 year (with reasonable functional status), even if other implantation criteria are met
  - ○ Patients with refractory VT or VF

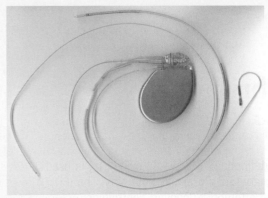

Figure 47-1 ICD and lead system (including superior vena cava lead, right ventricular lead, and coronary sinus lead). *(Courtesy Boston Scientific Corporation, Natick, MA.)*

- Patients with significant psychiatric illness that may be impacted by device implantation, or may impact patient's ability to follow up
- Patients with NYHA Class IV heart failure, refractory to drug therapy, who are not candidates for transplantation or cardiac resynchronization therapy
- Patients with syncope of undetermined cause, and no evidence of inducible ventricular tachyarrhythmias or structural heart disease
- Patients with VF/VT that can be treated with catheter or surgical ablation
- Patients with ventricular dysrhythmias due to a reversible disorder (such as electrolyte imbalance or medications) without evidence of structural heart disease
- A specific time period of guideline-driven medical therapy must be initiated before implantation of an ICD. The indication for implantation determines the necessary waiting period:
  - Patients with any cardiomyopathy not on optimal medical therapy must be reassessed for eligibility after 3 months.
  - Patients who are post-MI or ischemic cardiomyopathy and are revascularized with percutaneous coronary intervention or coronary artery bypass must be reassessed for eligibility after 3 months.
  - Patients who are post-MI without revascularization must be reassessed for eligibility after 40 days.
  - Patients with any cardiomyopathy who have been on guideline-directed medical therapy for the required interval can be referred for ICD implantation.[12]
- The ICD system is composed of a pulse generator and a lead system. The pulse generator is titanium and contains the capacitors, circuitry, and a lithium battery (Fig. 47-1).
- Battery longevity may be greater than 5 years, depending on the number of times therapies are delivered and the frequency of pacing.[15,16] The pulse generator is typically located in a pectoral subcutaneous pocket.
- The leads are insulated wires that sense the patient's intrinsic rhythm and can pace or deliver therapies (Fig. 47-2). Leads are classified as atrial or ventricular, endocardial (transvenous) or epicardial (myocardial), unipolar

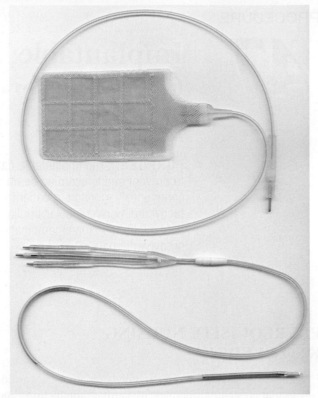

Figure 47-2 *Top,* ICD patch that is placed on the right ventricle. *Bottom,* Superior vena cava lead. *(Courtesy Boston Scientific Corporation, Natick, MA.)*

or bipolar, and active or passive fixation. The lead systems may be single, double, or multiple.
- Leads may be attached to the heart via active or passive fixation. Active fixation leads use a screw, barb, or hook at the tip that is embedded into the myocardium to ensure stability of the lead. Passive fixation leads use tines or fins at the tip that allow the lead to attach to trabeculae of the myocardium.
- Most leads are endocardial (transvenous) leads and are inserted transvenously through the subclavian, cephalic, or axillary veins.
- Epicardial leads are less common but are used in special circumstances. Epicardial pacing leads may be placed on the outside of the left ventricle to provide biventricular pacing when coronary sinus placement of the LV lead has been unsuccessful. Epicardial patches may be placed on the outside of the heart, both anteriorly and posteriorly. Epicardial patches provide a greater surface area for defibrillation (see Fig. 47-2).
- All leads have a cathode (negative pole) and an anode (positive pole). A unipolar lead uses one conductor wire, with a distal electrode as cathode and the metal can as the anode. This configuration produces a large electrical circuit and a large pacing artifact on electrocardiography (ECG). Because of the large area covered, this configuration is susceptible to stimulation of chest muscles and also to electromagnetic interference. A bipolar lead uses two electrodes on the distal end of the lead to form the circuit. The cathode is located at the distal tip, and the anode

several millimeters proximal to the tip. Because of the closer circuitry, a smaller pacing artifact is seen on ECG.

- All ICDs function as pacemakers. Some ICDs are also biventricular pacemakers. Cardiac resynchronization therapy (CRT) paces the right and left ventricles together to establish synchrony in an effort to improve LV function.[11] Biventricular pacing must be as close to 100% as possible for the greatest benefit. Biventricular pacing leads are placed in the right atrium, the right ventricle, and an epicardial vein on the surface of the left ventricle accessed through the coronary sinus. Patients must be on guideline-based medical therapy before placement of a device for CRT. Indications for biventricular pacing, based on the 2012 Update of the American College of Cardiology (ACC)/American Heart Association (AHA)/Heart Rhythm Society (HRS) guidelines[8]:
  - ❖ Class I: Indicated in:
    - ○ Patients with LVEF less than or equal to 35%, left bundle branch block (LBBB) with a QRS duration greater than or equal to 150 ms, NYHA class II-IV symptoms, and sinus rhythm
  - ❖ Class IIa: May be useful in:
    - ○ Patients with LVEF less than or equal to 35%, LBBB with a QRS duration 120 to 149 ms or non-LBBB pattern with QRS duration greater than or equal to 150 ms, NYHA class II-IV symptoms, and sinus rhythm
    - ○ Patients with ejection fraction less than or equal to 35% who require ventricular pacing for other reasons
    - ○ Patients with ejection fraction less than or equal to 35% who are undergoing new or replacement device placement and are expected to have ventricular pacing greater than 40% of the time
  - ❖ Class IIb: May be considered in:
    - ○ Patients with ischemic cardiomyopathy, LVEF less than or equal to 30%, LBBB with a QRS greater than or equal to 150 ms, NYHA class I symptoms, and sinus rhythm
    - ○ Patients with LVEF of less than or equal to 35%, a non-LBBB pattern with QRS 120 to 149 ms, NYHA class III/IV symptoms, and sinus rhythm
    - ○ Patients with LVEF of less than or equal to 35%, a non-LBBB pattern with QRS greater than or equal to 150 ms, NYHA class II symptoms, and sinus rhythm

- ❖ Class III: Not indicated in:
  - ○ Patients with a non-LBBB pattern and QRS duration less than 150 ms who have NYHA class I/II symptoms
  - ○ Patients whose expected survival with good functional capacity is less than 1 year
- The ICD detects tachydysrhythmias, delivers antitachycardia pacing (ATP) or electrical therapy (shock), and provides bradycardia pacing. ATP attempts to convert monomorphic VT by pacing at a rate faster than the VT rate, thereby terminating the dysrhythmia. ATP is a painless way of treating VT, sometimes avoiding shock therapy altogether. The PainFree II trial demonstrated that compared with shocks, empirical ATP for fast VT was highly effective, equally safe, and improved quality of life.[19] Cardioversion is generally referred to as synchronized electrical therapy. Defibrillation is not synchronized and is generally used to convert ventricular dysrhythmias.[6]
- The ICD therapies may be programmed from one to three zones. In the first zone (e.g., rates 182 to 200 beats per minute), the device may be programmed to differentiate between supraventricular tachycardia (SVT) and VF/VT. A delay of 30 to 40 beats allows the device to differentiate between rhythms and initiate appropriate therapy. Additional zones based on heart rates (201 to 250 and >250) allow for more aggressive management of tachyarrythmias. Zones may be programmed for sequential therapies of ATP followed by electrical defibrillation if ATP is unsuccessful. Programming of multiple zones helps to reduce inappropriate defibrillator shocks.[10,14,18,23]
- A defibrillator code was developed in 1993 by the North American Society of Pacing and Electrophysiology and the British Pacing and Electrophysiology Group to describe the capabilities and operation of ICDs. The defibrillator code is patterned after the pacemaker code; however, it has some important differences (Table 47-1).[3] The defibrillator code offers less information about the ICD's antibradycardia pacing function but more specific information about the shock functions.
- A magnet applied over an ICD disables the device therapies of ATP and electrical cardioversion/defibrillation but does not affect pacemaker function. The magnet is used during procedures that may cause electromagnetic interference (EMI). EMI from cautery devices, for example,

TABLE 47-1	NASPE/BPEG Defibrillator Code		
Position I	**Position II**	**Position III**	**Position IV**
Shock Chamber	**Antitachycardia Pacing Chamber**	**Tachycardia Detection**	**Antibradycardia Pacing Chamber**
0 = none	0 = none	E = electrogram	0 = none
A = atrium	A = atrium	H = hemodynamic	A = atrium
V = ventricle	V = ventricle		V = ventricle
D = dual (A + V)	D = dual (A + V)		D = dual (A + V)

NASPE/BPEG, North American Society of Pacing and Electrophysiology/British Pacing and Electrophysiology Group.
From Bernstein AD, et al. The NASPE/BPEG defibrillator code (NBD code). Pacing Clin Electrophysiol, 16, 1776, 1993.

may be improperly sensed as a tachydysrhythmia, causing inappropriate device shock. In most models, removal of the magnet restores normal ICD function. Some models, however, do not resume previous settings once the magnet is removed.[17] Checking with the manufacturer before magnet use is best to determine the specific recommendations for each ICD. If a device programmer and trained personnel are available, device tachydysrhythmia detection and therapies can be disabled through the programmer for the duration of the procedure.

- Emotional adjustments vary with each patient and family. Patients may experience depression, anxiety, fear, and anger. Some patients view the device as an activity restriction, and others see it as a life-saving device that allows normal life to resume. Preimplantation psychological variables, such as degree of optimism or pessimism, and an anxious personality style may place patients at a higher level of risk for difficulty adjusting to the ICD.[17] Support groups may serve a vital role for ICD recipients who are anxious and for patients who may need additional support. Education interventions with patients and family members help to reduce psychosocial distress. Delivery of shock is shown to increase the risk of posttraumatic stress disorder in patients with ICDs.[7]
- The option of ICD deactivation should be discussed before the device is implanted.[21] Early discussions of device deactivation facilitate later discussions and are an important part of the informed consent process.[13,22]

EQUIPMENT

- ECG monitor and recorder
- ECG electrodes

Additional equipment, to have available as needed, includes the following:

- ICD programmer (commonly obtained from the electrophysiology department or specific manufacturer)
- Magnet (doughnut or bar type)
- 12-lead ECG machine
- Analgesia and sedation as prescribed
- Emergency medications and resuscitation equipment
- Antidysrhythmia medications as prescribed

PATIENT AND FAMILY EDUCATION

- Assess learning needs, readiness to learn, and factors that influence learning. *Rationale:* This assessment allows the nurse to individualize teaching in a meaningful manner.
- Assess patient and family understanding of ICD therapy and the reason for its use. *Rationale:* This assessment provides information regarding knowledge level and necessity of additional teaching.
- Provide information about the normal conduction system, such as structure of the conduction system, source of the heartbeat, normal and abnormal heart rhythms, symptoms of abnormal heart rhythms, and the potentially life-threatening nature of VT and VF. *Rationale:* Understanding of the conduction system and dangerous dysrhythmias assists the patient and family in recognizing the seriousness of the patient's condition and the need for ICD therapy.

- Provide information about ICD therapy, including the reason for the ICD, device operation, location of the device, types of therapy given by the device, risks and benefits of the device, and follow-up. *Rationale:* Understanding of ICD functioning assists the patient and family in developing realistic perceptions of ICD therapy.
- Discuss postimplant incision care, including inspection of the incision and pocket. The incision is kept dry for several days after the procedure. *Rationale:* The nurse or physician needs to know whether any of the following signs or symptoms of infection appear: redness, edema, warmth, drainage, and/or fever.
- Discuss postoperative activity. For the first 4 to 6 weeks after implant: (1) no lifting of the arm on the side of the ICD above the shoulder or extending the arm to back (including activities such as swimming, golfing, and bowling); (2) no lifting of items heavier than 10 lb; and (3) no excessive pushing, pulling, or twisting. *Rationale:* The activity restrictions help to prevent new leads from dislodgment.
- Provide patients with an identification card (temporary cards are usually given to patients at the time of implant, and permanent cards are sent to patients by the manufacturer several weeks later). Encourage the patient to wear Medic Alert identification and to carry the identification card at all times. *Rationale:* This identification ensures that appropriate information is available to anyone caring for the patient.
- If patients are prescribed antidysrhythmic medication, stress the importance of continuing the medication. *Rationale:* Antidysrhythmic medications suppress dysrhythmias and may limit potential ICD shocks.
- Discuss the need for patients to keep a current list of medications in their wallets. *Rationale:* The patient or other family members should be prepared to provide necessary information to healthcare providers in an emergency situation.
- Encourage family members to learn community CPR. *Rationale:* Family members may be more prepared for an emergency situation (e.g., if the ICD does not convert a life-threatening rhythm or the ICD malfunctions).
- Educate patients and families about what to do for a device shock. The shock varies in intensity from mild to severe pain. If patients have received an isolated shock and are asymptomatic afterward, they should call their healthcare provider to determine further action (usually an appointment for device interrogation). If patients have received multiple shocks in a short period of time (within minutes to hours), or if they have had one shock and do not feel well, they should activate the emergency medical services (EMS) system by calling 911 to seek emergency evaluation at an emergency room.[4] *Rationale:* Repeated shocks may indicate conditions that necessitate prompt treatment, such as electrolyte imbalance or ischemia. They may also indicate malfunction of the device sensing, which may occur with lead fracture.
- Inform patients to call their healthcare provider if they hear an audible tone emitted from the device. An audible tone may indicate battery depletion or signal device

parameter alerts (such as lead impedance out of normal range). Some devices use vibratory alerts in place of audible tones to signal an alert condition. *Rationale:* The ICD should be interrogated to determine the reason for the tone and to ensure safe device function.

- Inform patients and families that family members are not harmed if they touch the patient when a shock is delivered. *Rationale:* This information prepares the patient and family and may decrease anxiety.
- Driving restrictions vary from state to state and among physicians. Each patient should discuss plans for long trips and driving restrictions with the physician. Current guidelines prohibit anyone with an ICD from obtaining a commercial driver's license.[9] *Rationale:* These restrictions are intended to prevent motor vehicle accidents from sudden loss of consciousness while driving.
- Educate patients and families that the terms "elective replacement indicated" (ERI) and "end of life" (EOL) are used to describe the status of the battery. At ERI, the battery is able to function for approximately another 2 to 3 months. A generator change is done as soon as possible during that time period. At EOL, the generator must be changed promptly. *Rationale:* This teaching prepares patients and families for generator changes, alleviates misunderstanding, and may decrease anxiety.
- Inform patients and family members about follow up device checks or "interrogations." Stress the importance of keeping these appointments. Devices are checked every 3 to 6 months (but may be more frequent if any issues arise that necessitate monitoring). Many follow-up checks are now done remotely, through Internet-based systems. A transmitter device is mailed to the patient from the device manufacturer.[15] *Rationale:* Routine interrogation maintains optimal functioning of the ICD and alerts providers of dysrhythmias.
- Inform the patient and family of potential sources of EMI to the ICD. In the hospital, EMI include magnetic resonance imaging, diathermy, computed tomography, lithotripsy, electrocautery, radiation therapy, and nerve stimulators. Outside the hospital, these include handheld wands used by airport security, arc welders, large transformers or motors, antitheft devices at stores or libraries, cellular phones less than 6 inches away from the pulse generator, the antenna of an operating citizens' band or ham radio, improperly grounded electrical equipment, and handheld tools less than 12 inches away from the pulse generator. Cellular phones should be positioned on the opposite side of device.[1] *Rationale:* EMI can deactivate ICD therapies.
- Explore the patient's feelings about having an ICD. Provide education to the patient and family members about the device implantation. *Rationale:* Acknowledging these stressors may alleviate the most common psychological disturbances after ICD implantation, which include stress, anxiety, depression, and fear.[17]
- Inform patients to notify their physicians if the device begins to wear through the skin or the device site becomes reddened, warm, painful, or has discharge. *Rationale:* These signs and symptoms identify problems (e.g., infection) that need additional medical care.

PATIENT ASSESSMENT AND PREPARATION

Patient Assessment

- Assess the patient's cardiac rate and rhythm. *Rationale:* This assessment establishes baseline data.
- Presurgical instructions usually include maintaining nothing by mouth (NPO) for at least 8 hours before the procedure and obtaining complete blood cell count (CBC), chemistries, prothrombin time (PT), and partial thromboplastin time (PTT) for baseline data. *Rationale:* All these actions ensure patient safety to prevent complications such as excessive bleeding and aspiration.
- For patients prescribed oral anticoagulation, review with the physician who will be implanting the device whether the anticoagulation medication should be continued or bridged with a short acting anticoagulant such as heparin. *Rationale:* Historically, warfarin has been held for several days before the implant procedure with heparin as a bridge to surgery. Recent research shows a lower incidence with continuation of warfarin rather than bridging with heparin.[5]
- Assess the patency of the patient's intravenous access. *Rationale:* Intravenous access should be ensured for administration of prescribed medications.
- Administer antibiotics as prescribed. *Rationale:* Antibiotics are administered to reduce infection from skin microorganisms such as *Staphylococcus aureus* (cause of early infection) and *Staphylococcus epidermidis* (cause of later infection).[2]
- Identify the manufacturer of the ICD and how it is programmed. *Rationale:* Interrogation of the device provides important information: battery voltage and impedance, charge time, dysrhythmias detected by device (logbook) and any therapies given (ATP or shock), pacing and sensing thresholds, and impedances for all leads, percent of pacing and sensing in each chamber, and review of programmed parameters.[20,21] Interrogation usually also reveals device and lead information (models and serial numbers), implant date, and implanting physician information. See Figure 47-3 for an example of an ICD interrogation report.

Patient Preparation

- Verify that the patient is the correct patient using two identifiers. *Rationale:* Before performing a procedure, the nurse should ensure the correct identification of the patient for the intended intervention.
- Ensure that the patient and family understand preprocedural teaching. Answer questions as they arise, and reinforce information as needed. *Rationale:* Understanding of previously taught information is evaluated and reinforced.
- Ensure that informed consent has been obtained (before ICD insertion). *Rationale:* Informed consent protects the rights of the patient and makes a competent decision possible for the patient.
- Perform a preprocedure verification and time out (before ICD insertion). *Rationale:* Ensures patient safety.
- Provide analgesia or sedatives as prescribed and needed. *Rationale:* Analgesia and sedatives promote comfort and may decrease anxiety.

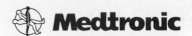

Medtronic **Quick Look**

Device: En Trust Serial Number: Date of Interrogation: -Feb-2007 16:08:52

Patient: Physician:

1	**Device Status (Implanted: 13-Jun-2006)**			**Measured on:**
	Battery Voltage (ERI=2.61 V)	3.17 V		24-Feb-2007
	Last Full Energy Charge	7.9 sec		13-Dec-2006
2		**Atrial(5076)**	**RV**	
	Pacing Impedance	488 ohms	504 ohms	24-Feb-2007
	Defibrillation Impedance		RV=76 ohms	24-Feb-2007
	Programmed Amplitude/Pulse Width	3 V / 0.4 ms	3 V / 0.4 ms	
3	Measured P/R Wave	3 mV	20 mV	24-Feb-2007
	Programmed Sensitivity	0.3 mV	0.45 mV	

4	**Parameter Summary**				
	Mode AAI<=>DDD	Lower Rate	60 bpm	Paced AV	180 ms
	Mode Switch 171 bpm	Upper Track	130 bpm	Sensed AV	150 ms
		Upper Sensor	130 bpm		

5	**Detection**		**Rates**	**Therapies**
	AT/AF	Monitor	>171 bpm	All Rx Off
	VF	On	>200 bpm	ATP During Charging, 25J, 35J × 5
	FVT	OFF		All Rx Off
	VT	On	171-200 bpm	Burst(3), Ramp(3), 20J, 35J × 3

Enhancements On: AF/All, Sinus Tach

	Clinical Status	**Since 24-Oct-2006**	
6	**Treated**		
	VF	0	
	FVT (Off)		
	VT	1	
	AT/AF (Monitor)		
7	**Monitored**		
	VT (Off)		
	VT-NS (>4 beats, >171 bpm)	3	
	SVT: VT/VF Rx Withheld	0	
	AT/AF	1	
	Time in AT/AF	<0.1 hr/day (<0.1%)	
	Longest AT/AF	2 hours	
	Functional	**Last Week**	
	Patient Activity	0.9 hr/day	

Cardiac Compass Trends (Jun-2006 to Feb-2007)

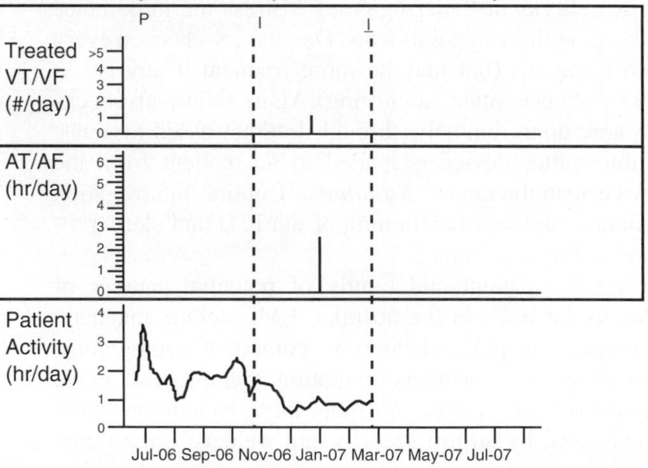

P
Treated VT/VF (#/day)
AT/AF (hr/day)
Patient Activity (hr/day)
Jul-06 Sep-06 Nov-06 Jan-07 Mar-07 May-07 Jul-07

9	**Therapy Summary**	**VT/VF**	**AT/AF**	**Pacing**	**(% of Time Since 24-Oct-2006)**	8
	Pace-Terminated Episodes	1 of 1	0	AS-VS	44.5%	
	Shock-Terminated Episodes	0	0	AS-VP	<0.1%	
	Total Shocks	0	0	AP-VS	55.4%	
	Aborted Charges	0	0	AP-VP	<0.1%	
				MVP	On	

10	**OBSERVATIONS (1)**
	Patient Activity less than 2 hr/day for 17 weeks.

Medtronic CareLink Network Confidential Patient Information 02-May-2007 16:27:07

A Copyright © 2001-2005 Medtronic, Inc Page 1

Figure 47-3 **A,** Printout from an ICD interrogation.

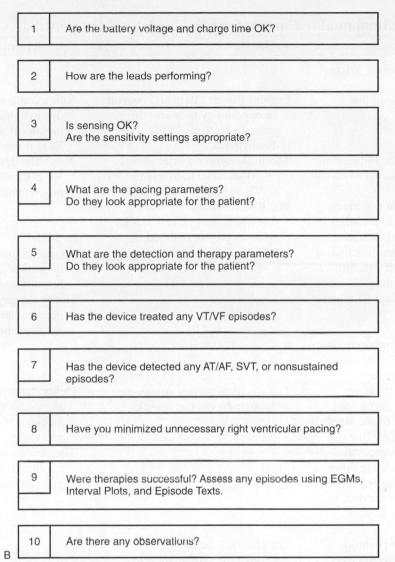

1	Are the battery voltage and charge time OK?

2	How are the leads performing?

3	Is sensing OK? Are the sensitivity settings appropriate?

4	What are the pacing parameters? Do they look appropriate for the patient?

5	What are the detection and therapy parameters? Do they look appropriate for the patient?

6	Has the device treated any VT/VF episodes?

7	Has the device detected any AT/AF, SVT, or nonsustained episodes?

8	Have you minimized unnecessary right ventricular pacing?

9	Were therapies successful? Assess any episodes using EGMs, Interval Plots, and Episode Texts.

10	Are there any observations?

B

Figure 47-3, cont'd B, Questions to consider during ICD interrogation. Healthcare providers trained at interpretation of results can gather this type of information from an ICD device check.

Procedure	**for Implantable Cardioverter-Defibrillator**	
Steps	**Rationale**	**Special Considerations**
1. **HH**		
2. **PE**		
3. Cleanse the skin for application of the ECG electrodes with cleansing pads or soap and water.	Proper skin preparation is essential to maintain appropriate skin-to-electrode contact.	Clipping of chest hair may be necessary to ensure good skin contact with the electrodes.
4. Attach the ECG leads to the electrodes, place the electrodes on the patient's chest, and record the ECG.	Assesses cardiac rhythm.	

Procedure continues on following page

Procedure	for Implantable Cardioverter-Defibrillator—*Continued*	
Steps	**Rationale**	**Special Considerations**
5. If the patient experiences VT or VF:		
A. Assess and stay with the patient.	Ensures patient safety and provides an opportunity to assess the patient's response to the dysrhythmia.	Run a continuous ECG strip of the dysrhythmia from the bedside monitor if possible; record a 12-lead ECG if possible.
B. Wait for the device to function: antitachycardia pacing or shock therapy.	The ICD requires a brief period (8–30 seconds) to assess the VT or VF and to initiate therapy.	Note: The device may not detect VT/VF if the rate of the VT is below the programmed detection rate.[23]
C. If the dysrhythmia continues, wait for the ICD to recharge and shock again if indicated.	The ICD reassesses the cardiac rhythm, recharges, and shocks again as preprogrammed.	
D. If the ICD has been functioning as preprogrammed and still does not convert the dysrhythmia, initiate BLS and ACLS.	Provides emergency care.	Assess the patient's response to VT; the patient's condition may be hemodynamically stable or unstable. Notify the physician or advanced practice nurse immediately and prepare emergency equipment.
E. Apply defibrillation electrodes (patches) or paddles in one of the two following ways:		
i. Place one electrode or paddle at the heart's apex just to the left of the nipple in the midaxillary line (at fifth to sixth intercostal space) and place the other electrode or paddle just below the right clavicle to the right of the sternum.	The electrical current passes through the cardiac muscle.	Defibrillator paddles and defibrillation electrodes should not be placed over medication patches or the ICD generator. The paddles and electrodes should be a minimum of 2 inches away from the generator when external shocks are delivered.
or		
ii. Apply anterior-posterior defibrillation electrodes or paddles. The anterior electrode or paddle is placed in the anterior left precordial area, and the posterior electrode or paddle is placed posteriorly behind the heart in the left infrascapular area.	The electrical current passes through the cardiac muscle.	
F. If the ICD does not convert VT/VF and the patient's condition is hemodynamically unstable, externally defibrillate the patient according to ACLS guidelines (see Procedure 36).	Provides emergency treatment.	ICDs have preprogrammed pacing capability; cardiac pacing is initiated by the ICD if the result of defibrillation is bradycardia or asystole. If external defibrillation is needed, the ICD should be interrogated to assess for potential damage to the device.

Procedure | **for Implantable Cardioverter-Defibrillator—*Continued***

Steps	Rationale	Special Considerations

ICD Deactivation
1. Prepare for deactivation of the ICD:
  A. Review the physician prescription.
  B. Obtain supplies.
	The ICD may need to be deactivated if it is defibrillating a cardiac rhythm that is not VT or VF, such as atrial fibrillation with a rapid ventricular response.
	The device also can be temporarily deactivated during surgical procedures where EMI may interfere with appropriate device function.
	The ICD may be deactivated if therapy is no longer effective or needed or is not desired.[15,21]
		If the device is functioning inappropriately, deactivation may be necessary to prevent harm to the patient.
		The following circumstances may necessitate ICD deactivation: lead dislodgment, lead migration, lead fracture, inappropriate identification of the rhythm, and inappropriate defibrillation threshold.
		Consider connecting the patient to an external defibrillator as indicated and desired.

2. **HH**		
3. **PE**		
4. Determine who will deactivate the ICD. This may include a physician, nurse, advance practice nurse, or other healthcare professional.	The ICD may be deprogrammed by personnel trained in use of the ICD programmer. Ensures that the device is deprogrammed as prescribed.	Follow institution standards regarding personnel who can deactivate the ICD with use of the programmer.

5. If the ICD programmer is unavailable, a magnet may be used to deactivate the device:
  A. Place a bar or doughnut magnet over the ICD generator.
  B. Follow the manufacturer's guidelines regarding removing the magnet or taping the magnet in place. **(Level M*)**
	Deactivation response to a magnet varies among manufacturers.
	Some ICDs are deactivated when the magnet is placed on the skin above the generator, and then the magnet can be removed.
	Other ICDs are deactivated only when the magnet remains on the skin over the generator.
		Follow the institution's standards regarding personnel who can deactivate the ICD with a magnet.
		A magnet applied over an ICD disables the device therapies of ATP and electrical cardioversion/defibrillation, but it does not turn off pacemaker function. The magnet may initiate asynchronous pacing.
		If information about a patient's ICD model and magnet features is unknown or is not clear, contact the personnel responsible for ICDs in your institution or contact the manufacturer to determine this information.
		Some ICDs emit a synchronous tone that occurs with each R wave when the device is activated and a constant tone when the ICD is deactivated. Knowledge of which manufacturers have this ability and whether the feature is turned on is important; not all devices emit a synchronous tone.

6. Remove gloves, discard used supplies, and ensure equipment is cleaned.	Reduces the transmission of microorganisms; Standard Precautions.	
7. **HH**		

*Level M: Manufacturer's recommendations only.

Procedure continues on following page

Procedure	for Implantable Cardioverter-Defibrillator—*Continued*	
Steps	**Rationale**	**Special Considerations**

ICD Reactivation

1. 🔲
2. 🔲

3. Determine who will reactivate the ICD. This may include a physician, nurse, advance practice nurse, or other healthcare professional.	The ICD may be reprogrammed by personnel trained in use of the ICD programmer. Ensures that the device is reprogrammed as prescribed.	Follow the institution's standards regarding personnel who can reactivate the ICD with use of the programmer.
4. If the ICD programmer is not available: A. If a bar or doughnut magnet is over the ICD generator, remove the magnet. B. If a bar or doughnut magnet is not over the ICD generator, place one there and then remove the magnet. (**Level M***)	When the magnet is removed, most ICDs automatically reactivate.	Follow the manufacturer's recommendations regarding magnet features. Some ICDs emit a synchronous tone that occurs with each R wave when the device is activated and a constant tone when the ICD is deactivated. Knowledge of which manufacturers have this ability and whether the feature is turned on is important; not all devices emit a synchronous tone.
5. Remove gloves, discard used supplies, and ensure equipment is cleaned.	Reduces the transmission of microorganisms; Standard Precautions.	
6. 🔲		

*Level M: Manufacturer's recommendations only.

Expected Outcomes

- ICD detects life-threatening VT or VF
- ICD delivers appropriate therapy, including antitachycardia pacing and defibrillation as necessary
- Cardiac rhythm is converted to a hemodynamically stable rhythm
- ICD provides bradycardia pacing as needed

Unexpected Outcomes

- Failure of the ICD to detect VT or VF
- Failure of the ICD to convert life-threatening dysrhythmia despite appropriate therapy and defibrillation attempts
- Failure of the backup pacing system to pace if bradycardia or asystole is the result of defibrillation
- Inappropriate defibrillation
- Infection at the ICD pulse generator site, leads, or myocardium
- Lead fracture or migration
- Pulse generator migration
- Pulse generator pocket hematoma
- Loosened set screw in device header (this screw holds the lead circuitry in place in the device header); loose set screws usually manifest as improper device function and occur generally immediately after implant
- Air embolism
- Venous thrombosis
- Cardiac tamponade
- Skin erosion
- Pneumothorax
- Frozen shoulder on operative side
- Twiddler's syndrome (manipulation of the device in the device pocket by a patient, either intentionally or unintentionally, which may lead to dislodgement)

Patient Monitoring and Care

Steps	Rationale	Reportable Conditions
		These conditions should be reported if they persist despite nursing interventions.
1. Monitor the ECG continuously.	Detects dysrhythmias.	• Dysrhythmias
2. Monitor the ICD for antitachycardia pacing, cardioversion, and defibrillation.	Detects functioning of the ICD.	• Ventricular dysrhythmias • ICD therapy • Defibrillation • ICD malfunction
3. Assess the patient's response to ICD defibrillation, including cardiac rate and rhythm, level of consciousness, and vital signs.	Determines patient status and necessity for additional treatment.	• Cardiac rate and rhythm before and after defibrillation • Level of consciousness • Vital signs
4. Follow institution standard for assessing pain. Administer analgesia as prescribed.	Identifies need for pain interventions.	• Continued pain despite pain interventions
5. Monitor for signs and symptoms of infection.	Placement of an invasive device may result in infection.	• Redness • Edema • Drainage • Increased white blood cell count • Increased temperature
6. Monitor for signs of bleeding and hematoma at ICD insertion site.	Placement of an invasive device may result in untoward bleeding.	• Bleeding at incision • Edema around ICD site

Documentation

Documentation should include the following:
- Device interrogation information: battery voltage and charge time, dysrhythmias detected by device and any therapies given, status of leads, programmed parameters (see Figs. 47-3, *A* and 47-3, *B*)
- Patient and family education
- Adjustment to device
- All rhythm strip recordings
- Patient response to ICD therapy
- Pain assessment, interventions, and effectiveness
- Anxiety assessment, interventions, and effectiveness
- Occurrence of any unexpected outcomes
- Additional interventions

References and Additional Readings

For a complete list of references and additional readings for this procedure, scan this QR code with any freely available smartphone code reader app, or visit http://booksite.elsevier.com/9780323376624.

48 Permanent Pacemaker (Assessing Function)

Valerie Spotts

PURPOSE: The purpose of permanent pacing is to electrically stimulate myocardial contraction and to restore and maintain an appropriate heart rate or ventricular synchrony when a chronic conduction or impulse-formation disturbance exists in the cardiac conduction system. Assessment of the permanent pacemaker is important in maintaining proper function.

PREREQUISITE NURSING KNOWLEDGE

- Knowledge of the normal anatomy and physiology of the cardiovascular system, cardiac conduction, and basic dysrhythmia interpretation is necessary.
- Knowledge of pacemaker function and patient response to pacemaker therapy is needed.
- Advanced cardiac life support (ACLS) knowledge and skills are needed.
- Permanent pacing is indicated for the following clinical conditions[5]:
  - ❖ Symptomatic sinus node dysfunction
  - ❖ Acquired atrioventricular (AV) block in adults
  - ❖ Chronic bifascicular and trifascicular block
  - ❖ AV block associated with acute myocardial infarction
  - ❖ Hypersensitive carotid sinus and neurocardiogenic syncope
  - ❖ Specific conditions related to cardiac transplantation, neuromuscular diseases, sleep apnea syndromes, or infiltrative and inflammatory diseases such as cardiac sarcoidosis
  - ❖ Prevention and termination of supraventricular tachycardia via pacing
  - ❖ Hypertrophic cardiomyopathy with sinus node dysfunction or AV block
  - ❖ Certain congenital heart defects
  - ❖ Certain cases of left-ventricular dysfunction, to restore ventricular synchrony (cardiac resynchronization therapy [CRT])[1,3,11]
- Relative contraindications to permanent pacemakers include the following:
  - ❖ Active infection (e.g., endocarditis, positive blood culture results)
  - ❖ Bleeding with abnormal coagulation laboratory results
- Components of the pacemaker are the pulse generator and the leads. The pulse generator weighs less than 1 oz and is typically implanted subcutaneously in a pectoral pocket. The outer casing is made of titanium and contains the electronic components and the battery (Fig. 48-1). Typical battery life is 5 to 10 years and is dependent on variables such as output values, impedance, and the percentage of

pacing. A transvenous pacing lead may be positioned in the right atrium, the right ventricle, or a cardiac vein supplying the left ventricle (or a combination of these), depending on the type of pacing needed.

- Unipolar pacing involves a relatively large electrical circuit. The distal tip of the pacing lead is the negative electrode and is in contact with the myocardium. The positive electrode encompasses the metallic pacemaker case, located in the soft tissue. Energy is delivered from the negative electrode to the positive electrode, causing myocardial depolarization. The electrocardiogram (ECG) tracing shows a large, easily visible spike.
- Bipolar pacing uses a smaller electrical circuit in which the distal tip of the pacing lead is the negative electrode in contact with the myocardium. The pacing lead has a second positive electrode that is located within 1 cm of the negative electrode. Energy is delivered from the negative electrode to the positive electrode, causing myocardial depolarization. The ECG tracing may show small spikes, or the spikes may not be visible on a surface ECG.
- Basic principles of cardiac pacing include sensing, pulse generation, capture, and impedance (Table 48-1 lists definitions).[6]
- Depending on the type of pacemaker, the pacemaker lead may be placed in the atrium, the right ventricle, or the left ventricle. A standard code exists to describe pacemakers (Table 48-2).[2] The nurse must know the programmed mode with the pacemaker code to determine whether the device is functioning appropriately. Refer to Table 48-3 to review different programmed modes for pacemakers.
- Dual-chamber pacemakers contain pacing leads that are located in the atrium and the ventricle. Pacing and sensing occur in both chambers when programmed in DDD or DDI modes. Pacing is inhibited by sensed atrial or ventricular activity. Sensed or paced atrial activity triggers a ventricular paced response in the absence of intrinsic ventricular activity within a programmed AV interval.[4]
- Biventricular pacemakers (CRT) contain leads in the right atrium and the right ventricle and on the surface of the left ventricle and simultaneously pace the right and left ventricles (Fig. 48-2).

- Some pacemaker systems also include an implantable cardioverter-defibrillator (see Procedure 47).
- Some pacemakers can be programmed to switch modes (e.g., DDD mode to DDI mode) to avoid pacing at the upper rate in patients who experience intermittent atrial dysrhythmias in which rapid atrial rates are generated.
- Certain pacemakers can be programmed with pacing therapies for atrial dysrhythmias. This programming is called antitachycardia pacing, in which the device paces faster

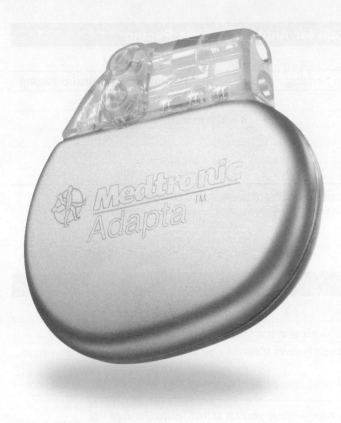

Figure 48-1 Permanent pacemaker pulse generator. *(Reproduced with permission of Medtronic, Inc.)*

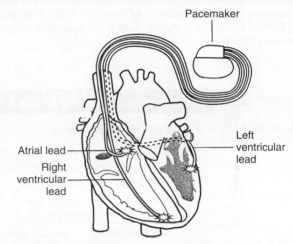

Figure 48-2 Biventricular pacemaker (cardiac resynchronization therapy). *(Courtesy Medtronic, Inc, Minneapolis, MN.)*

TABLE 48-1	**Pertinent Definitions Related to Pacemakers**
Sensing	Ability of the pacemaker to detect intrinsic myocardial electrical activity. The pacemaker is either inhibited from delivering a stimulus or initiates an electrical impulse based on the programmed response.
Pulse generation	Occurs when the pacemaker produces a programmed electrical current for a programmed duration. This energy travels through the transvenous lead wires to the myocardium. The electrical impulse is seen as a line or spike on the ECG recording (pacemaker spikes are shown in Fig. 48-4).
Capture	Successful stimulation of the myocardium by the pacemaker impulse that results in depolarization. Two settings are used to ensure capture: amplitude and pulse width. Evidenced on the ECG by a pacemaker spike/stimulus followed by either an atrial or ventricular complex, depending on the chambers being paced (see Fig. 48-4).
Lead impedance	Opposition to flow of electrical current by the leads, electrodes, the electrode-myocardial interface, and body tissues.[6] Measured in ohms, normally between 200 and 1200 ohms. A lead insulation break can cause impedance to fall below 200 ohms. A lead fracture can cause impedance to exceed 2000 ohms.
Failure of pulse generation	The pacemaker does not discharge a pacing stimulus to the myocardium at its programmed time. Evidenced by the absence of a pacemaker spike on the ECG where expected (see Fig. 48-5).
Failure to sense	The pacemaker has either detected extraneous signals that mimic intrinsic cardiac activity (oversensing) or has not accurately identified intrinsic activity (undersensing). Oversensing is recognized on the ECG by pauses where paced beats were expected and prolongation of the interval between paced beats (see Fig. 48-6). Oversensing leads to underpacing. Undersensing is recognized on the ECG by inappropriate pacemaker spikes relative to the intrinsic electrical activity (pacemaker spikes occurring where they are not needed) and shortened distances between paced beats (see Fig. 48-7). Undersensing leads to overpacing. Spikes may appear during the QRS complex as part of normal pacemaker function seen with fusion and pseudofusion beats.
Failure to capture	Pacemaker has delivered a pacing stimulus that was unable to initiate depolarization and contraction of the myocardium. Evidenced on the ECG by pacemaker spikes that are not followed by a P wave for atrial pacing or spikes not followed by a QRS complex for ventricular pacing (see Fig. 48-8).

TABLE 48-2   Revised NASPE/BPEG Generic Code for Antibradycardia Pacing

I	II	III	IV	V
Chambers Paced	**Chambers Sensed**	**Response to Sensing**	**Rate Modulation**	**Multisite Pacing**
0 = None	0 = None	0 = None	0 = None	0 = None
A = Atrium	A = Atrium	T = Triggered	R = Rate modulation	A = Atrium
V = Ventricle	V = Ventricle	I = Inhibited		V = Ventricle
D = Dual (A + V)	D = Dual (A + V)	D = Dual (T + I)		D = Dual (A + V)
S = Single (A or V)*	S + Single (A or V)*			

*Manufacturer's designation only. NASPE, North American Society of Pacing and Electrophysiology; BPEG, British Pacing and Electrophysiology Group.
(From Bernstein AD, Daubert JC, Fletcher RD, et al: The revised NASPE/BPEG generic code for antibradycardia, adaptive-rate, and multisite pacing, Pacing Clin Electrophysiol 25:261, 2002.)

TABLE 48-3   Programmed Pacing Modes

Pacemaker Code	Pacemaker Response
AOO	Atrial pacing; no sensing; asynchronous mode → paces atria at fixed, preprogrammed rate.
AAI	Atrial pacing, atrial sensing and inhibition; intrinsic P waves inhibit atrial pacing; if no sensed atrial events → paces in atria at preprogrammed rate.
AAIR	Atrial pacing; atrial sensing; intrinsic P waves inhibit atrial pacing; if no sensed atrial events → paces in atria; rate response to patient's activity.
VOO	Ventricular pacing; no sensing; asynchronous mode → paces ventricle at fixed, preprogrammed rate.
VVI	Ventricular pacing: ventricular sensing; intrinsic QRS inhibits ventricular pacing; if no sensed events → paces in ventricle at preprogrammed rate.
VVIR	Ventricular pacing: ventricular sensing; intrinsic QRS inhibits ventricular pacing; if no sensed events → paces in ventricle; rate response to patient's activity.
DOO	Atrial and ventricular pacing: no sensing; asynchronous mode → paces atria and ventricles at fixed, preprogrammed rate.
DDI	Atrial and ventricular pacing; atria and ventricular sensing; no tracking of atria: sensed atrial events inhibit atrial pacing/do not trigger a ventricular pacing pulse; sensed atrial events with absent ventricular event inhibit atrial pacing but do pace ventricle at preprogrammed rate; if both atrial and ventricular events absent → AV sequential pacing results at preprogrammed rate.
DDIR	Atrial and ventricular pacing; atrial and ventricular sensing; no tracking of atria (as described previously in DDI); AV sequential rate modulation.
DDD	Atrial and ventricular pacing; atrial and ventricular sensing; intrinsic P wave and intrinsic QRS can inhibit pacing; intrinsic P wave can trigger a paced QRS (tracks the atrium). May see four possible combinations in DDD mode: 1, atrial sensed/ventricular sensed; 2, atrial sensed/ventricular paced; 3, atrial paced/ventricular sensed; 4, atrial paced/ventricular paced.
DDDR	Atrial and ventricular pacing; atrial and ventricular sensing; tracks the atrium: intrinsic P wave and intrinsic QRS can inhibit pacing, intrinsic P wave can trigger a paced QRS; AV sequential rate modulation.

than a patient's heart rate in an attempt to convert the rhythm.

- Rate-responsive pacemakers include a sensor and are designed to mimic normal changes in heart rate based on physiological needs. Most commonly, the sensor reacts to motion and vibration or respirations and initiates an appropriate change in the pacing rate, depending on metabolic activity. These patients have a set pacemaker rate range.
- Inappropriate pacemaker function includes failure of pulse generation, failure to sense, and failure to capture (see Table 48-1 for definitions).[6]

- Electromagnetic interference (EMI) may interfere with pacemaker function and includes electrocautery, cardioversion and defibrillation, magnetic resonance imaging (which is relatively contraindicated for patients with pacemakers),[7] diathermy, and transcutaneous nerve stimulators. Magnetic resonance imaging–conditional pacemakers and leads have recently become available. Other outside causes of EMI include welding equipment less than 24 inches from the device, electrical motors, chain saws, battery-powered cordless power tools and drills less than 12 inches from the device, magnetic mattresses and chairs, and airport wands for security checks. Household appliances such as microwave ovens rarely cause EMI. Cell phones may cause EMI and should be used on the ear opposite the device. The cell phone should be carried on the opposite side of the body, with at least 6 inches maintained between the cell phone and the device.[12] Patients who are pacemaker-dependent may experience dizziness, lightheadedness, near syncope, or syncope if EMI inhibits proper sensing and therefore inhibits pacing.

- A pacemaker programmer appropriate for the pacemaker make and model is required for a device check or "interrogation." Note that some situations may require notification of the device manufacturer to obtain the proper interrogation equipment (the device programmer). Manufacturer information can be found on the patient's pacemaker identification card and via chest radiography.

EQUIPMENT

- ECG monitor and recorder with paper
- ECG cable and electrodes

Additional equipment, to have available as needed, includes the following:

- Pacemaker magnet
- Pacemaker programmer appropriate for the pacemaker manufacturer and model

PATIENT AND FAMILY EDUCATION

- Assess learning needs, readiness to learn, and factors that influence learning. *Rationale:* This assessment allows the nurse to individualize teaching in a meaningful manner.
- Provide information about the normal conduction system, such as structure of the conduction system, source of heartbeat, normal and abnormal heart rhythms, and symptoms of abnormal heart rhythms. Patients with cardiomyopathy and heart failure need further information about ventricular dyssynchrony. *Rationale:* Understanding of the normal conduction system and pumping function assists the patient and family in recognizing the need for permanent pacemaker therapy.
- Provide information about permanent pacing, including the reason for pacing; explanation of the equipment; what to expect during permanent pacing; precautions and restrictions in activities of daily living; signs and symptoms of complications; instructions on when to call the physician, advanced practice nurse, or pacemaker clinic; and information on expected follow-up. *Rationale:* Understanding of pacemaker functioning and expectations after discharge assists the patient and family in developing realistic perceptions of permanent pacing therapy. Information may improve compliance with restrictions and promote effective lifestyle management after discharge.
- Provide information about required device follow-up, including in-clinic evaluation, transtelephonic monitoring, or remote monitoring. *Rationale:* Periodic pacemaker checks are essential for routine device monitoring and evaluation of changes in patient condition related to the pacemaker. Current guidelines[11] recommend the following minimum frequency of routine device checks: within 72 hours of device implant (in person) then 2 to 12 weeks after implantation (in person), followed by every 3 to 12 months (in person or remote), annually, and then every 1 to 3 months at signs of battery depletion (in person or remote). Devices may be checked more frequently as needed (e.g., if a change occurs in antidysrhythmia medications or heart failure therapies).

- Instruct patients to carry their identification cards at all times. Patients receive identification cards from the manufacturer at the time of implant. These cards identify the model of pacemaker used. Also encourage patients to wear Medic Alert information. *Rationale:* This instruction ensures that appropriate identifying information is available to other healthcare providers, if needed.

PATIENT ASSESSMENT AND PREPARATION

Patient Assessment

- Identify the manufacturer of the pacemaker. This information may be found on the patient's identification card. If no card is available, the make of the device may be identified on chest radiography. *Rationale:* Identification of the manufacturer ensures that the correct programmer is used to review the programmed pacemaker parameters.
- Identify the programmed mode of the pacemaker. *Rationale:* Knowledge of how the pacemaker is intended to respond is necessary to detect appropriate and inappropriate function.
- Identify the reason for permanent pacemaker support. *Rationale:* Knowledge of the clinical indication (e.g., complete heart block) provides the nurse with baseline data, such as pacemaker dependency, when evaluating pacemaker function and patient response.
- Determine the patient's pacemaker history: date of insertion; last battery change; most recent pacemaker check; any problems with the pacemaker or pacemaker site; and any unexpected symptoms such as dizziness, chest pain, shortness of breath, palpitations, or activity intolerance. *Rationale:* The pacemaker history provides information useful for determining any problems that may occur.
- Assess the patient's ECG for appropriate pacemaker function. *Rationale:* Evidence of inappropriate function determines the need for further testing.
- Assess the patient's hemodynamic response to the paced rhythm. *Rationale:* The patient's hemodynamic response indicates how effective the pacemaker is in maintaining an adequate cardiac output in response to the patient's physiological needs. Evidence of inadequate cardiac output may be exhibited as decreased level of consciousness, fatigue, dizziness, shortness of breath, pallor, diaphoresis, chest pain, or hypotension.
- Patients with new biventricular pacemakers should also be assessed for signs and symptoms of dehydration. *Rationale:* Patients on long-term diuretics may have over-diuresis after pacemaker implantation as a result of improved circulation and hemodynamics[9].

Patient Preparation

- Verify the correct patient with two patient identifiers. *Rationale:* Before performing a procedure, the nurse should ensure the correct identification of the patient for the intended intervention.
- Ensure that the patient and family understand teaching. Answer questions as they arise, and reinforce information as needed. *Rationale:* This communication evaluates and reinforces understanding of previously taught information.
- Pacemaker interrogation may be performed with the patient either sitting or in the supine position. *Rationale:* This position prepares the patient for pacemaker interrogation.

Procedure	**for Assessing Function of Permanent Pacemaker**	
Steps	**Rationale**	**Special Considerations**
1. ▨HH		
2. ▨PE		
3. Prepare skin with cleansing pads or soap and water for the application of ECG electrodes.	Proper skin preparation is essential to maintain appropriate skin-to-electrode contact.	
4. Attach the ECG leads to the electrodes, and place the electrodes on the patient's chest (see Procedure 54).	Attaching the leads to the electrodes first and then placing the electrodes on the chest produces less discomfort.	
5. Record an ECG rhythm strip.	Allows for evaluation of the patient's intrinsic rhythm and aids in assessment of pacemaker function.	
6. Follow institutional standards for recording a rhythm strip with a magnet placed over the pacemaker (**Level M***):		
A. Place the pacemaker magnet on top of the pacemaker generator.	A magnet placed over the pacemaker causes the pacemaker to pace at the preprogrammed parameters.	Follow institutional standards to ensure that a nurse can use the pacemaker magnet.
B. Record the ECG rhythm strip.	This is needed to assess the rhythm and for documentation.	
C. Remove the magnet.	After the magnet is removed, the ECG rhythm represents the patient's current status (intrinsic rhythm, paced rhythm, or a combination).	
D. Assess the ECG rhythm.	Determines the patient's inherent rhythm.	
7. Inspect the ECG rhythm strip for pacemaker spikes, and evaluate for evidence of failure to sense or failure to capture (Figs. 48-3 through 48-8).	Determines whether the pacemaker is functioning adequately and assesses electrical activity of the atria and ventricles.	Depending on the type of lead and programming, pacemaker spikes may be difficult to detect on the surface ECG.
A. Identify atrial activity. Is the pacemaker programmed to detect atrial activity? Was the atrial activity sensed? What is the pacemaker programmed to do when atrial activity is sensed? If the pacemaker is programmed to trigger ventricular pacing with sensed atrial activity, is a ventricular-paced complex seen at the programmed AV interval? If not, did an intrinsic QRS complex occur before the programmed AV interval?	Determines the presence of atrial activity in response to the pacemaker settings.	Different AV intervals may be programmed for sensed and paced events.

*Level M: Manufacturer's recommendations only.

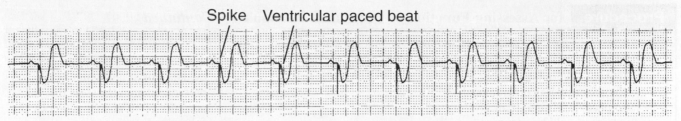

Figure 48-3 DDD pacing, normal operation: atrial activity sensed, ventricle paced.

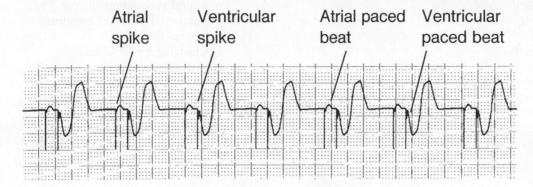

Figure 48-4 Dual-chamber DDD pacing, normal operation: atrial paced, ventricle paced.

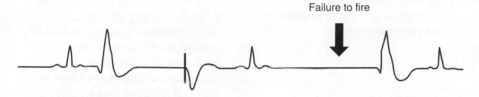

Figure 48-5 Failure of pulse generation.

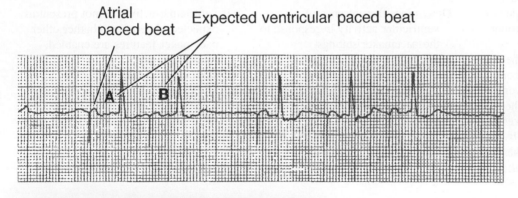

Figure 48-6 Ventricular oversensing and possibly ventricular pulse-generation failure. Ventricular spike expected at 150 ms. Ventricular spike and corresponding ventricular depolarization did not occur at points *A* and *B*. Also, atrial timing reset by oversensed ventricular activity resulted in erratic atrial pacing (suspicious for fracture of ventricular lead).

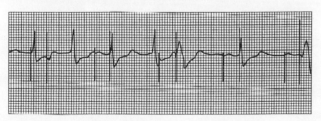

Figure 48-7 Ventricular undersensing. Pacemaker appears to be firing asynchronously. The third and sixth ventricular complexes represent concurrent intrinsic ventricular depolarization overlaid by inappropriate pacemaker fire.

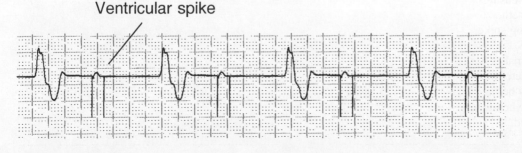

Figure 48-8 DDD system with failure to capture or sense ventricular activity. All ventricular spikes show absence of corresponding ventricular depolarization. No timing circuit reset by intrinsic ventricular complexes.

Procedure   for Assessing Function of Permanent Pacemaker—*Continued*

Steps	Rationale	Special Considerations
B. If no intrinsic atrial activity is present, determine whether the pacemaker is programmed to pace the atrium. If atrial pacing should be occurring, determine the lower rate limit at which the pacemaker stimulates atrial activity. Evaluate whether the pacemaker is firing at this rate.		If a pacemaker spike is present but evidence of atrial capture is not present, attempt to assess the presence of atrial contraction by the following: 1. Looking for the "*a*" wave in the central venous pressure (or right-atrial pressure) waveform (if available). 2. Changing the ECG lead. 3. Listening to the heart sounds (S_1 becomes softer in the absence of atrial contraction because left-ventricular contractility affects the loudness of S_1).[3] 4. Examine a 12-lead ECG tracing, which may show pacemaker spikes not seen on a monitor strip.
C. Identify ventricular activity. Is the pacemaker programmed to detect intrinsic activity? Is it sensed appropriately? What is the pacemaker programmed to do when ventricular activity is sensed? Does inhibition of ventricular pacing occur?	Determines the presence of ventricular activity in response to the pacemaker settings.	Failure of ventricular capture can be a life-threatening situation. With biventricular pacing, the loss of capture in one ventricle may be seen only by a change in the patient's condition or a change in the QRS width or appearance.[8]
D. If no intrinsic ventricular activity is found, determine whether the pacemaker is programmed to pace the ventricles. If pacing should occur, identify the lower rate limit and determine whether ventricular pacing spikes are occurring at this rate. If ventricular pacing spikes are occurring at intervals that are longer than the lower rate limit, evaluate for oversensing of unwanted signals. If ventricular pacing spikes are occurring at intervals that are shorter than the lower rate limit, is the pacemaker in a rate-responsive mode? Is hidden atrial activity triggering a ventricular output? Is atrial oversensing found? Determine whether each ventricular pacing spike is followed by a QRS complex. If the pacemaker has an upper rate limit, determine whether the patient is being paced appropriately when that limit has been reached.	Determines the presence of ventricular activity in response to the pacemaker settings.	If ventricular activity is not present as expected, determine whether other pacemaker features are enabled, such as programming to minimize ventricular pacing or hysteresis.

Procedure for Assessing Function of Permanent Pacemaker—*Continued*

Steps	Rationale	Special Considerations
E. If antitachycardia pacing is programmed, determine whether the tachycardia detection criterion has been met and whether the pacemaker intervened appropriately.	Determines appropriate pacemaker function.	
F. If the patient has a biventricular pacemaker, verify that the ventricles are consistently paced.[8,10]	The purpose of biventricular pacing is to pace both ventricles simultaneously to restore ventricular synchrony. If the patient is not consistently being paced in the ventricles, the system is not working properly.	Detailed interrogation of function is needed because a surface ECG rhythm strip does not provide enough information to assess proper function adequately. Fig. 48-9 illustrates various aspects of biventricular pacing.

Procedure continues on following page

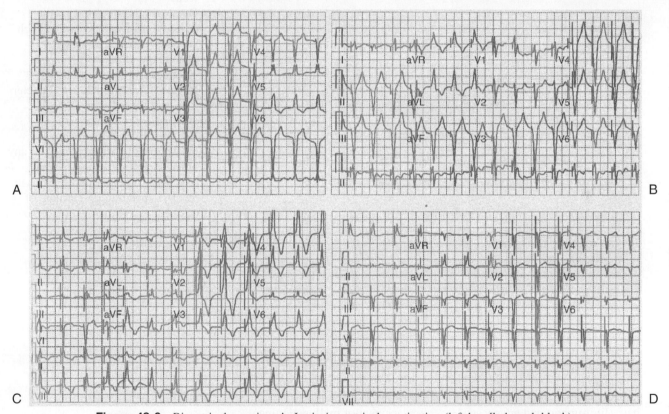

Figure 48-9 Biventricular pacing. **A**, Intrinsic ventricular activation (left bundle branch block). **B**, Right-ventricular pacing. **C**, Left-ventricular pacing. **D**, Biventricular pacing. *(Ellenbogen KA, Wood MA: Cardiac pacing & ICDs, ed 5, Oxford, 2008, Blackwell Publishing, 1095. Used with permission.)*

Procedure for Assessing Function of Permanent Pacemaker—*Continued*

Steps	Rationale	Special Considerations
8. Perform a check of the pacemaker using the manufacturer's programmer (only done by trained personnel), when available and as prescribed: A. Place the wand attached to the programmer over the patient's pacemaker. B. Perform testing of sensing, capture thresholds, and lead impedances.	Determines appropriate pacemaker function. The wand retrieves and transmits the programmed information. Allows for determination of pacemaker function, programmed parameters, dysrhythmias, and alerts.	Follow institutional standards regarding training required before use of the pacemaker programmer. Some devices have a wireless connection to the programmer and a wand is not used. Pacemaker device check with the programmer provides the following information[13,14]: • Battery voltage (and impedance) • Magnet rate (varies by manufacturer) • Pacing and sensing thresholds for atrium and right ventricle, and pacing threshold for left ventricle • Pacing lead impedance for all leads • Dysrhythmias detected by the device (e.g., mode switches, high ventricular rate episodes) • Percentage of pacing in each chamber • Review of programmed parameters • Review of any "safety" or automatic device alerts • Review of hemodynamic measurements or recordings of any other programmed parameters (e.g., heart rate variability, activity level), depending on the type of device
C. Determine whether the pacemaker needs to be reprogrammed.	Ensures proper programming.	
9. Assess the patient's vital signs and hemodynamic response.	The patient may have the electrical activity of pacing without the associated mechanical activity of cardiac contraction (e.g., pulseless electrical activity).	
10. If inappropriate pacemaker function is detected, notify the physician or advanced practice nurse immediately and implement basic life support and advanced cardiac life support as needed.	Inappropriate pacemaker function may compromise cardiac output and necessitate immediate adjustment of settings or replacement of malfunctioning components.	
11. Remove gloves and discard used supplies in appropriate receptacle.	Reduces the transmission of microorganisms; Standard Precautions.	
12. **HH**		

Expected Outcomes

- Appropriate pacemaker functioning based on programmed parameters
- Adequate systemic tissue perfusion and cardiac output as evidenced by patient being alert, oriented, and normotensive, with no dizziness, shortness of breath, chest discomfort, or lightheadedness
- Minimal discomfort with new implant, no discomfort with preexisting implant
- No signs or symptoms of fluid or infection at the incision

Unexpected Outcomes

- Failure to sense (e.g., oversensing, undersensing) or failure to capture; failure to sense or capture in the immediate postimplant period may indicate lead dislodgment
- Lead perforation of the myocardium may occur within the first 24 hours of implant; signs and symptoms may include intermittent failure of pacing or sensing, distant heart sounds, pericardial rub, and in extreme cases hemodynamic instability
- Diaphragmatic stimulation may occur if high-voltage outputs are needed to pace the ventricles
- Hematoma
- Wound infection
- Venous thrombus

Patient Monitoring and Care

Steps	Rationale	Reportable Conditions
		These conditions should be reported if they persist despite nursing interventions.
1. Monitor the ECG continuously.	Determines whether the patient's cardiac rate and rhythm are consistent with the programmed pacemaker parameters.	- Failure of the pacemaker to perform as programmed - Oversensing - Undersensing - Failure to capture
2. Monitor the patient's vital signs and hemodynamic status.	Determines the patient's response to pacemaker therapy.	- Abnormal vital signs - Hemodynamic instability
3. Assess the pacemaker pocket in the acute postimplant phase.	Determines healing and the presence of fluid.	- Bleeding at incision - Edema around pacemaker site - Increased pain at incision site
4. Assess for signs and symptoms of infection.	Identifies infection.	- Redness - Edema - Drainage - Elevated white blood cell count - Elevated temperature - Increased pain or tenderness at the pacemaker site
5. Follow institutional standards for assessing pain. Administer analgesia as prescribed.	Identifies need for pain interventions.	- Continued pain despite pain interventions

Documentation

Documentation should include the following:
- Device indications and device type
- Patient education and evaluation of patient and family understanding
- Programmed parameters
- ECG rhythm strip recordings
- Evaluation of pacemaker function
- Physical assessment, including vital signs and hemodynamic response
- Unexpected outcomes
- Interventions needed and evaluation of interventions
- Pain assessment, interventions, and effectiveness

References and Additional Readings

For a complete list of references and additional readings for this procedure, scan this QR code with any freely available smartphone code reader app, or visit http://booksite.elsevier.com/9780323376624.

Temporary Transcutaneous (External) Pacing

Valerie Spotts

PURPOSE: Transcutaneous or external pacing stimulates myocardial depolarization through the chest wall. External pacing is used as a temporary measure when normal cardiac conduction fails to produce myocardial contraction and the patient experiences hemodynamic instability.

PREREQUISITE NURSING KNOWLEDGE

- Knowledge of cardiac anatomy and physiology is needed.
- Knowledge of cardiac monitoring is necessary.
- The ability to interpret dysrhythmias is needed.
- Knowledge of temporary pacemaker function and expected patient responses to pacemaker therapy is necessary.
- Clinical and technical competence in the use of the external pacing equipment (Fig. 49-1) is needed.
- Indications for transcutaneous pacing are as follows:[1-3]
  ❖ Symptomatic bradycardia unresponsive to medications
  ❖ In standby mode for the following rhythms in the acute myocardial infarction setting:[3,4]
    ○ Symptomatic sinus node dysfunction
    ○ Mobitz type II second-degree heart block
    ○ Third-degree heart block
    ○ Newly acquired left, right, or alternating bundle-branch block or bifascicular block
- Temporary transvenous pacing is indicated when prolonged pacing is needed.
- Contraindications for transcutaneous pacing are as follows:[2,7]
  ❖ Severe hypothermia
  ❖ Asystole (as presenting rhythm)
- Pacing is contraindicated in severe hypothermia because cold ventricles are more prone to ventricular fibrillation and are more resistant to defibrillation.[7]
- External cardiac pacing is a temporary method of stimulating ventricular myocardial depolarization through the chest wall via two large pacing electrodes (patches). The electrodes are placed on the anterior and posterior chest wall (Figs. 49-2 and 49-3) or anterior and lateral chest wall (Fig. 49-4) and are attached by a cable to an external pulse generator. The external pulse generator delivers energy (milliamps) to the myocardium based on the set pacing rate, output, and sensitivity. Some models of external pulse generators are combined with an external defibrillator, and the electrodes of these models may be used for pacing and defibrillation.
- *Sensitivity* refers to the ability of the pacemaker to detect intrinsic myocardial activity.

- In the nondemand or asynchronous mode, pacing occurs at the set rate regardless of the patient's intrinsic rate. In the demand or synchronous mode, the pacemaker senses intrinsic myocardial activity and paces when the intrinsic cardiac rate is lower than the set rate on the external pulse generator.
- *Pacing* occurs when the external pulse generator delivers enough energy through the pacing electrodes to the myocardium, which is known as pacemaker firing and is represented as a spike on the electrocardiograph (ECG) tracing.
- *Electrical capture* occurs when the pacemaker delivers enough energy to the myocardium so that depolarization occurs. Capture is seen on the ECG with a pacemaker spike followed by a ventricular complex. The ventricular complex occurs after the pacemaker spike, and the QRS is wide (greater than 0.11 seconds), with the initial and terminal deflections in opposite directions. In Figure 49-5, complexes 2 and 3 begin with a downward (negative) deflection and end with an upward (positive) direction. *Mechanical capture* occurs when a paced QRS complex results in a palpable pulse.
- *Standby pacing* is when the pacing electrodes are applied in anticipation of possible use but pacing is not needed at the time.

EQUIPMENT

- Nonsterile gloves
- Blood pressure monitoring equipment
- External pulse generator
- Pacing cable
- Pacemaker electrodes (patches)
- ECG electrodes
- ECG monitor
- ECG cable

Additional equipment, to have available as needed, includes the following:
- Emergency cart
- Medications including sedatives and analgesics
- Scissors
- Transvenous pacing equipment

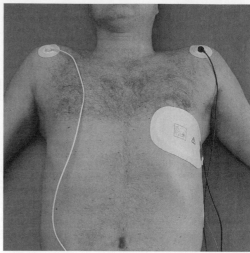

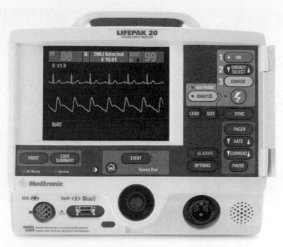

Figure 49-1   Provides defibrillation, monitoring, and external pacing. (*Reproduced with permission of Medtronic Inc.*)

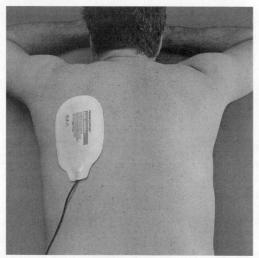

Figure 49-2   Location of the posterior (back) pacing electrode. (*Aehlert B:* ACLS study guide, *ed 3, St Louis, 2007, Mosby, 229.*)

PATIENT AND FAMILY EDUCATION

- Assess learning needs, readiness to learn, and factors that influence learning. *Rationale:* This assessment reveals the patient's and family's knowledge so that teaching can be individualized to be meaningful to the patient and family.
- Discuss basic facts about the normal conduction system, the reason external cardiac pacing is indicated, and what happens to the patient when pacing occurs. *Rationale:* This discussion assists the patient and family in recognizing the need for external pacing and what to expect when pacing occurs.
- Discuss interventions to alleviate discomfort. *Rationale:* This discussion provides the patient with an opportunity to validate perceptions. It gives the patient and family knowledge that interventions are used to minimize the level of discomfort.
- If indicated, inform the patient and family of the possibility of the need for transvenous or permanent pacing support. *Rationale:* This information prepares the patient and family for the possibility of additional therapy. If permanent pacing is necessary, the patient and family

Figure 49-3   Location of the anterior (front) pacing electrode. (*Aehlert B:* ACLS study guide, *ed 3, St Louis, 2007, Mosby, 229.*)

need further instruction about possible lifestyle modifications and follow-up visits, and information about the pacemaker to be implanted.

PATIENT ASSESSMENT AND PREPARATION

Patient Assessment

- Assess the patient's cardiac rate and rhythm for the presence of dysrhythmias that indicate the need for external cardiac pacing. *Rationale:* Recognition of a dysrhythmia is the first step in determining the need for external cardiac pacing or placing the external pacemaker on standby.
- Determine the patient's hemodynamic response to the dysrhythmia, such as the presence or absence of a pulse; presence of hypotension; altered level of consciousness; dizziness; shortness of breath; nausea and vomiting; cool, clammy, diaphoretic skin; or the development of chest pain. *Rationale:* The decision to initiate pacing depends on the effect of the dysrhythmia on the patient's cardiac output.

Patient Preparation

- Verify that the patient is the correct patient using two identifiers. *Rationale:* Before performing a procedure, the nurse should ensure the correct identification of the patient for the intended intervention.
- Ensure that the patient and family understand preprocedural teaching. Answer questions as they arise, and reinforce information as needed. *Rationale:* This communication evaluates and reinforces understanding of previously taught information.
- Maintain bedside ECG monitoring. *Rationale:* External pacing units do not provide central monitoring or dysrhythmia detection.
- Establish or ensure patency of intravenous access. *Rationale:* Medication administration may be necessary.
- Assist the patient to the supine position and expose the patient's torso while maintaining modesty. *Rationale:* This positioning prepares for electrode (patch) placement.

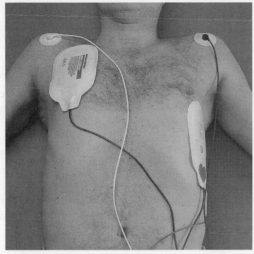

Figure 49-4 Location of anterior-lateral pacing electrodes. *(Aehlert B: ACLS study guide, ed 3, St Louis, 2007, Mosby, 229.)*

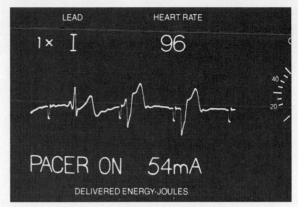

Figure 49-5 Electrocardiograph tracing of external pacing. *(From Zoll Medical Corporation, Burlington, MA.)*

Procedure	**for Temporary Transcutaneous (External) Pacing**	
Steps	**Rationale**	**Special Considerations**
1. [HH]		
2. [PE]		
3. Administer sedative or analgesic medications as prescribed.	Decreases discomfort associated with external cardiac pacing.[6,7]	Not indicated for patients who are unconscious with hemodynamically unstable conditions. Not indicated for standby because pacing may not be needed.
4. Turn on the pulse generator and monitor.	Provides the power source.	Many devices work on battery or alternating current (AC) power.
5. Prepare the skin on the patient's chest and back by washing with nonemollient soap and water.	Removal of skin oils, lotion, and moisture improves electrode adherence and maximizes delivery of energy through the chest wall.	Optional step in an emergency. Dry thoroughly. Trim body hair with scissors, if necessary. Avoid use of flammable liquids to prepare the skin (e.g., alcohol, benzoin) because of the increased potential for burns.[7] Avoid shaving the chest hair because the presence of nicks in the skin under the pacing electrodes can increase patient discomfort. Remove any medication patches applied to the chest area.
6. Apply the ECG electrodes to the ECG leads.	Prepares the equipment.	

Procedure continues on following page

Procedure for Temporary Transcutaneous (External) Pacing—*Continued*

Steps	Rationale	Special Considerations
7. Connect the ECG cable to the monitor inlet of the pulse generator. **(Level M*)**	Prepares the equipment.	Follow the manufacturer's recommendations. Attachment of the ECG electrodes to the ECG leads and the ECG cable to the pacemaker monitor is optional for some manufacturers in an emergency. If the ECG leads are not placed, the pacemaker may function in the asynchronous mode. The pacemaker may not function unless both the ECG monitoring connection and the pacing electrode connection are both connected to the pacemaker.
8. Apply the ECG electrodes to the patient (see Procedure 54).	Displays the patient's intrinsic rhythm on the monitor.	
9. Adjust the ECG lead and size to the maximum R wave size. Look for an indicator that the pacemaker is sensing the QRS complexes on the intrinsic rhythm, usually seen as a marker above each native QRS complex.	Detection of the intrinsic rhythm is necessary for the demand mode of pacing.	Lead II usually provides the most prominent R wave.
10. Apply the back (posterior, +) pacing electrode between the spine and left scapula at the level of the heart (see Fig. 49-2).	Placement of the pacing electrodes in the recommended anatomical location enhances the potential for successful pacing.	Avoid placing the pacing electrodes over bone because this increases the level of energy needed to pace, increases patient discomfort, and increases the possibility of noncapture.
11. Apply the front (anterior, −) pacing electrode at the left, fourth intercostal space, midclavicular line (see Fig. 49-3). **(Level M*)**	Placement of the pacing electrodes in the recommended anatomical locations enhance the potential for successful pacing.	For women, adjust the position of the pacing electrode below and lateral to breast tissue to ensure optimal adherence. Avoid placement of the pacing electrodes over the bedside monitor ECG electrodes and permanently placed devices, such as implantable cardioverter-defibrillators or permanent pacemakers.
12. If the patient's condition is hemodynamically unstable, the back (posterior) electrode may be placed over the patient's right sternal area at the second or third intercostal space. The front (anterior) electrode is maintained at the apex (fourth or fifth intercostal space, midclavicular line; see Fig. 49-4).	Facilitates ease of electrode placement for emergent pacing.	Pacing may be less effective with this method of electrode placement.[7,8]
13. Connect the pacing electrodes to the pacemaker cable and connect the pacemaker cable to the external pulse generator. **(Level M*)**	Necessary for the delivery of electrical energy.	

*Level M: Manufacturer's recommendations only.

Procedure	**for Temporary Transcutaneous (External) Pacing—*Continued***	
Steps	**Rationale**	**Special Considerations**
14. Set the pacemaker rate, level of energy (output, mA) (Fig. 49-6).	Each patient needs different pacemaker settings to provide safe and effective external pacing.	Follow institutional standards regarding who can initiate external cardiac pacing. The demand mode is used as long as the ECG leads are attached to the pacemaker monitor.
A. Set the demand or the synchronous mode.	The demand mode is used to prevent competition from the patient's intrinsic rhythm.	In the asynchronous mode, the pacemaker fires regardless of the intrinsic rhythm and rate.
B. Set the rate.	Pacing should be at a rate that maintains adequate cardiac output but does not induce ischemia.	The pacemaker may have a default setting (e.g., 80 bpm) that can be adjusted as needed.
C. Set the mA. i. Slowly increase the mA setting (output) until capture is present. ii. Set the mA slightly higher than the capture threshold (an additional 2 mA).[1,7]	Use the lowest amount of energy that consistently results in myocardial capture and contraction to minimize discomfort.[1]	The pacemaker may have a default setting that can be adjusted as needed, or the pacemaker may turn on at 0 mA and will need to be increased for pacing to occur. The average adult usually can be paced with a current of 40–70 mA.

Procedure continues on following page

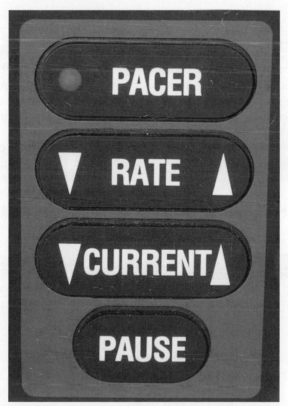

Figure 49-6   Controls for external pacemaker settings.

Procedure for Temporary Transcutaneous (External) Pacing—*Continued*

Steps	Rationale	Special Considerations
15. When the pacemaker fires, observe that each pacemaker spike is followed by a wide ventricular complex and a T wave in the opposite deflection of the QRS (see Fig. 49-5).	Identifies appropriate functioning of the pacemaker.	If a pacemaker spike occurs and is not followed by a ventricular complex, slowly increase the energy (mA) level. Artifact from skeletal muscle twitching may make an ECG tracing difficult to interpret. Skeletal muscle twitching occurs at lower mA settings, before capture of the myocardium.[1,7] Confirm mechanical capture by assessing pulse.
16. Palpate the patient's pulse (e.g., femoral pulse, right brachial pulse, radial pulse).	Ensures adequate blood flow with paced complexes.	The carotid pulses usually are not palpated because the electrical stimulation from the pacemaker may mimic a pulse.[1,2]
17. Evaluate the patient's vital signs and hemodynamic response to pacing.	The patient's hemodynamic response should improve with pacing if symptoms were related to bradycardia.[1,3]	If symptoms do not improve with pacing, assess for other causes such as electrolyte abnormalities.
18. Remove **PE** and discard used supplies in appropriate receptacles.	Reduces the transmission of microorganisms; Standard Precautions.	
19. **HH**		

Expected Outcomes

- Adequate systemic tissue perfusion and cardiac output as evidenced by blood pressure greater than 90 mm Hg systolic (or resolution of hypotension), return to baseline mental status, absence of dizziness or syncope, absence of shortness of breath, absence of nausea and vomiting, and absence of ischemic chest pain
- Stable cardiac rate and rhythm
- Appropriate sensing, pacing, and capture present

Unexpected Outcomes

- Failure of the pacemaker to sense the patient's underlying rhythm with the possibility of R-on-T phenomenon (initiation of ventricular tachydysrhythmias as a result of an improperly timed spike on the T wave)
- Failure of the pacemaker to capture the myocardium
- Failure of the pacemaker to pace
- Discomfort, including skin burns from the delivery of high levels of energy through the chest wall, painful sensations, and skeletal muscle twitching

Patient Monitoring and Care

Steps	Rationale	Reportable Conditions
		These conditions should be reported if they persist despite nursing interventions.
1. Monitor vital signs every 15 minutes until stable, then hourly or more frequently as needed.	Ensures adequate tissue perfusion with paced beats. Adjustments in the pacing rate may need to be made based on vital signs. Continuous assessment is needed because pacing thresholds may change and response to the pacemaker settings can change over time.	- Change in vital signs - Hemodynamic instability

Patient Monitoring and Care —*Continued*

Steps	Rationale	Reportable Conditions
2. Continue to monitor the patient's cardiac rate and rhythm through the central monitoring system. The pacing spike may obscure or mimic the QRS complex, making ventricular capture difficult to see.[5] Select a lead that minimizes the size of the pacing spike and maximizes the QRS complex.[5] Set the pacemaker option on the central monitoring system.	Provides an alarm system. Of note, if ECG leads are disconnected from the pacemaker monitor, pacing reverts to asynchronous, which could compete with the native rhythm.	• Changes in capture or sensing • Dysrhythmias
3. Monitor level of comfort and sedation level: A. Assess the patient's level of comfort and sedation level following institution standard. B. Administer prescribed analgesic and sedative medications as needed. C. Adjust the level of energy to the lowest level for capture. D. Evaluate the patient's response to interventions.	The external delivery of energy through the chest wall may cause varying degrees of discomfort.[1,2,7,8]	• Continued pain despite interventions to alleviate pain • Patient intolerance of the prescribed medications (e.g., nausea, hypotension, decreased respirations)
4. Obtain an ECG recording strip to document pacing function on initiation of pacing, every 4–8 hours, and as needed or according to institutional standards.	Documents cardiac rate, rhythm, and pacemaker activity.	• Dysrhythmias • Failure to capture • Failure to pace
5. Obtain blood samples for laboratory analysis as prescribed.	Acidosis and electrolyte abnormalities need to be corrected for an effective response to pacing.	• Electrolyte abnormalities • Acidosis
6. Evaluate pacemaker function (capturing and sensing) with any change in patient condition or vital signs.	Ensures continued functioning of the pacemaker.	• Inability to maintain appropriate sensing and capture • Changes in patient condition that affect appropriate pacemaker function
7. Monitor the patient's cardiac rate and rhythm for resolution of the dysrhythmia that necessitates pacemaker intervention. A. This monitoring may necessitate turning the pacemaker off, if prescribed, to assess the patient's underlying rate and rhythm. Do not turn the pacemaker off if the patient is 100% paced. B. When assessing the patient's intrinsic rate and rhythm, reduce the pacing rate slowly.	Determines whether the dysrhythmia has subsided. A sudden cessation of pacing can lead to asystole because the intrinsic rate and rhythm may be suppressed by continuous pacing.[7]	• Worsening of the baseline cardiac rate and rhythm (e.g., change from symptomatic second-degree heart block to complete heart block)

Procedure continues on following page

Patient Monitoring and Care —*Continued*

Steps	Rationale	Reportable Conditions
8. Check the adherence of the pacing electrodes to the skin at least every 4 hours. If pacing is not occurring, assess the skin integrity under the pacing electrodes.	Changes in skin integrity caused by burns or skin breaks significantly alter the patient's level of comfort and exposes the patient to possible infection.	• Changes in skin integrity • Burns
9. Change the electrodes at least every 24 hours or after 8 hours of continuous pacing.[8] **(Level M*)**	Pacing electrodes should not be used once they have been out of the package for 24 hours.[7]	

*Level M: Manufacturer's recommendations only.

Documentation

Documentation should include the following:

- Patient and family education
- Patient preparation
- Date and time external cardiac pacing is initiated
- Description of events that warranted intervention
- Vital signs and physical assessment before and after external cardiac pacing
- ECG recordings before and after pacing
- Pain assessment, interventions, and effectiveness

- Medications administered
- Pacing rate, mode, mA
- Percentage of the time the patient is paced if in the demand mode
- Status of skin integrity when the pacing electrodes are changed
- Unexpected outcomes
- Additional interventions

References and Additional Readings

For a complete list of references and additional readings for this procedure, scan this QR code with any freely available smartphone code reader app, or visit http://booksite.elsevier.com/9780323376624.

50 Temporary Transvenous AP Pacemaker Insertion (Perform)

Nikki Taylor

PURPOSE: The purpose of temporary cardiac pacing is to ensure or restore an adequate heart rate and rhythm. A transvenous pacemaker is inserted as a temporary measure when the normal conduction system of the heart fails to produce or conduct an electrical impulse, resulting in hemodynamic compromise or other debilitating symptoms.

PREREQUISITE NURSING KNOWLEDGE

- Knowledge of the normal anatomy and physiology of the cardiovascular system, principles of cardiac conduction, and basic and advanced dysrhythmia interpretation is needed.
- Knowledge of temporary pacemaker function and expected patient responses to pacemaker therapy is necessary.
- Clinical and technical competence in central line insertion, temporary transvenous pacemaker insertion, and suturing is needed.
- Knowledge of the principles of sterile technique is essential.
- Clinical and technical competence related to the use of temporary pacemakers is necessary.
- Competence in chest radiograph interpretation is needed.
- Advanced cardiac life support (ACLS) knowledge and skills are needed.
- Principles of general electrical safety apply with use of temporary invasive pacing.
- Gloves always should be worn when handling pacemaker electrodes to prevent microshock because even small amounts of electrical current can cause serious dysrhythmias if they are transmitted to the heart.[2,7,9,10]
- Knowledge of the care of the patient with central venous catheters (see Procedures 67 and 82).
- The insertion of a temporary transvenous pacemaker is performed in emergency and elective clinical situations. Temporary transvenous pacing may be used for the following:
  - ❖ Stimulate the myocardium to contract in the absence of an intrinsic rhythm
  - ❖ Establish adequate cardiac output and blood pressure
  - ❖ Ensure tissue perfusion to vital organs

- ❖ Reduce the possibility of ventricular dysrhythmias in the presence of bradycardia
- ❖ Supplement an inadequate rhythm, such as when transient decreases in heart rate occur (e.g., chronotropic incompetence in shock)
- ❖ Allow the administration of medications that may cause a rhythm or conduction abnormalities (e.g., beta blockers).
- Temporary transvenous pacing is indicated for the following:
  - ❖ Third-degree atrioventricular (AV) block
  - ❖ Type II AV block
  - ❖ Dysrhythmias that may occur in the setting of an acute myocardial infarction (e.g., symptomatic bradycardia, complete heart block, new bundle-branch block with transient complete heart block, alternating bundle-branch block)
  - ❖ Sinus node dysfunction (e.g., symptomatic bradydysrhythmias, treatment of bradycardia-tachycardia syndromes, sick sinus syndrome)
  - ❖ Ventricular standstill or cardiac arrest
  - ❖ Long QT syndrome with ventricular dysrhythmias
  - ❖ Drug toxicity
  - ❖ Postoperative cardiac surgery
  - ❖ Prophylaxis with cardiac diagnostic or interventional procedures
  - ❖ Chronotropic incompetence in the setting of cardiogenic shock
  - ❖ Malfunction/infection of permanent cardiac pacemaker
- When temporary transvenous pacing is used, the pulse generator is attached externally to one or more pacing leads that are inserted through a vein into the right atrium and/or right ventricle.
- Veins used for the insertion of a transvenous pacing lead wire include the subclavian, femoral, brachial, internal jugular, or external jugular.
- Single-chamber ventricular pacing is the most appropriate method in an emergency because the goal is to establish a heart rate as quickly as possible.
- The transvenous pacing lead is an insulated wire with one or two electrodes at the tip of the wire (Fig. 50-1).

AP This procedure should be performed only by physicians, advanced practice nurses, and other healthcare professionals (including critical care nurses) with additional knowledge, skills, and demonstrated competence per professional licensure or institutional standard.

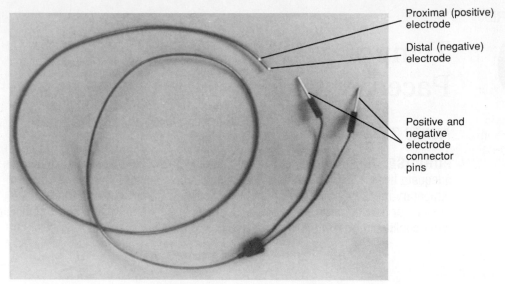

Proximal (positive) electrode

Distal (negative) electrode

Positive and negative electrode connector pins

Figure 50-1   Bipolar lead wire.

- The pacing lead can be a hard-tipped or a balloon-tipped pacing catheter that is placed in direct contact with the endocardium. Most temporary leads are bipolar with the distal tip electrode (seen as a metal ring) separated from the proximal electrode by 1 to 2 cm of pacing catheter (also seen as a metal ring; see Figs. 50-1 and 51-1).
- Basic principles of cardiac pacing include sensing, pacing, and capture.
- Sensing refers to the ability of the pacemaker device to detect intrinsic myocardial electrical activity. Sensing occurs if the pulse generator is in the synchronous or demand mode. The pacemaker either is inhibited from delivering a stimulus or initiates an electrical impulse in response to a sensed event.
- Pacing occurs when the temporary pulse generator is activated and the programmed level of energy travels from the pulse generator through the temporary pacing lead wire to the endocardium. This is known as pacemaker firing and is exhibited as a vertical line or spike on the electrocardiogram (ECG) recording.
- Capture refers to the successful conduction of the pacemaker impulse through the myocardium, resulting in depolarization. Capture is evidenced on the ECG by a pacemaker spike followed by either an atrial or a ventricular complex, depending on the chamber being paced. The healthcare provider can assess whether the electrical depolarization resulted in mechanical activity by observing pressure waveforms for evidence of contraction (right or left atrial, pulmonary artery, or arterial) or by palpating a pulse.
- Pulse generators can be used for single-chamber pacing with one set of terminals at the top of the pulse generator, into which the pacing wires are inserted (via a connecting cable). A dual-chamber pacemaker requires two sets of terminals, one each for the atrial and ventricular wires.
- The temporary pulse generator houses the controls and the energy source for pacing. Different models of pacemakers use either dials or touch pads to adjust the following settings:
  - ❖ Pacing rate adjusts the number of pacing stimuli delivered per minute.
  - ❖ Pacing output determines the amount of energy delivered to the endocardium in milliamperes (mA). Dual-chamber pacing requires that mA are set for both the atria and the ventricle.
  - ❖ AV interval on a dual-chamber pacemaker controls the amount of time between atrial and ventricular stimulation (electronic PR interval).
  - ❖ Sensitivity determines the size of the intrinsic activity in millivolts (mv) that will be detected by the generator.
- The ability of the pacemaker to detect the patient's intrinsic rhythm is determined by the pacing mode. In an asynchronous mode, the pacemaker functions as a fixed-rate pacemaker and is not able to sense any of the patient's inherent cardiac electrical activity. In a synchronous mode, the pacemaker is able to sense the patient's inherent cardiac electrical activity.
- The ability of the pacemaker to depolarize the myocardium depends on many variables: position of the electrode and degree of contact with viable endocardial tissue; level of energy delivered through the pacing wire; presence of hypoxia, acidosis, or electrolyte imbalances; fibrosis around the tip of the catheter; and concomitant medication therapy.[3,5]
- All electrical equipment in the patient's room must be properly grounded to prevent interference from occurring.
- Exposed pacing leads should be insulated when not in use to prevent microshock.[2,7,9,10]

EQUIPMENT

- Antiseptic skin preparation solution (e.g., 2% chlorhexidine-based solution)
- Sterile drapes, gloves and gowns, and towels
- Masks, head cover, goggles, or face shields
- Balloon-tipped pacing catheter and insertion tray
- Pacing lead wire
- Pulse generator

- 9-V battery for pulse generator
- Connecting cables
- Alligator clips or wires with connecting pins
- ECG monitor and recorder
- Supplies for dressing at insertion site

Additional equipment, to have available as needed, includes the following:

- Local anesthetic
- Percutaneous introducer needle or 14-gauge needle
- Introducer sheath with dilator
- Guidewire (per physician or advanced practice nurse choice)
- Suture, syringes, needles, and scalpel
- Emergency equipment (i.e., automated external defibrillator [AED], defibrillator)
- Portable ultrasound scan equipment
- Fluoroscopy
- Lead aprons or shields
- 12-lead ECG machine

PATIENT AND FAMILY EDUCATION

- Assess learning needs, readiness to learn, and factors that influence learning. *Rationale:* This assessment enables teaching to be individualized in a manner that is meaningful to the patient and the family.
- Discuss basic facts about the normal conduction system, such as structure and function of the conduction system, normal and abnormal heart rhythms, and symptoms and significance of abnormal heart rhythms. *Rationale:* The patient and family should understand the conduction system, why the procedure is necessary, and what potential risks and benefits are associated with this invasive procedure.
- Provide a basic description of the temporary transvenous pacemaker insertion procedure. *Rationale:* The patient and family should be informed of the invasive nature of the procedure and any risks associated with the procedure. An understanding of the procedure may reduce anxiety associated with the procedure.
- Describe the precautions and restrictions required while the temporary pacemaker is in place, such as limitation of movement, avoiding handling the pacemaker or touching exposed portions of the electrodes, and situations in which the nurse should be notified (e.g., if the dressing becomes damp, if the patient experiences dizziness). *Rationale:* Understanding potential limitations may improve the patient's cooperation with restrictions and precautions.

PATIENT ASSESSMENT AND PREPARATION

Patient Assessment

- Assess the patient's cardiac rhythm for the presence of the dysrhythmia that necessitates the initiation of temporary cardiac pacing. *Rationale:* This assessment determines the need for invasive cardiac pacing.
- Assess the patient's hemodynamic response to the dysrhythmia. Rhythm disturbances may reduce cardiac output significantly, with detrimental effects on perfusion of vital organs. *Rationale:* This assessment determines the urgency of the procedure. It may indicate the need for temporizing measures (e.g., vasopressors or transcutaneous pacing).
- Review current medications. *Rationale:* Medications may be implicated as a cause of the dysrhythmia that led to the need for pacemaker therapy, or medications may need to be held as a result of concomitant effect. Other medications, such as antidysrhythmics, may alter the pacing threshold. Review of medications could also determine whether reversal agents could be used as an alternative to pacemaker therapy.
- Review the patient's current laboratory study results, including chemistry, electrolyte profile, arterial blood gases, coagulation profile, platelet count, and cardioactive medication levels. *Rationale:* This review assists in determining whether inserting the pacemaker was precipitated by metabolic disturbances or medication toxicity and establishes the pacing milieu. The review provides the healthcare provider with information regarding the risk for abnormal bleeding during or after the procedure is performed.

Patient Preparation

- Verify that the patient is the correct patient using two identifiers. *Rationale:* Before performing a procedure, the nurse should ensure the correct identification of the patient for the intended intervention.
- Ensure that the patient and family understand preprocedural teaching. Answer questions as they arise and reinforce information as needed. *Rationale:* Evaluates and reinforces understanding of previously taught information.
- Obtain informed consent. *Rationale:* Informed consent protects the rights of the patient and makes a competent decision possible for the patient; however, in emergency circumstances, time may not allow a consent form to be signed.
- Perform a preprocedure verification and time out, if nonemergent. *Rationale:* Ensures patient safety.
- Connect the patient to a 5-lead monitoring system or to a 12-lead ECG machine. *Rationale:* This monitoring facilitates the placement of the balloon-tipped catheter by indicating the position of the catheter during its placement. Also, it allows for monitoring of the patient's cardiac rhythm during the procedure.
- Prescribe and ensure that pain medication and/or sedation is administered. *Rationale:* Medication may be indicated depending on the patient's level of anxiety and pain. Sedation or pain medication may not be possible if the patient's condition is hemodynamically unstable.

Procedure for Performing Temporary Transvenous Pacemaker Insertion

Steps	Rationale	Special Considerations
1. **HH**		
2. **PE**		
3. Connect the patient to the bedside monitoring system, and monitor the ECG continuously (see Procedure 54).	Monitors the patient's intrinsic heart rate and rhythm during and after the procedure to evaluate for adequate rate and pacemaker function.	If the monitoring system is not a 5-lead system, also connect the patient to the 12-lead ECG machine (see Procedure 57).
4. Dispose of used supplies and wash hands.	Minimizes the risk of infection.	
5. Check the placement of the central venous access with chest radiography before starting the procedure.	Central venous access is needed as the transvenous pacing catheter is passed through the central venous system.	If central venous access is needed, refer to Procedure 82.
6. Assess functioning of the temporary pacemaker, and insert a new battery into the pulse generator before beginning therapy. **(Level M*)**	Ensures a functional pacemaker pulse generator.	Different ways to assess battery function depend on the model and manufacturer; check manufacturer's recommendations for specific instructions.
7. Attach the connecting cable to the pulse generator, connecting the "positive" on the cable to the "positive" on the pulse generator and the "negative" on the cable to the "negative" on the pulse generator.	Prepares the pacing system; the pacing stimulus travels from the pulse generator to the negative terminal, and energy returns to the pulse generator via the positive terminal.	Some lead wires are labeled distal and proximal; distal connects to negative, and proximal connects to positive. Some lead wires may not have negative and positive marked on them. Polarity is established when the wires are placed in the connecting cable. Two connecting cables are needed with both atrial and ventricular pacing.
8. All personnel performing and assisting with the procedure should wash hands and apply **PE** and sterile equipment (e.g., masks, head covers, goggles or face shields, sterile gowns, and gloves).	Minimizes the risk of infection and maintains standard and sterile precautions.	Gloves should be worn whenever the pacing electrodes are handled to prevent microshock.[2,7,9,10]
9. Cleanse the site with antiseptic solution (e.g., 2% chlorhexidine-based preparation).	Minimizes the risk of infection.	
10. Drape the site with the sterile drapes.	Provides a sterile field and reduces the transmission of microorganisms.	
11. Insert the balloon-tipped pacing catheter through the introducer, and slowly advance the pacing lead, using one of the following insertion techniques:	The transvenous pacing catheter is threaded through the central venous system, using one of four methods to confirm proper placement.	For transvenous, ventricular pacing, the negative pacing electrode is positioned in the endocardium (at the apex) of the right ventricle.
A. Blind technique: i. Continue advancing the pacing lead.	This technique can be used to quickly achieve pacing in unstable patients.	If premature ventricular contractions or runs of ventricular tachycardia occur, deflate the balloon and withdraw the catheter a little.
ii. The balloon can be inflated when the tip of the pacing lead is in the vena cava, approximately at the 20 cm marking.	The balloon allows blood flow to facilitate catheter advancement.	Once capture is identified on ECG, mechanical contraction should be confirmed with palpation of a pulse.

*Level M: Manufacturer's recommendations only

Procedure	for Performing Temporary Transvenous Pacemaker Insertion—*Continued*	
Steps	**Rationale**	**Special Considerations**

B. Ultrasound guided technique **(Level E*)**:
   i. Obtain ultrasound equipment.
   ii. Continue advancing the pacing lead.
   iii. The balloon can be inflated when the tip of the pacing lead can be visualized in the vena cava.
   iv. Advance the pacing lead to the desired intracardiac position guided by ultrasound.
	Transcutaneous ultrasound scan visualization of the pacing lead as it is being passed through the central venous system may ensure a quicker and more accurate placement of the pacing electrode within the endocardium of the right ventricle.[1,4,6]	

C. Fluoroscopy guided technique:
   i. Obtain fluoroscopy equipment.
   ii. Continue advancing the pacing lead.
   iii. The balloon can be inflated when the tip of the pacing lead can be visualized in the vena cava.
   iv. Advance the pacing catheter to the desired intracardiac position guided by fluoroscopy.
	Fluoroscopy may be needed to permit direct visualization of the pacing electrode.	If fluoroscopy is used, all personnel must be shielded from the radiation with lead aprons or be positioned behind lead shields. A lead sheet or apron should also be placed below the patient's waist.

D. ECG-guided technique:
   i. The V lead of a 5-lead system or a 12-lead ECG machine can be used.
   ii. Connect the patient to the limb leads of the 12-lead ECG machine if this method is used.
   iii. Attach the V lead of the ECG monitoring system or the 12-lead ECG machine to the negative electrode connector pin (distal pin) of the pacing lead wire.
   iv. An alligator clip or a wire with connector pins can be used if needed (see Fig. 50-2).
   v. Set the monitoring system to record the V lead continuously.
   vi. Continue advancing the pacing lead.
   vii. The balloon can be inflated when the tip of the pacing lead is in the vena cava, approximately at the 20 cm marking.
   viii. Advance the pacing lead and observe the ECG for ST segment elevation in the V lead (see Fig. 50-3).
   ix. Observe for left bundle-branch block pattern and left-axis deviation that usually can be identified.
	When an ECG is obtained directly from the pacing electrode, proper position of the catheter tip is verified by visualization of the ST-segment elevation indicating catheter contact with the endocardium.	As a result of the temporary pacing catheter transmission of impulses from within the right ventricle, conduction of the impulse throughout the ventricles occurs via cellular conduction of the impulse rather than transmission down the bundle branches.

*Level E: Multiple case reports, theory-based evidence from expert opinions, or peer-reviewed professional organizational standards without clinical studies to support recommendations.

Procedure continues on following page

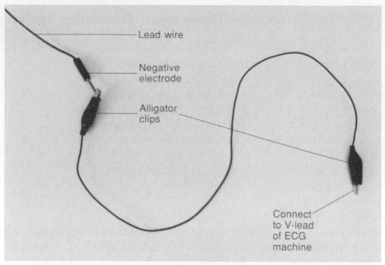

Figure 50-2   Alligator clips. ECG, electrocardiogram.

Procedure	for Performing Temporary Transvenous Pacemaker Insertion—*Continued*	
Steps	Rationale	Special Considerations
12. After the electrodes are properly positioned: A. Deflate the balloon. B. Connect the pacing lead external electrode pins to the pulse generator via the connecting cables. C. Ensure that the positive and negative electrodes are connected to the respective positive and negative terminals on the pulse generator via the connecting cables.	Energy from the pulse generator is directed to the negative electrode in contact with the ventricle. The pacing circuit is completed as energy reaches the positive electrode. The lead wires must be connected securely to the pacemaker to ensure appropriate sensing and capture and to prevent inadvertent disconnection.	A bridging connecting cable is recommended for use between the pacing lead and the pulse generator.
13. Set the pacemaker settings and initiate pacing (refer to Procedure 51).	Initiates pacemaker therapy.	
14. Suture the pacing lead in place.	Minimizes the risk of dislodgment.	
15. Apply a sterile occlusive dressing over the site.	Minimizes the risk of infection.	
16. Secure the pacemaker equipment such as strapping the pulse generator to the patient's torso or securing the pulse generator in a carrying device.	The pulse generator should be protected from falling or becoming inadvertently detached by patient movement. Disconnection or tension on the pacing electrodes may lead to pacemaker malfunction.	Pinning the generator to the patient's sheets or pillow is not recommended because if the patient moves, sits up, or gets out of bed, the pacing lead may be inadvertently disconnected.
17. Remove **PE** and discard used supplies in appropriate receptacles.	Reduces the transmission of microorganisms; Standard Precautions.	
18. **HH**		
19. Obtain a chest radiograph.	In the absence of fluoroscopy, a chest radiograph is essential to detect potential complications associated with insertion and to visualize lead position.	

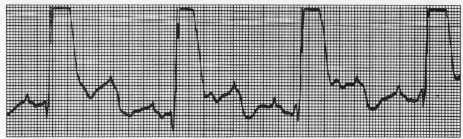

Figure 50-3 Electrocardiogram rhythm recorded in the right ventricle; elevated ST segments when the pacing electrode is wedged against the endocardial wall of the right ventricle. *(From Meltzer LE, Pinneo R, Kitchell JR:* Intensive coronary care, *ed 4, Bowie, MD, 1983, Robert J. Brady Co.)*

Expected Outcomes

- Paced rhythm on ECG consistent with parameters set on the pacemaker, as evidenced by appropriate heart rate, proper sensing, and proper capture
- Patient exhibits hemodynamic stability, as evidenced by systolic blood pressure greater than 90 mm Hg, mean arterial blood pressure greater than 60 mm Hg, alert and oriented condition, and no syncope or ischemia
- Pacemaker leads securely connected to the pulse generator

Unexpected Outcomes

- Inability to achieve proper placement of the pacing catheter
- Failure of the pacemaker to sense, causing competition between the pacemaker-initiated impulses and the patient's intrinsic cardiac rhythm
- Failure of the pacemaker to capture the myocardium
- Pacemaker oversensing that causes the pacemaker to be inappropriately inhibited
- Stimulation of the diaphragm that causes hiccupping, possibly related to pacing the phrenic nerve, perforation, wire dislodgment, or excessively high pacemaker mA setting
- Phlebitis, thrombosis, embolism, or bacteremia
- Ventricular dysrhythmias
- Arterial puncture, pneumothorax, hemothorax, pneumomediastinum, or the development of subcutaneous emphysema from the insertion procedure[3,5]
- Myocardial perforation, cardiac tamponade, or postpericardiotomy syndrome from the insertion procedure and electrode placement
- Air embolism
- Lead dislodgment
- Pain

Patient Monitoring and Care

Steps	Rationale	Reportable Conditions
		These conditions should be reported if they persist despite nursing interventions.
1. Monitor vital signs and hemodynamic response to pacing following institutional standards and as often as the patient's condition warrants.	The goal of cardiac pacing is to improve cardiac output by increasing heart rate or by overriding life-threatening dysrhythmias.	• Change in vital signs associated with signs and symptoms of hemodynamic deterioration
2. Evaluate the ECG for the presence of the paced rhythm or resolution of the initiating dysrhythmia.	Proper pacemaker functioning is assessed by observing the ECG for pacemaker activity consistent with the parameters set.	• Dysrhythmias • Inability to obtain capture • Oversensing • Undersensing

Procedure continues on following page

Patient Monitoring and Care —*Continued*

Steps	Rationale	Reportable Conditions
3. Follow institutional standards for assessing pain. Prescribe analgesia.	Promotes comfort.	• Continual hiccups (may indicate wire perforation or phrenic nerve stimulation) • Continued pain despite pain interventions
4. Check and document sensitivity and threshold at least every 24 hours. Threshold may be checked by physicians or advance practice nurses in patients at high risk (e.g., if pacemaker dependent). Follow institutional standards.	Ensures proper pacemaker functioning. Prevents unnecessarily high levels of energy delivery to the myocardium. Threshold may be checked more frequently if the patient's condition changes or pacemaker function is questioned.	• Problems with sensitivity or threshold
5. Replace gauze dressings every 2 days and transparent dressings at least every 7 days.[8] Cleanse the site with an antiseptic solution (e.g., 2% chlorhexidine-based preparation). Follow institutional standards. **(Level D*)**	Although guidelines specific to pacing leads do not exist, the Centers for Disease Control and Prevention (CDC) recommend replacing dressings on intravascular catheters when the dressing becomes damp, loosened, or soiled, or when inspection of the site is necessary.[8]	• Increased temperature • Increased white blood cell count • Purulent drainage at the insertion site • Warmth, redness, discoloration, or pain at the site
6. Monitor for other complications.	Early recognition leads to prompt treatment.	• Embolus • Thrombosis • Perforation of the myocardium • Pneumothorax • Hemothorax • Phlebitis
7. Monitor electrolyte levels.	Electrolyte imbalances may precipitate dysrhythmias.	• Abnormal electrolyte values
8. Ensure that all pacemaker connections are secure.	Maintenance of tight connections is necessary to ensure proper sensing, to ensure impulse conduction, and to minimize the risk of microshock conduction to the heart.	• Inability to maintain tight connections with available equipment, jeopardizing pacing therapy

*Level D: Peer-reviewed professional and organizational standards with the support of clinical study recommendations.

Documentation

Documentation should include the following:
- Description of the events that warranted intervention
- Patient and family education and response to education
- Signed informed consent form
- Universal Protocol requirements, if nonemergent
- Date and time of insertion
- Date and time of initiation of pacing
- Type of pacing wire inserted and location of insertion
- Pacemaker settings: mode, rate, output, sensitivity setting, threshold measurements, and whether pacemaker is on or off
- ECG monitoring strip recording before and after pacemaker insertion, with interpretation
- Vital signs and hemodynamic parameters before, during, and after the procedure
- Proper placement confirmed with chest radiography
- Patient response to procedure
- Complications and interventions
- Occurrence of unexpected outcomes and interventions taken
- Pain assessment, interventions, and patient response to medication
- Date and time pacing was discontinued
- Adjustment to monitoring system to ensure detection of paced rhythms

References and Additional Readings

For a complete list of references and additional readings for this procedure, scan this QR code with any freely available smartphone code reader app, or visit http://booksite.elsevier.com/9780323376624.

51 Temporary Transvenous and Epicardial Pacing

Valerie Spotts

PURPOSE: The purpose of temporary cardiac pacing is to ensure or restore an adequate heart rate and rhythm. Transvenous and epicardial pacing are initiated as temporary measures when a failure of the normal conduction system of the heart to produce an electrical impulse results in hemodynamic compromise.

PREREQUISITE NURSING KNOWLEDGE

- Knowledge of the normal anatomy and physiology of the cardiovascular system, principles of cardiac conduction, and basic dysrhythmia interpretation is needed.
- Understanding of temporary pacemakers is needed to evaluate pacemaker function and the patient's response to pacemaker therapy.
- Clinical and technical competence related to use of temporary pacemakers is needed.
- Advanced cardiac life support (ACLS) knowledge and skills are necessary.
- Basic principles of hemodynamic monitoring are essential in the assessment of the efficacy of temporary pacing therapy.
- Knowledge of the pulmonary artery (PA) catheter function and its use relative to hemodynamic monitoring with use of a PA catheter with pacing function is necessary (see Procedure 72).
- Knowledge of the care of patients with central venous catheters (see Procedure 66) is needed.
- Principles of general electrical safety apply, with the use of temporary invasive pacing methods, must be understood. Gloves always should be worn when handling electrodes to prevent microshock. In addition, the exposed proximal ends of the pacing wires should be insulated when not in use to prevent microshock.[3,11-13]
- The insertion of a temporary pacemaker is performed in emergent and elective clinical situations.
- Temporary pacing may be used to stimulate the myocardium to contract in the absence of an intrinsic rhythm, establish an adequate cardiac output and blood pressure to ensure tissue perfusion to vital organs, reduce the possibility of ventricular dysrhythmias in the presence of bradycardia, supplement an inadequate rhythm with transient decreases in heart rate (e.g., chronotropic incompetence in shock), or allow the administration of medications (e.g., beta blockers) to treat ischemia or tachydysrhythmias in the presence of conduction system dysfunction or bradycardia.

- Temporary invasive pacing is indicated for the following:[7,8,10]
  - Symptomatic third-degree atrioventricular (AV) block
  - Symptomatic second-degree heart block
  - Dysrhythmias that complicate acute myocardial infarction
  - Symptomatic bradycardia or bradydysrhythmias
  - New bundle-branch block with transient complete heart block
  - Alternating bundle-branch block
  - Symptomatic sinus node dysfunction
  - Treatment of bradycardia-tachycardia syndrome (sick sinus syndrome)
  - Ventricular standstill or cardiac arrest
  - Long QT syndrome with ventricular dysrhythmia
  - Medication toxicity or adverse effects of a medication
  - Postoperative cardiac surgery
  - Low cardiac output states
  - Prophylaxis with cardiac diagnostic, interventional, or surgical procedures
  - Chronotropic incompetence in the setting of cardiogenic shock
- The three primary methods of invasive temporary pacing are transvenous endocardial pacing, pacing via a PA catheter, and epicardial pacing.
- Transvenous pacing:
  - In temporary transvenous pacing, the pulse generator is externally attached to a pacing lead that is inserted through a vein into the right atrium or ventricle.
  - Veins used for insertion of the pacing lead are the subclavian, femoral, brachial, internal jugular, or external jugular veins.
  - Single-chamber ventricular pacing is the most common method used in an emergency because the goal is to establish a heart rate as quickly as possible.
  - Temporary atrial or dual-chamber pacing can be initiated if the patient needs atrial contraction for improvement in hemodynamics.
  - The pacing lead is an insulated wire with one or two electrodes at the tip of the wire (Fig. 50-1).

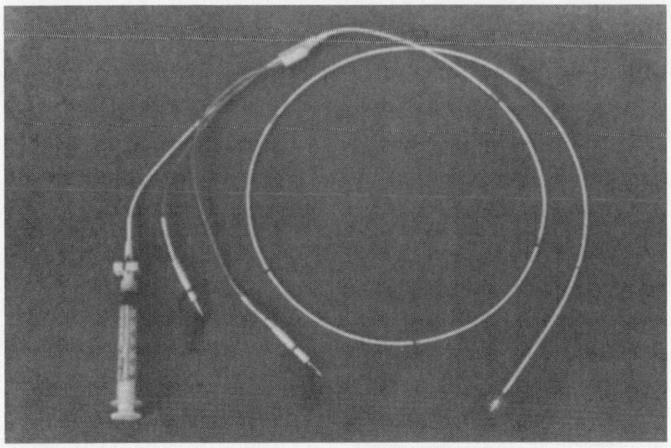

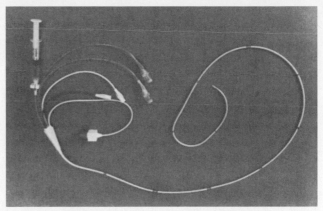

Figure 51-1 Balloon-tipped bipolar lead wire for transvenous pacing.

Figure 51-2 Pulmonary artery catheter with atrial and ventricular pacing lumens.

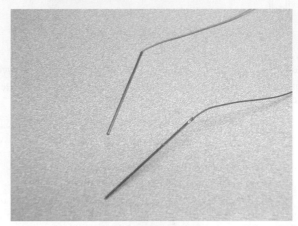

Figure 51-3 Epicardial wires.

- ❖ The pacing lead can be a hard-tipped or balloon-tipped pacing catheter that is placed in direct contact with the endocardium (Fig. 51-1). Most temporary leads are bipolar, with the distal tip electrode separated from the proximal ring by 1 to 2 cm (see Fig. 50-1).
- ❖ An external temporary pulse generator is connected to the transvenous pacing wire via a bridging or connecting cable.
- Pacing via a PA catheter:
  - ❖ Temporary atrial or ventricular pacing via a thermodilution PA catheter can be done with combination catheters that are specifically designed for temporary pacing.
  - ❖ PA pacing catheters feature atrial and ventricular ports for the introduction of the pacing lead wires (Fig. 51-2).
  - ❖ Use of a PA catheter combines the capabilities of PA pressure monitoring, thermodilution cardiac output measurement, fluid infusion, mixed venous oxygen sampling, and temporary pacing.
  - ❖ One limitation of these multifunction catheters is that the simultaneous measurement of pulmonary artery occlusion pressure (PAOP) and pacing is usually not possible. Balloon inflation can cause repositioning of the pacing electrode with catheter movement; measurement of the PAOP may cause pacing to become intermittent.[10]
- Temporary epicardial pacing:
  - ❖ Temporary epicardial pacing is a method of stimulating the myocardium through the use of polytetrafluoroethylene (PTFE)–coated, unipolar or bipolar stainless steel wires that are sutured loosely to the epicardium after cardiac surgery (Fig. 51-3).
  - ❖ The epicardial wires may be attached to the right atrium for atrial pacing, the right ventricle for ventricular pacing, or both for AV pacing.
  - ❖ Each pacing wire is brought through the chest wall before the chest is closed.
  - ❖ Epicardial wires can be placed in a unipolar or bipolar configuration.

- ○ Bipolar is more common. With bipolar placement, both leads are connected to the myocardium and both are able to function as negative poles.
- ○ Unipolar placement has one lead on the myocardium (negative) and another lead placed on the chest wall (positive). This positive lead is sometimes referred to as a ground or skin lead.
- ❖ Typically, the atrial wires are located on the right of the sternum, and the ventricular wires exit to the left of the sternum (Figs. 44-1 and 51-4).
- ❖ If a minimally invasive surgery was performed the pacing wires may be in different locations; discuss and label the pacing wires so that it is clear which wires are apical and which are ventricular.
- ❖ An external temporary pulse generator (Figs. 51-5, 51-6, and 51-7) is connected to the epicardial pacing wires via a bridging or connecting cable (Fig. 51-8).
- ❖ Atrial and ventricular thresholds for epicardial wires increase by the fourth postoperative day.[4]
- Basic principles of cardiac pacing include sensing, pacing, and capture.
  - ❖ Sensing refers to the ability of the pacemaker device to detect intrinsic myocardial electrical activity. Sensing occurs if the pulse generator is in the synchronous or demand mode. The pacemaker either is inhibited from delivering a stimulus or initiates an electrical impulse.

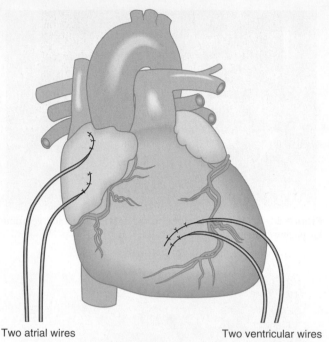

Two atrial wires   Two ventricular wires

Figure 51-4 Location of atrial and ventricular epicardial lead wires.

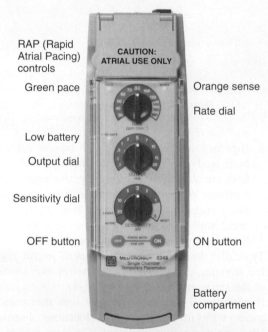

RAP (Rapid
Atrial Pacing)
controls

Green pace

Low battery

Output dial

Sensitivity dial

OFF button

CAUTION:
ATRIAL USE ONLY

Orange sense

Rate dial

ON button

Battery
compartment

Figure 51-5 Single-chamber temporary pulse generator. *(Reproduced with permission of Medtronic, Inc.)*

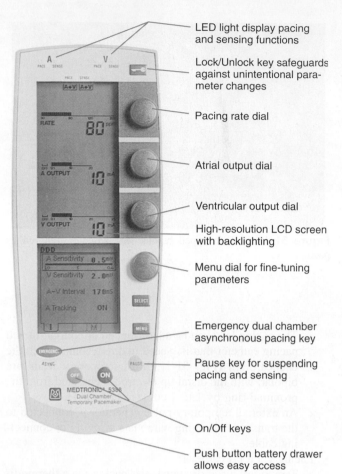

LED light display pacing
and sensing functions

Lock/Unlock key safeguards
against unintentional parameter changes

Pacing rate dial

Atrial output dial

Ventricular output dial

High-resolution LCD screen
with backlighting

Menu dial for fine-tuning
parameters

Emergency dual chamber
asynchronous pacing key

Pause key for suspending
pacing and sensing

On/Off keys

Push button battery drawer
allows easy access

Figure 51-6 Dual-chamber temporary pulse generator, model 5388. *LED, light-emitting diode; LCD, liquid crystal display. (Reproduced with permission of Medtronic, Inc.)*

* Pacing occurs when the temporary pulse generator is activated and the requisite level of energy travels from the pulse generator through the temporary wires to the myocardium, which is known as pacemaker firing and is represented as a line or spike on the electrocardiogram (ECG) recording.
* Electrical capture refers to the successful stimulation of the myocardium by the pacemaker, resulting in depolarization. Capture is evidenced on the ECG as an atrial or ventricular complex following the pacemaker

spike, depending on the chamber being paced. Mechanical capture is evidenced by generation of a pulse.
* Temporary pulse generator:
  ❖ The temporary pulse generator houses the controls and energy source for pacing.
  ❖ Some pulse generators are for single-chamber pacing only and have one set of terminals at the top of the pulse generator into which the pacing wires are inserted (via connecting cable; see Fig. 51-5).
* A dual-chamber pacemaker requires two sets of terminals for the atrial and ventricular wires (see Figs. 51-6, 51-7, and 51-9). A dual-chamber pacemaker can be used for single-chamber pacing, but settings for the chamber not being paced should be programmed to off to avoid any signal interference.[8]
* Different models of pacemakers use either dials or touch pads to change the settings.
  ❖ The pacing rate is determined by the rate dial or touch pad.
  ❖ The AV interval dial or pad on a dual-chamber pacemaker controls the amount of time between atrial and ventricular stimulation (electronic PR interval).
  ❖ The energy delivered to the myocardium is determined by setting the output (milliampere [mA]) dial or pad on the pulse generator.

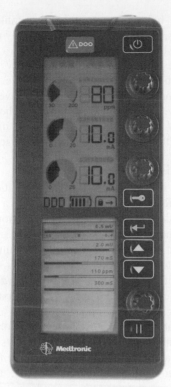

Figure 51-7 Dual-chamber temporary pulse generator, model 5392. *(Reproduced with permission of Medtronic, Inc.)*

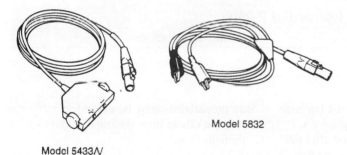

Model 5832

Model 5433/V
5433V

Figure 51-8 Connecting cables. *(Reproduced with permission of Medtronic, Inc.)*

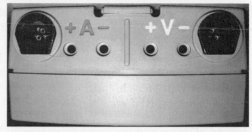

Figure 51-9 Pulse generator terminals to connect cables from atrial and ventricular leads.

EQUIPMENT

- Antiseptic solution (e.g., 2% chlorhexidine-based preparation)
- Nonsterile gloves
- Pacing lead wires
- Pulse generator
- Battery/batteries for pulse generator (usually 9 V or AA)
- Connecting cables
- ECG monitoring equipment
- Dressing supplies

Additional equipment, to have available as needed, includes the following:

- Central venous catheter insertion supplies (see Procedure 82)
- Alligator clips or wire with connector pins
- Suture, needles, syringes
- Emergency equipment
- Fluoroscopy
- Lead aprons or shields
- Multiple-pressure transducer system, with use of PA catheter (see Procedure 75)
- 12-lead ECG machine
- Local anesthetic
- Sterile drapes, towels, masks, goggles or face shields, gowns, caps
- Insulating material for epicardial wires (e.g., finger cots, glove, needle caps, ear plugs)

PATIENT AND FAMILY EDUCATION

- Assess learning needs, readiness to learn, and factors that influence learning. ***Rationale:*** This assessment enables teaching to be individualized in a manner that is meaningful to the patient and family.
- Discuss basic information about the normal conduction system, such as structure and function of the conduction system, normal and abnormal heart rhythms, signs, symptoms, and the significance of abnormal heart rhythms. ***Rationale:*** The patient and family should understand the conduction system and why the procedure is necessary.
- Provide a basic description of the temporary pacemaker insertion procedure. ***Rationale:*** The patient and family should be informed of the invasive nature of the procedure and any risks associated with it. An understanding of the procedure may reduce anxiety.
- Describe the precautions and restrictions required while the temporary pacemaker is in place, such as limitation of

❖ Dual-chamber pacing requires that mA be set for the atria and the ventricle.
- The ability of the pacemaker to detect the patient's intrinsic rhythm is determined by the pacing mode and sensitivity setting. In the asynchronous mode, the pacemaker functions as a fixed-rate pacemaker and is not able to sense any of the patient's inherent cardiac activity. In the synchronous mode, the pacemaker is able to sense the patient's inherent cardiac activity.
- The ability of the pacemaker to depolarize the myocardium depends on many variables: the position of the electrodes and degree of contact with viable myocardial tissue; the level of energy delivered through the pacing wire; the presence of hypoxia, acidosis, or electrolyte imbalances; fibrosis around the tip of the catheter; and concomitant medication therapy.[10,12]

movement, avoidance of handling the pacemaker or touching exposed portions of the electrodes, and when to notify the nurse (e.g., if the dressing becomes wet, if the patient experiences dizziness). *Rationale:* Understanding limitations may improve patient cooperation with restrictions and precautions. The patient and family also will alert nurses to potential problems.

PATIENT ASSESSMENT AND PREPARATION

Patient Assessment

- Assess the patient's baseline cardiac rhythm for the presence of the dysrhythmia that necessitates temporary cardiac pacing. *Rationale:* This assessment determines the need for invasive cardiac pacing.
- Assess the patient's hemodynamic response to the dysrhythmia. Rhythm disturbances may reduce cardiac output significantly with detrimental effects on perfusion to vital organs. *Rationale:* This assessment determines the urgency of the procedure. It may indicate the need for temporizing measures, such as vasopressors or transcutaneous pacing.
- Review the patient's current medications. *Rationale:* Medications may be a cause of the dysrhythmia that led to the need for pacemaker therapy, or medications may

need to be held because of concomitant effect. Other medications, such as antidysrhythmics, may alter the pacing threshold.
- Review the patient's current laboratory study results, including chemistry or electrolyte profile, arterial blood gases, and/or cardioactive medication levels. *Rationale:* This review assists in determining whether the need for pacing was precipitated by metabolic disturbances or medication toxicity and establishes the pacing milieu.

Patient Preparation

- Verify that the patient is the correct patient using two identifiers. *Rationale:* Before performing a procedure, the nurse should ensure the correct identification of the patient for the intended intervention.
- Ensure that the patient and family understand preprocedural teaching. Answer questions as they arise, and reinforce information as needed. *Rationale:* This communication evaluates and reinforces understanding of previously taught information.
- Confirm that informed consent has been obtained. *Rationale:* Informed consent protects the rights of the patient and makes a competent decision possible for the patient; however, in emergency circumstances, time may not allow the consent form to be signed.
- Perform a preprocedure verification and time out, if non-emergent. *Rationale:* Ensures patient safety.

Procedure	for Temporary Transvenous and Epicardial Pacing		
Steps	**Rationale**	**Special Considerations**	

Initiating Temporary Pacing
1. ▩HH▩
2. ▩PE▩

Steps	Rationale	Special Considerations
3. Connect the patient to the bedside monitoring system and monitor the ECG continuously (see Procedure 54).	Monitors the patient's intrinsic rhythm and the patient's rhythm during and after the procedure to evaluate for adequate pacemaker function.	Skin preparations may be needed to remove oils to improve impulse transmission.[2]
4. Assess pacemaker functioning and insert a new battery into the pulse generator before beginning therapy. **(Level M*)**	Ensures a functional pacemaker pulse generator.	Different ways to assess battery function depend on the model and manufacturer; check the manufacturer's recommendations for specific instructions.
5. Prepare the pacing system: A. Ensure that the pulse generator is turned off. B. Attach the connecting cable to the pulse generator. C. The atrial cable connects into the socket labeled "A." D. The ventricular cable connects into the socket labeled "V."	Prepares equipment; the pacing stimulus travels from the pulse generator to the negative terminal, and energy returns to the pulse generator via the positive terminal.	Connecting cables are specific to either transvenous or epicardial wires. Some lead wires are labeled distal and proximal; distal connects to negative, and proximal connects to positive. Some lead wires may not have negative and positive marked on them. Polarity is established when the wires are placed in the connecting cable. Two connecting cables are needed with both atrial and ventricular pacing.

*Level M: Manufacturer's recommendations only.

Procedure	for Temporary Transvenous and Epicardial Pacing—*Continued*	
Steps	**Rationale**	**Special Considerations**

Assisting With Initiation of Temporary Transvenous Pacing

Steps	Rationale	Special Considerations
1. Follow **Steps 1 through 5** in Initiating Temporary Pacing.		
2. If a central venous catheter is not in place, assist as needed with catheter insertion (see Procedures 82 and 83).	A central line is needed for transvenous pacing.	An introducer sheath is used that fits the pacemaker wire that is being inserted.
3. Assist as needed with insertion of the transvenous pacing lead wire.	Provides needed assistance.	
4. All personnel performing and assisting with the procedure should apply **PE** and sterile equipment (e.g., masks, head covers, goggles or face shields, sterile gowns, and sterile gloves).[9]	Minimizes the risk of infection, maintains sterility, and maintains standard and sterile precautions.	
5. Assist as needed with cleansing the insertion site with antiseptic solution (e.g., 2% chlorhexidine-based preparation).	Minimizes the risk of infection.	Gloves should be worn whenever handling the pacing electrodes to prevent microshock.[3,11–13]
6. Assist as needed with draping the insertion site.	Provides a sterile field and reduces the transmission of microorganisms.	
7. Assist as needed as the pacing lead is passed through the introducer.	Facilitates the insertion process.	If a balloon-tipped pacing lead is used, balloon inflation occurs when the tip of the pacing lead is in the vena cava. The air-filled balloon allows the blood flow to carry the catheter tip into the desired position in the right ventricle.
8. Assist with verifying the position of the transvenous pacing lead wire:	For transvenous, ventricular pacing, the negative pacing electrode is positioned in the endocardium (at the apex) of the right ventricle.	
A. Ultrasound scan	Transcutaneous ultrasound may be used to assist with insertion of the pacing electrode.	
B. Fluoroscopy	Fluoroscopy may be used to assist with visualization of the pacing electrode.	If fluoroscopy is used, all personnel must be shielded from the radiation with lead aprons or be positioned behind lead shields.
C. Chest radiography	X-ray may be used to confirm the placement of the pacing electrode.	

Procedure continues on following page

Procedure for Temporary Transvenous and Epicardial Pacing—*Continued*

Steps	Rationale	Special Considerations

D. Bedside monitoring system or 12-lead ECG machine
  i. Connect the patient to the limb leads.
  ii. Attach the V lead of the ECG monitoring system or the 12-lead ECG machine to the negative electrode connector pin (distal pin) of the pacing lead wire (an alligator clip or wire with connector pins may be needed; see Fig. 50-2).
  iii. Set the monitoring system to record the V lead continuously.
  iv. Observe the ECG for ST-segment elevation in the V lead recording (see Fig. 50-3).
  v. Observe for left bundle-branch block pattern and left-axis deviation that usually can be identified.
	The ECG is derived directly from the pacing electrode, and the position of the catheter tip is verified by the internal electrical recording, which shows ST-segment elevation when in contact with the myocardium.	Determine that the ECG monitoring system meets all safety requirements.
		As a result of the temporary pacing catheter transmission of impulses from within the right ventricle, conduction of the impulse throughout the ventricles occurs via cellular conduction of the impulse rather than transmission down the bundle branches.

9. After the pacing lead wire is properly positioned: A. Connect the external electrode pins to the pulse generator via the connecting cables. B. Ensure that the positive and negative electrode connector pins are connected to the respective positive and negative terminals on the pulse generator (see Fig. 51-9) via the connecting cables (Fig. 51-10). C. Ensure all connections are secure.	Energy from the pulse generator is directed to the negative electrode in contact with the ventricle. The pacing circuit is completed as energy reaches the positive electrode. The lead wires must be connected securely to the pacemaker to ensure appropriate sensing and capture and to prevent inadvertent disconnection.	A connecting cable is recommended for use between the pacing wires and the pulse generator. Some lead wires are labeled distal and proximal; distal connects to negative, and proximal connects to positive. Some lead wires may not have negative and positive marked on them. Polarity is established when the wires are placed in the connecting cable.

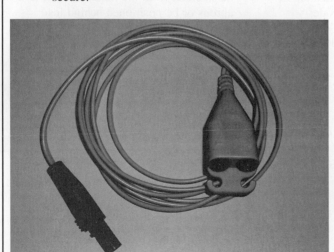

Figure 51-10 Transvenous cable that connects to transvenous pacemaker leads with shrouded pins. *(Reproduced with permission of Medtronic, Inc.)*

Procedure for Temporary Transvenous and Epicardial Pacing—*Continued*

Steps	Rationale	Special Considerations

10. For AV demand pacing, when an atrial lead is placed in addition to a ventricular lead:
  A. Connect the atrial electrodes to the atrial terminals via the connecting cable.
  B. Connect the ventricular electrodes to the ventricular terminals via the connecting cable.
  C. The connecting cable(s) should already be connected to the pulse generator for each chamber that is being paced (see Fig. 51-9).
	Ensures that the atrial electrodes are connected correctly to the pulse generator.
	Ensures that the ventricular electrodes are connected correctly to the pulse generator.
	The pacing stimulus travels from the pulse generator to the negative terminal, and energy returns to the pulse generator via the positive terminal.
		Transvenous temporary atrial leads may be placed short term for procedures and then removed.

Assisting With Initiating Temporary Pacing via a Pulmonary Artery Catheter

Steps	Rationale	Special Considerations
1. Follow **Steps 1 through 5** in Initiating Temporary Pacing.	Prepares equipment.	
2. Assist the physician, advanced practice nurse, or other provider with insertion of the PA catheter (see Procedure 72).	Provides assistance as needed.	Pacing electrodes may be inserted at the time of PA catheter insertion, or they may be inserted at a later time, when temporary pacing is needed because of a change in the patient's condition.
3. Obtain the appropriate pacing lead for insertion.	Only probes specifically manufactured for use with the PA catheter should be used; check specific manufacturer's recommendations.	Continuous monitoring of the right-ventricular pressure waveform via the pacing lumen is recommended before insertion of the electrode to ensure correct placement of the right ventricular port 1–2 cm distal to the tricuspid valve.
4. Assist as needed with insertion of the pacing lead wire.	Close monitoring of the ECG during insertion of the pacing lead is necessary to detect dysrhythmias.	Follow specific manufacturer's instructions regarding pacing lead insertion and securing the pacing lead in place within the catheter lumen.

5. After the pacing lead wire is properly positioned:
  A. Connect the positive and negative electrode connector pins to the pulse generator via the connecting cable.
  B. Ensure that the positive and negative electrodes are connected to the respective positive and negative terminals on the pulse generator via the connecting cables.
  C. Ensure all connections are secure.
	Energy from the pulse generator is directed to the negative electrode.
	The pacing circuit is completed as energy reaches the positive electrode.
	The pacing electrode needs to be securely connected to the pulse generator to ensure appropriate sensing and capture and to prevent inadvertent disconnection.
		Gloves should be worn whenever handling the pacing electrodes to prevent microshock.[3,11–13]

6. Check institutional policy or obtain specific provider prescription regarding not wedging the PA catheter.	Intermittent capture has been noted during the wedging procedure as a result of movement of the electrode with catheter migration into the wedge position.[6]	Usually, the PA catheter is not wedged during pacing therapy.[6]

Procedure continues on following page

Procedure for Temporary Transvenous and Epicardial Pacing—*Continued*

Steps	Rationale	Special Considerations
Epicardial Pacing		
1. Follow **Steps 1 through 5** in Initiating Temporary Pacing.		

2. Expose the epicardial pacing wires (Fig. 51-3) and identify the chamber of origin (see Figs. 44-1 and 51-4).
  A. Epicardial wires that exit to the right of the sternum are atrial in origin.
  B. Epicardial wires that exit to the left of the sternum are ventricular in origin.
	Identifies the correct chamber for pacing.	Gloves should be worn whenever handling the epicardial wires to prevent microshock.[3,11-13]

3. Set-up the system:
  A. Connect the epicardial wires to the pulse generator via the connecting cables (See step 4 below).
  B. Ensure that the positive and negative electrodes are connected to the respective positive and negative terminals on the pulse generator via the connecting cables.
  C. Ensure all connections are secure.
	Energy from the pulse generator is directed to the negative electrode in contact with the myocardium.
	The pacing circuit is completed as energy reaches the positive electrode.
	The epicardial wires must be connected securely to the pacemaker to ensure appropriate sensing and capture and to prevent inadvertent disconnection.	

4. Determine what type of pacing will be initiated:
  A. Unipolar pacing
  B. Bipolar pacing
	In a unipolar pacing system, only one epicardial pacing electrode is in contact with the chamber being paced (the negative electrode). The positive, or indifferent (ground), electrode may be an ECG electrode patch, may be an epicardial wire sewn to the subcutaneous tissue of the chest wall, or may be a subcutaneous needle inserted into the chest wall.
	In a bipolar pacing system, two epicardial pacing electrodes are in direct contact with the myocardial tissue of the chamber being paced.
		With unipolar pacing (one electrode in contact with the heart), the epicardial wire must be the negative electrode, and the ECG patch, skin wire, or subcutaneous needle is the positive electrode.
		With AV demand pacing, both atrial epicardial wires are connected to the atrium (via the connecting cable) and the ventricular epicardial wires are connected to the terminal labeled ventricle (via the connecting cable).

All Methods of Temporary Pacing		
1. Determine the mode of pacing desired.	The pacing mode chosen should be the one that best achieves the goal of pacing therapy. Possibilities include atrial, ventricular, or AV asynchronous (fixed rate) pacing or atrial, ventricular, or AV synchronous (demand) pacing.	Asynchronous pacing in the presence of an intrinsic rhythm may result in R-on-T phenomenon, leading to a lethal dysrhythmia, and should be used only in the absence of an intrinsic rhythm.[6,8,10]

Procedure for Temporary Transvenous and Epicardial Pacing—*Continued*

Steps	Rationale	Special Considerations
2. Set the pacemaker mode, pacemaker rate, and level of energy (output or mA) as prescribed or as determined by sensitivity and stimulation threshold testing (see subsequent **Steps 3, 4, and 5**).	Prepares pacemaker equipment.	Follow institutional standards regarding whether critical care nurses can set the pacemaker mode and energy level, and test the sensitivity and stimulation threshold levels. The demand or the synchronous mode is recommended to avoid competition between the pacemaker-initiated beats and the patient's intrinsic rhythm. Output is set to ensure capture of the myocardium. In AV pacing, separate output settings are used to ensure capture of the atrium and the ventricle.
3. Depending on the pulse generator, turn all settings to the lowest level, then turn on the pulse generator. **(Level M*)**	Prepares the equipment.	Follow the manufacturer's recommendations. Settings cannot be adjusted on some pulse generators until after the pulse generator is turned on. Other pulse generators turn on at default settings, after a self-test, and the settings can be adjusted at that time.
4. Determine the sensitivity threshold (for each chamber as appropriate). Set the rate for 10 beats/min below the patient's intrinsic rate.[1,7,8] **(Level M*)**	Sensitivity threshold is the level at which intrinsic myocardial activity is recognized by the sensing electrodes. Setting the pacemaker rate lower than the intrinsic rate avoids competition between the pacemaker and the patient's intrinsic rhythm. For demand pacing, the sensitivity must be measured and set.	This step is omitted if the patient has no intrinsic rhythm. In determining a sensitivity threshold, the mA should be turned to the lowest level to avoid the possibility of a pacemaker stimulus falling on the T wave (R-on-T phenomenon) and inducing a potentially lethal dysrhythmia.[5]
A. Gradually turn the sensitivity dial counterclockwise (or to a higher numeric setting) and observe the sense indicator light for flashing. The sense indicator light stops flashing when the device is unable to sense the patient's intrinsic rhythm.		After the sensitivity threshold is determined, some physicians and advanced practice nurses prefer to set the sensitivity settings all the way to the demand mode (most sensitive), regardless of the sensitivity threshold. Follow institutional standards.
B. Slowly turn the sensitivity dial clockwise (or to a lower numeric setting) until the sense indicator light flashes with each complex and the pace indicator light stops. This value is the sensing threshold.		If the sensitivity is set to the most sensitive, the pacemaker may be inappropriately inhibited because it may detect and interpret extramyocardial activity (e.g., muscle movement, artifact) as actual myocardial activity.

*Level M: Manufacturer's recommendations only.

Procedure continues on following page

Procedure for Temporary Transvenous and Epicardial Pacing—*Continued*

Steps	Rationale	Special Considerations
C. Set the sensitivity dial to the number that was half the sensing threshold to provide a 2:1 safety margin.[1,7,8]		
5. Determine the stimulation threshold (for each chamber as necessary).[1,7,8] Follow institution standard.	The output dial regulates the amount of electrical current (mA) that is delivered to the myocardium to initiate depolarization. The output (mA) is set at least two times above the stimulation threshold to allow for increases in the stimulation threshold without loss of capture.[1,7,8] The output (mA) is recommended to be ≤15 mA to prevent fibrosis at the lead/myocardium interface.[2]	This step should be performed by a physician or advanced practice nurse in a patient who is pacemaker dependent for bradydysrhythmia. Individual institutional policies govern when threshold determination should be done and whether a nurse may test the stimulation threshold; thresholds may not be determined if sensitivity is poor or if the patient's inherent heart rate is >90 beats/min. Threshold may increase or decrease within hours of electrode placement as a result of fibrosis at the tip of the catheter, medication administration (e.g., some antidysrhythmics), alteration of position, or underlying pathology.[1,5,7,8,10] In the case of dual-chamber pacing, the threshold for each chamber is assessed. Pacing rates vary depending on the indication for pacing.
A. Set the pacing rate approximately 10 beats/min above the patient's intrinsic rate.		
B. Gradually decrease the output from 20 mA until capture is lost.		
C. Gradually increase the mA until 1:1 capture is established. This is the stimulation threshold. The pace light will be flashing.		
D. Set the mA at least two times higher than the stimulation threshold.[1,7,8,13]	The output (mA) is recommended to be ≤15 mA to prevent fibrosis at the lead/myocardium interface.[2]	This output setting is sometimes referred to as the maintenance threshold.
6. Set the prescribed pacemaker rate.	Ensures adequate cardiac output.	
7. Assess the cardiac rate and rhythm for appropriate pacemaker function:	The ECG tracing should reflect appropriate response to the pacemaker settings if functioning properly.	
A. Capture: is there a QRS complex for every ventricular pacing stimulus? Is there also a P wave for every atrial pacing stimulus (Fig. 51-11)?	Sometimes atrial activity may not be visible because of low-voltage amplitude. If the patient is paced solely via atrial pacing, ventricular tracking and response should follow the atrial rate setting.	

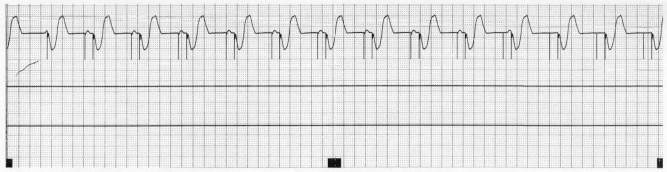

Figure 51-11 Pacemaker electrocardiogram (ECG) strip of atrioventricular pacing. Note the atrial pacing spike before each P wave and the ventricular pacing spike before each QRS complex.

Procedure	**for Temporary Transvenous and Epicardial Pacing—*Continued***	
Steps	**Rationale**	**Special Considerations**
B. Rate: is the rate at or above the pacemaker rate if in the demand mode?		
C. Sensing: does the sense light indicate that every QRS complex is sensed?		
8. After the settings are adjusted for optimal patient response, place the protective plastic cover over the pacemaker controls, or place the controls in the locked position.	Pacemaker settings may be inadvertently altered by patient movement or handling if the controls are not covered or locked.	The patient may need to be reminded not to touch the pulse generator.
9. Assess the patient's response to pacing, including blood pressure, level of consciousness, heart rhythm, and other hemodynamic parameters.	Pacemaker settings are determined by patient response.	
10. Apply a sterile occlusive dressing over the insertion site.	Prevents infection.	The epicardial electrodes and the insertion sites may be covered with a 4 × 4-inch dressing and taped to the chest.[5,13] The wires may be placed over the dressing and covered with gauze.
11. Secure the necessary equipment to provide some stability for the pacemaker, such as hanging the pulse generator on an intravenous pole, strapping the pulse generator to the patient's torso, hanging the pulse generator around the patient's neck, or securing the pulse generator under a draw sheet.	The pulse generator should be protected from falling or becoming inadvertently detached by patient movement.	Exposed wires should be secured in an insulated material (e.g., finger cots, glove, plastic needle cap, ear plugs).[11-13] Care must be taken to avoid bending or kinking the wires because this can lead to fractured wires.
12. Remove gloves and discard used supplies in appropriate receptacles.	Reduces the transmission of microorganisms; Standard Precautions.	
13. 🖐		
14. Obtain a chest radiograph as prescribed.	In the absence of fluoroscopy, a radiograph is essential to detect potential complications associated with insertion and to visualize lead position.	Not necessary for epicardial pacing.
15. Selectively restrict patient mobility depending on the insertion site.	Prevents electrode dislodgment.	Follow institutional policy regarding ambulation for the patient with a temporary pacemaker.

Procedure continues on following page

Expected Outcomes

- Paced rhythm on ECG consistent with parameters set on the pacemaker, as evidenced by appropriate heart rate, sensing, and capture
- Patient exhibits hemodynamic stability, as evidenced by a systolic blood pressure >90 mm Hg, a mean arterial blood pressure >60 mm Hg, baseline mental status, and no syncope or ischemia
- All pacemaker wires are securely connected to the pulse generator

Unexpected Outcomes

- Failure of the pacemaker to sense, causing competition between the pacemaker-initiated impulses and the patient's intrinsic cardiac rhythm
- Failure of the pacemaker to capture the myocardium
- Pacemaker oversensing that causes the pacemaker to be inappropriately inhibited
- Stimulation of the diaphragm that causes hiccupping, which may be related to pacing the phrenic nerve, perforation, wire dislodgment, or an excessively high pacemaker mA setting
- Phlebitis, thrombosis, embolism, or bacteremia
- Ventricular dysrhythmias
- Pneumothorax or hemothorax
- Myocardial perforation and cardiac tamponade
- Air embolism
- Lead dislodgment
- Pacemaker syndrome as a result of loss of AV synchrony
- Continual hiccups (may indicate wire perforation)
- Pain

Patient Monitoring and Care

Steps	Rationale	Reportable Conditions
		These conditions should be reported if they persist despite nursing interventions.
1. Monitor vital signs and hemodynamic response to pacing following institution standard and as often as the patient condition warrants.	The goal of cardiac pacing is to improve cardiac output by increasing heart rate or by overriding life-threatening dysrhythmias.	• Abnormal vital signs associated with signs and symptoms of hemodynamic deterioration
2. Evaluate the ECG for the presence of the paced rhythm or resolution of the initiating dysrhythmia.	Proper pacemaker functioning is assessed by observing the ECG for pacemaker activity consistent with the parameters set.	• Inability to obtain a paced rhythm (loss of capture or failure to capture) • Oversensing • Undersensing
3. Follow institutional standards for assessing pain. Administer analgesia as prescribed.	Identifies need for pain interventions.	• Continued pain despite pain interventions • Continual hiccups
4. Check and document sensitivity and stimulation threshold according to institutional standards (e.g., usually at least every 24 hours).[10,11] The threshold may be checked by physicians and/or advanced practice nurses in patients at high risk (e.g., if pacemaker dependent).	Ensures proper pacemaker functioning and prevents high levels of energy delivery to the myocardium. The threshold may be checked more frequently if the patient's condition changes or pacemaker function is questioned.	• Problems or significant changes with sensitivity or threshold

Patient Monitoring and Care —*Continued*

Steps	Rationale	Reportable Conditions
5. Replace gauze dressings every 2 days and transparent dressings at least every 7 days.[9] Cleanse the site with an antiseptic solution (e.g., 2% chlorhexidine-based preparation). Follow institutional standards. **(Level D*)**	Although guidelines specific to epicardial wires and transvenous pacemaker sites do not exist, the Centers for Disease Control and Prevention (CDC) recommend replacing dressings on intravascular catheters when the dressings become damp, loosened, or soiled or when inspection of the site is necessary.[9]	• Increased temperature • Increased white blood cell count • Drainage at the insertion site • Warmth or pain at the insertion site
6. Monitor for other complications.	Early recognition leads to prompt treatment.	• Embolus • Thrombosis • Perforation of the myocardium • Pneumothorax • Hemothorax • Phlebitis
7. Monitor electrolyte levels as prescribed.	Electrolyte imbalances may precipitate dysrhythmias or change stimulation thresholds.	• Abnormal electrolyte values
8. Ensure that all connections are secure and the low-battery indicator is not present.	Maintenance of tight connections is necessary to ensure proper pacemaker functioning. Battery life varies with the amount of pacing energy needed. Follow institutional guidelines for assessing the low-battery indicator.	• Inability to maintain tight connections with available equipment, jeopardizing pacing therapy
9. If the pulse generator is no longer needed for a patient with epicardial pacing wires, isolate and contain the tips to avoid microshocks (e.g., finger cot, needle cap, needle barrel, glove, ear plug).[11–13]	Microshocks can lead to lethal dysrhythmias. Epicardial wires are often left in place after pacing is no longer needed (generator is disconnected).	• Microshocks

*Level D: Peer-reviewed professional and organizational standards with the support of clinical study recommendations.

Documentation

Documentation should include the following:

- Patient and family education
- Signed informed consent form
- Universal Protocol requirements
- Date and time of initiation of pacing
- Description of events that warranted intervention
- Vital signs and hemodynamic parameters before, during, and after the procedure
- ECG monitoring strip recording before and after pacemaker insertion
- Type of pacemaker wire inserted and location
- Pacemaker settings: mode, rate, output, sensitivity, threshold measurements, and whether the pacemaker is on or off

- Presence of underlying rhythm
- Patient response to the procedure
- Complications and interventions
- Medications administered and patient response to the medications
- Pain assessment, interventions, and patient response
- Date and time of battery-status assessments
- Date and time pacing was discontinued
- Adjustment to monitoring system settings to ensure detection of paced rhythms

References and Additional Readings

For a complete list of references and additional readings for this procedure, scan this QR code with any freely available smartphone code reader app, or visit http://booksite.elsevier.com/9780323376624.

PROCEDURE

52 Intraaortic Balloon Pump Management

John P. Harper

PURPOSE: Intraaortic balloon pump therapy is designed to increase coronary artery perfusion, which increases myocardial oxygen supply, and decrease afterload and myocardial workload, which decreases myocardial oxygen demand.

PREREQUISITE NURSING KNOWLEDGE

- Knowledge of the anatomy and physiology of the cardiovascular system is needed.
- Understanding of the principles of hemodynamic monitoring, electrophysiology, dysrhythmias, and coagulation is necessary.
- Clinical and technical competence related to the use of the intraaortic balloon pump (IABP) is needed.
- Advanced cardiac life support knowledge and skills are necessary.
- Indications for IABP therapy are as follows:
  - ❖ Cardiogenic shock
  - ❖ Refractory unstable angina
  - ❖ Acute myocardial infarction (MI) complicated by left-ventricular failure[3,13,28,30]
  - ❖ Recurrent ventricular dysrhythmias as a result of ischemia[18]
  - ❖ Support before, during, and after coronary artery bypass graft surgery[2,31]
  - ❖ Support before, during, and after coronary artery angioplasty or additional interventional cardiology procedures for patients at high risk[4,11]
  - ❖ Mechanical complications of acute MI, including aortic stenosis, mitral stenosis, mitral valvuloplasty, mitral insufficiency, ventricular septal defect, and left-ventricular aneurysm
  - ❖ Intractable ventricular dysrhythmias[14,20]
  - ❖ Bridge to cardiac transplantation, ventricular-assist devices, or total artificial hearts
  - ❖ Cardiac injury, including contusion and coronary artery tears
  - ❖ Septic shock
  - ❖ Patient at high risk undergoing noncardiac surgery[20,31]
- Contraindications to IABP therapy are as follows:
  - ❖ Moderate to severe aortic insufficiency
  - ❖ Thoracic and abdominal aortic aneurysms
- The relative value of IABP therapy in the presence of severe aortoiliac disease, major coagulopathies, and terminal disease should be evaluated individually.

- IABP therapy is an acute short-term therapy for patients with reversible left-ventricular failure or an adjunct to other therapies for irreversible heart failure. Cardiac assistance with the IABP is performed to improve myocardial oxygen supply and reduce myocardial workload. Intraaortic balloon (IAB) pumping is based on the principles of counterpulsation (Fig. 52-1).
- The events of the cardiac cycle provide the stimulus for balloon function, and the movement of helium gas between the balloon and the control console gas source produces inflation and deflation of the balloon.
- Recognition of the R wave or the QRS complex on the electrocardiogram (ECG) is the most commonly used trigger source.
- Inflation occurs during ventricular diastole and causes an increase in aortic pressure. This increased pressure displaces blood proximally to the coronary arteries and distally to the rest of the body. The result is an increase in myocardial oxygen supply and subsequent improvement in cardiac output.
- Deflation occurs just before ventricular systole or ejection, which decreases the pressure within the aortic root, reducing afterload and myocardial workload.
- Insertion and placement verification:
  - ❖ The IAB catheter is commonly placed in the femoral artery via percutaneous puncture or arteriotomy.
  - ❖ The IAB catheter can also be placed in the left-axillary artery.[16,17]
  - ❖ The IAB catheter lies approximately 2 cm inferior to the left subclavian artery and superior to the renal arteries. This position allows for maximum balloon effect without occlusion of other arterial supplies (Fig. 52-2).
  - ❖ The IAB should not fully occlude the aorta during inflation. It should be 85% to 90% occlusive.
  - ❖ Fluoroscopy is recommended to aid in IAB catheter positioning, especially for patients with a tortuous aorta.
  - ❖ Correct catheter position is verified via radiography if fluoroscopy is not used during catheter insertion. The visibility of the IAB catheter tip may be enhanced

431

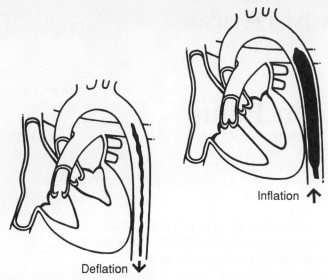

Figure 52-1 Counterpulsation. *(Courtesy Datascope Corp, Montvale, NJ.)*

when the IABP is temporarily placed on standby (follow manufacturer's guidelines).

❖ The central lumen of many IAB catheters provides a means for monitoring aortic pressure.

❖ Some IAB catheters use fiberoptic technology. These catheters have a fiberoptic sensor located at the tip of the IAB catheter. The sensor transmits the pressure signal to the IAB console where it is displayed as an aortic pressure waveform.[33]

• Timing methods of IABP therapy vary slightly from manufacturer to manufacturer. With the traditional or conventional method, the IAB deflates at the QRS complex, before isovolumetric contraction. The IAB also deflates at the QRS complex with the real-time method. An important principle of real timing is the duration of the balloon deflation during cardiac systole. During real timing, the IAB is timed to deflate at the onset of each QRS complex and to remain deflated throughout systole. A constant diastolic interval is not necessary for real timing.[5,6,21,24]

• The development of fiberoptic catheters and changes in the design of the IABP console has produced timing algorithms that automatically adjust timing. The algorithms identify markers, including the initial trigger event, the dicrotic notch, and end-diastolic pressure. The timing algorithms are updated on a continual basis, allowing for optimal inflation and deflation. Timing adapts to changes in both heart rate and ECG rhythm on a beat-to-beat basis.[12,33]

• The mechanics of the IABP control console vary from manufacturer to manufacturer.

• Specific information concerning controls, alarms, troubleshooting, and safety features is available from each manufacturer and should be read thoroughly by the nurse before use of the equipment.

EQUIPMENT

• IABP, helium gas supply
• ECG and arterial pressure monitoring supplies

• IAB catheter (size range, 7 to 10 Fr for adults; balloon catheters vary in balloon volumes, 25 to 50 mL)
• IAB catheter insertion kit
• Antiseptic solution (e.g., 2% chlorhexidine-based preparation)
• Caps, goggles or face shields, masks, sterile gowns, gloves, and drapes
• Sterile dressing supplies
• O-silk suture on a cutting needle or a sutureless securement device
• No. 11 scalpel, used for skin entry
• 1% lidocaine without epinephrine, one 30-mL vial
• Stopcocks, one two-way and one three-way
• One Luer-Lok plug
• 500 mL of normal saline flush solution (add heparin if prescribed or according to institutional standards)
• Single-pressure transducer system (see Procedure 75)

Additional equipment, to have available as needed, includes the following:

• Analgesics and sedatives as prescribed
• Lead apron/collar and radiation dosimeter badge (needed if procedure is performed with fluoroscopy)

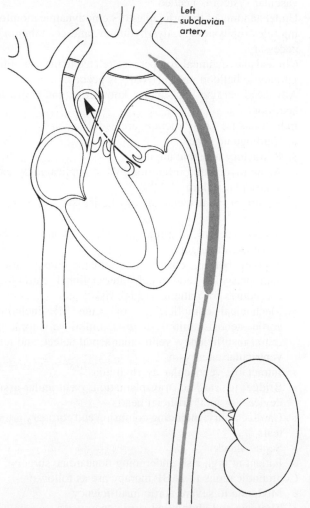

Left subclavian artery

Figure 52-2 Intraaortic balloon positioned in the descending thoracic aorta, just below the left subclavian artery but above the renal artery. *(From Quaal SJ: Comprehensive intraaortic balloon counterpulsation, ed 2, St Louis, 1993, Mosby.)*

- Intravenous (IV) solutions as prescribed
- Emergency medications and resuscitation equipment
- Vasopressors as prescribed
- Antibiotics as prescribed
- Heparin infusion or dextran if prescribed

PATIENT AND FAMILY EDUCATION

- Assess patient and family understanding of IABP therapy and the reason for its use. *Rationale:* Clarification or reinforcement of information is an expressed family need.
- Explain the standard care to the patient and family, including the insertion procedure, IABP sounds, frequency of assessment, alarms, dressings, need for immobility of the affected extremity, expected length of therapy, and parameters for discontinuation of therapy. *Rationale:* This explanation encourages the patient and family to ask questions and prepares the patient and family for what to expect.
- After catheter removal, instruct the patient to report any warm or wet feeling on the leg and any dizziness or light-headedness. *Rationale:* These feelings may be indicative of bleeding at the insertion site.

PATIENT ASSESSMENT AND PREPARATION

Patient Assessment

- Assess the patient's medical history, specifically related to competency of the aortic valve, aortic disease, or peripheral vascular disease. *Rationale:* This assessment provides baseline data regarding cardiac functioning and identifies contraindications to IABP therapy.
- Assess the patient's cardiovascular, hemodynamic, peripheral vascular, and neurovascular status. *Rationale:* This assessment provides baseline data.
- Assess the extremity for the intended IAB catheter placement for the quality and strength of the femoral, popliteal, dorsalis pedal, and posterior tibial pulses.[7,29]
- Assess the ankle/arm index as follows. *Rationale:* The IAB catheter is inserted into the vasculature of the extremity that exhibits the best perfusion. Also, this assessment provides baseline data related to peripheral blood flow, which may be compromised by the IAB.
  - ❖ Record the brachial systolic pressure with a Doppler scan signal.
  - ❖ Locate the posterior tibial or dorsalis pedal pulse with a Doppler scan signal.
  - ❖ Apply the blood pressure cuff around the ankle, above the malleolus.
  - ❖ Inflate the cuff to 20 mm Hg above the brachial systolic pressure.
  - ❖ Note the reappearance of the Doppler scan signal as the cuff deflates.

  - ❖ Divide the ankle systolic pressure by the brachial systolic pressure to determine the ankle/arm index (normal range, 0.8 to 1.2).
- Assess the patient's current laboratory profile, including complete blood count, platelet count, prothrombin time, international normalized ratio, partial thromboplastin time, and bleeding time. *Rationale:* Provides baseline data. Baseline coagulation studies are helpful in determining the risk for bleeding. Platelet function may be affected by the mechanical trauma from balloon inflation and deflation.
- Assess for signs and symptoms of heart failure that necessitate IABP therapy, including the following. *Rationale:* Physical signs and symptoms result from the heart's inability to adequately contract and from inadequate coronary or systemic perfusion.
  - ❖ Unstable angina[4]
  - ❖ Altered mental status
  - ❖ Heart rate greater than 110 beats/min
  - ❖ Dysrhythmias
  - ❖ Systolic blood pressure less than 90 mm Hg
  - ❖ Mean arterial pressure (MAP) less than 70 mm Hg with vasopressor support
  - ❖ Cardiac index less than 2.4[3]
  - ❖ Pulmonary artery occlusion pressure (pulmonary capillary wedge pressure) greater than 18 mm Hg
  - ❖ Decreased mixed venous oxygen saturation (Svo_2)
  - ❖ Inadequate peripheral perfusion
  - ❖ Urine output less than 0.5 mL/kg/hr

Patient Preparation

- Verify that the patient is the correct patient using two identifiers. *Rationale:* Before performing a procedure, the nurse should ensure the correct identification of the patient for the intended intervention.
- Ensure that the patient and family understand preprocedural teaching. Answer questions as they arise, and reinforce information as needed. *Rationale:* Understanding of previously taught information can be evaluated and reinforced.
- Validate that the informed consent form has been signed. *Rationale:* Informed consent protects the rights of the patient and makes a competent decision possible for the patient; however, in emergency circumstances, time may not allow the form to be signed.
- Perform a preprocedure verification and final time out. *Rationale:* Ensures patient safety.
- Validate the patency of central and peripheral intravenous access. *Rationale:* Central access is needed for vasopressor administration; peripheral access is needed for fluid administration.
- Assist the patient to a supine position. *Rationale:* Positions the patient for IAB insertion.

Procedure　for Assisting with IAB Catheter Insertion

Steps	Rationale	Special Considerations
1. **HH**		
2. **PE**		
3. Turn on the IABP console and the helium gas.	Provides power source and activates the gas that drives the IABP.	Follow the manufacturer's recommendations.
4. Sedate the patient as prescribed and as needed; the affected extremity may need to be restrained.	Movement of the lower extremity may inhibit insertion of the catheter or contribute to catheter kinking once the IAB is in place.	A knee immobilizer or a sheet placed over the affected leg and tucked in may minimize movement of the affected leg.
5. Establish ECG input to the IABP console and obtain an ECG configuration with optimal R wave amplitude and absence of artifact. Indirect ECG input can be obtained via a "slave" of the bedside ECG to the IABP console.	The R wave is the preferred trigger signal from which the IABP can reference systole and diastole and therefore establish inflation and deflation points.	Usually, one set of ECG electrodes connects to the bedside monitoring system and the second set of ECG electrodes connects to the IABP console. With use of a slave signal, refer to the bedside monitor manufacturer instructions for optimizing the ECG and pacemaker recognition.
6. Assist with placement of hemodynamic monitoring catheters if they are not already present (refer to Procedure 72).	Hemodynamic monitoring aids in the assessment and management of the patient who needs IABP therapy.	A radial arterial catheter is commonly inserted.[27]
7. Complete the IABP console preparation. Refer to the instruction manual. **(Level M*)**	Ensures adequate functioning of the IABP device.	Models of the pump console vary. Review of manufacturer instructions is recommended.
8. All personnel performing and assisting with the procedure should apply personal and protective sterile equipment (e.g., masks, head covers, goggles or face shields, sterile gowns, and gloves).	Minimizes the risk of infection and maintains standard and sterile precautions.	
9. Wear lead apron/collar and radiation dosimeter badge if inserted under fluoroscopy.	Lead apron/collar minimizes radiation exposure. Radiation dosimeter badges track radiation exposure.	
10. Assist if needed with prepping and draping the intended insertion site with the sterile drapes.	Provides a sterile field and reduces the transmission of microorganisms.	
11. Assist as needed with removing the IAB catheter from the sterile packing and place the catheter and insertion tray on the sterile field.	Makes supplies available and maintains sterility.	Catheters vary in balloon volumes. An adequate volume is necessary to achieve optimal hemodynamic effects from IABP therapy. Patient height may be used as a guideline for selection of balloon volume. Clinical judgment and patient factors, such as patient torso length, are considered.[11]

*Level M: Manufacturer's recommendations only.

Procedure for Assisting with IAB Catheter Insertion—*Continued*		
Steps	**Rationale**	**Special Considerations**
12. Administer a heparin bolus before arterial puncture, if clinically indicated and prescribed.	Anticoagulation therapy may decrease the incidence of thromboemboli related to the indwelling IAB catheter.	Systemic anticoagulation therapy may not be used in all patients.[32]
13. Attach the supplied one-way valve to the Luer-tip of the distal end of the balloon helium lumen.	Creates a device for removing air from the balloon catheter.	
14. Pull back slowly on the syringe until all the air is aspirated.	Removes air from the balloon, creating a vacuum.	Maintains the wrap of the balloon for insertion.
15. Disconnect the syringe only, leaving the one-way valve in place.	Prevents air entry back into the balloon.	
16. Follow the manufacturer recommendations for lubricating the catheter before insertion. **(Level M*)**	May decrease the drag on the catheter during insertion.	Not all IAB catheters need lubrication. Review manufacturer instructions.
17. Flush the inner lumen of the IAB catheter before insertion.	Removes air from the central lumen.	If the catheter is not flushed before insertion, allow the backflow of arterial blood before connection to the flush system.[25] Follow institutional policy or physician or advanced practice nurse prescription regarding the use of heparinized normal saline solution.
18. Assist as needed with the introducer sheath or dilator assembly and insertion.	Prepares for balloon catheter entry.	Some IABs are inserted without a sheath. If the IAB is inserted via the sheathless method, only the vessel dilator is used.[9,10]
19. Assist with balloon catheter insertion.	Catheter placement is a necessary part of IAB setup.	Some fiberoptic IABP catheters need to be calibrated before insertion. Follow manufacturer's guidelines.
20. Assist with removal of the one-way valve according to the manufacturer's recommendations.	Releases the vacuum and readies the balloon for counterpulsation.	
21. If the inner lumen of a double-lumen catheter is used to monitor arterial pressure, attach a three-way stopcock with a single-pressure transducer system (see Procedure 75) connected to the monitor and set the alarms.	Monitors the arterial pressure.	Follow institutional policy or physician or advanced practice nurse prescription regarding the use of heparinized normal saline solution. The inner lumen, if used, must be attached to an alarm system because undetected disconnection could result in life-threatening hemorrhage. The proximal tip of the inner lumen used for arterial pressure monitoring is at the level of the left subclavian artery, not at the aortic arch; therefore, this location is not the same as a central line placed at the aortic root.[25,26]

*Level M: Manufacturer's recommendations only.

Procedure continues on following page

Procedure for Assisting with IAB Catheter Insertion—*Continued*		
Steps	Rationale	Special Considerations
22. Avoid fast flush and blood sampling from the central aortic lumen.	Air may enter the system during fast flush and also during blood sampling, resulting in air emboli.	Some manufacturers and institutions recommend hourly fast flush of central lumen lines. If fast flush is required and prescribed, ensure that the IABP is on standby (not pumping) during the flush. However, the risk of air embolus entry or dislodging a thrombus at the lumen tip is a major concern. Refer to institutional policy in regard to fast flush of central lumen catheters.
23. Attach the helium tubing to the balloon helium lumen and connect the helium tubing to the IABP console.	Attachment is necessary to initiate therapy.	The helium tubing is packaged with the IAB.
24. Follow the steps for timing, troubleshooting, and patient monitoring.	Provides for appropriate operation of counterpulsation.	Many IABP consoles have features for automatic timing. Refer to specific manufacturer's instructions.
25. Conventional IAB: A. Level the air-fluid interface of the stopcock. B. Zero the hemodynamic monitoring system.	Ensures accurate arterial pressure measurement. Negates the effects of atmospheric pressure.	
26. Fiberoptic IAB: A. Calibrate the system. B. Follow the manufacturer's instructions for calibration.[23,27]	Prepares the equipment. Prepares the equipment.	Refer to specific manufacturer's instructions for fiberoptic IAB catheters. Some fiberoptic IAB catheters perform automatic in vivo calibration.
27. Ensure that a portable chest radiograph is obtained. Note: Temporarily place the IABP on standby while obtaining the chest radiograph.	Correct IAB catheter position must be confirmed to prevent complications associated with the interference of the arterial blood supply. Placing the IABP on standby enhances the visibility of the balloon on the radiograph. Some IAB catheters have radiopaque markers at the tip and base of the IAB membrane to identify the position of the catheter.	If fluoroscopy is used for insertion of the catheter, a radiograph immediately after placement is not necessary. Some patients may have hemodynamic instability when the IABP is on standby for more than a few seconds; assess each patient's hemodynamic response to IABP therapy.
28. Ensure that the IAB is secured to the patient's skin.	Maintains optimal position and reduces the risk of IAB catheter migration.	The IAB catheter may be sutured or a sutureless securement device may be used to secure the catheter.
29. Assist as needed with applying a sterile dressing to the catheter-insertion site.	Minimizes the risk of infection.	The IAB catheter may have a sleeve to allow for repositioning of the IAB catheter under aseptic conditions.
30. Ensure sharps are discarded in a sharp container; remove **PE** and sterile equipment and discard used supplies in appropriate receptacles.	Reduces the risk of injury and the transmission of microorganisms; Standard Precautions.	
31. **HH**		

Procedure for Timing of the IABP

Steps	Rationale	Special Considerations
1. Select an ECG lead that optimizes the R wave. (**Level M***)	The R wave of the ECG is the preferred trigger source for identifying the cardiac cycle.	Refer to manufacturer instructions for trigger options.
2. Assess the timing of the IABP with the arterial waveform.	The arterial waveform assists in identifying accurate IAB inflation and deflation.[23,25,26]	Refer to specific manufacturer's instructions for automatic timing.
3. Set the IABP to auto mode.	The IABP console automatically adjusts timing of inflation and deflation.	Some IABP consoles have this feature. Fiberoptic catheters have a sensor at the tip of the IAB catheter that transmits the pressure signal back to the IABP console, producing an aortic pressure waveform. Timing algorithms adjust inflation and deflation automatically.[33]
4. Timing can be checked by setting the IABP frequency to the every-other-beat setting (1:2 or 50%; Fig. 52-3).	Comparison can be made between the assisted and unassisted arterial waveforms.	

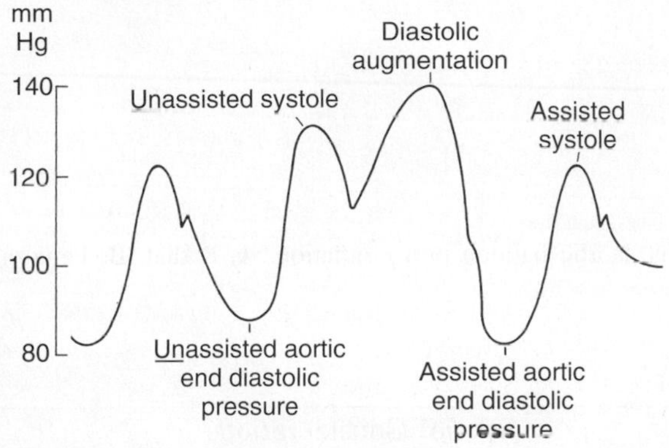

Figure 52-3 Intraaortic balloon pump frequency of 1:2. (*Courtesy Datascope Corp, Fairfield, NJ.*)

Steps	Rationale	Special Considerations
5. Inflation:	The dicrotic notch represents closure of the aortic valve.	
A. Identify the dicrotic notch of the assisted systolic waveform (see Fig. 52-3).		
B. Adjust inflation later to expose the dicrotic notch.	Identifies the landmark for accurate inflation.	
C. Slowly adjust inflation earlier until the dicrotic notch disappears and a sharp V wave forms (see Fig. 52-3).	Balloon augmentation should occur after the aortic valve closes.[5,12,24]	A sharp V wave may not be seen in patients with low systemic vascular resistance.
D. Compare the augmented pressure with the patient's unassisted systolic pressure.	Balloon augmentation ideally is equal to or greater than the patient's unassisted systolic blood pressure.[11]	If balloon augmentation is less than the patient's systolic pressure, consider the possibility that the patient is hypovolemic or tachycardic, the balloon is positioned too low, or the balloon volume is set too low.[27] Low volume may also be the result of an inadequate fill volume or an IAB catheter that is too small for the patient.

*Level M: Manufacturer's recommendations only.

Procedure continues on following page

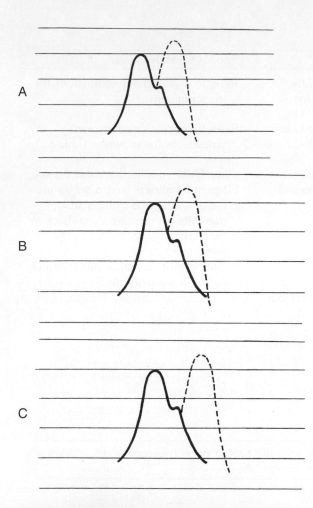

Figure 52-4   Intraaortic balloon pump inflation. **A,** Radial. **B,** Femoral. **C,** Central aortic.

Procedure	**for Timing of the IABP—*Continued***	
Steps	**Rationale**	**Special Considerations**
E. Adjust inflation if needed.	Necessary to achieve optimal diastolic augmentation.	Timing of inflation varies slightly depending on the location of the arterial catheter and resulting physiological delays.[24,26] Radial: Inflate 40–50 ms before the dicrotic notch. Femoral: Inflate 120 ms before the dicrotic notch (Fig. 52-4). The radial artery is recommended for use for pressure monitoring for IABP timing.[24,26]
6. Deflation: A. Identify the assisted and unassisted aortic end-diastolic pressures and the assisted and unassisted systolic pressures (see Fig. 52-3).[5,6]	These landmarks are important in determination of accurate IAB deflation.	IABP frequency is set at 1:2 (50%).
B. Set the balloon to deflate so that the assisted aortic end-diastolic pressure is as low as possible (lower than the patient's unassisted diastolic pressure) while still maintaining optimal diastolic augmentation and not impeding the next systole (the assisted systole).	The assisted systolic pressure is less than the unassisted systolic pressure as a result of a decrease in afterload, thus reducing the myocardial workload.[12,24]	Reduction of afterload decreases the energy required by the heart during systole. Afterload reduction without diminishment of diastolic augmentation is important to achieve.

1:1 IABP Frequency

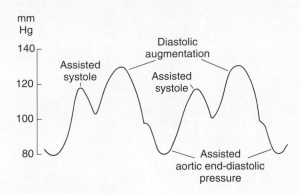

Figure 52-5 Correct intraaortic balloon pump timing (1:1). *(Courtesy Datascope Corp, Fairfield, NJ.)*

Procedure	**for Timing of the IABP—*Continued***	
Steps	**Rationale**	**Special Considerations**
7. Set the IABP frequency to 1:1 (100%; Fig. 52-5).	Ensures that each heartbeat is assisted.	
8. Assess timing every hour, whenever the heart rate changes by more than 10 beats/min, and when the rhythm changes.	Inappropriate timing prevents effective IABP therapy.	Many IABP models use algorithms to automatically adjust timing for changes in heart rate and rhythm. Refer to the specific manufacturer guidelines for a description of automatic timing modes and their specific features.
9. Assess and intervene to correct inappropriate timing.	Ensures accurate timing and optimal functioning of the IABP.	
A. Problem: early inflation (Fig. 52-6). Intervention: move inflation later.	Inflation occurs before closure of the aortic valve, leading to premature aortic valve closure, increased left-ventricular volume, and decreased stroke volume.[12]	Early inflation is the worst timing error, reducing left-ventricular performance and IABP efficiency.[12]
B. Problem: late inflation (Fig. 52-7). Intervention: adjust inflation earlier.	A delay in inflation leads to a decrease in coronary artery perfusion.	
C. Problem: early deflation (Fig. 52-8). Intervention: adjust deflation later.	Deflation occurs before the aortic valve opens, leading to decreased balloon augmentation and less or no afterload reduction; coronary artery perfusion may also be decreased.	Note the sharp diastolic wave after augmentation and the increase in the assisted systolic pressure.
D. Problem: late deflation (Fig. 52-9). Intervention: adjust deflation earlier.	Deflation occurs after the aortic valve has opened, leading to an increase in the aortic end-diastolic pressure and an increase in afterload.	Note the delayed diastolic wave after augmentation and the diminished assisted systole. Late deflation is identified by a diminished assisted systolic pressure, an increase in heart rate, an increase in filling pressures, a decrease in cardiac output and cardiac index, and an increased afterload. Maintaining a reliable trigger minimizes the risk of late deflation.[5,6,11,23]

Timing Errors
Early Inflation

Inflation of the IAB prior to aortic valve closure

Waveform Characteristics:
- Inflation of IAB prior to dicrotic notch
- Diastolic augmentation encroaches onto systole (may be unable to distinguish)

Physiologic Effects:
- Potential premature closure of aortic valve
- Potential increased in LVEDV and LVEDP or PCWP
- Increased left ventricular wall stress or afterload
- Aortic regurgitation
- Increased MVo$_2$ demand

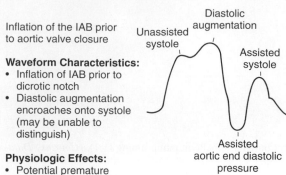

Figure 52-6 Early inflation. *(Courtesy Datascope Corp, Fairfield, NJ.)*

Timing Errors
Late Inflation

Inflation of the IAB markedly after closure of the aortic valve

Waveform Characteristics:
- Inflation of the IAB after the dicrotic notch
- Absence of sharp V
- Suboptimal diastolic augmentation

Physiologic Effects:
- Suboptimal coronary artery perfusion

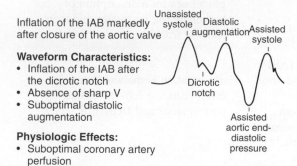

Figure 52-7 Late inflation. *(Courtesy Datascope Corp, Fairfield, NJ.)*

Timing Errors
Early Deflation

Premature deflation of the IAB during the diastolic phase

Waveform Characteristics:
- Deflation of IAB is seen as a sharp drop following diastolic augmentation
- Suboptimal diastolic augmentation
- Assisted aortic end diastolic pressure may be equal to or less than the unassisted aortic end diastolic pressure
- Assisted systolic pressure may rise

Physiologic Effects:
- Suboptimal coronary perfusion
- Potential for retrograde coronary and carotid blood flow
- Angina may occur as a result of retrograde coronary blood flow
- Suboptimal afterload reduction
- Increased MVo$_2$ demand

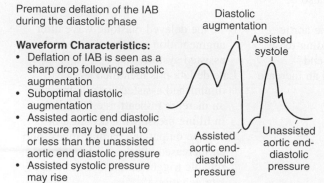

Figure 52-8 Early deflation. *(Courtesy Datascope Corp, Fairfield, NJ.)*

Timing Errors
Late Deflation
Deflation of the IAB late in diastolic phase as aortic valve is beginning to open
Waveform Characteristics:
• Assisted aortic end-diastolic pressure may be equal to or greater than the unassisted aortic end diastolic pressure
• Rate of rise of assisted systole is prolonged
• Diastolic augmentation may appear widened
Physiologic Effects:
• Afterload reduction is essentially absent
• Increased MVO_2 consumption due to the left ventricle ejecting against a greater resistance and a prolonged isovolumetric contraction phase
• IAB may impede left ventricular ejection and increase the afterload
Diastolic augmentation
Unassisted systole
Prolonged rate of rise of assisted systole
Widened appearance
Assisted aortic end-diastolic pressure

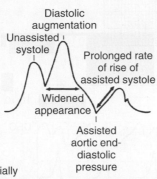

Figure 52-9 Late deflation. *(Courtesy Datascope Corp, Fairfield, NJ.)*

Procedure for Balloon-Pressure Waveform

Steps	Rationale	Special Considerations
1. Determine whether the IABP console has a balloon-pressure waveform.	Helium is shuttled in and out of the IAB catheter, and the balloon-pressure waveform represents this movement.	Refer to the specific manufacturer's instructions regarding the balloon-pressure waveform.
2. Assess the balloon-pressure waveform.	Reflects pressure that is in the IAB.	
3. Determine whether the balloon pressure waveform is normal (Fig. 52-10). A normal balloon pressure waveform:	A normal balloon-pressure waveform reflects that the IAB is inflating and deflating properly.[22]	
A. Has a fill pressure (baseline pressure) slightly above zero.	Reflects pressure in the tubing between the IAB and the IABP driving mechanism.	
B. Has a sharp upstroke.	Occurs as helium inflates the IAB catheter.	
C. Has peak inflation artifact.	This overshoot pressure artifact is caused by helium gas pressure in the pneumatic line.[1]	
D. Has a pressure plateau.	This plateau is created as the IAB remains inflated during diastole.	The plateau indicates the length of time of inflation and whether full inflation (volume) has been delivered to the IAB. If no plateau pressure is found, the IAB may not be fully inflated.
E. Has a rapid deflation.	Helium is quickly shuttled from the IAB.	

4
5
3
6
1
2
7

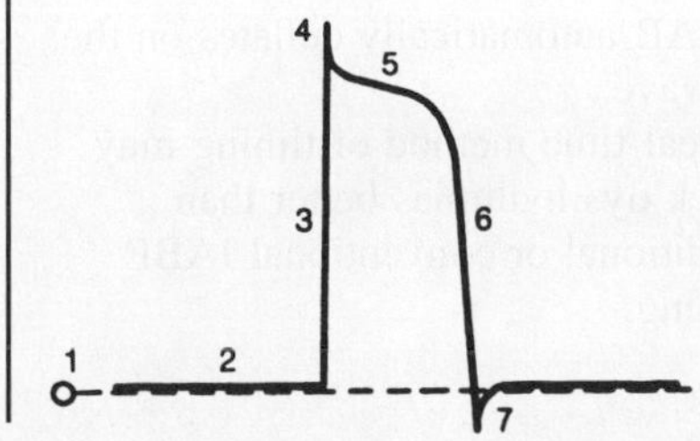

Figure 52-10 Normal balloon gas waveform. *1,* zero baseline; *2,* fill pressure; *3,* rapid inflation; *4,* peak inflation artifact; *5,* plateau pressure or inflation plateau pressure; *6,* rapid deflation; *7,* peak deflation pressure and return to fill pressure. *(Courtesy Arrow International.)*

Procedure continues on following page

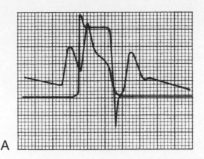

A

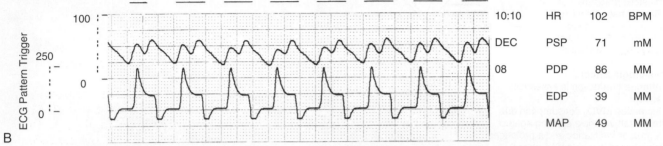

B

		10:10	HR	102	BPM
		DEC	PSP	71	mM
		08	PDP	86	MM
			EDP	39	MM
			MAP	49	MM

ECG Pattern Trigger

100

250

0

0

Figure 52-11 **A,** Balloon-pressure waveform superimposed on the arterial pressure waveform. **B,** Actual recording of an arterial pressure waveform *(top)* and balloon gas waveform *(bottom)* from a patient with balloon pump. *(Courtesy Arrow International.)*

Procedure   for Balloon-Pressure Waveform—*Continued*

Steps	Rationale	Special Considerations
F. Has a negative deflection below baseline and then returns to baseline.	Helium returns to the IABP console and then stabilizes within the system.	
4. Compare the balloon-pressure waveform with the arterial pressure waveform (Fig. 52-11).	Demonstrates the relationship between the balloon-pressure waveform and the arterial waveform. Reflects the effect of the balloon on the augmented arterial pressure.	Note the similarity in the width of the balloon-pressure waveform and the augmented arterial waveform.[18]
5. Determine whether the balloon pressure waveform meets the previous description.	Abnormal balloon-pressure waveforms may indicate restriction to helium shuttle.	Refer to the specific manufacturer's instructions regarding troubleshooting abnormal balloon-pressure waveforms.

Procedure   for Troubleshooting

Steps	Rationale	Special Considerations
1. Atrial fibrillation: A. Assess and treat the underlying cause.	The underlying cause of the dysrhythmia should be treated.	
B. Set the IABP to inflate and deflate most of the patient's beats.		Inflation of the IAB should correspond to the diastolic interval of each cardiac cycle. The IAB automatically deflates on the R wave.
C. Refer to manufacturer's instructions for the appropriate IABP console settings for atrial fibrillation (e.g., the atrial fibrillation trigger mode).	Select a mode on the IABP console for optimal R wave tracking.	The real-time method of timing may track dysrhythmias better than traditional or conventional IABP timing.[22]

Procedure	for Troubleshooting—*Continued*	
Steps	**Rationale**	**Special Considerations**

2. Tachycardia:
  A. Assess and treat the underlying cause.
  B. Set the timing and the frequency of the IABP to optimize hemodynamic response.
	The underlying cause of the tachycardia should be treated.
	IAB timing and frequency should be set to optimize coronary perfusion and afterload reduction.
		Because diastole is shortened during tachycardia, the IAB inflation time also is shortened.
		The IABP may need to be changed to a 1:2 frequency.
		Pumping every other beat may improve the patient's hemodynamic status.
		Some IABPs with automatic timing can track rates as high as 220 beats/min.

3. Asystole:
  A. Switch the trigger to arterial pressure.
 	
  B. If the IABP console is not in the auto-operation mode:
    i. Set inflation to provide diastolic augmentation.
    ii. Set deflation to occur before the upstroke of the next systole.
  C. If chest compressions do not provide an adequate trigger:
    i. Turn or push the control to internal trigger.
 	
    ii. Set the rate at 60–80 beats/min.
    iii. Set the IABP frequency to 1:2.
 	
    iv. Turn the balloon augmentation down to 50%.
 	
  D. If the IABP console is in the auto-timing mode, the console automatically attempts to self-time if an arterial pressure is generated, or switches to an internal trigger.
	This trigger can be used if an arterial pressure is generated from chest compressions.
	Sets the IABP timing.
	
	The internal trigger keeps the IAB catheter moving so that clot formation is minimized.[22]
	Maintains consistent movement of IAB catheter.
	A 1:2 frequency is adequate to prevent thrombus formation on the IAB catheter.
	Slight inflation and deflation of the IAB catheter prevents clot formation.
	Sets the IABP timing and maintains consistent movement of the IAB catheter.
		Follow advanced cardiac life support (ACLS) standards for emergency care.
		Refer to the manufacturer's manual.
		Preliminary research suggests that when used during cardiopulmonary resuscitation, IAB counterpulsation increases cerebral and coronary perfusion.[2,11]
		
		Refer to manufacturer's guidelines for recommendations for minimal balloon volume.

4. Ventricular tachycardia or ventricular fibrillation:
  A. Assess and treat the underlying cause.
  B. Cardiovert or defibrillate as necessary (see Procedures 35 and 36).
	The underlying cause of the tachycardia should be treated.
	Attempts to convert the dysrhythmia.
		Follow ACLS standards for emergency care.
		Ensure that personnel are cleared from the patient and equipment before cardioversion or defibrillation.
		The IABP console is electrically isolated.

5. Loss of vacuum or IABP failure: A. Check and tighten the connections on the pneumatic tubing.	A loose connection may contribute to a loss of vacuum.	

Procedure continues on following page

Procedure for Troubleshooting—*Continued*

Steps	Rationale	Special Considerations
B. Check the compressor power source.	Ensures that power is available to drive the helium.	
C. Hand inflate and deflate the balloon every 5 minutes if necessary. **(Level M*)**	Prevents clot formation along the dormant balloon.	Refer to specific manufacturer's guidelines for manually inflating and deflating the IAB. Ensure that the correct syringe is kept with the IABP console for this emergency; check manufacturer's guidelines for frequency of hand inflation.
D. Change the IAB console. **(Level M*)**	Establishes a power source and effective IABP therapy.	
6. Suspected balloon perforation:		
A. Observe for loss of augmentation.	Helium may be gradually leaking from the balloon catheter.	Set the alarm limits so the alarms sound with a decrease of 10 mm Hg in diastolic augmentation.
B. Check for blood in the balloon lumen tubing.	Blood or any discoloration in the helium tubing indicates that the balloon has perforated and that arterial blood is present.	It is possible for a balloon leak to be self-sealing as a result of the surface tension between the inside and the outside of the IAB membrane. This may be evidenced by the presence of dried blood in the balloon lumen tubing. The dried blood may appear as a brownish, coffee-ground–like substance.
C. Assess for changes or lack of a normal balloon-pressure waveform.	The balloon-pressure waveform may be absent if the balloon is unable to retain helium, or the pressure plateau may gradually decrease if the IAB is leaking helium.	
7. Balloon perforation:		
A. Place the IABP on standby.	Prevents further IAB pumping and continued helium exchange.	Some IABP consoles automatically shut off if a leak is detected. The IAB catheter should be removed within 15–30 minutes.[8]
B. Clamp the IAB catheter.	Prevents arterial blood backup.	
C. Disconnect the IAB catheter from the IABP console.	Prevents blood from backing up into the IABP console.	
D. Notify the physician or advanced practice nurse.	The IAB catheter needs to be removed or replaced immediately.	If the IAB leak has sealed itself off, this may result in entrapment of the IAB in the vasculature. Surgical removal may be necessary.
E. Prepare for IAB catheter removal or replacement.	The IAB catheter should not lie dormant for longer than 30 minutes.	Do not manually inflate and deflate the IAB if balloon perforation is suspected. Perforation of a balloon membrane may indicate that the patient's vascular condition may induce abrasion or perforation in subsequent balloon membranes.
F. Discontinue anticoagulation therapy as prescribed.	Clotting occurs more readily if anticoagulation therapy is stopped (necessary if removing the catheter).	

*Level M: Manufacturer's recommendations only.

Procedure   for Weaning and IAB Catheter Removal

Steps	Rationale	Special Considerations
1. **HH**		
2. **PE**		
3. Assess clinical readiness for weaning.	Optimal clinical and hemodynamic parameters validate readiness for weaning.	Patient hemodynamic status should be optimal before weaning from IABP therapy. Signs of clinical readiness include the following: no angina, heart rate <110 beats/min, absence of unstable dysrhythmias, MAP >70 mm Hg with minimal or no vasopressor support, pulmonary artery occlusion pressure <18 mm Hg, cardiac index >2.4 mixed venous oxygen saturation between 60% and 80%, capillary refill <2 seconds, and urine output >0.5 mL/kg/hr.
4. Change the assist ratio to 1:2 (50%), and monitor the patient's response for 1–6 hours, as prescribed, or per the institution's protocol.	The length of time required to wean from IABP therapy depends on the hemodynamic response of the patient and the length of time the patient has received IABP therapy.[13,29]	Follow physician or advanced practice nurse prescription or institutional policy on IABP weaning.
5. If hemodynamic parameters remain stable, further change the ratio (depending on the patient and the balloon-console assist frequencies, or as prescribed).	IABP consoles vary in assist ratios.	Follow physician or advanced practice nurse prescription or institutional policy on IABP weaning.
6. Discontinue heparin or dextran 4–6 hours before IAB catheter removal, or reverse heparin with protamine (as prescribed) just before catheter removal.	Decreases the likelihood of bleeding after balloon removal.	
7. Turn the IABP to standby or off and disconnect the IAB from the console.	Ensures deflation of the IAB catheter.	The patient's arterial pressure collapses the balloon membrane in preparation for withdrawal.
8. Assist with removing sutures or the sutureless securement device.	Prepares for IAB removal.	
9. Assist the physician or advanced practice nurse with removal of the percutaneous catheter.	Facilitates removal.	The IAB catheter is not withdrawn into the sheath but removed as an entire unit to avoid shearing the balloon.
10. Ensure that pressure is held on the insertion site for 30–45 minutes after the IAB catheter is withdrawn.	Ensures that hemostasis is obtained and decreases the incidence of bleeding and hematoma formation.	A femoral compression system can be used to achieve hemostasis (see Procedure 76). Pressure may be needed for a longer period of time if the patient has been receiving anticoagulant therapy or if coagulation study results are abnormal.
11. Assess the insertion site for signs of bleeding or hematoma formation before application of a sterile pressure dressing.	Assists in the detection of bleeding.	
12. Apply a pressure dressing to the insertion site for 2–4 hours or as prescribed.	Minimizes bleeding from the insertion site.	

Procedure continues on following page

Procedure for Weaning and IAB Catheter Removal—*Continued*

Steps	Rationale	Special Considerations
13. Obtain vital signs and hemodynamic parameters every 15 minutes × 4, every 30 minutes × 2, then every hour as the patient's condition warrants, or as prescribed.	Determines patient stability or instability.	
14. Assess the quality of perfusion to the decannulated extremity immediately after removal and every 1 hour × 2, then every 2 hours, or as prescribed.	Removal of the IAB catheter may dislodge thrombi on the catheter and lead to arterial occlusion.	
15. Maintain immobility of the decannulated extremity and maintain bed rest with the head of the bed no greater than 30 degrees for 8 hours, as prescribed or according to institutional protocol.	Promotes healing and decreases stress at the insertion site.	
16. Remove **PE** and discard used supplies in appropriate receptacle.	Reduces the transmission of microorganisms and body secretions; Standard Precautions.	
17. **HH**		

Expected Outcomes

- Increased myocardial oxygen supply
- Decreased myocardial oxygen demand
- Increased cardiac output
- Increased tissue perfusion, including cerebral, renal, and peripheral circulation

Unexpected Outcomes

- Impaired perfusion to the extremity with the IAB catheter in place
- Balloon perforation
- Inappropriate IAB placement
- Pain
- Bleeding or coagulation disorders
- Aortic dissection
- Infection

Patient Monitoring and Care

Steps	Rationale	Reportable Conditions
		These conditions should be reported if they persist despite nursing interventions.
1. Perform systematic cardiovascular, peripheral vascular, and hemodynamic assessments every 15–60 minutes as patient status requires or as prescribed.		
A. Level of consciousness	Assesses for adequate cerebral perfusion; thrombi may develop and dislodge during IABP therapy; the IAB may migrate, decreasing blood flow to the carotid arteries.	• Change in level of consciousness
B. Vital signs and pulmonary artery pressures	Demonstrates effectiveness of IABP therapy.	• Unstable vital signs • Significant changes in hemodynamic pressures • Lack of response to IABP therapy

Patient Monitoring and Care —*Continued*

Steps	Rationale	Reportable Conditions
C. Arterial and balloon pressures	Ensures effectiveness of IABP timing and therapy.	• Difficulty achieving effective IABP therapy
D. Cardiac output, cardiac index, and systemic vascular resistance values	Demonstrates effectiveness of IABP therapy.	• Abnormal cardiac output, cardiac index, and systemic vascular-resistance values
E. Circulation to extremities	Determines peripheral perfusion. If reportable conditions are found, they may indicate catheter or embolus obstruction of perfusion to the extremity. Specifically, decreased perfusion to the left arm may indicate misplacement of the IAB catheter.[2,8,15,29]	• Capillary refill >2 seconds • Diminished or absent pulses (e.g., antecubital, radial, femoral, popliteal, tibial, pedal) • Color pale, mottled, or cyanotic • Diminished or absent sensation • Pain • Diminished or absent movement • Cool or cold to the touch
F. Urine output	Determines perfusion to the kidneys.	• Urine output <0.5 mL/kg/hr
2. Assess heart and lung sounds every 4 hours and as needed.	Abnormal heart and lung sounds may indicate the need for additional treatment. Special note: When the patient's condition permits, place the IABP on standby to accurately auscultate heart and lung sounds because IABP therapy creates extraneous sounds and impairs heart and lung sound assessment.	• Abnormal heart and lung sounds
3. Maintain the head of the bed at less than 45 degrees.	Prevents kinking of the IAB catheter and migration of the catheter.	
4. Monitor for signs of balloon perforation by assessing the balloon tubing on a regular basis for evidence of discoloration or blood in the tubing.	In the event of balloon perforation, a very small amount of helium could be released into the aorta, potentially causing an embolic event. Because of pressure gradients in the aorta, blood is more likely to enter the balloon membrane and be dehydrated by the helium.	• Blood or brown flecks in the tubing • Loss of IABP augmentation • Control-console alarm activation (e.g., gas loss)
5. Maintain accurate IABP timing.	If timing is not accurate, cardiac output may decrease rather than increase.	• Signs and symptoms of hemodynamic instability
6. Log-roll the patient every 2 hours. Prop up pillows to support the patient and to maintain alignment. Consider use of pressure-relief devices. **(Level E*)**	Promotes comfort and skin integrity and prevents kinking of the IAB catheter. Special note: log-rolling may not be tolerated in patients with severe hemodynamic compromise; low-pressure beds are necessary for these patients. Low-pressure beds can decrease the occurrence of pressure ulcers in patients who need IABP therapy.[4,25]	

*Level E: Multiple case reports, theory-based evidence from expert opinions, or peer-reviewed professional organizational standards without clinical studies to support recommendations.

Procedure continues on following page

Patient Monitoring and Care —*Continued*

Steps	Rationale	Reportable Conditions
7. Immobilize the cannulated extremity with a draw sheet tucked under the mattress or with a soft ankle restraint or a knee immobilizer as prescribed.	Prevents dislodgment and migration of the IAB catheter. Special note: assess skin integrity and perfusion distal to the restraint every hour.	• Alteration in skin integrity • Alteration in peripheral perfusion
8. Initiate passive and active range-of-motion exercises every 2 hours to extremities that can be mobilized.	Prevents venous stasis and muscle atrophy.	
9. Assess the area around the IAB catheter insertion site every 2 hours and as needed for evidence of hematoma or bleeding.	IAB catheter inflation and deflation traumatizes red blood cells and platelets.	• Bleeding at insertion site • Hematoma at insertion site
10. Maintain anticoagulation therapy as prescribed; monitor coagulation studies.	Prophylactic anticoagulation therapy may be used to prevent thrombi and emboli development. Anticoagulation therapy may alter hemoglobin, hematocrit, and coagulation values.[32]	• Abnormal coagulation study results • Abnormal hemoglobin and hematocrit study results
11. Monitor patient for systemic evidence of bleeding or coagulation disorders.	Hematologic and coagulation profiles may be altered as a result of blood loss during balloon insertion, anticoagulation, and platelet dysfunction as a result of mechanical trauma by balloon inflation and deflation.[32]	• Bleeding from IAB insertion site • Bleeding from incisions or mucous membranes • Petechiae or ecchymosis • Guaiac-positive nasogastric aspirate or stool • Hematuria • Decreased hemoglobin or hematocrit • Decreased filling pressures • Increased heart rate • Retroperitoneal hematoma • Pain in the lower abdomen, flank, thigh, or lower extremity
12. Follow institutional standards for assessing pain. Administer analgesia as prescribed.	Promotes comfort.	• Continued pain despite pain interventions
13. Replace gauze dressings at the IAB catheter site every 2 days and transparent dressings at least every 7 days. Cleanse the site with an antiseptic solution (e.g., 2% chlorhexidine solution). **(Level D*)**	Decreases the incidence of infection and allows an opportunity for site assessment. Although guidelines do not exist specifically for IAB site dressings, the Centers for Disease Control and Prevention (CDC)[19] recommend replacing invasive line dressings when the dressing becomes damp, loosened, or soiled, or when inspection of the site is necessary.	• Signs or symptoms of infection

*Level D: Peer-reviewed professional and organizational standards with the support of clinical study recommendations.

Patient Monitoring and Care —*Continued*

Steps	Rationale	Reportable Conditions
14. Assess for balloon migration.	The IAB should be positioned 2 cm below the left subclavian artery and just above the renal arteries. If the IAB migrates proximally, it may occlude the subclavian or carotid arteries. If the IAB migrates too low, it could occlude the renal or mesenteric arteries.	• Signs of possible subclavian artery occlusion: unequal or absent radial pulse and dampening or loss of the arterial pressure waveform in the ipsilateral radial artery (radial artery on the same side as the IAB catheter) • Signs of possible carotid artery occlusion include change in level of consciousness and orientation or unilateral neurological deficit • Signs of renal artery occlusion: oliguria or anuria, back or flank pain, nausea, and anorexia • Signs of mesenteric artery occlusion: abdominal pain, diarrhea, nausea, and decreased bowel sounds
15. Identify parameters that demonstrate clinical readiness to wean from IABP therapy.	Close observation of the patient's tolerance to weaning procedures is necessary to ensure that the body's oxygen demands can be met. The presence of these reportable conditions indicates that consideration should be given to weaning the patient from the IABP.	• No angina • Heart rate <110 beats/min • Absence of unstable dysrhythmias • MAP >70 mm Hg with little or no vasopressor support • Pulmonary artery occlusion pressure <18 mm Hg • Cardiac index >2.4 • Svo_2 between 60% and 80% • Capillary refill <2 seconds • Urine output >0.5 mL/kg/hr

Documentation

Documentation should include the following:
- Patient and family education
- Informed consent
- Universal protocol requirements
- Insertion of the IAB catheter (including size of catheter used and balloon volume)
- Peripheral pulses and neurovascular assessment of the affected extremity
- Any difficulties with insertion
- IABP frequency
- Patient response to the procedure and to IABP therapy

- Assessment of pain, interventions, and response to interventions
- Confirmation of placement (e.g., chest radiograph)
- Insertion site assessment
- Hemodynamic status
- IABP pressures (unassisted end-diastolic pressure, unassisted systolic pressure, balloon-augmented pressure, assisted systolic pressure, assisted end-diastolic pressure, and MAP)
- Occurrence of unexpected outcomes
- Additional nursing interventions taken

References and Additional Readings

For a complete list of references and additional readings for this procedure, scan this QR code with any freely available smartphone code reader app, or visit http://booksite.elsevier.com/9780323376624.

53 Ventricular Assist Devices ᴬᴾ

Mark Puhlman and Angela Bingham

PURPOSE: Ventricular assist devices, depending on the device, can be used for cardiogenic shock and postcardiotomy support to allow for myocardial recovery, for bridge to cardiac transplantation, or for destination therapy (permanent implantation in those patients who are not transplant candidates). Temporary devices are used as a bridge from one device to another, as a bridge to a decision for cardiac transplant, or as a bridge to recovery. Patients should be in New York Heart Association class IIIB or IV heart failure, have a left ventricular ejection fraction of 25% or less, an oxygen treadmill test of 14 or less, or be inotrope-dependent for 14 days or intraaortic balloon pump–dependent for 7 days.[1–4,10,14–17,25,27,28]

PREREQUISITE NURSING KNOWLEDGE

- Understanding of the normal anatomy and physiology of the cardiovascular, peripheral vascular, and pulmonary systems is important.
- Understanding of the management of heart failure is essential.
- Knowledge of the principles of hemodynamic monitoring, cardiopulmonary bypass, electrophysiology and dysrhythmias, and coagulation is needed.
- Clinical and technical competence related to use of ventricular assist devices (VADs) is necessary.
- Advanced cardiac life support knowledge and skills are needed.
- Knowledge is necessary of the complications of VAD therapy, including, but not limited to, bleeding, cardiac tamponade, right ventricular failure, myocardial infarction, cardiac arrhythmias, hepatic dysfunction, pulmonary dysfunction, renal dysfunction, infection, neurological dysfunction, thrombosis, and VAD malfunction.[1,2,8,9]
- Knowledge of the effect of preload, afterload, right ventricular failure, cardiac tamponade, and cardiac dysrhythmias on the function of the device is necessary.
- Knowledge of the interaction between the patient and the device is needed.
- Specific information concerning controls, alarms, troubleshooting, and safety features is available from each manufacturer and should be read thoroughly by the nurse before use of the equipment. Please refer to the operator's instructions for use (IFU), which are available for each system, for more details.
- Knowledge and understanding of anticoagulation needs specific to the VAD that is being used are necessary, and demonstrated competence in testing coagulability and titrating medication to maintain optimal anticoagulation according to institutional standards is required.
- Indications for VAD therapy include the following:[5]
  - ❖ Inability to wean from cardiopulmonary bypass
  - ❖ Bridge to cardiac transplant
  - ❖ Destination therapy: New York Heart Association class IIIB or IV status in a patient whose condition does not respond to optimal medical therapy and who is not a transplant candidate[18,19]
  - ❖ Bridge to myocardial recovery after cardiogenic shock
- Relative contraindications of VAD therapy include the following[4,25]:
  - ❖ Body surface area (BSA) less than 1.2 m² (HeartMate II left ventricular assist device [LVAD; St. Jude/Thoratec Corporation, Pleasanton, CA])[23]
  - ❖ BSA less than 1.2 m² (HeartWare left ventricular assist device, HeartWare Corporation, Framingham, MA)[6]
  - ❖ Patients with irreversible end-stage organ damage[4,25]
  - ❖ Unrepairable ventricular septal defect or free wall rupture with those receiving an LVAD alone[4,25]
  - ❖ Comorbidity that limits life expectancy to less than 3 years (cancer, liver disease, etc.)[4,25]
  - ❖ Active infection (valvular endocarditis, implantable cardioverter defibrillator [ICD] infection with bacteremia)[4,25]
  - ❖ Diabetes-related proliferative retinopathy, very poor glycemic control, or severe nephropathy, vasculopathy, or peripheral neuropathy[4,25]
  - ❖ Active pregnancy[4,25]
  - ❖ Active psychiatric illness that requires long-term institutionalization or a patient's inability to care for or maintain the device[4,25]
  - ❖ Neuromuscular disease that severely compromises a patient's ability to use and care for the external system components or to ambulate or exercise[4,25]
  - ❖ Psychosocial and cognitive conditions may limit the use of a VAD except in bridge to recovery because the

---

ᴬᴾ This procedure should be performed only by physicians, advanced practice nurses, and other healthcare professionals (including critical care nurses) with additional knowledge, skills, and demonstrated competence per professional licensure or institutional standard.

patient needs to have the cognitive skills to manage the VAD[4,25]

- ❖ Significant caregiver burden or lack of any caregiver[4,25]
- ❖ Active substance abusers[4,25]
- ❖ Medical noncompliance
- Impella (temporary):[11–13]
  - ❖ The Impella systems are nonpulsatile microaxial flow devices that deliver 2.5 L (Impella LP 2.5), 3.5 L (Impella CP), or 5.0 L (Impella LP 5.0) of blood flow.[2]
  - ❖ The pumps are implanted percutaneously or via sternotomy.
  - ❖ The Impella 5.0 is implanted directly via a sternotomy or via a surgical cut down to expose the femoral artery.
  - ❖ Once in position, the Impella sits across the aortic valve, with the inlet area in the left ventricle and the outlet area in the ascending aorta.
  - ❖ Transthoracic echocardiography is used to confirm proper placement.
  - ❖ The console continuously monitors pump placement and alerts the physician, advanced practice nurses, and other healthcare professionals to issues with catheter displacement and other alarm states.
  - ❖ The Impella RP has been approved in the United States as a humanitarian device exception (HDE) for right-sided support.
- The CentriMag Ventricular Assist Device (St. Jude/ Thoratec Corp., Pleasanton, CA) (temporary)[24,26]:
  - ❖ The CentriMag VAD is a continuous centrifugal flow device that delivers up to 10 L of blood flow.[24]
  - ❖ The pump is placed via catheters by a thoracotomy approach.[24]
  - ❖ The CentriMag operates via an electromagnetic rotor that operates at a range of 0 to 5500 rpm.[24]
  - ❖ The pump is driven by a primary console.[24] Intraoperative cannulation can be accomplished via left atrial or left ventricular cannulation (inflow) to the aorta (outflow), accomplishing left ventricular support for short-term use.[24]
  - ❖ Intraoperative cannulation can also be accomplished via right atria (inflow) to pulmonary artery (outflow), accomplishing right ventricular support for short-term use.[24]
  - ❖ Using two devices, biventricular support can be accomplished.[24]
- The Tandem Heart (TandemLife Corp., Pittsburgh, PA) (temporary):[21,22]
  - ❖ The Tandem Heart is a continuous centrifugal flow device that delivers up to 5 L of blood flow at 7500 rpm.[21] This device is a left-atrial-to-femoral bypass system for short-term use.
  - ❖ The pump is implanted via a percutaneous approach.[21]
  - ❖ A 21-Fr cannula is inserted from the right atrium via a transseptal cannulation to the left atrium. Blood is drawn into the centrifugal pump and returned to the femoral artery.[21]
  - ❖ The Tandem Heart operates via an electromagnetic rotor that operates at a range of 3000 to 7500 rpm.[21]
  - ❖ The pump is driven by a microprocessor controller.[21]
  - ❖ The Tandem Heart has a dual-chamber pump. The upper housing allows for the movement of blood. The

lower housing communicates with the controller and contains a continuous flow of saline to decrease the risk of thrombus formation and provide lubrication.[21]
  - ❖ Using the ProtekDuo RA-PA catheter, percutaneous right ventricular support can be achieved.
- The HeartMate II Left Ventricular Assist System (LVAS) (Thoratec/St Jude Corporation, Pleasanton, CA):[23]
  - ❖ The HeartMate II LVAS[20] is a continuous axial flow pump and is approved as a bridge to transplant and destination therapy in patients with advanced heart failure.
  - ❖ The LVAD is implanted just below the diaphragm in the abdomen.
  - ❖ The HeartMate II is made of titanium and weighs approximately 160 g. Blood flows from the left ventricle through the pump and back to the patient's circulation via the outflow graft.
  - ❖ Continuous flow is generated by a small rotor inside the pump. The speed of the pump is set by the LVAD team and does not change in response to preload.
  - ❖ A driveline is passed underneath the skin and exits the right or left upper quadrant of the abdomen. The driveline connects the LVAD to a controller and a power source (batteries or power module).
- The HeartWare LVAS (HeartWare Corporation, Framingham, MA):[6]
  - ❖ The HeartWare Left Ventricular Assist System consists of a continuous flow centrifugal force blood pump with an integrated, partially centered inflow cannula; a 10-mm diameter gel-impregnated polyester outflow graft; and a percutaneous driveline.
  - ❖ The pump has one moving part, an impeller, which spins blood to generate up to 10 L/min of flow.
  - ❖ A short integrated inflow cannula is inserted into the left ventricle, and the outflow graft connects the pump to the aorta.
  - ❖ The device is implanted in the thoracic cavity.
  - ❖ The controller is a microprocessor unit that controls and manages the HeartWare System operation. The controller sends power and operating signals to the blood pump and collects information from the pump.
  - ❖ The device is approved as a bridge to transplant in patients with advanced heart failure listed for a cardiac transplant. This device is under study for permanent implantation (destination therapy).

EQUIPMENT

- VAD drive console/unit or monitor
- Connection cables (specific to device)
- Backup drive console/unit/monitor, batteries, and controller
- Device-specific equipment
- Impella Percutaneous Ventricular Assist Device
  - ❖ Impella Device
  - ❖ Automated Impella controller
  - ❖ Impella purge cassette
  - ❖ Purge fluid (dextrose/heparin solution prepared by pharmacy)
  - ❖ Normal saline 500 mL infusion bag
  - ❖ Straight IV tubing (nonpump tubing)

- ❖ Pressure bag
- ❖ Knee immobilizer (if Impella is placed femorally)
- ❖ Sterile gauze
- ❖ Straight IV tubing in the cage of the Impella controller
- ❖ Connector cable
- ❖ Impella "instructions for use" with alarm explanation
- Centrimag Ventricular Assist Device
  - ❖ CentriMag device
  - ❖ Automated CentriMag dontroller
  - ❖ Backup CentriMag controller
  - ❖ Two chest tube clamps
  - ❖ CentriMag "instructions for use" with alarm explanation
- TandemHeart Ventricular Assist Device
  - ❖ TandemHeart device
  - ❖ TandemHeart controller
  - ❖ Backup TandemHeart controller
  - ❖ 1000-mL bag of normal saline (NS) solution
  - ❖ TandemHeart infusion tubing
  - ❖ Two chest tube clamps
  - ❖ Kelly clamp
  - ❖ TandemHeart "instructions for use" with alarm explanation
- Heartmate II and Heartware
  - ❖ Power base unit (power module) with cable
  - ❖ Battery charger
  - ❖ System monitor
  - ❖ Display monitor
  - ❖ Controller
  - ❖ Controller cell
  - ❖ Large batteries
  - ❖ Battery clips

Additional equipment, to have available as needed, includes the following:

- Emergency equipment and medications
- Knee immobilizer
- Sterile dressing supplies for acute dressing change:
  - ❖ Preslit 4 × 4 sterile gauze pads (alternatively, round preslit island dressing)
  - ❖ Sterile 2 × 2 sterile gauze
  - ❖ Chrorprep applicator, 3 mL in size
  - ❖ Tape, 1-inch and 2-inch
  - ❖ Sterile gloves
  - ❖ Head covers (until driveline ingrowth occurs)
  - ❖ Masks (until driveline ingrowth occurs)
  - ❖ Sterile gowns (until driveline ingrowth occurs)
  - ❖ Sterile drapes
  - ❖ Driveline fixation device
  - ❖ Suture removal kit to remove circumferential suture postop
- Sterile dressing supplies for chronic dressing change:
  - ❖ Prepackaged driveline management system consisting of:
    - ○ Sterile 4 × 4 sterile gauze
    - ○ Chlorprep 3-mL applicator
    - ○ Sterile gloves
    - ○ Masks
    - ○ Driveline fixation device
    - ○ Biopatch
    - ○ Clear Tegaderm dressing shield

PATIENT AND FAMILY EDUCATION

- Assess patient and family understanding of VAD therapy and the reason for its use. *Rationale:* Clarification or reinforcement of information is an expressed patient and family need during times of stress and anxiety.
- Explain the environment and planned care to the patient and family, including the frequency of assessment, sounds and function of equipment, placement of the device, explanation of alarms, dressings and therapy, anticoagulation needs, decreased or assisted mobility, and parameters for discontinuation of therapy. *Rationale:* This communication provides information and encourages the patient and family to ask questions or voice concerns or fears related to the therapy.
- Before surgery, a meeting with another patient on a VAD may be helpful for the patient and family, if both patients agree. *Rationale:* Meeting with another patient with a VAD provides social support.
- If appropriate, begin discharge teaching to include operation of the VAD, dressing changes, battery changes, placement of self on and off of the battery and the power module, changing of the controller, and appropriate bathing techniques with use of shower equipment (when approved by the VAD team). It is recommended that patients and their families be provided with comprehensive education regarding the care and maintenance of their VAD with the expectation they will be able to perform a return demonstration of these key components. *Rationale:* This teaching provides information and ensures that the patient will be safe at home. It also allows the patient and family to ask questions as needed.

PATIENT ASSESSMENT AND PREPARATION
Patient Assessment

- Assess the patient's medical history, history of heart failure, competency of the aortic/pulmonic valves, competency of the mitral/tricuspid valves, pulmonary hypertension, right ventricular function, left ventricular function, and peripheral vascular disease. *Rationale:* This assessment provides baseline data regarding cardiac functioning and facilitates decision making regarding insertion of the appropriate device and postoperative management.
- Perform a cardiovascular, hemodynamic, peripheral vascular, neurovascular, and psychosocial assessment and assessment of body mass index (height, weight, BSA). *Rationale:* These assessments provide baseline data and help with determination of the type of device to use.
- Assess the current laboratory profile, including the complete blood cell count, platelet count, prothrombin time, partial thromboplastin time (PTT), international normalized ratio (INR), blood chemistry, liver profile, protein, and albumin levels. *Rationale:* This assessment provides baseline data and may indicate end-organ dysfunction related to low-flow state. It also may be used to predict the patient's risk of bleeding.

Patient Preparation

- Verify that the patient is the correct patient with two identifiers. *Rationale:* Before performing a procedure, the nurse should ensure the correct identification of the patient for the intended intervention.
- Ensure that the patient and family understand preoperative teaching. Answer questions as they arise, and reinforce information as needed. *Rationale:* This communication evaluates and reinforces understanding of previously taught information.
- Ensure that an informed consent form has been signed (if it is known before surgery that the VAD will be placed). *Rationale:* Informed consent protects the rights of the patient and makes a competent decision possible for the patient and family.
- Perform a preprocedure verification and time out. *Rationale:* This ensures patient safety.
- Provide emotional support to the patient and family. *Rationale:* The patient and family are under an extreme amount of stress.

Procedure for Ventricular Assist Devices (Temporary/Short Term)		
Steps	**Rationale**	**Special Considerations**
Impella Percutaneous LVAD (Abiomed Corporation)		
1. Verify the presence of the backup motor and console.	In the event of device failure, support can rapidly be reestablished.	
2. **HH**		
3. **PE**		
4. Once the patient is stable after admission to the critical care unit, transition from initial setup to standard configuration on the Impella controller:	Prepares the system.	
A. Attach normal saline (NS) with straight tubing to the red side arm of the Impella CP catheter.		
B. Pressurize the normal saline with the pressure bag to 300 mm Hg (do not use pressure tubing).		
C. Press "PURGE SYSTEM" on the Impella CP controller then select "Transfer to Standard Configuration."		
D. Create a slow drip from the pressurized NS to flood the Luer-Lok connector of the red pressure side arm and make a wet-to-wet connection.		
E. Fully open the roller clamp once connected.		
F. Select OK to confirm transfer.		
5. Change the purge fluid as prescribed or based on institution standard (e.g., heparin 25,000 units/D5W 500 mL).	Heparin and dextrose are specific to the function of the Impella device and longevity of the catheter.	The rate will be preset by the Automatic Impella Controller (AIC) flow rate. Change purge cassette, pressurized NS bag, and tubing every 96 hours; follow institutional standards.
6. Check the ACT as prescribed (e.g., 2 hours after the purge solution is initiated).	Determines whether the desired level of anticoagulation is achieved.	Additional heparin may be needed in the purge fluid to achieve the desired ACT range. The range will be determined by the physician or advanced practice nurse.

Procedure continues on following page

Procedure for Ventricular Assist Devices (Temporary/Short Term)—*Continued*		
Steps	**Rationale**	**Special Considerations**
7. Ensure the Impella device is in the proper position.		
A. Ensure that a transthoracic echocardiogram is obtained as prescribed.	Determines whether the device is across the aortic valve.	
B. Ensure the Tuohy-Borst valve is locked.	Maintains the position of the device across the aortic valve.	May need to remove the initial dressing to assess whether the valve is locked. Follow institutional standards. Document the centimeter marker on the Impella CP catheter closest to the sheath.
C. Apply the knee immobilizer (for femoral insertion).	Prevents catheter migration.	
D. Assess Impella position using the "Placement Signal" as displayed by the Automatic Impella.	Ensures the catheter has not migrated.	
8. Confirm the mode of operation is P-level mode.	Ensures equipment is set as prescribed.	Verify the prescribed P-level.
9. If the P-level needs to be changed, push the menu button and choose P-level mode.		
10. Ensure the white introducer side arm is capped off and marked "DO NOT USE."	Accessing the introducer could compromise the position of the Impella.	
11. Troubleshooting:		
A. Resuscitation:		
i. For CPR, decrease the performance level to P2.		
ii. Defibrillate as needed.		No need to stop or disconnect the device.
iii. Compressions may be contraindicated.	Compressions may dislodge cannulation, causing loss of support and/or bleeding.	Provide compressions only if prescribed by the physician or advanced practice nurse. Follow institutional standards.
iv. If the patient survives the resuscitation:		
a. Verify the position of the device with echocardiogram as prescribed.	Determines whether the position of the device is correct.	
b. Resume P-level as prescribed.	Continues treatment as prescribed.	
B. Respond to device alarms:	Corrects the alarm condition.	Refer to the IFU for specific interventions needed for each alarm.
i. Rapidly assess the alarm condition.		
ii. Respond to each alarm.		For technical support, call Abiomed Clinical Support Center (1-800-422-8666)
iii. Notify the physician or advanced practice nurse if assistance is needed.		

Procedure for Ventricular Assist Devices (Temporary/Short Term)—*Continued*

Steps	Rationale	Special Considerations
12. Weaning and removal:		Discontinue anticoagulation as prescribed.
A. Follow the weaning process as prescribed. Follow insitutional standards.		
B. Decrease the performance level by 2 P-levels every 3 hours, or as prescribed, until at P2.		
C. Maintain the Impella at P2 for the prescribed amount of time.		This is typically at least 2 hours.
D. Assess the patient's response to P2.		
E. Assist as needed with device removal.	The patient must demonstrate ventricular recovery before removal.	
F. Assist as needed as pressure is maintained at the insertion site.		Manual pressure may be maintained at the insertion site for a minimum of 20 minutes or until hemostasis is achieved. Follow institutional standards.
G. Compression devices may be utilized after manual compression.		
H. Monitor for hematoma formation or overt bleeding at the site.		
I. Assess for retroperitoneal bleeding (HCT dropping, abdominal/flank pain) or hemodynamic compromise.		
13. Remove **PE** and discard used supplies.	Reduces the transmission of microorganisms; Standard Precautions.	
14. **HH**		

CentriMag Ventricular Assist Device (Left, Right, or Biventricular Device) (St Jude/Thoratec Corporation)

Steps	Rationale	Special Considerations
1. Verify the presences of the backup motor, console, and chest tube clamps.	In the event of device failure, support can rapidly be established.	
2. **HH**		
3. **PE**		
4. Assess pump function.	Ensures the device is functioning appropriately.	
5. Assess the pump insertion site.	Determines whether bleeding or hematoma is present.	
6. Assess for VAD chatter.	VAD chatter indicates that the device is running too fast for the amount of blood being delivered to it.	Assess for volume, VAD rate, right ventricular function, arrhythmia, and position of the cannula.
7. Adjust the flow probe 1 cm every 8 hours, ensuring that the arrows on the probe point in the direction of blood flow.	The flow probe can contribute to thrombus formation if left in place too long.	
8. Anticoagulation:		
A. Administer anticoagulation as prescribed (e.g., heparin 25,000 units/500 mL D5W).	Maintains the patency of the device and decreases thrombus formation.	

Procedure continues on following page

Procedure	for Ventricular Assist Devices (Temporary/Short Term)—*Continued*	
Steps	**Rationale**	**Special Considerations**
B. Check the ACT as prescribed (e.g., hourly).	Determines whether the desired level of anticoagulation is achieved.	
C. Additional anticoagulation may be needed as prescribed.	The ACT range will be determined by the physician or advanced practice nurse.	
9. Troubleshooting:		
A. CPR: Compressions may be contraindicated.	Compressions may dislodge the cannula(ae).	Only provide compressions if prescribed by the physician or advanced practice nurse. Follow institutional standards.
B. Defibrillate as necessary.		No need to stop or disconnect the device.
C. Respond to device alarms:		
i. Rapidly assess the alarm condition.	If the device is stopped for longer than 5 minutes, it may not be safe to restart.	Refer to the IFU for specific interventions needed for each alarm.
		For technical support, call Thoratec HeartLine at 800-456-1477.
ii. Respond to each alarm.		
iii. Notify the physician or advanced practice nurse if assistance is needed.		
iv. If an equipment change is necessary, clamp the return tubing before switching to the backup equipment.	Prevents backflow of the device.	
v. Always unclamp the tubing after restarting the device.		
10. Weaning and removal:		Discontinue anticoagulation as prescribed.
A. Follow physician or advanced practice nurse prescription for weaning.		
B. Decrease the device rate as prescribed.		
C. Assess the patient's response to the decrease in the device rate.	The patient needs to demonstrate ventricular recovery before removal.	
D. The device will be removed in the operating room.		
E. Assess for bleeding, hematoma, and hemodynamic status after return from the operating room.	Determines patient stability.	
11. Remove 🅿🅴 and discard used supplies.	Reduces the transmission of microorganisms; Standard Precautions.	
12. 🅷🅷		
Tandem Ventricular Assist System (Left, Right, or Biventricular Device) (TandemLife Corporation)		
1. Verify the presence of the backup console and tubing clamps.	In the event of device failure, support can be rapidly reestablished.	
2. 🅷🅷		
3. 🅿🅴		
4. Assess pump function.	Ensures the device is functioning appropriately.	
5. Assess the pump insertion site.	Determines whether bleeding or hematoma is present.	

Procedure for Ventricular Assist Devices (Temporary/Short Term)—*Continued*

Steps	Rationale	Special Considerations
6. Assess the VAD for chatter.	VAD chatter indicates that the device is running too fast for the amount of blood being delivered to it.	Assess for volume, VAD rate, right ventricular function, arrhythmia, and malposition of cannula
7. Assess the insertion depth.	Determines the position of the cannula(ae).	
8. Immobilize the affected limb.	Prevents catheter migration.	
9. Anticoagulation:		
A. Administer anticoagulation as prescribed (e.g., heparin 25,000 units/500 mL D5W).	Maintains the patency of the device and decreases thrombus formation.	A heparin infusion is prescribed along with the TandemHeart infusate.
B. Check the activated clotting time as prescribed (e.g., hourly).	Determines whether the desired level of anticoagulation is achieved.	
C. Additional anticoagulation may be needed as prescribed.	The ACT range will be determined by the physician or advanced practice nurse.	
D. Heparin may also be used as an infusate through the device.	Maintains the patency of the device and decreases thrombus formation.	Do not use heparin in D5W through the device.
10. Troubleshooting:		
A. CPR: Compressions may be contraindicated.	Compressions may dislodge the cannula(ae).	Only provide compressions if prescribed by the physician or advanced practice nurse. Follow institution standard.
B. Defibrillate as necessary.		No need to stop or disconnect the device.
C. Respond to device alarms:		
i. Rapidly assess the alarm condition.	If the device is stopped for longer than 5 minutes, it may not be safe to restart.	Refer to the IFU for specific interventions needed for each alarm.
		For technical support, call CardiacAssist/Technical Support at 1-800-373-1607.
ii. Respond to each alarm.		
iii. Notify the physician or advanced practice nurse if assistance is needed.		
iv. If an equipment change is necessary, clamp the return tubing before switching to the backup equipment.	Prevents backflow of blood into the device.	
v. Always unclamp the tubing after restarting the device.		
11. Weaning and removal:		Discontinue anticoagulation as prescribed.
A. Follow the weaning process as prescribed. Follow institutional standards.		
B. Decrease the device rate as prescribed.		
C. Assess the patient's response to the decrease in device rate.	The patient must demonstrate ventricular recovery before removal.	
D. Assist as needed with device removal.		

Procedure continues on following page

Procedure	**for Ventricular Assist Devices (Temporary/Short Term)—*Continued***	
Steps	Rationale	Special Considerations
E. Assist as needed as pressure is maintained at the insertion site.		Manual pressure may be maintained at the insertion site for a minimum of 20 minutes or until hemostasis is achieved.
		Follow institutional standards.
F. Compression devices may be utilized after manual compression.		
G. Monitor for hematoma formation or overt bleeding at site.		
H. Assess for retroperitoneal bleeding (HCT decreasing, abdominal/flank pain) or hemodynamic compromise.		
12. Remove **PE** and discard used supplies.	Reduces the transmission of microorganisms; Standard Precautions.	
13. **HH**		

Procedure	**for (Durable/Long Term)**	
Steps	Rationale	Special Considerations

HeartMate II LVAS (St Jude/Thoratec Corporation)

1. **HH**		
2. **PE**		
3. Changing from the power module to batteries:		
A. Check the battery life by pushing down the alarm silence button.	Ensures that the battery is charged.	Batteries are fully charged when four green lights appear. Batteries are changed when one green light is lit.
B. Place a battery into each battery clip by lining up the arrow on the large battery and battery clip and inserting until the battery clicks securely into the holder.	Allows patient ambulation.	
C. Disconnect the white controller cable from the power module cable by loosening the white nut and then pulling them apart.	An alarm sounds once per second, and a yellow crescent flashes, indicating disconnection from the power module.	Do not disconnect both power sources at the same time.
D. Connect the white controller cable to the battery clip.	The alarm is resolved.	
E. Disconnect the black controller cable from the power module cable by loosening the black nut and then pulling them apart.	An alarm sounds once per second, and the yellow crescent flashes, indicating disconnection from the power module. The alarm resolves after the cable is connected properly.	

Procedure   for (Durable/Long Term)—*Continued*

Steps	Rationale	Special Considerations
4. Changing from batteries to the power module:		
A. Disconnect the white controller cable from the battery clip.	An alarm sounds once per second, and the yellow crescent flashes, indicating disconnection from the battery.	Do not disconnect both cables at the same time because power failure may occur, resulting in the need to use the emergency backup battery.
B. Connect the white controller cable to the white power module cable connection.		The alarm is resolved.
C. Disconnect the black controller cable from the battery clip.	An alarm sounds once per second, and the yellow crescent flashes, indicating disconnection from the power module.	
D. Connect the black controller cable to the black power module cable connection.	Returns the power connection to the power module cable to allow power to be obtained from an AC source.	The alarm is resolved.
E. Remove the batteries from the clips and place the batteries back into the universal battery charger.	Allows the batteries to recharge.	
5. Troubleshooting (general):		
A. Power module alarm: AC fail:	The external power to the power module is off. The internal battery of the power module powers the pump for 30 minutes.	The power module emits a steady tone.
i. Change the power source.		
ii. Switch from the power module to the batteries.		
iii. Ensure that the power module is plugged into an outlet with emergency power backup.		
B. Power module alarm: Low battery:	The power module internal battery is almost depleted.	This alarm is a steady tone.
i. Change the power source.		
ii. Switch from the power module to batteries.		
C. Power module alarm: Alarm reset:	Used to silence the power module fail alarm.	If the patient is connected to the power module, all alarms sound at the power module and controller; both need to be silenced.
i. Press the alarm reset switch.		
ii. The AC fail alarm is silenced and does not come back on.		
6. Troubleshooting (HeartMate II controller alarms):		Always check the patient, then check connections from the patient to the controller, and then check connetions from the controller to the patient. If the patient is on the monitor, the alarm is visible on the monitor.
A. Alarm: Red heart:	The VAD may not be functioning adequately.	Emits a steady tone. Call physician and LVAD team.

Procedure continues on following page

Procedure for (Durable/Long Term)—*Continued*

Steps	Rationale	Special Considerations
i. Check whether the LVAD is still pumping by listening for a VAD hum with a stethoscope and look for the green power light on the controller.	If the VAD is not functioning adequately, emergency interventions may be needed.	"RED HEART: GREEN POWER LIGHT ON" can occur if the LVAD flow is <2.5 L/min. If the pump is running, administer IV fluids and treat arrhythmias and hypertension as prescribed. If the pump is not running, change the controller per the IFU procedure. If the pump is not running and the patient is in cardiovascular arrest, begin basic life support (BLS) and advanced cardiac life support (ACLS). (Do not start compressions without a specific order.)
ii. Check that the controller is connected securely to the driveline.		
iii. Change the power source: change batteries or, if on the power module, switch to battery source.		
B. Alarm: Red battery:	Fewer than 5 minutes of battery power remain. After the batteries are depleted, the emergency battery will give an additional 15 minutes of power.	Emits a steady tone. Batteries should not be permitted to get this low.
i. Immediately replace the batteries. *Or* ii. Change to an alternate power source.		
C. Alarm: Yellow diamond:	Fewer than 15 minutes of battery power remain.	Emits 1 beep per second.
i. Change batteries. *Or* ii. Change to power module.		
D. Alarm: Yellow wrench:	Assess for interruption of the driveline (driveline fault), emergency battery not installed or expired, or controller not synchronized with monitor time.	Refer to the IFU for specific interventions.
i. Read the LCD screen and follow instructions. ii. Consult your hospital contact or Thoratec representative.		
7. Self-test:		
A. Place the patient on the power module, then hold down the battery button until all the lights on the controller light and a loud alarm sounds.	A self-test is done each day to check the function of the pump, controller, and the emergency backup battery.	

Procedure for (Durable/Long Term)—*Continued*

Steps	Rationale	Special Considerations
B. All lights should go off except for the power light, and all alarms should silence if the controller passes the test.		
8. Changing the controller:		Refer to the IFU for specific interventions.
A. Lay out the new controller next to the old controller.	Eases the changing of the controllers.	The patient should be in a sitting or lying position.
B. Open the latch on the back of the controller. Push the red button down and pull the driveline out of the controller at the same time.	Allows for the controller change.	The device will stop when you disconnect the patient from the controller. Monitor the patient closely.
C. Connect the driveline to the new controller by lining up the "black triangles or black lines" and pushing to engage. Close the controller lock to ensure the driveline stays engaged.	Allows the power to be restored.	The controller will have the backup battery powering the controller but must have both batteries replaced to continue safely. The controller starts the pump at the preset rate.
D. Connect the batteries to the new controller.	Restores power.	
E. The original controller must be placed in standby mode by pushing and holding the battery button for a count of five after both power cables have been disconnected.	This silences the alarms on the disconnected controller.	The controller will stop alarming.
9. Remove **PE** and discard used supplies	Reduces the transmission of microorganisms; Standard Precautions.	
10. **HH**		

HeartWare LVAS (HeartWare Corporation)

Steps	Rationale	Special Considerations
1. **PE**		
2. **HH**		
3. Changing from the AC power to batteries:		
A. Assure that the battery to which you are connecting is fully charged by pressing the battery button.	Ensures that the backup battery will power the LVAD during disconnect from the AC source.	Batteries are fully charged when four green lights appear. Make certain that the backup battery is available and is fully charged.
B. Remove the AC power cable from the controller by turning the connector toward the arrow and pulling straight out.		
C. Connect the new battery to the controller by grasping the connector of the battery, lining up the arrows, and pushing straight in.	The patient is now on total battery power.	There will be an audible click when the battery is engaged.
4. Changing from batteries to AC power:		
A. Connect the power cable to the AC outlet (be sure that it is grounded).	Ensures safety.	
B. Remove one of the batteries from the controller by turning the connector toward the arrow and pulling straight out.		

Procedure continues on following page

Procedure	**for (Durable/Long Term)—*Continued***

Steps	Rationale	Special Considerations
C. Connect the AC power cable to the controller by grasping at the connector of the battery, lining up the arrows, and pushing straight in.	Connects the VAD to AC power.	There will be an audible click when the battery is engaged. One battery will remain connected to the controller as a backup.
5. Troubleshooting HeartWare Alarms:		
A. VAD Stopped		Assess the patient and implement emergency care if needed.
B. Look at the LED screen. The LED screen displays "connect driveline" and the red alarm indicator will be flashing red.	If the driveline disconnects, the device will stop.	
C. Check connections.		
D. Reconnect the driveline to the controller	Continues VAD function.	
E. If the LED screen displays, "change controller" or "controller failure.		
F. Immediately change the controller.	Replaces equipment.	Notify the VAD coordinator.
6. Battery alarms:		
A. If the alarm is "Critical Battery 1 or 2," change the battery that is depleted.	Ensures that the battery is fully charged.	
B. If there is a continuous high-pitched alarm with no LED message, replace the power immediately.	All power has been lost, necessitating a new power source.	This will result in the VAD stopping. Assess the patient and implement emergency care if needed.
7. Changing the controller:		Refer to the IFU.
A. Place the new controller next to the old controller.	Eases the transition when connecting the new controller.	The patient should lie or sit down because the patient will lose support momentarily as the controller is changed.
B. Connect the backup power source to the new controller.	Provides power to the new controller.	The power-disconnect alarm and the VAD-stopped alarm will sound until the controller is connected to the driveline.
C. Pull back the white driveline cover on the old controller's silver connector.	Exposes the driveline connector to the controller.	
D. Grasp the driveline connector and pull straight out to disconnect the patient from the controller.		The device will stop when the driveline is disconnected from the controller. Monitor the patient closely.
E. Align the black dot on the driveline connector with the black dot on the new controller driveline port and push in until a click is heard.	The device will restart.	
F. Replace the second battery on the new controller.		
G. Replace the white driveline cover over the silver connector.		

Procedure for (Durable/Long Term)—*Continued*

Steps	Rationale	Special Considerations
H. Place the red adapter into the old controller and remove all power.		The controller should stop alarming.
I. If no red alarm adapter is available, press both the alarm silence and the scroll buttons together for 5 seconds.		
8. Remove **PE** and discard used supplies.	Reduces the transmission of microorganisms; Standard Precautions.	
9. **HH**		

Procedure for Acute Driveline Dressing[4]

Steps	Rationale	Special Considerations
1. Gather supplies and protective equipment for dressing change.	Prepares for the procedure.	
2. **HH**		
3. **PE**		
4. Create a sterile field with the sterile drape.		
5. Drop sterile dressing supplies onto the sterile drape.		
6. Place a mask on the patient unless the patient is intubated.	Decreases contamination of the wound.	Everyone in the room should apply a mask. This is required until tissue ingrowth occurs.
7. Apply a cap.	Prepares for the procedure.	This is required until tissue ingrowth occurs.
8. Remove gloves, wash hands, and apply clean gloves	Prepares for the procedure.	
9. Carefully remove the old dressing.		
10. Assess the driveline site for drainage and redness.	Determines early signs of infection.	
11. Remove clean gloves and wash hands.		
12. Apply sterile gloves	Prepares for sterile procedure.	
13. Gently clean around the exit site from the center out with antiseptic solution (e.g., 2% chlorhexidine-based preparation).	Deceases the risk of infection.	
14. Allow the antiseptic solution to dry.	Increases the effectiveness of the antiseptic.	
15. Never use Betadine ointment, skin prep, Uni-Solve, or acetone around the driveline.	These products can cause damage to the driveline.	
16. Place a folded 2 × 2 gauze pad under the driveline.	This relieves pressure at the edge of the exit site under the driveline preventing erosion.	
17. Apply a preslit 4 × 4 gauze pad (for excessive drainage) or preslit island dressing (for normal drainage).	Decreases strikethrough.	

Procedure continues on following page

Procedure for Acute Driveline Dressing—*Continued*		
Steps	**Rationale**	**Special Considerations**
18. Use breathable tape to secure the 4 × 4 or to close the preslit island dressing.	Decreases strikethrough.	
19. Secure the driveline with a driveline fixation device or an abdominal binder.	An immobilized driveline allows for faster tissue ingrowth and decreases the risk of infection.	
20. Remove **PE** and discard used supplies.	Reduces the transmission of microorganisms; Standard Precautions.	
21. **HH**		

Procedure for Chronic Driveline Dressing[4]		
Steps	**Rationale**	**Special Considerations**
1. Gather supplies and protective equipment for dressing change.		Use the acute dressing if any drainage or redness appears.
2. **HH**		
3. **PE**		
4. Open the dressing kit.		
5. Place a mask on the patient unless the patient is intubated.	Decreases contamination of the wound.	Everyone in the room should apply a mask.
6. Remove gloves, wash hands, and apply clean gloves.		
7. Remove the old dressing.		
8. Assess the driveline site for drainage and redness.	Determines whether signs of infection are present.	
9. Remove clean gloves, wash hands, and apply sterile gloves.	Prepares for the procedure.	
10. Gently clean around the exit site from the center out with antiseptic solution (e.g., 2% chlorhexidine-based preparation).	Decreases the risk of infection.	
11. Allow the antiseptic solution to dry.	Increases the effectiveness of the antiseptic.	
12. Never use Betadine ointment, skin prep, Uni-Solve, or acetone around the driveline.	These products can cause damage to the driveline.	
13. Place a Biopatch around driveline. Follow institution standard.	May decrease the risk of infection.	Placing the Biopatch on damp skin can cause irritation. The stie must be dry.
14. Place a clear dressing (e.g., Tegaderm) over the driveline exit site.		
15. Secure the driveline with a driveline fixation device or abdominal binder.		
16. Remove **PE** and discard used supplies.	Reduces the transmission of microorganisms; Standard Precautions.	
17. **HH**		

Expected Outcomes

- Increased myocardial oxygen supply and decreased myocardial oxygen demand
- Increased cardiac output and index
- Increased tissue perfusion
- Safe bridge to heart transplant
- Improved activity tolerance and quality of life

Unexpected Outcomes

- Device failure
- VAD infection
- Neurological dysfunction
- Bleeding and coagulation disorders
- Multisystem organ failure
- Thrombotic event
- Pain

Patient Monitoring and Care

Steps	Rationale	Reportable Conditions
		These conditions should be reported if they persist despite nursing interventions.
1. Perform systematic cardiovascular, respiratory, peripheral vascular, and hemodynamic assessments as patient status necessitates. Follow institutional standards.		
A. Level of consciousness.	Assesses for the adequacy of cerebral perfusion; thrombi may develop and dislodge during VAD therapy.	• Decreased level of consciousness • Agitation • Confusion
B. Vital signs and pulmonary artery pressures.	Demonstrates the effectiveness of VAD therapy and evaluates ventricular function.	• Unstable vital signs • Hemodynamic instability
C. VAD flow and mixed venous oxygen saturation.	Demonstrates the effectiveness of VAD therapy.	• Abnormal values
D. Circulation to the extremities.	Demonstrates adequate peripheral perfusion. If reportable conditions are found, they may indicate thrombotic or embolic obstruction of perfusion to an extremity. Nonpalpable pulses may be a normal finding in the continuous flow devices. Doppler should be used in these cases to verify continuous flow. May only have "wind tunnel" pulses if continuous flow pump (e.g., Impella).	• Extremities: Cool or cold to the touch • Capillary refill >2 seconds • Diminished or absent pulses (radial, popliteal, tibial, pedal) • Color pale, mottled, or cyanotic • Diminished or absent sensation • Pain • Diminished or absent movement
E. Urine output.	Demonstrates adequate perfusion to the kidneys.	• Urine output <0.5 mL/kg/hr.
2. Assess VAD, heart, and lung sounds every 4 hours and as needed. Follow institutional standards.	Abnormal VAD, heart, and lung sounds may indicate the need for additional treatment.	• Abnormal VAD sounds, such as grinding or sputtering • Diastolic murmur • Crackles or rhonchi
3. Monitor for signs and symptoms of inadequate preload.	Adequate VAD function depends on an appropriate volume status.	• Inadequate VAD output • Abnormal hemodynamic data
4. Logroll the patient every 2 hours until hemodynamic stability is obtained, and then advance activity as prescribed and tolerated. Prop pillows or positioning wedge to support the patient and to maintain alignment. Consider specialty beds as needed.	Promotes comfort and skin integrity and prevents kinking of the VAD drivelines.	• Disruption of skin integrity

Procedure continues on following page

Patient Monitoring and Care —*Continued*

Steps	Rationale	Reportable Conditions
5. Initiate passive and active range-of-motion exercises every 2 hours.	Prevents venous stasis and muscle atrophy.	• Mobility concerns • Developing contractures • Bleeding from the driveline exit site • Any signs of cracking or wear in the driveline
6. Assess the area around the VAD cannulae/drivelines exit site(s) for evidence of bleeding. Ensure that each driveline is positioned properly and secured. Use of a VAD driveline securement device or stabilizer belt may help. Follow institutional standards.	Anticoagulation therapy increases the risk of bleeding.	
7. Assess prothrombin time, PTT, INR, CBC, platelet, haptoglobin, and plasma-free hemoglobin as prescribed.	Monitors for coagulation problems and hemolysis. All VADs require prophylactic anticoagulation therapy to prevent thrombi and emboli development.	• Bleeding from cannulation sites, mucus membranes, or wounds • Abnormal laboratory values and coagulation levels outside of goal range • Signs and symptoms of emboli • Signs and symptoms of infection • Alterations in wound healing
8. Change the VAD site dressing per institutional standards. Do not use prophylactic topical agents because they may increase maceration and increase the risk of resistant microorganisms.[4,7,21]	Decreases the incidence of infection and allows an opportunity for site assessment. Special note: Most manufacturers do not recommend the use of povidone-iodine because of degradation of the drivelines. In addition, no acetone should be in the patient's room. Patients with an open sternotomy may need a physician or an advanced practice nurse at the bedside during dressing changes.	
9. Follow institutional standards for assessing pain. Administer analgesia as prescribed.	Identifies the need for pain interventions.	• Continued pain despite pain interventions.

Documentation

Documentation should include the following:
- Patient and family education
- Universal protocol requirements
- Informed consent
- VAD parameters (e.g., flow, pump speed)
- VAD power source
- Patient response to the VAD
- Confirmation of placement
- Hemodynamic status
- Pain assessment, interventions, and effectiveness
- Activity level

- Unexpected outcomes
- Additional interventions
- Assessment of driveline site
- Backup equipment (e.g., drive console, controllers)
- Dressing changes
- Skin integrity
- Device-specific documentation:
  - HeartMate II: pump speed, flow, motor power, and pulse index
  - HeartWare: pump speed, flow, and motor power

References and Additional Readings

For a complete list of references and additional readings for this procedure, scan this QR code with any freely available smartphone code reader app, or visit http://booksite.elsevier.com/9780323376624.

PROCEDURE

54

Cardiac Monitoring and Electrocardiographic Leads

Michele M. Pelter, Teri M. Kozik, and Mary G. Carey

PURPOSE: Continuous physiological monitoring is performed routinely for patients with acute and critical illnesses. A key component of physiological monitoring is electrocardiographic or ECG monitoring. The electrocardiogram provides a graphic picture of cardiac electrical activity, and can be used continuously to assess dynamic changes. The electrocardiogram is used for diagnostic purposes and to guide treatment.

PREREQUISITE NURSING KNOWLEDGE

- Knowledge of the anatomy and physiology of the cardiovascular system, principles of cardiac conduction, principles of electrophysiology, electrocardiographic lead placement, basic dysrhythmia interpretation, and electrical safety is necessary. Knowledge of cardiac pathophysiology is also required.
- Electrocardiographic monitoring is indicated for patients in critical care units and for those in select acute-care settings, including progressive care, medical surgical units, postanesthesia care units, operating rooms, and emergency departments to list a few. Electrocardiographic monitoring may also be used during patient transport in the acute-care setting.
- Electrocardiographic monitoring is designed to provide clinicians with a graphic display of the electrical activity of the heart and is generated by depolarization and repolarization of cardiac tissue. Cardiac depolarization and repolarization is the result of electrolytes shifting in and out of the myocardial cells, which is captured on the body surface in the form of an ECG. Both normal and abnormal cardiac activity can be assessed with the ECG.
- Hardwire ECG monitors display the ECG using skin electrodes that are placed on the patient's torso and lead wires that are attached to the skin electrodes. This type of monitoring system means patients cannot exceed the length of the lead wires; consequently patients are tethered to the monitoring system, which may be bedside or portable (Fig. 54-1). ECG abnormalities generate an audible alarm and are transmitted and stored in a central monitoring system, which may or may not be assessed by a dedicated monitor observer. Alarms can and should be adjusted for each patient from either the bedside monitor or central monitoring station to minimize false alarms.[5]

- Telemetry ECG monitoring systems also use skin electrodes and leads wires, but are designed to transmit the ECG waveforms, via telemetry, to a central monitoring system for analysis (Figs. 54-2 and 54-3). This wireless system allows patients to ambulate freely. Some telemetry systems can monitor patients' ECGs during transport to other hospital units such as radiology, the cardiac catheterization laboratory, and other diagnostic areas of the hospital.
- With both hardwire and telemetry monitoring systems it is important to appreciate that ECG waveforms can be altered from body-position changes and artifact, which can cause false alarms.[4,7] Because of this, careful human oversight is required.
- Electrocardiographic leads are placed at specific locations on the torso to "view" different aspects of the heart. The number of ECG leads available varies by manufacturer and age of the ECG system; there are 3-, 5-, 6- or even 12-lead systems. Some ECG monitoring systems "derive" more views of the heart using a reduced number of lead wires, and then mathematically generate additional views of the heart. One example is the EASI lead configuration, which uses five lead wires to generate a "derived" 12-lead ECG (Phillips Healthcare, Andover, MA). EASI derived 12-lead ECGs and their measurements are approximations to standard 12-lead ECGs and should not be used for diagnostic interpretations; instead, a standard 12-lead ECG that applies electrodes on the wrist and ankles should be obtained.
- Accurate ECG interpretation is based on precise placement of skin electrodes on the torso; hence, correct and consistent placement of skin electrodes during ECG monitoring is critical. Incorrect placement of skin electrodes can distort the appearance of the ECG waveform enough that misdiagnosis and therefore inappropriate treatment can occur. Fig. 54-4 illustrates the location of skin electrodes for three- and five-lead ECG systems, which are

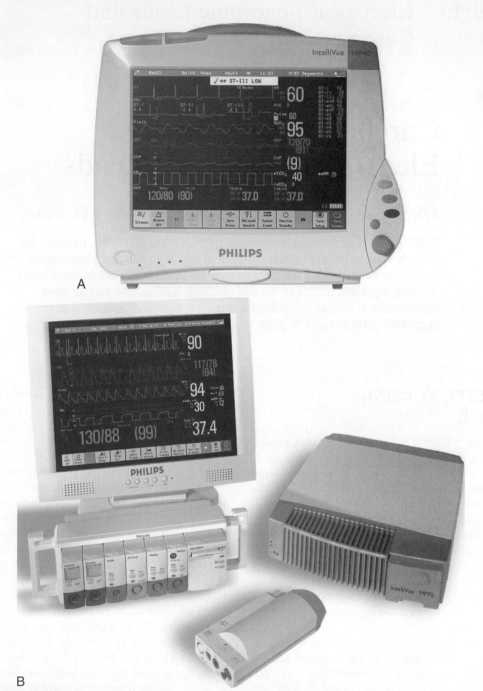

Figure 54-1 **A,** Bedside monitoring system. **B,** Networked patient monitor with portal technology for critical and intermediate care. *(Courtesy Philips Medical System, Andover, MA.)*

shown because these two lead systems are commonly used in the hospital setting.

• Correct attachment of the lead wires to the skin electrodes is of critical importance as well. Lead wires are labeled by the manufacturer to assist with placement. Labels typically used are RA (right arm), RL (right leg), LA (left arm), LL (left leg), and V or C (V or precordial vector and C or chest lead) in systems that provide this lead(s). Lead wires may also be color coded, but these can vary by manufacturer. Figures 54-5 and 54-6 show lead wires for three- and five-lead systems.

• Electrocardiographic waveforms are described as either positive (i.e., upward direction) or negative (i.e., downward direction). The factors that determine the direction of the ECG waveforms are (1) lead location, (2) lead polarity (positive or negative), and (3) the direction of the cardiac impulse generated by the heart. Normal cardiac conduction proceeds from the atria (superior part of the heart) to the ventricles (inferior part of the heart). When cardiac conduction flows toward a positive electrode, an upright QRS complex, or positive, waveform is produced (Fig. 54-7A).

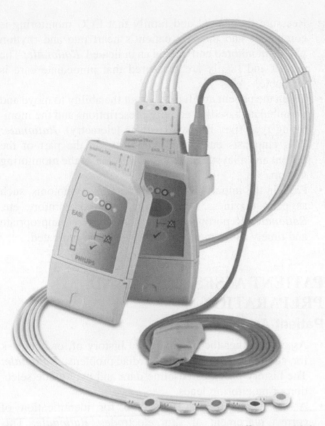

Figure 54-2 Telemetry monitoring system. (*Courtesy Philips Medical Systems, Andover, MA.*)

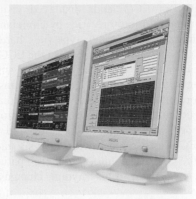

Figure 54-3 Central station. (*Courtesy Philips Medical Systems, Andover, MA.*)

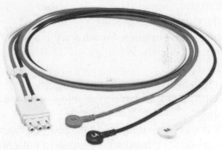

Figure 54-5 Three-lead wire system. (*Courtesy Philips Medical Systems, Andover, MA.*)

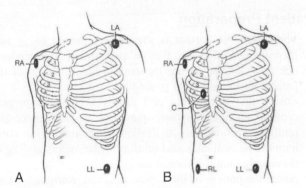

Figure 54-4 **A, B,** Three- and five-lead system lead locations on the torso.

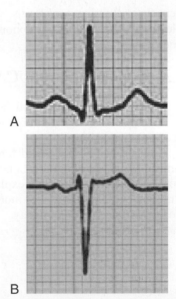

Figure 54-7 Shows positive and negative waveforms.

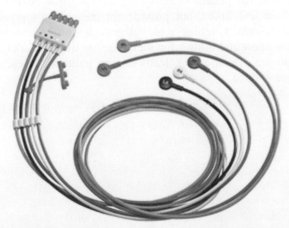

Figure 54-6 Five-lead wire system. (*Courtesy Philips Medical Systems, Andover, MA.*)

- The number of ECG leads displayed visually on the bedside or central monitor varies by clinician preference, manufacturer, or lead system type (i.e., hardwire versus telemetry). It is important to note that the ECG monitoring system may analyze more leads than are visible on the monitoring screen, thus providing clinicians with more ECG information. Variations among cardiac monitors should be communicated in the unit's educational program and included in each unit's policies and procedures. Optimal ECG lead selection for analysis and display is based on the goals of monitoring for each patient's clinical situation (i.e., heart rate, rhythm changes, ischemia, etc.).[3,5,7,8]

EQUIPMENT

- ECG monitor (i.e., hardwire or telemetry), which may also include transport ECG monitor
- ECG lead wires, which may or may not be disposable
- Skin electrodes, pregelled and disposable
- Nonsterile gloves
- Skin-preparation supplies, which vary based on the hospital protocol, to include
  - ❖ Dry gauze pads
  - ❖ Terrycloth with soap and water

Additional equipment, to have available as needed, includes the following:

- Pouch or pocket gown to hold telemetry device
- Clippers or scissors, used with caution in patients on anticoagulants, to clip hair from the chest as needed to ensure adequate adhesion of skin electrodes.
- Black indelible marker to mark precordial sites where skin electrodes are placed, to ensure electrodes are replaced in the correct location and thus maintain consistent lead locations.
- ECG calipers for measuring waveforms, which may be available electronically via the central monitor.
- Telemetry batteries

PATIENT AND FAMILY EDUCATION

- Assess the readiness of the patient and family to learn. *Rationale:* Anxiety and concerns of the patient and family may inhibit the ability to learn.
- Provide explanation to the patient and family regarding ECG equipment, the purpose of ECG monitoring, and the possibility of alarms. *Rationale:* These explanations assist in making the patient and family feel more comfortable with monitoring and may reduce anxiety.

- Reassure the patient and family that ECG monitoring is continuous and that the patient's heart rate and rhythm will be monitored and treated as indicated. *Rationale:* The patient and family are reassured that immediate care is available.
- Teach the patient and family about the ability to move and or ambulate based on activity prescriptions and the monitoring type (i.e., hardwire versus telemetry). *Rationale:* This emphasis encourages mobility on the part of the patient and allays fears about disruption of the monitoring system.
- Explain the importance of reporting any symptoms, such as pain, dizziness, palpitations, chest discomfort, etc. *Rationale:* Reporting of symptoms ensures appropriate and timely assessment and intervention if indicated.

PATIENT ASSESSMENT AND PREPARATION

Patient Assessment

- Assess whether the patient has a history of, or is at risk for, cardiac dysrhythmias or cardiac problems. *Rationale:* The history provides baseline data and may guide selection of monitoring leads.
- Assess landmarks on the torso for identification of correct placement of skin electrodes. *Rationale:* This assessment ensures accurate ECG data will be obtained for interpretation.

Patient Preparation

- Verify that the patient is the correct patient using two identifiers. *Rationale:* Before performing a procedure, clinicians should ensure the correct identification of the patient for the intended procedure.
- Ensure that the patient and family understand preprocedural teaching. Answer questions as they arise, and reinforce information as needed. *Rationale:* This communication evaluates and reinforces the understanding of previously taught information.
- Assist the patient to the supine position. *Rationale:* This position enables easy access to the chest for electrode placement.
- Assist the patient in removing clothing that covers the chest and limbs, but provide for the patient's privacy. *Rationale:* Clothing removal provides a clear view of the chest and allows for identification of landmarks and proper placement of leads as the patient's privacy is maintained.

Procedure for Cardiac Monitoring: Hardwire and Telemetry

Steps	Rationale	Special Considerations
1. **HH**		
2. Verify that the central monitor system is on, if applicable.	When activated, the central monitoring system will turn on ECG software that will sound an alarm when ECG parameters are exceeded.	When an alarm is generated, the nurse must assess the patient to confirm findings, verify patterns, and carefully evaluate computer software interpretations for accuracy.
3. For telemetry monitoring, insert a battery (or batteries) into the telemetry device.	Batteries can fail if left sitting for long periods of time in the unit.	Refer to manufacturer recommendations regarding battery storage and replacement.
4. Check the cable and lead wires for fraying, broken wires or discoloration.	Detects conditions that may interfere with the ECG signal.	Safety must be maintained; if equipment is damaged, obtain alternative equipment and notify the biomedical engineer for repair. Disposable lead wires systems are available.
5. Plug the patient cable into the monitor. Identify the number of lead wires available for the system being used.	Assists with determining placement of skin electrodes and the number of lead wires available for monitoring.	Optimal lead selection should be based on the type of lead system available and the goals of monitoring for each patient's clinical situation (i.e., heart rate, arrhythmia, ischemia, QT-interval monitoring).[3,5,7,8]
A. Three-lead systems use the following lead wires; RA, LA, and LL (Figs. 54-4A and 54-5).	Assists with determining placement of skin electrodes and lead wires available.	The three-lead system is the simplest ECG monitoring lead system. With this lead configuration, leads I, II, or III can be displayed. This system is often used for portable monitor defibrillators.
B. Five-lead systems use the following lead wires; RA, LA, RL, LL, and a chest lead labeled "C" or "V" (Figs. 54-4B and 54-6).	Assists with determining placement of skin electrodes and lead wires available.	This lead system provides the following leads; the six limb leads I, II, III, aVR (augmented unipolar [vector] right arm), aVL (augmented unipolar [vector] left arm), aVF (augmented unipolar [vector] foot [i.e., left leg]), and one precordial or chest lead labeled V unipolar [vector] or C (chest). Select the V or chest lead based on goals of ECG monitoring.[3,7,8]
6. If lead wires are designed with a "snap" connection, connect the lead wires to the each electrode before placing the skin electrode on the patient's torso.	Prepares monitoring.	Pushing the snap type lead wires onto the skin electrodes already placed on the torso can be uncomfortable for the patient.
7. **HH**		
8. **PE**		

Procedure continues on following page

Procedure for Cardiac Monitoring: Hardwire and Telemetry—*Continued*

Steps	Rationale	Special Considerations
9. Identify skin electrode locations (Fig. 54-4A and B), then clean and slightly abrade the skin where the electrodes will be applied. A. Wash the skin with soap and water. B. Abrade the skin with a gauze pad. C. Ensure that the skin is dry before skin electrodes are applied. D. Clipping of chest hair may be necessary to ensure that adequate skin contact with the skin electrodes is made. **(Level C*)**	Removes dead skin cells, promoting impulse transmission. Moist skin is not conducive to electrode adherence. Failure to properly prepare the skin may cause artifacts and interfere with interpretation.[1,3]	Clipping hair should be done with caution in patients at risk for bleeding. Quality improvement projects have shown that changing skin electrodes daily can reduce artifacts,[1,2] but considerations for skin breakdown should be made.
10. If possible, mark any precordial location with a black indelible marker.	Ensures that skin electrodes are replaced to the correct location to maintain consistent lead locations.	
11. Remove the backing from the pregelled electrodes and assess the center of the pads for moistness.	The gel should be moist to allow for maximal impulse transmission.	Skin electrodes should be stored in a dry area and not exposed to direct sunlight because this can dry out the conductive gel.
12. Apply electrodes to the correct location on the torso. Ensure the skin electrodes are completely adhering to the skin.	Electrodes must be applied firmly to the skin to prevent external influences from affecting the ECG.	Electrode failure due to loss of contact with the skin or dried-out gel can results in excessive false alarms.[1,2,5]

13. Place electrodes as follows:
A. Three-lead system (Figs. 54-4A, 54-5):
  • Apply RA electrode just below the clavicle close to the junction of the right arm and torso.
  • Apply LA electrode just below the clavicle close to the junction of the left arm and torso.
  • Apply LL electrode below the level of the umbilicus, on the left abdominal region.
(Level C*)
	Proper positioning is essential to ensure accurate waveforms are generated for analysis.[3,4,7,8]	Lead selection for display and analysis by the central monitoring station is based on the aims of cardiac monitoring and chest wall constraints (i.e., wounds, dressings, etc.).[3,4,7,8]

*Qualitative studies, descriptive or correlational studies, integrative reviews, systematic reviews, or randomized controlled trials with inconsistent results.

Procedure	**for Cardiac Monitoring: Hardwire and Telemetry—*Continued***	
Steps	**Rationale**	**Special Considerations**
B. Five-lead system (Figs. 54-4B, 54-6): • Apply RA electrode just below the clavicle close to the junction of the right arm and torso. • Apply LA electrode just below the clavicle close to the junction of the left arm and torso. • Apply RL electrode below the level of the umbilicus, on the right abdominal region. • Apply LL electrode below the level of the umbilicus, on the left abdominal region. • Apply the chest (precordial) lead electrode to the selected site based on the goals of monitoring: Lead V_1 is the single best chest, or precordial lead for arrhythmia monitoring.[1] This lead is located in the 4th intercostal space on the right sternal border. Lead V_6 can be substituted when V_1 cannot be applied (e.g., dressings, wounds, etc.). Lead V_6 is located at the midaxillary in the 5th intercostal space. Lead V_3 is the single best precordial lead for detection of transient myocardial ischemia.[3] On the central monitoring station, ensure that the chest lead placed on the patient is correctly identified on the monitor. **(Level D*)**	Arm electrodes that are not placed on the outer chest and under the clavicle or leg electrodes that are placed above the umbilicus can alter the ECG waveforms and result in inaccurate recordings.[7,8] In five-lead systems only one precordial lead can be selected. The central monitoring station should be programed to indicate the chest (precordial) lead selected.	Many hospitals set the default precordial lead to V_1. If another chest lead is selected, the central monitoring station should be edited to reflect the correct chest lead being monitored because the V lead selected will be printed on any rhythm strips printed or stored.
14. Reduce tension on the lead wires and cables.	Decreased tension on the lead wires will minimize the leads becoming disconnected. This will also minimize pulling on the electrodes, which can be uncomfortable for the patient.	Software analysis will cease when the lead wires are not connected, or the skin electrodes are not in contact with the torso.
15. For telemetry monitoring, secure the recorder in a pouch or pocket in the patient's gown.	The recorder must be secure so that it is not dropped or damaged, and to minimize pulling on the electrodes.	

*Level D: Peer-reviewed professional and organizational standards with the support of clinical study recommendations.

Procedure continues on following page

Procedure   for Cardiac Monitoring: Hardwire and Telemetry—*Continued*

Steps	Rationale	Special Considerations
16. Examine the ECG tracing on the monitor for quality waveforms.	The QRS complex should be approximately twice the height of the other waveforms (e.g., P wave, T wave, etc.) to ensure proper detection of heart rate by the ECG software. If the T wave is nearly equal to the R wave, each complex may be double counted, resulting in false heart rate alarms.	Most calibration is set to default settings by each facility's biomedical department. Typically, calibration of the ECG should be set to 10 mm/mV; at this calibration, 1 mV is expected to produce a rectangle of 10 mm height and 5 mm width. Calibration for ECG time (speed of paper recording) is typically set to 25 mm/sec. Some cardiac monitors have size adjustments that can be used to increase or decrease the size (gain) of complexes, and speed adjustments to slow or speed up the rate of the paper recording of the ECG. Alteration of these settings can affect waveform analysis; it should be done with careful consideration and noted in the medical record.
17. Obtain a baseline ECG strip and interpret for rhythm, heart rate, presence of P waves, length of PR interval, width of QRS complexes, ST-segment deviation, presence of T waves, and length of QT interval.	Review the normal conduction sequence and identify abnormalities that may necessitate further evaluation or treatment.	
18. Set alarm parameters. Upper and lower alarm limits are set on the basis of the patient's current clinical status and heart rate.	For hard-wire monitoring systems, alarms can be adjusted at the bedside or at the central monitoring station. For telemetry monitoring systems, alarm parameters are typically adjusted at the central monitoring station.	Monitoring systems allow for setting and adjusting alarms at the bedside or the central console. The types of alarms may include heart rate (i.e., high or low), abnormal rhythms or waveforms, pacemaker recognition, and others, depending on the manufacturer. Caution: alarms should not be disabled except in specific circumstances (i.e., anticipated end of life). To reduce alarm burden (false alarms), alarms should be adjusted according to the known clinical status of the patient to minimize false alarms.[3,5]
19. Set ST-segment parameters if indicated (see Procedure 56).	Transient myocardial ischemia can be assessed with ST-segment software in select patients when indicated.	ST-segment monitoring should not be used in patients with left bundle branch block, or ventricular pacing because a high number of false alarms are likely to occur.[3]
20. Remove **PE** and discard used supplies in appropriate receptacles.	Reduces the transmission of microorganisms; Standard Precautions.	
21. **HH**		

Expected Outcomes	**Unexpected Outcomes**

- Properly applied skin electrodes and lead wires
- A clear ECG tracing displayed (Fig. 54-8)
- Alarms are adjusted to the patient's current clinical status
- Prompt identification of heart rate changes, arrhythmias, ischemia, and lengthening of the QT-interval based on the goals of monitoring
- False alarms that require human overreading

- Altered skin integrity
- Alternating current interference, also called 60-cycle interference (Fig. 54-9)
- Wandering baseline (Fig. 54-10)
- Artifact (Fig. 54-11)

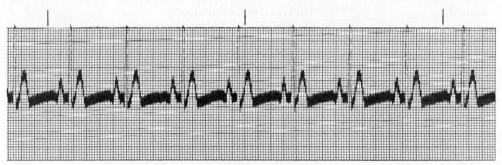

Figure 54-8   Monitor strip of clear ECG pattern.

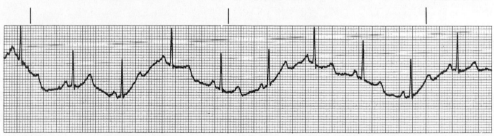

Figure 54-9   Monitor strip with 60-cycle interference.

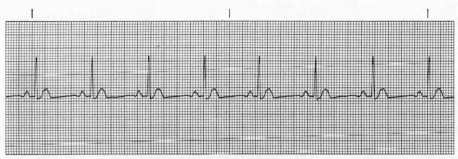

Figure 54-10   Monitor strip with wandering baseline.

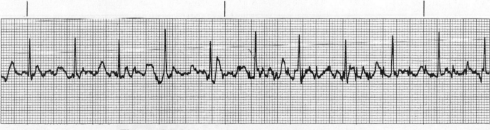

Figure 54-11   Monitor strip with motion artifact.

Procedure continues on following page

Patient Monitoring and Care

Steps	Rationale	Reportable Conditions
		These conditions should be reported if they persist despite nursing interventions.
1. Evaluate the ECG routinely for the presence of P waves, QRS complexes, clear interpretable baseline, and absence of artifact or distortion. Obtain and analyze visually a rhythm strip on admission, every shift (as per institution protocol), and following any changes from the patient's baseline.	Continuous evaluation of ECG waveforms and following any changes can promptly identify alterations in a patient's condition so treatment can be initiated if indicated.[3,6-8]	• Abnormal ECG waveforms, heart rate changes from a patient's baseline level, and rhythm changes
2. Evaluate the ECG pattern continually for arrhythmias, assess patient clinical tolerance following any changes, and provide prompt nursing intervention.	Changes in the ECG pattern may indicate significant problems for the patient and may necessitate immediate intervention or additional diagnostic tests, such as a 12-lead ECG, or laboratory tests.	• Abnormal cardiac rate and rhythm • Hemodynamic instability
3. Evaluate skin integrity around the electrodes on a daily basis, and change the electrodes according to institutional standards.	Skin integrity must be maintained in patients while ensuring that ECG quality is high. Replace electrodes quickly so that continuous monitoring is ensured. Skin electrodes may require slight relocation if skin integrity is compromised. Place the skin electrode as close to the correct site as possible, and note this in the medical record.	• Alteration in skin integrity
4. Verify accurate electrode placement and that lead wires are correctly attached every shift or when leads are removed (i.e., following transport to another department, shower, etc.).	Accurate interpretation of waveforms and arrhythmias depends on proper placement of the electrodes and knowledge of leads being viewed.	

Documentation

Documentation should include the following:
• Patient and family education
• An initial or baseline ECG strip
• Routine ECG strips according to institutional protocol
• An ECG strip should be printed and placed in the medical record following changes in heart rate or rhythm, when the patient experiences symptoms, when

there is a change in lead placement, when there are changes in electrolytes, or following administration of medications that can affect the QT interval.[2]
• Unexpected outcomes

References and Additional Readings

For a complete list of references and additional readings for this procedure, scan this QR code with any freely available smartphone code reader app, or visit http://booksite.elsevier.com/9780323376624.

55 Extra Electrocardiographic Leads: Right Precordial and Left Posterior Leads

Shu-Fen Wung

PURPOSE: Extra electrocardiographic (ECG) leads are used in conjunction with the standard 12-lead ECG to provide additional diagnostic information.

PREREQUISITE NURSING KNOWLEDGE

- Understanding of the anatomy and physiology of the cardiovascular system, principles of electrophysiology, ECG lead placement, basic rhythm interpretation, and electrical safety is necessary.
- Advanced cardiac life support (ACLS) knowledge and skills are needed.
- The right ventricular (RV) leads V_{1R} through V_{6R} and left posterior leads V_7 through V_9 are unipolar leads in which the chest electrode serves as the "exploring" electrode or positive pole of the lead. These precordial leads view the heart from the vantage point of their electrode positions on the chest, similar to the standard precordial leads V_1 through V_6.
- For recordings of RV or left posterior leads, the three limb electrodes (right arm [RA], left arm [LA], left leg [LL]) also are required to create a central terminal (negative pole); the one limb electrode (right leg [RL]) serves as the ground lead and is used to stabilize the ECG recording.
- Accurate identification of electrode positions for the standard 12-lead ECG is needed because the same anatomical landmarks are used to locate the RV and left posterior leads.
- Right precordial leads are useful in diagnosing an RV myocardial infarction (MI). These RV leads are important because they enable clinicians to identify patients with an acute MI who are at high risk of atrioventricular (AV) conduction disturbances, to predict the site of coronary artery occlusion, and to guide appropriate hemodynamic monitoring and interventions.
- Left posterior leads are used to aid in the detection of posterior wall MI and to facilitate timely reperfusion treatment. Recording of left posterior leads also can help in the differential diagnosis of tall R waves in leads V_1 and V_2.[1]
- Patients with an acute inferior MI and RV involvement, determined by ST-segment elevation in the right precordial leads, are at high risk for high-degree AV block. Nurses should monitor patients closely for conduction disturbances and anticipate the need for temporary pacing.

Patients with RV infarction are prone to hypotension and shock that responds to treatment with fluid resuscitation.

- Indications for recording a right-precordial ECG are as follows:
  - Evaluation and treatment of suspected acute MI, especially patients with inferior-wall MI (ST-segment elevation in leads II, III, and augmented vector foot [aVF])
  - Evaluation of the risk for AV node conduction disturbances and anticipation of treatment plans
  - Prediction of the site of coronary artery occlusion (RV infarction occurs with proximal right coronary artery [RCA] occlusion)[2]
  - Determination of the risk of "volume-responsive" shock, in which case fluid resuscitation is warranted and vasodilators (e.g., nitroglycerin) are contraindicated
- Indications for recording a left-posterior ECG are as follows:
  - Evaluation and treatment of acute or suspected MI, especially patients with isolated ST-segment depression in the precordial leads V_1 through V_3 and patients with a nondiagnostic ECG
  - Presence of chest pain or anginal-equivalent symptoms (e.g., jaw, left shoulder or arm discomfort, or shortness of breath) or ST-segment depression in the left precordial leads V_1 through V_3 after percutaneous coronary interventions of the left circumflex artery
  - Any of these ECG characteristics are indicative of posterior MI (inferobasal MI) in lead V_1: R waves ≥ 6 mm in height, R wave ≥ 40 ms in duration, R/S ratio (R wave amplitude in mm over S wave amplitude in mm) ≥ 1, or S wave ≤ 3 mm. In lead V_2, R wave ≥ 15 mm in height, R wave ≥ 50 ms in duration, R/S ratio ≥ 1.5, or S wave ≤ 4 mm.[3]
  - Differentiation of true posterior MI from other conditions that can cause tall R waves in lead V_1, such as RV hypertrophy, right bundle-branch block, Wolff-Parkinson-White syndrome, and ventricular septal hypertrophy
- In patients with RV infarction who exhibit shock, volume expansion is used to provide adequate RV and left ventricular filling pressures and to restore arterial pressure

and peripheral blood flow. Positive inotropic agents also may be indicated to augment the residual contractile force of the damaged RV. Use of vasodilators (e.g., nitroglycerin) should generally be avoided because they cause venous dilation and reduced preload. Use of diuretics (e.g., furosemide) should be avoided because they reduce preload and left ventricular filling.[4]

EQUIPMENT

- 12-lead ECG machine with patient cable and lead wires
- ECG electrodes

Additional equipment, to have available as needed, includes the following:

- Gauze pads or terrycloth washcloth
- Cleansing pads or nonemollient soap and water
- Skin preparation solution (e.g., skin barrier wipe or tincture of benzoin)
- Indelible marker
- Clippers or scissors to clip hair from chest if needed

PATIENT AND FAMILY EDUCATION

- Describe the procedure and reasons for obtaining extra ECG leads. Reassure the patient that the procedure is painless. *Rationale:* This communication clarifies information, reduces anxiety, and gains cooperation from the patient.
- Explain the patient's role in assisting with the ECG recording and emphasize actions that improve the quality of the ECG tracing, such as relaxing, avoiding conversation and body movement, and breathing normally. *Rationale:* This explanation ensures the patient's cooperation to improve the quality of the tracing and avoids unnecessary repeating of the ECG because of muscle artifacts.

PATIENT ASSESSMENT AND PREPARATION
Patient Assessment

- Assess for the presence of anginal symptoms, such as chest pain, pressure, tightness, heaviness, fullness, or squeezing sensation; radiated pain; shortness of breath; nausea; and extreme fatigue. *Rationale:* This evaluation correlates ECG changes with patient symptoms.
- Assess the patient's history of cardiac conditions and medications. *Rationale:* Knowledge about the patient's cardiac history and medications can help in interpretation of ECG recordings. For example, digitalis therapy causes chronic ST-segment depression that does not indicate acute myocardial ischemia. A normal-looking isoelectric ST segment in a patient on digitalis therapy may indicate acute myocardial ischemia (Fig. 55-1).
- Interpret the patient's standard 12-lead ECG for any signs of myocardial ischemia or MI and dysrhythmias. *Rationale:* Nurses should be able to evaluate the standard 12-lead ECG for the location of myocardial ischemia or infarction and assess the possibility of RV and posterior involvement (Fig. 55-2).

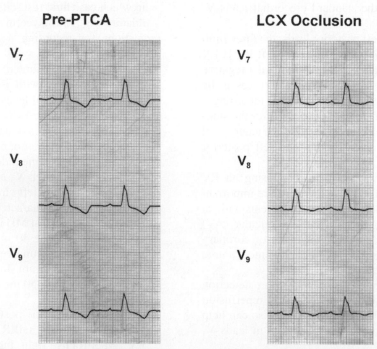

Pre-PTCA   **LCX Occlusion**

Figure 55-1   Baseline ST-segment deviation as a result of left bundle-branch block before percutaneous coronary intervention (*left panel,* before angioplasty). During angioplasty balloon inflation of the proximal left circumflex (LCX) coronary artery (*right panel,* LCX occlusion), the patient developed myocardial ischemia with chest pain radiating to the left arm. ST segments in the left posterior leads (V₇, V₈, and V₉) became elevated compared with the baseline preangioplasty tracing to produce a normal-looking, isoelectric ST segment. This pseudonormalization of the ST segment during ischemia can be misinterpreted as normal without assessment of the baseline ECG.

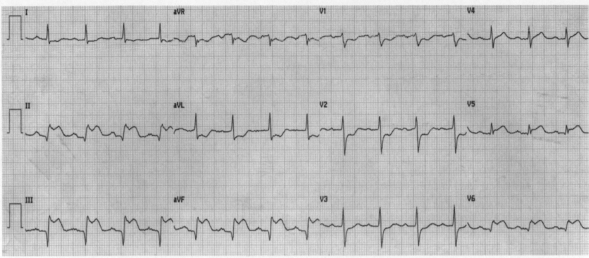

Figure 55-2   Initial ECG in a patient admitted to the emergency department with an acute inferior MI (elevated ST segments and Q waves in leads II, III, and aVF) with apical involvement (elevated ST segment in leads V_4, V_5, and V_6). ST-segment depression in leads V_1, V_2, and V_3 suggests posterior involvement. Left posterior and right precordial leads should be recorded to assess posterior and RV involvement.

Patient Preparation

- Verify that the patient is the correct patient using two identifiers. *Rationale:* Before performing a procedure, the nurse should ensure the correct identification of the patient for the intended intervention.
- Ensure that the patient and family understand preprocedural teaching. Answer questions as they arise, and reinforce information as needed. *Rationale:* This com-

munication evaluates and reinforces the understanding of previously taught information.

- Assist the patient to the supine position and expose the patient's torso while maintaining the patient's modesty. *Rationale:* This position enables the recording of the ECG and allows comparison of serial ECGs and comparison with standard waveforms. Body positional changes, such as elevation and rotation, can change recorded amplitudes and axes.

Procedure   for Extra Electrocardiographic Leads

Steps	Rationale	Special Considerations
1. **HH**		
2. Check cables and lead wires for fraying or broken wires.	Detects faulty equipment.	If the equipment is damaged, obtain alternative equipment and notify a biomedical engineer for repair.
3. Check the lead wires for accurate labels.	Obtains accurate ECG recordings and proper placement of leads.	
4. Plug the ECG machine into a grounded alternating current (AC) wall outlet or ensure functioning if battery operated.	Maintains electrical safety.	Follow manufacturer's recommendations and institutional protocol on electrical safety per the biomedical department.
5. Turn the ECG machine on and program the ECG machine: paper speed, 25 mm/sec; calibration, 10 mm/mV; filter settings, 0.05–100 Hz. **(Level E*)**	Equipment may require self-test and warm-up time. Verify equipment setting in accordance with clinical practice and recommendation by the American Heart Association (AHA).[5] Multichannel machines may require input of information (e.g., data about the patient) to store the ECG appropriately.	Manufacturers provide a calibration check in the machine to identify the sensitivity setting. Most machines have automatic settings.
6. **PE**		

*Level E: Multiple case reports, theory-based evidence from expert opinions, or peer-reviewed professional organizational standards without clinical studies to support recommendations.

Procedure continues on following page

Procedure for Extra Electrocardiographic Leads—*Continued*

Steps	Rationale	Special Considerations
7. Place the patient in a supine position. (**Level B***)	Provides adequate support for limbs so that muscle activity is minimal. Body-position changes can cause ST-segment deviation and QRS waveform alteration.[6-9]	ECGs should be recorded in the same body position to ensure ECG changes are not caused by a change in body position. If another position is clinically necessary, note the altered position on the ECG recording.
8. Expose only the necessary body parts of the patient (legs, arms, and chest) for electrode placement.	Provides privacy and warmth, which reduces shivering.	Ensuring privacy may reduce anxiety. Shivering may interfere with the quality of recording.
9. Identify the electrode locations.	Ensures the accuracy of the lead placement.	
Limb Leads (Fig. 57-4) • RA: inside right forearm • LA: inside left forearm. • RL: anywhere on the body; by convention, usually on the right ankle or inner aspect of the calf • LL: left ankle or inner aspect of the calf	Accurate electrode placement is essential for obtaining valid and reliable data for ECG recordings. The RL electrode is a ground electrode that does not contribute to the ECG tracings.	Limb leads should be placed in fleshy areas; bony prominences should be avoided. The limb leads need to be placed equidistant from the heart and should be positioned in approximately the same place on each limb.
Right Precordial Leads (Fig. 55-3) • V_{1R}: fourth intercostal space (ICS) at the left sternal border (same as V_2) • V_{2R}: fourth ICS at the right sternal border (same as V_1) • V_{3R}: halfway between V_{2R} and V_{4R}	All patients with an acute inferior wall MI should have right precordial leads recorded in addition to precordial leads V_1 through V_6.	These right precordial leads are placed across the right precordium with the same landmarks that are used for the precordial leads V_1 through V_6.[10]

***Level B:** Well-designed controlled studies with results that consistently support a specific action, intervention, or treatment.

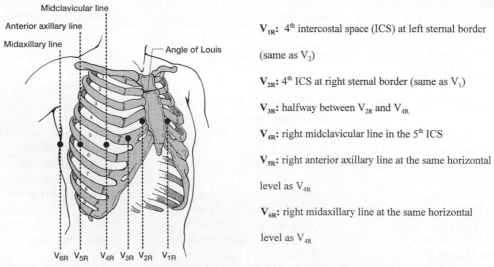

V_{1R}: 4th intercostal space (ICS) at left sternal border (same as V_2)

V_{2R}: 4th ICS at right sternal border (same as V_1)

V_{3R}: halfway between V_{2R} and V_{4R}

V_{4R}: right midclavicular line in the 5th ICS

V_{5R}: right anterior axillary line at the same horizontal level as V_{4R}

V_{6R}: right midaxillary line at the same horizontal level as V_{4R}

Figure 55-3   Electrode locations for recording a right precordial ECG. (*From Drew BJ, Ide B: Right ventricular infarction, Prog Cardiovasc Nurs 10:46, 1995.*)

Conventional 12-Lead ECG

Right Precordial Leads

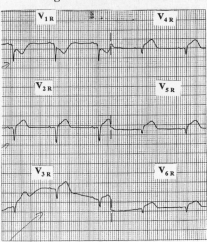

Figure 55-4 ST-segment elevation in leads II, III, and aVF indicates acute inferior wall MI. These characteristics on the standard 12-lead electrocardiogram (ECG) *(left panel)* suggest RV infarction: diagnosis of an inferior MI; ST-segment elevation in lead III exceeding that of lead II; ST-segment elevation confined to V_1 without elevation in the remaining precordial leads; and ST depression in lead aVL.[15] Definitive diagnosis of RV infarction is made by observing ST-segment elevation greater than or equal to 1 mm in one or more of the right precordial leads. In the *right panel*, ST-segment elevation is seen in V_{2R} (V_1) through V_{6R}. *(From Drew BJ, Ide B: Right ventricular infarction, Prog Cardiovasc Nurs 10:46, 1995.)*

Procedure for Extra Electrocardiographic Leads—*Continued*

Steps	Rationale	Special Considerations
• V_{4R}: right midclavicular line in the fifth ICS • V_{5R}: right anterior axillary line at the same horizontal level as V_{4R} • V_{6R}: right midaxillary line at the same horizontal level as V_{4R}	Slight alterations in the position of one precordial electrode may distort significantly the appearance of the cardiac waveforms and can have a significant impact on the diagnosis.[11,12]	V_{1R} is at the same location as V_2, and V_{2R} is at the same location as V_1 in the standard 12-lead ECG (see Fig. 55-4). The redundancy of V_1 (or V_{2R}) and V_2 (or V_{1R}) can be used to ensure that the ECGs are recorded accurately. Identify the sternal notch and move downward to locate the angle of Louis; the second ICS is located right below the angle of Louis.
Left Posterior Leads (Fig. 55-5) • V_7: posterior axillary line at the same level as V_4 through V_6 • V_8: halfway between V_7 and V_9 • V_9: left paraspinal line at the same level as V_4 through V_6	Left posterior leads are placed to view the posterior wall of the left ventricle. Left posterior leads should be recorded in patients admitted with a suspected posterior MI or known to have left circumflex artery disease.	Help the patient turn to the right side to expose the left side of the back. Ensure the patient is safely turned. Leads V_4 through V_6 are located at the midclavicular line in the fifth ICS; leads V_7 through V_9 are at the same horizontal level as V_4 through V_6.

Procedure continues on following page

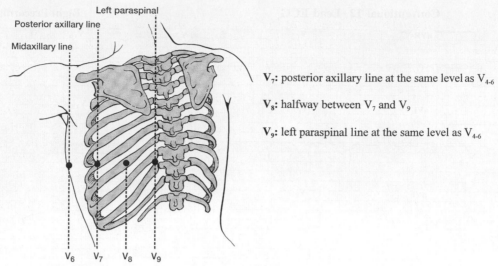

Left paraspinal
Posterior axillary line
Midaxillary line

V_7: posterior axillary line at the same level as V_{4-6}

V_8: halfway between V_7 and V_9

V_9: left paraspinal line at the same level as V_{4-6}

V_6 V_7 V_8 V_9

Figure 55-5   Electrode locations for recording a left posterior electrocardiogram.

Procedure   for Extra Electrocardiographic Leads—*Continued*

Steps	Rationale	Special Considerations
10. Clean and slightly abrade the skin where the electrodes will be applied. A. Wash the skin with soap and water if needed. B. Abrade the skin with a gauze pad or abrader. C. Ensure that the skin is dry before skin electrodes are applied. D. Clipping of chest hair may be necessary to ensure that adequate skin contact with the skin electrodes is made. **(Level C*)**	Removes dead skin cells, promoting impulse transmission.[13-15] Moist skin is not conducive to electrode adherence.	Failure to properly prepare the skin may cause artifact.
11. Identify the electrode sites and mark with an indelible marker.	Minimizes ECG changes caused by altered electrode placement.[16]	After accurate identification of the locations, an indelible marker should be used to mark the electrode sites if serial ECGs are anticipated.
12. For pregelled electrodes, remove the backing and test for moistness. For adhesive electrodes, remove the backing and check each adhesive pad, as each should be sticky or moist.	Allows for appropriate conduction of impulses.	Gel must be moist. If pregelled electrodes are not moist or adhesive electrodes are not sticky, replace the electrodes.
13. Apply the electrodes securely and place the electrodes on the marked locations.	Electrodes must be secure to prevent external influences from affecting the ECG. Secure the electrodes to obtain quality ECG recordings.	If limb plate electrodes are used, do not overtighten to minimize discomfort.

*Level C: Qualitative studies, descriptive or correlational studies, integrative reviews, systematic reviews, or randomized controlled trials with inconsistent results.

Procedure for Extra Electrocardiographic Leads—*Continued*

Steps	Rationale	Special Considerations
14. Identify the number of available ECG channels for simultaneous recording in the ECG machine.	Newer multiple-channel machines can record 16 leads at a time, which allows simultaneous recording of a standard 12-lead ECG and four channels of RV leads V_{3R} through V_{6R} or three channels of left posterior leads V_7 through V_9.	If the ECG machine can record only 12 leads, record three separate ECGs: (1) standard 12-lead with precordial leads, (2) RV leads, and (3) left posterior leads. Some newer-generation ECG machines may allow recording more than 12 leads. If the machine can record 16 leads, you can record two ECGs: (1) standard 12-lead plus RV leads (V_{3R} through V_{6R}), then (2) standard 12-lead plus left posterior leads (V_7 through V_9). Follow institutional protocol for recording these extra leads so that a consistent method is used to avoid confusion.
15. Connect the lead wires to the electrodes and record the ECG. Correctly label the ECG tracings, with the extra leads noted.	Identifies RV and posterior leads.	Make a notation on the ECG tracing that these are RV leads or posterior leads. Labels on the ECG printout depend on the connected lead wire and the location of the electrode.

A. For recording RV leads with a 12-lead ECG machine, connect as follows:
    • V_1 wire to electrode V_{1R}
    • V_2 wire to electrode V_{2R}
    • V_3 wire to electrode V_{3R}
    • V_4 wire to electrode V_{4R}
    • V_5 wire to electrode V_{5R}
    • V_6 wire to electrode V_{6R}
	When the unipolar precordial lead wires V_1 through V_6 are connected to the RV or left posterior electrodes, the ECG machine records signals from where the electrodes are placed.	Change the labels on the ECG printouts from V_1 to V_{1R}, V_2 to V_{2R}, V_3 to V_{3R}, V_4 to V_{4R}, V_5 to V_{5R}, and V_6 to V_{6R}.

B. For recording of left posterior leads with a 12-lead ECG machine, connect as follows:
    • V_4 wire to electrode V_7
    • V_5 wire to electrode V_8
    • V_6 wire to electrode V_9
		Make a notation of "left posterior leads" and relabel appropriately on the printouts: change V_4 to V_7, V_5 to V_8, and V_6 to V_9.

16. Assess the quality of the tracing.	Ensures a clear tracing is obtained and no lead is off.	
17. Disconnect the equipment; clean the gel off the patient (if necessary), remove **PE**, discard used supplies, and prepare the equipment for future use.	Reduces the transmission of microorganisms; Standard Precautions.	Some pregelled electrodes can be left in place for repeat ECGs. Follow the manufacturer's directions and hospital policy for electrode use and removal in these cases.
18. **HH**		

Procedure continues on following page

Expected Outcomes

- Clear and accurate recording of ECG tracings that allows clinicians to diagnose dysrhythmias and ischemia
- Institutional protocol developed for recording the extra posterior and RV leads according to the availability and type of ECG machine so that the recording method is consistent

Unexpected Outcomes

- Inaccurate lead placement: electrode misplacement or incorrect lead connection
- Failure to identify the recordings as either RV or left posterior ECGs and to change the ECG leads to their correct labels; this could lead to misdiagnosis
- Poor ECG tracing caused by electrical artifacts from external or internal sources
- External artifact introduced by line current (60-cycle interference), which may be minimized by disconnecting nearby electrical devices, unplugging the ECG machine and operating on battery, improving grounding, or replacing lead wires
- Internal artifact may result from body movement, shivering, muscle tremors, and hiccups

Patient Monitoring and Care

Steps	Rationale	Reportable Conditions
		These conditions should be reported if they persist despite nursing interventions.
1. Evaluate the ECG recordings for acute RV or posterior myocardial ischemia or infarction (Fig. 55-6). Record whether the patient has chest pain on the ECG tracing. Use a 0–10 score to quantify pain severity (e.g., 8/10 chest pain).	Promptly initiates appropriate interventions, such as reperfusion treatment or vasodilators. A criterion of 0.5 mm ST elevation in V_{7-9} may suggest acute myocardial ischemia in the posterior wall of the left ventricle.[10]	• Abnormal ST-segment deviation (elevation or depression) may indicate acute myocardial ischemia, injury, or infarction

Standard 12-Lead ECG

Left Posterior Leads

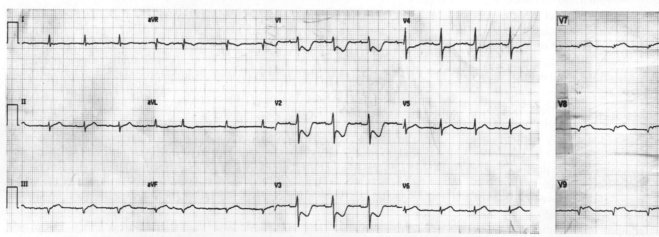

Figure 55-6 An electrocardiogram (ECG) recorded in a 76-year-old patient with diabetes during occlusion of the left circumflex artery. ST-segment depression is observed in precordial leads V_1 to V_4, which suggests a posterior MI *(left panel)*. Left posterior leads V_7 to V_9 are helpful in recording ST-segment elevation that confirms posterior myocardial ischemia *(right panel)*. Observing ST-segment elevation in the contiguous posterior leads allows patients with an acute MI to benefit from thrombolytic therapy, which would be denied based on analysis of the standard 12-lead ECG alone.

Patient Monitoring and Care —*Continued*

Steps	Rationale	Reportable Conditions
2. Assess the presence of chest pain or anginal equivalent symptoms (e.g., jaw, left shoulder or arm discomfort, or shortness of breath).	Ischemia caused by decreased coronary blood flow or increased myocardial oxygen demand may produce anginal symptoms.	• Angina
3. Evaluate the patient's ECG for signs of AV node conduction disturbances in patients with RV infarction (e.g., second-degree or third-degree AV block).	The RCA supplies blood to the AV node in 90% of patients. Occlusion of the RCA proximal to the RV branch decreases the blood supply to the AV nodal artery. The incidence rate of high-degree AV block in patients with inferior MI with RV involvement is significantly higher (48%) than in patients without RV MI (13%).[18]	• Patients with an acute MI with RV involvement, as evidenced by a QRS pattern or ST-segment elevation greater than or equal to 1 mm in the right precordial leads.[17]
4. Assess the patient's hemodynamic status.	Hypotension and reduced cardiac output in patients with RV infarction could be attributed to inadequate left ventricular filling.[4]	• Cardiovascular and hemodynamic changes associated with RV ischemia, injury, or infarction (e.g., elevated mean atrial pressure, reduced cardiac output, hypotension, and prominent venous engorgement).

Documentation

Documentation should include the following:
- Patient and family education
- The reason the extra leads are recorded (e.g., suspected RV infarction, posterior MI)
- Description of associated symptoms
- Interpretation of the ECGs recorded
- Interventions as indicated from the recorded ECG
- Occurrence of unexpected outcomes
- Assessment of pain, interventions, and response to interventions
- Additional interventions

References and Additional Readings

For a complete list of references and additional readings for this procedure, scan this QR code with any freely available smartphone code reader app, or visit http://booksite.elsevier.com/9780323376624.

56 ST-Segment Monitoring (Continuous)

Mary G. Carey and Michele M. Pelter

PURPOSE: Bedside ST-segment monitoring provides ongoing surveillance for detection of transient myocardial ischemia. This technology should be applied to patients who are being evaluated or are diagnosed with acute coronary syndrome (ACS), including acute myocardial infarction and unstable angina. For these patients, continuous ST-segment monitoring is valuable in detecting recurrent or transient ischemia and in determining the success of thrombolytic therapy and percutaneous coronary intervention.

PREREQUISITE NURSING KNOWLEDGE

- Understanding of the anatomy and physiology of the cardiovascular system, coronary arteries and associated location of the heart perfused by the coronary arteries, principles of cardiac conduction, electrocardiogram (ECG) lead placement, basic dysrhythmia interpretation, ECG leads and location of each lead or lead views, and electrical safety is needed.
- Understanding of ACS and associated terms is necessary: (1) ST-elevation myocardial infarction (STEMI), (2) non-STEMI, and (3) unstable angina.
- Advanced cardiac life support (ACLS) knowledge and skills are needed.
- Continuous monitoring of the ECG for ischemic ST-segment changes is more reliable than patient symptoms because more than three quarters of ECG-detected ischemic events are clinically silent.[2,9,14,15,18] Patients who have transient ischemia detected with continuous ST-segment monitoring are more likely to have unfavorable outcomes, including myocardial infarction (MI) and death, compared with patients without such events.[2,3,9,11,12,14,15,18]
- Given the dynamic, unpredictable, and silent nature of myocardial ischemia, continuous ECG monitoring of patients for ischemia is essential.[16] Clinicians should monitor over time the trend of the ST segments and the part of the ECG that changes during acute ischemia and evaluate any ST-segment changes (elevation or depression) for possible myocardial ischemia[19] (Fig. 56-1).
- Nonischemic ST-segment changes can occur and should be considered when evaluating ST-segment trend changes, and they include movement of the skin electrodes, dysrhythmias, intermittent bundle-branch block pattern, body position changes, and ventricular paced rhythms.[1,9,13]
- One type of myocardial ischemia seen in patients with ACS is supply-related ischemia, which results from complete coronary artery occlusion. Coronary occlusion is brought on by disruption of an atherosclerotic plaque followed by cycles of plaque rupture, coronary vasospasm, platelet stimulation, and thrombus formation with resultant loss of blood flow.[5,7,15] Because this type of ischemia threatens the entire thickness (transmural) part of the myocardium, immediate treatment to reestablish blood flow to the heart is essential. The typical ECG manifestation of total supply-related ischemia is ST-segment elevation visible in the ECG leads that lie directly over the ischemic myocardial zone.

- Occlusion of the right coronary artery typically produces ST-segment elevation in leads II, III, and aVF (Fig. 56-2). Occlusion of the left anterior descending coronary artery typically produces ST-segment elevation in leads V_2, V_3, and V_4 (Fig. 56-3). Diagnosis of total coronary occlusion of the left circumflex coronary artery (LCX) is more complex because placement of the standard ECG electrodes is on the anterior chest, opposite the wall that this coronary artery supplies. Occlusion of the LCX may produce ST-segment depression in leads V_1, V_2, or V_3, which reflects the reciprocal, or mirror image, ST-segment elevation occurring in the posterior wall of the left ventricle. In some patients ST-segment changes may also be seen in leads I and aVL.[21]

- A second type of ischemia for which patients with ACS or stable angina are at risk is demand-related ischemia. This type of ischemia occurs when the demand for oxygen (i.e., exercise, tachycardia, or stress) exceeds the flow capabilities of a coronary artery. Patients with this type of ischemia are likely to have a stable atherosclerotic plaque. The ST-segment pattern of demand-related ischemia is ST-segment depression, often appearing in several ECG leads (Fig. 56-4).

- Ideally, diagnosis of myocardial ischemia should be done with continuous monitoring of all 12 ECG leads because the mechanism of ischemia may vary (i.e., supply- [occlusion] versus demand-related ischemia), resulting in distinctly different ST-segment patterns (e.g., elevation or depression) in specific ECG leads. If only two ECG leads

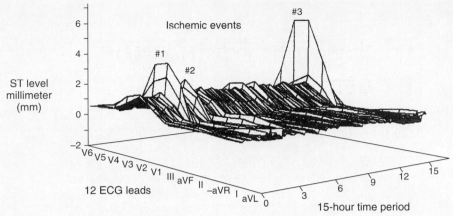

Figure 56-1 The importance of assessing the trend of the ST segments over time. The three-dimensional image illustrates ST-segment deviation in millimeters *(Y-axis)* in all 12 electrocardiograph leads *(X-axis)* over a 15-hour period *(Z-axis)*. Illustrated are three separate ischemic events, characterized by ST-segment elevation, in leads V_3 to V_5. *(Adapted from Pelter MM, Adams MG, Drew BJ: Transient myocardial ischemia is an independent predictor of adverse in-hospital outcomes in patients with acute coronary syndromes treated in the telemetry unit,* Heart Lung *32:71–78, 2003.)*

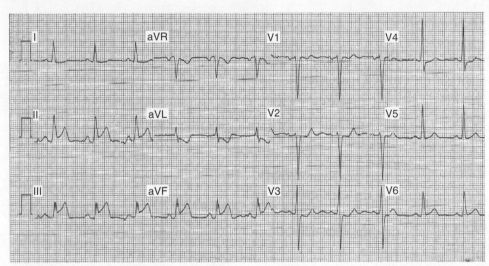

Figure 56-2 The typical ST-segment pattern of supply-related ischemia in the inferior wall. The right coronary artery is likely occluded, resulting in ST-segment elevation in leads II, III, and aVF.

are available, however, the best two for ischemia detection are leads III and V_3.[9] Patient-specific monitoring also may be done if a prior 12-lead ECG was obtained during acute ischemia (i.e., STEMI, percutaneous coronary intervention [PCI], or treadmill test). In this scenario, the ECG lead(s) showing maximal ST-segment deviation should be selected for continuous monitoring to detect recurrent ischemia.

- According to current consensus statements,[9,10] multilead ST-segment monitoring is indicated in most patients with the following diagnoses:
  - ❖ Early phase of acute MI (STEMI, non-ST STEMI, "rule-out"): patients should be monitored for a minimum of 24 hours until they remain event-free for 12 to 24 hours.
  - ❖ Chest pain (or anginal equivalent) that prompts a visit to the emergency department: ST-segment monitoring for 8 to 12 hours in combination with testing serum

biomarkers of injury may be a cost-effective way to triage patients who arrive at the emergency department with chest pain.
  - ❖ After nonurgent PCI procedures with suboptimal results, monitoring should be initiated immediately postprocedure and continue for 24 hours or longer if arrhythmias or ST-segment–deviation events occur.
  - ❖ Variant angina resulting from coronary vasospasm
- According to these same guidelines,[9,10] ST-segment monitoring may be of benefit for the following cases:
  - ❖ Postacute MI
  - ❖ After nonurgent uncomplicated PCI
  - ❖ With high risk for ischemia after cardiac or noncardiac surgery
- ST-segment monitoring may not be appropriate for certain patient groups because current software cannot reliably interpret ST-segment changes resulting from myocardial ischemia and leads to false-positive alarms, contributing

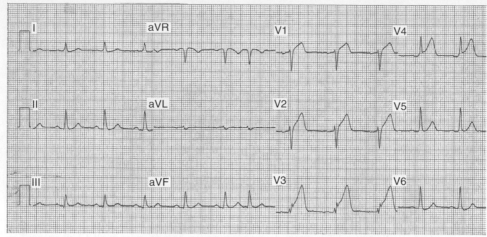

Figure 56-3 The typical ST-segment pattern of supply-related ischemia in the anterior wall. The left anterior descending artery is likely occluded, resulting in ST-segment elevation in leads V_2 to V_4.

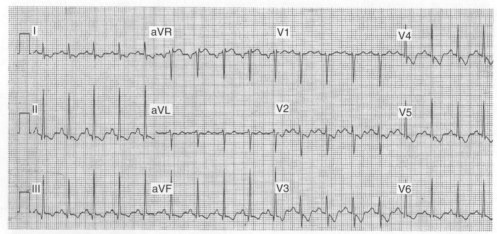

Figure 56-4 The typical ST-segment pattern of demand-related ischemia. Note the ST-segment depression appearing in nearly every ECG lead, with the exception of V_1 and aVR. Note also that this patient is experiencing tachycardia, a common cause of demand-related ischemia.

to alarm fatigue.[9,10,15] Specifically, it may not be suitable to monitor patients with the following:

* Left bundle-branch block
* Ventricular paced rhythm
* Confounding dysrhythmias that obscure the ST segment
* Agitation causing excessive artifact
- A variety of bedside and telemetry cardiac monitors are currently available for use in clinical practice. Not all monitoring systems are equipped with ST-segment monitoring software, however. Clinicians must determine whether their cardiac monitoring system has ST-segment monitoring capabilities.

EQUIPMENT

- ECG monitor with ST-segment monitoring capacity
- ECG lead wires, which may or may not be disposable
- Skin electrodes, pregelled and disposable
- Nonsterile gloves
- Skin-preparation supplies, which vary based on the hospital protocol; these may include a wash cloth, soap and water, or gauze pads

Additional equipment, to have available as needed, includes the following:

- Clippers or scissors, used with caution in patients on anticoagulants, to clip hair from the chest as needed to ensure adequate adhesion of skin electrodes
- Black indelible marker to mark precordial sites where skin electrodes are placed to maintain consistent lead locations by ensuring electrodes are replaced to the correct locations.
- ECG calipers for measuring waveforms (may be available electronically via the central monitor)

PATIENT AND FAMILY EDUCATION

- Explain the purpose of ST-segment monitoring. ***Rationale:*** This explanation decreases patient and family anxiety.
- Encourage the patient to report any symptoms of chest pain or anginal equivalent (e.g., arm pain, jaw pain, shortness of breath, or nausea). ***Rationale:*** This education heightens the patient's awareness of cardiac sensations and encourages communication of anginal symptoms.

PATIENT ASSESSMENT AND PREPARATION

Patient Assessment

- Assess if the patient is at high risk for ischemia. *Rationale:* Patients at risk for myocardial ischemia need to be identified.
- Assess the patient's cardiac rhythm. *Rationale:* This assessment provides baseline data and ensures the patient has a cardiac rhythm suitable for ST-segment monitoring.
- Identify the patient's baseline ST-segment levels before initiating ST-segment monitoring. *Rationale:* The patient's baseline ST-segment level is identified for comparison with subsequent changes.

Patient Preparation

- Verify that the patient is the correct patient using two identifiers. *Rationale:* Before performing a procedure, the nurse should ensure the correct identification of the patient for the intended intervention.
- Ensure that the patient and family understand preprocedural teaching. Answer questions as they arise, and reinforce information as needed. *Rationale:* This communication evaluates and reinforces understanding of previously taught information.
- Place the patient in a resting supine position in bed, and expose the patient's torso while maintaining modesty. *Rationale:* This preparation provides access to the patient's chest for electrode placement and ensures that an artifact-free ECG is obtained.

Procedure	for Continuous ST-Segment Monitoring	
Steps	**Rationale**	**Special Considerations**
1. 🅷🅷		
2. 🅿🅴		
3. Identify accurate electrode placement (Fig. 56-5).	Ensures accurate ECG data.	Electrodes (V_3 to V_5) should be placed immediately below a pendulous breast so that the breast lies on top of the electrode, preventing motion artifact.

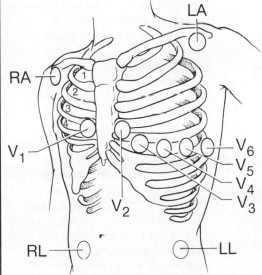

Figure 56-5 Correct lead placement for 12-lead ST segment monitoring. Limb electrodes must be located as close as possible to the junction of the limb and the torso. To ensure an inferior view of the myocardium, the left leg *(LL)* electrode must be placed well below the level of the umbilicus. For V_1, the electrode is located at the fourth intercostal space to the right of the sternum. V_2 is in the same fourth intercostal space just to the left of the sternum, and V_4 is in the fifth intercostal space on the midclavicular line. Placement of lead V_3 is halfway on a straight line between leads V_2 and V_4. Leads V_5 and V_6 are positioned on a straight line from V_4, with V_5 in the anterior axillary line and V_6 in the midaxillary line. *RA*, right arm; *LA*, left arm; *RL*, right leg.

Procedure continues on following page

Procedure   for Continuous ST-Segment Monitoring—*Continued*

Steps	Rationale	Special Considerations

4. Clean and slightly abrade the skin where the electrodes will be applied.
  A. Wash the skin with soap and water.
  B. Abrade the skin with a gauze pad.
  C. Ensure that the skin is dry before skin electrodes are applied.
  D. Clipping chest hair may be necessary to ensure that adequate skin contact with the skin electrodes is made. (**Level C***)
	Removes dead skin cells, promoting impulse transmission. Moist skin is not conducive to electrode adherence. Failure to properly prepare the skin may cause artifacts and interfere with interpretation.[4,9,17]	Clipping hair should be done with caution in patients at risk for bleeding. Quality improvement projects have shown that changing skin electrodes daily can reduce artifacts.[4,6]

5. If possible, mark any precordial locations with a black indelible marker.	Ensures that skin electrodes are replaced to the correct location to maintain consistent lead locations.	Continuous ST-segment monitoring trends depend on stable electrode placement. Sudden changes in ST-segment trends often indicate electrode movement.
6. Remove the backing from the pregelled electrodes and assess the center of the pads for moistness.	Gel should be moist to allow for maximal impulse transmission.	Skin electrodes should be stored in a dry area and not exposed to direct sunlight because this can dry out the conductive gel.
7. Connect the ECG leads to the electrodes before placing the electrodes on the patient.	Prepares the monitoring system and prevents unnecessary pressure on the patient's chest when connecting the lead wires to the electrodes.	
8. Select the monitoring leads.	Although any ECG lead can be used for ST-segment monitoring, monitoring of all 12 ECG leads or the selection of a lead or leads based on the myocardial zone at risk is desirable (e.g., inferior or anterior).[9]	If continuous 12-lead ECG monitoring is unavailable, lead-specific ischemia monitoring is encouraged. Lead III is sensitive to inferior ischemia, and V_3 is sensitive to anterior or posterior ischemia.[9,10]
9. If required by the bedside monitor manufacturer, identify the ECG complex landmarks and select the J point + 60-ms landmark.[9,10] (**Level M***)	Prepares the monitoring system and ensures accurate monitoring.	Refer to manufacturer's recommendations.
10. Set the ST-segment alarm.	Maximizes the sensitivity and specificity of ST-segment monitoring and may reduce unnecessary false alarms.	For bedside cardiac monitoring, the alarm threshold should be set 1–2 mm above and below the patient's baseline ST-segment level (Fig. 56-6).[9,10] Recently, a wider threshold of 2 mm for triggering an alarm has been used to reduce false positives and alarm fatigue. Establishing a patient-specific ST-segment level, rather than an isoelectric ST-segment level, is important because the patient's baseline ST-segment level is rarely isoelectric.[9,10,13]

*Level C: Qualitative studies, descriptive or correlational studies, integrative reviews, systematic reviews, or randomized controlled trials with inconsistent results.
*Level M: Manufacturer's recommendations only.

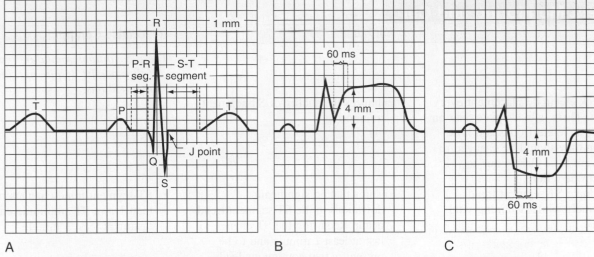

Figure 56-6   A, Normal electrocardiograph complex. Measurement points used in ST-segment analysis are indicated. The PR segment is used to identify the isoelectric line. The ST segment begins at the J point, which is the end of the QRS complex. The ST-segment measurement point can be measured at 60 or 80 ms past the J point. **B,** ST-segment elevation. The ST segment shown measures +4 mm. **C,** ST-segment depression. The ST segment shown measures −4 mm. *(Adapted from Tisdale LA, Drew BJ: ST segment monitoring for myocardial ischemia,* AACN Clin Issues Crit Care Nurs *4:36, 1993.)*

Procedure for Continuous ST-Segment Monitoring—*Continued*

Steps	Rationale	Special Considerations
11. Print the baseline ECG tracing to evaluate the quality of the signal and secure for future reference.	Ensures a quality baseline ECG for comparing subsequent changes because ST-segment monitoring is based on continuous trending.	Verify that lead wires are not reversed, especially the limb leads.
12. If possible, obtain an ECG with the patient in right- and left-side–lying positions and secure these for future reference.	Comparison of side-lying ECGs with ECGs from subsequent alarms may prevent interpreting as ischemia false-positive ST-segment deviations caused by changes in body position.[1,8,18]	
13. Remove **PE** and discard used supplies in appropriate receptacles.	Reduces the transmission of microorganisms; Standard Precautions.	
14. **HH**		

Expected Outcomes

- Accurate ECG monitoring that allows clinicians to detect and interpret ST-segment changes
- Timely detection of myocardial ischemia
- An increase in the number of bedside alarms when the ST-segment software is initiated which may be caused by actual ischemia, body-position changes, transient dysrhythmias, heart rate changes, artifacts, or lead misplacement[13]

Unexpected Outcomes

- Altered skin integrity
- Alternating current (AC) interference, also called 60-cycle interference (see Fig. 54-9)
- Wandering baseline (see Fig. 54-10)
- Artifacts (see Fig. 54-11)
- Inappropriate diagnosis of ischemia in nonischemic conditions (i.e., bundle-branch block, early repolarization)[20]
- Inappropriate intervention based on a false ST-segment alarm[8]

Procedure continues on following page

Patient Monitoring and Care

Steps	Rationale	Reportable Conditions
		These conditions should be reported if they persist despite nursing interventions.
1. Check electrode placement every shift. There is inadequate data on disposable electrodes and how often they should be changed to prevent false alarms due to electrode failure.	Enhances the quality of ST-segment monitoring.	
2. Evaluate ST-segment trends routinely while obtaining vital signs.	Ensures that no significant deviations in the ST-segment trend occur. Requiring the ST change to last at least 1 minute and to be present in two contiguous leads may drastically reduce the number of false ST-segment monitor alarms. Contiguous (side-by-side) leads in the limb leads, should be defined using the following sequence: aVL, I, minus aVR, II, aVF, III. ST changes in two of these side-by-side leads would meet the criteria for ischemia.	• ST-segment trend changes more than 1 mm ST amplitude change lasting at least 1 minute[8]
3. Interpret all ST-segment alarms and determine the cause. If actual ischemia is noted, assess the patient for signs and symptoms that suggest acute ischemia, anginal equivalents, hemodynamic changes, or dysrhythmias, and then obtain a 12-lead ECG.	Ensures accurate interpretation. A 12-lead resting ECG assists with determining ischemia location and type (i.e., supply versus demand). Determines the patient's response to ischemia.	• ST-segment changes • Onset of symptoms or anginal equivalent
4. Assess the patient for signs and symptoms that suggest acute ischemia, even if no new ST-segment changes are identified, and obtain a 12-lead ECG as needed.	Determines the presence of ischemia. Because ischemia can be clinically silent, a 12-lead ECG assists with determining ischemia location and type (i.e., supply versus demand).	• ST-segment changes • Onset of symptoms or anginal equivalent
5. Follow institutional standards for assessing pain. Administer analgesia and nitrates as prescribed.	Identifies need for pain interventions.	• Continued pain despite pain interventions

Documentation

Documentation should include the following:
- Patient and family education
- Initiation of ST-segment bedside monitoring
- Initial ECG strip with baseline ST segment
- Any ST-segment changes or any symptoms that suggest acute ischemia

- Presence and intensity of chest pain or anginal equivalent, interventions, and effectiveness
- Additional interventions taken
- Unexpected outcomes

References and Additional Readings

For a complete list of references and additional readings for this procedure, scan this QR code with any freely available smartphone code reader app, or visit http://booksite.elsevier.com/9780323376624.

PROCEDURE

57

Twelve-Lead Electrocardiogram

Shu-Fen Wung

PURPOSE: A 12-lead electrocardiogram (ECG) provides information about the electrical activity of the heart from 12 different views or leads. The ECG is the most commonly performed cardiovascular diagnostic procedure.[1] Common uses of a 12-lead ECG include diagnosis of acute coronary syndromes, identification of arrhythmias, and determination of the effects of medications, electrolytes, or structural abnormalities on the electrical system of the heart.

PREREQUISITE NURSING KNOWLEDGE

- Understanding of the anatomy and physiology of the cardiovascular system, principles of electrophysiology, ECG lead placement, basic rhythm interpretation, and electrical safety is necessary.
- Advanced cardiac life support (ACLS) knowledge and skills are needed.
- A 12-lead ECG provides different views or leads of the electrical activity of the heart. The 12 standard leads include six limb leads (I, II, III, augmented vector right [aVR], augmented vector foot [aVF], and augmented vector left [aVL]), and six chest leads (V_1 to V_6).
- The limb leads view the heart from the frontal or vertical plane (Fig. 57-1), and the chest leads view the heart from the horizontal plane (Fig. 57-2).
- The basic ECG waveforms are labeled with P, Q, R, S, and T waves, which represent electrical activity within the heart.
- Accuracy in identification of anatomical landmarks for location of electrode sites and knowledge of the importance of accurate electrode placement are needed. Accurate ECG interpretation is possible only when the recording electrodes are placed in the proper positions. Slight alterations of the electrode positions may distort significantly the appearance of the ECG waveforms and can lead to misdiagnosis.[2] Reliable comparison of serial (more than two ECGs recorded at different times) ECG recordings relies on accurate and consistent electrode placement. An indelible marker is recommended for clear identification of the electrode locations to ensure that the same electrode locations are selected when serial ECGs are recorded.
- Nurses should be aware of body-positional changes that can alter ECG recordings. Serial ECGs should be recorded with the patient in a supine position to ensure that all recordings are done in a consistent manner. Side-lying positions and elevation of the torso may change the position of the heart within the chest and can change the waveforms on the ECG recording.[3,4] If a position other than supine is clinically necessary, notation of the altered position should be made on the tracing.

- Nurses should be able to operate the 12-lead ECG machine. Calibration of 1 mV equals 10 mm and paper speed of 25 mm/sec are standards used in clinical practice. For ST-segment analysis, filter settings of 0.05 to 100 Hz are recommended by the American Heart Association.[5] Any variation used for particular clinical purposes should be noted on the tracing. Specific information regarding configuring the ECG machine, troubleshooting, and safety features is available from the manufacturer and should be read before use of the equipment.
- Nurses should be able to interpret recorded ECGs for the presence or absence of myocardial ischemia/infarction and arrhythmias so that patients can be treated appropriately.
- Advances in technology have allowed for online or wireless transmission, networking capabilities, and computerized interpretation of the 12-lead ECG (Fig. 57-3). The 12-lead ECG cable is attached to a processing device that digitizes the 12-lead ECG recording and transfers the information to the wireless device, which transmits the information to the medical record. This increases access to the 12-lead ECG for review and can assist with rapid interpretation and treatment of the patient.

EQUIPMENT

- 12-lead ECG machine with patient cable and lead wires
- ECG electrodes

Additional equipment, to have available as needed, includes the following:

- Gauze pads or terrycloth washcloth
- Cleansing pads or nonemollient soap and water
- Skin preparation solution (e.g., skin barrier wipe or tincture of benzoin)
- Indelible marker
- Clippers or scissors to clip hair from the patient's chest if needed

PATIENT AND FAMILY EDUCATION

- Describe the procedure and reasons for obtaining the 12-lead electrocardiogram. Reassure the patient that the procedure is painless. ***Rationale:*** This communication

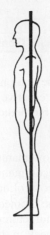

Figure 57-1   Vertical plane leads: I, II, III, aVR, aVL, aVF.

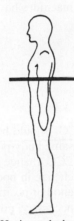

Figure 57-2   Horizontal plane leads: V₁ to V₆.

clarifies information, reduces anxiety, and gains cooperation from the patient.

- Explain the patient's role in assisting with the ECG recording and emphasize actions that improve the quality of the ECG tracing, such as relaxing, avoiding conversation and body movement, and breathing normally. *Rationale:* This explanation ensures the patient's cooperation to improve the quality of the tracing and avoids unnecessary repeating of the ECG because of muscle artifact.

PATIENT ASSESSMENT AND PREPARATION

Patient Assessment

- Interpret previously recorded ECGs. *Rationale:* Each patient has an individual baseline ECG. Previous ECG

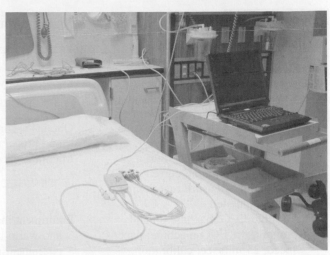

Figure 57-3   Example of a wireless electrocardiograph (ECG) device. The 12-lead cable is attached to a processing device that can then be transmitted to the medical record.

recordings can help clinicians determine whether a change is acute or chronic.

- Assess for the presence of anginal symptoms, such as chest pain, pressure, tightness, heaviness, fullness, or squeezing sensation; radiated pain; or shortness of breath, nausea, and extreme fatigue. *Rationale:* This evaluation correlates ECG changes with patient symptoms.
- Assess the patient's history of cardiac conditions and review medication history. *Rationale:* Knowledge about the patient's cardiac history and medications can help in interpretation of ECG recordings.

Patient Preparation

- Verify that the patient is the correct patient using two identifiers. *Rationale:* Before performing a procedure, the nurse should ensure the correct identification of the patient for the intended intervention.
- Ensure that the patient and family understand preprocedural teaching. Answer questions as they arise, and reinforce information as needed. *Rationale:* This communication evaluates and reinforces the understanding of previously taught information.
- Assist the patient to the supine position and expose the patient's torso while maintaining the patient's modesty. *Rationale:* This position enables the recording of a standard 12-lead ECG and allows comparison of serial ECGs and comparison with standard waveforms. Body-positional changes, such as elevation and rotation, can change recorded amplitudes and axes.

Procedure for 12-Lead Electrocardiogram

Steps	Rationale	Special Considerations
1. 🅷🅷		
2. Check cables and lead wires for fraying or broken wires.	Detects faulty equipment.	If the equipment is damaged, obtain alternative equipment and notify a biomedical engineer for repair.
3. Check the lead wires for accurate labels.	Obtains accurate ECG recordings and proper placement of leads.	
4. Plug the ECG machine into a grounded alternating current (AC) wall outlet or ensure functioning if battery operated.	Maintains electrical safety.	Follow manufacturer's recommendations and institutional protocol on electrical safety per the biomedical department.
5. Turn the ECG machine on and program the ECG machine: paper speed, 25 mm/sec; calibration, 10 mm/mV; filter settings, 0.05–100 Hz. **(Level E*)**	Equipment may require self-test and warm-up time. Verify equipment settings in accordance with clinical practice and recommendations by the American Heart Association (AHA).[5] Multichannel machines may require input of information (e.g., data about the patient) to store the ECG appropriately.	Manufacturers provide a calibration check in the machine to identify the sensitivity setting. Most machines have automatic settings.
6. 🅿🅴		
7. Place the patient in a supine position. **(Level B*)**	Provides adequate support for limbs so that muscle activity is minimal. Body-position changes can cause ST-segment deviation and QRS waveform alteration.[3,4,6]	ECGs should be recorded in the same body position to ensure ECG changes are not caused by a change in body position. If another position is clinically necessary, note the altered position on the ECG recording.
8. Expose only the necessary body parts of the patient (legs, arms, and chest) for electrode placement.	Provides privacy and warmth, which reduces shivering.	Ensuring privacy may reduce anxiety. Shivering may interfere with the quality of recording.
9. Identify skin electrode locations. A. Limb leads (Fig. 57-4).	Ensures the accuracy of the lead placement.	

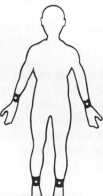

Figure 57-4   Limb lead placement in 12-lead ECG.

---

*Level B: Well-designed, controlled studies with results that consistently support a specific action, intervention, or treatment.

*Level E: Multiple case reports, theory-based evidence from expert opinions, or peer-reviewed professional organizational standards without clinical studies to support recommendations.

Procedure	for 12-Lead Electrocardiogram—*Continued*	
Steps	**Rationale**	**Special Considerations**

• Right arm (RA): inside right forearm
• Left arm (LA): inside left forearm
• Right leg (RL): anywhere on the body; by convention, usually on the right ankle or inner aspect of the calf
• Left leg (LL): left ankle or inner aspect of the calf
 	
B. Precordial Leads (Fig. 57-5)
• Identify the sternal notch. Slide fingers down the center of the sternum to the obvious bony prominence, angle of Louis, which identifies the second rib and provides a landmark for noting the second intercostal space (ICS).
  ❖ V$_1$: fourth ICS at right sternal border
  ❖ V$_2$: fourth ICS at left sternal border
  ❖ V$_4$: fifth ICS at midclavicular line
  ❖ V$_3$: halfway between V$_2$ and V$_4$
  ❖ V$_5$: horizontal level to V$_4$ at the anterior axillary line
  ❖ V$_6$: horizontal level to V$_4$ at the midaxillary line
	Accurate electrode placement is essential for obtaining valid and reliable data for ECG recordings. The RL electrode is a ground electrode that does not contribute to the ECG tracings.
	
	The angle of Louis assists with identifying the second rib for correct placement of precordial leads in the appropriate ICS. Slight alterations in the position of any of the precordial leads may alter the ECG significantly and can affect diagnosis and treatment.[2,7,8]
		Limb leads should be placed in fleshy areas; bony prominences should be avoided. The limb leads need to be placed equidistant from the heart and should be positioned in approximately the same place on each limb.
		
		Variations in precordial lead placement of as little as 2 cm can result in important diagnostic errors, particularly in anteroseptal infarction and ventricular hypertrophy.[6]
		If precordial leads cannot be accurately placed because of chest wounds, placement of defibrillator pads, or other reasons, the alternative site should be clearly documented on the ECG.[9]
		It is recommended that electrodes be placed under the breast in women until additional studies are available.[5]

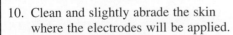

Figure 57-5 Precordial or chest lead placement.

10. Clean and slightly abrade the skin where the electrodes will be applied. A. Wash the skin with soap and water, if needed. B. Abrade the skin with a gauze pad or abrader. C. Ensure that the skin is dry before skin electrodes are applied. D. Clipping of chest hair may be necessary to ensure that adequate skin contact with the skin electrodes is made. **(Level C*)**	Removes dead skin cells, promoting impulse transmission.[10-12] Moist skin is not conducive to electrode adherence.	Failure to properly prepare the skin may cause artifacts and interfere with interpretation.

*Level C: Qualitative studies, descriptive or correlational studies, integrative reviews, systematic reviews, or randomized controlled trials with inconsistent results.

Procedure continues on following page

Procedure	**for 12-Lead Electrocardiogram—*Continued***	
Steps	**Rationale**	**Special Considerations**
11. Identify the electrode sites and mark them with an indelible marker.	Minimizes ECG changes caused by altered electrode placement.[2,6]	After accurate identification of the locations, an indelible marker should be used to mark the electrode sites if serial ECGs are anticipated.
12. For pregelled electrodes, remove the backing and test for moistness. For adhesive electrodes, remove the backing and check each adhesive pad, as each should be sticky or moist.	Allows for appropriate conduction of impulses.	Gel must be moist. If pregelled electrodes are not moist or adhesive electrodes are not sticky, replace the electrodes.
13. Apply the electrodes securely and place the electrodes on the marked locations.	Electrodes must be secure to prevent external influences from affecting the ECG. Secure the electrodes to obtain quality ECG recordings.	If limb plate electrodes are used, do not overtighten to minimize discomfort.
14. Fasten the lead wires to the limb electrodes, avoiding bending or strain on the wires, and use the correct lead-to-electrode connection.	Provides for correct lead-to-limb connection.	
15. Identify the multiple-channel machine recording setting (Fig. 57-6).	Multiple-channel machines run several leads simultaneously and can be set to run leads in different configurations.	

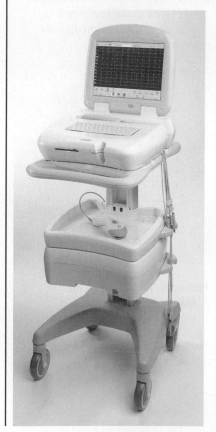

Figure 57-6 Multiple-channel ECG machine. (*Courtesy Philips Medical Systems, Andover, MA.*)

Procedure for 12-Lead Electrocardiogram—*Continued*

Steps	Rationale	Special Considerations
16. Obtain a 12-lead ECG recording. Most systems record each lead for 3–6 seconds and automatically mark the correct lead.	Three to six seconds are all that is needed for a permanent record; a longer strip may be obtained if a rhythm strip is needed.	A multiple-channel machine runs the limb and chest leads simultaneously.
17. Examine the quality of the 12-lead ECG tracing.	While the patient is still connected to the machine, the nurse should examine the ECG to see whether any leads need to be repeated.	Reviews the normal conduction sequence and identifies abnormalities that may necessitate further evaluation or treatment.
18. Disconnect the equipment; clean the gel off the patient (if necessary), remove **PE**, discard used supplies, and prepare the equipment for future use.	Increases patient comfort. Reduces the transmission of microorganisms; Standard Precautions.	Some pregelled electrodes can be left in place for repeat ECGs. Follow the manufacturer's directions and hospital policy for electrode use and removal in these cases.
19. **HH**		

Expected Outcomes

- A clear and accurate 12-lead ECG recording that allows clinicians to diagnose dysrhythmias and ischemia (Fig. 57-7)
- Prompt identification of abnormalities

Unexpected Outcomes

- Altered skin integrity
- Inaccurate lead placement or connection (Fig. 57-8)
- AC interference, also called 60-cycle interference (see Fig. 54-9)
- Wandering baseline (see Fig. 54-10)
- Artifact or waveform interference (see Fig. 54-11)

Procedure continues on following page

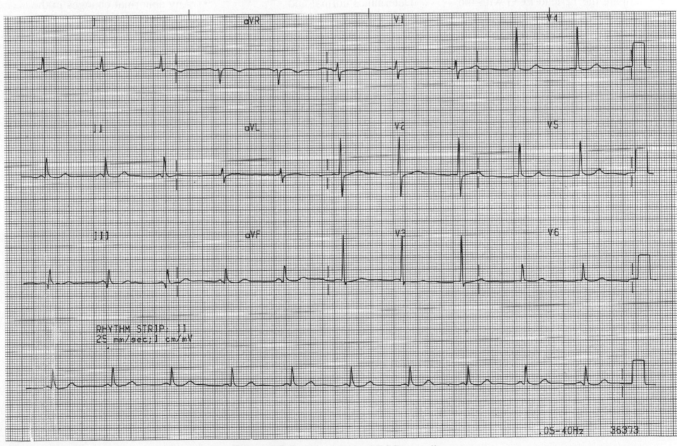

Figure 57-7 Clear 12-lead ECG recording.

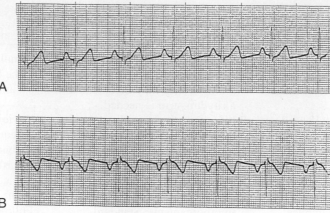

Figure 57-8   Limb lead reversal on 12-lead electrocardiograph (ECG) in lead I. **A,** Correct placement. **B,** Incorrect placement.

Patient Monitoring and Care

Steps	Rationale	Reportable Conditions
		These conditions should be reported if they persist despite nursing interventions.
1. Obtain a 12-lead ECG as prescribed and as needed (e.g., for angina or arrhythmias).	Provides determination of myocardial ischemia, injury, and infarction. Aids in diagnosis of arrhythmias.	• Angina • Arrhythmias • Abnormal 12-lead ECG
2. Compare the 12-lead ECG with the previous 12-lead ECGs.	Determines normal and abnormal findings.	• Any abnormal changes in the 12-lead ECG
3. Follow institutional standards for assessing pain. Administer analgesia and nitrates as prescribed.	Promotes comfort.	• Continued pain despite pain interventions

Documentation

Documentation should include the following:

- Patient and family education
- The fact that a 12-lead ECG was obtained
- The reason for the 12-lead ECG
- Any altered lead placement and reason
- Symptoms that the patient experienced (e.g., chest pain, syncope, dizziness, or palpitations)

- Pain assessment, interventions, and patient response to interventions
- Follow-up to the 12-lead ECG as indicated
- Unexpected outcomes
- Additional interventions

References and Additional Readings

For a complete list of references and additional readings for this procedure, scan this QR code with any freely available smartphone code reader app, or visit http://booksite.elsevier.com/9780323376624.

PROCEDURE

58   Arterial Catheter Insertion AP (Perform)

Hillary Crumlett and Alex Johnson

> **PURPOSE:** Arterial catheters are used for continuous monitoring of blood pressure, assessment of cardiovascular effects of vasoactive drugs, and frequent arterial blood gas and laboratory sampling. In addition, arterial catheters provide access to blood samples that support the diagnostics related to oxygen, carbon dioxide, and bicarbonate levels (oxygenation, ventilation, and acid-base status).

PREREQUISITE NURSING KNOWLEDGE

- Knowledge of anatomy and physiology of the vasculature and adjacent structures is needed.
- Nurses must be adequately prepared to insert arterial catheters. This preparation should include specific educational content about arterial catheter insertion and opportunities to demonstrate clinical competency.
- Knowledge of the principles of sterile technique is essential.
- Understanding the principles of hemodynamic monitoring is necessary.
- Clinical competence in suturing is needed.
- Conditions that warrant the use of arterial pressure monitoring include patients with the following:
  - ❖ Frequent blood sampling:
    - ○ Respiratory conditions requiring arterial blood gas monitoring (oxygenation, ventilation, acid-base status)
    - ○ Bleeding, actual or potential
    - ○ Electrolyte or glycemic abnormalities, actual or potential
    - ○ Metabolic abnormalities (acid-base, tissue perfusion), actual or potential
    - ○ Monitoring serum levels related to therapeutic interventions (renal replacement therapy, chemotherapy, biotherapy, apheresis therapy, etc.)
  - ❖ Continuous blood pressure monitoring:
    - ○ Hypotension or hypertension
    - ○ Shock: cardiogenic, septic, hypovolemic, neurogenic

- ○ Mechanical cardiovascular support
- ○ Vasoactive medication administration
- Noninvasive indirect blood pressure measurements determined with auscultation of Korotkoff sounds distal to an occluding cuff consistently average 10 to 20 mm Hg lower than simultaneous direct measurement.[11]
- Arterial waveform inspection can help with rapid diagnosis of the presence of valvular disorders, and determine the effects of dysrhythmias on perfusion, the effects of the respiratory cycle on blood pressure, and the effects of intraaortic balloon pump therapy or ventricular assist device therapy on blood pressure.
- The most common complications associated with arterial puncture include pain, vasospasm (artery spasm), hematoma formation, thrombosis, embolism, infection, hemorrhage, vascular insufficiency, ischemia, direct nerve trauma, and fistula formation.[3] It has been found that major complications occurred in less than 1% of patients with arterial catheters, regardless of site selection.[17] Arterial catheter sites are a source of bloodstream infections, with the femoral site being more heavily associated with colonization compared with other sites. The infective potential of the arterial catheter is equivalent to the short-term central venous device regarding colonization and bloodstream infections, and should be assessed together for signs and symptoms of infection.[8]
- Causes of failure to cannulate the artery include a tangential approach to the artery, tortuosity of the artery, arterial spasm, and impingement of the needle tip on the posterior wall.[18]
- Site selection should include the following considerations:
  - ❖ The preferred artery for arterial catheter insertion is the radial artery.[12] Although this artery is smaller than the ulnar artery, it is more superficial and can be more easily stabilized during the procedure.[8] Conduct a modified Allen's test before performing an arterial puncture

AP   This procedure should be performed only by physicians, advanced practice nurses, and other healthcare professionals (including critical care nurses) with additional knowledge, skills, and demonstrated competence per professional licensure or institutional standard.

on the radial artery (see Fig. 81-3). Normal palmar blushing is complete before 7 seconds, indicating a positive result; 8 to 14 seconds is considered equivocal; and 15 or more seconds indicates a negative test result. Doppler flow studies or plethysmography can also be performed to ensure the presence of collateral flow. Research shows these studies to be more reliable than the modified Allen's test.[1,18] Thrombosis of the arterial cannula is a possible complication. Ensuring collateral flow distal to the puncture site is important for prevention of ischemia. Puncture of both the radial and ulnar arteries on the same hand is never recommended, to prevent compromising blood supply to the hand.[4,13]

❖ The brachial artery is a potential insertion site. Before use of this site consider that the brachial artery is the main artery supplying the arm; it branches into the radial and ulnar arteries, and it has no collateral circulation.[16] Hemostasis after arterial cannulation is enhanced by its proximity to the bone if the entry point is approximately 1.5 inches above the antecubital fossa.

❖ Use the femoral artery in the case of cardiopulmonary arrest or altered perfusion to the upper extremities. The femoral artery is a large superficial artery located in the groin. It is easily palpated and punctured; however, risk is associated with accessing the arterial vessel due to the proximity of the femoral artery to the femoral vein (see Fig. 81-2). Complications related to femoral artery puncture include hemorrhage and hematoma formation (because bleeding can be difficult to control), inadvertent puncture of the femoral vein (because of its close proximity to the artery), infection (because aseptic techniques are difficult to maintain in the groin area), and limb ischemia (if the femoral artery is damaged).

❖ The dorsalis pedis and posterior tibial arteries are typically avoided when selecting an arterial catheter site; however, they may be considered because they are supported by collateral circulation, which can prevent an ischemic injury.[9] The dorsalis pedis is typically avoided due to the risk of dislodgement and inability to secure the catheter well. The posterior tibial artery has been associated with ischemic injuries that have resulted in amputation.[16]

• In adults, the use of the radial, brachial, or dorsalis pedis sites is preferred over the femoral or axillary sites of insertion to reduce the risk of infection.[12,15]

• Ultrasound guidance is recommended to place arterial catheters if the technology is available.[12]

EQUIPMENT

• 2-inch, 20-gauge, nontapered Teflon cannula-over-needle or prepackaged kit that includes a 6-inch, 18-gauge Teflon catheter with appropriate introducer and guidewire (or the specific catheter for the intended insertion site)
• Pressure module and cable for interface with the monitor
• Pressure transducer system, including flush solution recommended according to institutional standards, a pressure bag or device, pressure tubing with transducer, and flush device (see Procedure 75)
• Dual-channel recorder

• Nonsterile gloves, head covering, goggles, and mask
• Sterile gloves and large sterile fenestrated drape
• Skin antiseptic solution (e.g., 2% chlorhexidine-based preparation)
• Sterile 4 × 4 gauze pads
• Transparent occlusive dressing
• 1% lidocaine without epinephrine, 1 to 2 mL
• Sterile sodium chloride 0.9%
• 3-mL syringe with 25-gauge needle
• Sheet protector
• Bedside ultrasound machine with vascular probe
• Sterile ultrasound probe cover
• Sterile ultrasound gel

Additional equipment, to have available as needed, includes the following:
• Sterile gown and full drape
• Bath towel
• Small wrist board
• Sutureless securement device
• Chlorhexidine-impregnated sponge
• Additional transparent adhesive dressing with tapes (if dressing has no tape, consider the use of $\frac{1}{2}$-inch Steri-Strips)
• Transducer holder, intravenous pole, and laser lever for pole-mounted arterial catheter transducers
• Suture material

PATIENT AND FAMILY EDUCATION

• Explain the procedure and the purpose of the arterial catheter. *Rationale:* This explanation decreases patient and family anxiety.
• Explain to the patient that the procedure may be uncomfortable but that a local anesthetic will be used first to alleviate most of the discomfort. *Rationale:* Patient cooperation is elicited, and insertion is facilitated.
• Explain the patient's role in assisting with catheter insertion. *Rationale:* This explanation elicits patient cooperation and facilitates insertion.

PATIENT ASSESSMENT AND PREPARATION
Patient Assessment

• Obtain the patient's medical history, including history of diabetes, hypertension, peripheral vascular disease, vascular grafts, arterial vasospasm, thrombosis, or embolism. Obtain the patient's history of coronary artery bypass graft surgery in which radial arteries were removed for use as conduits or presence of arteriovenous fistulas or shunts. *Rationale:* Extremities with any of these problems should be avoided as sites for cannulation because of the potential for complications. Patients with diabetes mellitus or hypertension are at higher risk for arterial or venous insufficiency. Previously removed radial arteries are a contraindication for ulnar artery cannulation.
• Assess the patient's medical history of coagulopathies, use of anticoagulant therapy, vascular abnormalities, or peripheral neuropathies. *Rationale:* This assessment assists in determining the safety of the procedure and aids in site selection.

- Assess the patient's allergy history (e.g., allergy to lidocaine, topical anesthetic cream, antiseptic solutions, or tape). *Rationale:* This assessment decreases the risk for allergic reactions.
- Assess the patient's current anticoagulation therapy, known blood dyscrasias, and pertinent laboratory values (e.g., platelet levels, partial thromboplastin time, prothrombin time, and international normalized ratio) before the procedure. *Rationale:* Anticoagulation therapy, blood dyscrasias, or alterations in coagulation studies could increase the risk for hematoma formation or hemorrhage.
- Assess the intended insertion site for the presence of a strong pulse. *Rationale:* Identification and localization of the pulse increases the chance of a successful arterial cannulation.
- Presence of collateral flow to the area distal to the arterial catheter should be evaluated before the artery is cannulated. For radial arterial lines, a modified Allen's test should be performed. *Rationale:* This assessment determines the presence of collateral flow to the hand to reduce vascular complications including ischemia.
- If available, assess the intended artery with a Doppler ultrasound scan. *Rationale:* This assessment aids in determination of the patency of the artery and blood flow.[1,2] Identification and localization of the artery to be cannulated increases the chance of a successful cannulization and reduces the complication rate and need for multiple attempts at placement.[14]

Patient Preparation

- Verify that the patient is the correct patient using two identifiers. *Rationale:* Before performing a procedure, the nurse should ensure the correct identification of the patient for the intended intervention.
- Perform a preprocedure verification and time out, if nonemergent. *Rationale:* Ensures patient safety.
- Ensure that the patient and family understand preprocedural teaching. Answer questions as they arise and reinforce information as needed. *Rationale:* Understanding of previously taught information is evaluated and reinforced.
- Obtain informed consent. *Rationale:* Informed consent protects the rights of the patient and makes a competent decision possible for the patient; however, in emergency circumstances, time may not allow the form to be signed.
- Place the patient supine with the head of the bed at a comfortable position. The limb into which the arterial catheter will be inserted should be resting comfortably on the bed. *Rationale:* This placement provides patient comfort and facilitates insertion.
- If the radial artery is selected, position the hand to allow for palpation of the artery (a pillow or towel may be used to support the wrist). *Rationale:* This placement positions the arm and brings the artery closer to the surface.
- If the brachial artery is selected, elevate and hyperextend the patient's arm and palpate the artery (a pillow or towel may be used to support the arm). *Rationale:* This action increases accessibility of the artery.
- If the femoral artery is selected, position the patient supine with the head of the bed at a comfortable angle. The patient's leg should be straight with the femoral area easily accessible and palpate the artery (a small towel may be needed to support the hip in some cases). *Rationale:* This position is the best for localizing the femoral artery pulse.

Procedure	for Performing Arterial Catheter Insertion	
Steps	**Rationale**	**Special Considerations**
1. Obtain ultrasound equipment.	Prepares equipment.	Assistance may be needed from radiology.
2. Ensure that a single-pressure transducer system is prepared (see Procedure 75).	Prepares equipment.	
3. **HH**		
4. **PE**		
5. Place a waterproof pad under the selected site.	Avoids soiling of bed linens.	
6. Determine the anatomy of the artery. **(Level E*)**	Helps ensure proper placement of the arterial catheter and guides the area to be prepped.[12]	

*Level E: Multiple case reports, theory-based evidence from expert opinions, or peer-reviewed professional organizational standards without clinical studies to support recommendations.

Procedure continues on following page

Procedure	for Performing Arterial Catheter Insertion—*Continued*	
Steps	**Rationale**	**Special Considerations**
7. If the radial artery is to be used, the modified Allen's test should be performed before arterial catheter insertion (see Fig. 81-3). **(Level C*)**	Although evidence is found in support of and against the use of the modified Allen's test, the test can be performed before a radial artery puncture in an attempt to assess the patency of the ulnar artery and to assess for an intact superficial palmar arch.[3–5,7,13,14]	The modified Allen's test does not always ensure adequate flow through the ulnar artery. A Doppler ultrasound flow indicator can also be used to further verify blood flow.[1,5]
A. With the patient's hand held overhead, instruct the patient to open and close the hand several times.	Forces the blood from the hand.	
B. With the patient's fist clenched, apply direct pressure on both the radial and the ulnar arteries.	Obstructs the flow of blood to the hand.	If the patient is unconscious or unable to perform the procedure, clench the fist passively for the patient.
C. Instruct the patient to lower and open the hand.	Allows observation for pallor.	Performed passively if the patient is unconscious or unable to assist.
D. While maintaining pressure on the radial artery, release the pressure over the ulnar artery and observe the hand for the return of color.	Return of color within 7 seconds indicates patency of the ulnar artery and an intact superficial palmar arch; this is interpreted as normal Allen's test results. If color returns between 8 and 14 seconds, the test is considered equivocal and the healthcare provider must consider the risk and benefits of continuing with performing this procedure. If 15 or more seconds are needed for color to return, test results are considered abnormal and another site should be considered.	If the test results are abnormal, the modified Allen's test should be performed on the opposite hand. If results for both hands are abnormal, consider use of a site other than the radial arteries.
8. **HH**		
9. **PE**	Reduces the transmission of microorganisms.	
10. Prepare the site with the antiseptic solution (e.g., 2% chlorhexidine-based preparation).	Limits the introduction of potentially infectious skin flora into the vessel during the puncture.	
A. Cleanse the site with a back-and-forth motion while applying friction for 30 seconds.		
B. Allow the antiseptic solution to dry.		
11. Remove gloves and perform **HH**		
12. Open the arterial cannula insertion kit.	Prepares for the procedure.	
13. Apply sterile gloves.	Arterial catheter insertion is a sterile procedure.	Personnel protective equipment (e.g., head cover, mask, goggles) is needed as well as sterile equipment. If the arterial catheter will be placed in a femoral artery, a sterile gown should be worn.[15]

*Level C: Qualitative studies, descriptive or correlational studies, integrative reviews, systematic reviews, or randomized controlled trials with inconsistent results.

Procedure	for Performing Arterial Catheter Insertion—*Continued*	
Steps	**Rationale**	**Special Considerations**
14. Drape the area around the site with sterile drapes.	Provides a sterile field and minimizes the transmission of organisms.	A large sterile fenestrated drape should be used during peripheral arterial catheter insertion.[12,15] Maximal sterile barrier precautions should be used for femoral artery catheter insertion.[12,15]
15. Locally anesthetize the puncture site.[4,7,9,10,13] **(Level C*)**	Provides local anesthesia for the arterial puncture.	Most patients experience pain during arterial puncture.[6,7]
A. Use a 1-mL syringe with a 25-gauge needle to draw up 0.5 mL of 1% lidocaine without epinephrine.	Minimizes vessel trauma. Absence of epinephrine decreases the risk for peripheral vasoconstriction.	Medications such as lidocaine ointment, amethocaine gel, and EMLA cream may reduce pain.[8,11,13,19] If these medications are used, manufacturer's recommendations should be followed.
B. Aspirate before injecting the local anesthetic.	Determines whether or not a blood vessel has been inadvertently entered.	
C. Inject intradermally and then with full infiltration around the intended arterial insertion site. Use approximately 0.2–0.3 mL for an adult.	Decreases the incidence of localized pain during injection of all skin layers. Patients report reduced pain when a local intradermal anesthetic agent is used before arterial puncture.	
16. Perform the percutaneous puncture of the selected artery.		Use of ultrasound scan technology may be used to assist with catheter insertion.
A. Palpate and stabilize the artery with the index and middle fingers of the nondominant hand.	Increases the likelihood of correctly locating the artery and decreases the chance of the vessel rolling.	
B. With the needle bevel up and the syringe at a 30-degree to 60-degree angle to the radial or brachial artery, puncture the skin slowly. Adjust the angle to a 60-degree to 90-degree angle to the femoral artery.	A slow, gradual thrust promotes entry into the artery without inadvertently passing through the posterior wall.	
17. Advance the needle and the cannula until a blood return is noted in the hub, then slowly advance the catheter about $\frac{1}{4}$–$\frac{1}{2}$ inch farther to ensure that the cannula is in the artery.	Advancing the cannula farther ensures that the entire cannula is in the artery and not just the tip of the stylet.	
18. If, on initial insertion, a blood return is not noted, a 3-mL syringe may be placed at the end of the cannula. While advancing the catheter, gentle withdrawing of the syringe plunger may be performed in an effort to determine proper placement in the artery.	Some arteries may vasospasm as a result of sudden insertion of the catheter. Taking the time to place a syringe on the catheter and withdrawing slightly during insertion may allow the artery to relax and help to determine whether proper placement within the artery has been achieved.	

*Level C: Qualitative studies, descriptive or correlational studies, integrative reviews, systematic reviews, or randomized controlled trials with inconsistent results.

Procedure continues on following page

Procedure for Performing Arterial Catheter Insertion—*Continued*

Steps	Rationale	Special Considerations
19. Level the catheter to the skin; then continue to advance the cannula to its hub with a steady rotary action.	The rotary action helps to advance the catheter through the skin.	If an over the wire catheter is used, advance the wire completely to the hub and then advance the catheter over the wire.
20. Once positioning is confirmed, remove the stylet and connect the catheter to the single-pressure transducer system and flush the system.	Maintains catheter patency and prepares the system for arterial blood pressure monitoring.	Arterial blood is pulsatile.
21. Observe the arterial waveform.	Confirms arterial catheter placement.	
22. Secure the arterial catheter in place.	Maintains arterial catheter positioning; reduces the chance of accidental dislodgment.	The catheter may be sutured in place, or a sutureless securement device may be used to secure the catheter. Follow institutional standards.
23. Apply an occlusive, sterile dressing to the insertion site.	Reduces the risk for infection.	Follow institutional standards for application of a chlorhexidine-impregnated sponge.
24. Level the air-fluid interface (zeroing stopcock) to the phlebostatic axis, zero the monitoring system, verify the arterial waveform through a square wave test, and activate the alarm system (see Procedure 59).	Prepares the monitoring system.	
25. Remove **PE** and discard used supplies in appropriate receptacles; dispose of needles and other sharp objects in appropriate containers.	Reduces the transmission of microorganisms; Standard Precautions. Safely removes sharp objects.	
26. **HH**		

Expected Outcomes

- Successful cannulation of the artery
- Ability to obtain blood samples from the arterial catheter
- Peripheral vascular and neurovascular systems intact
- Alterations in blood pressure stability identified and treated accordingly

Unexpected Outcomes

- Pain
- Complications of puncture or vasospasm
- Complications after the procedure, such as change in color, temperature, sensation, or movement of the extremity cannulated; hematoma, hemorrhage, infection, or thrombus at the insertion site
- Inability to cannulate the artery

Patient Monitoring and Care

Steps	Rationale	Reportable Conditions
		These conditions should be reported if they persist despite nursing interventions.
1. Observe the insertion site for signs of hemostasis after the procedure.	Postinsertion bleeding can occur in any patient but is more likely to occur in patients with coagulopathies or patients undergoing anticoagulation therapy.	• Bleeding • Hematoma • Changes in vital signs
2. Assess the arterial catheter insertion site and involved extremity for signs of postinsertion complications.[13]	Arterial catheter insertion can result in peripheral vascular and neurovascular compromise of the extremity distal to the puncture site.	• Changes in pulse, color, size, temperature, sensation, or movement in the extremity used for the arterial catheter insertion

Patient Monitoring and Care —*Continued*

Steps	Rationale	Reportable Conditions
3. Ensure that the catheter is clearly labeled as "arterial."	Alerts physicians, advanced practice nurses, and other healthcare professionals that the catheter is arterial not venous.	
4. Assess the arterial catheter insertion site for signs or symptoms of infection.	Determines necessity for catheter removal and further treatment.	• Erythema, warmth, hardness, tenderness, or pain at the arterial line insertion site • Presence of purulent drainage from the arterial line insertion site
5. Follow institutional standards for assessing pain. Administer analgesia as prescribed.	Identifies need for pain interventions.	• Continued pain despite pain interventions

Documentation

Documentation should include the following:
- Patient and family education
- Performance of the modified Allen's test before insertion and its results (when using the radial artery)
- Preprocedure verifications and time out
- Signed consent form
- Arterial site accessed
- Insertion of the arterial catheter (date, time, and initials marked on the dressing itself)
- Size of cannula-over-needle catheter used

- Any difficulties in the insertion; number of attempts
- Patient tolerance of the procedure
- Pain assessment, interventions, and effectiveness
- Appearance of the site
- Appearance of the limb, color, pulse, sensation, movement, capillary refill time, and temperature of the extremity after insertion is complete
- Occurrence of unexpected outcomes
- Nursing interventions taken

References and Additional Readings

For a complete list of references and additional readings for this procedure, scan this QR code with any freely available smartphone code reader app, or visit http://booksite.elsevier.com/9780323376624.

59 Arterial Catheter Insertion (Assist), Care, and Removal

Hillary Crumlett and Alex Johnson

PURPOSE: Arterial catheters are used for continuous monitoring of blood pressure, assessment of cardiovascular effects of vasoactive drugs, and frequent arterial blood gas and laboratory sampling. In addition, arterial catheters provide access to blood samples that support the diagnostics related to oxygen, carbon dioxide, and bicarbonate levels (oxygenation, ventilation, and acid-base status).

PREREQUISITE NURSING KNOWLEDGE

- Knowledge of the anatomy and physiology of the vasculature and adjacent structures is needed.
- Knowledge of the principles of hemodynamic monitoring is necessary.
- Understanding of the principles of aseptic technique is needed.
- Conditions that warrant the use of arterial pressure monitoring include patients with the following:
  - ❖ Frequent blood sampling:
    - ○ Respiratory conditions requiring arterial blood gas monitoring (oxygenation, ventilation, acid-base status)
    - ○ Bleeding, actual or potential
    - ○ Electrolyte or glycemic abnormalities, actual or potential
    - ○ Metabolic abnormalities (acid-base, tissue perfusion), actual or potential
    - ○ Monitoring serum levels related to therapeutic interventions (renal replacement therapy, chemotherapy, biotherapy, apheresis therapy, etc.)
  - ❖ Continuous blood pressure monitoring:
    - ○ Hypotension or hypertension
    - ○ Shock: cardiogenic, septic, hypovolemic, neurogenic
    - ○ Mechanical cardiovascular support
    - ○ Vasoactive medication administration
- Arterial pressure represents the forcible ejection of blood from the left ventricle into the aorta and out into the arterial system. During ventricular systole, blood is ejected into the aorta, generating a pressure wave. Because of the intermittent pumping action of the heart, this arterial pressure wave is generated in a pulsatile manner (Fig. 59-1). The ascending limb of the aortic pressure wave (anacrotic limb) represents an increase in pressure because of left-ventricular ejection. The peak of this ejection is the peak systolic pressure, which should be less than 120 mm Hg in adults.[21] After reaching this peak, the ventricular pressure declines to a level below aortic pressure and the

aortic valve closes, marking the end of ventricular systole. The closure of the aortic valve produces a small rebound wave that creates a notch known as the dicrotic notch. The descending limb of the curve (diastolic downslope) represents diastole and is characterized by a long declining pressure wave, during which the aortic wall recoils and propels blood into the arterial network. The diastolic pressure is measured as the lowest point of the diastolic downslope, which should be less than 80 mm Hg in adults.[21]
- The difference between the systolic and diastolic pressures is the pulse pressure, with a normal value of about 40 mm Hg.
- Arterial pressure is determined by the relationship between blood flow through the vessels (cardiac output) and the resistance of the vessel walls (systemic vascular resistance). The arterial pressure is therefore affected by any factors that change either cardiac output or systemic vascular resistance.
- The average arterial pressure during a cardiac cycle is called the mean arterial pressure (MAP). MAP is not the average of the systolic plus the diastolic pressures because, during the cardiac cycle, the pressure remains closer to diastole than to systole for a longer period (at normal heart rates). The MAP is calculated automatically by most patient monitoring systems; however, it can be calculated with the following formula:

$$MAP = \frac{(systolic\ pressure) + (diastolic\ pressure \times 2)}{3}$$

- MAP represents the driving force (perfusion pressure) for blood flow through the cardiovascular system. MAP is at its highest point in the aorta. As blood travels through the arterial system away from the aorta, systolic pressure increases and diastolic pressure decreases, with an overall decline in the MAP (Fig. 59-2).
- The location of arterial catheter placement depends on the condition of the arterial vessels and the presence of other catheters (i.e., the presence of a dialysis shunt is a contraindication for placement of an arterial catheter in the same extremity). Once inserted, the arterial catheter causes little

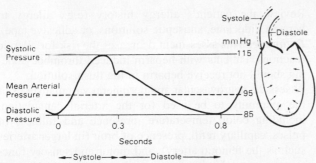

Figure 59-1 The generation of a pulsatile waveform. This is an aortic pressure curve. During systole, the ejected volume distends the aorta and aortic pressure rises. The peak pressure is known as the aortic systolic pressure. After the peak ejection, the ventricular pressure falls; when it drops below the aortic pressure, the aortic valve closes, which is marked by the dicrotic notch, the end of the systole. During diastole, the pressure continues to decline and the aortic wall recoils, pushing blood toward the periphery. The trough of the pressure wave is the diastolic pressure. The difference between the systolic and diastolic pressure is the pulse pressure. *(From Smith JJ, Kampine JP: Circulating physiology. Baltimore, 1980, Williams & Wilkins, 55.)*

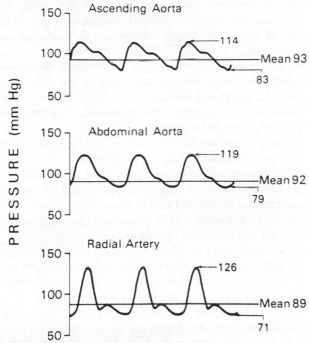

Figure 59-2 Arterial pressure from different sites in the arterial tree. The arterial pressure waveform varies in configuration, depending on the location of the catheter. With transmission of the pressure wave into the distal aorta and large arteries, the systolic pressure increases and the diastolic pressure decreases; with a resulting heightening of the pulse, pressure declines steadily. *(From Smith JJ, Kampine JP: Circulating physiology. Baltimore, 1980, Williams & Wilkins, 57.)*

or no discomfort to the patient and allows continuous blood pressure assessment and intermittent blood sampling. If intraaortic balloon pump therapy is necessary, arterial pressure may be directly monitored from the tip of the balloon catheter in the aorta.

- The radial artery is the most common site for arterial pressure monitoring. When arterial pulse waveforms are recorded from a peripheral site (compared with a central site), the waveform morphology changes. The anacrotic limb becomes more peaked and narrowed, with increased amplitude; therefore, the systolic pressure in peripheral sites is higher than the systolic pressure recorded from a more central site (see Fig. 59-2). In addition, the diastolic pressure decreases, the diastolic downslope may show a secondary wave, and the dicrotic notch becomes less prominent from distal sites.
- Vasodilators and vasoconstrictors may change the appearance of the waveforms from distal sites. Vasodilators may cause the waveform to take on a more central appearance. Vasoconstrictors may cause the systolic pressure to become more exaggerated because of enhanced resistance in the peripheral arteries.
- Several potential complications are associated with arterial pressure monitoring. Infection at the insertion site can develop and cause sepsis. Clot formation in the catheter can lead to arterial embolization. The catheter can cause a pseudoaneurysm or vessel perforation with extravasation of blood and flush solution into the surrounding tissue. Finally, the distal extremity can develop circulatory or neurovascular impairment.
- Ultrasound guidance is recommended to place arterial catheters if the technology is available.[8]

EQUIPMENT

- 2-inch, 20-gauge, nontapered Teflon cannula-over-needle or prepackaged kit that includes a 6-inch, 18-gauge Teflon catheter with appropriate introducer and guidewire (or the specific catheter for the intended insertion site)
- Pressure module and cable for interface with the monitor
- Pressure transducer system, including flush solution recommended according to institutional standards, a pressure bag or device, pressure tubing with transducer, and flush device (see Procedure 75)
- Dual-channel recorder
- Nonsterile gloves, head covering, goggles, and mask
- Sterile gloves and large sterile fenestrated drape
- Skin antiseptic solution (e.g., 2% chlorhexidine-based preparation)
- Sterile 4 × 4 gauze pads
- Transparent occlusive dressing
- 1% lidocaine without epinephrine, 1 to 2 mL
- Sterile sodium chloride 0.9%
- 3-mL syringe with 25-gauge needle
- Sheet protector
- Bedside ultrasound machine with vascular probe
- Sterile ultrasound probe cover
- Sterile ultrasound gel

Additional equipment, to have available as needed, includes the following:
- Sterile gown and full drape
- Bath towel
- Small wrist board
- Sutureless securement device
- Suture material

- Chlorhexidine-impregnated sponge
- Additional transparent adhesive dressing with tapes (if dressing has no tape, consider the use of ½-inch Steri-Strips)
- Transducer holder, intravenous (IV) pole, and laser lever for pole-mounted arterial catheter transducers

PATIENT AND FAMILY EDUCATION

- Explain the procedure and the purpose of the arterial catheter. *Rationale:* This explanation decreases patient and family anxiety.
- Explain the standard of care to the patient and family, including insertion procedure, alarms, dressings, and length of time the catheter is expected to be in place. *Rationale:* This explanation encourages the patient and family to ask questions and voice concerns about the procedure and decreases patient and family anxiety.
- Explain the patient's expected participation during the procedure. *Rationale:* Patient cooperation during insertion is encouraged.
- Explain the importance of keeping the affected extremity immobile. *Rationale:* This explanation encourages patient cooperation to prevent catheter dislodgment and maintains catheter patency and function.
- Instruct the patient to report any warmth, redness, pain, or wet feeling at the insertion site at any time. *Rationale:* These symptoms may indicate infection, bleeding, or disconnection of the tubing or catheter.

PATIENT ASSESSMENT AND PREPARATION

Patient Assessment

- Obtain the patient's medical history, including history of diabetes, hypertension, peripheral vascular disease, vascular grafts, arterial vasospasm, thrombosis, or embolism. Obtain the patient's history of coronary artery bypass graft surgery in which radial arteries were removed for use as conduits or presence of arteriovenous fistulas or shunts. *Rationale:* Extremities with any of these problems should be avoided as sites for cannulation because of the potential for complications. Patients with diabetes mellitus or hypertension are at higher risk for arterial or venous insufficiency. Previously removed radial arteries are a contraindication for ulnar artery cannulation.
- Review the patient's current anticoagulation therapy, history of blood dyscrasias, and pertinent laboratory values (prothrombin time [PT], international normalized ratio [INR], partial thromboplastin time [PTT], and platelets) before the procedure. *Rationale:* Anticoagulation therapy, blood dyscrasias, or alterations in coagulation studies could increase the risk of hematoma formation or hemorrhage.

- Review the patient's allergy history (e.g., allergy to heparin, lidocaine, antiseptic solutions, or adhesive tape). *Rationale:* This assessment decreases the risk for allergic reactions. Patients with heparin-induced thrombocytopenia should not receive heparin in the flush solution.
- Assess the neurovascular and peripheral vascular status of the extremity to be used for the arterial cannulation, including color, temperature, presence and fullness of pulses, capillary refill, presence of bruit (in larger arteries such as the femoral artery), and motor and sensory function (compared with the opposite extremity). Note: A modified Allen's test should be performed before cannulation of the radial artery (see Fig. 81-3). *Rationale:* This assessment may help identify any neurovascular or circulatory impairment before cannulation to avoid potential complications.[2,3,20]

Patient Preparation

- Verify that the patient is the correct patient using two identifiers. *Rationale:* Before performing a procedure, the nurse should ensure the correct identification of the patient for the intended intervention.
- Ensure that the patient and family understand preprocedural teaching. Answer questions as they arise, and reinforce information as needed. *Rationale:* Understanding of previously taught information is evaluated and reinforced.
- Ensure that informed consent is obtained. *Rationale:* Informed consent protects the rights of the patient and allows a competent decision to be made by the patient; however, in emergency circumstances, time may not allow the form to be signed.
- Perform a preprocedure verification and time out, if nonemergent. *Rationale:* Ensures patient safety.
- Place the patient supine with the head of the bed at a comfortable position. The limb into which the arterial catheter will be inserted should be resting comfortably on the bed. *Rationale:* This placement provides patient comfort and facilitates insertion.
- If the radial artery is selected, position the hand to allow for palpation of the artery (a pillow or towel may be used to support the wrist). *Rationale:* This placement positions the arm and brings the artery closer to the surface.
- If the brachial artery is selected, elevate and hyperextend the patient's arm and palpate the artery (a pillow or towel may be used to support the arm). *Rationale:* This action increases accessibility of the artery.
- If the femoral artery is selected, position the patient supine with the head of the bed at a comfortable angle. The patient's leg should be straight with the femoral area easily accessible and palpate the artery (a small towel may be needed to support the hip in some cases). *Rationale:* This position is the best for localizing the femoral artery pulse.

Procedure	for Assisting With Insertion of an Arterial Catheter	
Steps	**Rationale**	**Special Considerations**
1. **HH**		
2. Prepare the flush solution (see Procedure 75). A. Use an IV solution of normal saline. B. Follow institutional standards for adding heparin to the IV solution, if heparin is not contraindicated. **(Level B*)**	Heparinized flush solutions are commonly used to minimize thrombi and fibrin deposits on catheters that might lead to thrombosis or bacterial colonization of the catheter.	Although heparin may prevent thombosis,[9,14,17] it has been associated with thrombocytopenia and other hematologic complications.[6] Other factors that promote patency of the arterial line besides heparinized saline solution include male gender, longer arterial catheters, larger vessels cannulated, patients receiving other anticoagulants or thrombolytics, and short-term use of the catheter.[1]
3. Consider the use of a blood-conservation arterial line system. **(Level B*)**	Reduces the risk of nosocomial anemia.[5,11,16,18,19]	
4. Prime or flush the entire single-pressure transducer system (see Procedure 75).	Removes air bubbles. Air bubbles introduced into the patient's circulation can cause air embolism. Air bubbles within the tubing dampen the waveform.	Air is more easily removed from the hemodynamic tubing when the system is not under pressure.
5. Apply and inflate the pressure bag or device to 300 mm Hg.	Each flush device delivers 1–3 mL/hr to maintain patency of the hemodynamic system.	
6. Connect the pressure cable to the bedside monitor.	Connects the pressure transducer system to the bedside monitoring system.	
7. Set the scale on the bedside monitor for the anticipated pressure waveform.	Prepares the bedside monitor.	
8. Level the air-fluid interface (zeroing stopcock) to the phlebostatic axis (see Figs. 75-7 and 75-9).	Leveling ensures that the air-fluid interface of the monitoring system is level with a reference point on the body. The phlebostatic axis reflects central arterial pressure.[13]	Use a pole mount or patient mount according to institutional protocol (see Procedure 75). The tip of the arterial catheter is not used as the reference point because it measures transmural pressure of a specific area in the arterial tree, which may be increased by hydrostatic pressure.[13]
9. Zero the system by turning the stopcock off to the patient, opening it to air, and zeroing the monitoring system (see Procedure 75).	Prepares the monitoring system.	
10. **HH**		
11. **PE**		
12. Assist as needed with skin preparation.	Provides help to the provider inserting the catheter.	

*Level B: Well-designed, controlled studies with results that consistently support a specific action, intervention, or treatment.

Procedure continues on following page

Procedure	for Assisting With Insertion of an Arterial Catheter—*Continued*	
Steps	**Rationale**	**Special Considerations**
13. Assist as needed with immobilizing the extremity during catheter insertion.	Facilitates insertion.	Personal protective equipment (e.g., head cover, mask, goggles) is needed, as well as sterile equipment. Maximal sterile barrier precautions should be used for femoral artery catheter insertion.[8,14]
14. Connect the pressure cable from the arterial transducer to the bedside monitor.	Connects the arterial catheter to the bedside monitoring system.	
15. Reassess accurate leveling, and secure the transducer (see Procedure 75).	Ensures that the air-filled interface (zeroing stopcock) is maintained at the level of the phlebostatic axis. If the air-fluid interface is above the phlebostatic axis, arterial pressures are falsely low. If the air-fluid interface is below the phlebostatic axis, arterial pressures are falsely high.	Leveling ensures accuracy. The point of the phlebostatic axis should be marked with an indelible marker, especially when the transducer is secured in a pole-mount system.
16. Zero the system again (see Procedure 75).	Ensures accuracy of the system with the established reference point.	
17. Turn the stopcock off to the top port of the stopcock. Place a sterile cap or a needleless cap on the top port of the stopcock.	Prepares the system for monitoring and ensures a closed system.	
18. Observe the waveform and perform a dynamic response test (square wave test; Fig. 59-3).	Determines whether the system is damped. This will ensure that the pressure waveform components are clearly defined. This aids in accurate measurement.	The square wave test can be performed by activating and quickly releasing the fast flush. A sharp upstroke should terminate in a flat line at the maximal indicator on the monitor. This should be followed by an immediate rapid downstroke extending below the baseline with 1–2 oscillations within 0.12 second and a quick return to baseline (see Fig. 59-3).
19. Ensure that the provider inserting the catheter has secured the arterial catheter in place.	Maintains arterial catheter position; reduces the chance of accidental dislodgement.	A sutureless securement device can be used.
20. Ensure that the provider inserting the catheter has applied an occlusive, sterile dressing to the insertion site.	Reduces the risk of infection.	
21. Apply an arm board, if necessary.	Ensures the correct position of the extremity for an optimal waveform.	
22. Set the alarm parameters according to the patient's current blood pressure.	Activates the bedside and central alarm system.	
23. Remove PE and discard used supplies in appropriate receptacles; ensure that all needles and other sharp objects are disposed of in appropriate containers.	Reduces the transmission of microorganisms; Standard Precautions. Safely removes sharp objects.	
24. HH		

When the fast flush of the continuous flush system is activated and quickly released, a sharp upstroke terminates in a flat line at the maximal indicator on the monitor and hard copy. This is then followed by an immediate rapid downstroke extending below baseline with just 1 or 2 oscillations within 0.12 second (minimal ringing) and a quick return to baseline. The patient's pressure waveform is also clearly defined with all components of the waveform, such as the dicrotic notch on an arterial waveform, clearly visible.

Square wave test configuration

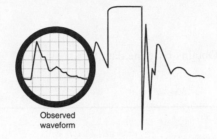

Observed
waveform

Intervention

A   There is no adjustment in the monitoring system required.

The upstroke of the square wave appears somewhat slurred, the waveform does not extend below the baseline after the fast flush and there is no ringing after the flush. The patient's waveform displays a falsely decreased systolic pressure and false high diastolic pressure as well as poorly defined components of the pressure tracing such as a diminished or absent dicrotic notch on arterial waveforms.

Square wave test configuration

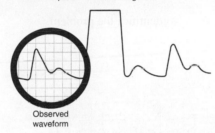

Observed
waveform

Intervention

To correct for the problem:
1. Check for the presence of blood clots, blood left in the catheter following blood sampling, or air bubbles at any point from the catheter tip to the transducer diaphragm and eliminate these as necessary.
2. Use low compliance (rigid), short (less than 3 to 4 feet) monitoring tubing.
3. Connect all line components securely.
B 4. Check for kinks in the line.

The waveform is characterized by numerous amplified oscillations above and below the baseline following the fast flush. The monitored pressure wave displays false high systolic pressures (overshoot), possibly false low diastolic pressures, and "ringing" artifacts on the waveform.

Square wave test configuration

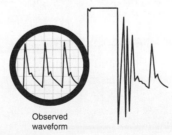

Observed
waveform

Intervention

C   To correct the problem, remove all air bubbles (particularly pinpoint air bubbles) in the fluid system, use large-bore, shorter tubing, or use a damping device.

Figure 59-3 Dynamic response test (square wave test) using the fast flush system. **A**, Optimally damped system. **B**, Overdamped system. **C**, Underdamped system. *(From Darovic GO, Zbilut JP: Fluid-filled monitoring systems. In Hemodynamic monitoring, ed 3. Philadelphia, 2002, Saunders, 122.)*

Procedure | for Assisting With Insertion of an Arterial Catheter—*Continued*

Steps	Rationale	Special Considerations
25. Compare the manual (noninvasive) blood pressure with the arterial (invasive) blood pressure.	Obtains baseline data.	No direct relationship exists between noninvasive and invasive blood pressures because noninvasive techniques measure blood flow and invasive techniques measure pressure.[13]
26. Run a waveform strip and record the patient's baseline arterial pressures.	Obtains baseline data.	Digital values are not used because they are averaged calculations.

Procedure | for Troubleshooting an Overdamped Waveform

Steps	Rationale	Special Considerations
1. **HH**		
2. **PE**		
3. Identify the overdamped waveform (Fig. 59-4).	Identifies the problem.	An overdamped waveform results in a falsely low systolic pressure and a falsely high diastolic pressure.

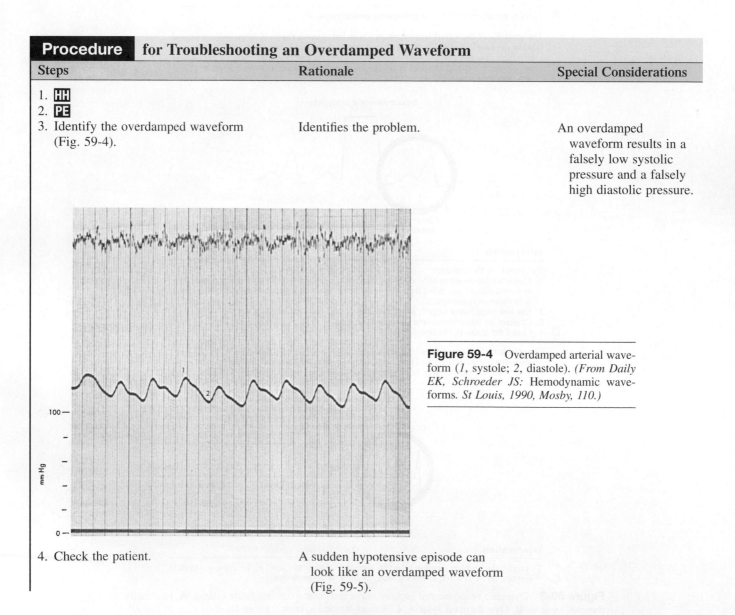

Figure 59-4 Overdamped arterial waveform (*1*, systole; *2*, diastole). *(From Daily EK, Schroeder JS: Hemodynamic waveforms. St Louis, 1990, Mosby, 110.)*

4. Check the patient.	A sudden hypotensive episode can look like an overdamped waveform (Fig. 59-5).	

Procedure for Troubleshooting an Overdamped Waveform—*Continued*

Steps	Rationale	Special Considerations

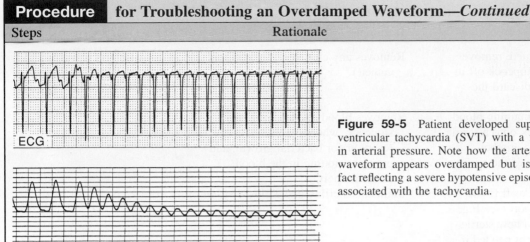

Figure 59-5 Patient developed supraventricular tachycardia (SVT) with a fall in arterial pressure. Note how the arterial waveform appears overdamped but is in fact reflecting a severe hypotensive episode associated with the tachycardia.

Steps	Rationale	Special Considerations
5. If the waveform is overdamped, follow these steps:		
A. Check the arterial line insertion site for catheter positioning.	Wrist movement in the radial site or leg flexion in the femoral site can cause catheter kinking or dislodgment, resulting in an overdamped waveform.	
B. Check the system for air bubbles and eliminate them if they are found.	Air bubbles can be a cause of an overdamped system; air bubbles can also cause emboli.	
C. Check the tubing system for leaks or disconnections, and correct the problem if it is found.	Ensures all connections are tight.	
D. Check the flush bag to ensure fluid is present in the bag and that pressure is maintained at 300 mm Hg.	An empty flush bag or a pressure of less than 300 mm Hg may result in an overdamped system.	
E. A catheter with an overdamped waveform should always be aspirated before flushing.	Use of the fast-flush device or flushing with a syringe first may force a clot at the catheter tip into the arterial circulation.	
Attempt to aspirate and flush the catheter as follows:	Assists with the withdrawal of air in the tubing or clots that may be at the catheter tip.	
• Using the stopcock closest to the patient, remove the nonvented cap from the blood sampling port or cleanse the needleless port and attach a 5- or 10-mL syringe to the top port of the stopcock (see Fig. 61-1).	A 5-mL syringe generates less pressure and may prevent arterial spasm in smaller arteries (e.g., radial artery).	A 10-mL syringe may be needed for larger arteries (e.g., the femoral artery). A needleless system can also be used.
• Turn the stopcock off to the flush solution (see Fig. 61-4B).	Opens the system from the patient to the syringe. Assesses catheter patency. Normally, blood should be aspirated into the syringe without difficulty.	
• Gently attempt to aspirate; if resistance is felt, reposition the extremity and reattempt aspiration.		
• If resistance is still felt, stop and notify the physician or advanced practice nurse.		

Procedure continues on following page

Procedure   for Troubleshooting an Overdamped Waveform—*Continued*

Steps	Rationale	Special Considerations
• If blood is aspirated, remove 3 mL, turn the stopcock off to the patient, and discard the 3-mL sample.	Removes any clotted material within the catheter.	All blood wastes should be disposed using Standard Precautions.
• Fast-flush the remaining blood from the stopcock onto a sterile gauze pad or into another syringe and remove the syringe.	Removes blood residue from the stopcock, where it could be a reservoir for bacterial growth, and prevents clotting in the blood sampling port.	
• Turn the stopcock off to the blood sampling port (see Fig. 61-1) and place a new sterile nonvented cap (not needed if using a needleless port).	Maintains sterility and a closed system.	
• Use the fast-flush device to clear the line of blood.	Prevents the arterial line from clotting.	
6. Remove **PE** and discard used supplies in the appropriate receptacles.	Reduces the transmission of microorganisms; Standard Precautions.	
7. **HH**		

Procedure   for Troubleshooting an Underdamped Waveform

Steps	Rationale	Special Considerations
1. **HH**		
2. **PE**		
3. Identify the underdamped waveform.	Identifies the problem.	An underdamped waveform results in a falsely high systolic pressure and a falsely low diastolic pressure.
4. Check the system for air bubbles and eliminate them if they are found.	Air bubbles can contribute to underdamping; air bubbles can also cause emboli.	
5. Check the length of the tubing of the pressure transducer system.	Ensures that the tubing length is minimized.	
6. Observe the waveform and perform a dynamic response test (square wave test; Fig. 59-3).	Determines whether the system is damped. This will ensure that the pressure waveform components are clearly defined. This aids in accurate measurement.	
7. Remove **PE** and discard used supplies in appropriate receptacles.	Reduces the transmission of microorganisms; Standard Precautions.	
8. **HH**		

Procedure	**for Arterial Catheter Dressing Change**	
Steps	**Rationale**	**Special Considerations**
1. HH		
2. PE		
3. Carefully remove and discard the arterial line dressing.	Removes the previous dressing without disrupting the integrity of the catheter.	If present, remove the securement device.
4. Inspect the catheter, insertion site, and surrounding skin.	Assesses for signs of infection, catheter dislodgement, or leakage.	
5. Remove nonsterile gloves, discard dressings, and perform hand hygiene.	Reduces the transmission of microorganisms	
6. Don sterile gloves	Maintains aseptic and sterile technique.	
7. Cleanse the skin and catheter with 2% chlorhexidine-based preparation.[14]	Reduces the rate of recolonization of skin flora. Decreases the risk for bacterial growth at the insertion site.	Allow time for the solution to air dry.
8. Apply a new stabilization device.	Secures the catheter.	
9. Apply a chlorhexidine-impregnated sponge to the site.[12,14] **(Level D*)**	Reduces the transmission of microorganisms.	Follow institutional standards. A chlorhexidine-impregnated sponge dressing is recommended if an institution's central line–associated bloodstream infection rate is not decreasing despite adherence to basic prevention measures, including education and training, appropriate use of chlorhexidine for skin antisepsis, and maximum sterile barrier.[8,12,14] Use with caution in patients predisposed to local skin necrosis, such as burn patients or patients with Stevens-Johnson syndrome.[22]
10. Apply a sterile air-occlusive dressing. Dressings may be a sterile gauze or a sterile, transparent, semipermeable dressing.[14]	Provides a sterile environment.	Write the date and time of the dressing change on a label and tape it to the dressing.
11. Remove gloves and discard used supplies in appropriate receptacles.	Reduces the transmission of microorganisms; Standard Precautions.	
12. HH		

*Level D: Peer-reviewed professional and organizational standards with the support of clinical study recommendations.

Procedure continues on following page

Procedure for Removal of the Arterial Catheter

Steps	Rationale	Special Considerations
1. Review the patient's coagulation profile (PT, INR, PTT, platelets) and anticoagulation medication profile before removal of the arterial catheter.	Elevated PT, INR, PTT, and decreased platelets affect time to hemostasis.	If laboratory values are abnormal, pressure needs to be applied for a longer period to achieve hemostasis.
2. **HH**		
3. **PE**		
4. Turn off the arterial monitoring alarms.	The alarm system is no longer needed.	
5. Remove the dressing.	Prepares for catheter removal.	
6. Remove the stabilizing device.	Prepares for catheter removal.	
7. Turn the stopcock off to the flush solution (see Fig. 61-4B).	Turns the monitoring system off to the flush solution.	
8. Apply pressure 1–2 finger widths above the insertion site.	The arterial puncture site is above the skin puncture site because the catheter enters the skin at an angle.	
9. Remove the arterial catheter and place a sterile 4 × 4 gauze pad over the catheter site.	Prevents splashing of blood.	
10. Continue to hold proximal pressure and immediately apply firm pressure over the insertion site as the catheter is removed.	Prevents bleeding.	
11. Continue to apply pressure for a minimum of 5 minutes for the radial artery.	Achieves hemostasis.	Follow institutional standards. Longer periods of direct pressure may be needed to achieve hemostasis (e.g., patients receiving systemic heparin or thrombolytics, patients with catheters in larger arteries such as the femoral artery, or patients with abnormal coagulation values).
12. Apply a pressure dressing to the insertion site.	A pressure dressing helps prevent rebleeding.	The dressing should not encircle the extremity (prevents ischemia of the extremity).
13. Remove **PE** and discard used supplies in appropriate receptacles.	Reduces the transmission of microorganisms; Standard Precautions.	
14. **HH**		

Expected Outcomes

- Successful cannulation of the artery
- Peripheral vascular and neurovascular systems intact
- Alterations in blood pressure identified and treated
- Able to continuously monitor blood pressure
- Maintenance of baseline hemoglobin and hematocrit levels
- Adequate circulation to the involved extremity
- Adequate sensory and motor function to the involved extremity
- Maintenance of catheter site without infection
- Removal of catheter when no longer needed

Unexpected Outcomes

- Pain
- Insertion complications
- Inability to cannulate the artery
- Change in color, temperature, sensation; movement of the extremity used for insertion
- Hematoma, hemorrhage, infection, or thrombosis at the insertion site
- Decreased hemoglobin and hematocrit values
- Catheter disconnection with significant blood loss
- Presence of a new bruit
- Impaired sensory or motor function of the extremity
- Elevated temperature or elevated white blood cell count
- Redness, warmth, edema, or drainage at or from the insertion site

Patient Monitoring and Care

Steps	Rationale	Reportable Conditions
		These conditions should be reported if they persist despite nursing interventions.
1. Assess the neurovascular and peripheral vascular status of the cannulated extremity immediately after catheter insertion and every 4 hours, or more often if warranted, according to institutional standards.	Validates adequate peripheral vascular and neurovascular integrity. Changes in sensation, motor function, pulses, color, temperature, or capillary refill may indicate ischemia, thrombosis, arterial spasm, or neurovascular compromise.	• Diminished or absent pulses • Pale, mottled, or cyanotic appearance of the distal extremity • Extremity that is cool or cold to the touch • Capillary refill time of greater than 2 seconds • Diminished or absent sensation or pain at the site or distal extremity • Diminished or absent motor function
2. Check the arterial line flush system every 4 hours to ensure the following: • Pressure bag or device is inflated to 300 mm Hg. • Fluid is present in the flush solution.	Ensures that approximately 1–3 mL/hr of flush solution is delivered through the catheter, thus maintaining patency and preventing backflow of blood into the catheter and tubing. The risk of catheter occlusion related to fibrin sheath or clot formation increases if the flush solution is not continuously infusing.	
3. Perform a dynamic response test (square wave test) at the start of each shift, with a change of the waveform, or after the system is opened to air (see Fig. 59-3).	An optimally damped system provides an accurate waveform.	• Overdamped or underdamped waveforms that cannot be corrected with troubleshooting procedures
4. Monitor for overdamped or underdamped waveforms. An overdamped waveform is characterized by a flattened waveform, a diminished or absent dicrotic notch, or a square wave that does not fall to baseline or below baseline (see Fig. 59-4). An underdamped waveform is characterized by catheter fling or artifacts on the waveform (see Fig. 59-3,C).	An optimally damped system provides an adequate waveform which facilitates accuracy of blood pressure monitoring. An overdamped waveform can result in inaccurate blood pressure measurement. The patient's blood pressure measure may be inaccurately low. An overdamped system can be caused by air bubbles in the system; use of compliant tubing versus stiff, loose tubing connections in the system; too many stopcocks in the system; a cracked tubing or stopcock; arterial catheter occlusion or a kink; the catheter tip being against the arterial wall; blood in the transducer; and insufficient pressure of the flush solution. An underdamped waveform can also result in inaccurate blood pressure measurement. The patient's blood pressure measure may be inaccurately high. Common causes of an underdamped waveform include excessive tubing length, movement of the catheter in the artery, patient movement, and air bubbles in the system.	• Overdamped or underdamped waveforms that cannot be corrected with troubleshooting procedures

Procedure continues on following page

Patient Monitoring and Care —*Continued*

Steps	Rationale	Reportable Conditions
5. Zero the transducer during the initial setup, after insertion, if disconnection occurs between the transducer and the monitoring cable, if disconnection occurs between the monitoring cable and the monitor, and when the values obtained do not fit the clinical picture. Follow manufacturer recommendations for disposable systems.	Ensures accuracy of the hemodynamic monitoring system.	
6. Recheck the level of the air-fluid interface (zeroing stopcock) to the phlebostatic axis whenever patient position changes (see Procedure 75).	Ensures accurate reference point for the left atrium and accuracy of blood pressure measurements.	
7. Place sterile injectable or noninjectable caps on all stopcocks. Replace with new sterile caps whenever the caps are removed.	Stopcocks can be a source of contamination. Stopcocks that are part of the initial setup are packaged with vented caps. Vented caps need to be replaced with sterile injectable or noninjectable caps to maintain a closed system and reduce risk of contamination and infection.	
8. Continuously monitor the arterial catheter values and waveform.	Provides for continuous waveform analysis and assessment of patient status.	
9. Observe the insertion site for signs and symptoms of infection.	Infected catheters must be removed as soon as possible to prevent bacteremia. The CDC does not recommend routinely replacing peripheral arterial catheters to prevent catheter-related infections.[14]	• Redness at the site • Purulent drainage • Tenderness or pain at the insertion site • Elevated temperature • Elevated white blood cell count
10. Change the pressure transducer system (flush solution, pressure tubing, transducers, and stopcocks) every 96 hours. **(Level B*)** The flush solution may need to be changed more frequently.	The CDC[14] and the Infusion Nurses Society[8] and research findings[10,15] recommend that the hemodynamic flush system can be used safely for 96 hours. This recommendation is based on research conducted with disposable pressure monitoring systems used for peripheral and central lines.	
11. Label the tubing: A. Arterial B. Date and time prepared	Identifies that the catheter is arterial and when the system needs to be changed.	
12. Maintain the pressure bag or device at 300 mm Hg.	Maintains catheter patency.	

*Level B: Well-designed, controlled studies with results that consistently support a specific action, intervention, or treatment.

Patient Monitoring and Care —*Continued*

Steps	Rationale	Reportable Conditions
13. Print a strip of the arterial pressure waveform and obtain measurement of the arterial pressures. Note if there are respiratory variations.	Ensures accurate blood pressure measurement.	
14. Obtain an arterial pressure waveform strip to place on the patient's chart at the start of each shift and whenever a change is found in the waveform.	The printed waveform allows assessment of the adequacy of the waveform, damping, or respiratory variation.	
15. Monitor hemoglobin or hematocrit values daily or as prescribed.	Allows assessment of nosocomial anemia.	• Abnormal hemoglobin values • Abnormal hematocrit values
16. Replace gauze dressings every 2 days and transparent dressings at least every 5–7 days and more frequently as needed.[7,8,14,22] **(Level D*)**	Decreases the risk for infection at the catheter site. The CDC[14] and the Infusion Nurses Society[7,8] recommends replacing the dressing when it becomes damp, loosened, or soiled or when inspection of the site is necessary.	
17. Print a strip of the arterial waveform to place on the patient's chart at the start of each shift and whenever a change in the waveform occurs.	The printed waveform allows assessment of the adequacy of the waveform and the presence of damping.	
18. Assess the need for the arterial catheter daily. **(Level D*)**	The CDC[14] does not recommend routine replacement of arterial catheters. Catheters should be removed when no longer needed and should be replaced when there is a clinical indication.	• Signs and symptoms of infection at the arterial catheter insertion site
19. Follow institutional standards for assessing pain. Administer analgesia as prescribed.	Identifies need for pain interventions.	• Pain at the catheter site.

*Level D: Peer-reviewed professional and organizational standards with the support of clinical study recommendations.

Documentation

Documentation should include the following:
- Patient and family education
- Completion of informed consent
- Preprocedure verifications and time out
- Performance of the modified Allen's test before insertion and its results (when using the radial artery)
- Insertion of the arterial catheter
- Size of the arterial catheter inserted
- Number of insertion attempts
- Date and time of arterial catheter site care and dressing change
- Pain assessment, interventions, and effectiveness

- Site assessment
- Arterial site dressing change
- Intake of flush solution volume
- Printed strip of the arterial pressure waveform
- Appearance of the limb, color, pulse, sensation, movement, capillary refill time, and temperature of the extremity after insertion is complete
- Arterial pressures
- Waveforms
- Occurrence of unexpected outcomes and interventions

References and Additional Readings

For a complete list of references and additional readings for this procedure, scan this QR code with any freely available smartphone code reader app, or visit http://booksite.elsevier.com/9780323376624.

60 Arterial Pressure–Based Cardiac Output Monitoring

Susan Scott

PURPOSE: Arterial pressure–based cardiac output monitoring is a minimally invasive technology that can be used to obtain hemodynamic data on a continuous basis.

PREREQUISITE NURSING KNOWLEDGE

- Knowledge of the anatomy and physiology of the cardiovascular system is necessary.
- Knowledge of the anatomy and physiology of the vasculature and adjacent structures is needed.
- Understanding of the pathophysiologic changes that occur in heart disease and affect flow dynamics is necessary.
- Understanding of aseptic technique is needed.
- Understanding of the hemodynamic effects of vasoactive medications and fluid resuscitation is needed.
- Understanding of the principles involved in hemodynamic monitoring is necessary.
- Knowledge of invasive cardiac output monitoring is needed.
- Knowledge of arterial waveform interpretation is needed.
- Knowledge of definitions and norms for cardiac output, cardiac index, systemic vascular resistance, stroke volume, stroke index, preload, afterload, and contractility and stroke volume variation is necessary.
- Arterial pressure represents the forcible ejection of blood from the left ventricle into the aorta and out into the arterial system. During ventricular systole, blood is ejected into the aorta, generating a pressure wave. Because of the intermittent pumping action of the heart, this arterial pressure wave is generated in a pulsatile manner (see Fig. 59-1). The ascending limb of the aortic pressure wave (anacrotic limb) represents an increase in pressure because of left-ventricular ejection. The peak of this ejection is the peak systolic pressure, which is normally 100 to 140 mm Hg in adults. After reaching this peak, the ventricular pressure declines to a level below aortic pressure and the aortic valve closes, marking the end of ventricular systole. The closure of the aortic valve produces a small rebound wave that creates a notch known as the dicrotic notch. The descending limb of the curve (diastolic down slope) represents diastole and is characterized by a long declining pressure wave, during which the aortic wall recoils and propels blood into the arterial network. The diastolic pressure is measured at the lowest point of the diastolic down slope and is normally 60 to 80 mm Hg.

- The difference between the systolic and diastolic pressures is called the pulse pressure, with a normal value of 40 mm Hg.
- Arterial pressure is determined by the relationship between blood flow through the vessels (cardiac output), the compliance of the aorta and larger vessels, and the resistance of the more peripheral vessel walls (systemic vascular resistance). The arterial pressure is therefore affected by any factors that change either cardiac output, compliance, or systemic vascular resistance.
- The average arterial pressure during a cardiac cycle is called the mean arterial pressure (MAP). It is not the average of the systolic plus the diastolic pressures, because at normal heart rates systole accounts for $\frac{1}{3}$ of the cardiac cycle and diastole accounts for $\frac{2}{3}$ of the cardiac cycle. The MAP is calculated automatically by most patient monitoring systems; however, it can be calculated manually using the following formula:

$$\frac{\text{Systolic pressure} + (\text{diastolic pressure} \times 2)}{3}$$

- MAP represents the driving force (perfusion pressure) for blood flow through the cardiovascular system. MAP is at its highest point in the aorta. As blood travels through the circulatory system, systolic pressure increases and diastolic pressure decreases, with an overall decline in the MAP (see Fig. 59-2).
- Arterial pressure–based cardiac output (APCO) is obtained from an arterial catheter.[10–12]
- APCO technology measures the rate of flow (cardiac output).[10–12]
- Stroke volume and heart rate are key determinants of cardiac output.
- Although systemic vascular resistance affects cardiac output, the location of that effect is global and not limited by location of that measurement because cardiac output is measured as flow per minute throughout the body. Manufacturers of the arterial pressure–based cardiac output systems have factored in variance for both radial artery catheters and femoral artery catheters.[9]
- Ultrasound guidance is recommended to place arterial catheters if the technology is available.[7]

EQUIPMENT

- Invasive arterial catheter and insertion kit
- Specialized sterile transducer and sensor kit (manufacturer specific)
- Intravenous (IV) pole and transducer holder (manufacturer specific)
- Pressure-transducer system, including flush solution recommended according to institutional standards, a pressure bag or device, pressure tubing with transducer, and flush device
- Pressure module and cable for interface with the monitor
- Normal saline-flush solution
- Monitoring system (central and bedside monitor)
- Special monitor to interface with the bedside monitor for trending and display of hemodynamic values (manufacturer specific)
- Dual-channel recorder
- Indelible marker
- Nonvented (noninjectable) caps
- Leveling device (low-intensity laser or carpenter level)
- Sterile and nonsterile gloves

Additional equipment, to have available as needed, includes the following:

- Heparin if prescribed
- 3-mL syringe
- Dressing supplies
- Tape
- Sterile ultrasound probe cover
- Sterile ultrasound gel

PATIENT AND FAMILY EDUCATION

- Explain the rationale for arterial line insertion, including how the arterial pressure is displayed on the bedside monitor. *Rationale:* This explanation may decrease patient and family anxiety and increase understanding.
- Explain the standard of care to the patient and family, including insertion procedure, alarms, dressings, and length of time the catheter is expected to be in place. *Rationale:* This explanation encourages the patient and family to ask questions and voice concerns about the procedure and may decrease patient and family anxiety.
- Explain the patient's expected participation during the procedure. *Rationale:* Patients will know how they can help with the procedure.
- Explain the importance of keeping the affected extremity immobile. *Rationale:* This explanation encourages patient cooperation to prevent catheter dislodgment and ensures a more accurate waveform.
- Instruct the patient to report any warmth, redness, pain, numbness, or wet feeling at the insertion site at any time, including after catheter removal. *Rationale:* These symptoms may indicate infection, bleeding, or disconnection of the tubing or catheter.

PATIENT ASSESSMENT AND PREPARATION

Patient Assessment

- Obtain the patient's medical history, including a history of peripheral vascular disease, diabetes, and hypertension. *Rationale:* These conditions increase the patient's risk for arterial or venous insufficiency.
- Obtain the patient's medical history for peripheral vascular disease, vascular grafts, arteriovenous fistulas or shunts, arterial vasospasm, thrombosis, or embolism. In addition, obtain the patient's history of coronary artery bypass graft surgery in which radial arteries were removed for use as conduits. *Rationale:* Extremities with any of these problems should be avoided as sites for cannulation because of the potential for complications.
- Assess the neurovascular and peripheral vascular status of the extremity to be used for the arterial cannulation, including color, temperature, presence and fullness of pulses, capillary refill, presence of bruit, and motor and sensory function (compared with the opposite extremity). Note: A modified Allen's test may be performed before cannulation of the radial artery (see Fig. 81-3). *Rationale:* This assessment may identify neurovascular or circulatory impairment, so potential complications related to radial artery cannulation may be avoided.
- Assess the patient's vital signs and compliance factors (e.g., age, gender, height, weight). *Rationale:* This assessment provides baseline data. The compliance factors allow for the individual variables that ultimately dictate pulse pressure and its relevance (proportionality) to stroke volume.

Patient Preparation

- Verify that the patient is the correct patient using two identifiers. *Rationale:* Before performing a procedure, the nurse should ensure the correct identification of the patient for the intended intervention.
- Ensure that the patient and family understand preprocedural teaching. Answer questions as they arise, and reinforce information as needed. *Rationale:* Understanding of previously taught information is evaluated and reinforced.
- Ensure that informed consent has been obtained. *Rationale:* Informed consent protects the rights of the patient and makes a competent decision possible for the patient.
- Perform a preprocedure verification and time out, if nonemergent. *Rationale:* Ensures patient safety.
- Validate the patency of IV access. *Rationale:* Access may be needed for administration of emergency medications or fluids.
- Place the patient's extremity in the appropriate position with adequate lighting of the insertion site. *Rationale:* This placement prepares the site for cannulation and facilitates an accurate insertion.

Procedure for Arterial Pressure–Based Cardiac Output Monitoring

Steps	Rationale	Special Considerations
Initiating the Procedure 1. HH 2. PE		
3. If the radial artery is to be used, perform the modified Allen's test before the puncture (see Fig. 81-3). **(Level C*)**	The modified Allen's test has been recommended before a radial artery puncture to assess the patency of the ulnar artery and an intact superficial palmar arch.[3,14]	The modified Allen's test does not always ensure adequate flow through the ulnar artery. A Doppler ultrasound flow indicator can also be used to further verify blood flow.[1,2,4,7]
4. Prepare the flush solution (see Procedure 75). A. Use an IV solution of normal saline. B. Follow institutional standards for adding heparin to the IV solution, if heparin is not contraindicated. **(Level B*)**	Heparinized flush solutions are commonly used to minimize thrombi and fibrin deposits on catheters that might lead to thrombosis or bacterial colonization of the catheter.	Although heparin may prevent thrombosis,[8,13,15] it has been associated with thrombocytopenia and other hematologic complications.[5] Other factors that promote patency of the arterial line besides heparinized saline solution include male gender, longer arterial catheters, larger vessels cannulated, patients receiving other anticoagulants or thrombolytics, and short-term use of the catheter.[1]
5. Gather the equipment needed for obtaining an arterial pressure–based cardiac output.	Prepares supplies.	Refer to the specific manufacturer for additional required equipment for setup and maintenance. Some technologies require additional calibration procedures and equipment.[10]
6. Obtain the patient's baseline compliance factors (e.g., age, gender, height, weight). **(Level M*)**	This information may be needed to allow for the individual variables that ultimately dictate pulse pressure and its relevance (proportionality) to stroke volume.	Follow manufacturer guidelines. Some manufacturers require calibration. Manufacturers that do not require calibration use age, gender, height, and weight to determine vascular compliance. An accurate height and weight reflecting perfused tissue is important in the determination of body surface area (BSA) and cardiac index. Fluid weight gain often is discounted because it is not perfused tissue. Medications are generally based on perfused weight in the case of morbidly obese patients. Because adipose tissue is highly vascular, actual weight and height are necessary to determine BSA. BSA is needed for calculating indexed values.
7. Remove PE and discard used supplies.	Reduces the transmission of microorganisms; Standard Precautions.	
8. HH		

*Level B: Well-designed, controlled studies with results that consistently support a specific action, intervention, or treatment.

*Level C: Qualitative studies, descriptive or correlational studies, integrative reviews, systematic reviews, or randomized controlled trials with inconsistent results.

*Level M: Manufacturer's recommendations only.

Procedure continues on following page

Procedure for Arterial Pressure–Based Cardiac Output Monitoring—*Continued*

Steps	Rationale	Special Considerations
Setting Up the Arterial Pressure–Based Cardiac Output (APCO) System		
1. ▢		
2. ▢		
3. Open the APCO sensor kit.	Prepares equipment.	Follow manufacturer recommendations.
4. Secure all connections.	Tight connections ensure the integrity of the system.	Vented caps are standard with transducer sets and kits, and allow for initial priming of the system.
5. Insert the APCO sensor into the transducer holder that is secured on the IV pole next to the patient.	Stabilizes the sensor.	
6. Level the vent port near the sensor to the phlebostatic axis.	The reference point is the phlebostatic axis because it accurately reflects central arterial pressure.	
7. Prime or flush the entire APCO system:	Removes air bubbles.	Prime the system using gravity to minimize small bubbles.
A. Activate the flush device to deliver the flush solution through the sensor and out through the vent port.	Removes air from the system.	
B. Close the vent port by turning the stopcock to the neutral position.		
C. Place a sterile nonvented (noninjectable) cap on the top of the stopcock.	Maintains a closed sterile system.	
D. Purge air from the remaining part of the tubing.	Prepares the monitoring system.	
8. Inflate the pressure bag or device to 300 mm Hg.	Inflating the pressure bag to 300 mm Hg allows approximately 1–3 mL/hr of flush solution to be delivered through the catheter, thus maintaining catheter patency and minimizing clot formation.	
9. Assist as needed with insertion of the arterial catheter (See Procedures 58 & 59).	Provides needed assistance.	
10. Connect the bedside monitor cable to the APCO sensor (Fig. 60-1).	Information can then be transferred from the sensor to the monitor.	Follow manufacturer guidelines. Some cables are color coded.
11. Enter the patient's gender, age, height, and weight. **(Level M*)**	This information is needed to allow for the individual variables that ultimately dictate pulse pressure and its relevance (proportionality) to stroke volume. The result is stroke volume variability.	Follow manufacturer guidelines. Some manufacturers require calibration.
12. Set up the monitor.	Prepares equipment.	Follow the manufacturer's guidelines as the setup may vary.
13. Observe the cardiac output (CO) display.	Provides assessment data.	The cardiac output value is updated regularly based on the manufacturer.

*Level M: Manufacturer's recommendations only.

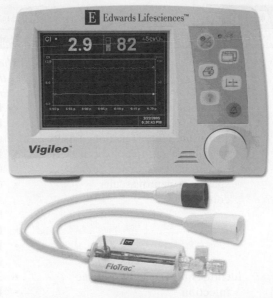

Figure 60-1   FloTrac sensor and Vigileo monitor. *(Courtesy of Edwards Lifesciences, LLC, 2009.)*

Procedure   for Arterial Pressure–Based Cardiac Output Monitoring—*Continued*

Steps	Rationale	Special Considerations
14. Set the alarm parameters according to the patient's current blood pressure.	Activates the bedside and central alarm system.	Follow manufacturer guidelines.
15. Remove **PE** and discard used supplies in appropriate receptacles.	Reduces the transmission of microorganisms; Standard Precautions.	Ensure sharps are safely disposed.
16. **HH**		

Expected Outcomes

- Accurate measurement of cardic output (CO)
- Maintenance of catheter patency
- Minimal discomfort from the arterial catheter
- Maintenance of baseline hemoglobin and hematocrit levels
- Adequate circulation to the involved extremity
- Adequate sensory and motor function of the extremity
- Maintenance of the catheter site without infection

Unexpected Outcomes

- Poor-quality arterial pressure wave leading to the inability to obtain an accurate CO
- Infection
- Impaired peripheral tissue perfusion (e.g., edema, coolness, pain, paleness, or slow capillary refill of the fingers of the cannulated extremity)
- Perforated or lacerated artery
- Hematoma at the insertion site
- Pain or discomfort from the arterial catheter insertion site
- Decreased hemoglobin and hematocrit values
- Catheter disconnection with significant blood loss

Procedure continues on following page

Patient Monitoring and Care

Steps	Rationale	Reportable Conditions
		These conditions should be reported if they persist despite nursing interventions.
1. Assess the neurovascular and peripheral vascular status of the cannulated extremity immediately after catheter insertion and every 4 hours, or more often if needed. Follow institutional standards.	Determines peripheral vascular and neurovascular integrity. Changes in sensation, motor function, pulses, color, temperature, or capillary refill may indicate ischemia, arterial spasm, or neurovascular compromise.	• Diminished or absent pulses • Pale, mottled, or cyanotic appearance of the extremity • Extremity that is cool or cold to the touch • Capillary refill time of more than 2 seconds (or longer than patient's baseline) • Diminished or absent sensation • Diminished or absent motor function
2. Assess the arterial catheter insertion site for signs and symptoms of infection.	Identifies the possibility of site infection.	• Redness at the site • Purulent drainage • Tenderness or pain at the insertion site • Elevated temperature • Elevated white blood cell count
3. Continuously monitor heart rate, blood pressure, and cardiac indices.	Provides assessment of patient status.	• Abnormal vital signs • Abnormal cardiac output • Abnormal cardiac index
4. Follow institutional standards for assessing pain. Administer analgesia as prescribed.	Identifies need for pain interventions.	• Continued pain despite pain interventions
5. Assess the patient's response to prescribed interventions.	The hemodynamic management of the patient requires close monitoring and interventions based on the parameters obtained from the APCO data.	• Abnormal cardiac output • Abnormal cardiac index • Abnormal vital signs
6. Replace gauze dressings every 2 days and transparent dressings at least every 5–7 days and more frequently as needed.[6,7,13,16] **(Level D*)**	Decreases the risk for infection at the catheter site. The Centers for Disease Control and Prevention (CDC)[13] and the Infusion Nurses Society[6,7] recommend replacing the dressing when the dressing becomes damp, loosened, or soiled, or when inspection of the site is necessary.	

*Level D: Peer-reviewed professional and organizational standards with the support of clinical study recommendations.

Documentation

Documentation should include the following:
- Patient and family education
- Informed consent
- Preprocedure verification and time out
- Patient tolerance of the procedure
- Peripheral vascular and neurovascular assessment before and after the procedure
- Assessment of the insertion site
- Patient response to the insertion procedure
- Pain assessment, interventions, and effectiveness
- Type of flush used
- Amount of flush solution on intake and output record
- Vital signs, cardiac output, cardiac index, and other hemodynamic parameters
- Positive flow by modified Allen's test if the radial artery is used
- Site assessment
- Unexpected outcomes
- Additional nursing interventions

References and Additional Readings

For a complete list of references and additional readings for this procedure, scan this QR code with any freely available smartphone code reader app, or visit http://booksite.elsevier.com/9780323376624.

61

Blood Sampling from an Arterial Catheter

Hillary Crumlett and Alex Johnson

PURPOSE: Blood sampling from an arterial catheter is performed to obtain blood specimens for arterial blood gas analysis or other laboratory testing.

PREREQUISITE NURSING KNOWLEDGE

- Knowledge of aseptic and sterile technique is necessary.
- Knowledge of the vascular anatomy and physiology is needed.
- Understanding of gas exchange and acid-base balance is necessary.
- Technique for specimen collection and labeling should be understood.
- Principles of hemodynamic monitoring are necessary.
- Knowledge about the care of patients with arterial catheters (see Procedure 59) and stopcock manipulation (see Procedure 75) is needed.
- Understanding of the closed arterial line blood sampling system is necessary.
- Closed blood-sampling systems provide the opportunity to reinfuse blood to the patient after the laboratory sample is obtained to help reduce the risk of nosocomial anemia.[3,7,10,14,15]

EQUIPMENT

- Nonsterile gloves
- Sterile 4 × 4 gauze pads
- Arterial blood gas kit and blood specimen tubes
- Labels with the patient's name and appropriate identifying data
- Laboratory form and specimen labels
- Goggles or fluid shield face mask
- Needleless blood-sampling access device (blood-transfer device)
- Extra blood-specimen tube (for discard)
- Sterile injectable or noninjectable caps
- Antiseptic solution (i.e., 2% chlorhexidine–based preparation)
- Specimen transport bag(s)

Additional equipment, to have available as needed, includes the following:

- Bag of ice
- Syringes, 5 and 10 mL
- Needleless cannula (for closed arterial blood-sampling system)

PATIENT AND FAMILY EDUCATION

- Explain the procedure to the patient and family. *Rationale:* Teaching provides information and may reduce anxiety and fear.
- Explain the importance of keeping the affected extremity immobile. *Rationale:* This explanation encourages patient cooperation during blood withdrawal.
- Explain the patient's expected participation during the procedure. *Rationale:* Patient cooperation during insertion is encouraged.

PATIENT ASSESSMENT AND PREPARATION

Patient Assessment

- Assess the patency of the arterial catheter. *Rationale:* This ensures a functional arterial catheter.
- Assess the patient's previous laboratory results. *Rationale:* This assessment provides data for comparison.

Patient Preparation

- Verify that the patient is the correct patient using two identifiers. *Rationale:* Before performing a procedure, the nurse should ensure the correct identification of the patient for the intended intervention.
- Ensure that the patient and family understand preprocedural teaching. Answer questions as they arise, and reinforce information as needed. *Rationale:* Understanding of previously taught information is evaluated and reinforced.
- Expose the stopcock to be used for blood sampling, and position the patient's extremity so that the site can easily be accessed. *Rationale:* This prepares the site for blood withdrawal.

Procedure | for Blood Sampling From an Arterial Catheter

Steps	Rationale	Special Considerations
1. **HH**		
2. **PE**		
3. When obtaining an ABG sample, open the ABG kit and use the plunger to rid the excess heparin and air from the syringe.	Prepares the ABG syringe.	Heparin is usually in powdered form. If prepackaged ABG kits are not available, draw 0.5 mL of a 1:1000 dilution of heparin in a 3-mL syringe. Pull back on the plunger to coat the inside of the syringe and the needle. Rid the excess heparin and air from the syringe.[2]
4. Temporarily suspend the arterial alarms.	Prevents the alarm from sounding as the pressure waveform is lost during the blood draw.	

Blood Sampling With a Needleless Blood-Sampling Access Device (Blood-Transfer Device) or a Syringe

Steps	Rationale	Special Considerations
1. Arterial stopcock:		
A. Remove the sterile cap from the port of the three-way stopcock closest to the patient and attach the needleless blood-sampling access device (blood-transfer device) (Fig. 61-1, *A*) or syringe (Fig. 61-1, *B*) to the stopcock.	Prepares for blood sampling.	
Or		
B. Cleanse the injectable cap at the top of the stopcock closest to the patient with an antiseptic solution[1,9] **(Level B*)** and attach the needleless blood-sampling access device (blood-transfer device) (Fig. 61-2).		
2. Turn the stopcock off to the flush solution (Fig. 61-3).	The needleless blood-sampling access device (blood-transfer device) or syringe is then in direct contact with the blood in the arterial catheter.	
3. When using a needleless blood-sampling access device (blood-transfer device), engage the blood specimen tube to obtain the discard volume or, if using a syringe, slowly and gently aspirate the discard volume.	Clears the catheter of flush solution.	
A. When obtaining blood for an ABG sample, discard a blood sample that is two times the dead-space volume. **(Level B*)**	The discard volume includes the dead space and the blood diluted by the flush solution (e.g., dead space of 0.8 mL = 1.6 mL discard).[11,12]	The dead space is the space between the tip of the arterial catheter to the top port of the stopcock.

*Level B: Well-designed, controlled studies with results that consistently support a specific action, intervention, or treatment.

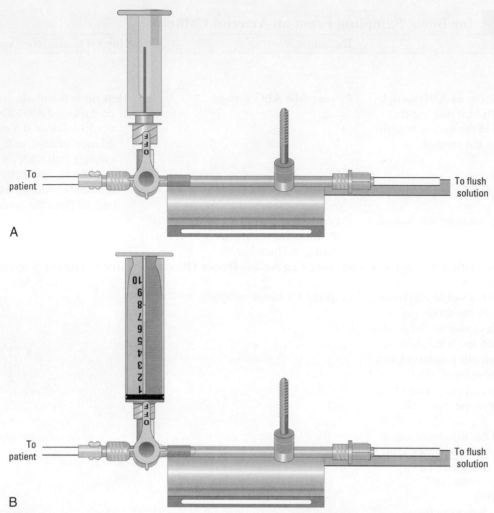

To patient

To flush solution

A

10
9
8
7
6
5
4
3
2
1

To patient

To flush solution

B

Figure 61-1　**A,** The needleless blood-sampling access device (blood-transfer device) attached to the port of the three-way stopcock. The stopcock is turned "off" to the port of the stopcock. **B,** A syringe attached to the port of the three-way stopcock. The stopcock is turned "off" to the port of the stopcock). *(Drawing by Paul W. Schiffmacher, Thomas Jefferson University Hospital, Philadelphia, PA.)*

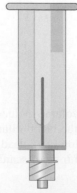

Figure 61-2　Needleless blood-sampling access device (blood-transfer device). *(Drawing by Paul W. Schiffmacher, Thomas Jefferson University Hospital, Philadelphia, PA.)*

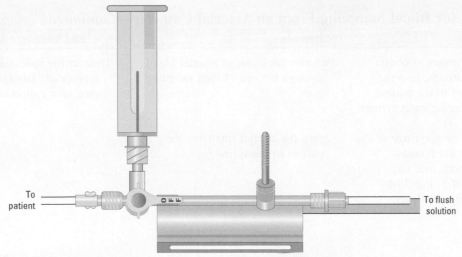

Figure 61-3   The needleless blood-sampling access device (blood-transfer device) attached to the port of the three-way stopcock. The stopcock is turned "off" to the flush solution. (*Drawing by Paul W. Schiffmacher, Thomas Jefferson University Hospital, Philadelphia, PA.*)

Procedure   for Blood Sampling From an Arterial Catheter—*Continued*

Steps	Rationale	Special Considerations
B. When obtaining blood for coagulation studies (particularly activated partial thromboplastin time) from a heparinized arterial line, use a discard volume of six times the dead-space volume. **(Level B*)**	Additional discard is needed to prevent contamination of the specimen with heparin in order to ensure accurate laboratory results (e.g., dead space of 0.8 mL = 4.8 mL discard).[4-6,8,13]	This recommendation does not apply to patients undergoing systemic heparin therapy. More research is needed with this patient population.
4. Turn the stopcock off to the syringe.	Stops blood flow and closes the top port of the stopcock.	Not necessary if using a needleless blood-sampling device.
5. Remove the syringe or the blood-specimen tube and discard in the appropriate receptacle.	Removes and safely disposes of the discard.	If unable to dispose of the discard specimen immediately, place it away from the field so it is not mistaken for the actual blood specimen(s) for laboratory analysis.
6. Obtain the blood sample:	Obtains the appropriate blood specimens.	If obtaining laboratory specimens in addition to an ABG and coagulation studies, obtain the routine laboratory studies first and then obtain the ABG and coagulation studies to minimize the heparin effect. Specimen size should be the amount required for the blood test(s).
A. If using the needleless system, the stopcock should remain off to the flush solution as each blood specimen tube is engaged.	The needleless blood-sampling access device (blood-transfer device) is a nonvented system, so no backflow of arterial blood from the patient occurs.	

*Level B: Well-designed, controlled studies with results that consistently support a specific action, intervention, or treatment.

Procedure continues on following page

Procedure	**for Blood Sampling From an Arterial Catheter—*Continued***	
Steps	**Rationale**	**Special Considerations**
B. If using syringes to obtain blood specimens, turn the stopcock off to the patient before changing each syringe (Fig. 61-4, *A*).	Prevents backflow of arterial blood through the open blood sampling port.	Transfer the specimen to the appropriate laboratory tubes or specimen collection containers.
After each new syringe is attached to the blood-sampling port, turn the stopcock off to the flush solution (Fig. 61-4, *B*).	Opens the arterial line from the patient to the syringe.	

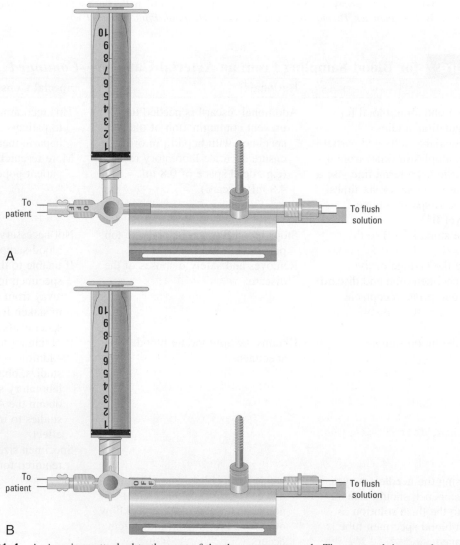

Figure 61-4   **A,** A syringe attached to the port of the three-way stopcock. The stopcock is turned "off" to the patient. **B,** A syringe attached to the top of the three-way stopcock. The stopcock is turned "off" to the flush solution. *(Drawing by Paul W. Schiffmacher, Thomas Jefferson University Hospital, Philadelphia, PA.)*

Procedure	**for Blood Sampling From an Arterial Catheter—*Continued***	
Steps	**Rationale**	**Special Considerations**
C. When obtaining an ABG sample, turn the stopcock off to the patient and attach the ABG syringe directly to the top port of the stopcock or place the ABG syringe inside of the needleless access device.	Prepares for connection of the ABG syringe.	
D. Turn the stopcock off to the flush solution.	Opens the arterial line to the ABG syringe.	
E. Gently aspirate the ABG sample.	Obtains the ABG sample while minimizing vessel trauma.	
F. Turn the stopcock off to the patient before removing the ABG syringe.	Prevents the backflow of arterial blood.	
G. Expel any air bubbles from the ABG syringe and cap the syringe.	Ensures accuracy of the ABG results.	
7. After the last specimen is obtained, turn the stopcock off to the patient.	Detaches the specimen and ensures no backflow of arterial blood from the patient.	
8. Using the fast flush device, flush the remaining blood from the top port of the stopcock onto a sterile gauze pad, into a discard syringe, or into a blood-specimen tube.	Clears blood from the system.	Follow institution standard.
9. Turn the stopcock off to the top port of the stopcock.	Opens the system up for continuous arterial pressure monitoring.	Remove the needleless blood-sampling access device (blood-transfer device) if used.
10. Place a new, sterile, injectable or noninjectable cap to the top port of the stopcock.	Maintains a closed sterile system.	
11. Using the fast flush device, flush the remaining blood in the arterial catheter back into the patient.	Promotes patency of the arterial catheter.	
Blood Sampling With a Closed Arterial Blood-Sampling System		
1. Slowly and gently pull back on the blood-withdrawal reservoir plunger until it fills to full capacity (Fig. 61-5).	Withdraws and stores blood from the patient until it is ready to be reinfused after blood sampling is complete.	Temporarily silence the arterial alarm.
2. Close the stopcock by turning it perpendicular to the tubing (Fig. 61-6).	Closes the system.	
3. Attach a needleless cannula (Fig. 61-7) to the needleless blood-sampling access device (blood-transfer device) (Fig. 61-8, *A*) or a syringe (Fig. 61-8, *B*).	Prepares for blood sampling.	
4. Cleanse the blood-sampling port with an antiseptic solution.[1,9] **(Level B*)**	Prepares for blood sampling and reduces the risk for infection.	Follow institutional standards.

*Level B: Well-designed, controlled studies with results that consistently support a specific action, intervention, or treatment.

Procedure continues on following page

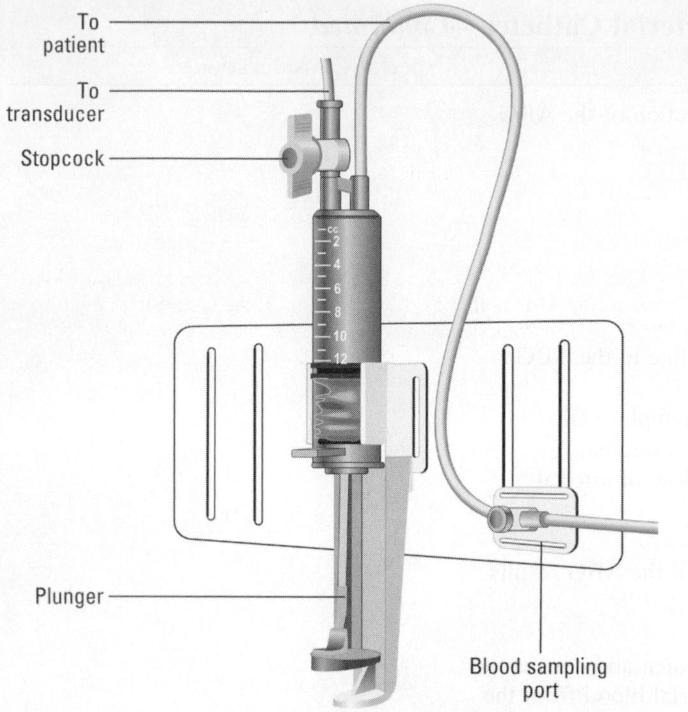

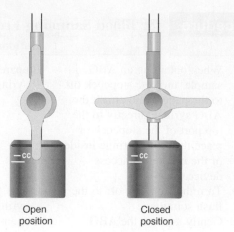

To
patient

To
transducer

Stopcock

Plunger

Blood sampling
port

Figure 61-5   Closed blood-sampling system. *(Drawing by Paul W. Schiffmacher, Thomas Jefferson University Hospital, Philadelphia, PA.)*

Open
position

Closed
position

Figure 61-6   The stopcock of the closed blood-sampling system in the open and closed position. *(Drawing by Paul W. Schiffmacher, Thomas Jefferson University Hospital, Philadelphia, PA.)*

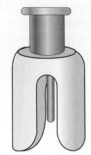

Figure 61-7   The needleless cannula for the closed blood-sampling system. *(Drawing by Paul W. Schiffmacher, Thomas Jefferson University Hospital, Philadelphia, PA.)*

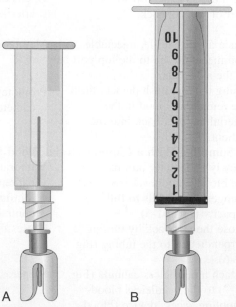

A

B

Figure 61-8   **A,** The needleless cannula attached to a needleless blood-sampling access device. **B,** The needleless cannula attached to a syringe. *(Drawing by Paul W. Schiffmacher, Thomas Jefferson University Hospital, Philadelphia, PA.)*

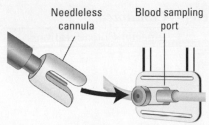

Figure 61-9 Attachment of the needleless cannula into the blood-sampling port of the closed blood-sampling system. *(Drawing by Paul W. Schiffmacher, Thomas Jefferson University Hospital, Philadelphia, PA.)*

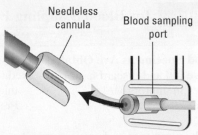

Figure 61-10 Removal of the needleless cannula from the blood-sampling port of the closed blood-sampling system. *(Drawing by Paul W. Schiffmacher, Thomas Jefferson University Hospital, Philadelphia, PA.)*

Procedure	**for Blood Sampling From an Arterial Catheter—*Continued***	
Steps	**Rationale**	**Special Considerations**
5. While holding the base of the blood sampling port, engage (push) the needleless cannula (with the attached needleless blood-sampling access device or syringe) into the blood-sampling port (Fig. 61-9).	Prepares for blood sampling.	
6. Engage each blood tube into the needleless blood-sampling access device (blood-transfer device) or obtain an ABG sample.	Obtains the sample.	If obtaining both blood samples and an ABG sample, remove the entire unit (needleless cannula with the needleless blood-sampling access device) before engaging the needleless cannula with the ABG syringe.
7. After the blood samples are obtained, hold the base of the blood-sampling port and remove the needleless cannula (with attached needleless blood-sampling access device or ABG syringe) from the sampling port by pulling it straight out (Fig. 61-10).	Removes the needleless cannula.	
8. Open the stopcock by turning it to the open position (parallel to the tubing) (see Fig. 61-6).	Opens the system to prepare for reinfusion of the stored withdrawn blood sample.	
9. Slowly and smoothly reinfuse the discard volume.[3,7,10,14,15] **(Level B*)**	Returns blood to the patient to help reduce the risk of nosocomial anemia.	
10. Swab the blood-sampling port with antiseptic solution.	Removes excess blood and fluid from the sampling port to prevent bacterial growth.	
11. Flush the system with the fast flush device.	Promotes the patency of the arterial catheter.	

*Level B: Well-designed, controlled studies with results that consistently support a specific action, intervention, or treatment.

Procedure continues on following page

Procedure   for Blood Sampling From an Arterial Catheter—*Continued*

Steps	Rationale	Special Considerations
After Blood Specimens Are Obtained		
1. Remove **PE** and discard used supplies in appropriate receptacles.	Reduces the transmission of microorganisms; Standard Precautions.	
2. **HH**		
3. Turn the alarms on and ensure that the waveform returns.	Provides accurate waveform and safe blood pressure monitoring.	
4. Label the specimens and place in a transport bag. Complete the laboratory form per institutional protocol.	Properly identifies the patient and laboratory tests to be performed.	Confirm identifying information. For ABG samples, note the time the specimen was drawn and the percentage of oxygen therapy and any other data required by institutional protocol.
5. Send the specimens for analysis.	Allows the laboratory to conduct the analysis.	Follow institutional standards regarding the use of ice for ABG samples.

Expected Outcomes

- Adequate blood sample with minimal blood loss
- No hemolysis of specimens
- No arterial spasm
- Arterial line patency maintained

Unexpected Outcomes

- Inadequate blood sample
- Hemolysis of specimens
- Arterial spasm
- Dilution of specimens that causes inaccurate laboratory results
- Anemia
- Clotting of the arterial catheter

Patient Monitoring and Care

Steps	Rationale	Reportable Conditions
		These conditions should be reported if they persist despite nursing interventions.
1. Use the minimal volume of blood discard.	Helps prevent nosocomial anemia.	• Decrease in hemoglobin or hematocrit levels
2. Monitor hemoglobin or hematocrit daily or as prescribed.	Allows early detection of nosocomial anemia.	• Decrease in hemoglobin or hematocrit levels
3. Attempt to group blood draws together whenever possible.	Diminishes the number of times the system is entered to help minimize the risk for infection.	• Signs of catheter-related infection
4. Before and after the blood withdrawal, assess and evaluate the arterial waveform.	Ensures accurate arterial pressure monitoring.	
5. Turn on arterial blood pressure alarms after blood withdrawal and review parameters.	Ensures safe arterial pressure monitoring.	
6. Obtain laboratory specimen results.	Monitors test results.	• Abnormal specimen results

Documentation

Documentation should include the following:
- Patient and family education
- Date, time, and type of specimen drawn
- Unexpected outcomes
- Additional nursing interventions
- Results of laboratory tests, when available

References and Additional Readings

For a complete list of references and additional readings for this procedure, scan this QR code with any freely available smartphone code reader app, or visit http://booksite.elsevier.com/9780323376624.

62 Blood Sampling from a Central Venous Catheter

Kathleen M. Cox

PURPOSE: To obtain blood from the central venous catheter for laboratory analysis.

PREREQUISITE NURSING KNOWLEDGE

- Knowledge of anatomy and physiology of the cardiovascular system is needed.
- Understanding principles and performance of sterile and aseptic technique and infection control is necessary.
- Understanding the technique for specimen collection and labeling is required.
- Knowledge and significance of signs and symptoms of catheter-related infection and sepsis is necessary.
- Central line–associated bloodstream infection (CLABSI) is linked to increased mortality of up to 25% and greater than $1 billion in associated costs.[5,6,10]
- Knowledge of strategies to prevent catheter-related infections is essential.
- Skill and knowledge of caring for patients with central venous catheters (CVCs) is needed (see Procedure 83).
- Understanding of the principles of hemodynamic monitoring is necessary.
- Awareness of the effect of heparin and hemolysis on various blood tests and understanding of the need for appropriate discard volumes are required.
- Alternate routes of blood withdrawal such as venipuncture or arterial catheters should be considered to minimize the risk of CLABSI.[3,6,10]
- Ideally a needleless system should be used for capping and accessing CVC ports. Needleless systems reduce needlestick injuries and risk of blood-borne infection transmission to physicians, advanced practice nurses, and other healthcare professionals and may also reduce CLABSI.[10]

EQUIPMENT

- Nonsterile gloves
- Goggles or fluid shield face mask
- Antiseptic solution (e.g., 2% chlorhexidine–based solution)
- Needleless blood-sampling access device (blood-transfer device)
- Blood specimen tubes
- 10-mL syringe
- Sterile normal saline solution for injection
- Extra blood-specimen tube for discard
- Laboratory form and patient identification specimen labels
- 2 × 2 and 4 × 4 gauze pads
- Needleless caps (injectable caps)
- Specimen transport bag(s)

Additional equipment, to have available as needed, includes the following:

- Additional syringes

PATIENT AND FAMILY EDUCATION

- Explain the purpose for blood sampling to the patient and family. *Rationale:* Provision of information helps the patient and family make informed decisions, reduces anxiety, and facilitates cooperation.
- Explain the patient's expected participation during the procedure. *Rationale:* Discussion of the patient's participation supports patient autonomy and sense of control, and increases patient cooperation.[1]

PATIENT ASSESSMENT AND PREPARATION

Patient Assessment

- Assess the patency of the CVC. *Rationale:* Ensures function of the CVC catheter.
- Evaluate previous laboratory results. *Rationale:* These results provide baseline data for comparison.
- Determine whether intravenous solutions or medications are infusing through the CVC. *Rationale:* Intravenous solutions and medication must be temporarily discontinued before blood sampling to reduce interference with the laboratory analysis.[14] Critical infusions (i.e., vasoactive medications) may not be able to be stopped; additional blood access sites need to be considered.

Patient Preparation

- Verify that the patient is the correct patient using two identifiers. *Rationale:* Before performing a procedure, the nurse should ensure the correct identification of the patient for the intended intervention.
- Confirm that the patient and family understand preprocedural teaching by having them verbalize understanding.

Clarify key points by reinforcing important information and answer all questions. ***Rationale:*** Preprocedure communication provides a framework of patient expectations, enhances cooperation, and reduces anxiety.[1]

• Position the patient so that the intended blood sampling port is exposed. ***Rationale:*** Optimal positioning improves the ease of obtaining the blood sample and reduces potential contamination of the port.

Procedure	for Blood Sampling from Central Venous Catheters	
Steps	**Rationale**	**Special Considerations**

1. HH		
2. PE		
Blood Sampling From the CVC Hemodynamic Monitoring System		
1. Cleanse the needleless cap (injectable cap) on the hemodynamic monitoring system stopcock with an antiseptic solution and allow to dry.[3,8,10,12,13] **(Level B*)**	Reduces the risk for infection.	Follow institutional standards.
2. Attach the needleless blood sampling device (blood transfer device) to the stopcock of the hemodynamic monitoring system (Fig. 62-1).	Prepares for blood sampling.	
3. Temporarily suspend the right-atrial pressure/central venous pressure (RAP/CVP) monitoring alarm.	Prevents the alarm from sounding because the RAP/CVP waveform is lost during the blood sampling.	

*Level B: Well-designed, controlled studies with results that consistently support a specific action, intervention, or treatment.

Procedure continues on following page

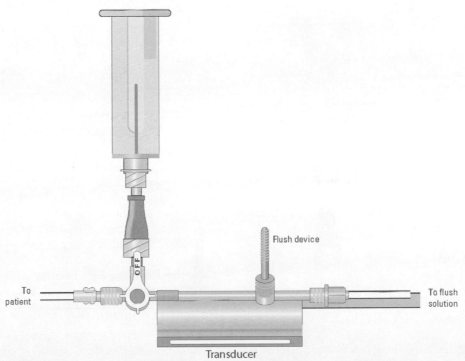

Figure 62-1 Needleless blood-sampling device (blood-transfer device) attached to the needleless (injectable) capped stopcock of the hemodynamic monitoring system. The stopcock is open to the transducer system. *(Drawing by Paul W. Schiffmacher, Thomas Jefferson University, Philadelphia, PA.)*

Procedure   for Blood Sampling from Central Venous Catheters—*Continued*

Steps	Rationale	Special Considerations
4. Turn the stopcock off to the monitoring system and flush solution (Fig. 62-2).	The needleless blood sampling device is now in contact with the central venous blood.	
5. Insert a blood-specimen tube into the blood-sampling device (blood-transfer device) to obtain the discard volume.[3,13] (**Level B***)	Clears the catheter of flush solution. The discard volume includes the dead space (from the tip of the lumen to the top port of the needleless capped stopcock) and the blood diluted by the flush solution (e.g., 3.5 mL).[2–4,11,14]	Dead-space information for a catheter is usually listed in the information that comes with the catheter.
6. Remove the discard blood-specimen tube and discard in the appropriate receptacle.	Removes discard safely.	
7. Insert the blood-specimen tube into the blood-sampling device to obtain the specimen.	Obtains the blood specimen.	
8. After obtaining the specimen, detach the blood-sampling device from the capped stopcock and discard it in appropriate receptacle.	Removes and safely discards equipment.	The blood in the needleless cap can be cleared by fast flushing the blood into a blood-specimen tube or syringe (Fig. 62-3).

*Level B: Well-designed, controlled studies with results that consistently support a specific action, intervention, or treatment.

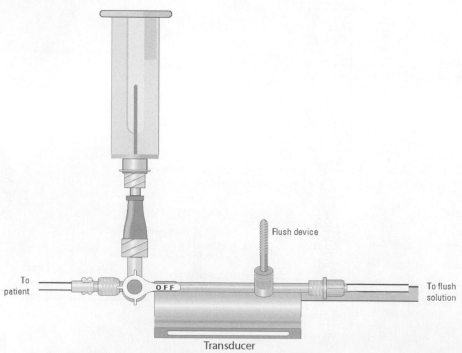

Figure 62-2 Needleless blood-sampling device (blood-transfer device) attached to the needleless (injectable) capped stopcock of the hemodynamic monitoring system. The stopcock is turned "off" to the monitoring system and flush solution. (*Drawing by Paul W. Schiffmacher, Thomas Jefferson University, Philadelphia, PA.*)

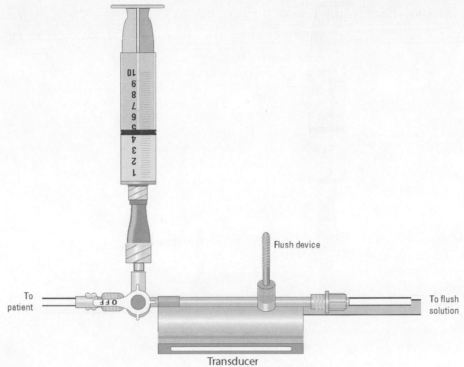

Figure 62-3 A syringe attached to the port of the three-way stopcock. The stopcock is turned "off" to the patient. The system is open between the flush solution and the syringe attached to the needleless cap. *(Drawing by Paul W. Schiffmacher, Thomas Jefferson University, Philadelphia, PA.)*

Procedure	for Blood Sampling from Central Venous Catheters—*Continued*	
Steps	**Rationale**	**Special Considerations**
9. Cleanse the needleless cap at the top of the stopcock with an antiseptic solution and allow to dry.[3,8,10,12,13] **(Level B*)**	Reduces the risk for infection.	Follow institutional standards.
10. Attach a 10-mL syringe filled with sterile normal saline solution to the needleless (injectable) capped stopcock.	Prepares flush solution.	
11. Gently flush the normal saline solution into the needleless (injectable) cap (Fig. 62-4).	Clears blood from the needleless cap and the stopcock.	
12. Turn the stopcock off to the blood-sampling device (blood-transfer device).[7]	This opens the system for continuous RAP/CVP pressure monitoring.	
13. Fast flush the remaining blood in the CVC back into the patient.	Promotes patency of the CVC.	
14. Observe the monitor for return of the RAP/CVP waveform.	Ensures continuous monitoring of the waveform.	
15. Remove **PE** and discard used supplies in appropriate receptacles.	Reduces the transmission of microorganisms; Standard Precautions.	
16. **HH**		
17. Turn the alarms back on.	Activates the alarm system.	

*Level B: Well-designed, controlled studies with results that consistently support a specific action, intervention, or treatment.

Procedure continues on following page

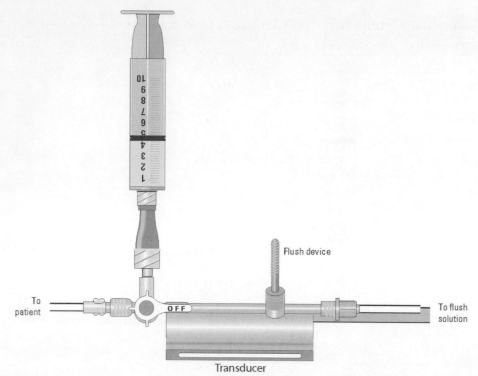

Figure 62-4 A syringe attached to the port of the three-way stopcock. The stopcock is turned "off" to the monitoring system and flush solution. The system is open between the patient and the syringe attached to the needleless (injectable) cap. (*Drawing by Paul W. Schiffmacher, Thomas Jefferson University, Philadelphia, PA.*)

Procedure	**for Blood Sampling from Central Venous Catheters—*Continued***	
Steps	Rationale	Special Considerations
18. Label the specimen and place in a transport bag. Complete the laboratory form.	Properly identifies the patient and laboratory tests to be performed.	Confirm identifying information.
19. Send the specimen for analysis.	Ensures analysis.	
Blood Sampling From a Single CVC Port That Is Not Monitored		
1. 🔲		
2. 🔲		
3. Temporarily discontinue intravenous solutions and medications before blood sampling.	Minimizes the risk of diluting the blood specimen, which may affect the accuracy of the laboratory results.[14]	If the blood sample is obtained from a multiple-lumen catheter (e.g., triple lumen), stop intravenous and medication infusions from all of the CVC ports, and ensure that temporarily stopping intravenous medications does not affect hemodynamic stability. Obtain the blood sample from the distal lumen.
4. Remove and cap the intravenous solution infusing through the intended blood-sampling port.	Prepares equipment and maintains asepsis of the intravenous system.	

Procedure for Blood Sampling from Central Venous Catheters—*Continued*

Steps	Rationale	Special Considerations
5. Cleanse the needleless cap (injectable cap) at the end of the CVC sampling port with an antiseptic solution and allow to dry.[3,8,10,12,13] **(Level B*)**	Reduces the risk for infection.	Follow institutional standards.
6. Attach the needleless blood-sampling device (blood-transfer device) to the needleless cap (injectable cap) of the CVC port (Fig. 62-5).	Prepares for blood sampling.	
7. Insert a blood-specimen tube into the blood-sampling device to obtain the discard volume.	Clears the catheter of flush solution. The discard volume includes the dead space (from the tip of the lumen to the top port of the needleless capped stopcock) and the blood diluted by the flush solution (e.g., 3.5 mL).[3,14]	Dead-space information for a catheter is usually listed in the information that comes with the catheter.
8. Remove the discard blood-specimen tube and discard in the appropriate receptacle.	Removes discard safely.	
9. Insert the blood-specimen tube into the blood-sampling device to obtain the specimen.	Obtains the blood specimen.	Obtain additional specimens as prescribed. Specimen size should be the amount required for the blood test(s).
10. After obtaining the specimen, detach the blood-sampling device from the capped stopcock and discard it in the appropriate receptacle.	Removes and safely discards equipment.	
11. Cleanse the needleless cap (injectable cap) of the CVC port with an antiseptic solution and allow to dry.[3,8,10,12,13] **(Level B*)**	Reduces the risk for infection.	Follow institutional standards.
12. Attach a 10-mL syringe filled with sterile normal saline solution to the needleless cap (injectable cap) of the CVC port.	Prepares flush solution.	

*Level B: Well-designed, controlled studies with results that consistently support a specific action, intervention, or treatment.

Procedure continues on following page

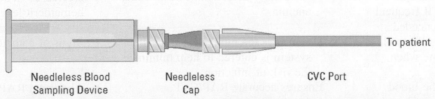

Figure 62-5 The needleless blood-sampling device (blood-transfer device) attached to the needleless (injectable) cap of the central venous catheter (CVC) port. *(Drawing by Paul W. Schiffmacher, Thomas Jefferson University, Philadelphia, PA.)*

Procedure   for Blood Sampling from Central Venous Catheters—*Continued*

Steps	Rationale	Special Considerations
13. Gently flush the normal saline solution into the needleless cap (injectable cap).	Clears blood from the needleless cap (injectable cap) and the CVC port.	
14. Remove the normal saline solution syringe and discard it in the appropriate receptacle.	Removes and safely discards equipment.	
15. Cleanse the needleless cap (injectable cap) of the CVC port with an antiseptic solution.[3,8,10,12,13] **(Level B*)**	Reduces the risk for infection.	Follow institutional standards.
16. Reattach and resume the intravenous solution or medication infusion.	Continues treatment.	
17. Remove **PE** and discard used supplies in appropriate receptacles.	Reduces the transmission of microorganisms; Standard Precautions.	
18. **HH**		
19. Label the specimen and place in a transport bag. Complete the laboratory form.	Properly identifies the patient and laboratory tests to be performed.	Confirm identifying information.
20. Send the specimen for analysis.	Allows the laboratory to conduct the analysis.	

*Level B: Well-designed, controlled studies with results that consistently support a specific action, intervention, or treatment.

Expected Outcomes

- Catheter remains patent with good waveform if monitoring system is used
- Catheter site remains free from infection
- Adequate blood sample with minimal blood loss
- No hemolysis of the specimen

Unexpected Outcomes

- Clotting of the CVC
- Catheter-related infection
- Inability to obtain blood sample
- Hemolysis of specimens
- Dilution of specimens that causes inaccurate laboratory results

Patient Monitoring and Care

Steps	Rationale	Reportable Conditions
		These conditions should be reported if they persist despite nursing interventions.
1. Use the minimal volume of blood discard.[14]	Helps prevent nosocomial anemia.	• Decreased hemoglobin level and hematocrit level
2. Monitor hemoglobin and hematocrit values if frequent blood sampling is needed.	Allows early detection of nosocomial anemia.	• Decreased hemoglobin level and hematocrit level
3. Attempt to obtain all blood samples at one time when possible.[9]	Diminishes the number of times the system is entered to help minimize the risk of infection.	• Signs of catheter-related sepsis
4. Before and after the blood withdrawal, assess and evaluate the RAP/CVP waveform if monitored.	Ensures accurate RAP/CVP monitoring.	• Abnormal RAP/CVP waveforms
5. Obtain laboratory specimen results.	Assesses patient condition.	• Abnormal specimen results

Documentation

Documentation should include the following:
- Patient and family education
- Time and type of specimen drawn
- Results of laboratory tests when available

- Unexpected outcomes
- Inability to obtain sample

References and Additional Readings

For a complete list of references and additional readings for this procedure, scan this QR code with any freely available smartphone code reader app, or visit http://booksite.elsevier.com/9780323376624.

63 Blood Sampling from a Pulmonary Artery Catheter

Kathleen M. Cox

PURPOSE: To obtain blood from the pulmonary artery (PA) catheter for determination of mixed venous oxygen saturation.

PREREQUISITE NURSING KNOWLEDGE

- Knowledge of anatomy and physiology of the pulmonary and cardiovascular system is needed.
- Understanding principles and performance of sterile and aseptic technique and infection control is necessary.
- Physiological gas exchange and acid-base balance should be understood.
- Technique for specimen collection and labeling should be known.
- Principles of hemodynamic monitoring need to be understood.
- Knowledge about the care of patients with PA catheters (see Procedure 72) and stopcock manipulation (see Procedure 75) is needed.
- The most frequent blood specimen obtained from the PA is one for mixed venous oxygen saturation (Svo_2) analysis.[9,10]
- Svo_2 measures the oxygen saturation of the venous blood in the PA (see Procedure 16).
- Svo_2 samples may be obtained to calibrate the equipment when continuously monitoring Svo_2 values.
- Routine blood sampling from the PA catheter is not recommended because entry into the sterile system may increase the incidence of catheter-related infection.[2,6,7]

EQUIPMENT

- Nonsterile gloves
- Goggles or fluid shield face mask
- Antiseptic solution (e.g., 2% chlorhexidine-based solution)
- Needleless blood sampling access device (blood-transfer device)
- Two 10-mL syringes
- Blood-specimen tubes
- Blood gas sampling syringe
- Needleless cap (injectable cap) or nonvented cap (noninjectable cap)
- Laboratory form and specimen label
- Specimen transport bag(s)

Additional equipment, to have available as needed, includes the following:
- Additional syringes
- Bag of ice
- Sterile 4 × 4 gauze pad

PATIENT AND FAMILY EDUCATION

- Explain the purpose for blood sampling to the patient and family. **Rationale:** Provision of information helps the patient and family make informed decisions, reduces anxiety, and facilitates cooperation.
- Explain the patient's expected participation during the procedure. **Rationale:** Discussion of the patient's participation supports patient autonomy and sense of control and increases patient cooperation.[1]

PATIENT ASSESSMENT AND PREPARATION
Patient Assessment

- Assess the patient's cardiopulmonary and hemodynamic status, including abnormal lung sounds, respiratory distress, dysrhythmias, decreased mentation, agitation, and skin color changes. **Rationale:** These signs and symptoms could necessitate blood sampling for venous oxygenation.
- Assess for a decrease in cardiac output related to changes in preload, afterload, or contractility. **Rationale:** Mixed venous blood samples are used to evaluate changes in cardiopulmonary function.
- Assess the hemodynamic waveforms. **Rationale:** Determines that the PA catheter is in the proper position.
- Assess for a decrease in cardiac output related to changes in preload, afterload, or contractility. **Rationale:** Mixed venous blood samples are used to evaluate changes in cardiopulmonary function.

Patient Preparation

- Verify that the patient is the correct patient using two identifiers. **Rationale:** Before performing a procedure, the nurse should ensure the correct identification of the patient for the intended intervention.
- Confirm that the patient and family understand preprocedural teaching by having them verbalize understanding. Clarify key points by reinforcing important information and answer all questions. **Rationale:** Understanding of previously taught information is evaluated and reinforced.
- Position the patient so that the intended blood sampling port is exposed. **Rationale:** Optimal positioning improves the ease of obtaining the blood sample and reduces potential contamination of the port.

Procedure for Blood Sampling from a Pulmonary Artery Catheter

Steps	Rationale	Special Considerations
1. **HH**		
2. **PE**		
3. When drawing a mixed venous oxygen (SvO₂) sample, open the arterial blood gas (ABG) kit and expel the excess air and heparin from the syringe.	Prepares the ABG syringe.	Heparin is usually in powdered form.
4. Temporarily suspend the PA alarms.	Prevents the alarm from sounding because the PA waveform is lost during the blood draw.	
5. PA distal stopcock:		
A. Remove the nonvented cap (noninjectable cap) from the stopcock of the distal lumen of the PA catheter.	Prepares the line for blood sampling.	
or		
B. Cleanse the needleless cap (injectable cap) at the top of the stopcock of the distal lumen of the PA catheter with an antiseptic solution and allow to dry.[2,4,7,8] **(Level B*)**	Prepares the line for blood sampling and reduces the risk for infection.	Follow institutional standards.
6. Place a sterile syringe or a needleless blood sampling access device (blood-transfer device) into the top port of the stopcock of the distal lumen of the PA catheter (see Figs. 62-1 and 63-1).	Prepares for blood sampling.	

*Level B: Well-designed, controlled studies with results that consistently support a specific action, intervention, or treatment.

Procedure continues on following page

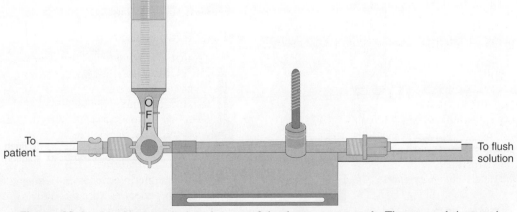

Figure 63-1 A syringe attached to the port of the three-way stopcock. The stopcock is turned "off" to the port of the stopcock. (*Drawing by Paul W. Schiffmacher, Thomas Jefferson University, Philadelphia, PA.*)

Procedure for Blood Sampling from a Pulmonary Artery Catheter—*Continued*

Steps	Rationale	Special Considerations
7. Turn the stopcock off to the flush solution (see Figs. 62-2 and 63-2).	The syringe or needleless blood-sampling access device is then in direct contact with the blood in the PA.	
8. With a syringe, slowly and gently aspirate the discard volume or, if using a needleless blood-sampling access device, engage the blood specimen tube to obtain the discard volume. **(Level B*)**	Clears the catheter of flush solution. The discard volume includes the dead space (from the tip of the distal lumen to the top port of the stopcock) and the blood diluted by the flush solution (e.g., 3.5 mL).[2,3,5,10–12]	If additional laboratory studies are needed, larger discard volumes may be necessary for accurate results.[12]
9. Turn the stopcock off to the syringe or the needleless blood-sampling access device (see Figs. 62-1 and 63-1).	Stops blood flow and closes the top port of the stopcock.	
10. Remove the syringe or the blood specimen tube and discard in the appropriate receptacle.	Removes and safely disposes of the discard.	
11. Insert an ABG syringe into the stopcock or insert the ABG syringe into the needleless blood-sampling access device.	Prepares for removal of a blood sample.	
12. Turn the stopcock off to the flush system (see Figs. 62-2 and 63-2).	Prepares for blood sampling.	

*Level B: Well-designed, controlled studies with results that consistently support a specific action, intervention, or treatment.

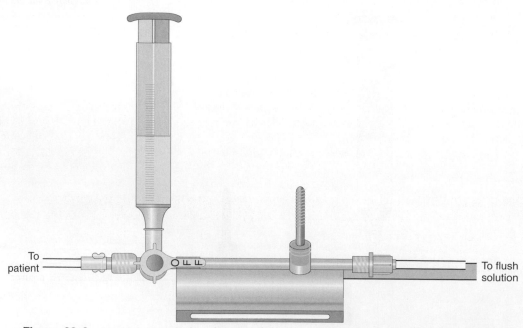

Figure 63-2 A syringe attached to the port of the three-way stopcock. The stopcock is turned "off" to flush solution. (*Drawing by Paul W. Schiffmacher, Thomas Jefferson University, Philadelphia, PA.*)

Procedure | for Blood Sampling from a Pulmonary Artery Catheter—*Continued*

Steps	Rationale	Special Considerations
13. Slowly aspirate the SvO₂ sample (e.g., 1 mL).	Slow aspiration is important to prevent contamination of the mixed venous sample with arterial blood from the pulmonary capillaries, which will falsely elevate the SvO_2 value.[11]	
14. Turn the stopcock off to the syringe or the needleless blood sampling access device (see Figs. 62-1 and 63-1).	Prevents bleeding.	
15. Remove the ABG syringe.	Detaches the specimen.	
16. Expel any air bubbles from the ABG syringe and cap the syringe.	Ensures the accuracy of the SvO_2 results.	
17. Turn the stopcock off to the patient.	Prepares the system.	
18. Fast flush the remaining blood from the top port of the stopcock: A. Remove the nonvented or noninjectable cap. B. Flush the blood onto a sterile gauze pad, into a discard syringe, or into a blood specimen tube.	Clears blood from the system.	
19. Turn the stopcock off to the top port of the stopcock (see Figs. 62-1 and 63-1).	Opens the system up for continuous PA pressure monitoring.	Remove the needleless blood-sampling access device if used.
20. Attach a new sterile nonvented cap (noninjectable cap) or cleanse the needleless cap (injectable cap) with antiseptic solution.	Maintains a closed sterile system.	
21. Flush the remaining blood in the PA catheter back into the patient.	Promotes patency of the PA catheter.	
22. Observe the monitor for return of the PA waveform.	Ensures continuous monitoring of the PA waveform.	
23. Remove PE and discard used supplies.	Reduces the transmission of microorganisms; Standard Precautions.	
24. 🖐		
25. Turn the alarms back on.	Activates the alarm system.	
26. Label the specimen and place in a transport bag. Complete the laboratory form.	Properly identifies the patient and laboratory tests to be performed.	Confirm identifying information. Label the blood-gas laboratory slip as a mixed venous sample.
27. Send the specimen for analysis.	Needed for ABG analysis.	Follow institutional policy regarding use of ice for ABG samples.

Expected Outcomes

- Adequate blood sample with minimal blood loss
- PA catheter patency maintained
- SvO₂ value and trends within normal range (60–80%)

Unexpected Outcomes

- Inability to obtain SvO₂ sample
- Clotting of the PA catheter
- Arterial sample obtained as a result of rapid withdrawal of blood from the pulmonary capillaries instead of mixed venous oxygen sample for blood-gas analysis

Procedure continues on following page

Patient Monitoring and Care

Steps	Rationale	Reportable Conditions
		These conditions should be reported if they persist despite nursing interventions.
1. Before and after the blood withdrawal, assess and evaluate the PA waveform.	Ensures that the PA catheter is properly positioned.	• Abnormal PA waveforms or values
2. Correlate the SvO_2 results with the measured cardiac output.	Changes in the SvO_2 indicate changes in cardiac output and hemodynamic status.	• Abnormal mixed venous oxygen saturation, preload, afterload, cardiac output, and cardiac index
3. Correlate the SvO_2 results with the clinical assessment data.[2,10]	SvO_2 decreases with: • Increased oxygen consumption • Decreased oxygen delivery SvO_2 increases with: • Decreased tissue oxygen consumption • Increased oxygen delivery	• Fever • Shivering • Seizures • Agitation • Pain • Decreased cardiac output • Decreased hemoglobin • Decreased arterial oxygen saturation • Hypothermia

Documentation

Documentation should include the following:
- Patient and family education
- Time and date of the SvO_2 sample
- SvO_2 results
- Any difficulties with PA catheter blood sampling
- Nursing interventions performed
- Unexpected outcomes

References and Additional Readings

For a complete list of references and additional readings for this procedure, scan this QR code with any freely available smartphone code reader app, or visit http://booksite.elsevier.com/9780323376624.

PROCEDURE

64

Cardiac Output Measurement Techniques (Invasive)

Susan Scott

PURPOSE: Cardiac output (CO) measurements are used to assess and monitor cardiovascular status. CO monitoring can be used in the evaluation of patient responses to various therapies, including fluid management interventions, vasoactive and inotropic medication administration, and mechanical assist devices. CO measurements can be obtained either continuously or intermittently via a pulmonary artery (PA) catheter. CO measurements provide data that may be useful in directing and/or improving the care for critically ill patients with hemodynamic instability.

PREREQUISITE NURSING KNOWLEDGE

- Understanding of normal anatomy and physiology of the cardiovascular system and pulmonary system is necessary.
- Understanding of basic dysrhythmia recognition and treatment of life-threatening dysrhythmias is needed.
- Pathophysiologic changes associated with structural heart disease (e.g., ventricular dysfunction from myocardial infarction, diastolic or systolic changes, and valve dysfunction) should be understood.
- Understanding of the principles of aseptic technique is necessary.
- Understanding of the PA catheter (see Fig. 72-1), lumens and ports, and the location of the PA catheter in the heart and PA (see Fig. 72-2) is needed.
- Pressure transducer systems (see Procedure 75) should be understood.
- Competence in the use and clinical application of hemodynamic waveforms and values obtained with a PA catheter including assessing normal and abnormal waveforms and values for right atrial pressure (RAP), pulmonary artery pressure (PAP), and pulmonary artery occlusion pressure (PAOP) is needed. PAOP may also be termed pulmonary artery wedge pressure (PAWP).
- Knowledge of vasoactive and inotropic medications and their effects on cardiac function, ventricular function, coronary vessels, and vascular smooth muscles is needed.
- CO is defined as the amount of blood ejected by the left ventricle (LV) per minute and is the product of stroke volume (SV) and heart rate (HR). It is measured in liters per minute.

$$CO = SV \times HR$$

- Normal CO is 4 to 8 L/min. The four physiological factors that affect CO are preload, afterload, contractility, and heart rate.

- Stroke volume is the amount of blood volume ejected from either ventricle per contraction. Left ventricular stroke volume is the difference between left ventricular end-diastolic volume and left ventricular end-systolic volume. Left ventricular stroke volume is normally 60 to 100 mL/contraction. Major factors that influence stroke volume are preload, afterload, and contractility.
- Right heart preload refers to the pressure in the right ventricle (RV) at the end of diastole and is measured by the RAP or CVP. Elevations in left heart filling pressures may be accompanied by parallel changes in RAP, especially in patients with left systolic ventricular dysfunction. Other factors that affect RAP are venous return, intravascular volume, vascular capacity, and pulmonary pressure. Right heart preload is increased in right heart failure, right ventricular infarction, tricuspid regurgitation, pulmonary hypertension, and fluid overload. Right heart preload is decreased in hypovolemic states.
- Left heart preload refers to the pressure in the LV at the end of diastole and is measured by the PAOP. When LV preload or end-diastolic volume increases, the muscle fibers are stretched. The increased tension or force of contraction that accompanies an increase in diastolic filling is called the Frank-Starling law. According to the Frank-Starling law the heart adjusts its pumping ability to accommodate various levels of venous return. Note: In patients with advanced chronic LV dysfunction and remodeled hearts (spherical or globular shaped LV instead of the normal elliptical-shaped LV), the Frank-Starling law does not apply. In these patients, muscle fibers of the heart are already maximally lengthened; as a result, the heart cannot respond significantly to increased filling or stretch with increased force of contraction.
- Afterload refers to the force the ventricular myocardial fibers must overcome to shorten or contract. It is the force that resists contraction. The amount of force the LV must overcome influences the amount of blood ejected into the systemic circulation. Afterload is influenced by peripheral

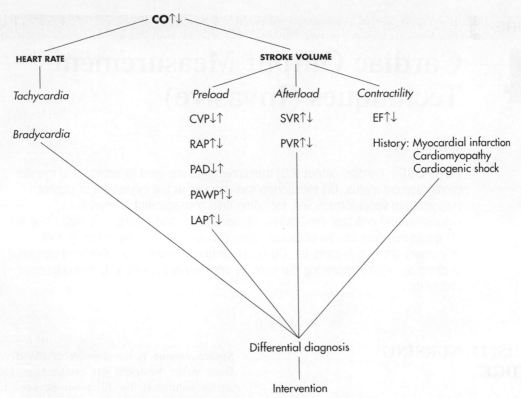

Figure 64-1   Systematic assessment of the determinants of cardiac output may assist the clinician in defining the etiological factors of cardiac output alteration more precisely. *(From Whalen DA, Keller R: Cardiovascular patient assessment. In Kinney MR, et al, editors:* AACN clinical reference for critical care nurse, *ed 4, St. Louis, 1998, Mosby, 227-319)*

vascular resistance (the force opposing blood flow within the vessels), systolic blood pressure, systolic stress, and systolic impedance. Peripheral resistance is affected by the length and radius of the blood vessel, arterial blood pressure, and venous constriction or dilation. The systolic force of the heart is increased in conditions that cause vasoconstriction (increased afterload), including aortic stenosis, hypertension, or hyperviscosity of blood (e.g., polycythemia). The systolic force of the heart is decreased in conditions that cause vasodilation or decrease the viscosity of blood (e.g., anemia). Right ventricular afterload is calculated as pulmonary vascular resistance. Left ventricular afterload is calculated as systemic vascular resistance.

- Contractility is defined as the ability of the myocardium to contract and eject blood into the pulmonary or systemic vasculature. Contractility is increased by sympathetic neural stimulation, and the release of calcium and norepinephrine is decreased by parasympathetic neural stimulation, acidosis, and hyperkalemia. Contractility and heart rate can be influenced by neural, humoral, and pharmacological factors.
- In addition to stroke volume, CO is affected by heart rate. Normally, nerves of the parasympathetic and sympathetic nervous system regulate heart rate through specialized cardiac electrical cells. Heart rate and rhythm are influenced by neural humoral, and pharmacological factors. Decreased heart rate can be the result of factors such as increased parasympathetic neural stimulation, decreased

sympathetic neural stimulation, or decreased body temperature. Increased heart rate can be triggered by factors that cause catecholamine release, such as hypoxia, hypotension, pain, or anxiety. The more rapid the heart rate, the less time is available for adequate diastolic filling, which can result in a decreased CO. Because multiple factors regulate cardiac performance and affect CO, these factors must be assessed (Fig. 64-1).

- Cardiac index adjusts the CO to an individual's body size (square meter of body surface area), making it a more precise measurement than CO.
- Refer to Table 64-1 for normal hemodynamic values and calculations.
- At the bedside, CO measurements are obtained through a PA catheter via the intermittent bolus CO method or the continuous CO method.
- Thermodilution CO measures right ventricular outflow; therefore, intracardiac right-to-left shunts, as well as tricuspid and pulmonic valve insufficiency, can result in inaccurate measurements.[3,38]
- The thermodilution cardiac output (TDCO) method: an injectate solution of a known volume (10 mL) and temperature (room or cold temperature) is injected into the right atrium (RA) through the proximal port of the PA catheter. The injectate exits the catheter into the RA, where it mixes with blood and flows through the RV to the PA. A thermistor located at the tip of the PA catheter detects the change in blood temperature as the blood passes the tip of the catheter in the PA. The CO is

TABLE 64-1 Hemodynamic Parameters

Parameters	Calculations	Normal Value
Body surface area (BSA)	Weight (kg) × height (cm) × 0.007184	Varies with size (range = 0.58–2.9 m²)
CO	HR × SV	4–8 L/min
Stroke volume (SV)	CO × 1000 / HR	60–100 mL/beat
Stroke volume index (SVI)	SV / BSA	30–65 mL/beat/m²
Cardiac index (CI)	CO / BSA	2.5–4.5 L/min/m²
Heart rate (HR)		60–100 beats/min
Preload		
Central venous pressure (CVP) or RAP		2–6 mm Hg
Left atrial pressure (LAP)		4–12 mm Hg
Pulmonary artery diastolic pressure (PADP)		5–15 mm Hg
PAOP		4–12 mm Hg
RVEDP		0–8 mm Hg
LVEDP		4–10 mm Hg
Afterload		
Systemic vascular resistance (SVR)	MAP – CVP/RAP × 80 / CO	900–1400 dynes/s/cm⁻⁵
SVR index (SVRI)	MAP – CVP/RAP × 80 / CI	2000–2400 dynes/s/cm⁻⁵/m²
Pulmonary vascular resistance (PVR)	PAMP – PAOP × 80 / CO	100–250 dynes/s/cm⁻⁵
PVR index (PVRI)	PAMP – PAOP × 80 / CI	255–315 dynes/s/cm⁻⁵/m²
Systolic blood pressure		100–130 mm Hg
Contractility		
Ejection fraction (EF):		
Left	LVEDV × 100 / SV	60–75%
Right	RVEDV × 100 / SV	45–50%
Stroke work index:		
Left	SVI (MAP – PAOP) × 0.0136	50–62 g-m/m²/beat
Right	SVI (MAP – CVP) × 0.0136	5–10 g-m/m²/beat
Pressures:		
MAP	DBP + ⅓ (SBP – DBP)	70–105 mm Hg
PAMP	PADP + ⅓ (PASP – PADP)	9–16 mm Hg

CO, Cardiac output; *DBP*, diastolic blood pressure; *MAP*, mean arterial pressure; *LVEDP*, left ventricular end-diastolic pressure; *RVEDP*, right ventricular end-diastolic pressure; *PAMP*, pulmonary artery mean pressure; *PAOP*, pulmonary artery occlusion pressure; *LVEDV*, left ventricular end-diastolic volume; *RVEDV*, right ventricular end-diastolic volume; *PASP*, pulmonary artery systolic pressure; *PADP*, pulmonary artery diastolic pressure; *SBP*, systolic blood pressure.
Adapted from Tuggle D: Optimizing hemodynamics: Strategies for fluid and medication titration in shock. In Carlson K, editor: AACN advanced critical care nursing, *St Louis, 2009, Saunders, 1106; and Ahrens T: Hemodynamic monitoring,* Crit Care Nurs Clin N Am *11:19-31, 1999.*

calculated as the difference in temperatures on a time versus temperature curve.
- CO can be calculated from PA catheters with two types of thermistors:
  - A single thermistor has one inline temperature sensor near the tip of the catheter that lies in the PA when in proper position.
  - A dual thermistor has two inline temperature sensors, one in the right atrium/superior caval vein (immediately above the injectate port opening) and one near the tip of the catheter (same position as single thermistor). Because a temperature sensor is located in the right atrium, there is no need to enter a "correction factor" or "computation constant" into the computer to account for the loss in thermal indicator (heat) from the hub of the RA injectate port to the RA. Investigators found that

the second thermistor improved accuracy compared with Fick CO measurements and also improved precision or repeatability of CO measurements in both cold and room temperature.[4,26] In one study, cold injectate had excellent precision with the standard single-thermistor PA catheter. Researchers concluded that the dual-thermistor PA catheter provided the greatest benefit in decreasing measurement variability when room temperature injections were used to measure CO.[4]
- The change in temperature over time is plotted as a curve and displayed on the bedside monitor screen. CO is mathematically calculated from the area under the curve and is displayed digitally and graphically on the monitor screen (Fig. 64-2). The area under the curve is inversely proportional to the rate of blood flow. Thus a high CO is associated with a small area under the curve, whereas a low CO

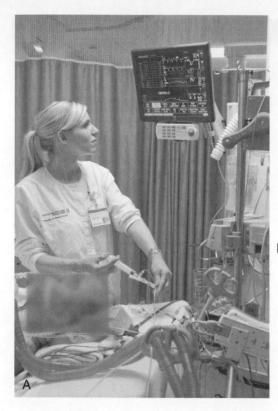

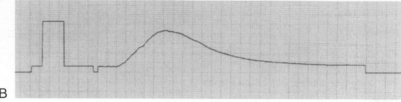

B

Figure 64-2   A, Examining cardiac output curves to establish reliability of values. B, Normal cardiac output curve with rapid upstroke and smooth progressive decrease in temperature sensing. (B: *From Ahrens T: Hemodynamic monitoring,* Crit Care Nurs Clin North Am *11[1]:28, 1999.*)

is associated with a large area under the curve (Fig. 64-3, A).

- The thermistor near the distal tip of the catheter detects the temperature change and sends a signal to the CO computer and bedside monitor. The computer calculates the CO with the modified Stewart-Hamilton equation, and the CO number is displayed on the monitor screen. The average result of three to five measurements is used to determine CO.

- Accuracy of TDCO is dependent on adequate mixing of blood and injectate, forward blood flow, steady baseline temperature in the PA, and appropriate procedural technique.[3,19] In addition, loss of thermal indicator (heat), respiratory artifact, and hemodynamic instability can cause variability from one injection to another.[19,29,32]

- Traditionally cardiac output measurements have been recommended to be performed at end-expiration, though there is research suggesting that this is not necessary.[20,24] Additional research is needed.

- Commercially available closed-system delivery sets (CO-Set, Edwards Lifesciences, LLC, Irvine, CA) can be used with both cold and room temperature injectate (Figs. 64-4 and 64-5).

- The Continuous Cardiac Output (CCO) method proceeds as follows:
  - ❖ Continuous measurement of CO can be performed without the need for injected fluid. The CO can be obtained with a heat-exchange CO catheter. This catheter has a membrane that allows for heat to exchange with blood in the right atrium.
  - ❖ The PA catheter with CCO capability contains a 10-cm thermal filament located close to the injection port (15 to 25 cm from the tip of the catheter, near the

proximal lumen port). When a PA catheter is properly placed, the thermal filament section of the catheter is located in the RV. This filament emits a pulsed low heat energy signal in a 30- to 60-second pseudorandom binary (on/off) sequence, which allows blood to be heated and the heat signal adequately processed over time as blood passes through the ventricle. A bedside computer constructs thermodilution curves detected from the pseudorandom heat impulses and measures CO automatically. The computer screen displays digital readings updated every 30 to 60 seconds that reflect the average CO of the preceding 3 to 6 minutes. The CCO eliminates the need for fluid boluses, reduces contamination risk, and provides a continuous CO trend.[1,2,32]

- ❖ Because the CCO computer constantly displays and frequently updates the CO, treatment decisions can be expedited. Derived hemodynamic calculations (e.g., cardiac index and systemic vascular resistance) can be obtained with greater frequency, thereby providing up-to-time information in assessment of response to therapies that affect hemodynamics.[1]

- CCO has been compared with TDCO, transesophageal Doppler scan technique, and aortic transpulmonary technique to determine its precision. Study results all show small bias, limits of agreement, and 95% confidence limits, reflecting that CCO provides accurate measurement of CO and is a reliable method.[1,2,6,22,32,39,50]

- Adequate mixing of blood and indicator (heat) is necessary for accurate CCO measurements. Conditions that prevent appropriate mixing or directional flow of the indicator or blood include intracardiac shunts or tricuspid regurgitation.

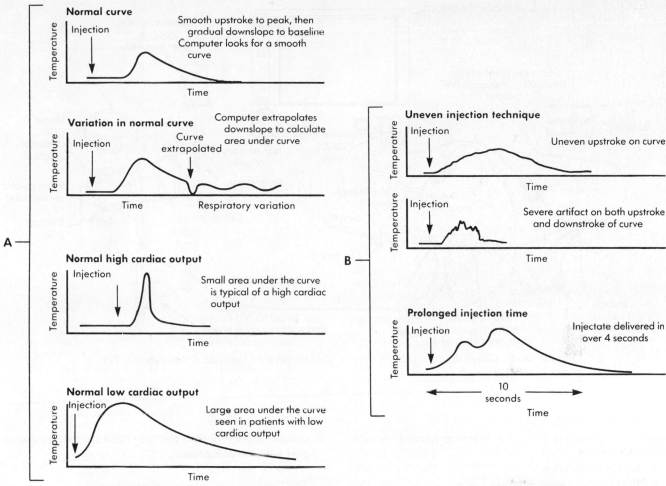

Figure 64-3 **A,** Variations in the normal cardiac output curve seen in certain clinical conditions. **B,** Abnormal cardiac output curves that produce an erroneous cardiac output value. *(From Urden LD, Stacy KM, Lough ME:* Critical care nursing: Diagnosis and management, *ed,7, St Louis, 2014, Mosby.)*

- The CCO method is based on the same physiological principle as the TDCO method (indicator-dilution technique).
- The TDCO method uses a bolus of injectate as the indicator for measurement of CO. The CCO method uses heat signals produced by the thermal filament as the indicator. The CCO computer provides a time-averaged rather than instantaneous CO reading. CCO values are influenced by the same principles as TDCO.
- The heated thermal filament has a temperature limit to a maximum of 44 °C (111.2 °F). When calibrated by the manufacturer, CCO computers produce reliable calculations within a temperature range of 30 to 40 °C (86 to 104 °F) or 31 to 43 °C (87.8 to 109.4 °F). An error message appears if the temperature in the PA is out of range. Follow manufacturer's guidelines.
- Infusions through proximal lumens should be limited to maintenance of patency of the lumen. Concomitant infusions through the proximal lumen can theoretically affect CCO measurements by altering the PA temperature. Studies have shown that such infusions can cause variations in TDCO measurements.[19,47]
- To date, no published data describing the effect of concurrent central line infusions on the accuracy of CCO

measurements are available, but large infusions of fluid are discouraged.[8,15]
- Because bolus injections are not needed with the CCO method, the prevalence of user error is theoretically reduced.[14]
- The CCO catheter can be used to obtain both CCO and TDCO measurements.
- The CCO does not reflect acute changes in CO values because the updated value on the monitor display is an average of 3 to 6 minutes of data. A delay of approximately 10 or more minutes to detect a change of 1 L/min in CO may occur. When monitoring a patient with an unstable condition that is being aggressively treated with medication or other therapies, one should be aware of the delay in data displayed.

EQUIPMENT

- Nonsterile gloves
- Cardiac monitor
- Hemodynamic monitoring system (see Procedure 75)
- PA catheter (in place)
- CO computer or module
- Connecting cables

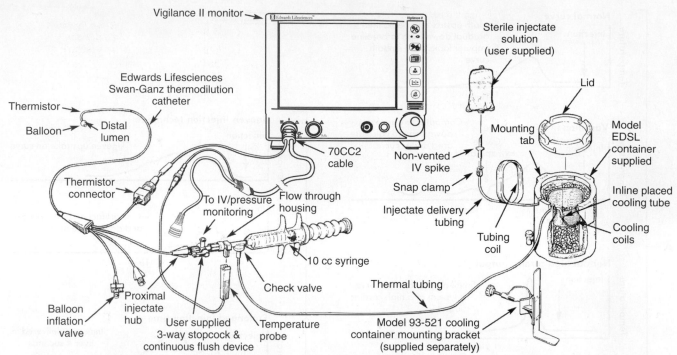

Figure 64-4 Closed injectate delivery system. Cold temperature injectate. *(From Edwards Life-sciences, LLC, Irvine, CA.)*

Additional equipment, to have available as needed, includes the following:
- Bolus thermodilution
  - ❖ Injectate temperature probe
  - ❖ Injectate solution
  - ❖ 10-mL prefilled syringes
  - ❖ Injectate solution bag with intravenous (IV) tubing and three-way Luer-Lok stopcock
  - ❖ Closed CO injectate system
  - ❖ Ice (for cold injectate only)
  - ❖ Nonvented caps for stopcocks
- Setup for CCO
- Syringe holder or automatic injector device
- Printer
- Dispensing port

PATIENT AND FAMILY EDUCATION

- Explain the procedure for CO and the reason for its measurement. Include expectations related to sensations during the procedure. (The patient should not experience pain or discomfort.) *Rationale:* Explanation decreases patient and family anxiety. Preparatory information of sensations decreases patient fear of the impending procedure.
- Explain the monitoring equipment involved, the frequency of measurements, and the goals of therapy. *Rationale:* Explanation encourages the patient and family to ask questions and voice specific concerns about the procedure.
- Explain any potential variations in temperature the patient may or may not experience if a cold injectate is used. *Rationale:* This explanation acknowledges the varying physical responses to the injectate and the possible per-

ception of cold solution and may decrease anxiety associated with the procedure.

PATIENT ASSESSMENT AND PREPARATION
Patient Assessment

- Assess the patient's history of medication therapy, including medication allergies, recent bolus therapies, and current medications. *Rationale:* Medications can influence CO measurements.
- Assess the patient's medical history for the presence of coronary artery disease, valvular heart disease, and left or right ventricular dysfunction. *Rationale:* Medical history provides baseline information regarding cardiovascular performance.
- Assess current intracardiac waveforms (e.g., PAP, RAP, PAOP). *Rationale:* This assessment ensures the PA catheter is positioned properly.
- Assess the patient's vital signs, fluid balance, heart and lung sounds, skin color, temperature, level of consciousness, peripheral pulses, cardiac rate and rhythm, and hemodynamic values. In patients with advanced systolic heart failure, assess for pulsus alternans (alternating strong and weak pulses). *Rationale:* Clinical information provides data regarding blood flow and tissue perfusion. Abnormalities can influence the variability of CO measurements.
- Ensure that no medication is being infused via the proximal port. *Rationale:* Medications infused via this port will be bolused into the patient if the bolus CO method is utilized. This is not an issue with the CCO method.

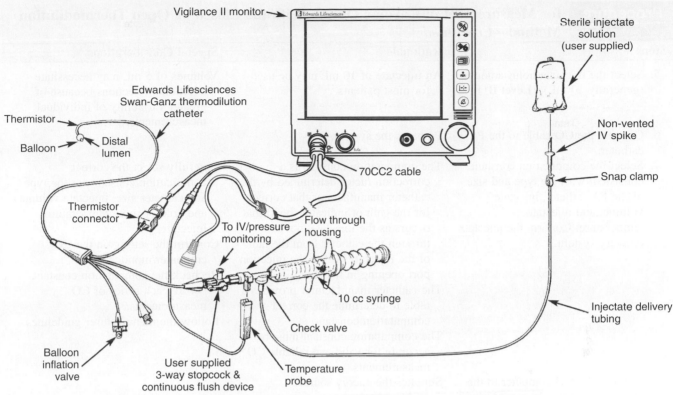

Figure 64-5 Closed injectate delivery system. Room temperature injectate. *(From Edwards Life-sciences, LLC, Irvine, CA.)*

Patient Preparation

- Verify that the patient is the correct patient using two identifiers. ***Rationale:*** Before performing a procedure, the nurse should ensure the correct identification of the patient for the intended intervention.

- Ensure that the patient and family understand preprocedural information. Answer questions as they arise, and reinforce information as needed. ***Rationale:*** Understanding of previously taught information is evaluated and reinforced.

- Assist the patient to the supine position. ***Rationale:*** CO measurements are most accurate in the supine position.

Procedure	for Measurement of Cardiac Output With the Closed or Open Thermodilution Method	
Steps	**Rationale**	**Special Considerations**
1. **HH**		
2. **PE**		
3. Select the injectate delivery system: open or closed method. **(Level B*)**	Both systems are reliable.[32,37,40]	A closed system may eliminate cost and time expenditures of individual syringe preparation. The closed system has infection control benefits because of reduction of multiple entries into the system.[34]
4. Select cold or room temperature injectate. **(Level B*)**	Room temperature injectate may be used for most patients. Research on room temperature versus cold injectate supports the accuracy of either method.[7,9,12,23,41,42,45,48] Cold injectate may improve the accuracy of CO measurement for patients with low or high CO.[45]	The acceptable temperature range for cold and room temperature injectate varies by system (manufacturer). Generally, room temperature is 18–25 °C, and cold is 0–12 °C.

*Level B: Well-designed, controlled studies with results that consistently support a specific action, intervention, or treatment.

Procedure continues on following page

Procedure for Measurement of Cardiac Output With the Closed or Open Thermodilution Method—*Continued*

Steps	Rationale	Special Considerations
5. Select the injectate bolus amount (generally 10 mL). **(Level B*)**	An injectate of 10 mL may be used for most patients.[12,31,36]	Volumes of 5 mL may necessitate additional injections because of greater variability of individual measurements.[31]
6. Connect the CO cable to the PA catheter.	Prepares the system.	
7. Select the computation constant consistent with the type and size of the PA catheter, injectate volume, and injectate temperature. Confirm the injectate delivery system.	The computation constant is a correction factor determined by the catheter manufacturer that corrects for the gain of indicator (heat) that occurs as the injectate moves through the catheter from the hub of the injectate port to the injection port opening in the RA. The catheter manufacturer provides a table to determine the correct computation constant. The computation constant must be accurate for valid and reliable CO measurements.	Carefully select the correct computation constant for the type and catheter size, injectate volume, and cold or room temperature injectate. Confirm the setting on the CO computer/monitor. Recheck the computation constant before each series of CO measurements. Follow the manufacturer guidelines.
8. Connect the CO computer to the power source if it is a stand-alone device or turn on the CO computer or module.	Supplies the energy source.	
9. Note the temperature of the injectate (on the computer or monitor screen).	The injectate temperature should be at least 10°C less than the patient's core temperature.[27]	Follow manufacturer's recommendations.
10. Position the patient supine, with the head of the bed elevated no more than 20 degrees. **(Level B*)**	Studies of patients in the supine position with the head of bed flat or elevated up to 20 degrees have not shown significant differences in TDCO measurements.[18,21,25,50] Consistency in patient position may increase stability in consecutive CO readings.	CCO values may be accurate with the patient's head of the bed elevated to 45 degrees.[11,17] The patient's medical condition and level of instability may determine positioning. Position should be documented and communicated. Consistent positioning when obtaining CO measurements over time decreases measurement variability. Cautiously use CO values obtained from lateral positions. The lateral recumbent position increases variability in CO measurements.[10,51]
11. Verify the position of the PA catheter by assessing both the RA and PA waveforms for proper waveform contours.	Proper positioning of the PA catheter ensures that the distal thermistor is located in the PA. The distal thermistor sensor calculates the time-temperature data. Excessive coiling of the PA catheter in the RA or RV can result in poor positioning of the distal thermistor in relation to the injectate port.[22]	Improper positioning of the PA catheter tip may result in false values.[14,15,22,28]

*Level B: Well-designed, controlled studies with results that consistently support a specific action, intervention, or treatment.

Procedure	for Measurement of Cardiac Output With the Closed or Open Thermodilution Method—*Continued*		
Steps	**Rationale**	**Special Considerations**
12. Observe the patient's cardiac rate and rhythm.	A rapid heart rate or dysrhythmias may decrease CO and lead to variability in CO measurements.	
13. If possible, consider restricting infusions delivered through the introducer or other central lines. **(Level C*)**	TDCO measurements obtained during administration of other infusions can cause variability in CO measurements (by as much as 40% higher).[19,50]	
14. Remove ▣PE and discard used supplies.	Reduces the transmission of microorganisms; Standard Precautions.	
15. ▣HH		

*Level C: Qualitative studies, descriptive or correlational studies, integrative reviews, systematic reviews, or randomized controlled trials with inconsistent results.

Procedure	for Closed-Method of Syringe Preparation and Cardiac Output Determination		
Steps	**Rationale**	**Special Considerations**

Follow Steps 1–13 of the Procedure for Measurement of CO

Steps	Rationale	Special Considerations
1. ▣HH		
2. ▣PE		
3. Obtain the injectate solution		
4. Aseptically connect the IV tubing to the injectate solution.	Prepares the system.	
5. Hang the IV injectate solution on an IV pole; prime the tubing.	Eliminates air from the tubing.	
6. Remove the sterile cap from the proximal lumen of the PA catheter.	Prepares for the injectate connection.	
7. Connect the injectate tubing to the proximal lumen of the PA catheter via a three-way Luer-Lok stopcock (see Figs. 64-4 and 64-5).	Connects the injectate solution to the PA catheter.	
8. Connect the injectate syringe to the three-way stopcock (see Figs. 64-4 and 64-5).	The syringe is used for solution injection.	Connect the system so that the CO syringe is in a straight line with the PA catheter to decrease resistance with injection of solution. To ensure accurate readings, when using a multiport PA catheter the proximal port should be used rather than the venous infusion port.[38]
9. Connect the inline temperature probe (see Figs. 64-4 and 64-5).	Measures the injectate temperature.	Verify temperature.
10. If using cold injectate, set up the cold injectate system (e.g., CO-Set closed injectate system; see Fig. 64-4).	If using cold injectate, cool the injectate solution to 0–12°C (32–53°F).	Refer to manufacturer's recommendations. Cold injectate may be proarrhythmic in some patients.[35,46]
11. Turn the stopcock so that it is open to the injectate solution (closed to the patient) and withdraw 10 mL of the injectate solution into the syringe.	Prepares for injection.	

Procedure continues on following page

Procedure	**for Closed-Method of Syringe Preparation and Cardiac Output Determination—*Continued***	
Steps	**Rationale**	**Special Considerations**
12. Turn the stopcock so that it is closed to the injectate solution and open to the patient. Support the stopcock with the palm of the nondominant hand to aid in injectate administration.	Minimal handling (<30 seconds) of the syringe is recommended to avoid thermal indicator variation that may introduce error into the CO calculation.[5,8,28]	Syringe holders or automatic injector devices are available and can be used.
13. Activate the CO computer, and wait for the "ready" message.	The CO computer or module needs to be ready before injection of solution.	Follow manufacturer's guidelines.
14. Before administering the bolus injectate, observe for a steady baseline temperature (e.g., the line before the CO curve begins should be flat without undulations) on the monitor screen (see Figs. 64-2B and 64-3A).	An abnormal baseline may increase variability in CO measurements and introduce error.[1]	Patients with advanced systolic heart failure (low ejection fraction) are more susceptible to a wavering initial baseline from unstable PA blood temperature.
15. Observe the patient's respiratory pattern. Prepare to begin administering the injectate at end expiration to decrease variance in CO measurements from the respiratory cycle **(Level C*)**	End expiration is defined as the phase of the respiratory cycle preceding the start of inspiration. Significant variations in transthoracic pressure during respiration can affect CO by altering venous return.[20,40,44,45]	Follow institution standard.
16. Administer the bolus injectate rapidly and smoothly in 4 seconds or less.	Prolonged injection time may result in false low CO. Rates of 2–4 seconds for injection of 5–10 mL of injectate yield accurate results.[5,13,43]	A prolonged injection time interferes with time and temperature calculations. One respiratory cycle is generally <4 seconds. One ventilation cycle on a ventilator is generally 4 seconds.
17. Assess the CO curve and value on the monitor screen (see Figs. 64-2 and 64-3).	The CO curve must be a normal curve. A normal curve starts at baseline (baseline must be a straight, flat, nonwavering line) with a smooth upstroke and a gradual downstroke. If the CO curve is not normal, the CO measurement obtained from the injection should be discarded. Abnormal contours of the curve may indicate improper catheter position. An abnormal CO curve may represent technical error.	Normal CO is 4–8 L/min. Abnormal CO curves may also provide information about the patient's clinical condition, such as tricuspid valve regurgitation.
18. Repeat Steps 3 through 17 (up to three times total for cold injectate and up to five times total for room temperature injectate).	Discard all CO measurements that do not have normal CO curves or have wandering baselines.	Allow 60 seconds between each CO measurement to ensure consistency and accuracy.

*Level C: Qualitative studies, descriptive or correlational studies, integrative reviews, systematic reviews, or randomized controlled trials with inconsistent results.

Procedure for Closed-Method of Syringe Preparation and Cardiac Output Determination—*Continued*

Steps	Rationale	Special Considerations
19. Determine the CO measurement by calculating the average of three measurements within 10% of a middle (median) value. **(Level E*)**	Determines accurate CO value.[49]	
20. Return the proximal stopcock at the RA lumen to the original position.	Resumes RA monitoring.	
21. Continue infusions delivered through the introducer or other central lines.	Continues therapy.	
22. Observe the PA and RA waveforms on the monitor.	Continues hemodynamic monitoring.	
23. Remove **PE** and discard used supplies in appropriate receptacles.	Reduces the transmission of microorganisms; Standard Precautions.	
24. **HH**		
25. Determine the hemodynamic calculations.	Assesses cardiac performance and hemodynamic status.	Compare the values with prior values and determine whether the plan of care requires alterations.

*Level E: Multiple case reports, theory-based evidence from expert opinions, or peer-reviewed professional organizational standards without clinical studies to support recommendations.

Procedure for Open Method of Syringe Preparation and Cardiac Output Determination

Steps	Rationale	Special Considerations
Follow Steps 1–13 of the Procedure for Measurement of Cardiac Output		
1. **HH**		
2. **PE**		
3. Prepare syringes or obtain manufactured prefilled syringes for CO determination.	Prepares the injectate for CO measurements.	Prefilled syringes may decrease variability related to injectate volume.
A. Clean the injectate port of the D5W IV bag with an alcohol wipe.		Manufactured prefilled syringes may be stored per manufacturer's recommendations.
B. Apply a dispensing port to the bag's injectate port		Solutions drawn up should be used immediately for CO measurements.
C. Aseptically withdraw the injectate solution from the IV bag into three to five 10-mL syringes and cap securely.		Solution drawn up in the clinical area (as opposed to under a laminar flow area) that has no preservative, should not be stored for later use. A dispensing port negates the use of needles and reduces the incidence of accidental needlesticks.
4. Cold injectate: Cool the syringes in ice.	Iced slush is used to cool syringes.	Place syringes in a bag in the container, not directly into the slush. Handling of a cold syringe causes warming and hampers validity of CO measurements.[5,8,28] Cold injectate may be proarrhythmic.[35,46]

Procedure continues on following page

Procedure	for Open Method of Syringe Preparation and Cardiac Output Determination—*Continued*	
Steps	**Rationale**	**Special Considerations**
5. Remove the nonvented cap from the proximal lumen stopcock of the PA catheter.	Prepares the stopcock.	
6. Aseptically connect one of the sterile CO injectate syringes onto the proximal lumen stopcock of the PA catheter.	Reduces the risk of introducing microorganisms into the system.	
7. Turn the stopcock so that it is closed to the flush solution and open between the injectate syringe and the patient. Support the stopcock with the palm of the nondominant hand.	Prepares the system for injectate administration.	Minimize handling (<30 seconds)
8. Connect the inline temperature probe (see Figs. 64-4 and 64-5).	Measures the injectate temperature.	
9. Activate the CO computer, and wait for the "ready" message.	The CO computer or module needs to be ready before injection of solution.	Follow manufacturer's guidelines.
10. Before administering the bolus injectate, observe for a steady baseline temperature (e.g., the line before the CO curve begins should be flat without undulations) on the monitor screen (see Figs. 64-2B and 64-3A).	An abnormal baseline may increase variability in CO measurements and introduce error.[1]	Patients with advanced systolic heart failure (low ejection fraction) are more prone to a wavering initial baseline from unstable PA blood temperature.
11. Observe the patient's respiratory pattern. Prepare to begin administering the injectate at end expiration to decrease variance in CO measurements from the respiratory cycle **(Level C*)**	End expiration is defined as the phase of the respiratory cycle preceding the start of inspiration. Significant variations in transthoracic pressure during respiration can affect CO by altering venous return.[20,40,44,45]	Follow institution standard.
12. Administer the bolus injectate rapidly and smoothly in 4 seconds or less.	Prolonged injection time may result in false low CO. Rates of 2–4 seconds for injection of 5–10 mL of injectate yield accurate results.[5,13,43]	A prolonged injection time interferes with time and temperature calculations. One respiratory cycle is generally <4 seconds. One ventilation cycle on a ventilator is generally 4 seconds.
13. Assess the CO curve and value on the monitor screen (see Figs. 64-2 and 64-3).	The CO curve must be a normal curve. A normal curve starts at baseline (baseline must be a straight, flat, nonwavering line) with a smooth upstroke and a gradual downstroke. If the CO curve is not normal, the reading should be discarded. Abnormal contours of the curve may indicate improper catheter position. An abnormal CO curve may represent technical error.	Normal CO is 4–8 L/min. Abnormal CO curves may also provide information about the patient's clinical condition, such as tricuspid valve regurgitation.

*Level C: Qualitative studies, descriptive or correlational studies, integrative reviews, systematic reviews, or randomized controlled trials with inconsistent results.

Procedure	for Open Method of Syringe Preparation and Cardiac Output Determination—*Continued*	
Steps	**Rationale**	**Special Considerations**
14. Repeat Steps 6 through 13 (up to three times total for cold injectate and up to five times total for room temperature injectate).	Obtains CO measurements. Discard all CO measurements that do not have normal CO curves or have wandering baselines.	Allow 60 seconds between each CO measurement to ensure consistency and accuracy. Asepsis is essential as the stopcock is turned and syringes are exchanged between CO measurements.
15. Determine the CO measurement by calculating the average of three measurements within 10% of a middle (median) value. **(Level E*)**	Determines accurate CO value.[49]	
16. After the last injectate is completed: A. Turn the right atrial lumen stopcock of the PA catheter so that the system is open between the patient and the transducer. B. Aseptically remove the last injectate syringe. C. Place a new, sterile, nonvented cap on the stopcock port.	Closes the system; maintains the sterility of the system.	
17. Observe the PA and RA waveforms on the monitor.	Continues hemodynamic monitoring.	
18. Remove **PE** and discard used supplies in appropriate receptacles.	Removes and safely discards used supplies.	
19. **HH**		
20. Determine hemodynamic calculations.	Assesses cardiac performance and hemodynamic status.	Compare values with prior values and determine whether the plan of care requires alterations.

*Level E: Multiple case reports, theory-based evidence from expert opinions, or peer-reviewed professional organizational standards without clinical studies to support recommendations.

Procedure	for Measurement of Cardiac Output With Continuous Cardiac Output Method	
Steps	**Rationale**	**Special Considerations**
1. **HH**		
2. **PE**		
3. Turn on the CO computer or module.	Provides energy.	
4. Connect the CO cable to the PA catheter.	Prepares equipment.	
5. Observe PA waveforms (e.g., RA, PA).	Determines whether the PA catheter is in the correct position.	The thermal filament should float freely in the RV to prevent the loss of indicator (heat) into the cardiac tissue. If the loss of indicator occurs, the CO value is overestimated, giving erroneous readings. Follow manufacturer's guidelines. The device may not measure CO if the PA catheter is malpositioned.

Procedure continues on following page

Procedure	for Measurement of Cardiac Output With Continuous Cardiac Output Method—*Continued*	

Steps	Rationale	Special Considerations
6. Position the patient supine with the head of the bed elevated up to 45 degrees. (**Level C***)	CCO measurements are most accurate in a supine position, but head-of-bed angle can be varied for comfort, between 0 and 45 degrees.[16]	Additional studies are needed to determine the effect of patient body position on CCO measurements. Document body position at the time of hemodynamic data collection.
7. Check the heat signal indicator on the CO computer or module per manufacturer's recommendations.	CCO systems assess the quality of the measured thermal signal. Relationships are in response to thermal noise or signal-to-noise ratio.	CCO monitors provide messages for troubleshooting signal-to-noise ratio interferences. Refer to manufacturer recommendations. Technologic advances suppress the effects of blood thermal noise.[52]
8. Note that the CCO values reflect an average of the preceding 3–6 minutes of data collection.	CCO measurements are averaged over the preceding 3–6 minutes and are not individual measurements.	CCO values are updated every 30–60 seconds. Continuous data collection reflects phasic changes in the respiratory cycle. CCO measurements are not timed to the respiratory cycle.
9. When documenting CCO values, also document other hemodynamic findings.	Provides data regarding hemodynamic status.	
10. Compare the CCO value with the patient's current clinical status and hemodynamic findings.	CCO is a global assessment parameter and must be appreciated as part of the patient's total hemodynamic profile at a given time.	The CCO method eliminates many of the potential user-related and technique-related errors associated with the intermittent bolus CO method. Research shows clinically acceptable correlation between the TDCO technique and the CCO method in the steady state.[1,6,30,32,33] Future studies are needed to determine efficacy in patients in various phases of acute hemodynamic instability and in specific patient populations. Also, the effects of changes in positioning need to be studied further, especially in patients with structural or functional heart damage.
11. Note: The CCO catheter system can be used to obtain TDCO by following Steps 1–13 of the Procedure for Measurement of Cardiac Output with the Closed or Open Thermodilution Method CO and then follow the steps for either the Closed or Open Method of Syringe Preparation and Cardiac Output Determination.		
12. Remove **PE** and discard used supplies in appropriate receptacles.	Removes and safely discards used supplies.	
13. **HH**		

*Level C: Qualitative studies, descriptive or correlational studies, integrative reviews, systematic reviews, or randomized controlled trials with inconsistent results.

Expected Outcomes

- Accurate CO measurement are obtained
- Hemodynamic profile and derived parameters are obtained with accuracy, whether through the continuous or intermittent method
- Sterility and patency of the PA catheter is maintained

Unexpected Outcomes

- Inability to accurately measure CO
- Erroneous readings because of technical, equipment, or operator error
- Contamination of the system
- Occlusion of the proximal PA lumen

Patient Monitoring and Care

Steps	Rationale	Reportable Conditions
		These conditions should be reported if they persist despite nursing interventions.
1. Maintain patency of the PA catheter.	PA catheter patency is essential for accurate monitoring.	• Inability to maintain PA catheter patency
2. Monitor RA and PA waveforms for confirmation of proper catheter position.	Proper placement determines accurate hemodynamic and CO measurement.	• Abnormal RA or PA waveforms or values
3. Maintain the sterility of the PA catheter.	Reduces the risk for catheter-related infections.	• Fever, site redness, drainage, or symptoms consistent with infection
4. Calculate cardiac index, systemic vascular resistance, and other parameters as prescribed or indicated.	Determines cardiac performance and current hemodynamic status.	• Abnormal cardiac index, systemic vascular resistance, or other hemodynamic values
5. Monitor vital signs and respiratory status hourly and as indicated.	Changes in vital signs or respiratory status may indicate hemodynamic compromise.	• Changes in vital signs • Changes in respiratory status
6. Include the fluid volume used in the TDCO in the patient's total fluid volume intake.	Additional volume given intermittently should be included in the total intake for accurate fluid volume assessment.	• Signs or symptoms of fluid overload (e.g., respiratory distress, crackles, increased PADP or PAOP, elevated jugular venous pressure, new or worsening S3 gallop, worsening edema)
7. Assess the patient's response to therapies.	Hemodynamic monitoring may expedite treatment decisions.	• Significant worsening or improvement in CO and hemodynamic parameters. • Pulmonary vascular resistance (PVR) and systemic vascular resistance (SVR)
8. If using a closed system delivery set (CO set), change the system components (tubing, syringe, stopcocks, and IV solution) every 96 hours with the hemodynamic monitoring system (see Procedure 75).	Reduces the incidence of infection.	

Procedure continues on following page

Documentation

Documentation should include the following:
- Patient and family education
- CO, cardiac index, SVR, volume indicators (PAOP and RAP)
- CO curves
- Baseline PA blood temperature
- Continuous or intermittent bolus method
- Volume and temperature of injectate
- Concurrent headrest elevation, vital signs, and hemodynamic measurements
- Titration or administration of medications that affect contractility (e.g., dobutamine, milrinone, dopamine, epinephrine), vascular resistance (e.g., intravenous nitrates or arterial vasodilator therapy [e.g., nitroprusside, nicardipine, or nesiritide]), and intravascular volume (e.g., diuretics)
- Significant medical therapies or nursing interventions that affect CO (e.g., intraaortic balloon pump or ventricular assist device therapies, volume expanders, position changes), vascular resistance, or intravascular volume (e.g., sedation, blood/blood products, headrest elevation, fluid restriction, sodium restriction)
- Unexpected outcomes
- Additional interventions, including psychosocial or emotional/psychiatric interventions that might influence hemodynamic trends

References and Additional Readings

For a complete list of references and additional readings for this procedure, scan this QR code with any freely available smartphone code reader app, or visit http://booksite.elsevier.com/9780323376624.

65 Central Venous Catheter Removal

Jillian Hamel

PURPOSE: Central venous catheters are removed when therapy is completed, when complications occur, or when the patient has a catheter-related infection.

PREREQUISITE NURSING KNOWLEDGE

- Knowledge of the normal anatomy and physiology of the vasculature and cardiovascular system is necessary.
- Knowledge of normal coagulation values is needed.
- Principles of aseptic technique should be known.
- Advanced cardiac life support (ACLS) knowledge and skills are necessary.
- Clinical and technical competence in central venous catheter (CVC) removal is necessary.
- Knowledge of the state nurse practice act is important because some states do not allow this intervention to be performed by a registered nurse.
- Knowledge of potential complications associated with the removal of the CVC is needed.
- An air embolism can occur during or after the removal of the catheter as a result of air drawn in along the subcutaneous tract and into the vein. During inspiration, negative intrathoracic pressure is transmitted to the central veins. Any opening external to the body to one of these veins may result in aspiration of air into the central venous system. The pathological effects depend on the volume and rate of air aspirated. Signs and symptoms include: respiratory distress, agitation, cyanosis, gasp reflex, sucking sound, hypotension, petechiae, cardiac dysrhythmias, altered mental status, and cardiac arrest.

EQUIPMENT

- Fluid-shield face mask or goggles
- Gowns, nonsterile gloves
- Antiseptic solution (e.g., 2% chlorhexidine-based preparation)
- 4 × 4 gauze pads
- Petroleum-based ointment
- One roll of 2-inch tape
- Two moisture-proof absorbent pads

Additional equipment, to have available as needed, includes the following:

- Additional dressing supplies (e.g., semipermeable transparent dressing)
- Sterile scissors
- Sterile specimen container (needed if a culture of the catheter tip will be obtained)
- Suture removal kit
- Emergency equipment

PATIENT AND FAMILY EDUCATION

- Explain the procedure to the patient and family and the reason for catheter removal. *Rationale:* This explanation provides information and decreases anxiety.
- Explain the importance of patient participation during the catheter removal. *Rationale:* This explanation ensures patient cooperation and facilitates safe removal of the catheter.
- Instruct the patient and family to report any signs and symptoms of shortness of breath, bleeding, or discomfort at the site of catheter removal. *Rationale:* Identifies patient discomfort and early recognition of complications.

PATIENT ASSESSMENT AND PREPARATION

Patient Assessment

- Assess vital signs and the neurovascular status of the extremity distal to the catheter insertion site. *Rationale:* This assessment provides baseline data.
- Assess the patient's current coagulation values. *Rationale:* If the patient has abnormal coagulation study results, hemostasis may be difficult to obtain. Abnormal coagulation results should be discussed with the physician or advance practice nurse before catheter removal.
- Assess the catheter site for redness, warmth, tenderness, or presence of drainage. *Rationale:* Determines whether signs or symptoms of infection are present.

Patient Preparation

- In collaboration with the physician or advance practice nurse, determine when the CVC should be removed. *Rationale:* The invasive catheter is removed when it is no longer indicated.
- In collaboration with the physician or advance practice nurse, determine whether the tip of the catheter will be

cultured. *Rationale:* This discussion determines additional supplies that may be needed.

- Verify that the patient is the correct patient using two identifiers. *Rationale:* Before performing a procedure, the nurse should ensure the correct identification of the patient for the intended intervention.
- Ensure that the patient and family understand preprocedural teaching. Answer questions as they arise, and reinforce information as needed. *Rationale:* Understanding of previously taught information is evaluated and reinforced.
- Place the patient in a supine position with the head of the bed in a slight Trendelenburg's position (or flat if Tren-

delenburg's position is contraindicated or not tolerated by the patient). *Rationale:* The patient should be positioned so that the catheter exit site is at or below the level of the heart.[5,6] A normal pressure gradient exists between atmospheric air and the central venous compartment that promotes air entry if the compartment is open. The lower the site of entry below the heart, the lower the pressure gradient, thus minimizing the risk of air being drawn in and thus a venous air embolism.

- Start a new peripheral intravenous (IV) line or ensure that an existing peripheral IV line is patent. *Rationale:* IV access is established for fluids or medications.

Procedure for Central Venous Catheter Removal

Steps	Rationale	Special Considerations
1. HH		
2. PE		All physicians, advanced practice nurses, and other healthcare professionals in the room should wear personal protective equipment including a face mask.
3. Transfer or discontinue the IV solution.	Prepares the catheter for removal and ensures IV fluids are infusing in another site.	
4. Open the sterile scissors or suture removal kit and sterile gauze pads.	Prepares supplies for use.	
5. Place a moisture-proof absorbent pad under the patient's upper torso and another close to the catheter site.	Collects blood and body fluids associated with removal; serves as a receptacle for the contaminated catheter.	
6. Place the patient supine in slight Trendelenburg's position.[1,3,4,7–10,13,16] **(Level E*)**	Minimizes the risk for venous air embolus by increasing the pressure in the large veins above atmospheric pressure, thus reducing the risk of air aspiration. The patient should be positioned so that the catheter exit site is at or below the level of the heart.[5,6]	Place the patient flat if Trendelenburg's position is contraindicated or not tolerated by the patient or a femoral CVC will be removed. If the CVC is in the femoral vein, extend the patient's leg and ensure the groin area is adequately exposed. Cases have been reported of venous air embolus occurring after removal of CVCs when patients were not in a supine slight Trendelenburg position.
7. Have the patient turn his or her head away from the catheter site (if removing an internal jugular or subclavian catheter).	Decreases the risk for contamination.	This step is not needed if a femoral catheter is removed.
8. Remove the catheter dressing and discard.	Prepares for removal.	
9. Remove the nonsterile gloves, perform hand hygiene, and apply a pair of sterile gloves.	Decreases the risk for contamination.	
10. Remove the securing device or, if present, cut sutures and gently pull the sutures through the skin.	Allows for removal of the catheter.	Ensure that the entire suture is removed. Retained sutures can form epithelialized tracts that can lead to infection.

*Level E: Multiple case reports, theory-based evidence from expert opinions, or peer-reviewed professional organizational standards without clinical studies to support recommendations.

Procedure for Central Venous Catheter Removal—*Continued*

Steps	Rationale	Special Considerations
11. Ask the patient to take a deep breath in and hold it if removing an internal jugular or subclavian catheter.[12,14,16,17] **(Level E*)**	Minimizes the risk for venous air embolus.	If the patient is receiving positive pressure ventilation, withdraw the catheter during the inspiratory phase of the respiratory cycle or when a breath is delivered via a bag-valve device.
12. Withdraw the catheter, pulling parallel to the skin and using a steady motion.	Minimizes trauma.	If resistance is met, do not continue to remove the catheter. Notify the advanced practice nurse or physician immediately.
13. As the catheter exits the site, apply pressure with a gauze pad.	Minimizes the risk for venous air embolus and promotes hemostasis.	The distal end of a multilumen catheter should be removed quickly because the exposed proximal and medial openings could permit the entry of air.
14. Instruct the patient to exhale after the catheter is removed.	Once the catheter is removed the patient can breathe normally.	
15. Lay the catheter on the moisture-proof absorbent pad. Check to be sure that all of the catheter was removed.	Ensures the removal of the entire catheter.	If the introducer tip will be cultured, have another provider assist with cutting the tip with sterile scissors and placing it in a sterile specimen container before placing the catheter on the moisture-proof absorbent pad. Routine culturing of tips upon removal is not recommended.[6]
16. Continue applying firm, direct pressure over the insertion site with the gauze pad until bleeding has stopped.	Ensures hemostasis.	Because CVCs are placed in large veins, hemostasis may take up to 10 minutes to occur. Pressure may be needed for a longer period of time if the patient has been receiving anticoagulant therapy or if coagulation studies are abnormal.
17. Apply an occlusive dressing, consisting of sterile petroleum-based ointment, sterile gauze, and cover with tape or a transparent semipermeable membrane dressing.[1,2,5,6,8,10,13] **(Level E*)**	Decreases the risk for infection at the insertion site and minimizes the risk for venous air embolus.	Label the dressing with the date, time, and your initials.
18. Maintain the patient in the supine position for 30 minutes after catheter removal.[5]	May decrease the risk of a postprocedure venous air embolism.	
19. Remove **PE** and discard used supplies in appropriate receptacles	Reduces the transmission of microorganisms; Standard Precautions.	
20. **HH**		

*Level E: Multiple case reports, theory-based evidence from expert opinions, or peer-reviewed professional organizational standards without clinical studies to support recommendations

Procedure continues on following page

Expected Outcomes

- The catheter is removed intact
- Hemostasis is achieved at the catheter site

Unexpected Outcomes

- Inability to remove the catheter
- Catheter not removed intact
- Venous air emboli
- Persistent bleeding
- Hematoma
- Infection
- Broken catheter/fragmentation
- Pain

Patient Monitoring and Care

Steps	Rationale	Reportable Conditions
		These conditions should be reported if they persist despite nursing interventions.
1. Assess the patient's vital signs, pulse oximetry, and level of consciousness before and after the CVC is removed.	Provides baseline data and data that identify changes in patient condition.	• Abnormal vital signs • Shortness of breath or tachypnea • Cyanosis or decreased oxygen saturation • Changes in mental status
2. If signs and symptoms of venous air embolus are present, immediately place the patient in the left lateral Trendelenburg's position.	Venous air embolus is a potentially life-threatening complication. The left lateral Trendelenburg's position prevents air from passing into the left side of the heart and traveling into the arterial circulation.	• Respiratory distress • Dyspnea • Coughing • Tachypnea • Altered mental status (agitation, restlessness) • Cyanosis • Gasp reflex • Sucking sound near the site of the catheter insertion/air entrainment • Petechiae • Chest pain • Cardiac dysrhythmias • Hypotension
3. After removal of the CVC, assess the site for signs of bleeding every 15 minutes × 2, every 30 minutes × 2, and then 1 hour later.	Bleeding or a hematoma can develop if there is still bleeding from the vessel.	• Bleeding • Hematoma development
4. Remove the dressing and assess for site closure 24 hours after CVC removal.	Verifies healing and closure of the site.	• Abnormal healing

Patient Monitoring and Care —*Continued*

Steps	Rationale	Reportable Conditions
5. Daily assess the need for the CVC. If long-term use of the CVC is needed, frequently reassess the necessity of the line. **(Level C*)**	The Centers for Disease Control and Prevention (CDC)[11] do not have specific recommendations regarding routine replacement of CVCs. Researchers conducting one study recommend that CVCs do not need to be changed more frequently than every 7 days.[2] There are no specific recommendations regarding routine replacement of CVCs that need to be in place for >7 days.[2,15] Guidewire exchanges should not be used routinely. A guidewire exchange should only be used to replace a catheter that is malfunctioning.[11]	• Signs and symptoms of infection at the CVC catheter insertion site • Signs and symptoms of sepsis
6. Follow institutional standards for assessing pain. Administer analgesia as prescribed.	Identifies need for pain interventions.	• Continued pain despite pain interventions

*Level C: Qualitative studies, descriptive or correlational studies, integrative reviews, systematic reviews, or randomized controlled trials with inconsistent results.

Documentation

Documentation should include the following:
- Patient and family education
- Date and time of catheter removal
- Site assessment
- Pain assessment, interventions, and effectiveness
- Application of air occlusive dressing
- Patient tolerance of the procedure
- Unexpected outcomes and interventions

References and Additional Readings

For a complete list of references and additional readings for this procedure, scan this QR code with any freely available smartphone code reader app, or visit http://booksite.elsevier.com/9780323376624.

66 Central Venous Catheter Site Care

Jillian Hamel

PURPOSE: Site care of the central venous catheter allows for assessment and care of the catheter-insertion site.

PREREQUISITE NURSING KNOWLEDGE

- Understanding of the principles of aseptic technique is needed.
- Knowledge of the signs and symptoms of catheter-related infection and sepsis is necessary.
- Most serious catheter-related infections are associated with central venous catheters (CVCs), especially those that are placed in the intensive-care setting.[6]
- Bloodstream infections related to the use of CVCs are an important cause of patient morbidity, mortality, and increased healthcare costs.[2]
- Topical antibiotic ointment or creams are not recommended on the catheter insertion site. The use of antibiotic ointment or cream can potentially promote fungal infections and antimicrobial resistance.[6]
- CVCs do not need to be routinely replaced to prevent catheter-related infections.[6] Clinical judgment should be used to determine the appropriateness of removing the catheter.[6]

EQUIPMENT

- Nonsterile gloves
- Prepackaged sterile dressing kit or separate supplies as listed below
- Sterile gloves
- Face mask
- Transparent semipermeable dressing or sterile 4 × 4 gauze
- Roll of 2-inch tape
- Antiseptic solution (e.g., 2% chlorhexidine-based preparation)

Additional equipment, to have available as needed, includes the following:
- Securement device (used with nonsutured central venous catheters)
- Chlorhexidine gluconate–impregnated sponge

PATIENT AND FAMILY EDUCATION

- Explain the dressing change procedure. *Rationale:* Explanation prepares the patient and decreases patient anxiety.

- Explain the importance of patient positioning during the dressing change. *Rationale:* Patient cooperation is increased; the potential for contamination is decreased.

PATIENT ASSESSMENT AND PREPARATION

Patient Assessment

- Assess the patient's arm, shoulder, neck, and chest on the same side as the catheter insertion site for signs of pain, swelling, or tenderness. Assess the patient's leg size and assess for signs of pain, swelling, or tenderness on the same side as the catheter insertion site if the CVC is placed in the femoral vein. *Rationale:* Assessment evaluates for thrombophlebitis or venous thrombosis.
- Assess for signs and symptoms of infection. Signs and symptoms may include redness, swelling, and drainage at the catheter site or fever, chills, and positive blood cultures. *Rationale:* Infection is a potential complication of any invasive catheter.
- Assess the patient's history for sensitivity to antiseptic solutions. *Rationale:* Assessment decreases the risk for allergic reactions.

Patient Preparation

- Verify that the patient is the correct patient using two identifiers. *Rationale:* Before performing a procedure, the nurse should ensure the correct identification of the patient for the intended intervention.
- Ensure that the patient and family understand preprocedural teaching. Answer questions as they arise, and reinforce information as needed. *Rationale:* Understanding of previously taught information is evaluated and reinforced.
- If the patient is on ventilatory support, assess the patient's need for suctioning before beginning the procedure. Femoral catheter sites need to be inspected for potential contamination with urine or stool. *Rationale:* The risk for catheter site contamination by secretions or excretions is minimized.

Procedure for Central Venous Catheter Site Care

Steps	Rationale	Special Considerations
1. **HH**		
2. **PE**		
3. Prepare supplies.	Prepares equipment.	
4. Position the patient so that the CVC site is easily accessible.	Prepares for dressing change.	If the CVC is in the femoral vein, extend the patient's leg and ensure the groin area is adequately exposed while maintaining patient privacy and comfort.
5. Have the patient turn his or her head away from the catheter insertion site (if performing site care on an internal jugular or subclavian catheter).	Decreases the risk for site contamination.	
6. Apply a face mask.	Reduces the transmission of microorganisms.	
7. Remove and discard the CVC dressing.	Exposes the catheter site for inspection and site care.	
8. Remove the securement device if it is present.	The securement device should be changed with each dressing change.[3]	
9. Inspect the catheter, insertion site, and surrounding skin.	Assesses for signs of infection, catheter dislodgment, leakage, or loose sutures.	
10. Remove and discard gloves in the appropriate receptacle.	Removes and safely discards used supplies.	
11. **HH**		
12. Apply sterile gloves.	Maintains aseptic and sterile technique.	
13. Cleanse the skin, catheter, and stabilizing device with 2% chlorhexidine-based preparation.[1-4,6,7] **(Level A*)**	Reduces the rate of recolonization of skin flora.	Allow the solution to dry. When cleansing, a back-and-forth motion should be used for at least 30 seconds.[3]
14. Apply a new stabilization device.	Secures the catheter.	
15. Apply a chlorhexidine-impregnated sponge to the site.[4,6] **(Level D*)**	Reduces the transmission of microorganisms.	Follow institutional standards. A chlorhexidine-impregnated sponge dressing is recommend if an institution's central line–associated bloodstream infection rate is not decreasing despite adherence to basic prevention measures, including education and training, appropriate use of chlorhexidine for skin antisepsis and MSB.[4,5] Use with caution in patients predisposed to local skin necrosis, such as burn patients or patients with Stevens-Johnson syndrome.[8]

*Level A: Meta-analysis of quantitative studies or metasynthesis of qualitative studies with results that consistently support a specific action, intervention, or treatment (including systematic review of randomized controlled trials).
*Level D: Peer-reviewed professional and organizational standards with the support of clinical study recommendations.

Procedure continues on following page

Procedure for Central Venous Catheter Site Care—*Continued*

Steps	Rationale	Special Considerations
16. Apply a sterile air occlusive dressing. Dressings may be a sterile gauze or a sterile, transparent, semipermeable dressing.[6]	Provides a sterile environment.	If the patient is diaphoretic or if the site is bleeding or oozing, a gauze dressing is preferred.[4,6] Topical antibiotic ointment and creams should be avoided.[6]
17. Remove **PE** and discard used supplies in appropriate receptacles.	Reduces the transmission of microorganisms; Standard Precautions.	
18. Document date and time of changes of the external dressing.	Indicates when the dressing was changed.	
19. **HH**		

Expected Outcomes

- Dressing remains dry, sterile, and intact
- Catheter site remains free of infection
- Catheter remains in place without dislodgment

Unexpected Outcomes

- Catheter-associated bloodstream infection
- Infection at the catheter site
- Accidental removal or dislodgement of the catheter
- Impaired integrity of the skin under the dressing

Patient Monitoring and Care

Steps	Rationale	Reportable Conditions
		These conditions should be reported if they persist despite nursing interventions.
1. Assess the catheter site daily and as needed by palpation through an intact dressing.	If there is tenderness at the insertion site, fever without obvious source, or other signs and symptoms of a local or bloodstream infection, the dressing should be removed to allow thorough examination of the site.[4,6]	- Signs and symptoms of infection at the catheter insertion site - Signs and symptoms of sepsis
2. Replace gauze dressings every 2 days and transparent dressings at least every 5–7 days and more frequently as needed.[3,4,6,7] **(Level D*)**	Decreases the risk for infection at the catheter site. The Centers for Disease Control and Prevention (CDC) and the Infusion Nurses Society recommend replacing the dressing when it becomes damp, loosened, or soiled, or when inspection of the site is necessary.[3,4,6]	
3. Follow institutional standards for assessing pain. Administer analgesia as prescribed.	Identifies need for pain interventions.	- Continued pain despite pain interventions

*Level D: Peer-reviewed professional and organizational standards with the support of clinical study recommendations

Documentation

Documentation should include the following:
- Patient and family education
- Date and time of the procedure
- Assessment of the catheter site
- Type of dressing applied
- Date and time of dressing change
- Unexpected outcomes
- Additional interventions
- Pain assessment, interventions, and effectiveness

References and Additional Readings

For a complete list of references and additional readings for this procedure, scan this QR code with any freely available smartphone code reader app, or visit http://booksite.elsevier.com/9780323376624.

67 Central Venous/Right Atrial Pressure Monitoring

Reba McVay

PURPOSE: Central venous/right-atrial pressure monitoring provides information about the patient's intravascular volume status and right-ventricular preload. The central venous pressure (CVP) or the right atrial pressure (RAP) allows for evaluation of right-sided heart hemodynamics and evaluation of patient response to therapy. CVP and right-atrial pressure are used interchangeably.

PREREQUISITE NURSING KNOWLEDGE

- Knowledge of the normal anatomy and physiology of the cardiovascular system is needed.
- Knowledge of the principles of aseptic technique and infection control is necessary.
- Knowledge is needed of the principles of hemodynamic monitoring.
- The CVP/RAP represents right-sided heart preload or the volume of blood found in the right ventricle at the end of diastole.
- CVP/RAP influences and is influenced by venous return and cardiac function. Although the CVP/RAP is used as a measure of changes in the right ventricle, the relationship is not linear because the right ventricle has the ability to expand and alter its compliance, changes in volume can occur with little change in pressure.
- The CVP/RAP normally ranges from 2 to 6 mm Hg in the adult.
- The central venous catheter is inserted in a central vein with the tip of the catheter placed in the proximal superior vena cava.
- Knowledge is needed of the setup, leveling, and zeroing of the hemodynamic monitoring system (see Procedure 75).
- Interpretation of RA/CVP waveforms including identification of *a, c,* and *v* waves is important. The *a* wave reflects right-atrial contraction. The *c* wave reflects closure of the tricuspid valve. The *v* wave reflects passive filling of the atria during right-ventricular systole. The CVP/RAP measurement is the mean of the *a* wave.
- CVP/RAP values are useful in evaluating volume status, effect of medication therapy (especially medication that decreases preload), and cardiac function (Box 67-1).
- Monitoring parameters from the femoral catheter is not recommended. The catheter is too distant from the right atrium to produce reliable data.

EQUIPMENT

- Pressure transducer system, including flush solution recommended according to institutional standards, a pressure bag or device, pressure tubing with transducer, and flush device (see Procedure 75)
- Pressure module and cable for interface with the monitor
- Dual-channel recorder
- Leveling device (low-intensity laser or carpenter level)
- Nonsterile gloves
- Sterile injectable or noninjectable caps

Additional equipment (to have available depending on patient need) includes the following:

- Indelible marker

PATIENT AND FAMILY EDUCATION

- Discuss the purpose of the central venous catheter and monitoring with both the patient and family. *Rationale:* This discussion reduces anxiety and includes the patient and family in the plan of care.
- Explain the patient's expected participation during the procedure. *Rationale:* The explanation encourages patient assistance.

PATIENT ASSESSMENT AND PREPARATION

Patient Assessment

- Determine hemodynamic, cardiovascular, and peripheral vascular status. *Rationale:* This assessment provides baseline data.
- Determine the patient's baseline pulmonary status. If the patient is mechanically ventilated, note the type of support, ventilator mode, and presence or absence of positive end-expiratory pressure (PEEP) or continuous positive airway pressure (CPAP). *Rationale:* The pres-

BOX 67-1 Central Venous Pressure (CVP)

CONDITIONS CAUSING INCREASED CVP
Elevated intravascular volume
Depressed right-sided cardiac function (RV infarct, RV failure)
Cardiac tamponade
Constrictive pericarditis
Pulmonary hypertension
Chronic left-ventricular failure

CONDITIONS CAUSING DECREASED CVP
Reduced intravascular volume*
Decreased mean arterial pressure
Venodilation

---

*Although the measured CVP is low, cardiac function may be depressed, normal, or hyperdynamic when there is reduced vascular volume.
RV, Right ventricular.

ence of mechanical ventilation alters hemodynamic waveforms and pressures.
- Assess for signs and symptoms of fluid volume deficit. Signs and symptoms may include thirst, oliguria, tachy-cardia, and dry mucous membranes. *Rationale:* Assessment data should correlate with a decreased CVP/RAP value.
- Assess for signs and symptoms of fluid volume excess. Signs and symptoms may include dyspnea, abnormal breath sounds (i.e., crackles), S_3 heart sound, peripheral edema, tachycardia, and jugular vein distention. *Rationale:* Assessment data should correlate with an increased CVP/RAP value.

Patient Preparation

- Verify that the patient is the correct patient using two identifiers. *Rationale:* Before performing a procedure, the nurse should ensure the correct identification of the patient for the intended intervention.
- Ensure that the patient and family understand teaching. Answer questions as they arise, and reinforce information as needed. *Rationale:* Understanding of previously taught information is evaluated and reinforced.
- Place the patient in the supine position with the head of the bed flat or elevated up to 45 degrees. *Rationale:* This positioning prepares the patient for hemodynamic monitoring.

Procedure for Central Venous/Right-Atrial Pressure Monitoring

Steps	Rationale	Special Considerations
1. **HH**		
2. **PE**		
3. Position the patient in the supine position with the head of the bed at 0–45 degrees. **(Level B*)**	Studies have determined that the CVP/RAP is accurate in this position.[3–5,7,12,14,16,27,28]	CVP/RAP may be accurate for patients in the supine position with the head of the bed elevated up to 60 degrees,[5,16] but additional studies are needed to support this. Only one study[13] supports the accuracy of hemodynamic values for patients in the lateral positions; other studies do not.[3,9,12,20,26] The majority of studies support the accuracy of hemodynamic monitoring for patients in the prone position.[1,2,8,11,15,21,25] Two studies demonstrated that prone positioning caused an increase in hemodynamic values.[22,24]
4. Level the air-fluid interface of the monitoring system to the phlebostatic axis (see Procedure 75 and Figs. 75-7 and 75-9).	The phlebostatic axis is at approximately the level of the atria and should be used as the reference point for the air-fluid interface.	Mark the location of the phlebostatic axis if not already identified.
5. Zero the transducer (see Procedure 75).	Allows the monitor to use atmospheric pressure as a reference for zero.	

---

*Level B: Well-designed, controlled studies with results that consistently support a specific action, intervention, or treatment.

Procedure continues on following page

Procedure	for Central Venous/Right-Atrial Pressure Monitoring—*Continued*	
Steps	**Rationale**	**Special Considerations**
6. Observe the waveform and perform a dynamic response test (square wave test).	Determines whether the system is damped. This will ensure that the pressure waveform components are clearly defined. This aids in accurate measurement.	The square wave test can be performed by activating and quickly releasing the fast flush. A sharp upstroke should terminate in a flat line at the maximal indicator on the monitor. This should be followed by an immediate rapid downstroke extending below baseline with 1–2 oscillations within 0.12 second and a quick return to baseline (see Fig. 59-3).
7. Run a dual-channel strip of the electrocardiogram (ECG) and CVP/RAP waveform (Fig. 67-1).	Right-atrial pressures should be determined from the graphic recording so that end expiration can be properly identified.	Some monitors have the capability of "freeze framing" waveforms. A cursor can be used to determine pressure measurements.
8. Measure the CVP/RAP at end expiration.	Measurement is most accurate as the effects of intrathoracic pressure changes are minimized.	
9. With the dual-channel recorded strip, draw a vertical line from the beginning of the P wave of one of the ECG complexes down to the CVP/RAP waveform. Repeat this with the next ECG complex (see Fig. 72-7).	Compares electrical activity with mechanical activity. Usually, three waves are present on the CVP/RAP waveform.	At times, the *c* wave is not present.
10. Align the PR interval with the CVP/RAP waveform (see Fig. 72-7).	The *a* wave correlates with this interval.	

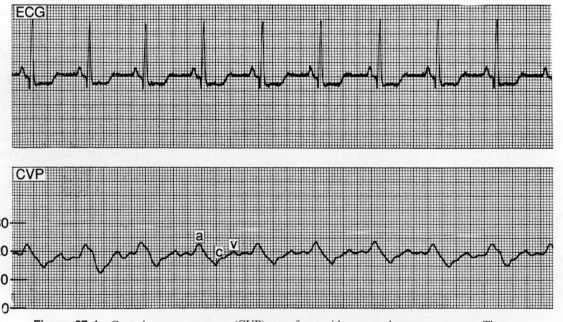

Figure 67-1 Central venous pressure (CVP) waveform with *a, c,* and *v* waves present. The *a* wave is usually seen just after the *p* wave of the electrocardiogram (ECG). The *c* wave appears at the time of the RST junction on the ECG. The *v* wave is seen in the TP interval.

Procedure | for Central Venous/Right-Atrial Pressure Monitoring—*Continued*

Steps	Rationale	Special Considerations
11. Identify the *a* wave (see Fig. 67-1).	The *a* wave is seen approximately 80–100 ms after the P wave. The *c* wave follows the *a* wave, and the *v* wave follows the *c* wave.	The *a* wave reflects atrial contraction. The *c* wave reflects closure of the tricuspid valve. The *v* wave reflects passive filling of the right atrium.
12. Identify the scale of the CVP/RAP tracing (see Figs. 67-1 and 67-2).	Aids in determining the pressure measurement.	The RAP scale commonly is set at 20 mm Hg. Scale settings may vary based on monitoring equipment.
13. Measure the mean of the *a* wave to obtain the RAP (see Fig. 67-2 and Fig. 72-8).	The *a* wave represents atrial contraction and reflects ventricular filling at end diastole.	
14. Remove PE and discard used supplies in appropriate receptacles.	Reduces the transmission of microorganisms; Standard Precautions.	
15. HH		

Expected Outcomes

- Accurate CVP/RAP measurements
- Adequate and appropriate waveforms
- CVP/RAP readings that correlate with physical findings
- Evaluation of information obtained to guide therapeutic interventions

Unexpected Outcomes

- Inaccurate readings
- CVP/RAP readings that do not correlate with physical findings
- Infection
- Sepsis
- Occluded catheter

Procedure continues on following page

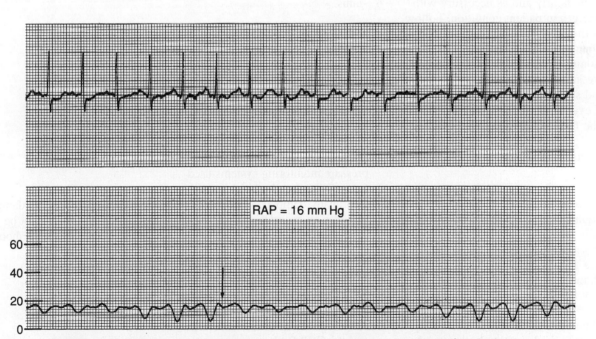

Figure 67-2 Reading the right-atrial pressure (RAP) from paper printout at end expiration in a spontaneously breathing patient. While observing the patient, identify inspiration. The point just before inspiration is end expiration. The *arrow* indicates the point of end expiration. Reading is taken as a mean value. The RAP value for this patient is 16 mm Hg.

Patient Monitoring and Care

Steps	Rationale	Reportable Conditions
		These conditions should be reported if they persist despite nursing interventions.
1. Recheck leveling whenever the patient position changes.	Ensures an accurate reference point at the phlebostatic axis.	
2. Zero the transducer during initial setup or before insertion, if disconnection occurs between the transducer and the monitoring cable, if disconnection occurs between the monitoring cable and the monitor, at least once per shift, and when the values obtained do not fit the clinical picture. Follow manufacturer's recommendations regarding routine zeroing of the system.	Ensures the accuracy of the hemodynamic monitoring system; minimizes the risk for contamination of the system.	
3. Monitor the pressure transducer system (pressure tubing, transducer, stopcocks, etc.) for air and eliminate air from the system.	Air emboli are potentially fatal.	
4. Assess central venous catheter patency every 8 hours and administer thrombolytics as prescribed if the catheter is occluded.[6,23] (**Level B***)	Ensures catheter patency.	• Occluded catheter
5. Continuously monitor the CVP/RAP waveform; obtain the hemodynamic value hourly and as necessary with changes in patient condition. Follow institutional standards.	Provides for continuous waveform analysis and assessment of patient status.	• Abnormal CVP/RAP values or waveforms
6. Change the hemodynamic monitoring system (flush solution, pressure tubing, transducer, and stopcocks) every 96 hours. (**Level B***) The flush solution may need to be changed more frequently if the volume of solution is decreased.	The Centers for Disease Control and Prevention (CDC),[18] the Infusion Nurses Society,[10] and research findings[17,19] recommend that the hemodynamic flush system can be used safely for 96 hours. This recommendation is based on research conducted with disposable pressure monitoring systems used for peripheral and central lines.	
7. Perform a dynamic response test (square wave test) at the start of each shift, with a change of the waveform, or when the system is opened to air (see Fig. 59-3).	An optimally damped system provides an accurate waveform.	• Overdamped or underdamped waveforms that cannot be corrected with troubleshooting procedures
8. Maintain the pressure bag or device at 300 mm Hg.	At 300 mm Hg, each flush device delivers approximately 1–3 mL/hr to maintain patency of the system.	
9. Obtain a CVP/RAP waveform strip to place on the patient's chart at the start of each shift and whenever there is a change in the waveform or patient condition.	Allows assessment of the waveform and the CVP/RAP measurement.	

*Level B: Well-designed, controlled studies with results that consistently support a specific action, intervention, or treatment.

Documentation

Documentation should include the following:
- Patient and family education
- CVP/RAP pressures and waveform
- Site assessment
- Occurrence of unexpected outcomes and interventions

References and Additional Readings

For a complete list of references and additional readings for this procedure, scan this QR code with any freely available smartphone code reader app, or visit http://booksite.elsevier.com/9780323376624.

68 Esophageal Cardiac Output Monitoring: Perform

Alexander Johnson and Hillary Crumlett

PURPOSE: Insertion of an esophageal probe for monitoring aortic blood flow is used to assess the hemodynamic condition of critically ill patients. Esophageal cardiac output monitoring or esophageal Doppler monitoring (EDM) uses Doppler ultrasound technology to provide information regarding left ventricular performance and patient fluid status.

PREREQUISITE NURSING KNOWLEDGE

- Knowledge of cardiovascular anatomy and physiology is needed.
- Understanding of the anatomy of the upper gastrointestinal tract is essential.
- It is important to understand the appropriateness, criteria, and contraindications of the insertion of an esophageal probe for monitoring aortic blood flow.
- The ability to recognize the EDM aortic waveforms by visual display and auditory pitch is necessary.
- An understanding of normal and associated values of aortic waveforms is important (Fig. 68-1 and Table 69-1).
- An understanding of additional waveforms that guide esophageal probe insertion is needed (Fig. 69-1).
- Clinical and technical competence in esophageal probe insertion and esophageal monitoring is essential.
- Clinical and technical competence in understanding the esophageal Doppler monitor functions and options are needed.
- Corrected flow time (FTc), peak velocity (PV), and stroke distance (SD) come directly from the Doppler velocity measurements; stroke volume (SV) and cardiac output (CO) are derived using an algorithm generated from the patient nomogram information (see Table 69-1).
- The base of the waveform is used as a marker of left ventricular preload and displayed as FTc.
- The waveform height is used as a marker of contractility and is displayed as PV.
- Minute distance (MD) is the distance (cm) moved by the column of blood through the aorta in 1 minute.
- SD is the distance (cm) moved by the column of blood through the aorta in one systolic period.
- A narrowed waveform base with decreased FTc may indicate hypovolemia.

- A widened waveform base with increased FTc may indicate euvolemia.
- A reduced waveform height with low PV may indicate left ventricular failure.
- An increased waveform height with increased PV may indicate a hyperdynamic state.
- A reduced waveform height with a narrow waveform base may indicate elevation in systemic vascular resistance (SVR).
- Indications for the EDM are as follows:
  - ❖ Potential status of hypoperfusion (e.g., hypovolemia, cardiogenic shock, hemorrhagic shock, septic shock)
  - ❖ Hemodynamic monitoring and evaluation of patients with major organ dysfunction (e.g., renal failure, respiratory failure, liver failure)
  - ❖ Differential diagnosis of hypotensive states
  - ❖ Aid in the diagnosis of heart failure, cardiogenic shock, papillary muscle rupture, mitral regurgitation, ventricular septal rupture, or cardiac rupture with tamponade
  - ❖ Management of high-risk cardiac patients undergoing surgical procedures during preoperative, intraoperative, and postoperative periods
- Contraindications to EDM include oral or upper gastrointestinal tract anomalies, coagulopathies, coarctation of the aorta, and intraaortic balloon pump therapy.
- Proper positioning of the esophageal probe is essential for accurate data collection and waveform monitoring.
- EDM technology utilizes a thin silicone probe, approximately 6 mm in diameter and 90 cm in length.
- Once the patient's age, height, and weight are entered into the monitor, they are burned into a memory chip within the probe. EDM nomogram limits are:
  - ❖ Age: 16 to 99 years
  - ❖ Weight: 66 to 330 pounds
  - ❖ Height: 59 to 83 inches
- When nomogram limits are surpassed, calculated data such as SVR, SV, stroke volume index (SVI), CO, and cardiac index (CI) are not obtainable. Velocity data such as FTc, PV, SD, and MD will still be measured. Refer to specific manufacturer's nomogram limits.

AP This procedure should be performed only by physicians, advanced practice nurses, and other healthcare professionals (including critical care nurses) with additional knowledge, skills, and demonstrated competence per professional licensure or institutional standard.

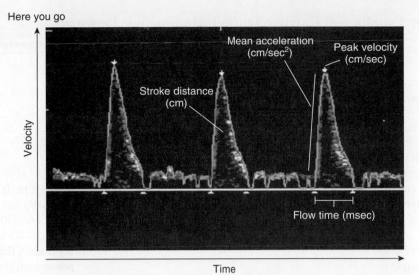

Figure 68-1 The EDM/EDM + waveform. *(From the* EDM *quick reference guide, with kind permission of Deltex Medical, Greenville, SC.)*

EQUIPMENT

- EDM monitor, patient interface cable, power cord
- EDM probe
- Water-soluble lubricant
- Nonsterile gloves
- Sedative or analgesic

Additional equipment, to have available as needed, includes the following:

- Topical lidocaine
- Tongue blade
- Supportive equipment if conscious sedation is necessary (e.g., oxygen, Ambu bag, suction, oral airway)
- Gown, mask, and goggles or face shield

PATIENT AND FAMILY EDUCATION

- Explain the procedure and the reason for the EDM monitoring. *Rationale:* This explanation increases patient understanding and may decrease patient anxiety.
- Explain that the procedure may stimulate gagging and that sedation may be given to promote comfort. *Rationale:* This explanation prepares the patient and may decrease his or her anxiety.
- Inform the patient of the risks and anticipated benefits of the esophageal monitoring probe. *Rationale:* This allows the patient to make an informed decision.

PATIENT ASSESSMENT AND PREPARATION

Patient Assessment

- Obtain the patient's medical history specifically related to oral or upper gastrointestinal anomalies (e.g., esophageal strictures, varices, oral surgery, trauma, ulcers). *Rationale:* This assesses for contraindications to insertion.
- Assess the patient's hemodynamic, cardiovascular, peripheral vascular, and neurovascular status. *Rationale:* This assessment provides baseline data that can be used for comparison with postinsertion data.
- Assess the patient's respiratory status. If the patient is mechanically ventilated, note the type of support: ventilator-assisted breathing and/or continuous positive airway breathing. *Rationale:* Determines the patient's baseline pulmonary status.
- If the patient currently has respiratory compromise or could develop respiratory compromise with the adjunct of conscious sedation, consider mechanical ventilation. *Rationale:* Protects airway and provides oxygenation. Sedation and/or local anesthesia may be needed for probe insertion and tolerance.
- Assess the patient's current laboratory profile, including electrolyte and coagulation studies. *Rationale:* Baseline coagulation studies are helpful in determining the risk for bleeding. Electrolyte abnormalities may contribute to cardiac irritability.

Patient Preparation

- Verify that the patient is correct patient using two identifiers. *Rationale:* Before performing a procedure, the nurse should ensure the correct identification of the patient for the intended intervention.
- Ensure that the patient and/or family understand the preprocedural information. Answer questions as they arise and reinforce information as needed. *Rationale:* This process evaluates and reinforces the understanding of previously taught information.
- Obtain informed consent. *Rationale:* Informed consent protects the rights of the patient and ensures that he or she can make a competent decision.
- Perform a preprocedure verification and time out. *Rationale:* This ensures patient safety.
- Consider administration of sedation or analgesics. *Rationale:* This decreases the anxiety and gagging that occurs with enhanced probe tolerance.

Procedure	for Esophageal Cardiac Output Monitoring: Perform	
Steps	**Rationale**	**Special Considerations**
1. 🅷🅷		
2. Plug the esophageal Doppler monitor into the wall outlet and turn it on.	Provides the energy source.	
3. Connect the interface cable to the esophageal Doppler monitor.	Prepares the equipment.	
4. Connect the esophageal probe to the interface cable.	Prepares the equipment.	
5. When prompted, enter the patient's age, weight, and height into the esophageal Doppler monitor. A. Turn the control knob to change the values. B. Press the control knob to enter the selected values. C. Push the keypad under the words "accept data." D. If any data are incorrect, press "change data" to return to the nomogram screen and change any data that have been incorrectly entered; then repress the "accept data" key pad. If the probe has been used previously, the patient information will appear on the screen. Probes are reusable by the same patient.	Prepares the monitor. The monitor will confirm data entry and change to the probe focus mode.	Data must be in these ranges: Age: 16–99 years Weight: 66–330 pounds Height: 59–83 inches If a patient's data are outside the nomogram limits, estimated values cannot be obtained but velocity data are available. Refer to the manufacturer's recommendations for nomograms.
6. Wash hands and don nonsterile gloves.		
7. Administer sedation if necessary.	Promotes patient comfort and ability to tolerate the esophageal probe insertion.	The esophageal probe may cause gagging. Topical lidocaine may be used to reduce gagging.
8. Apply a water-based lubricant on 6–10 cm of the distal end of the esophageal probe.	Minimizes mucosal injury and irritation during insertion; facilitates insertion and aids in signal acquisition.	It is important that only water-soluble lubricant be used in probe placement. Oil-soluble lubricant cannot be absorbed through the pulmonary mucosa and may cause respiratory complications should the probe be inadvertently placed in the lungs.
9. Insert the probe orally with the bevel edge toward the hard palate.	Begins the insertion process.	Nasal insertion may also be appropriate in select patients if oral insertion is contraindicated. Insertion should never be forced. Forceful insertion can cause mucosal damage to the posterior pharynx or the esophagus.
10. Utilize the depth markings on the esophageal probe to facilitate positioning.	Aids in proper probe depth adjustment.	Proper probe depth is essential to obtain optimal aortic signal. Generally the patient's incisors should be between the 35-cm and the 40-cm length markings.

Procedure	for Esophageal Cardiac Output Monitoring: Perform—*Continued*	
Steps	**Rationale**	**Special Considerations**
11. Observe the esophageal Doppler monitor and listen for an auditory signal to establish the optimal descending aortic waveform while rotating, inserting, and withdrawing the probe until the ideal waveform appears and is heard as the sharpest audible pitch (see Figs. 68-1 and 69-1). If unable to obtain an aortic waveform, consider that the probe may be in the trachea. If this occurs, remove the probe and attempt reinsertion.	Enhances the accuracy of the probe insertion.	The ideal waveform has a black center outlined with red and yellow. The sound pitch should be clear and should correspond with the aortic flow pattern noted on the monitor screen.
12. Observe the peak velocity display (PVD) on the monitor to assess for the greatest peak velocity achieved. **(Level M*)**	The highest peak velocity is usually associated with the best visual and auditory signal.	Use specific manufacturer's recommendation for PVD (e.g., sharp upstroke with moderately crisp peak to the waveform).
13. Press the filter button to activate the signal artifacts filter when appropriate. **(Level M*)**	Eliminates visual and auditory low frequency signals (usually due to excess heart valve or wall motion noise).	Use specific manufacturer's recommendations for noise filters.
14. Press the auto gain button for optimal amplification of the signal. **(Level M*)**	Optimizes amplification of the waveform.	Use specific manufacturer's recommendations for optimal waveform management.
15. Press the scale button to change the waveform scale. **(Level M*)**	Aids in visualization of the waveform display.	Use specific manufacturer's recommendations for optimal waveform visualization.
16. If activation of auto gain does not provide parameter display, press "run" after an optimal signal is obtained. A green line called the *follower* should hug the contour of the waveform. **(Level M*)**	Indicates initiation of monitoring.	A white arrow depicts the beginning and end of systole and the peak velocity of each cycle. Use manufacturer's recommendations for beginning the monitoring process.
17. Record the displayed data from the top of the EDM screen. **(Level M*)**	SD, PV, and FTc are direct measurements. All other data are calculated from these three measurements along with body surface area.	Use specific manufacturer's recommendations for obtaining and recording data.
18. Remove gloves and discard used supplies.	Reduces the transmission of microorganisms; Standard Precautions.	
19. 🅷🅷		
20. Compare SD, FTc, and PV values with normal values (see Table 69-1).	Determines hemodynamic status.	

*Level M: Manufacturer's recommendations only.

Procedure continues on following page

Expected Outcomes

- Accurate placement of the esophageal probe
- Adequate and appropriate waveforms
- Ability to obtain accurate information regarding hemodynamic parameters
- Evaluation of information obtained to guide therapeutic interventions

Unexpected Outcomes

- Oral, pharyngeal, or esophageal mucosal tears; ulceration; or infections
- Hematoma
- Hemoptysis
- Hemorrhage
- Probe placed into the trachea or bronchus
- Vagal response during insertion or from gagging
- Vomiting or aspiration
- Esophageal-tracheal fistula formation
- Pain

Patient Monitoring and Care

Steps	Rationale	Reportable Conditions
		These conditions should be reported if they persist despite nursing interventions.
1. Perform systematic cardiovascular and neurological assessments before, during, and after the insertion of the probe.	Obtains baseline data and assesses patient status. Assesses for signs of adequate perfusion. Evaluates patient response to the procedure and medications administered.	• Changes in level of consciousness • Changes in vital signs • Abnormal hemodynamic parameters
2. Monitor the patient's mouth for signs of trauma from the probe insertion.	Identifies skin breakdown.	• Redness, ulceration • Swelling, drainage • Foul odor • Bleeding • Skin breakdown
3. Perform oral care every 2 hours and as needed while the probe is in place. The esophageal probe may be left in place if tolerated; the probe usually does not require taping to maintain placement.	Oral tubes tend to cause mouth dryness and increase the potential for mucosal breakdown.	• Patient unable to tolerate esophageal probe placement (e.g., inability to relieve gagging, anxiety)
4. Follow institutional standards for assessing pain. Administer analgesia as prescribed.	Identifies need for pain interventions. Promotes patient comfort.	• Unrelieved patient discomfort
5. Monitor aortic waveforms while the esophageal probe is in place. Waveforms should be assessed when data collection is needed, such as every hour.	Ensures proper probe placement.	• Abnormal waveforms

Documentation

Documentation should include the following:

- Patient and family education
- Signed informed consent
- Appearance of waveforms
- Sedatives or analgesia administered

- Patient tolerance of the procedure
- Hemodynamic data obtained
- Occurrence of unexpected outcomes
- Nursing interventions taken

References and Additional Readings

For a complete list of references and additional readings for this procedure, scan this QR code with any freely available smartphone code reader app, or visit http://booksite.elsevier.com/9780323376624.

69 Esophageal Cardiac Output Monitoring: Assist, Care, and Removal

Alexander Johnson and Hillary Crumlett

PURPOSE: Esophageal Doppler monitoring of aortic blood flow is used to assess the hemodynamic condition of critically ill patients. Esophageal cardiac output or esophageal Doppler monitoring (EDM) uses Doppler ultrasound technology to provide information regarding left ventricular performance and patient fluid status.

PREREQUISITE NURSING KNOWLEDGE

- Knowledge of cardiovascular anatomy and physiology is needed.
- Understanding of the anatomy of the upper gastrointestinal tract is essential.
- The ability to recognize the EDM aortic waveforms by visual display and auditory pitch is necessary.
- An understanding of normal and associated values aortic waveforms is important (Table 69-1 and Fig. 68-1).
- An understanding of additional waveforms that guide esophageal probe insertion is needed (Fig. 69-1).
- Understanding of the technique and importance of obtaining an optimal signal is needed.
- Clinical and technical competence in understanding the esophageal Doppler monitor functions and options is needed.
- Corrected flow time (FTc), peak velocity (PV), and stroke distance (SD) come directly from the Doppler velocity measurements; stroke volume (SV) and cardiac output (CO) are derived using an algorithm generated from the patient nomogram information (see Table 69-1).
- The base of the waveform is used as a marker of left ventricular preload and displayed as FTc.
- The waveform height is used as a marker of contractility and is displayed as PV.
- Minute distance (MD) is the distance (cm) moved by the column of blood through the aorta in 1 minute.
- SD is the distance (cm) moved by the column of blood through the aorta in one systolic period.
- A narrowed waveform base with decreased FTc may indicate hypovolemia.
- A widened waveform base with increased FTc may indicate euvolemia.
- A reduced waveform height with low PV may indicate left ventricular failure.
- An increased waveform height with increased PV may indicate a hyperdynamic state.

- A reduced waveform height with a narrow waveform base may indicate elevation in systemic vascular resistance (SVR).
- Optimal positioning of the probe is essential for accurate data collection (refer to Procedure 68)
- EDM technology uses a thin silicone probe, approximately 6 mm in diameter and 90 cm in length.
- Once the patient's age, height, and weight are entered into the monitor, they are burned into a memory chip within the probe. EDM nomogram limits are:
  - ❖ Age: 16 to 99 years
  - ❖ Weight: 66 to 330 pounds
  - ❖ Height: 59 to 83 inches
- When nomogram limits are surpassed, calculated data such as SVR, SV, stroke volume index (SVI), CO, and cardiac index (CI) are not obtainable. Velocity data such as FTc, PV, SD, and MD will still be measured. Refer to specific manufacturer's nomogram limits.

EQUIPMENT

- EDM monitor, patient interface cable, power cord
- EDM probe
- Water-soluble lubricant
- Nonsterile gloves

Additional equipment, to have available as needed, includes the following:
- ❖ Topical lidocaine
- ❖ Tongue blade
- ❖ Supportive equipment if conscious sedation is necessary (e.g., oxygen, Ambu bag, suction, oral airway)
- ❖ Gown, mask, and goggles or face shield
- ❖ Sedatives or analgesics as necessary

PATIENT AND FAMILY EDUCATION

- Explain the procedure and the reason for the EDM monitoring. ***Rationale:*** This explanation increases patient understanding and may decrease patient anxiety.

TABLE 69-1	Normal Ranges for Measured Parameters Obtained From Esophageal Doppler Monitoring*	
Corrected Flow Time (FTc)	**Age**	**Peak Velocity (PV)[1,2]**
330–360 milliseconds	20 years	90–120 cm/sec
	30 years	85–115 cm/sec
	40 years	80–110 cm/sec
	50 years	70–100 cm/sec
	60 years	60–90 cm/sec
	70 years	50–80 cm/sec
	80 years	40–70 cm/sec
	90 years	30–60 cm/sec

*Note: Normal ranges should not be confused with a physiological target.
[1]Singer, M (1993). Esophageal Doppler monitoring of aortic blood flow: Beat-by-beat cardiac output monitoring. *Inter Anaesthesia Clin* 31; 99–125. Normal range values appear in bold.
[2]Gardin, J.M., Davidson, D.M., Rohan, M.K., et al. Relationship between age, body size, gender, and blood pressure and Doppler flow measurements in the aorta and pulmonary artery. *Am Heart J* 113; 101–109. Extrapolated values do not appear in bold.

- Explain that the procedure may stimulate gagging and that sedation may be given to promote comfort. ***Rationale:*** This explanation prepares the patient and may decrease his or her anxiety.
- Explain the monitoring and troubleshooting procedures to the patient and family. ***Rationale:*** This explanation keeps the patient and family informed and reduces their anxiety.
- Instruct the patient about signs and symptoms to report to the critical care nurse and staff, including oral bleeding, sore throat, and displacement of the probe. ***Rationale:*** This encourages the patient to report changes and problems.

PATIENT ASSESSMENT AND PREPARATION
Patient Assessment

- Assess the patient's hemodynamic, cardiovascular, peripheral vascular, and neurovascular status. ***Rationale:*** This assessment provides baseline data that can be used for comparison with postinsertion data.
- Assess the patient's current laboratory profile, including electrolyte and coagulation studies. ***Rationale:*** Baseline coagulation studies are helpful in determining the risk for bleeding. Electrolyte abnormalities may contribute to cardiac irritability.

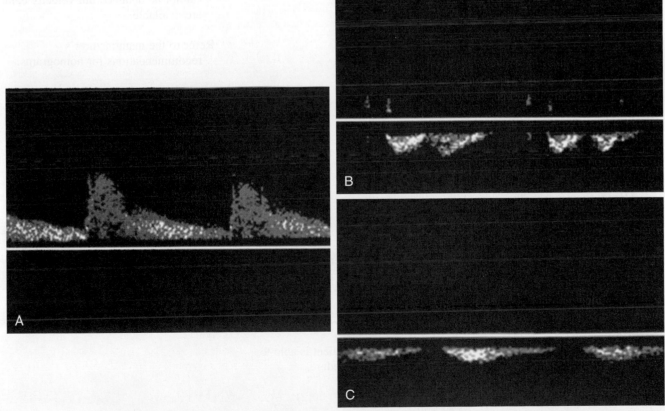

Figure 69-1 Additional waveforms that guide esophageal probe insertion. **A,** Celiac axis: Probe too low. **B,** Intracardiac: Rotate probe. Adjust depth as necessary. **C,** Azygos vein: Correct depth or slightly low. Rotate and/or withdraw probe slightly. (*From the* EDM Quick Reference Guide, *with kind permission of Deltex Medical, Greenville, SC.*)

Patient Preparation

- Verify that the patient is the correct patient using two identifiers. *Rationale:* Before performing a procedure, the nurse should ensure the correct identification of the patient for the intended intervention.
- Ensure that the patient and/or family understand the pre-procedural information. Answer questions as they arise and reinforce information as needed. *Rationale:* This process evaluates and reinforces understanding of previously taught information.
- Ensure that informed consent was obtained. *Rationale:* Informed consent protects the rights of the patient and ensures that he or she can make a competent decision.
- Administer sedation, analgesia, and local anesthetics as prescribed. *Rationale:* This may decrease the pain, anxiety and gagging that occurs with probe manipulation.

Procedure for Esophageal Cardiac Output Monitoring: Assist, Care, and Removal		
Steps	**Rationale**	**Special Considerations**
1. ▣		
2. Ensure that the esophageal Doppler monitor is plugged into the wall outlet and is turned on.	Provides the energy source.	
3. Ensure that the interface cable is connected to the esophageal Doppler monitor and that the esophageal probe is connected to the interface cable.	Prepares the equipment.	
4. If needed, assist with entering patient information into the esophageal Doppler (i.e., patient's age, weight, and height). If the probe has been used previously, the patient information will appear on the screen. Probes are reusable by the same patient.	Prepares the monitor. The monitor will confirm data entry and change to the probe focus mode.	Data must be in these ranges: Age: 16–99 years Weight: 66–330 pounds Height: 59–83 inches If a patient's data are outside the nomogram limits, estimated values cannot be obtained but velocity data are available.
A. Turn the control knob to change the values.		Refer to the manufacturer's recommendations for nomograms.
B. Press the control knob to enter the selected values.		
C. Push the keypad under the words "accept data." If any data are incorrect, press "change data" to return to the nomogram screen and change any data that have been incorrectly entered; then repress the "accept data" key pad.		
5. Wash hands and don nonsterile gloves.		
6. Administer sedation, analgesia, and topical anesthetics as prescribed and as needed.	Decreases the patient's anxiety, promotes patient comfort and the ability to tolerate the esophageal probe insertion.	The esophageal probe may cause gagging. Topical lidocaine may be used to reduce gagging.
7. Assist, if needed, with probe insertion.	Provides needed assistance.	
8. Monitor the patient's response to probe insertion.	Ensures that the patient is able to tolerate the procedure.	

Procedure	for Esophageal Cardiac Output Monitoring: Assist, Care, and Removal—*Continued*	
Steps	**Rationale**	**Special Considerations**
9. Assist as needed with comparing the EDM values to normal values and the patient's baseline values.	Increases and decreases in SD, PV, or FTc depict specific hemodynamic physiology.	Follow manufacturer's recommendations for normal values and interpretation. Normal values should not be confused with physiological targets (see Table 69-1).
10. Administer IV fluids and/or vasoactive agents as prescribed.	Provides interventions to improve cardiac output.	
11. Validate the effectiveness of medical therapy by obtaining values again after the prescribed therapy has been completed.	Values may show the need for therapy adjustments.	It is important that the probe is refocused before each patient assessment, ensuring an optimal signal.
12. If prescribed and tolerated by the patient, leave the probe in place throughout therapy adjustments.	Continues monitoring.	A physician, advanced practice nurse, or other healthcare professional may need to adjust the position of the esophageal probe. The probe can also be removed and replaced as needed. Follow institution standard.
13. Remove gloves and discard used supplies.	Reduces the transmission of microorganisms; Standard Precautions.	
14. ▣		
Finding the Maximum Flow		
1. ▣		
2. ▣		
3. Adjust the volume control knob on the esophageal Doppler monitor.	Auditory signals are necessary for accurate probe placement.	
4. Grasp the probe gently in one hand.	Manipulates the position of the esophageal probe.	
5. Rotate left and right and then slowly pull back and insert the probe while listening for the sharpest audible pitch associated with the highest peak velocity.	Facilitates locating the appropriate aortic signal.	A physician, advanced practice nurse, or other healthcare professional may need to adjust the position of the esophageal probe. Follow institution standard. The esophageal probe should be adjusted until the sharpest aortic waveform possible is obtained, in terms of both visual display and audible pitch.
6. Remove gloves and discard used supplies.	Reduces the transmission of microorganisms; Standard Precautions.	
7. ▣		
Troubleshooting the Absence of the Aortic Waveform		
1. ▣		
2. ▣		
3. Locate the depth markings to check that the probe has not been dislodged.	An optimal waveform is obtained when the distance to aortic flow is closest.	
4. Ensure the monitor, cable, and probe are all connected appropriately.	Loose connections will distort values.	

Procedure continues on following page

Procedure | **for Esophageal Cardiac Output Monitoring: Assist, Care, and Removal—*Continued***

Steps	Rationale	Special Considerations
5. Readjust the esophageal probe as needed according to the insertional procedure.	Ensures accurate positioning.	A physician, advanced practice nurse, or other healthcare professional may need to adjust the position of the esophageal probe. Follow institution standard.
6. Remove gloves and discard used supplies.	Reduces the transmission of microorganisms; Standard Precautions.	
7. **HH**		
Removal of the Esophageal Probe		
1. **HH**	Reduces transmission of microorganisms; Standard Precautions	A physician, advanced practice nurse, or other healthcare professional may need to remove the esophageal probe. Follow institution standard.
2. **PE**		
3. Gently pull the esophageal probe from the esophagus and mouth.	Careful removal decreases the possibility of causing mucosal tears.	
4. Place the probe in a clean container or wrap it for future reuse.	Probes may be used on an intermittent basis.	
5. Remove gloves and discard used supplies.	Reduces the transmission of microorganisms; Standard Precautions.	
6. **HH**		

Expected Outcomes

- Accurate placement of the esophageal probe
- Adequate and appropriate waveforms
- Ability to obtain accurate information regarding hemodynamic parameters
- Evaluation of information obtained to guide therapeutic interventions

Unexpected Outcomes

- Oral, pharyngeal, or esophageal mucosal tears; ulceration; or infections
- Hematoma
- Hemoptysis
- Hemorrhage
- Probe placed into the trachea or bronchus
- Vagal response during insertion or from gagging
- Vomiting or aspiration
- Esophageal-tracheal fistula formation
- Pain

Patient Monitoring and Care

Steps	Rationale	Reportable Conditions
		These conditions should be reported if they persist despite nursing interventions.
1. Perform systematic cardiovascular and neurological assessments before, during, and after the insertion of the probe.	Obtains baseline data and assesses patient status. Assesses for signs of adequate perfusion. Evaluates patient response to the procedure and medications administered.	• Changes in level of consciousness • Changes in vital signs • Abnormal hemodynamic parameters
2. Monitor the EDM waveforms while the esophageal probe is in place.	Provides assessment of proper placement of the probe; normal and abnormal waveforms.	• Abnormal waveforms

Patient Monitoring and Care —*Continued*

Steps	Rationale	Reportable Conditions
3. Monitor hemodynamic status as frequently as prescribed and as needed (e.g., SV, CO, CI, SVR, FTc, PV). Follow institution standard.	Guides therapy	• Changes in hemodynamic monitoring values
4. Assess EDM waveforms and values before and after troubleshooting. Assess waveforms when data collection is needed, such as every hour. Follow institution standard.	Identifies that troubleshooting has been successful.	• Unsuccessful troubleshooting attempts
5. Perform oral care every 2 hours and as needed while the probe is in place. The esophageal probe may be left in place if tolerated; the probe usually does not require taping to maintain placement.	Oral tubes tend to cause mouth dryness, which increases the potential for mucosal breakdown.	• Patient unable to tolerate esophageal probe placement (e.g., inability to relieve gagging, anxiety)
6. Follow institutional standards for assessing pain. Administer analgesia as prescribed.	Identifies need for pain interventions. Promotes patient comfort.	• Unrelieved patient discomfort

Documentation

Documentation should include the following:
- Patient and family education
- Appearance of waveforms
- Sedatives or analgesia administered
- Hemodynamic data obtained
- Patient tolerance
- Pain
- Site assessment
- Occurrences of unexpected outcomes and interventions

References and Additional Readings

For a complete list of references and additional readings for this procedure, scan this QR code with any freely available smartphone code reader app, or visit http://booksite.elsevier.com/9780323376624.

PROCEDURE

70 Noninvasive Cardiac Output Monitoring

Susan Scott

PURPOSE: Noninvasive cardiac output monitoring is a technology that can be used to obtain hemodynamic data on a continuous basis without the use of an invasive procedure.

PREREQUISITE NURSING KNOWLEDGE

- Knowledge of the anatomy and physiology of the cardiovascular system is necessary.
- Knowledge of the anatomy and physiology of the vasculature and adjacent structures is needed.
- Understanding of the pathophysiologic changes that occur in heart disease and affect flow dynamics is necessary.
- Understanding of the hemodynamic effects of vasoactive medications and fluid resuscitation is needed.
- Understanding of the principles involved in hemodynamic monitoring is necessary.[3]
- Understanding of the appropriateness, criteria, and contraindications of the use of noninvasive cardiac output is important.
- Knowledge of the principles of noninvasive cardiac output monitoring is essential.[3]
- Knowledge of definitions and norms for cardiac output, cardiac index, systemic vascular resistance, stroke volume, stroke index, preload, afterload, and contractility is necessary.
- Arterial pressure represents the forcible ejection of blood from the left ventricle into the aorta and out into the arterial system.
- Noninvasive cardiac output methods are easy to use and there is little if any risk associated with their application.
- Noninvasive cardiac output methods are typically compared with the thermodilution method because this is considered the "gold standard" for determining cardiac output.[12]
- One noninvasive cardiac output method is bioimpedance cardiography. This involves the application of electrodes placed on the skin or the endotracheal tube.[12] Bioimpedance cardiography is based on measurements of the resistance to the transmission of electrical currents.[1,9,10,12,15] In the body, blood and plasma are channels of low resistance to electrical current, whereas heart muscle, lungs, and fat have higher resistance.[1] When the current is applied, if blood is being ejected from the heart, the impedance to flow decreases. During diastole, when the heart is filling, impedance returns to baseline. Some bioimpedance devices involve obtaining whole body bioimpedance, whereas others use thoracic bioimpedance. Although this method

has been validated in postcardiac surgery patients,[10] care must be taken when interpreting data via this method with other patient populations because researchers have reported conflicting results.[4,7,8,11,16]

- Bioreactance, another method, estimates cardiac output noninvasively by analysis of the frequency spectra variations of a delivered oscillating current.
- Signal stability of both bioimpedance and bioreactance may fail after 24 hours.[15]
- Another method, ultrasonic cardiac output monitoring, uses a continuous wave Doppler monitor using a probe applied to the chest. The cardiac output is calculated from the cross-sectional area of either the aortic or pulmonic valve using a software nomogram. A report of a meta-analysis of this method revealed results comparable to that of thoracic bioimpedance in the perioperative and critical care settings.[5]
- A fourth type of noninvasive cardiac output device obtains a cardiac output based on arterial pressure pulse contour analysis. It works via an inflatable cuff wrapped around a finger, along with a device that measures the diameter of the arteries in the finger. With each systole, the device senses the increase in diameter of the arteries and inflates the cuff to keep the diameter of the arteries constant. The accuracy of this method has been validated during and after cardiac surgery.[1,4,5,11] Its reliability for tracking the effects of a fluid challenge has been questioned,[14] and although it is not interchangeable with transpulmonary thermodilution cardiac output, trending the values correlates well with it.[2,6,7,11,13]

EQUIPMENT

- Electrocardiographic (ECG) monitor (i.e., hardwire or telemetry); may also include transport ECG monitor
- ECG lead wires, which may or may not be disposable
- Skin electrodes, pregelled and disposable
- Noninvasive cardiac output monitor
- Noninvasive cardiac output cables
- Noninvasive electrodes and probes

Additional equipment, to have available as needed, includes the following:

- Emergency equipment and medications
- Arm board

PATIENT AND FAMILY EDUCATION

- Explain the rationale for noninvasive cardiac output monitoring, including how the reading is displayed at the bedside. *Rationale:* This explanation may decrease patient and family anxiety.
- Explain the standard of care to the patient and family, including application of the monitoring device, alarms, and length of time the technology is expected to be utilized. *Rationale:* This explanation encourages the patient and family to ask questions and voice concerns about the procedure and decreases patient and family anxiety.
- Explain the patient's expected participation during the procedure. *Rationale:* Patient cooperation during use of the device is encouraged.
- Explain the importance of keeping the affected extremity immobile based on the technology utilized. *Rationale:* This explanation helps the patient to understand the importance of the device and ensures an accurate waveform.
- Instruct the patient to report any discomfort related to the device. *Rationale:* There should be no to minimal discomfort associated with this technology.

PATIENT ASSESSMENT AND PREPARATION

Patient Assessment

- Obtain the patient's medical history, including any perfusion problems to the upper extremities. *Rationale:* This provides baseline information and may aid in selecting the extremity for monitoring. Decreased perfusion may impair the signal to the selected extremity.
- Assess the patient's vital signs and compliance factors (e.g., age, gender, height, weight). *Rationale:* This assessment provides baseline data and information that needs to be entered into the noninvasive cardiac output monitor.

Patient Preparation

- Ensure that the patient and family understand preprocedural teachings. Answer questions as they arise, and reinforce information as needed. *Rationale:* Understanding of previously taught information is evaluated and reinforced.
- Verify that the patient is the correct patient using two identifiers. *Rationale:* Before performing a procedure, the nurse should ensure the correct identification of the patient for the intended intervention.

Procedure	for Noninvasive Cardiac Output Monitoring	
Steps	**Rationale**	**Special Considerations**
Noninvasive Cardiac Output Monitoring Using the Bioimpedence or Bioreactance Method		
1. **HH**		
2. **PE**		
3. Apply the electrodes to the patient's chest, endotracheal tube if using endotracheal bioimpedance cardiography, and neck based on the manufacturer's instructions. **(Level M*)**	Proper electrode placement is needed for acquisition of accurate hemodynamic data.	Follow the manufacturer's guidelines regarding the exact locations for electrode placement.
4. Turn on the noninvasive cardiac output monitor.	Prepares the equipment.	
5. Input the specific patient data as required by the noninvasive cardiac output monitor. **(Level M*)**	The data are used to calculate hemodynamic parameters.	
6. Observe the waveforms and data displayed on the monitor. **(Level M*)**	Accurate hemodynamic calculations are dependent on quality input.	Follow manufacturer's guidelines.
7. Remove **PE** and discard used supplies.	Reduces the transmission of microorganisms; Standard Precautions.	
8. **HH**		

*Level M: Manufacturer's recommendations only.

Procedure continues on following page

Procedure for Noninvasive Cardiac Output Monitoring—*Continued*

Steps	Rationale	Special Considerations
Noninvasive Cardiac Output Monitoring Using the Arterial Pressure Contour Analysis Method		
1. **HH**		
2. **PE**		
3. Determine the correct finger cuff size and apply the cuff to the middle phalanx of either the index, middle, or ring finger. A. Apply the finger cuff snugly enough so that the cuff does not move. B. The image of the finger on the cuff should be just proximal to the fingernail. **(Level M*)**	Proper application of the pressure cuff is needed for acquisition of accurate hemodynamic data.	
4. Lead the cuff cable and the pneumatic hose around the finger to the dorsum of the hand.	Positions the cable and the hose to facilitate connection to the wrist unit.	
5. Apply the wrist unit and attach the connectors.	Secures the equipment.	The wrist unit can be applied to an arm board alongside the wrist. Avoid overtightening the arm board to the wrist.
6. Attach the pneumatic hose and the electronic connector to the wrist unit.	Prepares the equipment.	
7. Connect the heart reference sensor to its port on the wrist unit.	Prepares the equipment.	
8. Put the finger strap of the heart reference sensor on the index finger.	Prepares the equipment.	
9. Turn on the noninvasive cardiac output monitor.	Prepares the equipment.	
10. Enter the specific patient data as required by the noninvasive cardiac output monitor (i.e., gender, height, weight, and age). **(Level M*)**	These data are used to calculate hemodynamic data.	Press the measurement button to enter the data.
11. Zero the sensor: A. Place the heart end of the heart reference sensor next to the finger end of the sensor. B. Press the hand icon on the screen. C. Press the "zero HRS" key on the lower left-hand corner of the screen and press the "next" key, which appears in the dialogue box on the screen. Then press the "zero" button. Once zeroing is complete, press the "finish" button.	Prepares the system.	Keep the heart reference sensor next to the other end of the sensor that is on the patient's finger.

*Level M: Manufacturer's recommendations only.

Procedure   for Noninvasive Cardiac Output Monitoring—*Continued*

Steps	Rationale	Special Considerations
12. Attach the heart reference sensor to the patient at the level of the heart.	Prepares the system.	The sensor may also be attached to a stationary object at the level of the heart.
13. Press the "start" key at the lower right-hand corner of the screen and, after approximately 20 seconds, data will be displayed.	It takes 20 seconds for the noninvasive cardiac output monitoring device to provide accurate hemodynamic calculations.	Data are upgraded over five cardiac heartbeats and are updated every two cardiac heartbeats.
14. Set alarms.	Alerts the nurse to important hemodynamic changes.	
15. Tap on the display screen over a given parameter.	This permits the nurse to see each parameter value.	
16. Press "stop" to discontinue monitoring.	Stops all noninvasive cardiac output monitoring.	Do not remove the finger cuff before stopping the system. Removal while the system is still on can result in damage to the cuff.
17. Remove **PE** and discard used supplies.	Reduces the transmission of microorganisms; Standard Precautions.	
18. **HH**		

Expected Outcomes

- Generation of reliable, continuous hemodynamic data, including cardiac output, cardiac index, and systemic vascular resistance.
- Hemodynamic data are incorporated into patient assessment, diagnosis, and therapeutic interventions

Unexpected Outcomes

- Inability to accurately monitor hemodynamic parameters
- Hemodynamic data do not reflect clinical presentation

Patient Monitoring and Care

Steps	Rationale	Reportable Conditions
		These conditions should be reported if they persist despite nursing interventions.
1. Continuously monitor heart rate and rhythm.	Provides assessment of patient status.	• Abnormal heart rate • Dysrhythmias
2. Obtain vital signs per institutional standards and as needed.	Provides assessment of patient status.	• Abnormal heart rate • Abnormal blood pressure • Abnormal respirations
3. Obtain cardiac indices as prescribed or per institutional standards.	Provides assessment of patient's hemodynamic status.	• Abnormal cardiac output and cardiac index • Abnormal systemic vascular resistance

Documentation

Documentation should include the following:
- Patient and family education
- Peripheral vascular and neurovascular assessment
- Pain assessment, interventions, and effectiveness

- Vital signs, cardiac output, cardiac index, and other hemodynamic parameters
- Unexpected outcomes
- Additional nursing interventions

References and Additional Readings

For a complete list of references and additional readings for this procedure, scan this QR code with any freely available smartphone code reader app, or visit http://booksite.elsevier.com/9780323376624.

71 Pulmonary Artery Catheter **AP** Insertion (Perform)

Nikki Taylor

PURPOSE: Pulmonary artery (PA) catheters are used to determine hemodynamic status in critically ill patients. PA catheters provide information about right-sided and left-sided intracardiac pressures and cardiac output. Additional functions available are fiberoptic monitoring of mixed venous oxygen saturation (Svo_2), intracardiac pacing, and assessment of right-ventricular volumes and ejection fraction.

PREREQUISITE NURSING KNOWLEDGE

- Knowledge of the normal anatomy and physiology of the cardiovascular and pulmonary systems is needed.
- Knowledge of the normal anatomy and physiology of the vasculature and adjacent structures of the neck is necessary.
- Knowledge of the principles of sterile technique is essential.
- Clinical and technical competence in central line insertion and suturing is important.
- Clinical and technical competence in PA catheter insertion is essential. Competence in chest radiograph interpretation is needed.
- Basic dysrhythmia recognition and treatment of life-threatening dysrhythmias should be understood.
- Advanced cardiac life support (ACLS) knowledge and skills are needed.
- Understanding of PA pressure monitoring (see Procedure 72) is required.
- Hemodynamic information obtained with a PA catheter is routinely used to guide therapeutic interventions, including administration of fluids and diuretics, and titration of vasoactive and inotropic medications.[1–3,12,13]
- Interpretation of right-atrial pressure (RAP)/central venous pressure and pulmonary arterial occlusion pressure (PAOP) waveforms including identification of *a, c,* and *v* waves is needed. The *a* wave reflects atrial contraction. The *c* wave reflects closure of the atrioventricular valves. The *v* wave reflects passive filling of the atria during ventricular systole.
- Directly measured or calculated hemodynamic data obtained from the PA catheter include cardiac output (CO), cardiac index (CI), systemic vascular resistance (SVR), pulmonary vascular resistance (PVR), stroke volume/stroke index), Svo_2, right-heart pressures (pulmonary artery pressure [PAP] and RAP), and PAOP, a reflection of left-ventricular end-diastolic pressure and volume. Also, information regarding right-ventricular ejection fraction and end-diastolic volume can be determined with specific PA catheters.
- CO, CI, and Svo_2 can be measured intermittently or continuously.
- There are several types of PA catheters with different functions (e.g., pacing, Svo_2 monitoring, continuous CO, or right-ventricular volume monitoring). Catheter selection is based on patient need.
- The PA catheter contains a proximal lumen port, a distal lumen port, a thermistor connector, and a balloon inflation lumen port (see Fig. 72-1). Some catheters also have additional infusion ports that can be used for the infusion of medications and intravenous fluids.
- The distal lumen port is connected to a transducer system to monitor systolic, diastolic, and mean PA pressures, and can be accessed to obtain mixed venous blood samples for analysis or calibration of Svo_2 for continuous monitoring. The proximal lumen (or injectate lumen) port is connected to a transducer system to monitor the right-atrial pressure and is accessed to inject solution when measuring thermo-dilution cardiac outputs. The balloon inflation lumen port is accessed to inflate the balloon with air to advance (float) the catheter tip to occlude forward flow through the PA and measure PAOP or pulmonary artery wedge pressure.
- The standard 7.5 Fr PA catheter is 110 cm long, and has black markings at 10-cm increments and wide black markings at 50-cm increments to facilitate insertion and positioning (see Fig. 72-1). The catheter should reach the PA after advancing 40 to 55 cm from the internal jugular vein, 35 to 50 cm from the subclavian vein, 60 cm from the femoral vein, 70 cm from the right antecubital fossa, and 80 cm from the left antecubital fossa.
- Central venous access for PA catheter insertion may be obtained at a variety of sites (see Procedure 82).

AP This procedure should be performed only by physicians, advanced practice nurses, and other healthcare professionals (including critical care nurses) with additional knowledge, skills, and demonstrated competence per professional licensure or institutional standard.

- The right subclavian vein is a more direct route than the left subclavian vein for placement of a PA catheter because the catheter does not cross the midline of the thorax.[1,2,9,15]
- Use of an internal jugular vein minimizes the risk for a pneumothorax. The preferred site for catheter insertion is the right internal jugular vein. The right internal jugular vein is a "straight shot" to the right atrium.[15]
- Knowledge of West's lung zones helps identify optimal physiological zones to obtain data from the PA catheter (Fig. 71-1). The PA catheter tip should be positioned in lung zone 3, below the level of the left atrium in the dependent portion of the lung.[19] In lung zone 3, both pulmonary arterial and venous pressures exceed alveolar pressure, resulting in the PAOP reflecting left-atrial pressures rather than alveolar pressures.[19]
- Common indications for insertion of a PA catheter include the following:[1,2,7,8,10,11,14,16,18]
  - ❖ Acute coronary syndrome or myocardial infarction (MI) complicated by hemodynamic instability, heart failure, cardiogenic shock, mitral regurgitation, ventral septal rupture, subacute cardiac rupture with tamponade, postinfarction ischemia, papillary muscle rupture, or severe heart failure (e.g., cardiomyopathy, constrictive pericarditis)
  - ❖ Hypotension unresponsive to fluid replacement or with heart failure
  - ❖ Cardiac tamponade, significant dysrhythmias, right-ventricular infarct, acute pulmonary embolism, and tricuspid insufficiency

- ❖ Anesthesia in cardiac surgery with any of the following:
  - ○ Evidence of previous MI
  - ○ Resection of ventricular aneurysm
  - ○ Coronary artery bypass graft (reoperation)
  - ○ Coronary artery bypass graft (left main or complex coronary disease)
  - ○ Complex cardiac surgery (multivalvular surgery)
  - ○ High-risk surgery (e.g., pulmonary hypertension)
- ❖ General surgery:
  - ○ Vascular procedures (abdominal aneurysm repair, aortobifemoral bypass)
  - ○ Patients at high risk[1,15,17]
  - ○ Hypotensive anesthesia[1]
- ❖ Cardiac disorders:
  - ○ Unstable angina that necessitates vasodilator therapy
  - ○ Heart failure unresponsive to conventional therapy (cardiomyopathy)[1,2,18]
  - ○ Management of heart failure
  - ○ Cardiogenic shock
  - ○ Potentially reversible systolic heart failure, such as fulminant myocarditis and peripartum cardiomyopathy
  - ○ Pulmonary hypertension during acute medication therapy
  - ○ Distinguishing cardiogenic from noncardiogenic pulmonary edema
  - ○ Constrictive pericarditis or cardiac tamponade
  - ○ Evaluation of pulmonary hypertension for a precardiac transplant workup

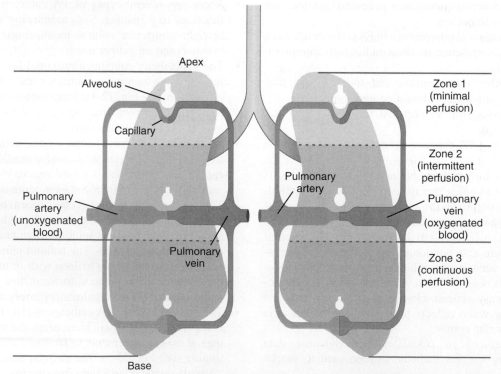

Figure 71-1 West's lung zones. Schema of the heart and lungs demonstrating the relationship between the cardiac chambers and the blood vessels and the physiological zones of the lungs. Zone 1 (PA > Pa > Pv): Absence of blood flow. Zone 2 (Pa > PA > Pv): Intermittent blood flow. Zone 3 (Pa > Pv > PA): Continuous blood flow, resulting in an open channel between the pulmonary artery catheter and the left atrium. *PA*, pulmonary artery; *Pa*, pressure arterial; *Pv*, pressure venous. (*From Copstead LC, Banasik JL:* Pathophysiology, *ed 5. Philadelphia, 2014, Saunders.*)

- ❖ Patients who need intraaortic balloon pump therapy
- ❖ Pulmonary disorders:
  - ○ Acute respiratory failure with chronic obstructive pulmonary diseases
  - ○ Cor pulmonale with pneumonia
  - ○ Optimization of positive end-expiratory pressure and volume therapy in patients with acute respiratory distress syndrome[1]
- ❖ Critically ill pregnant patients (e.g., severe preeclampsia with unresponsive hypertension, pulmonary edema, persistent oliguria)
- ❖ Severe shock states
- ❖ Major trauma or burn
- ❖ Systemic inflammatory response syndrome
- Relative contraindications to PA catheter insertion include the following:
  - ❖ Preexisting left bundle-branch block
  - ❖ Presence of fever (>101°F [38°C])
  - ❖ Mechanical tricuspid valve
  - ❖ Severe coagulopathy
  - ❖ Presence of an endocardial pacemaker
  - ❖ History of heparin-induced thrombocytopenia if only heparin-coated PA catheters are available

EQUIPMENT

- Percutaneous sheath introducer kit and sterile catheter sleeve
- PA catheter (non–heparin-coated catheters and latex-free PA catheters are available)
- Bedside hemodynamic monitoring system with pressure and cardiac output monitoring capability
- Pressure modules and cables for interface with the monitor
- Cardiac output cable with a thermistor/injectate sensor
- Pressure transducer system, including flush solution recommended according to institutional standards, a pressure bag or device, pressure tubing with transducers, and flush device (see Procedure 75)
- Dual-channel recorder
- Sterile normal saline intravenous fluid for flushing the introducer and catheter-infusion ports
- Antiseptic solution (e.g., 2% chlorhexidine–based preparation)
- Head covering, fluid-shield masks, sterile gowns, sterile gloves, nonsterile gloves, and full sterile drapes
- 1% lidocaine without epinephrine
- Sterile basin or cup
- Sterile water or normal saline solution for checking balloon integrity
- Sterile dressing supplies
- Stopcocks (may be included with the pressure tubing systems)
- Sterile caps (injectable or noninjectable)
- Leveling device (low-intensity laser or carpenter level)

Additional equipment, to have available as needed, includes the following:
- Fluoroscope
- Emergency equipment
- Temporary pacing equipment
- Indelible marker
- Transducer holder and intravenous pole
- Heparin
- 3-mL syringe
- Chlorhexidine-impregnated sponge

PATIENT AND FAMILY EDUCATION

- Explain the procedure and the reason for the PA catheter insertion. *Rationale:* Explanation may decrease patient and family anxiety.
- Explain the need for sterile technique and explain that the patient's face may be covered. *Rationale:* The explanation decreases patient anxiety and elicits cooperation.
- Inform the patient of expected benefits and potential risks. *Rationale:* The patient is given information to make an informed decision.
- Explain the patient's expected participation during the procedure. *Rationale:* Patient assistance is encouraged.

PATIENT ASSESSMENT AND PREPARATION
Patient Assessment

- Determine the patient's medical history of cervical disk disease or difficulty with vascular access. *Rationale:* Baseline data are provided.
- Determine the patient's medical history of pneumothorax or emphysema. *Rationale:* Patients with emphysematous lungs may be at higher risk for puncture and pneumothorax depending on the approach.
- Determine the patient's medical history of anomalous veins. *Rationale:* Patients may have a history of dextrocardia or transposition of the great vessels, which leads to greater difficulty in catheter placement.
- Assess the intended insertion site. *Rationale:* Scar tissue may impede placement of the catheter.
- Assess the patient's cardiac and pulmonary status. *Rationale:* Some patients may not tolerate the supine position or Trendelenburg's position for extended periods.
- Assess vital signs and pulse oximetry. *Rationale:* Baseline data are provided.
- Assess for electrolyte imbalances (potassium, magnesium, and calcium). *Rationale:* Electrolyte imbalances may increase cardiac irritability.
- Assess the electrocardiogram (ECG) for left bundle-branch block. *Rationale:* Right bundle-branch block has been associated with PA catheter insertion. Caution should be used because complete heart block may ensue.[9,17]
- Assess for heparin and latex sensitivity or allergy. *Rationale:* PA catheters are heparin bonded and contain latex. If the patient has a heparin allergy or a history of heparin-induced thrombocytopenia, consider the use of a non–heparin-coated catheter.[17,19] If the patient has a latex allergy, use a latex-free PA catheter.
- Assess for a coagulopathic state and determine whether the patient has recently received anticoagulant or thrombolytic therapy. *Rationale:* These patients are more likely to have complications related to bleeding and may need interventions before insertion of the PA catheter.

Patient Preparation

- Verify that the patient is the correct patient using two identifiers. *Rationale:* Before performing a procedure, the inserting provider should ensure the correct identification of the patient for the intended intervention.
- Ensure that the patient understands preprocedural teaching. Answer questions as they arise, and reinforce information as needed. *Rationale:* Understanding of previously taught information is evaluated and reinforced.
- Obtain informed consent. *Rationale:* Informed consent protects the rights of a patient and makes a competent decision possible for the patient.

- Perform a preprocedure verification and time out. *Rationale:* Ensures patient safety.
- Prescribe sedation or analgesics as needed. *Rationale:* Sedation and analgesics minimize anxiety and discomfort. Movement of the patient may inhibit insertion of the PA catheter.
- If the patient is obese or muscular and the preferred site is the internal jugular vein or subclavian vein, place a towel posteriorly between the shoulder blades. *Rationale:* This action helps extend the neck and provide better access to the subclavian and internal jugular veins.

Procedure for Performing Pulmonary Artery Catheter Insertion

Steps	Rationale	Special Considerations
1. HH		
2. PE		
3. Place the patient in the supine position and prepare the area with the antiseptic solution (e.g., 2% chlorhexidine–based preparation).[15,17]	The site access is prepared for PA catheter insertion.	Ensure that the patient is in the Trendelenburg position (see Procedure 82).
4. Perform hand hygiene and apply sterile gown and gloves.	Minimizes the risk of infection and maintains standard and sterile precautions.	All healthcare personnel involved in the procedure need to apply head coverings, fluid-shield masks, sterile gowns, and gloves.
5. Place sterile drapes over the prepared area.	Prepares the sterile field.	Fully drape the patient with exposure of only the insertion site.
6. With assistance, open the sterile kits.	Prepares the equipment.	
7. Obtain central venous access with an introducer (see Procedure 82).	The PA catheter is inserted into a central vein.	
8. Hand off the ports of the PA catheter to the critical care nurse assisting with connection to the hemodynamic monitoring system (see Procedure 72).	Connects the ports to the flush system; connects the transducer systems to the bedside monitor.	
9. Flush all open lumens with normal saline and attach sterile injectable or noninjectable caps to retain the flush.	Removes air from the PA catheter.	
10. Insert the PA catheter through the sterile catheter sleeve. **(Level B*)**	Maintains sterility of the PA catheter to allow repositioning of the catheter.[4-6]	
11. Insert the recommended amount of air (1.5 mL) into the balloon port and immerse the inflated balloon in the sterile bowl with water or normal saline solution.	Checks for integrity of the balloon.	If an air leak is present, air bubbles are noted.
12. Remove the balloon syringe and let the balloon passively deflate; empty the syringe and reattach the syringe to the balloon port.	Prepares for insertion.	

*Level B: Well-designed, controlled studies with results that consistently support a specific action, intervention, or treatment.

Procedure	**for Performing Pulmonary Artery Catheter Insertion—*Continued***	
Steps	**Rationale**	**Special Considerations**
13. If a PA catheter with the ability to monitor Svo$_2$ is being inserted, the fiberoptics are calibrated before removal from the package (see Procedure 16). **(Level M*)**	Calibrates the system.	Calibrate the catheter according to manufacturer's guidelines.
14. Ensure that the critical care nurse has leveled and zeroed the hemodynamic monitoring system (see Procedure 75).	Prepares the monitoring system so that right-heart pressures and PA pressures can be visualized and measured during catheter insertion.	
15. Wiggle the PA catheter and observe the monitor. Wiggling (sometimes called whipping) the PA catheter will produce artifacts on the monitor screen.	Ensures the ability to see the waveform during insertion and ensures that there are no connection issues or catheter defects before insertion.	
16. While observing the monitor and the markings on the PA catheter (Fig. 71-2), follow these steps: A. Advance the catheter through the introducer to the superior vena cava into the right atrium. B. Slowly inflate the balloon with 1.5 mL of air after verifying a right-atrial waveform. C. Advance the catheter through the tricuspid valve, into the right ventricle. Assess for the right-ventricular waveform. D. Continue to advance the catheter from the right ventricle through the pulmonic valve into the PA and assess for the PA waveform. E. Advance the catheter until a PAOP waveform (*a, c, v* waves) is visualized to obtain a PAOP. F. Passively allow the balloon to deflate. G. Observe the waveform change from the PAOP waveform to the PA waveform.	Waveforms and pressure values change while moving from the superior vena cava to the right atrium to the right ventricle to the pulmonary artery and into the wedge position.	If there is any resistance when inflating the balloon, allow the balloon to deflate, advance the catheter another centimeter, and attempt to inflate the balloon again. The catheter should reach the PA after advancing 40–55 cm from the internal jugular vein, 35–55 cm from the subclavian vein, 60 cm from the femoral vein, 70 cm from the right antecubital fossa, and 80 cm from the left antecubital fossa. When inserting the PA catheter into the subclavian vein, have the patient bring his or her ear to the shoulder on the side of the insertion site. This creates a sharp angle between the jugular and subclavian veins and may help prevent misdirection of the catheter into the internal jugular vein. During insertion, monitor the ECG tracing for dysrhythmias. Run a graphic strip of the insertion waveforms. The balloon should only be inflated when advancing the catheter and should always be deflated when the catheter is withdrawn.[11]
17. Ensure proper placement by wedging the PA catheter again and print a graphic strip of the waveforms.	Ensures proper placement and accurate readings.	

*Level M: Manufacturer's recommendations only.

Procedure continues on following page

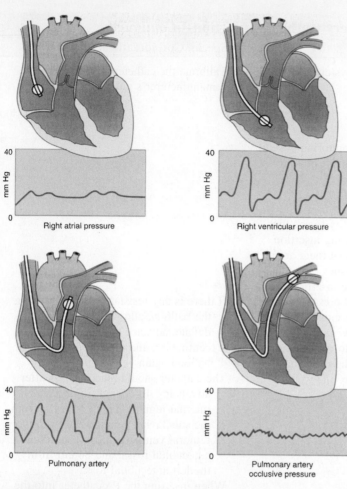

40 mm Hg / 0 — Right atrial pressure

40 mm Hg / 0 — Right ventricular pressure

40 mm Hg / 0 — Pulmonary artery

40 mm Hg / 0 — Pulmonary artery occlusive pressure

Figure 71-2 Pulmonary artery catheter advancing through the heart with appropriate waveforms. *(Adapted from Bucher L, Melander S: Critical care nursing. Philadelphia, 1999, Saunders.)*

Procedure   for Performing Pulmonary Artery Catheter Insertion—*Continued*

Steps	Rationale	Special Considerations
18. Extend the sterile catheter sleeve over the catheter and secure in place.	Maintains sterility of the PA catheter to allow repositioning of the catheter.[4-6]	The duration of catheter sterility in the sleeve is unknown. One team of researchers found that the catheter was thought to be sterile up to 4 days.[5] Another team of researchers also studied catheter sterility using the sleeve; they recommend that the PA catheter should not be repositioned after 4 hours.[6]
19. Apply an occlusive, sterile dressing and secure the catheter.	Reduces the incidence of infection and prevents dislodgement.	Dressings may be a sterile gauze or a sterile, transparent, semipermeable dressing.[15,17] Follow institutional standards for application of a chlorhexidine-impregnated sponge (see Procedure 66).
20. Note the centimeter marking at the introducer site.	Aids in ensuring placement and troubleshooting.	The tip of the PAC may migrate.
21. Obtain a chest radiograph.	Confirms the catheter tip is positioned in the PA.	
22. Remove sterile and **PE** and discard used supplies in appropriate receptacles.	Reduces the transmission of microorganisms; Standard Precautions.	
23. **HH**		

Expected Outcomes

- Accurate placement of the pulmonary artery catheter
- Adequate and appropriate waveforms
- Ability to obtain accurate information about cardiac pressures
- Evaluation of information to guide diagnosis and/or therapeutic interventions

Unexpected Outcomes

- Pneumothorax or hemothorax
- Infection or sepsis
- Ventricular dysrhythmias
- Misplacement (e.g., hepatic vein)
- Valvular damage
- Vessel wall erosion
- Hemorrhage
- Hematoma
- Pericardial or ventricular rupture
- Venous air embolism
- Cardiac tamponade
- Pulmonary artery infarction
- Pseudoaneurysms
- Catheter-site infection
- Air embolism
- PA rupture
- PA dissection
- PA catheter balloon rupture
- PA catheter knotting
- Heparin-induced thrombocytopenia or thrombosis
- Thromboembolism
- Pain
- Balloon rupture

Patient Monitoring and Care

Steps	Rationale	Reportable Conditions
		These conditions should be reported if they persist despite nursing interventions.
1. Perform systematic cardiovascular, peripheral vascular, and hemodynamic assessments before and immediately after insertion: A. Assess level of consciousness.	Assesses for signs of adequate perfusion; air embolism may present with restlessness; patient may present with decreased level of consciousness if the catheter is advanced into the carotid artery.	• Change in level of consciousness
B. Assess vital signs.	Demonstrates response to the procedure and effectiveness of therapies performed.	• Abnormal vital signs
C. Assess postinsertion hemodynamic values: PA systolic pressure, PA diastolic pressure (PADP), RAP, PAOP, CO, CI, SVR, and other parameters as needed.	Obtains baseline data and assesses patient status.	• Abnormal hemodynamic pressures or cardiac parameters
2. Assess the central line insertion site for hematoma or hemorrhage.	If coagulopathies are present, a pressure dressing may be needed.	• Bleeding that does not stop • Hematoma
3. Assess heart and lung sounds after PA catheter insertion.	Abnormal heart or lung sounds may indicate cardiac tamponade, pneumothorax, or hemothorax.	• Diminished or muffled heart sounds • Absent or diminished breath sounds unilaterally

Procedure continues on following page

Patient Monitoring and Care —*Continued*

Steps	Rationale	Reportable Conditions
4. Assess the results of the chest radiograph.	Ensures adequate placement in lung zone 3 below the level of the left atrium.	• Abnormal chest radiograph results
5. Monitor for signs and symptoms of cardiac tamponade and air embolism.	Identifies complications.	• Signs or symptoms of cardiac tamponade or air embolism
6. Monitor the centimeter marking at the introducer site.	Aids in determining if the position of the catheter has moved.	• Changes in the external centimeter marking • Abnormal PA waveforms
7. Follow institutional standards for assessing pain. Administer analgesia as prescribed.	Identifies need for pain interventions.	• Continued pain despite pain interventions

Documentation

Documentation should include the following:

- Patient and family education
- Completion of informed consent
- Universal Protocol requirements
- Insertion of PA catheter and sheath introducer
- Type and size of catheter placed
- Size of introducer sheath
- PA pressure values on insertion (RAP, right-ventricular systolic and diastolic pressures, PA systolic pressure, PADP, PAOP)
- Graphic strip of insertion
- Insertion site of the PA catheter

- Centimeter mark at the edge of the introducer
- Any difficulties encountered during placement (e.g., ventricular ectopy, new bundle-branch blocks)
- Patient tolerance
- Confirmation of placement (e.g., chest radiograph)
- Initial values after placement of the catheter (PAPs, PAOP, RAP, CO, CI, SVR, PVR, SvO_2)
- Occurrence of unexpected outcomes
- Additional interventions
- Pain assessment, interventions, and effectiveness

References and Additional Readings

For a complete list of references and additional readings for this procedure, scan this QR code with any freely available smartphone code reader app, or visit http://booksite.elsevier.com/9780323376624.

72 Pulmonary Artery Catheter Insertion (Assist) and Pressure Monitoring

Reba McVay

PURPOSE: Pulmonary artery (PA) catheters are used to determine hemodynamic status in critically ill patients. PA catheters provide information about right-sided and left-sided intracardiac pressures and cardiac output. Additional functions available are fiberoptic monitoring of mixed venous oxygen saturation, intracardiac pacing, and assessment of right-ventricular volumes and ejection fraction. Hemodynamic information obtained with a PA catheter is used to aid diagnosis and guide therapeutic intervention, including administration of fluids and diuretics and titration of vasoactive and inotropic medications.

PREREQUISITE NURSING KNOWLEDGE

- Knowledge of the normal cardiovascular and pulmonary anatomy and physiology is needed.
- Knowledge of principles of aseptic technique is essential.
- Basic dysrhythmia recognition and treatment of life-threatening dysrhythmias should be understood.
- Advanced cardiac life support (ACLS) knowledge and skills are needed.
- Knowledge of the components of the PA catheter (Fig. 72-1) and the location of the PA catheter in the heart and PA (Fig. 72-2) is necessary.
- Knowledge of the setup of the hemodynamic monitoring system (see Procedure 75) is needed.
- Understanding of normal hemodynamic values (see Table 64-1) is essential.
- The PA catheter contains a proximal injectate lumen port, a PA distal lumen port, a thermistor connector, and a balloon-inflation port with valve. Some catheters also have two infusion ports, right atrial (RA) and right ventricular (RV) lumens that can be used for infusion of medications and intravenous fluids.
- The PA distal lumen is used to monitor systolic, diastolic, and mean pressures in the PA. This lumen also allows for sampling of mixed venous blood. The proximal injectate lumen is used to monitor the RA pressure and inject the solution used to obtain cardiac output (CO). The balloon-inflation port is used to advance the PA catheter tip to the wedge position and measure the pulmonary artery occlusion pressure (PAOP).
- PAOP may be referred to as pulmonary artery wedge pressure or the pulmonary capillary wedge pressure.
- The PA diastolic pressure and the PAOP are indirect measures of left ventricular (LV) end-diastolic pressure.

Usually, the PAOP is approximately 1 to 4 mm Hg less than the pulmonary artery diastolic pressure (PADP). Because these two pressures are similar, the PADP is commonly followed, which minimizes the frequency of balloon inflation, thus decreasing the potential of balloon rupture and PA trauma.
- Differences between the PADP and the PAOP may exist for patients with pulmonary hypertension, chronic obstructive lung disease, acute respiratory distress syndrome, pulmonary embolus, and tachycardia.
- See Procedure 71 for common indications for insertion of a PA catheter.
- Hemodynamic monitoring with a PA catheter has no absolute contraindications, but an assessment of risk versus benefit to the patient should be considered. Relative contraindications to PA catheter insertion include presence of fever, presence of a mechanical tricuspid valve, presence of an endocardial pacemaker, and a coagulopathic state. A patient with left bundle-branch block may have a right bundle-branch block develop during PA catheter insertion, resulting in complete heart block. In these patients, a temporary pacemaker should be readily available.
- PA pressures may be elevated as a result of PA hypertension, pulmonary disease, mitral valve disease, LV failure, atrial or ventricular left-to-right shunt, pulmonary emboli, or hypervolemia.
- PA pressures may be low due to hypovolemia or low pulmonary vascular resistance (e.g., vasodilation).
- Transduced waveforms that are viewable during insertion include RA, RV, PA, and PA occlusion (PAO; Figs. 71-2 and 72-3).
- The RA and PAO waveforms have *a*, *c*, and *v* waves:
  ❖ The *a* wave reflects atrial contraction, the *c* wave reflects closure of the atrioventricular valve, and the *v* wave reflects passive filling of the atria during ventricular systole (Figs. 72-4 and 72-5).

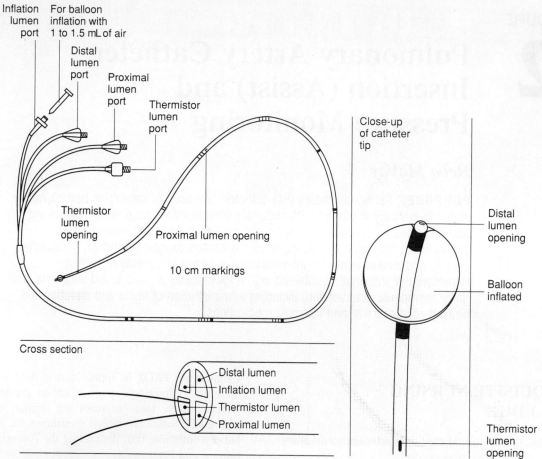

Inflation lumen port

For balloon inflation with 1 to 1.5 mL of air

Distal lumen port

Proximal lumen port

Thermistor lumen port

Thermistor lumen opening

Proximal lumen opening

10 cm markings

Close-up of catheter tip

Distal lumen opening

Balloon inflated

Thermistor lumen opening

Cross section

Distal lumen
Inflation lumen
Thermistor lumen
Proximal lumen

Figure 72-1 Anatomy of the pulmonary artery (PA) catheter. The standard 7.5-Fr thermodilution PA catheter is 110 cm in length and contains four lumens. It is constructed of radiopaque polyvinyl chloride. Black markings are on the catheter in 10-cm increments beginning at the distal end. At the distal end of the catheter is a latex rubber balloon of 1.5-mL capacity, which, when inflated, extends slightly beyond the tip of the catheter without obstructing it. Balloon inflation cushions the tip of the catheter and prevents contact with the right-ventricular wall during insertion. The balloon also acts to float the catheter into position and allows measurement of the pulmonary artery occlusion pressure. The *narrow black bands* represent 10-cm lengths, and the *wide black bands* indicate 50-cm lengths. *(From Visalli F, Evans P: The Swan-Ganz catheter: A program for teaching safe effective use,* Nursing *81[11]:1, 1981.)*

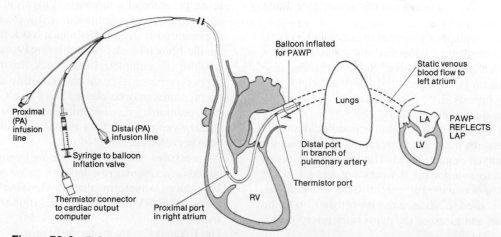

Balloon inflated for PAWP

Static venous blood flow to left atrium

Lungs

Proximal (PA) infusion line

Distal (PA) infusion line

Syringe to balloon inflation valve

Thermistor connector to cardiac output computer

Proximal port in right atrium

Distal port in branch of pulmonary artery

Thermistor port

RV

LA

LV

PAWP REFLECTS LAP

Figure 72-2 Pulmonary artery (PA) catheter location within the heart. Pulmonary artery occlusion pressure (PAOP) is an indirect measure of left-atrial (LA) and left-ventricular (LV) end-diastolic pressure. Pulmonary artery occlusion pressure (PAOP) is also referred to as pulmonary artery wedge pressure (PAWP). *(From Kersten LD:* Comprehensive respiratory nursing, *Philadelphia, 1989, Saunders.)*

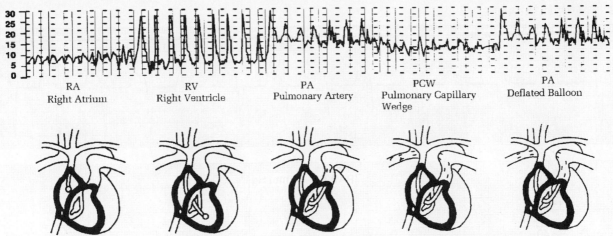

RA	RV	PA	PCW	PA
Right Atrium	Right Ventricle	Pulmonary Artery	Pulmonary Capillary Wedge	Deflated Balloon

Figure 72-3 Schematic of waveform progression as a pulmonary artery (PA) catheter is inserted through the various cardiac chambers. *(From Abbott Critical Care Systems, Mountain View, CA.)*

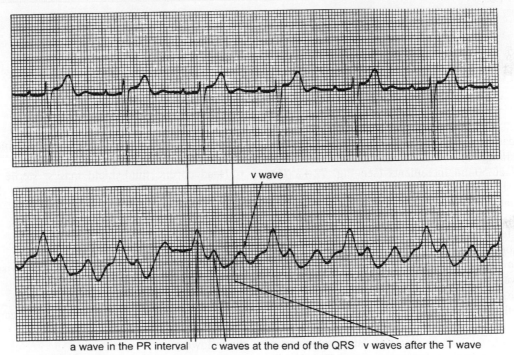

v wave

a wave in the PR interval   c waves at the end of the QRS   v waves after the T wave

Figure 72-4 Identification of *a*, *c*, and *v* waves in the waveform for right-atrial and central venous pressure. Atrial waveforms are characterized by three components: *a*, *c*, and *v* waves. The *a* wave reflects atrial contraction, the *c* wave reflects closure of the tricuspid valve, and the *v* wave reflects passive filling of the atria. *(From Ahrens TS, Taylor LK:* Hemodynamic waveform analysis, *Philadelphia, 1992, Saunders.)*

❖ The *a* wave reflects ventricular filling at end diastole. The mean of the *a* wave is determined by averaging the top and bottom values of the *a* wave.

❖ Elevated *a* and *v* waves may be evident in right atrial pressure (RAP/central venous pressure [CVP]) and in PAOP waveforms. These elevations may occur in patients with cardiac tamponade, constrictive pericardial disease, and hypervolemia.

❖ Elevated *a* waves in the RAP/CVP waveform may occur in patients with pulmonic or tricuspid valve stenosis, RV ischemia or infarction, RV failure, PA hypertension, and atrioventricular (AV) dissociation.

❖ Elevated *a* waves in the PAOP waveform may occur in patients with mitral valve stenosis, acute LV ischemia or infarction, LV failure, and AV dissociation.

❖ Elevated *v* waves in the RAP/CVP waveform may occur in patients with tricuspid valve insufficiency.

❖ Elevated *v* waves in the PAOP waveform may occur in patients with mitral valve insufficiency or a ruptured papillary muscle.

• Insertion and placement verification should occur as follows:

❖ The PA catheter is typically inserted through the subclavian, internal jugular, or femoral veins.

ECG

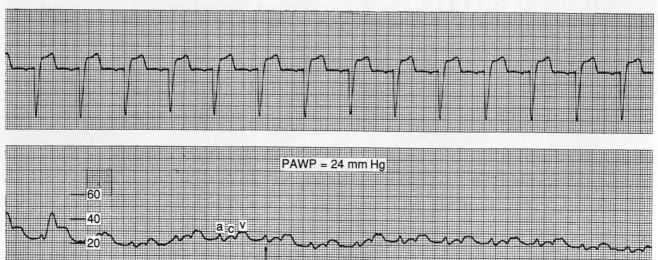

Figure 72-5   Normal pulmonary artery occlusion pressure (PAOP) waveform. Note the delay in the *a, c,* and *v* waves because of the time needed for the mechanical events to show a pressure change. This waveform is from a spontaneously breathing patient. The *arrow* indicates end expiration, where the mean of *a* wave pressure is measured. Pulmonary artery occlusion pressure (PAOP) is also referred to as pulmonary artery wedge pressure (PAWP).

- ❖ The standard 7.5 Fr PA catheter is 110 cm long and has black markings at 10-cm increments and wide black markings at 50-cm increments (see Fig. 72-1). The catheter should reach the PA after being advanced approximately 40 to 55 cm from the internal jugular vein, 35 to 50 cm from the subclavian vein, and 60 cm from the femoral vein.
- ❖ Verification of PA catheter position is validated with waveform analysis. Correct catheter position shows a PAO waveform when the balloon is inflated and a PA waveform when the balloon is deflated.
- ❖ Confirmation of the PA catheter position is also verified with chest radiography.
- ❖ The PA catheter balloon contains latex, which may cause allergic reactions. Latex-free catheters are available.

EQUIPMENT

- PA catheter (non–heparin-coated PA catheters and latex-free PA catheters are available)
- Percutaneous sheath introducer kit and sterile catheter sleeve
- Pressure modules and cables for interface with the monitor
- Cardiac output cable with a thermistor/injectate sensor and/or continuous CO monitor
- Pressure-transducer system, including flush solution recommended according to institutional standards, a pressure bag or device, pressure tubing with transducers, and flush device (see Procedure 75)
- Dual-channel recorder
- Sterile normal saline intravenous (IV) solution for flushing of the introducer and catheter infusion ports

- Antiseptic solution (e.g., 2% chlorhexidine–based preparation)
- Head covers, fluid-shield masks, sterile gowns, sterile gloves, nonsterile gloves, and full sterile drapes
- 1% lidocaine without epinephrine
- Sterile basin or cup
- Sterile water or normal saline solution
- Sterile dressing supplies
- Stopcocks (may be included in some pressure-tubing systems)
- Sterile injectable or noninjectable caps
- Leveling device (low-intensity laser or carpenter level)

Additional equipment, to have available as needed, includes the following:

- Fluoroscope or ultrasound machine
- Emergency resuscitation equipment
- Temporary pacing equipment
- Indelible marker
- Transducer holder and IV pole
- Heparin
- 3-mL syringe, slip tip and Luer-Lock
- Chlorhexidine-impregnated sponge

PATIENT AND FAMILY EDUCATION

- Provide the patient and family with information about the PA catheter, the reason for the PA catheter, and an explanation of the equipment. ***Rationale:*** The patient and family will understand the procedure, why it is needed, and how it will help manage care. Patient and family anxiety may decrease.
- Explain the patient's expected participation during the procedure. ***Rationale:*** This explanation will encourage patient assistance.

PATIENT ASSESSMENT AND PREPARATION

Patient Assessment

- Determine baseline hemodynamic, cardiovascular, peripheral vascular, and neurovascular status. ***Rationale:*** Assessment provides data that can be used for comparison with postinsertion assessment data and hemodynamic values.
- Determine the patient's baseline pulmonary status. If the patient is mechanically ventilated, note the type of support, ventilator mode, and presence or absence of positive end-expiratory pressure (PEEP) or continuous positive airway pressure. ***Rationale:*** The presence of positive pressure mechanical ventilation alters hemodynamic waveforms and pressures.
- Assess the patient's medical history specifically related to problems with venous access sites, cardiac anatomy, and pulmonary anatomy. ***Rationale:*** Identification of obstructions or disease should be made before the insertion attempt.
- Assess the patient's current laboratory profile, including electrolyte, coagulation, and arterial blood gas results. ***Rationale:*** Laboratory abnormalities are identified. Baseline coagulation studies are helpful in determination of the risk for bleeding. Electrolyte and arterial blood gas imbalances may increase cardiac irritability.

Patient Preparation

- Verify that the patient is the correct patient using two identifiers. ***Rationale:*** Before performing a procedure, the nurse should ensure the correct identification of the patient for the intended intervention.
- Ensure that the patient and family understand preprocedural teaching. Answer questions as they arise, and reinforce information as needed. ***Rationale:*** Understanding of previously taught information is evaluated and reinforced.
- Ensure that informed consent has been obtained. ***Rationale:*** Informed consent protects the rights of the patient and makes a competent decision possible for the patient.
- Perform a preprocedure verification and time out. ***Rationale:*** Ensures patient safety.
- Validate the patency of the alternate central or peripheral IV access catheter. ***Rationale:*** Access may be needed for administration of emergency medications or fluids.
- Assist the patient to the supine position. ***Rationale:*** This position prepares the patient for skin preparation, catheter insertion, and setup of the sterile field.
- Sedate the patient and/or give analgesics as prescribed and needed. ***Rationale:*** Movement of the patient may inhibit insertion of the PA catheter.

Procedure for Assisting With Pulmonary Artery Catheter Insertion and Pressure Monitoring

Steps	Rationale	Special Considerations
Assisting With PA Catheter Insertion		
1. 🅷🅷		
2. Prepare the flush solution for the pressure-transducer systems (see Procedure 75). A. Use an IV bag of normal saline. B. Follow institutional standards for adding heparin to the IV bag, if heparin is prescribed and not contraindicated. **(Level B*)**	Heparinized flush solutions are commonly used to minimize thrombi and fibrin deposits on catheters that might lead to thrombosis or bacterial colonization of the catheter.	Although heparin may prevent thrombosis,[24,29] it has been associated with thrombocytopenia and other hematologic complications.[5] Further research is needed regarding use of heparin versus normal saline to maintain PA catheter patency.
3. Prime or flush the pressure-transducer systems (see Procedure 75).	Removes air bubbles. Air bubbles introduced into the patient's circulation can cause air embolism. Air bubbles within the tubing dampen the waveform.	Air is more easily removed from the hemodynamic tubing when the system is not under pressure.
4. Apply and inflate the pressure bag or device to 300 mm Hg.	Each flush device delivers 1–3 mL/hr to maintain patency of the hemodynamic system.	
5. Connect the pressure cables (RA and PA) to the bedside monitor (see Fig. 75-2).	Connects the pressure-transducer systems to the bedside monitoring system.	

*Level B: Well-designed, controlled studies with results that consistently support a specific action, intervention, or treatment.

Procedure continues on following page

Procedure	for Assisting With Pulmonary Artery Catheter Insertion and Pressure Monitoring—*Continued*	
Steps	**Rationale**	**Special Considerations**
6. Set the scales on the bedside monitor for each anticipated pressure waveform.	Prepares the bedside monitor.	The scale for the RA/CVP pressure commonly is set at 20 mm Hg, and the PA scale commonly is set at 40 mm Hg. Scale settings may vary based on monitoring equipment. The scales can be adjusted if needed after the PA catheter is inserted based on patient pressures.
7. Level the RA (proximal) air-fluid interface (zeroing stopcock) and the PA (distal) air-fluid interface (zeroing stopcock) to the phlebostatic axis (see Figs. 75-7 and 75-9).	The phlebostatic axis approximates the level of the atria and is the reference point for patients in the supine position.	The reference point for the atria changes when a patient is in the lateral position (see Fig. 75-8).
8. Zero the system connected to the PA (distal) lumen and to the RA (proximal) lumen of the PA catheter by turning the stopcock of each system off to the patient, opening it to air, and zeroing the monitoring system (see Procedure 75).	Prepares each monitoring system so that pressures can be obtained during catheter insertion.	
9. **HH**		
10. **PE**		All healthcare personnel involved in the procedure need to apply head coverings, fluid-shield masks, and sterile gowns.
11. Assist the physician or advanced practice nurse as needed with opening the packaging of sterile drapes, and opening the PA catheter and introducer kits.	Aids in preparing for the procedure.	The patient will be fully draped with exposure of only the insertion site.
12. When the sheath introducer is in place, connect a normal saline IV solution to the infusion port.	Maintains the patency of the sheath introducer infusion port.	
13. Connect the pressure-transducer system to the PA distal and proximal ports of the PA catheter when the physician, advanced practice nurse, or other healthcare professional inserting the PA catheter hands them off to the critical care nurse.	Provides assistance in preparing the catheter.	
14. Flush the air from the catheter.	Removes air from the pulmonary artery catheter.	Flush additional infusion ports and attach sterile injectable or noninjectable caps.
15. If inserting a PA catheter with the ability to monitor mixed venous oxygenation, the fiberoptics are calibrated before removal from the package (see Procedure 16).	Calibrates the system before insertion.	Follow manufacturer guidelines for catheter calibration.
16. Observe as the physician or advanced practice nurse wiggles the PA catheter (sometimes called "whipping").	The movement of the catheter will be seen on the monitor. This ensures that there are no connection issues or catheter defects before insertion.	

Procedure	**for Assisting With Pulmonary Artery Catheter Insertion and Pressure Monitoring—*Continued***	
Steps	Rationale	Special Considerations
17. The physician or advanced practice nurse will insert the PA catheter through a sterile catheter sleeve (see Procedure 71).	Maintains sterility of the PA catheter to allow repositioning of the catheter.[8]	Additional research is needed to determine how long the sleeve remains sterile.
18. As insertion begins, continuously monitor and print the electrocardiogram (ECG) and PA distal pressure waveform strip.	Provides documentation of RA, RV, and PA pressures during insertion and dysrhythmia occurrence during insertion.	A dual-channel recorder is preferred so the ECG and the PA waveform can be simultaneously recorded.
19. After the tip of the PA catheter is in the right atrium, inflate the balloon with no more than 1.25–1.5 mL of air and close the gate valve or the stopcock (Fig. 72-6).	The inflated balloon helps to advance the PA catheter through the right side of the heart and into the PA, minimizing the chance of endocardial damage. Closing the gate valve or the stopcock holds air in the balloon during insertion.	The presence of the tip of the catheter in the right atrium is determined by observing the waveform (for RA/CVP waveform with *a, c, v* waves) from the catheter's distal lumen during insertion (see Fig. 72-3). Use the syringe from the PA insertion kit. It will not allow more than 1.5 mL of air to be used. Clearly communicate with the physician, advanced practice nurse, or other healthcare professional inserting the catheter: A. If the provider requests, "Inflate the balloon." B. The critical care nurse should respond, "Inflating the balloon" and "Balloon inflated and locked."
20. Observe for RA, RV, PA, and then PAO waveforms (see Fig. 72-3).	Placement in the PA is validated with waveform analysis.	Monitor the ECG tracing as the PA catheter is inserted because ventricular dysrhythmias may result from RV irritability. RV pressures are obtained only during insertion.
21. Verify that the PA catheter tip is in the proper position. A. When the balloon is deflated, the PA waveform is displayed on the monitor. B. When the balloon is inflated, the PAO waveform is displayed on the monitor.	When the balloon is inflated, the catheter floats from the PA to a smaller pulmonary arteriole.	The catheter usually reaches the PA after being advanced approximately 40–55 cm from the internal jugular vein, 35–50 cm from the subclavian vein, and 60 cm from the femoral vein. Placement may vary depending on patient size. A chest radiograph is obtained to verify catheter position.

Procedure continues on following page

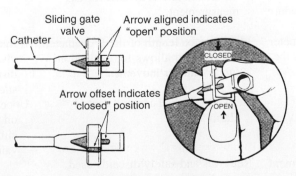

Figure 72-6 Pulmonary artery catheter gate valve. *Top left:* Gate valve in the open position. *Bottom left:* Gate valve in the closed position. *(From Baxter Edwards Corporation.)*

Procedure for Assisting With Pulmonary Artery Catheter Insertion and Pressure Monitoring—*Continued*

Steps	Rationale	Special Considerations
22. After the PA catheter is in place: A. Open the balloon inflation gate valve or stopcock. B. Remove the balloon syringe.	The gate valve or stopcock is closed during insertion to retain air in the balloon. The air is then passively released so that continuous monitoring of the PA waveform can be performed.	Air is expelled from the syringe, and the empty syringe is reconnected to the balloon inflation valve port. Clearly communicate with the physician, advanced practice nurse, or other healthcare professional inserting the catheter: A. If the physician, advanced practice nurse, or other healthcare professional requests, "Deflate the balloon." B. The critical care nurse should respond, "Deflating the balloon" and "Balloon deflated."
23. Reassess accurate leveling and secure the pressure transducer system (see Procedure 75).	Ensures that the air-filled interface (zeroing stopcock) is maintained at the level of the phlebostatic axis. If the air-fluid interface is above the phlebostatic axis, PA pressures are falsely low. If the air-fluid interface is below the phlebostatic axis, PA pressures are falsely high.	Leveling ensures accuracy. The point of the phlebostatic axis should be marked with an indelible marker, especially with use of a pole-mount setup.
24. Zero both the RA and PA pressure transducer systems (see Procedure 75).	Allows the monitor to use atmospheric pressure as a reference for zero.	
25. Observe the waveform and perform a dynamic response test (square wave test; see Fig. 59-3).	Determines whether the system is damped. This will ensure that the pressure waveform components are clearly defined and aids in accurate measurement.	The square wave test can be performed by activating and quickly releasing the fast flush. A sharp upstroke should terminate in a flat line at the maximal indicator on the monitor. This should be followed by an immediate rapid downstroke extending below baseline with 1–2 oscillations within 0.12 second and a quick return to baseline.
26. Assist if needed with applying an occlusive, sterile dressing to the insertion site (see Procedure 66).	Reduces the risk for infection.	Follow institutional standards for application of a chlorhexidine-impregnated sponge (see Procedure 66).
27. Connect the thermistor connector of the PA catheter to the CO monitor or module (see Procedure 64).	Allows the core temperature to be monitored and is needed for CO measurement.	
28. Document the external centimeter marking of the PA catheter at the introducer exit site.	Identifies the length of the PA catheter inserted and allows for evaluation of PA catheter movement.	If the centimeter marking is not visible at the exit site, measure the distance from the introducer exit site to the nearest visible marking.
29. Set the monitor alarms.	Activates the bedside and central alarm system.	Upper and lower alarm limits are set on the basis of the patient's current clinical status and hemodynamic values.
30. Remove **PE** and sterile equipment and discard used supplies in appropriate receptacles.	Removes and safely discards used supplies.	

Procedure	for Assisting With Pulmonary Artery Catheter Insertion and Pressure Monitoring—*Continued*	
Steps	**Rationale**	**Special Considerations**
31. 🅷🅷		
32. Ensure chest radiograph is completed.	Verifies PA catheter positioning.	

Obtaining PA Pressure Measurements
RA/CVP

1. Position the patient in the supine position with the head of the bed from 0 to 45 degrees. (**Level B***)	Studies have determined that the RA and PA pressures are accurate in this position.[3,6,7,10,18,20,22,34,35]	RA and PA pressures may be accurate for patients in the supine position with the head of the bed elevated up to 60 degrees,[7,22] but additional studies are needed to support this. Only one study[19] supports the accuracy of hemodynamic values for patients in the lateral positions; other studies do not.[3,13,18,26,34] The majority of studies support the accuracy of hemodynamic monitoring for patients in the prone position.[1,2,12,17,21,27,32] Two studies demonstrated that prone positioning caused an increase in hemodynamic values.[28,31]
2. Run a dual-channel strip of the ECG and RA waveform (Fig. 72-7).	RA pressures should be measured from the graphic strip because the effect of ventilation can be identified.	The digital monitor data can be used to measure RA pressure if ventilation does not cause respiratory variation of the RA pressure waveform. Some monitors have the capability of "freeze framing" waveforms. A cursor can be used to measure pressure measurements.
3. Measure RA pressure at end expiration.	The effects of intrathoracic pressure on the RAP is minimized at the end-expiration phase of the respiratory cycle.	

*Level B: Well-designed, controlled studies with results that consistently support a specific action, intervention, or treatment.

Procedure continues on following page

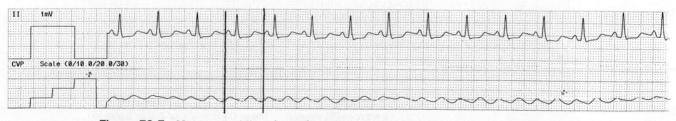

Figure 72-7 Note *vertical lines* drawn from the beginning of the P wave of two of the electrocardiogram complexes down to the right atrial (RA) waveform. The first positive deflection of the RA waveform is the *a* wave; the second positive deflection is the *v* wave. The *c* wave, which would lie between the *a* wave and the *v* wave, is not evident in this strip. CVP, central venous pressure.

Procedure	**for Assisting With Pulmonary Artery Catheter Insertion and Pressure Monitoring—*Continued***	
Steps	**Rationale**	**Special Considerations**
4. With the dual-channel recorded strip, draw a vertical line from the beginning of the P wave of one of the ECG complexes down to the RA waveform. Repeat this with the next ECG complex (see Fig. 72-7).	Compares electrical activity with mechanical activity. Usually three waves are present on the RA waveform.	At times, the *c* wave is not present.
5. Align the PR interval with the RA waveform.	The *a* wave correlates with this interval.	
6. Identify the *a* wave.	The *a* wave is seen approximately 80–100 ms after the P wave. The *c* wave follows the *a* wave, and the *v* wave follows the *c* wave.	The *a* wave reflects atrial contraction. The *c* wave reflects closure of the tricuspid valve. The *v* wave reflects passive filling of the atria.
7. Identify the scale setting of the RA waveform on the monitor (Fig. 72-8).	Optimizes the view of the waveform and aids in measurement of the pressure.	The RAP scale commonly is set at 20 mm Hg and may be adjusted to the patient's RAP to optimize the view of the waveform. Scale settings may vary based on monitoring equipment.
8. Measure the mean of the *a* wave to obtain the RAP (see Fig. 72-8).	The *a* wave represents atrial contraction and reflects right ventricular filling at end diastole.	

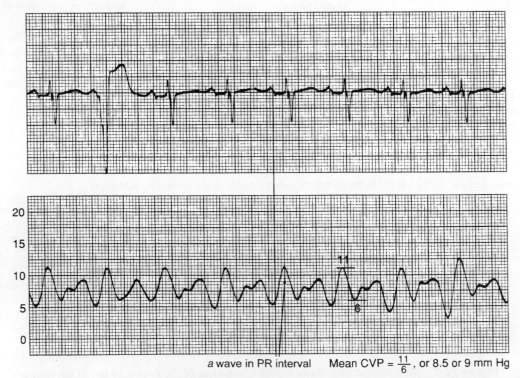

a wave in PR interval   Mean CVP = $\frac{11}{6}$, or 8.5 or 9 mm Hg

Figure 72-8 Obtaining measurements of right-atrial and central venous pressures (RA/CVP). Aligning the *a* wave on the RA/CVP waveform with the PR interval on the electrocardiogram facilitates accurate measurement of RA/CVP at end diastole. *(From Ahrens TS, Taylor LK:* Hemodynamic waveform analysis, *Philadelphia, 1992, Saunders.)*

Procedure	for Assisting With Pulmonary Artery Catheter Insertion and Pressure Monitoring—*Continued*	
Steps	**Rationale**	**Special Considerations**

PA Systolic and Diastolic Pressures

1. Position the patient in the supine position with the head of the bed from 0 to 45 degrees. **(Level B*)**	Studies have determined that the RA and PA pressures are accurate in this position.[3,6,7,10,18,20,22,34,35]	RA and PA pressures may be accurate for patients in the supine position with the head of the bed elevated up to 60 degrees,[7,22] but additional studies are needed to support this. Only one study[19] supports the accuracy of hemodynamic values for patients in the lateral positions; other studies[3,13,18,26,33] do not. The majority of the studies[1,2,12,17,21,27,32] support the accuracy of hemodynamic monitoring for patients in the prone position, yet two studies showed that prone positioning caused an increase in hemodynamic values.[28,31]
2. Print a dual-channel strip of the ECG and PA waveform (Fig. 72-9).	PA pressures are measured from the graphic strip when respiratory variation of the waveform is noted because the effect of ventilation can be identified.	Some monitors have the capability of "freeze framing" waveforms. A cursor can be used to measure pressures.

*Level B: Well-designed, controlled studies with results that consistently support a specific action, intervention, or treatment.

Procedure continues on following page

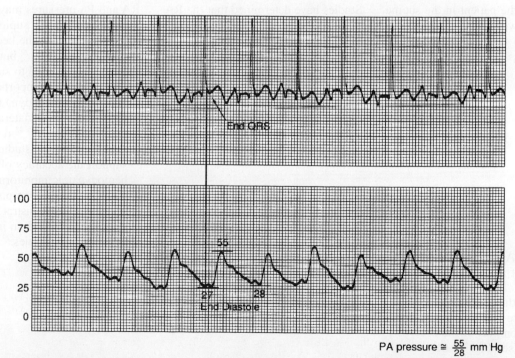

$$PA\ pressure \cong \frac{55}{28}\ mm\ Hg$$

Figure 72-9 Obtaining measurements of pressure in the pulmonary artery (PA). For systolic pressure, align the peak of the systolic waveform with the QT interval on the electrocardiogram. For PA diastolic pressure, use the end of the QRS as a marker to detect the PA diastolic phase. Obtain the reading just before the upstroke of the systolic waveform. (*From Ahrens TS, Taylor LK: Hemodynamic waveform analysis, Philadelphia, 1992, Saunders.*)

Procedure	for Assisting With Pulmonary Artery Catheter Insertion and Pressure Monitoring—*Continued*	
Steps	**Rationale**	**Special Considerations**
3. Measure the PA pressure at end expiration.	The effects of intrathoracic pressure on the PAP is minimized at the end-expiration phase of the respiratory cycle.	
4. Identify the QT interval on the ECG strip.	Represents ventricular depolarization.	
5. Align the QT interval with the PA waveform.	Allows comparison of cardiac electrical activity with mechanical activity.	
6. Identify the scale setting of the PA waveform on the monitor.	Optimizes the view of the waveform and aids in measurement of the pressure.	The PAP scale commonly is set at 40 mm Hg and may be adjusted to the patient's PAP to optimize the view of the waveform. Scale settings may vary based on monitoring equipment.
7. Measure the PA systolic pressure at the peak of the systolic waveform on the PA waveform (see Fig. 72-9).	Reflects the highest PA systolic pressure.	
8. Align the end of the QRS complex with the PA waveform (see Fig. 72-9).	Compares electrical activity with mechanical activity. The end of the QRS complex correlates with ventricular end-diastolic pressure.	
9. Measure the PA diastolic pressure at the point of the intersection of this line (see Fig. 72-9).	This point occurs just before the upstroke of the systolic pressure.	
PAOP		
1. Position the patient in the supine position with the head of the bed from 0 to 45 degrees. **(Level B*)**	Studies have determined that the RA and PA pressures are accurate in this position.[3,6,7,10,18,20,22,34,35]	RA and PA pressures may be accurate for patients in the supine position with the head of the bed elevated up to 60 degrees,[7,22] but additional studies are needed to support this. Only one study[19] supports the accuracy of hemodynamic values for patients in the lateral positions; other studies[3,13,18,26,33] do not. The majority of the studies[1,2,12,17,21,27,32] support the accuracy of hemodynamic monitoring for patients in the prone position, but two studies demonstrated that prone positioning caused an increase in hemodynamic values.[28,31]
2. Fill the PA balloon syringe with 1.5 mL of air.	More than 1.5 mL of air may rupture the PA balloon and the pulmonary arteriole.	
3. Connect the PA balloon syringe to the gate valve or stopcock of the balloon port of the PA catheter (see Fig. 72-6).	This port is designed for balloon air inflation.	

*Level B: Well-designed, controlled studies with results that consistently support a specific action, intervention, or treatment.

Procedure	for Assisting With Pulmonary Artery Catheter Insertion and Pressure Monitoring—*Continued*	
Steps	**Rationale**	**Special Considerations**
4. Print a dual-channel strip of the ECG and PA waveform.	The PAO pressures are measured from the graphic strip because the effect of ventilation can be identified.	Some monitors have the capability of "freeze framing" waveforms. A cursor can be used to measure pressures.
5. Slowly inflate the balloon with air until the PA waveform changes to a PAO waveform (Fig. 72-10).	A slight resistance is usually felt during inflation of the balloon. Only enough air needed to convert the PA waveform to a PAO waveform should be instilled. Thus the entire amount of 1.5 mL of air is not necessarily needed.	Avoid overinflation of the balloon because it can cause pulmonary arteriole infarction or rupture, resulting in potentially life-threatening hemorrhage.[14]
6. Inflate the balloon for no more than 8–15 seconds (2–4 respiratory cycles).	Prolonged inflation of the balloon can cause pulmonary arteriole infarction and/or rupture, with potentially life-threatening hemorrhage.[14]	
7. Disconnect the syringe from the balloon-inflation port to passively deflate the balloon. **(Level M*)**	Allows air to passively escape from the balloon.	Active withdrawal of air from the balloon can weaken the balloon, pull the balloon structure into the inflation lumen, and possibly cause balloon rupture.
8. Observe the monitor to verify the PAO waveform changes back to the PA waveform.	Ensures adequate balloon deflation and safe positioning of the PA catheter for continuous monitoring.	
9. Expel air from the balloon syringe.	The syringe should remain empty when reconnected so that accidental balloon inflation does not occur.	

*Level M: Manufacturer's recommendations only.

Procedure continues on following page

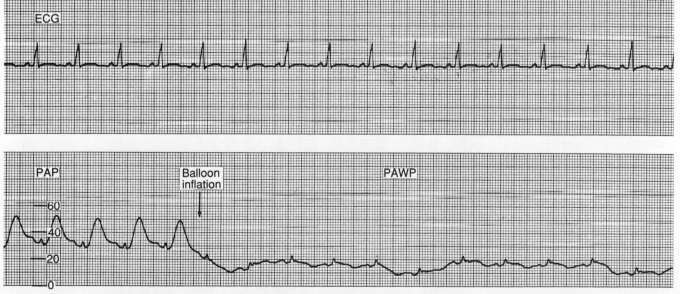

Figure 72-10   Change in pulmonary artery pressure (PAP) waveform to pulmonary artery occlusion pressure waveform with balloon inflation. The balloon is inflated while the bedside monitor is observed for change in the waveform. Balloon inflation *(arrow)* in patient with normal pulmonary artery occlusion pressure. Pulmonary artery occlusion pressure (PAOP) is also referred to as pulmonary artery wedge pressure (PAWP).

Procedure	**for Assisting With Pulmonary Artery Catheter Insertion and Pressure Monitoring—*Continued***	
Steps	**Rationale**	**Special Considerations**
10. Reconnect the empty balloon syringe to the balloon-inflation port.	The syringe that is manufactured for the PA catheter should be connected to the PA balloon port to avoid loss of the custom designed syringe. This syringe can be filled with only 1.5 mL of air, thus serving as a safety feature to minimize the chance of balloon overinflation.	
11. Follow institutional standard regarding keeping the gate valve or the stopcock open.	The most important considerations are that the balloon syringe is attached to the balloon-inflation port, the syringe is empty, and the PA distal waveform reflects a pulmonary artery waveform.	
12. With the dual-channel recorded strip, draw a vertical line from the beginning of the P wave of one of the ECG complexes down to the PAO waveform. Repeat this with the next ECG complex.	Compares cardiac electrical activity with mechanical activity. Two waves (*a* and *v*) to three waves (*a, c,* and *v* waves) will be present on the PAO waveform.	The *c* waves commonly are not present on PAO waveforms because of the distance the pressure needs to travel back to the transducer.
13. Align the end of a QRS complex of the ECG strip with the PAO waveform (Fig. 72-11).	Aligns relationship of cardiac electrical activity with mechanical activity	

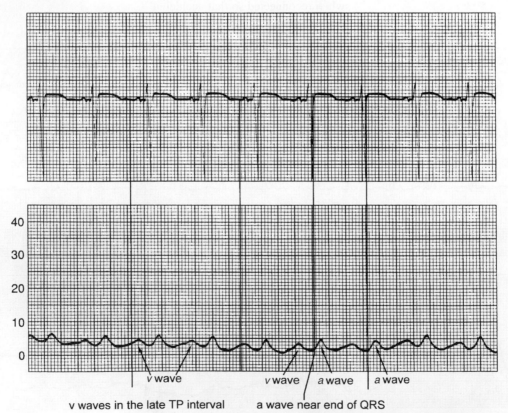

v waves in the late TP interval   a wave near end of QRS

Figure 72-11   Obtaining measurement of the pulmonary artery occlusion pressure (PAOP). For accurate readings, align the *a* wave from the PAO waveform with the end of the QRS on the electrocardiogram at end diastole. Pulmonary artery occlusion pressure (PAOP) is also referred to as pulmonary artery wedge pressure (PAWP). *(From Ahrens TS, Taylor LK:* Hemodynamic waveform analysis, *Philadelphia, 1992, Saunders.)*

Procedure	for Assisting With Pulmonary Artery Catheter Insertion and Pressure Monitoring—*Continued*	
Steps	**Rationale**	**Special Considerations**
14. Identify the *a* wave (see Fig. 72-11).	The *a* wave correlates with the end of the QRS complex. The *c* wave follows the *a* wave, and the *v* wave follows the *c* wave.	If only two waves are present, the first wave is the *a* wave and the second wave is the *v* wave.
15. Identify the scale of the PAO tracing.	Aids in determination of pressure measurement.	The PA scale commonly is set at 40 mm Hg.
16. Measure the mean of the *a* wave to obtain the PAOP (see Fig. 72-5).	The *a* wave represents atrial contraction and reflects LV filling at end diastole.	If PEEP is being used and the PEEP is more than 10 cm H_2O, adjustments in determination of the pressures may be necessary. Follow institutional standards.
17. Compare the PADP with the PAOP.	The PAOP is commonly 1–4 mm Hg less than the PADP. PADPs that correlate with PAOPs represent LV filling pressures.	Significant differences between PADP and PAOP may exist for patients with pulmonary hypertension, chronic obstructive lung disease, acute respiratory distress syndrome, pulmonary embolus, and tachycardia.
18. Follow PADP if a close correlation is found between PADP and PAOP.	Considered an accurate measurement of LV filling pressures.	Minimizes the number of times the PA balloon is inflated.
19. Follow the PAOP if >4 mm Hg of difference is found between PAOP and PADP.	Ensures the accuracy of measurements.	

Measurement of Hemodynamic Pressures at End Expiration

1. Measure all hemodynamic pressures at end expiration to ensure accuracy.	Atmospheric and alveolar pressures are approximately equal at end expiration. Intrathoracic pressure is closest to zero at end expiration. Measurement of hemodynamic pressures is most accurate at end expiration because pulmonary pressures have minimal effect on intracardiac pressures.	
2. Determine end expiration by observing the rise and fall of the chest during breathing and use of printed graphics of hemodynamic, respiratory, capnography, or continuous airway pressure waveforms.	Aids in the determination of the end expiratory phase of ventilation.	

Determining End Expiration for the Patient Breathing Spontaneously

1. Record a strip of the PA waveform.	A labeled recording aids in determination of accurate hemodynamic pressure values.	In patients who are breathing spontaneously, the normal inspiratory:expiratory ratio is approximately 1:2.
2. Note that the pressure waveform dips down during the inspiratory phase of spontaneous breathing (Fig. 72-12).	Intrapleural pressure decreases during spontaneous inspiration, and this decrease is reflected by a fall in cardiac pressures.	
3. Note that the pressure waveform elevates during the expiratory phase of breathing (see Fig. 72-12).	At end-expiration atmospheric and intrathoracic pressures (pleural and alveolar) are equalized; thus cardiac pressures are most accurately reflected.	

Procedure continues on following page

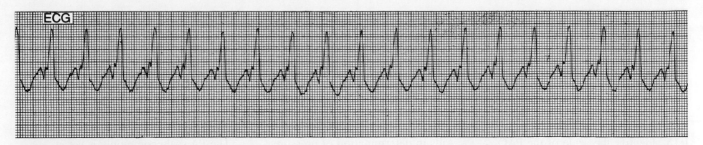

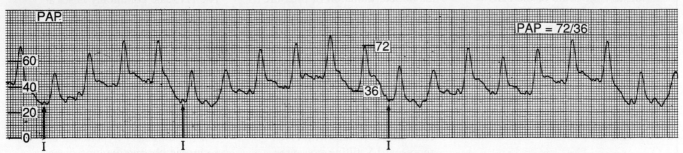

Figure 72-12   Respiratory fluctuations of pulmonary artery pressure (PAP) waveform in a spontaneously breathing patient. The location of inspiration *(I)* is marked on the waveform. The points just before inspiration are end expiration, where readings are taken.

Procedure	**for Assisting With Pulmonary Artery Catheter Insertion and Pressure Monitoring—*Continued***	
Steps	**Rationale**	**Special Considerations**
4. Measure the pressure at the end of the expiratory phase (see Fig. 72-12).	Ensures accurate and consistent pressure measurements.	
Determining End Expiration for the Patient Receiving Positive Pressure Mechanical Ventilation		
1. Record a strip of the PA waveform.	A labeled recording aids in determination of accurate hemodynamic pressure values.	
2. Note that the pressure waveform elevates as a breath is delivered by the ventilator (Fig. 72-13).	As the ventilator delivers a positive pressure breath to the lungs, an increase in intrathoracic pressure results. This increase in intrathoracic pressure causes an increase in cardiac pressures.	
3. Note that the pressure waveform dips down as the breath is exhaled (see Fig. 72-13).	As the mechanical breath is exhaled, intrathoracic pressures decrease and cardiac pressures are most accurately and consistently measured.	
Determining End Expiration for the Patient Receiving Intermittent Mandatory Mechanical Ventilation		
1. Record a strip of the PA waveform.	A labeled recording aids in determination of accurate hemodynamic pressure monitoring.	
2. If the patient is receiving intermittent mandatory ventilation, measure the pressure during the end expiration.	Aids in accuracy of pressure measurements.	
3. Note that the pressure waveform elevates as a breath is delivered by the ventilator (Fig. 72-14).	As the ventilator delivers a breath to the lungs, an increase in intrathoracic pressure results. This increase in pressure causes an increase in cardiac pressures.	

Procedure continues on following page

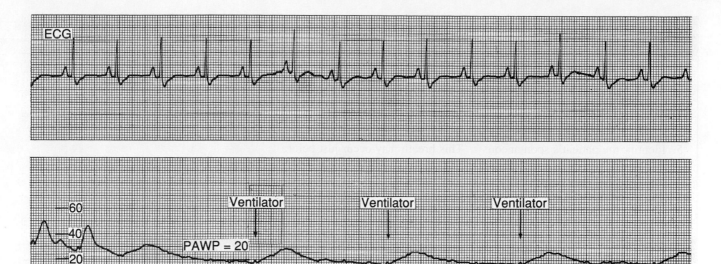

Figure 72-13 Patient on mechanical ventilation (on pressure support–type ventilator) who had no spontaneous respiration because of neuromuscular-blocking agent (vecuronium). The point of end expiration is located just before the ventilator artifact. Pulmonary artery occlusion pressure (PAOP) is also referred to as pulmonary artery wedge pressure (PAWP).

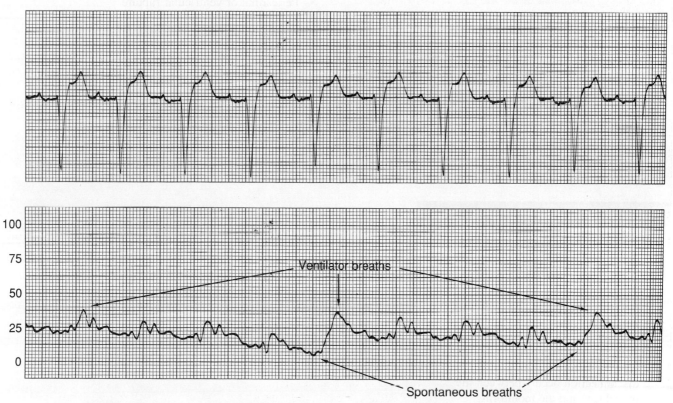

Figure 72-14 Intermittent mandatory ventilation mode of ventilation and the effect on the pulmonary artery waveform. *(From Ahrens TS, Taylor LK:* Hemodynamic waveform analysis, *Philadelphia, 1992, Saunders.)*

Procedure for Assisting With Pulmonary Artery Catheter Insertion and Pressure Monitoring—*Continued*

Steps	Rationale	Special Considerations
4. Note that the pressure waveform dips down as the breath is exhaled (see Fig. 72-14).	As the mechanical breath is exhaled, intrathoracic pressure decreases and cardiac pressures are more accurately reflected.	
5. Identify the patient's spontaneous breath (see Fig. 72-14).	This breath may occur just before triggered ventilator breaths.	
6. Determine end expiration.	Ensures accuracy of measurements.	Airway pressure waveforms can be used to facilitate identification of end expiration.

Expected Outcomes

- Accurate placement of the PA catheter
- Adequate and appropriate waveforms
- Ability to obtain accurate cardiac pressure measurements and associated hemodynamic data
- Evaluation of information obtained to guide diagnostic and therapeutic interventions

Unexpected Outcomes

- Pneumothorax or hemothorax
- Infection/sepsis
- Ventricular dysrhythmias
- Heart block
- Misplacement
- Hemorrhage
- Hematoma
- Pericardial or ventricular rupture
- Venous air embolism
- Cardiac tamponade
- PA infarction
- PA rupture
- PA catheter balloon rupture
- PA catheter knotting
- Pseudoaneurysm formation
- Heparin-induced thrombocytopenia
- Thrombosis
- Valvular damage
- Pain

Patient Monitoring and Care

Steps	Rationale	Reportable Conditions
		These conditions should be reported if they persist despite nursing interventions.
1. Recheck transducer leveling whenever patient position changes.	Ensures accurate reference point for the left atrium.	
2. Zero the transducer during initial setup or before insertion if disconnection occurs between the transducer and the monitoring cable, if disconnection occurs between the monitoring cable and the monitor, and when the values obtained do not fit the clinical picture.	Ensures accuracy of the hemodynamic monitoring system.	

Patient Monitoring and Care —*Continued*

Steps	Rationale	Reportable Conditions
3. Place sterile injectable or noninjectable caps on all stopcocks. Replace with new sterile caps whenever the caps are removed.	Stopcocks can be a source of contamination. Stopcocks that are part of the initial setup are packaged with vented caps. Vented caps need to be replaced with sterile injectable or noninjectable caps to maintain a closed system and reduce the risk of contamination and infection.	
4. Monitor the pressure-transducer system (pressure tubing, transducer, stopcocks, etc.) for air and eliminate air from the system.	Air in the transducer system affects the accuracy of pressure measurements. Air emboli are also potentially fatal.	• Suspected air emboli
5. Continuously monitor hemodynamic waveforms and obtain hemodynamic values (pulmonary artery systolic pressure, PADP, RAP) hourly and as necessary with condition changes and to evaluate therapy interventions. Follow institutional standards for obtaining hemodynamic values.	Provides for continuous waveform analysis and assessment of patient status.	• Abnormal hemodynamic waveforms or pressures
6. Obtain CO, cardiac index, and systemic vascular resistance and additional parameters after catheter insertion and as necessary per patient condition and interventions.	Monitors patient status and response to therapeutic interventions.	• Abnormal hemodynamic parameters or significant changes in hemodynamic parameters
7. Change the hemodynamic monitoring system (flush solution, pressure tubing, transducers, and stopcocks) every 96 hours. **(Level B*)** The flush solution may need to be changed more frequently if near empty of solution.	The Centers for Disease Control and Prevention (CDC),[23] the Infusion Nurses Society,[16] and research findings[23,25] recommend that the hemodynamic flush system can be used safely for 96 hours. This recommendation is based on research conducted with disposable pressure-monitoring systems used for peripheral and central lines.	
8. Perform a dynamic response test (square wave test) at the start of each shift, with a change of the waveform, or after the system is opened to air (see Fig. 59-3).	An optimally damped system provides an accurate waveform.	• Overdamped or underdamped waveforms that cannot be corrected with troubleshooting procedures
9. Label the tubing with the date and time the system was prepared.	Identifies when the system needs to be changed.	
10. Maintain the pressure bag or device at 300 mmHg.	At 300 mmHg, each flush device delivers approximately 1–3 mL/hr to maintain patency of the system.	

*Level B: Well-designed, controlled studies with results that consistently support a specific action, intervention, or treatment.

Procedure continues on following page

Patient Monitoring and Care —*Continued*

Steps	Rationale	Reportable Conditions
11. Do not fast flush the distal lumen of the PA catheter for longer than 2 seconds.[9]	PA rupture may occur with prolonged flushing of high-pressure fluid.	• Hemoptysis
12. Never flush the distal lumen of the PA catheter when the balloon is wedged in the pulmonary artery.	Excessive PA pressure may cause PA damage or rupture.	• Hemoptysis
13. Use aseptic technique when withdrawing from or flushing the PA catheter.	Prevents contamination of the system and related infection.	
14. Clear the system, including stopcocks, of all traces of blood after blood withdrawal.	Blood can become a medium for bacterial growth.[24] Clots also may be flushed into the catheter if all blood is not eliminated.	
15. Maintain sterility and integrity of the plastic sleeve covering the PA catheter.	Any tear in the sleeve breaks the sterile barrier, making catheter repositioning no longer possible.	• Defects in the integrity of the plastic sleeve
16. Blood products and albumin should never be infused through the PA catheter.	Viscous blood may occlude the catheter. The accuracy of the PA monitoring system may be adversely affected.	
17. IV fluids are never infused via the distal lumen of the PA catheter and are sometimes infused via the proximal lumen of the PA catheter when IV access is necessary.	PA monitoring is not possible, and a life-threatening situation can occur (e.g., undetected wedged PA catheter).	
18. Replace gauze dressings every 2 days and transparent dressings at least every 5–7 days and more frequently as needed.[15,16,24,30] **(Level D*)**	Decreases the risk for infection at the catheter site. The Centers for Disease Control and Prevention (CDC) and the Infusion Nurses Society recommend replacing the dressing when it becomes damp, loosened, or soiled or when inspection of the site is necessary.[15,16,24]	• Signs or symptoms of infection
19. Perform central venous catheter site care (see Procedure 66).	Ensures consistency of dressing change and indicates when the next change will occur.	
20. Print PA waveform strips to place on the patient's chart at the start of each shift and whenever a change in the waveform occurs.	The printed waveform allows assessment of the adequacy of the waveform, the presence of damping, and if respiratory variation is present.	

*Level D: Peer-reviewed professional and organizational standards with the support of clinical study recommendations.

Patient Monitoring and Care —*Continued*

Steps	Rationale	Reportable Conditions
21. Assess the need for the PA catheter daily. If long-term use of the PA catheter is needed, consider changing the PA catheter every 7 days. **(Level B*)**	The Centers for Disease Control and Prevention (CDC)[24] and research findings[4,11] recommend that PA catheters do not need to be changed more frequently than every 7 days. There are no specific recommendations regarding routine replacement of PA catheters that need to be in place for >7 days.[11,24] Guidewire exchanges should not be used routinely. A guidewire exchange should only be used to replace a catheter that is malfunctioning.[24]	• Signs and symptoms of infection at the PA catheter insertion site • Signs and symptoms of sepsis
22. Follow institutional standards for assessing pain. Administer analgesia as prescribed.	Identifies need for pain interventions.	• Continued pain despite pain interventions

*Level B: Well-designed, controlled studies with results that consistently support a specific action, intervention, or treatment.

Documentation

Documentation should include the following:
- Patient and family education
- Completion of informed consent
- Universal protocol requirements
- Insertion of the PA catheter
- External centimeter marking of PA catheter noted at exit site
- Patient tolerance of procedure
- Confirmation of PA catheter placement (e.g., waveforms, chest radiograph)
- Date and time of PA catheter site care and dressing change

- Pain assessment, interventions, and effectiveness
- Cardiac rhythm during PA catheter insertion and monitoring
- Site assessment
- PA pressures (RA/CVP, RV, PA systolic, diastolic, mean, and PAOP)
- Waveforms (RA/CVP, RV, pulmonary artery pressure, PAOP)
- CO/CI and systemic vascular resistance
- Occurrence of unexpected outcomes and interventions

References and Additional Readings

For a complete list of references and additional readings for this procedure, scan this QR code with any freely available smartphone code reader app, or visit http://booksite.elsevier.com/9780323376624.

73 Pulmonary Artery Catheter Removal

Nikki Taylor

PURPOSE: The pulmonary artery catheter is removed when hemodynamic monitoring is no longer clinically indicated, when complications occur (e.g., dysrhythmias, pseudoaneurysms), or when there is risk for infection associated with the prolonged use of intravascular catheters.

PREREQUISITE NURSING KNOWLEDGE

- Knowledge of the normal cardiovascular anatomy and physiology is necessary.
- Knowledge of normal values for intracardiac pressures is important.
- Knowledge of normal coagulation values is needed.
- Knowledge of normal waveform configurations for right-atrial pressure, right-ventricular pressure, pulmonary artery pressure, and pulmonary arterial occlusive pressure is necessary.
- Venous access routes should be known.
- Principles of aseptic technique should be known.
- Advanced cardiac life support knowledge and skills are needed.
- Potential complications associated with removal of the pulmonary artery (PA) catheter should be understood.
- Clinical and technical competence in PA catheter removal is necessary.
- Knowledge of the state nurse practice act is important to ensure that removal of a PA catheter is not prohibited.
- Air embolism can occur during the removal of the catheter. Air embolism after the removal of the catheter is the result of air drawn in along the subcutaneous tract and into the vein. During inspiration, negative intrathoracic pressure is transmitted to the central veins. Any opening external to the body to one of these veins may result in aspiration of air into the central venous system. The pathological effects depend on the volume and rate of air aspirated.
- Indications for the removal of the PA catheter include the following:
  - The patient's condition no longer necessitates hemodynamic monitoring.
  - Complications occur because of the presence of the PA catheter.
  - The patient shows evidence of a catheter-related infection that may be associated with the PA catheter.
- Contraindications to percutaneous removal of the PA catheter include the following:
  - The PA catheter is knotted (observed on chest radiograph).
  - A permanent pacemaker, temporary transvenous pacemaker, or implantable cardioverter defibrillator (ICD) is present (catheter should be removed by an advanced practice nurse or a physician).

EQUIPMENT

- 1.5-mL syringe
- Sterile and nonsterile gloves
- Gown
- Fluid-shield face mask or goggles
- 4 × 4 sterile gauze pads
- Central line dressing kit
- Two moisture-proof absorbent pads
- One roll of 2-inch tape

Additional equipment, to have available as needed, includes the following:

- Obturator/cap for introducer catheter port with hemostasis valve
- Additional dressing supplies (e.g., transparent dressing)
- Petroleum-based ointment
- Suture removal kit
- Scissors
- Sterile specimen container
- Emergency equipment

PATIENT AND FAMILY EDUCATION

- Explain the procedure and the reason for removal of the catheter. *Rationale:* This explanation provides information and decreases anxiety.
- Explain the importance of patient participation during the removal of the catheter. *Rationale:* The explanation ensures patient cooperation and facilitates safe removal of the catheter.
- Instruct the patient and family to report any shortness of breath, bleeding, or discomfort at the insertion site after removal of the catheter. *Rationale:* Identifies patient discomfort and early recognition of complications.

PATIENT ASSESSMENT AND PREPARATION

Patient Assessment

- Assess the electrocardiogram (ECG), vital signs, and neurovascular status of the extremity distal to the catheter insertion site. *Rationale:* This assessment serves as baseline data.
- If the introducer will also be removed, assess the current coagulation values of the patient. *Rationale:* If the patient has abnormal coagulation study results, hemostasis may be difficult to obtain after the introducer catheter is removed.
- Verify catheter position with waveform analysis or chest radiograph. *Rationale:* Accuracy of catheter position is ensured.
- Determine whether the patient has a permanent pacemaker, temporary transvenous pacemaker, or ICD. *Rationale:* PA catheter removal by a critical care nurse is contraindicated in the presence of a permanent pacemaker, temporary transvenous pacemaker, or ICD. Entanglement of the PA catheter and the pacemaker electrodes can occur.
- Assess the integrity of the PA catheter. *Rationale:* The PA catheter should be removed by an advanced practice nurse or physician if the integrity of the PA catheter or introducer is compromised (e.g., visible cracks are noted).
- Assess the catheter insertion site for redness, warmth, tenderness, or presence of drainage. *Rationale:* Signs and symptoms of infection are assessed.

Patient Preparation

- In collaboration with the physician and/or advance practice nurse, determine when the PA catheter should be removed. *Rationale:* The invasive catheter is removed when it is no longer indicated.
- Verify that the patient is the correct patient using two identifiers. *Rationale:* Before performing a procedure, the nurse or the provider removing the PA catheter should ensure the correct identification of the patient for the intended intervention.
- Ensure that the patient and family understand preprocedural teaching. Answer questions as they arise, and reinforce information as needed. *Rationale:* Understanding of previously taught information is evaluated and reinforced.
- Place the patient in a supine position with the head of the bed in a slight Trendelenburg's position (or flat if Trendelenburg's position is contraindicated or not tolerated by the patient). *Rationale:* The patient should be positioned so that the catheter exit site is at or below the level of the heart.[5,6] A normal pressure gradient exists between atmospheric air and the central venous compartment that promotes air entry if the compartment is open. The lower the site of entry below the heart, the lower the pressure gradient, thus minimizing the risk of air being drawn in and thus a venous air embolism.

Procedure for Pulmonary Artery Catheter Removal

Steps	Rationale	Special Considerations
1. **HH**		
2. **PE**		All physicians, advanced practice nurses, and other healthcare professionals in the room should wear personal protective equipment including a face mask.
3. Transfer or discontinue intravenous (IV) solution and flush solutions.	Prepares the catheter for removal.	Make sure the patient has the proper alternative IV access to transfer solutions/medications that were administered through the PA catheter before removal.
4. Place a moisture-proof absorbent pad under the patient's upper torso and another under the PA catheter.	Collects blood and body fluids associated with removal; serves as a receptacle for the contaminated catheter.	
5. Place the patient supine in a slight Trendelenburg's position.[3,7–9,14] **(Level E*)**	Minimizes the risk for venous air embolus. The patient should be positioned so that the catheter exit site is at or below the level of the heart.[5,6]	Place the patient flat if Trendelenburg's position is contraindicated, not tolerated by the patient, or a femoral PA catheter will be removed. If the PA catheter is in the femoral vein, extend the patient's leg and ensure the groin area is adequately exposed.

---

*Level E: Multiple case reports, theory-based evidence from expert opinions, or peer-reviewed professional organizational standards without clinical studies to support recommendations.

Procedure continues on following page

Procedure   for Pulmonary Artery Catheter Removal—*Continued*

Steps	Rationale	Special Considerations
6. Have the patient turn his or her head away from the PA catheter and insertion site.	Decreases the risk for contamination.	This step is not needed if a femoral PA catheter.
7. Open supplies.	Prepares for removal.	
8. Remove the syringe from the balloon inflation port, ensure that the gate valve or stopcock is in the open position, and observe the PA waveform (see Fig. 72-6).	Allows air to passively escape from the balloon and ensures adequate balloon deflation.	Myocardial or valvular tissues can be damaged if the PA catheter is removed with the balloon inflated.
9. Turn off all stopcocks to the patient.	Prepares for removal.	
10. Remove the old dressing.	Prepares for removal.	Signs of local or systemic infection may determine the need to send a culture of the catheter tip.
11. Unlock the sheath from the introducer catheter.	Prepares for removal.	
12. Discard nonsterile gloves in appropriate receptacle, perform hand hygiene, and apply sterile gloves.	Removes and safely discards used supplies. Reduces the transmission of microorganisms; Standard Precautions.	
13. If present, clip the sutures securing the PA catheter.	Frees the PA catheter for removal.	
14. Ask the patient to take a deep breath in and hold it.[11–15] (**Level E***)	Minimizes the risk for venous air embolus.	If the patient is receiving positive pressure ventilation, withdraw the catheter during the inspiratory phase of the respiratory cycle or while a breath is delivered via a bag-valve device.
15. While stabilizing the introducer catheter, gently withdraw the PA catheter with a constant, steady motion (Fig. 73-1).	Ensures the removal of an intact catheter.	Observe the ECG tracing rhythm and the waveforms from the distal lumen during removal. Dysrhythmias may occur during removal but are usually self-limiting.[1,11,13] If resistance is met, do not continue to remove the catheter; notify the advanced practice nurse or physician immediately. Resistance may be caused by catheter knotting, kinking, or wedging.

*Level E: Multiple case reports, theory-based evidence from expert opinions, or peer-reviewed professional organizational standards without clinical studies to support recommendations

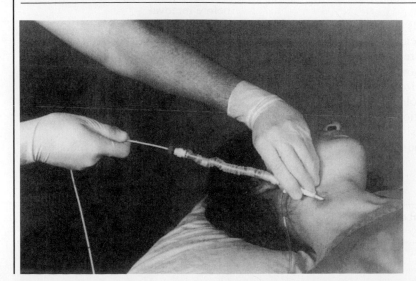

Figure 73-1   While stabilizing the introducer, gently withdraw the pulmonary artery catheter using a constant, steady motion. *(From Wadas TM: Pulmonary artery catheter removal, Crit Care Nurse 14:63, 1994.)*

Procedure	for Pulmonary Artery Catheter Removal—*Continued*	
Steps	**Rationale**	**Special Considerations**
16. Temporarily cover the hemostasis valve with a sterile-gloved finger until the sterile obturator/cap is attached.	The hemostasis valve must be occluded to minimize the risk for air embolus and blood loss.	The introducer may remain in place to provide central venous access.
17. Instruct the patient to exhale as soon as the PA catheter is removed.	Once the catheter is removed the patient can breathe normally.	
18. Place the PA catheter on the moisture-proof absorbent pad and inspect it to ensure that the entire catheter was removed.	Allows for assessment of the catheter.	If the catheter tip will be cultured, have another provider assist with cutting the tip with sterile scissors and placing it in a sterile specimen container before placing the PA catheter on the moisture-proof absorbent pad.
19. If the introducer remains in place, perform site care and apply a sterile dressing to the site per institutional standards.	Decreases the risk for infection at the insertion site.	
20. If the introducer is to be removed, clip the sutures or remove the securing device.	Frees the introducer for removal.	
21. Ensure that the patient is still supine in a slight Trendelenburg's position.[3,7-9,14] **(Level E*)**	Minimizes the risk for venous air embolus. The patient should be positioned so that the catheter exit site is at or below the level of the heart.[5,6]	Cases have been reported of venous air embolus occurring after removal of central venous catheters when patients were not in a supine slight Trendelenburg position.
22. Ask the patient to take a deep breath in and hold it.[9,11-13] **(Level E*)**	Minimizes the risk for venous air embolus.	If the patient is receiving positive pressure ventilation, withdraw the catheter during the inspiratory phase of the respiratory cycle or while a breath is delivered via a bag-valve device.
		If the introducer is in the femoral vein, extend the patient's leg and ensure the groin area is adequately exposed.
23. Withdraw the introducer, pulling parallel to the skin and using a steady motion.	Minimizes trauma.	If resistance is met, do not continue to remove the introducer. Notify the advanced practice nurse or physician immediately.
24. As the introducer exits the site, apply pressure with a gauze pad.	Minimizes the risk for venous air embolus and promotes hemostasis.	
25. Instruct the patient to exhale as soon as the introducer is removed.	Once the catheter is removed, the patient can breathe normally.	
26. Lay the introducer on the moisture-proof absorbent pad. Check to be sure that all of the introducer was removed.	Ensures the removal of the entire introducer.	If the introducer tip will be cultured, have another provider assist with cutting the tip with sterile scissors and placing it in a sterile specimen container before placing the introducer on the moisture-proof absorbent pad. Routine culturing of tips upon removal is not recommended.[6]

*Level E: Multiple case reports, theory-based evidence from expert opinions, or peer-reviewed professional organizational standards without clinical studies to support recommendations.

Procedure continues on following page

Procedure for Pulmonary Artery Catheter Removal—*Continued*

Steps	Rationale	Special Considerations
27. Continue applying firm, direct pressure over the insertion site with the gauze pad until bleeding has stopped.	Ensures hemostasis.	Because central venous catheters are placed in large veins, 10 minutes may be needed for hemostasis to occur. Pressure may be needed for a longer period of time if the patient has been receiving anticoagulant therapy or if coagulation study results are abnormal.
28. Apply an occlusive dressing, consisting of sterile petroleum-based ointment and sterile gauze, and cover with tape or a transparent semipermeable membrane dressing.[3,5–7,9,11] **(Level E*)**	Decreases the risk for infection at the insertion site and minimizes the risk for venous air embolus.	Mark the dressing with the date, time, and your initials. Indicates when the dressing was placed.
29. Maintain the patient in the supine position for 30 minutes after catheter removal.[5]	May decrease the risk of a postprocedure venous air embolism.	
30. Remove **PE** and discard used supplies in appropriate receptacles.	Reduces the transmission of microorganisms; Standard Precautions.	
31. **HH**		

*Level E: Multiple case reports, theory-based evidence from expert opinions, or peer-reviewed professional organizational standards without clinical studies to support recommendations.

Expected Outcomes

- The PA catheter is removed
- The introducer may or may not be removed

Unexpected Outcomes

- Dysrhythmias
- Valvular damage
- PA rupture
- Thrombosis
- Venous air emboli
- Uncontrolled bleeding
- Infection
- Inability to percutaneously remove the PA catheter because of knotting or kinking
- Pain
- Broken catheter/fragmentation

Patient Monitoring and Care

Steps	Rationale	Reportable Conditions
		These conditions should be reported if they persist despite nursing interventions.
1. Assess the need for the PA catheter daily. If long-term use of the PA catheter is needed; consider changing the PA catheter every 7 days. **(Level B*)**	The Centers for Disease Control and Prevention (CDC)[10] and research findings[2,4] recommend that PA catheters do not need to be changed more frequently than every 7 days. There are no specific recommendations regarding routine replacement of PA catheters that need to be in place for >7 days.[4,10] Guidewire exchanges should not be used routinely. A guidewire exchange should only be used to replace a catheter that is malfunctioning.[8]	• Signs and symptoms of infection at the PA catheter insertion site • Signs and symptoms of sepsis
2. Monitor the patient's vital signs, pulse oximetry, and level of consciousness before and after the PA catheter and/or introducer removal.	Provides baseline data and data that identify changes in patient condition.	• Abnormal vital signs • Persistent shortness of breath or tachypnea • Cyanosis or decreased oxygen saturation • Changes in mental status • Signs of acute cardiac ischemia (chest pain, ECG changes, etc.)
3. Monitor the patient's cardiac rate and rhythm during PA catheter withdrawal.	Ventricular dysrhythmias may occur as the PA catheter passes through the right ventricle.	• Ventricular dysrhythmias that occur after the PA catheter is removed
4. Monitor for signs and symptoms of venous air embolus and, if present, immediately place the patient in the left lateral Trendelenburg's position.	Venous air embolus is a potentially life-threatening complication. The left lateral Trendelenburg's position prevents air from passing into the left side of the heart and traveling into the arterial circulation.	• Respiratory distress • Dyspnea • Coughing • Tachypnea • Altered mental status (agitation, restlessness) • Cyanosis • Gasp reflex • Sucking sound near site of catheter insertion/air entrainment • Petechiae • Cardiac dysrhythmias • Chest pain • Hypotension
5. After removal of the introducer, assess the site for signs of bleeding every 15 minutes × 2, every 30 minutes × 2, and then 1 hour later.	Bleeding or a hematoma can develop if there is still bleeding from the vessel.	• Bleeding • Hematoma development
6. Remove the dressing and assess for site closure 24 hours after introducer removal.	Verifies healing and closure of the site.	• Abnormal healing
7. Follow institutional standards for assessing pain. Administer analgesia as prescribed.	Identifies need for pain interventions.	• Continued pain despite pain interventions

*Level B: Well-designed, controlled studies with results that consistently support a specific action, intervention, or treatment.

Procedure continues on following page

Documentation

Documentation should include the following:
- Patient and family education
- Patient assessment before and after removal of the PA catheter
- Patient's response to the procedure
- Pain assessment, interventions, and effectiveness
- Date and time of removal
- Occurrence of unexpected outcomes
- Nursing interventions taken
- Application of an air-occlusive dressing
- Site assessment

References and Additional Readings

For a complete list of references and additional readings for this procedure, scan this QR code with any freely available smartphone code reader app, or visit http://booksite.elsevier.com/9780323376624.

74 Pulmonary Artery Catheter and Pressure Lines, Troubleshooting

Reba McVay

PURPOSE: Troubleshooting of the pulmonary artery (PA) catheter is important to maintain catheter patency, to ensure that data from the PA catheter are accurate, and to prevent the development of catheter-related and patient-related complications.

PREREQUISITE NURSING KNOWLEDGE

- Knowledge of cardiovascular and pulmonary anatomy and physiology is needed.
- An understanding of basic dysrhythmia recognition and treatment of life-threatening dysrhythmias is important.
- Advanced cardiac life support (ACLS) knowledge and skills are needed.
- Knowledge of principles of aseptic technique is necessary.
- Understanding of the setup of the hemodynamic monitoring system (see Procedure 75) is needed.
- An understanding of the PA catheter (see Fig. 72-1) and the location of the PA catheter in the heart and pulmonary artery (see Fig. 72-2) is needed.
- Pulmonary artery occlusion pressure (PAOP) may be referred to as PA wedge pressure.
- After wedging of the PA catheter, air is passively removed by disconnecting the syringe from the balloon-inflation port. Active withdrawal of air from the balloon is avoided because it can weaken the balloon, pull the balloon structure into the inflation lumen, and possibly cause balloon rupture.
- The pulmonary artery diastolic pressure (PADP) and the PAOP are indirect measures of left-ventricular end-diastolic pressure. Usually, the PAOP is approximately 1 to 4 mm Hg less than the PADP. Because these two pressures are similar, the PADP is commonly followed, which minimizes the frequency of balloon inflation, thus decreasing the potential of balloon rupture.
- Differences between the PADP and the PAOP may exist for patients with pulmonary hypertension, chronic obstructive lung disease, adult respiratory distress syndrome, pulmonary embolus, and tachycardia.
- Pulmonary artery pressures (PAPs) may be elevated because of PA hypertension, pulmonary disease, mitral valve disease, left ventricular failure, atrial or ventricular left-to-right shunt, pulmonary emboli, or hypervolemia.
- PAPs may be decreased because of hypovolemia or low pulmonary vascular resistance (e.g., vasodilation).

- The waveforms that occur during insertion should be recognized, including right atrial (RA), right ventricular (RV), PA, and PA occlusion (PAO; see Fig. 72-3).
- The *a* wave reflects atrial contraction. The *c* wave reflects closure of the atrioventricular valves. The *v* wave reflects passive filling of the atria during ventricular systole (see Figs. 72-4 and 72-5).
- Knowledge of normal hemodynamic values (see Table 64-1) is needed.
- Elevated *a* and *v* waves may be evident in RA or central venous pressure (CVP) and in PAO waveforms. These elevations may occur in patients with cardiac tamponade, constrictive pericardial disease, and hypervolemia.
- Elevated *a* waves in the RA or CVP waveform may occur in patients with pulmonic or tricuspid stenosis, right-ventricular ischemia or infarction, right-ventricular failure, PA hypertension, and atrioventricular dissociation.
- Elevated *a* waves in the PAO waveform may occur in patients with mitral stenosis, acute left ventricular ischemia or infarction, left ventricular failure, and atrioventricular dissociation.
- Elevated *v* waves in the RA or CVP waveform may occur in patients with tricuspid insufficiency.
- Elevated *v* waves in the PAO waveform may occur in patients with mitral insufficiency or ruptured papillary muscle.

EQUIPMENT

- Nonsterile gloves
- Syringes (5 or 10 mL)
- Sterile injectable or noninjectable caps
- Sterile 4 × 4 gauze
- Stopcocks
- Needleless blood-sampling access device
- Pressure monitoring cables
- Pressure transducer system, including flush solution recommended according to institutional standards, a pressure bag or device, pressure tubing with transducers, and flush device
- Dual-channel recorder
- Leveling device (low-intensity laser or carpenter level)

Additional equipment (to have available depending on patient need) includes the following:

- Indelible marker
- Emergency equipment
- Blood-specimen tubes

PATIENT AND FAMILY EDUCATION

- Explain the troubleshooting procedures to the patient and family. *Rationale:* The patient and family are kept informed, and anxiety is reduced.
- Explain the patient's expected participation during the procedure. *Rationale:* This explanation will encourage patient assistance.
- Inform the patient and family of signs and symptoms to report to the critical care nurse, including chest pain, palpitations, new cough, tenderness at the catheter-insertion site, and chills. *Rationale:* The patient is encouraged to report signs of discomfort and potential PA catheter complications.

PATIENT ASSESSMENT AND PREPARATION

Patient Assessment

- Monitor PA waveforms continuously. *Rationale:* The PA catheter may migrate forward into a wedged position, may move back into the right ventricle, or may become dislodged with the catheter tip malpositioned in the RA or central vein.
- Assess the configuration of the PA catheter waveforms. *Rationale:* Thrombus formation at the tip of the catheter lumen may be evidenced by an overdamped waveform.
- Assess the patient's hemodynamic and cardiovascular status. *Rationale:* The patient's clinical assessment should correlate with the PA catheter derived hemodynamic data.
- Assess the patient and the PA catheter site for signs of infection. *Rationale:* Infection can develop because of the invasive nature of the PA catheter.

Patient Preparation

- Verify that the patient is the correct patient using two identifiers. *Rationale:* Before performing a procedure, the nurse should ensure the correct identification of the patient for the intended intervention.
- Ensure that the patient understands preprocedural teaching. Answer questions as they arise, and reinforce information as needed. *Rationale:* Understanding of previously taught information is evaluated and reinforced.
- Determine the patency of the patient's intravenous catheters. *Rationale:* Access may be needed for administration of emergency medication or fluids.

Procedure	for Pulmonary Artery Catheter and Pressure Lines, Troubleshooting	
Steps	**Rationale**	**Special Considerations**
1. **HH**		
2. **PE**		
Troubleshooting an Overwedged PA Catheter Balloon		
1. Identify an overwedged PA catheter balloon from the PA waveform analysis (Fig. 74-1).	The overwedged PA catheter balloon occurs when the PA catheter balloon is overinflated.	Overinflation of the balloon can cause pulmonary arteriole infarction or rupture, resulting in life-threatening hemorrhage.
2. Remove the syringe from the gate valve or the stopcock of the PA balloon inflation port.	Facilitates passive removal of air from the PA catheter balloon.	Ensure that the gate valve or stopcock is in the open position (see Fig. 72-6).
3. Note the change in the PA waveform from the overwedged waveform to the PA waveform.	As the balloon deflates the PA waveform returns.	
4. Fill the syringe with 1.5 mL of air and connect the syringe to the gate valve or stopcock of the balloon port of the PA catheter. Slowly inflate the balloon with air until the PA waveform changes to a PAO waveform (see Fig. 72-10) and note the amount of air used.	Determines the amount of air needed to convert the PA waveform to a PAO waveform.	
5. Disconnect the syringe from the balloon-inflation port to deflate the balloon and verify that the PAO waveform changes back to the PA waveform. **(Level M*)**	Allows air to passively escape from the balloon.	Active withdrawal of air from the balloon can weaken the balloon, pull the balloon structure into the inflation lumen, and possibly cause balloon rupture.

*Level M: Manufacturer's recommendations only.

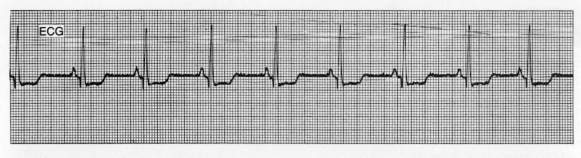

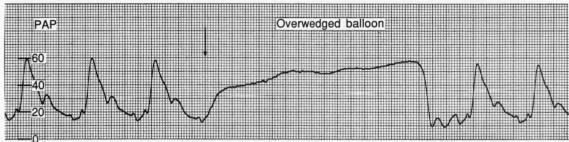

Figure 74-1 Balloon inflation *(arrow).* Overwedging of balloon (balloon has been overinflated). The danger of overinflating the balloon is that the pulmonary artery vessel may rupture from the pressure of the balloon. *ECG,* electrocardiogram; *PAP,* Pulmonary artery pressure.

Procedure	for Pulmonary Artery Catheter and Pressure Lines, Troubleshooting—*Continued*	
Steps	**Rationale**	**Special Considerations**
6. Expel air from the balloon syringe and reconnect the empty balloon syringe to the balloon-inflation port.	The syringe should remain empty when reconnected so that accidental balloon inflation does not occur.	The syringe that is manufactured for the PA catheter should be connected to the PA balloon port to avoid loss of the custom-designed syringe.
7. Follow institutional standards regarding keeping the gate valve or the stopcock open.	The most important considerations are that the balloon syringe is attached to the balloon-inflation port, the syringe is empty, and the PA distal waveform reflects a PA waveform.	
8. Note the external centimeter marking of the PA catheter at the introducer exit site.	Identifies whether the PA catheter has migrated forward from the previously documented measurement.	The advanced practice nurse or the physician may need to reposition the catheter.
9. Note and record the amount of air needed to wedge the PA catheter.	Prevents overinflation of the PA catheter balloon.	
Preventing an Overwedged PA Catheter		
1. Fill the syringe with 1.5 mL of air.	Instilling more than 1.5 mL of air may rupture the PA balloon and the pulmonary arteriole.	
2. Connect the PA balloon syringe to the gate valve or stopcock of the balloon-inflation port of the PA catheter.	This port is designed for PA balloon inflation.	The PA balloon syringe is designed so it will not hold more than 1.5 mL of air.
3. Slowly inflate the balloon with air until the PA waveform changes to a PAO waveform (see Fig. 72-10).	Only instill enough air needed to convert the PA waveform to a PAO waveform.	
4. Inflate the PA balloon for no more than 8–15 seconds (2–4 respiratory cycles).	Avoids prolonged pressure on the pulmonary arteriole.	

Procedure continues on following page

Procedure	for Pulmonary Artery Catheter and Pressure Lines, Troubleshooting—*Continued*	

Steps	Rationale	Special Considerations
5. Disconnect the PA balloon syringe from the balloon-inflation port for passive deflation of the balloon.	Allows air to passively exit from the balloon.	
6. Observe the monitor as the PAO waveform changes back to the PA waveform.	Ensures adequate balloon deflation.	
7. Expel air from the PA syringe.	The syringe should remain empty when reconnected so that accidental balloon inflation does not occur.	
8. Reconnect the empty PA balloon syringe to the balloon inflation port.	Retains the safety syringe.	
9. Follow institutional standards regarding keeping the gate valve or the stopcock open.	The most important considerations are that the balloon syringe is attached to the balloon-inflation port, the syringe is empty, and the PA distal waveform reflects a PA waveform.	

Troubleshooting an Absent Waveform

Steps	Rationale	Special Considerations
1. Check to see whether there is a kink in the PA catheter.	Kinks may inhibit waveform transmission.	
2. Ensure that all connections are tight.	Loose connections allow air into the system and can overdamp or eliminate the waveform.	
3. Ensure that the stopcock is open to the transducer (Fig. 74-2).	Stopcocks open to the transducer system allow waveform transmission from the cardiovascular system to the monitor; stopcocks closed to the transducer prevent waveform transmission to the monitor and oscilloscope.	
4. Check that the cables are in the appropriate pressure modules.	Necessary for signal transmission.	
5. Ensure that the pressure cables are securely plugged into the monitor.	No waveform is transmitted without proper connection.	
6. Ensure that the appropriate monitor parameters are turned on.	Necessary for specific parameter monitoring.	
7. Ensure the appropriate scale has been chosen for pressure being monitored (e.g., 40 mm Hg scale is used for PA monitoring).	A larger scale (e.g., 100 mm Hg) causes the waveform to be smaller and possibly not to be visible on the oscilloscope.	
8. Level and zero the monitoring system (see Procedure 75).	Ensures accurate setup and function of the monitoring system.	
9. Ensure that there is fluid in the flush bag and that the pressure on the flush bag or device is delivering 300 mm Hg.	Low pressure may result in a clotted catheter, resulting in loss of the waveform.	A square waveform test should not be done. A clotted catheter under pressure of flush may dislodge clots.
10. Aspirate through the stopcock that is closest to the catheter to check for blood return (see Fig. 63-2).	Ensures patency of the PA catheter.	A clotted/obstructed catheter has no waveform and no blood return when aspirated.

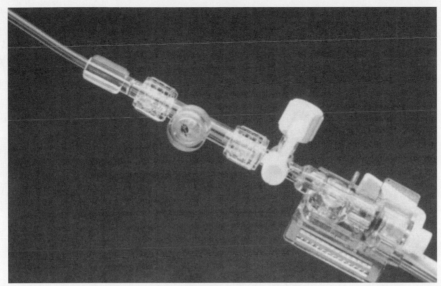

Figure 74-2   The stopcock is open to the transducer. *(From Ahrens TS, Taylor LK:* Hemodynamic waveform recognition, *Philadelphia, 1993, Saunders.)*

Procedure	for Pulmonary Artery Catheter and Pressure Lines, Troubleshooting—*Continued*	
Steps	**Rationale**	**Special Considerations**
11. Replace the monitoring cable.	A faulty cable can result in an absent waveform.	If the cable is changed, zero the monitoring system.
12. Replace the pressure transducer system.	A faulty transducer can result in an absent waveform.	If the pressure transducer system is changed, zero the new monitoring system.
13. Notify the advanced practice nurse or the physician if troubleshooting is unsuccessful.	The catheter may need to be removed or replaced.	
Troubleshooting an Overdamped Waveform		
1. Obtain a monitor strip of the overdamped waveform (Fig. 74-3).	The waveform can be compared with the previous waveforms.	
2. Ensure that all connections are tight.	Loose connections allow air into the system or loss of pressure from the system and can overdamp the waveform.	
3. Ensure that there is fluid in the flush bag and that the pressure on the flush bag or device is set at 300 mm Hg.	Low counterpressure from the flush solution bag results in an overdamped waveform.	

Procedure continues on following page

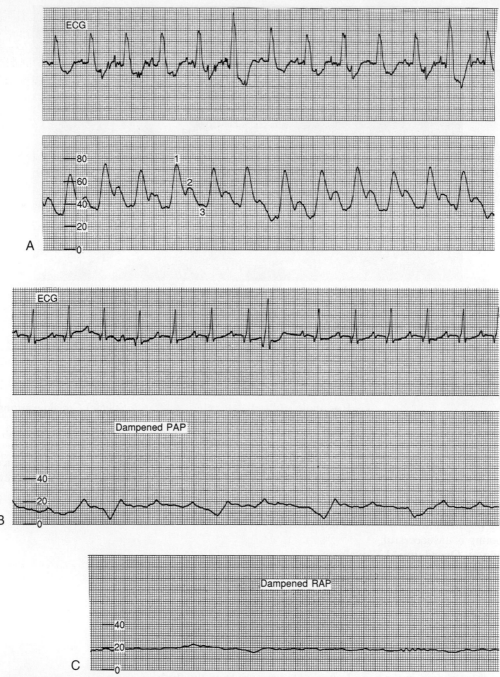

Figure 74-3   Effects of overdamping on pulmonary artery pressure (PAP) and right-atrial pressure (RAP) waveforms. **A,** Normal waveform with elevated pulmonary artery pressures *(1,* systole; *2,* dicrotic notch; *3,* diastole). **B,** Overdamped PAP waveform. **C,** Overdamping of RAP waveform. Overdamping of the waveform may result from clots at the catheter tip, catheter against vessel or heart wall, air in lines, stopcock partially closed, or deflated pressure bag. *ECG,* electrocardiogram.

Procedure	for Pulmonary Artery Catheter and Pressure Lines, Troubleshooting—*Continued*	
Steps	**Rationale**	**Special Considerations**
4. Check all tubing for air bubbles. If air exists within the transducer, follow these steps: A. Remove the noninjectable cap at the top port of the stopcock or cleanse the top of the injectable cap with an antiseptic solution. B. Insert a sterile syringe or a blood-sampling access device into the top port of the stopcock or the top of the injectable cap of the stopcock (see Figs. 62-1 and 63-1). C. Turn the stopcock off to the patient (see Figs. 62-3). D. Fast flush the air from the transducer and system into the syringe or insert a blood-specimen tube into the blood-sampling access device. E. Open the system to the transducer (see Figs. 62-1 and 63-1). F. Remove the syringe or the blood-sampling access device from the stopcock. G. Zero the hemodynamic monitoring system (see Procedure 75). H. If not using an injectable cap, place a new noninjectable cap on the top port of the stopcock. I. Evaluate and then monitor the waveform.	Removes air from the system, prevents the air from entering the patient, and ensures accurate monitoring of waveforms.	Check that the IV flush bag and pressure tubing drip chamber contain fluid.
5. If air exists between the pressure bag and a stopcock, follow these steps: A. Remove the noninjectable cap at the top port of the stopcock or cleanse the top of the injectable cap with an antiseptic solution. B. Insert a sterile syringe or a blood-sampling access device into the top port of the stopcock or the top of the injectable cap of the stopcock (see Figs. 62-1 and 63-1).	Removes air from the system, prevents the air from entering the patient, and prevents overdamping of the system to ensure accurate monitoring.	

Procedure continues on following page

Procedure	for Pulmonary Artery Catheter and Pressure Lines, Troubleshooting—*Continued*		
Steps	**Rationale**		**Special Considerations**

C. Turn the stopcock off to the patient (see Fig. 62-3).

D. Fast flush the air from the transducer and system into the syringe or insert a blood-specimen tube into the blood-sampling access device.

E. Open the system to the transducer (see Fig. 62-1 and 63-1).

F. Remove the syringe or the blood-sampling access device from the stopcock.

G. If not using an injectable cap, place a new sterile noninjectable cap on the top port of the stopcock.

H. Evaluate and monitor the PA waveform.

6. If the air is between the patient and a stopcock (Fig. 74-4), follow these steps:

   Removes air from the system, prevents the air from entering the patient, and ensures accurate monitoring of waveforms.

   A. Remove the noninjectable cap at the top port of the stopcock or cleanse the top of the injectable cap with an antiseptic solution.

   B. Insert a sterile syringe or a blood-sampling access device into the top port of the stopcock or the top of the injectable cap of the stopcock (see Figs. 62-1 and 63-1).

   C. Turn the stopcock off to the flush solution (see Figs. 62-2, 62-4, and 63-2.

   D. Gently pull the air back into the syringe or insert a blood-specimen tube into the injectable system.

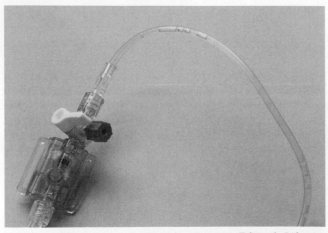

Figure 74-4   Air between the patient and stopcock. (*Courtesy Edwards Lifesciences, Irvine, CA.*)

Procedure	for Pulmonary Artery Catheter and Pressure Lines, Troubleshooting—*Continued*	
Steps	**Rationale**	**Special Considerations**
E. When all the air is removed, turn the stopcock off to the patient (see Fig. 62-3).		
F. Fast flush the blood from the top port of the stopcock.	Clears the tubing of blood.	
G. Open the system to the transducer (see Figs. 62-1 and 63-1).		
H. Remove the syringe or blood-sampling access device from the stopcock.		
I. Zero the hemodynamic monitoring system (see Procedure 75).		
J. If not using an injectable cap, place a new sterile noninjectable cap on the top port of the stopcock.		
K. Evaluate and then monitor the pressure waveform.		
7. Aspirate through the stopcock of the catheter to check for adequate blood return.	Ensures that blood flows easily within the catheter and assesses for the presence of clots.	
A. Remove the noninjectable cap at the top port of the stopcock or cleanse the top of the injectable cap with an antiseptic solution.		
B. Connect a 5–10-mL syringe to the stopcock or to the injectable cap.		
C. Turn the stopcock off to the flush solution (see Figs. 62-2, 62-4 and 63-2).		
D. Gently aspirate until blood enters the syringe.		
E. Turn the stopcock open to the transducer (see Figs. 62-1 and 63-1).		
F. Fast flush the blood in the tubing back into the patient.		
G. Turn the stopcock off to the patient (see Fig. 62-3) and fast flush the blood from the top port of the stopcock or the injectable cap into the syringe.		
H. Open the stopcock to the transducer (see Figs. 62-1 and 63-1).		
I. Remove the syringe from the top port of the stopcock or the injectable cap.		
J. Zero the hemodynamic monitoring system (see Procedure 75).		

Procedure continues on following page

Procedure	for Pulmonary Artery Catheter and Pressure Lines, Troubleshooting—*Continued*	
Steps	**Rationale**	**Special Considerations**
K. If not using an injectable cap, place a new sterile noninjectable cap on the top of the stopcock.		
L. Evaluate and then monitor the waveform.		
8. Check the transducer for the presence of blood. If blood is present, follow these steps:	Ensures accurate monitoring of waveforms.	The pressure-transducer system may need to be replaced.
A. Remove the noninjectable cap at the top port of the stopcock or cleanse the top of the injectable cap with an antiseptic solution.		
B. Turn the stopcock off to the patient (see Fig. 75-4).		
C. Connect a 5–10-mL syringe to the stopcock or to the injectable cap or insert a blood-sampling access device.		
D. Fast flush the blood from the transducer tubing into the syringe or insert a blood-specimen tube into the injectable access device.		
E. Remove the syringe or the blood-access device.		
F. Turn the stopcock open to the transducer (see Fig. 75-5).		
G. Zero the hemodynamic monitoring system (see Procedure 75).		
H. If not using an injectable cap, place a new sterile noninjectable cap on the top port of the stopcock.		
I. Evaluate and monitor the waveform.		
9. Observe the waveform and perform a dynamic response test (square-wave test).	Determines whether the system is damped. This will ensure that the pressure waveform components are clearly defined. This aids in accurate measurement.	The square-wave test can be performed by activating and quickly releasing the fast flush. A sharp upstroke should terminate in a flat line at the maximal indicator on the monitor. This should be followed by an immediate rapid downstroke extending below the baseline with 1–2 oscillations within 0.12 second and a quick return to baseline. (See Fig. 59-3).
10. Notify the advanced practice nurse or physician if troubleshooting is unsuccessful.	The catheter needs to be removed or replaced.	

Procedure	for Pulmonary Artery Catheter and Pressure Lines, Troubleshooting—*Continued*	
Steps	**Rationale**	**Special Considerations**

Troubleshooting a Continuously Wedged Waveform

1. Identify the wedged waveform (see Fig. 72-5).	Confirms the need for troubleshooting.	Continuous monitoring of the PA waveform is necessary to assess for the presence of the PA waveform. PA catheters should be wedged for no longer than 8–15 seconds (2–4 respiratory cycles) when obtaining a PAOP measurement.
2. Remove the PA balloon inflation syringe and ensure that the gate valve (see Fig. 72-6) or stopcock is open.	Ensures that air is not trapped within the PA balloon.	
3. Assist the patient in changing position, or if possible ask the patient to cough.	May help the catheter float out of the wedge position.	Monitor the PA waveform for a change from a PAO waveform to a PA waveform.
4. If troubleshooting is unsuccessful, notify the advanced practice nurse or physician.	Immediate repositioning of the catheter is necessary because prolonged wedging can lead to PA infarction.	The critical care nurse may withdraw the PA catheter according to institutional policy.
5. Never flush a wedged PA catheter.	Flushing the catheter in the wedged position may lead to PA rupture and hemorrhage.	

Troubleshooting a Catheter in the Right Ventricle

1. Identify the RV waveform (Fig. 74-5).	The RV waveform resembles the PA waveform. The RV waveform, however, does not have a dicrotic notch. In addition, the diastolic pressure of the RV waveform is lower than the PADP. The normal PADP is 8–15 mm Hg; the normal RV diastolic pressure is 0–8 mm Hg.	Note the external centimeter marking on the PA catheter.
2. Inflate the PA balloon with 1.5 mL of air.	The inflated PA balloon may readily float into position in the PA.	
3. Observe for a change in the waveform from RV to PA to PAO (see Fig. 72-3).	Waveform analysis aids in identification of PA catheter position.	The catheter may not advance to the PA or PAO waveforms.
4. Remove the syringe from the PA balloon inflation port.	Air passively is released from the PA balloon.	Expel the air from the PA balloon syringe, and then reconnect the empty syringe to the balloon inflation port.
5. Observe the PA waveform.	The waveform should change from the PAO waveform to a PA waveform.	
6. If the RV pressure waveform is still present, inflate the PA balloon inflation port with 1.5 mL of air.	An inflated PA balloon cushions the catheter tip and prevents endocardial irritation.	The PA catheter tip may cause ventricular dysrhythmias. If the PA balloon is inflated, the ventricular dysrhythmias may decrease because the inflated balloon may cause less irritation of the endocardium.

Procedure continues on following page

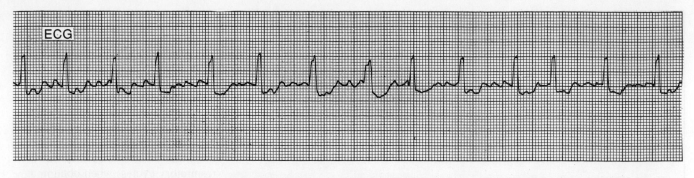

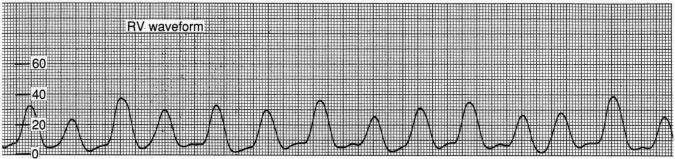

Figure 74-5   Right ventricular pressure (RVP) waveform. This waveform was seen coming from the pulmonary artery (PA; distal) lumen of a PA catheter. The catheter was coiled in the right ventricle (RV). *ECG,* electrocardiogram.

Procedure	for Pulmonary Artery Catheter and Pressure Lines, Troubleshooting—*Continued*

Steps	Rationale	Special Considerations
7. Assist the patient with a change of position.	The inflated PA catheter may float into the PA after a position change.	
8. Observe for change in waveform from RV to PA to PAO (see Fig. 72-3).	Waveform analysis aids identification of the PA catheter position.	
9. Remove the balloon syringe from the balloon port.	Deflates the PA balloon.	Expel air from the syringe.
10. If troubleshooting is unsuccessful, notify the advanced practice nurse or physician.	The PA catheter cannot remain in the right ventricle because it may trigger life-threatening ventricular dysrhythmias. Immediate repositioning is necessary.	If ventricular dysrhythmias are present, consider temporarily leaving the balloon inflated until the catheter is repositioned in the PA. If the balloon remains inflated, continuous visual monitoring is necessary in case the catheter floats into the wedge position. The critical care nurse may advance or remove the PA catheter according to institutional policy.
Troubleshooting an Inability to Wedge the PA Catheter		
1. Note the external centimeter marking of the PA catheter at the introducer exit site and compare this with the most recent documented marking.	Determines whether the catheter has moved from its previous location. Most PA catheters are in the correct position if the external markings of the catheter are between 45 and 55 cm. The PA catheter tip may not be distal enough in the PA to float into the wedge position.	The advanced practice nurse or physician may need to reposition the catheter.

Procedure	for Pulmonary Artery Catheter and Pressure Lines, Troubleshooting—*Continued*	

Steps	Rationale	Special Considerations
2. Ensure that the PA balloon is inflated with the maximum 1.5 mL of air.	The full 1.5 mL of air may be necessary to wedge some PA catheters.	Repositioning the patient may aid in changing the position of the catheter and may facilitate successful wedging of the PA catheter.
3. Resistance should be felt when inflating the PA balloon.	Resistance is present when the PA balloon is intact.	The balloon may rupture because of overinflation, frequent inflations, or repeated aspiration of air from the balloon rather than allowing it to passively deflate.
4. If no resistance is felt or if blood flows back from the balloon lumen, follow these steps: A. Immediately discontinue balloon inflation attempts. B. Remove the syringe. C. Close the gate valve or stopcock. D. Tape the balloon inflation port closed and label the tape that the balloon should not be used.	If the balloon is ruptured, no resistance is felt during an inflation attempt. Blood may also come back through the balloon lumen.	
5. If the balloon is ruptured or troubleshooting is unsuccessful, notify the advanced practice nurse or physician.	The PA catheter may be removed and/or replaced.	If the PA catheter remains in place, the PADP can be followed if the PADP correlated with the PAOP.

Troubleshooting Unexpected Changes in PAP

Steps	Rationale	Special Considerations
1. Ensure that the patient is in the supine position with the head of the bed from 0 to 45 degrees. **(Level B*)**	Studies have determined that the RA and the PA pressures are accurate in this position.[3–6,10,12,14,22,23]	RA and PA pressures may be accurate for patients in the supine position with the head of the bed elevated up to 60 degrees,[5,14] but additional studies are needed to support this. Only one study[11] supports the accuracy of hemodynamic values for patients in lateral positions; other studies do not.[3,8,10,16,21] The majority of studies support the accuracy of hemodynamic monitoring for patients in the prone position.[1,2,7,9,13,17,20] Two studies demonstrated that prone positioning caused an increase in hemodynamic values.[18,19]
2. Ensure that the air-fluid interface (zeroing stopcock) is level with the phlebostatic axis (see Procedure 75).	Ensures accurate pressure measurements. If the air-fluid interface is above the phlebostatic axis, PA pressures are falsely low. If the air-fluid interface is below the phlebostatic axis, PA pressures are falsely high.	

*Level B: Well-designed, controlled studies with results that consistently support a specific action, intervention, or treatment.

Procedure continues on following page

Procedure	for Pulmonary Artery Catheter and Pressure Lines, Troubleshooting—*Continued*	
Steps	**Rationale**	**Special Considerations**
3. Zero the transducer-monitoring system (see Procedure 75).	Ensures the accuracy of the monitoring system.	
4. Check for air bubbles in the pressure-monitoring system and eliminate bubbles if present.	Air contributes to an overdamped pressure transducer system, resulting in falsely low pressure measurements.	
5. Assess the patient's hemodynamic parameters and compare with assessment data.	Hemodynamic data and assessment data should correlate.	If the hemodynamic data and assessment data do not correlate, review hemodynamic measurement steps for potential sources of inaccuracy.
6. If the PAP changes and hemodynamic parameters are accurate, administer/titrate fluids or vasoactive agents as prescribed and/or notify the advanced practice nurse or physician.	Hemodynamic data guide therapeutic interventions.	

Troubleshooting Blood Backup into a PA Catheter or Pressure-Transducer System

1. Turn the stopcock off to the patient (see Fig. 75-4).	Prevents blood from going into the transducer.	If blood reaches the transducer, it may have to be replaced.
2. Ensure that the transducer system is closed and that all connections are tight and that all stopcocks are closed to air and have noninjectable or injectable caps.	Loose connections or open stopcocks cause a decrease in pressure within the fluid-filled system, and blood may exert a back pressure into the pressure tubing.	A crack in the system necessitates replacing the entire monitoring system.
3. Ensure that there is fluid in the flush solution bag and that the pressure on the flush bag or device is delivering 300 mm Hg.	Low pressure from the bag results in blood backup.	
4. Once the source of the problem is located and corrected, flush the entire line to remove blood from the system.	Prevents clot formation within the monitoring system. Blood can become a medium for bacterial growth.[15]	
5. Zero the hemodynamic monitoring system (see Procedure 75).	Ensures accuracy of the monitoring system.	
6. Observe the waveform and perform a dynamic response test (square-wave test).	Determines whether the system is damped. This will ensure that the pressure waveform components are clearly defined and aids in accurate measurement.	The square-wave test can be performed by activating and quickly releasing the fast flush. A sharp upstroke should terminate in a flat line at the maximal indicator on the monitor. This should be followed by an immediate rapid downstroke extending below baseline with 1–2 oscillations within 0.12 seconds and a quick return to baseline (see Fig. 59-3).
7. Evaluate and monitor the PA waveform.	Ensures presence of the correct waveform, location of PA catheter, and system functioning.	

Procedure for Pulmonary Artery Catheter and Pressure Lines, Troubleshooting—*Continued*

Steps	Rationale	Special Considerations
Troubleshooting When the Patient Develops Hemoptysis or Bloody Secretions from the Endotracheal Tube During PA Catheter Monitoring		
1. Notify the physician/advanced practice nurse immediately.	PA perforation with hemorrhage is a potentially lethal complication of a PA catheter.	
2. Maintain patency of the airway.	Prevents alterations in ventilation and oxygenation.	Prepare for intubation if the patient is not already intubated.
3. Remain with the patient for monitoring and reassurance.	Reduces anxiety and fear; provides essential assessment.	
4. Be prepared to follow these steps: A. Send blood specimens to assess coagulation status and to prepare for blood-product transfusions. B. Assist if needed with calling for a chest radiograph. C. Prepare the patient for transport to the procedural area/operating room as requested.	Blood loss from the PA can be fatal. Immediate surgical or interventional radiology repair of the PA may be necessary.	
After All Troubleshooting Interventions:		
1. Remove **PE** and discard used supplies.		
2. **HH**		

Expected Outcomes

- Normal pulmonary tissue perfusion
- Absence of PA catheter–related dysrhythmias and other complications
- Absence of signs of PA catheter–related infection
- Absence of discomfort associated with PA catheter
- Accurate PA waveform, pressure monitoring, and data

Unexpected Outcomes

- PA balloon rupture
- Pulmonary infarction and rupture
- PA catheter–related infection
- Discomfort at the PA catheter insertion site
- Ventricular tachycardia unresponsive to antidysrhythmic medications

Patient Monitoring and Care

Steps	Rationale	Reportable Conditions
		These conditions should be reported if they persist despite nursing interventions.
1. The PA waveform should be continuously monitored.	Provides assessment of proper placement of the PA catheter and abnormal waveforms such as PAO or RV waveforms.	• Abnormal waveforms (e.g., continued PAO waveform and RV waveforms)
2. Pressure alarms should be set and remain on at all times.	Alerts the critical care nurse to pressure changes and to disconnections in the pressure-monitoring system.	• Abnormal hemodynamic values
3. Evaluate the hemodynamic monitoring system and waveform configurations.	Ensures that the system is intact and functioning appropriately.	• Abnormal waveforms

Procedure continues on following page

Patient Monitoring and Care —*Continued*

Steps	Rationale	Reportable Conditions
4. Monitor hemodynamic status (PA, PAO, RA, cardiac output, cardiac index, systemic vascular resistance, etc.).	Guides diagnosis, appropriate therapeutic interventions, and evaluation of therapies.	• Abnormal hemodynamic monitoring values
5. Assess the hemodynamic waveforms and pressure values before and after troubleshooting.	Identifies that troubleshooting has been successful.	• Unsuccessful troubleshooting attempts
6. Follow institutional standards for assessing pain. Administer analgesia as prescribed.	Identifies need for pain interventions.	• Continued pain despite pain interventions

Documentation

Documentation should include the following:
- Patient and family education
- Troubleshooting intervention and outcome
- Occurrence of unexpected outcomes and interventions
- Pain assessment, interventions, and effectiveness

- Patient tolerance of procedure
- Site assessment
- External centimeter marking of PA catheter noted at exit site

References and Additional Readings

For a complete list of references and additional readings for this procedure, scan this QR code with any freely available smartphone code reader app, or visit http://booksite.elsevier.com/9780323376624.

75 Single-Pressure and Multiple-Pressure Transducer Systems

Reba McVay

PURPOSE: Single-pressure and multiple-pressure transducer systems provide a catheter-to-monitor interface so that intravascular and intracardiac pressures can be measured. The transducer detects a biophysical event and converts it to an electronic signal.

PREREQUISITE NURSING KNOWLEDGE

- Knowledge of the anatomy and physiology of the cardio-vascular system is needed.
- Knowledge of principles of aseptic technique is necessary.
- Fluid-filled pressure-monitoring systems used for bedside hemodynamic pressure monitoring are based on the principle that a change in pressure at any point in an unobstructed system results in similar pressure changes at all other points of the system.
- Pressure transducers detect the pressure waveform generated by ventricular ejection and converts that pressure wave into an electrical signal, which is transmitted to the monitoring equipment for representation as a waveform on the oscilloscope.
- Invasive measurement of intravascular (arterial) pressure requires insertion of a catheter into an artery.
- Invasive measurement of intracardiac (right atrial [RA] and pulmonary artery [PA]) pressures requires insertion of a catheter into the PA.
- Invasive measurement of central venous pressure/RA pressure can be monitored by insertion of a catheter into the internal jugular vein or subclavian vein or via a port of a PA catheter.
- A single-pressure transducer system is used to measure pressure from a single catheter (e.g., arterial catheter, central venous; Fig. 75-1).
- A double-pressure transducer system is used to measure pressure from two catheters (e.g., arterial and central venous) or two ports (e.g., PA and RA) from a single catheter (e.g., PA catheter; Fig. 75-2).
- A triple-pressure transducer system is commonly used to measure pressures from the arterial and PA catheters. With this system, arterial pressures, PA pressures, and RA pressures can be obtained (Fig. 75-3).
- For accuracy of the hemodynamic values obtained from any transducer system, leveling and zeroing are essential.
- All hemodynamic values (PA, RA, and arterial) are referenced to the level of the atria. The external reference point of the atria is the phlebostatic axis.

EQUIPMENT

- Invasive catheter (e.g., arterial, PA)
- Pressure modules and cables for interface with the monitor
- Cardiac output cable with a thermistor/injectate sensor for use with the PA catheter
- Pressure transducer system, including flush solution recommended according to institutional standards, a pressure bag or device, pressure tubing with transducers, and flush device
- Monitoring system (central and bedside monitor)
- Dual-channel recorder
- Sterile injectable or noninjectable caps
- Indelible marker
- Leveling device (low-intensity laser or carpenter level)

Additional equipment (to have available depending on patient need) includes the following:

- Heparin
- 3-mL syringe
- Stopcocks
- 4 × 4 gauze pads or hydrocolloid gel pad
- Tape
- Nonsterile gloves
- Transducer holder and intravenous (IV) pole

PATIENT AND FAMILY EDUCATION

- Assess patient and family understanding of hemodynamic monitoring and the reason for its use. *Rationale:* Clarification or reinforcement of information is an expressed patient and family need.
- Explain the procedure for hemodynamic monitoring. *Rationale:* This information prepares the patient and the family for what to expect and may decrease anxiety.

PATIENT ASSESSMENT AND PREPARATION
Patient Assessment

- Assess the patient for conditions that may warrant the use of a hemodynamic monitoring system, including hypotension or hypertension, cardiac failure, cardiogenic shock, cardiac arrest, hemorrhage, respiratory failure,

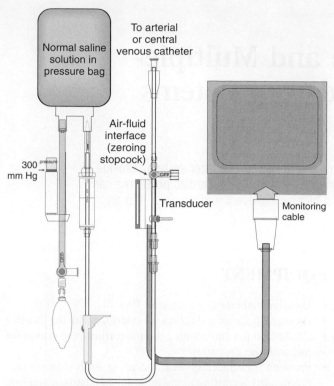

Figure 75-1 Single-pressure transducer system. *(Drawing by Paul W. Schiffmacher, Thomas Jefferson University, Philadelphia, PA.)*

fluid imbalances, oliguria, anuria, and sepsis. ***Rationale:*** Assessment provides data regarding signs and symptoms of hemodynamic instability.

• Obtain the patient's medical history of coagulopathies, use of anticoagulants, vascular abnormalities, cardiac valvular disease, pulmonary hypertension, and peripheral neuropathies. ***Rationale:*** The medical history assists in determining the safety of the procedure and aids in site selection.

Patient Preparation

• Verify the patient is the correct patient using two identifiers. ***Rationale:*** Before performing a procedure, the nurse should ensure the correct identification of the patient for the intended intervention.

• Ensure that the patient and the family understand preprocedural teaching. Answer questions as they arise, and reinforce information as needed. ***Rationale:*** Understanding of previously taught information is evaluated and reinforced.

• Position the patient in the supine position with the head of the bed flat or elevated up to 45 degrees. ***Rationale:*** This positioning prepares the patient for hemodynamic monitoring.

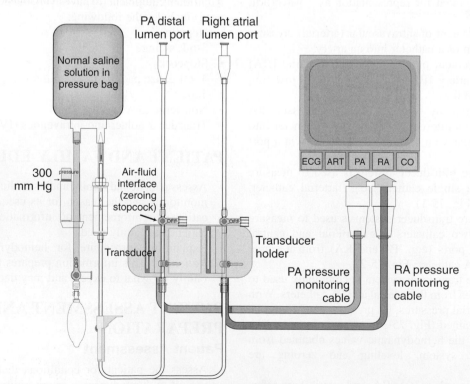

Figure 75-2 Double-pressure transducer system. ART, arterial; CO, cardiac output, *ECG,* electrocardiogram; *PA,* pulmonary artery; *RA,* right atrial. *(Drawing by Paul W. Schiffmacher, Thomas Jefferson University, Philadelphia, PA.)*

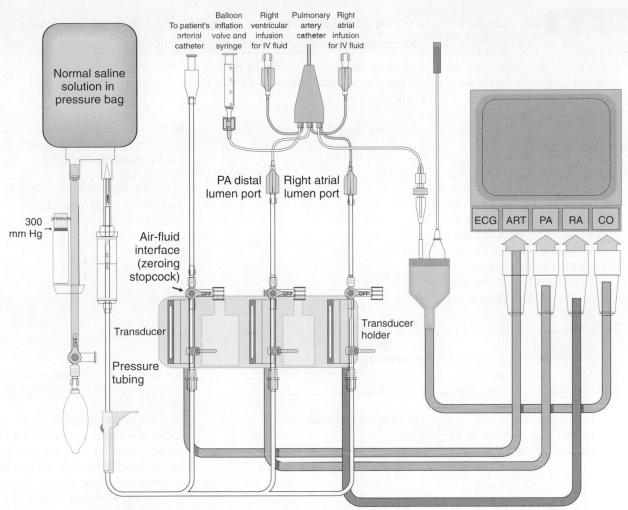

Figure 75-3 Triple-pressure transducer system. *ART,* arterial; *CO,* cardiac output, *ECG,* electrocardiogram; *PA,* pulmonary artery; *RA,* right atrial. *(Drawing by Paul W. Schiffmacher, Thomas Jefferson University, Philadelphia, PA.)*

Procedure	for Single-Pressure and Multiple-Pressure Transducer Systems	
Steps	**Rationale**	**Special Considerations**

Disposable Pressure Transducer System Setup

Steps	Rationale	Special Considerations
1. 🅷🅷		
2. Use an IV bag of normal saline solution. **(Level B*)**	Normal saline solution is preferred. Solutions containing dextrose increase the incidence of infection and should not be used.[7,15,26,28,38]	
3. Follow institutional standards for adding heparin to the flush solution. **(Level B*)**	Heparinized flush solutions are used to minimize thrombi and fibrin deposits on catheters that might lead to thrombosis or bacterial colonization of the catheter.	Although heparin may prevent thrombosis,[28,35] it has been associated with thrombocytopenia and other hematologic complications.[9] Arterial catheters flushed with heparinized saline solution are more likely than those flushed with nonheparinized saline solution to remain patent for up to 72 hours.[1,21] Further research is needed regarding use of heparin versus normal saline solution to maintain PA line patency.

---

*Level B: Well-designed, controlled studies with results that consistently support a specific action, intervention, or treatment.

Procedure continues on following page

Procedure **for Single-Pressure and Multiple-Pressure Transducer Systems—*Continued***

Steps	Rationale	Special Considerations
4. Label the IV bag, indicating the date and time the solution was hung, the dose of heparin (if used), and your initials.	Identifies the contents of the IV flush bag and identifies when the IV bag needs to be changed.	
5. Open the prepackaged pressure transducer kit with aseptic technique. A. A single-pressure tubing kit can be used for RA or arterial monitoring (see Fig. 75-1). B. A double-pressure tubing kit can be used for PA and RA monitoring (see Fig. 75-2). C. A triple-pressure tubing kit can be used for arterial, PA, and RA monitoring (see Fig. 75-3).	Provides the correct pressure tubing.	Assemble the pressure transducers, pressure tubing, and stopcocks if not preassembled by the manufacturer. Use the minimal number of stopcocks and tubing length to avoid underdamped waveforms.
6. Tighten all connections.	Prepares the system. Tightening the connections prevents air from entering the system and fluid leaks.	
7. Spike the outlet port of the IV solution with the pressure tubing.	Allows access to the IV flush solution.	Separate flush systems are needed if invasive catheters are inserted at different times.
8. Open the roller clamp and squeeze the drip chamber to fill the chamber half full.	Primes the drip chamber.	Filling the drip chamber at least halfway is important to prevent air bubbles from entering the tubing and allows the nurse to see that the solution is flowing when performing a manual flush of the invasive line.
9. Insert the IV bag into the pressure bag or device on the IV pole. Do not inflate the pressure bag.	Priming the tubing under pressure increases turbulence and may cause air bubbles to enter the tubing.	Air should never be allowed to develop in a hemodynamic system. Micro or macro air emboli can migrate to major organs and present a potentially life-threatening complication.
10. Flush the entire system, including transducer, stopcock, and pressure tubing with the flush solution. A. With the flush device, flush solution from the IV bag through to the tip of the pressure tubing. B. Turn the stopcock off to the patient end of the tubing (Fig. 75-4). C. With the flush device, flush solution from the IV bag through the stopcock. D. Replace the vented cap on the stopcock with an injectable or noninjectable cap. E. Open the stopcock to the transducer (Fig. 75-5).	Eliminates air from the system.	Vented caps are placed by the manufacturer and permit sterilization of the entire system. These vented caps need to be replaced with sterile injectable or noninjectable caps to prevent bacteria and air from entering the system.
11. With use of double-pressure or triple-pressure transducer systems, **repeat Step 10** with each of the pressure transducer systems.	Eliminates air from the systems.	

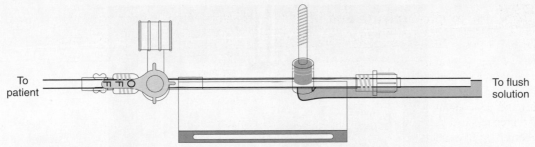

Figure 75-4 Stopcock off to the patient. *(Drawing by Paul W. Schiffmacher, Thomas Jefferson University, Philadelphia, PA.)*

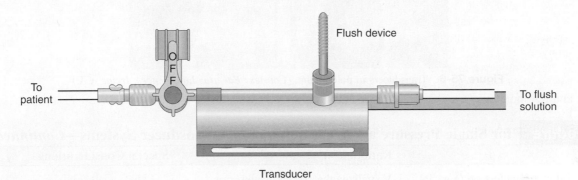

Figure 75-5 Stopcock open to the transducer. *(Drawing by Paul W. Schiffmacher, Thomas Jefferson University, Philadelphia, PA.)*

Procedure	**for Single-Pressure and Multiple-Pressure Transducer Systems—***Continued*	
Steps	**Rationale**	**Special Considerations**
12. Inflate the pressure bag or device to 300 mm Hg.	Inflating the pressure bag to 300 mm Hg allows approximately 1–3 mL/ hr of flush solution to be delivered through the catheter, thus maintaining catheter patency and minimizing clot formation.	
13. With use of a pole mount, insert the transducer into the pole-mount holder (sometimes called a transducer plate) (Fig. 75-6).	Secures each transducer.	Place each of the transducers into the space with the correct label (i.e., PA, RA/central venous, or arterial) (see Fig. 75-6).
14. With sterile technique, connect the end of each transducer tubing to the appropriate catheter port (e.g., PA, RA, arterial).	Allows for monitoring of pressures.	Before assisting with connections, protective equipment needs to be applied.
15. Remove **PE** and discard used supplies.		
16. **HH**		
17. Label the pressure tubing, indicating the date, time, and your initials.	Identifies when the pressure tubing needs to be changed.	
Monitor Setup		
1. Turn on the bedside monitor.	Prepares the monitor.	
2. Plug the pressure cables into the appropriate pressure modules in the bedside monitor (see Fig. 75-3).	Necessary for signal transmission to the monitor.	Some monitors are preprogrammed to display the waveform that corresponds to the module for cable insertion (e.g., first position, arterial; second position, pulmonary artery; third position, right atrial).

Procedure continues on following page

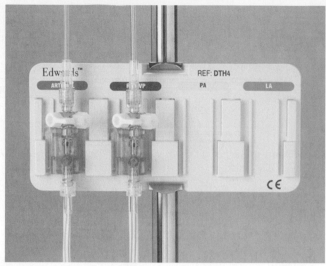

Figure 75-6   Transducers in pole mount. *(Courtesy Edwards Lifesciences, Irvine, CA.)*

Procedure   for Single-Pressure and Multiple-Pressure Transducer Systems—*Continued*

Steps	Rationale	Special Considerations
3. Turn the parameters on (e.g., PA, RA, arterial).	Visualizes the correct waveforms.	
4. Set the appropriate scale for the pressure being measured.	Necessary for visualization of the complete waveform and to obtain accurate readings. Waveforms vary in amplitude depending on the pressure within the system.	The scale for RA pressure is commonly set at 20 mm Hg. The scale for PA pressure is commonly set at 40 mm Hg. The scale for arterial blood pressure is commonly set at 180 mm Hg. Scales may vary based on monitoring equipment. Scales can be adjusted based on patient pressures.

Leveling the Transducer

1. HH
2. PE
3. Position the patient in the supine position with the head of the bed from 0 to 45 degrees. **(Level B*)** | Studies have determined that the RA and the PA pressures are accurate in this position.[8,10–12,17,22,24,42,43] | RA and PA pressures may be accurate for patients in the supine position with the head of the bed elevated up to 60 degrees,[11,24] but additional studies are needed to support this.
Only one study[19] supports the accuracy of hemodynamic values for patients in lateral positions; other studies do not.[4,8,14,17,30,37,41]
The majority of studies support the accuracy of hemodynamic monitoring for patients in the prone position.[3,6,13,16,23,32,40]
Two studies demonstrated that prone positioning caused an increase in hemodynamic values.[34,39]

*Level B: Well-designed, controlled studies with results that consistently support a specific action, intervention, or treatment.

Procedure	for Single-Pressure and Multiple-Pressure Transducer Systems—*Continued*	
Steps	**Rationale**	**Special Considerations**
4. Locate the phlebostatic axis for the supine position (Fig. 75-7).	The phlebostatic axis is at approximately the level of the atria and should be used as the reference point for the air-fluid interface.	The reference point for the left-lateral decubitus position is the fourth intercostal space (ICS) at the left parasternal border (Fig. 75-8).[18,31] The reference point for the right-lateral decubitus position is the fourth ICS at the midsternum (see Fig. 75-8).[18,31]

A. Identify the fourth ICS on the edge of the sternum.
  B. Draw an imaginary line along the fourth ICS laterally, along the chest wall.
  C. Draw a second imaginary line from the axilla downward, midway between the anterior and posterior chest walls.
  D. The point at which these two lines cross is the level of the phlebostatic axis.
  E. Mark the point of the phlebostatic axis with an indelible marker.		

5. Use a leveling device (low-intensity laser or carpenter's level) to align the air-fluid interface with the phlebostatic axis.	Ensures that the air-fluid interface is level with the phlebostatic axis. Leveling to the phlebostatic axis reflects accurate central arterial pressure values.	

Procedure continues on following page

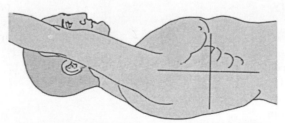

Figure 75-7 Phlebostatic axis in the supine position.

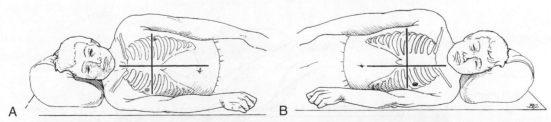

Figure 75-8 Reference points for the hemodynamic monitoring system for patients in lateral positions. **A,** For the right-lateral position, the reference point is the intersection of the fourth intercostal space and the midsternum. **B,** For the left-lateral position, the reference point is the intersection of the fourth intercostal space and the left-parasternal border. *(From Keckelsen M: Protocols for practice: Hemodynamic monitoring series: Pulmonary artery monitoring, Aliso Viejo, CA, 1997, American Association of Critical-Care Nurses.)*

Procedure	for Single-Pressure and Multiple-Pressure Transducer Systems—*Continued*	
Steps	**Rationale**	**Special Considerations**

Pole mount[2,36]:
Low-intensity laser:

A. Place the low-intensity laser leveling device next to the air-fluid interface (zeroing stopcock).	Ensures that the air-fluid interface is level with the phlebostatic axis. Leveling to the phlebostatic axis reflects accurate central arterial pressure values.	
B. Point the laser light at the phlebostatic axis.		
C. Move the pole mount holder up or down until the interface is level with the phlebostatic axis.		

Carpenter level:

A. Place one end of the carpenter level next to the air-fluid interface (zeroing stopcock).	Ensures that the air-fluid interface is level with the phlebostatic axis. Leveling to the phlebostatic axis reflects accurate central arterial pressure values.	
B. Place the other end of the carpenter level at the phlebostatic axis.		
C. Move the pole-mount holder up or down until the interface is level with the phlebostatic axis (Fig. 75-9).		
6. With patient mount:		
A. Place the pulmonary artery distal/PA air-fluid interface (zeroing stopcock) at the phlebostatic axis.	Ensures that the air-fluid interface is level with the phlebostatic axis. Leveling to the phlebostatic axis reflects accurate central arterial pressure values.	
B. Place the PA proximal (RA) and arterial air-fluid interfaces (zeroing stopcocks) directly next to the pulmonary artery distal/PA air-fluid interface.		Leveling the arterial interface to the tip of an arterial catheter reflects the transmural pressure of a particular point in the arterial tree (e.g., radial artery) and not central arterial pressure.[5,20,27,33]
C. Place a 4 × 4 gauze or hydrocolloid gel pad between each of the transducers and the patient's skin.	May prevent skin breakdown.	
D. Secure each of the systems in place with tape.		
7. Remove **PE** and discard.		
8. **HH**		

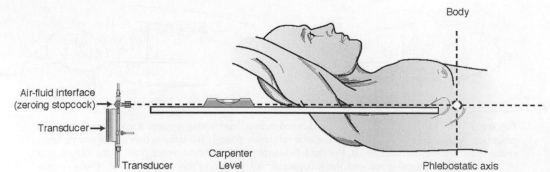

Figure 75-9 Air-fluid interface (zeroing stopcock) is level with the phlebostatic axis using a carpenter level. *(Drawing by Paul W. Schiffmacher, Thomas Jefferson University, Philadelphia, PA.)*

Procedure	for Single-Pressure and Multiple-Pressure Transducer Systems—*Continued*	
Steps	**Rationale**	**Special Considerations**

Zeroing the Transducer

1. 🆔 HH
2. 🆔 PE
3. Turn the stopcock off to the patient end of the tubing (see Fig. 75-4). | Prepares the system for the zeroing procedure. | |
4. Remove the nonvented cap from the stopcock, opening the stopcock to air. | Allows the monitor to use atmospheric pressure as a reference for zero. | |
5. Push and release the zeroing button on the bedside monitor. Observe the digital reading until it displays a value of zero. | The monitor automatically adjusts itself to zero. Zeroing negates the effects of atmospheric pressure. | Some monitors require that the zero be turned and adjusted manually. Some systems also may require calibration. Refer to manufacturer's guidelines for specific information. |
6. Place a new, sterile injectable or noninjectable cap on the stopcock. | Maintains sterility. | |
7. Turn the stopcock so that it is open to the transducer (see Fig. 75-5). | Permits pressure monitoring and maintains catheter patency. | |
8. Observe the waveform and perform a dynamic response test (square-wave test). | Determines whether the system is damped. This will ensure that the pressure waveform components are clearly defined and aids in accurate measurement. | The square-wave test can be performed by activating and quickly releasing the fast flush. A sharp upstroke should terminate in a flat line at the maximal indicator on the monitor. This should be followed by an immediate rapid downstroke extending below baseline with 1–2 oscillations within 0.12 second and a quick return to baseline (see Fig. 59-3). |
9. Remove 🆔 PE and discard used supplies in appropriate receptacles. | Reduces the transmission of microorganisms; Standard Precautions. | |
10. 🆔 HH

Expected Outcomes	Unexpected Outcomes

- The pressure-monitoring system is prepared aseptically
- The hemodynamic monitoring system remains intact with secure connections
- The phlebostatic axis is accurately identified
- The air-fluid interface of the transducer is leveled to the phlebostatic axis
- The pressure-monitoring system is zeroed

- Loose connections within the hemodynamic monitoring system
- Stopcocks left open to air without an injectable or noninjectable cap
- Air bubbles within the system
- Pressure bag inflated to <300 mm Hg

Procedure continues on following page

Patient Monitoring and Care

Steps	Rationale	Reportable Conditions
		These conditions should be reported if they persist despite nursing interventions.
1. Check the IV flush bag every 4 hours and as needed.	Ensures that the IV flush bag contains solution to maintain catheter patency.	
2. Check that the IV flush bag is maintained at 300 mm Hg every 4 hours and as needed.	Maintains catheter patency.	
3. Change the hemodynamic monitoring system (flush solution, pressure tubing, transducers, and stopcocks) every 96 hours. **(Level B*)** The flush solution may need to be changed more frequently if near empty of solution.	The Centers for Disease Control and Prevention (CDC),[28] the Infusion Nurses Society[15] and research findings[25,29] recommend that the hemodynamic flush system can be used safely for 96 hours. This recommendation is based on research conducted with disposable pressure monitoring systems used for peripheral and central lines.	
4. If a nonvented cap is removed from a stopcock it should be replaced with a new sterile injectable or noninjectable cap.	Reduces the risk of infection.	
5. Zero the hemodynamic monitoring system during initial setup or before insertion, after insertion, if disconnection occurs between the transducer and the monitoring cable, if disconnection occurs between the monitoring cable and the monitor, and when the values obtained do not fit the clinical picture. Follow manufacturer's recommendations for disposable systems.	Ensures the accuracy of the hemodynamic monitoring system.	
6. Perform a dynamic response test (square-wave test) at the start of each shift, with a change of the waveform, or when the system is opened to air (see Fig. 59-3).	An optimally damped system provides an accurate waveform.	Overdamped or underdamped waveforms that cannot be corrected with troubleshooting procedures.
7. Check the hemodynamic monitoring system every 4 hours and as needed.	Ensures that all connections are tightly secured and that there are no cracks in the system. Ensures that the system is closed with nonvented caps on all stopcocks. Ensures that the system is free of air bubbles.	
8. Set the hemodynamic monitoring system alarms.	Provides immediate alarm for high and low pressures.	

*Level B: Well-designed, controlled studies with results that consistently support a specific action, intervention, or treatment.

Documentation

Documentation should include the following:
- Patient and family education
- Date and time of hemodynamic monitoring system preparation
- Hemodynamic monitoring system leveling and zeroing
- Type of flush solution
- Unexpected outcomes
- Additional nursing interventions

References and Additional Readings

For a complete list of references and additional readings for this procedure, scan this QR code with any freely available smartphone code reader app, or visit http://booksite.elsevier.com/9780323376624.

PROCEDURE

76 Femoral Arterial and Venous **AP** Sheath Removal

Rose B. Shaffer

PURPOSE: Arterial and venous sheaths are placed for cardiac catheterizations and interventional procedures. Achieving and maintaining hemostasis after their removal is essential to prevent access site complications.

PREREQUISITE NURSING KNOWLEDGE

- Knowledge of the femoral artery and vein anatomy is important.
- The technique for the percutaneous approach to the insertion of the arterial and venous sheaths should be understood.
- Technical and clinical competence in removal of arterial and venous sheaths is needed.
- Knowledge about anticoagulation and antiplatelet therapy used during interventional procedures is essential.
- Understanding the technology (i.e., activated clotting time [ACT] machine) used to determine the timing of arterial sheath removal and knowledge of the institution's standards regarding the appropriate ACT level before arterial sheath removal is important.
- The importance of peripheral vascular and neurovascular assessment of the affected extremity (e.g., assessment of the quality and strength of the pulse to be accessed and the pulses distal to the access site, assessment for a bruit) should be understood.
- Knowledge about the variety of hemostasis options available should include the following:
  - ❖ Manual compression alone or in combination with non-invasive hemostasis pads (e.g., Syvek Patch [Marine Polymer Technologies, Inc., Danvers, MA]; D-Stat Dry [Vascular Solutions, Minneapolis, MN])
  - ❖ Mechanical compression devices (e.g., FemoStop [St. Jude Medical, St. Paul, MN; Fig. 76-1]; CompressAR C-clamp [Advanced Vascular Dynamics, Milwaukie, OR]).
  - ❖ Collagen plug devices (e.g., Angio-Seal [St. Jude Medical, St Paul, MN])

- ❖ Percutaneous suture-mediated closure devices (e.g., Perclose [Abbott Vascular Devices, Santa Clara, CA])
- ❖ Percutaneous staple/clip closure devices (e.g., Star-Close [Abbott Vascular Devices, Santa Clara, CA])
- Collagen plug devices, percutaneous suture-mediated closure devices, and percutaneous staple/clip closure devices are deployed into the artery by the physician at the end of the diagnostic catheterization or interventional procedure.
- Sheath removal can be associated with many complications, including the following:
  - ❖ External bleeding at the site
  - ❖ Internal bleeding (e.g., localized hematoma or retroperitoneal bleed)
  - ❖ Vascular complications (e.g., pseudoaneurysm, arteriovenous fistula, dissection, thrombus, or embolus)
  - ❖ Neurovascular complications (sensory or motor changes in the affected extremity)
  - ❖ Vasovagal complications

EQUIPMENT

- Cardiac monitoring system
- Blood pressure monitoring system
- Antiseptic solution (e.g., 2% chlorhexidine-based preparation)
- Nonsterile gloves
- Sterile gloves
- Protective eyewear
- Dressing supplies
- 10-mL syringe

Additional equipment, to have available as needed, includes the following:

- Selected hemostasis option (mechanical compression device or noninvasive hemostasis pad)
- Alcohol pads
- Indelible marker
- Selected analgesic and/or sedative as prescribed
- Portable Doppler ultrasound machine

AP   This procedure should be performed only by physicians, advanced practice nurses, and other healthcare professionals (including critical care nurses) with additional knowledge, skills, and demonstrated competence per professional licensure or institutional standard.

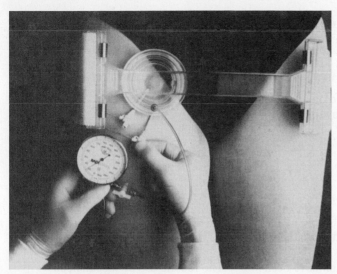

Figure 76-1 FemoStop in the correct position. *(From Barbiere C: A new device for control of bleeding after transfemoral catheterization,* Crit Care Nurse *15[1]:52, 1995.)*

- Suture removal kit
- ACT machine
- Readily available emergency medications (e.g., atropine), additional IV fluids, and resuscitation equipment

PATIENT AND FAMILY EDUCATION

- Explain the procedure to the patient and the family. *Rationale:* This explanation provides information and may help decrease anxiety and fear. This also encourages the patient to ask questions and voice concerns about the procedure.
- Explain the importance of bed rest, of not lifting the head off the pillow, of maintaining the head of the bed at no higher than 30 degrees, and of keeping the affected extremity straight after the procedure. *Rationale:* The patient is prepared for what to expect after the procedure, and patient cooperation is elicited to decrease the risk for bleeding, hematoma, and other vascular complications.
- Explain that the procedure may produce discomfort and that pressure will be felt at the site until hemostasis is achieved. Encourage the patient to report discomfort, and reassure the patient that analgesia and or sedation will be provided. *Rationale:* Explanation prepares the patient for what to expect and allays fears.
- After sheath removal, instruct the patient to report any warm, wet feeling, numbness, or pain at the puncture site. Also, instruct the patient to report any sensory or motor changes in the affected extremity. *Rationale:* This aids in the early recognition of complications and identifies the need for additional pain interventions.

PATIENT ASSESSMENT AND PREPARATION

Patient Assessment

- Assess the patient's medical history for bleeding disorders. *Rationale:* Bleeding disorders may increase the risk for bleeding or vascular complications.

- Assess the patient's platelet count, prothrombin time, with international normalized ratio, and partial thromboplastin time before sheath removal. *Rationale:* Laboratory results should be within acceptable limits (per institutional standards) to decrease the risk for bleeding after sheath removal.
- Assess the patient's complete blood count (CBC). *Rationale:* Assessment determines baseline data.
- Assess the patient's ACT before sheath removal. *Rationale:* Results should be within acceptable limits (per institutional standards) to decrease the risk for bleeding after sheath removal.
- Assess the patient's electrocardiographic rhythm and vital signs. *Rationale:* Baseline data are established. Collaborate with the physician or advanced practice nurse if the patient's blood pressure is elevated; elevated blood pressure may need to be treated before sheath removal to achieve and maintain hemostasis.
- Review the documented baseline assessment of the access site before vascular access, including assessment for presence or absence of bruit. *Rationale:* Baseline assessment data are established.
- Assess the extremity distal to the sheath for quality and strength of pulses, color, temperature, sensation, and movement. *Rationale:* Baseline assessment data are established before sheath removal.
- Assess for patency of the intravenous (IV) access and ensure that more than 500 mL of IV fluid remains in the IV bag or is readily available. *Rationale:* This assessment allows for emergency medication or fluids to be administered if necessary (e.g., vasovagal reaction).

Patient Preparation

- Verify that the patient is the correct patient using two identifiers. *Rationale:* Before performing a procedure, the nurse should ensure the correct identification of the patient for the intended intervention.
- Ensure that the patient and the family understand preprocedural teaching. Answer questions as they arise, and reinforce information as needed. *Rationale:* Understanding of previously taught information is evaluated and reinforced.
- Verify that the physician, advanced practice nurse, or other healthcare professional has placed an order stating when the femoral sheath can be removed. *Rationale:* Before performing a procedure, the nurse should determine the timing of removal of the femoral sheath.
- Mark the distal pulses with an indelible marker. *Rationale:* Marking facilitates the ability to locate pulses after the procedure.
- If a mechanical device is used to maintain pressure, position the device under the patient. *Rationale:* The device is positioned before sheath removal because patient movement must be minimized after sheath removal.

Procedure   for Arterial and Venous Sheath Removal

Steps	Rationale	Special Considerations
1. **HH**		
2. **PE**		
3. Place a blood pressure cuff on the patient's arm and obtain the patient's blood pressure.	Establishes a baseline blood pressure before sheath removal.	Monitor the patient's blood pressure every 5 minutes during arterial sheath removal until hemostasis is achieved. If possible, place the blood pressure cuff on the opposite arm of the IV to allow for uninterrupted flow of IV fluids.
4. Place the head of the patient's bed in the flat position.	Prepares the patient for the procedure and improves the ability to achieve hemostasis.	
5. Administer analgesia or sedation as prescribed. **(Level B*)**	Analgesia and sedation have been shown to reduce the discomfort associated with sheath removal.[15,31,34]	The routine use of subcutaneous lidocaine infiltrated around the catheter site has not been proven to reduce the discomfort associated with sheath removal.[8,15,31,34]
6. Turn off the arterial catheter alarm.	Monitoring is no longer needed; prevents the alarm from sounding.	
7. Open the suture-removal kit if the sheaths are sutured in place.	Prepares for sheath removal.	
8. If using a noninvasive hemostasis pad in conjunction with manual compression, open the pad using sterile technique.	Prepares for sheath removal and ensures sterility.	
9. Remove the arterial and venous sheath dressing.	Prepares for sheath removal.	
10. Clean the arterial and venous sites with an antiseptic solution (e.g., 2% chlorhexidine solution).	Decreases the risk for infection.[22]	Follow institutional standards.
11. Attach a 10-mL syringe to the blood-sampling port of the stopcock, turn the stopcock off to the flush bag, and gently draw back 5–10 mL of blood into the syringe.	Ensures there is no clot in the sheath.	Notify the physician or advanced practice nurse if unable to withdraw blood.
12. Remove and discard the nonsterile gloves and used supplies in the appropriate receptacle.	Removes and safely discards used supplies.	
13. **HH**		
14. Apply sterile gloves.	Maintains asepsis.	
15. Remove sutures, if present.	Prepares for sheath removal.	Additional stabilizing devices may be used and removed.
16. Palpate the femoral pulse.	Allows for more accurate positioning of the hemostasis option (manual or mechanical).	

*Level B: Well-designed, controlled studies with results that consistently support a specific action, intervention, or treatment.

Procedure	for Arterial and Venous Sheath Removal—*Continued*	
Steps	**Rationale**	**Special Considerations**
17. Determine the method that will be used to achieve hemostasis. **(Level B*)**	Both manual and mechanical compression devices are effective in achieving hemostasis and reducing the risk of groin complications.[5,7,13,23,24,27,33] Studies comparing arterial closure devices to either manual or mechanical compression are inconclusive regarding the optimal method of arterial closure in terms of vascular complications.[1,6,12,16,21,25,27,29]	Collagen plug devices, percutaneous suture-mediated closure devices, and percutaneous staple/clip closure devices are deployed into the artery by the physician at the end of the catheterization or interventional procedure.
18. Position the hemostasis option (manual or mechanical) 1–2 cm above the site where the arterial sheath enters the skin. (If using a noninvasive hemostasis pad in conjunction with manual pressure, **see Step 21.**) With manual pressure, ensure positioning with the arms straight down, directly over the femoral artery.	The arterial puncture site (arteriotomy) is superior and medial to the skin puncture site because the arterial sheath is inserted at a 45-degree angle. Body weight is used to apply firm pressure.	If the patient is obese or has a large abdomen, a second person may be needed to assist with sheath removal. Adjust the bed height for the comfort of the person holding manual pressure.
19. Simultaneously depress the hemostasis option (manual or mechanical) and gently remove the arterial sheath from the femoral artery during exhalation.	Prevents bleeding. Removing the arterial sheath during the exhalation phase of the respiratory cycle may prevent the patient from "bearing down" during arterial sheath removal.	Never withdraw the sheath if resistance is met. Notify the physician or advanced practice nurse.
20. Continue to apply firm pressure.	Firm pressure is needed to achieve hemostasis.	The distal pulse may decrease during application of full pressure but should not be completely obliterated. If manual compression is being performed, another person is needed to assess distal perfusion.
A. Maintain manual pressure above the arterial puncture site for approximately 20 minutes.	The length of time needed to achieve hemostasis depends on several factors, including the size of the sheath used; the type of procedure; the use of bivalirudin, heparin, or antiplatelet medications during the procedure; the ACT level at the time of sheath removal; and the patient's anatomy at the femoral insertion site. Patients who are hypertensive or obese may need a longer application of pressure.	Follow institution standard.

*Level B: Well-designed, controlled studies with results that consistently support a specific action, intervention, or treatment.

Procedure continues on following page

Procedure for Arterial and Venous Sheath Removal—*Continued*

Steps	Rationale	Special Considerations
B. Maintain the mechanical compression device. **(Level M*)**	Prevents bleeding.	With use of a mechanical device, set the pressure of the device according to manufacturer's recommendation and institutional standards. Tissue damage may occur if prolonged pressure is maintained (i.e., longer than 2–3 hours).[3] During mechanical compression, monitoring of the arterial puncture site and distal pulses is essential.
21. With use of a noninvasive hemostasis pad in conjunction with manual compression:		Follow manufacturer's guidelines.
A. Apply manual pressure 1–2 cm proximal to the skin insertion site **(see Step 18)**.	The arterial puncture site (arteriotomy) is superior and medial to the skin puncture site because the arterial sheath is inserted at a 45-degree angle.	
B. Place the noninvasive hemostasis pad directly over the puncture site before removing the sheath.	Prevents bleeding	
C. Remove the sheath.	Removes unneeded catheter.	
D. Reduce the proximal pressure to allow a small amount of blood from the arterial puncture site to moisten the noninvasive hemostasis pad; then quickly reapply the proximal manual pressure. **(Level M*)**	Noninvasive hemostasis pads must be moistened to activate the hemostatic mechanism.	
E. Hold firm manual pressure proximal to the skin insertion site and over the noninvasive hemostasis pad at the puncture site.	The arterial puncture site (arteriotomy) is superior and medial to the skin puncture site because the arterial sheath is inserted at a 45-degree angle.	
F. Gradually release the proximal pressure after 3–4 minutes; however, pressure should be maintained over the puncture site for at least 10 minutes.	Ensures hemostasis.	The total time of compression depends on the same factors listed for manual compression **(see Step 20 A)**.
G. Place a new sterile gauze over the hemostasis pad and cover with a sterile dressing.	Maintains asepsis.	The noninvasive hemostasis pad is left in place for 24 hours.
22. While achieving hemostasis, assess the circulation of the extremity distal to the site of the arterial sheath removal.	Verifies adequate circulation while hemostasis is achieved.	The pulse may decrease during application of full pressure but should not be completely obliterated. If manual compression is being performed, another person is needed to assess distal perfusion.

*Level M: Manufacturer's recommendations only.

Procedure	**for Arterial and Venous Sheath Removal—*Continued***	
Steps	**Rationale**	**Special Considerations**
23. With use of manual compression or mechanical compression, discontinue pressure once hemostasis is achieved.	Pressure is no longer needed.	With use of a mechanical device, follow manufacturer's recommendations, institutional standards, or physician prescription regarding the gradual reduction of pressure from the device. Notify the physician or advanced practice nurse if unable to achieve hemostasis.
24. When a venous sheath is in place, remove the venous sheath approximately 5–10 minutes after removal of the arterial sheath and maintain manual pressure over both sites for approximately 10 additional minutes or until hemostasis is achieved.[2,18]	Achieves both arterial and venous hemostasis. The arterial sheath is removed first because pressure needs to be applied to the arterial site longer than the venous site to achieve hemostasis. In addition, the venous line may be used to give additional IV fluids or medications, if needed (e.g., vasovagal reaction).	Follow manufacturer's guidelines and institutional standards. For example, if the FemoStop device is used, the venous sheath is removed first to reduce the risk of arteriovenous fistula formation.
		Collagen plug devices, percutaneous suture-mediated devices, and percutaneous staple/clip closure devices are not used for venous punctures.
		If a collagen plug device, a percutaneous suture-mediated or a staple/clip closure device is deployed in the arteriotomy immediately after the procedure, the venous sheath must still be removed with manual pressure applied for at least 10 minutes.
		Noninvasive hemostasis pads may be used in conjunction with manual pressure to achieve hemostasis for venous punctures.
25. After hemostasis is achieved, palpate the area around the arterial site.	Determines whether bleeding or a hematoma has occurred around the arterial site.	If bleeding or a hematoma is noted around the arterial site after hemostasis is achieved, apply manual pressure and notify the physician or advanced practice nurse.
26. Apply a sterile dressing to the arterial and/or venous sites.	Maintains asepsis.	Follow institutional standards for type of sterile dressing to be applied (transparent vs. pressure dressing). A sterile transparent dressing allows for easier assessment of the puncture site for bleeding or hematoma formation.[2,19]
27. Remove **PE** and sterile equipment and discard used supplies in appropriate receptacles.	Reduces the transmission of microorganisms; Standard Precautions.	
28. **HH**		

Procedure continues on following page

Expected Outcomes

- Arterial and venous sheaths removed with hemostasis achieved
- Adequate peripheral vascular and neurovascular integrity of the extremity distal to the site of sheath removal (positive sensation, movement, capillary refill, color, temperature, pulse)
- No evidence of peripheral vascular or neurovascular complications
- Cardiovascular and hemodynamic stability

Unexpected Outcomes

- Inability to remove the arterial or venous sheaths
- Inability to achieve hemostasis
- Impaired perfusion to the extremity distal to the site of sheath removal
- Impaired motor/sensory status of the extremity distal to the site of sheath removal
- Loss of arterial pulses distal to the site of sheath removal.
- Development of a hematoma or new bruit
- Development of a retroperitoneal bleed
- Development of a pseudoaneurysm or arteriovenous fistula
- Vasovagal response during the removal of the arterial sheath
- Hemodynamic instability
- Angina or shortness of breath
- Decrease in hemoglobin >2 g compared with preprocedure values
- Unrelieved pain

Patient Monitoring and Care

Steps	Rationale	Reportable Conditions
		These conditions should be reported if they persist despite nursing interventions.
1. Assess the peripheral vascular and neurovascular status of the affected extremity after arterial sheath removal: every 15 minutes × 4, every 30 minutes × 2, and then every 60 minutes × 4.	A thrombus, embolus, or dissection may precipitate changes in peripheral vascular or neurovascular status, necessitating early intervention.	• Change in strength of pulses in the affected extremity (diminished or absent) • Coldness or coolness of the distal extremity • Paresthesia in the affected extremity • Pallor, cyanosis of the affected extremity • Pain in the affected extremity • Decrease in mobility of the affected extremity
2. Obtain vital signs after removal of the arterial sheath every 15 minutes × 4, every 30 minutes × 2, and then every 60 minutes × 4.	Changes in vital signs may occur because of a vasovagal response or blood loss.	• Abnormal vital signs
3. Assess the puncture site every 15 minutes × 4, every 30 minutes × 2, and then every 60 minutes × 4, including assessment of presence or absence of bruit.	Detects presence of bleeding, hematoma, or bruit.	• Bleeding at arterial or venous sites • Hematoma development • New bruit • Pain at the access site
4. Monitor the electrocardiographic data during and after sheath removal.	Detects the presence of dysrhythmias. Bradydysrhythmias are common with vasovagal reactions.	• Dysrhythmias
5. After hemostasis is achieved, the head of the patient's bed can be elevated up to 30 degrees. **(Level B*)**	Minimizes back discomfort and does not increase vascular complications.[9,26]	• Occurrence of bleeding • Hematoma development • Abnormal vital signs • New bruit • Changes in peripheral vascular or neurovascular status • Back pain not relieved with position changes or analgesics

*Level B: Well-designed, controlled studies with results that consistently support a specific action, intervention, or treatment.

Patient Monitoring and Care —*Continued*

Steps	Rationale	Reportable Conditions
6. Maintain bed rest for 1–6 hours after hemostasis obtained when manual or mechanical pressure is used. **(Level B*)** With collagen plug devices, percutaneous suture-mediated closure devices, percutaneous staple/clip closure devices, and noninvasive hemostasis pads, the bed rest time is decreased to between 1 and 4 hours, depending on the manufacturer's recommendations; follow institutional standards.	Minimizes back discomfort, minimizes complications of prolonged bed rest, and does not increase vascular complications.[4,10,11,14,17,20,28,30,32,35] Bed rest times vary depending on the size of sheath used; the type of procedure; the use of bivalirudin, heparin, or antiplatelet medications during the procedure; and institutional standards.	• Occurrence of bleeding • Hematoma development • Abnormal vital signs • New bruit • Changes in peripheral vascular or neurovascular status • Back pain not relieved with position changes or analgesics
Maintain bed rest for 1–4 hours after venous sheath removal. Follow institutional standards.	Patients with venous punctures need less time in bed than with arterial punctures because the venous system is a lower-pressure system, so the incidence of vascular complications is decreased.	
7. Follow institutional standards for assessing pain. Administer analgesia as prescribed and reassess per institutional standards.	Identifies need for pain interventions.	• Continued pain despite pain interventions

*Level B: Well-designed, controlled studies with results that consistently support a specific action, intervention, or treatment.

Documentation

Documentation should include the following:
- Patient and family education
- Date and time of sheath removal
- Site of arterial and venous sheath removal
- Quality of arterial and venous sheaths removed (e.g., intact, cracked)
- Any difficulties with removal
- Patient tolerance of the procedure
- Pain assessment, interventions, and effectiveness
- Any medications administered
- Time hemostasis is obtained

- Method of hemostasis
- Site assessment after hemostasis is obtained, including presence or absence of a bruit
- Heart rate and rhythm, blood pressure, and respiratory rate
- Peripheral vascular and neurovascular checks to the affected extremity
- Occurrence of unexpected outcomes
- Nursing interventions
- Evaluation of any nursing intervention

References and Additional Readings

For a complete list of references and additional readings for this procedure, scan this QR code with any freely available smartphone code reader app, or visit http://booksite.elsevier.com/9780323376624.

77 Radial Arterial Sheath Removal

Rose B. Shaffer

PURPOSE: Radial arterial sheaths are placed for cardiac catheterizations and interventional procedures. Achieving and maintaining hemostasis after their removal is essential to prevent access-site complications.

PREREQUISITE NURSING KNOWLEDGE

- Knowledge of the radial and ulnar artery anatomy is important.
- Knowledge and skill regarding how to perform and interpret a modified Allen's test using plethysmography and oximetry is needed.
- The technique for the percutaneous insertion of the radial artery sheath should be understood.
- The importance of peripheral vascular and neurovascular assessment of the affected extremity should be understood.
- Knowledge that the radial artery access is sometimes associated with procedure failure (i.e., inability to access the radial artery or advance catheters) so that the femoral site may also be prepared for possible access.
- Knowledge that the radial artery sheath is removed with the use of a radial compression device at the end of the diagnostic or interventional procedure.
- Knowledge of the concept of patent hemostasis.
- Commercially available radial compression devices are available to assist achieving hemostasis. One device is the TR Band™, Radial Compression Device (Terumo Medical Corporation, Somerset, NJ) (Fig. 77-1).
- Technical and clinical competence in removal of the radial compression device is needed.
- Conditions that may influence the choice for radial access include the presence of bleeding disorders, current anticoagulant use, morbid obesity, and severe peripheral arterial disease.
- Contraindications to a radial approach include abnormal modified Allen's test (Barbeau test), absence of a radial pulse, the presence of a dialysis fistula, planned intraaortic balloon pump insertion, and severe vasospastic disease such as Raynaud's disease.
- Complications of radial artery sheath removal include the following:
  - ❖ External bleeding at the site
  - ❖ Internal bleeding (e.g., localized hematoma)
  - ❖ Vascular complications (e.g., radial artery occlusion from thrombus, embolus, dissection, or spasm; pseudoaneurysm; arteriovenous fistula; radial artery perforation)
  - ❖ Neurovascular complications (sensory or motor changes in the affected extremity)
  - ❖ Compartment syndrome

EQUIPMENT

- Cardiac monitoring system
- Blood pressure monitoring system
- Pulse oximeter sensor with monitor
- Antiseptic solution (e.g., 2% chlorhexidine-based preparation)
- Nonsterile gloves
- Protective eyewear
- Dressing supplies
- Commercially available inflatable bladder-based radial compression device
- 10-mL syringe or syringe supplied with the radial compression device

Additional equipment, to have available as needed, includes the following:
- Alcohol pads
- Selected analgesia and/or sedative as prescribed
- Portable Doppler ultrasound machine
- Armboard

PATIENT AND FAMILY EDUCATION

- Explain the procedure to the patient and the family. ***Rationale:*** This explanation provides information and may help decrease anxiety and fear. This also encourages the patient and family to ask questions and voice concerns about the procedure.
- Explain the importance of keeping the radial compression device on the affected wrist after the procedure for the prescribed timeframe to maintain hemostasis after the procedure. ***Rationale:*** The patient is prepared for what to expect after the procedure, and patient cooperation is elicited to decrease the risk for bleeding, hematoma, and other vascular complications.
- Explain that the procedure may produce discomfort and that pressure will be felt at the site until hemostasis is achieved. Encourage the patient to report discomfort, and reassure the patient that analgesia will be provided if needed. ***Rationale:*** Explanation prepares the patient for what to expect and allays fears.
- After radial arterial sheath removal, instruct the patient to report any warm, wet feeling or pain at the puncture site. Also, instruct the patient to report any sensory or motor changes in the affected extremity. ***Rationale:*** This aids in

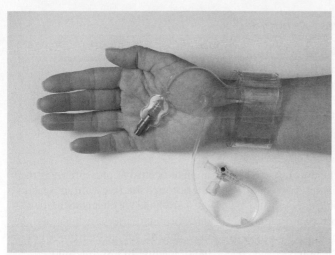

Figure 77-1 TR Band radial compression device. *(Courtesy Terumo Medical Corporation, Somerset, NJ.)*

the early recognition of complications and identifies the need for additional pain interventions.

PATIENT ASSESSMENT AND PREPARATION

Patient Assessment

- Assess the patient's complete blood count, platelet count, prothrombin time, with international normalized ratio, and partial thromboplastin time. *Rationale:* Laboratory results should be within acceptable limits (per institutional standard) to decrease the risk for bleeding after sheath removal.
- Assess the patient's electrocardiographic rhythm and vital signs. *Rationale:* Baseline data are established and determine hemodynamic stability.
- Review the documented baseline assessment of the extremity distal to the sheath for color, temperature, sensation, movement, and pulse oximetry waveform. *Rationale:* Baseline assessment data are established.

Patient Preparation

- Verify that the patient is the correct patient using two identifiers. *Rationale:* Before performing a procedure, the nurse should ensure the correct identification of the patient for the intended intervention.
- Ensure that the patient and the family understand preprocedural teaching. Answer questions as they arise, and reinforce information as needed. *Rationale:* Understanding of previously taught information is evaluated and reinforced.
- Ensure that the physician, advanced practice nurse, or other healthcare professional has placed an order stating when to begin removing air from the radial compression device. *Rationale:* Before performing a procedure, the nurse should determine when to begin removing air from the radial compression device.

Procedure	for Radial Arterial Sheath Removal	
Steps	**Rationale**	**Special Considerations**
1. HH		
2. PE		
3. At the completion of both diagnostic and interventional procedures, the radial artery compression device is placed around the wrist per manufacturer's recommendation (see Fig. 77-1).	Early discontinuation of the radial sheath can help reduce the risk of complications such as ischemia or thrombosis, which can lead to radial artery occlusion.[1]	There is no need to obtain an activated clotting time because the radial artery is more superficial and easier to compress than the femoral artery.[1,3,4]
4. Using a syringe, a prescribed amount of air is injected into the port to inflate the bladder (per physician preference and manufacturer guidelines), as the radial sheath is removed. Once the sheath is out, air is slowly removed using the syringe until a flash of blood is seen at the radial insertion site. Then another 1–2 cm³ of air is reinjected into the port.	Enough pressure is applied over the radial arteriotomy site to achieve patent hemostasis.	Some radial compression devices come with a special syringe only used for that specific device. Each compression device has a maximum amount of air that can be injected into the bladder. Do not exceed manufacturer guidelines for inflation. The patient will leave the procedure room with the compression device in place and the bladder inflated. An arm board may be used to prevent hyperflexion and hyperextension of the wrist.

Procedure continues on following page

Procedure   for Radial Arterial Sheath Removal—*Continued*

Steps	Rationale	Special Considerations
5. Place a blood pressure cuff on the opposite extremity to obtain the patient's blood pressure.	Avoids an increase in pressure on the affected radial artery.	
6. Place a pulse oximeter sensor on the thumb or index finger of the affected extremity and observe the waveform on the monitor.	Aids in determining adequate perfusion to the distal digits.	
7. Determine whether an adequate pulse oximetry waveform is present. **(Level B*)**	Patent (nonocclusive) hemostasis allows enough radial artery compression to result in hemostasis as well as maintain forward radial artery flow, to help reduce the risk of radial artery occlusion.[1,5–8]	Complete occlusive pressure over the arteriotomy site (e.g., a tight elastic pressure bandage) leads to higher rates of radial artery occlusion and may impede venous return to the hand, leading to swelling and discoloration of the hand and/or fingers.[2,3,8]
		If the waveform is dampened or absent, release air from the bladder using the syringe, per institutional standards or manufacturer guideline, until the waveform returns.
		If bleeding occurs during this time, reinflate the bladder to achieve hemostasis and immediately notify the physician or the advanced practice nurse.
8. Compress the ulnar artery of the affected extremity. If the waveform continues, blood flow in the radial artery is confirmed.	Absence of the waveform with ulnar artery compression confirms diminished or absent blood flow in the radial artery.	If the waveform is lost with ulnar artery compression, immediately notify the physician or the advanced practice nurse.
9. Determine the time the bladder of the radial compression device was inflated in the procedure room and the amount of air that was placed in the bladder.	Establishes baseline information and provides hand-off communication to the next physician, advanced practice nurse, or other healthcare professional for when to begin releasing the air (pressure) from the bladder.	A flow sheet may be used as a communication tool. Air (pressure) is released from the bladder at specific time increments.
10. Maintain the initial bladder compression for the prescribed time. **(Level M*)**	Maintains initial hemostasis.	Follow institutional standard and manufacturer guidelines for how long to maintain the initial bladder compression before beginning to release air from the bladder. The initial bladder compression may be longer for interventional procedures than for diagnostic procedures based on factors such as the amount of anticoagulation used and the sheath size. Initial bladder compression time may vary from 30 minutes to 2 hours.

*Level B: Well-designed, controlled studies with results that consistently support a specific action, intervention, or treatment.
*Level M: Manufacturer's recommendations only.

Procedure for Radial Arterial Sheath Removal—*Continued*

Steps	Rationale	Special Considerations
11. If no bleeding is noted, using the syringe, release the prescribed amount of air from the bladder at the specified intervals (i.e., remove 3 cm³ of air every 15 minutes) until all of the air is removed. **(Level M)**	Gradually decreases pressure and assesses the progress of hemostasis.	Follow institutional standards and manufacturer guidelines for time intervals and the amount of air to be released. When attaching the syringe to the connector, keep a finger on the plunger so that all the air does not escape at once. Some devices have a safety mechanism to prevent this from occurring.
12. If bleeding occurs at any point during the release of air from the bladder, reinject the specified amount of air (i.e., 3 cm³) for the specified time period (i.e., 15 minutes) and reassess hemostasis. If there is no bleeding after reinflation (i.e., 15 minutes), resume releasing air from the bladder (i.e., 3 cm³ of air every 15 minutes) according to institutional protocol or manufacturer guideline until all of the air is removed from the bladder.	Maintains hemostasis.	Follow manufacturer guideline and institutional standards.
13. When all the air is removed from the bladder and hemostasis is obtained, monitor the site for another 5 minutes with the compression device in place.	Determines that hemostasis is maintained.	If bleeding recurs, the bladder can be reinflated with the prescribed amount of air to achieve hemostasis.
14. Carefully remove the radial compression device.	Removes equipment.	
15. Clean the area with antiseptic solution and apply a dry sterile dressing.	Maintains asepsis.	Follow institutional standards.
16. The dressing should not encircle the entire wrist.	Avoids impaired arterial circulation and impaired venous return.	
17. Assess the area.	Determines whether there is any bleeding or hematoma.	If bleeding or hematoma is noted around the arterial site, apply manual pressure and notify the physician, advanced practice nurse, or physician assistant.
18. Remove **PE** and discard used supplies in the appropriate receptacles.	Reduces the transmission of microorganisms; Standard Precautions.	
19. **HH**		

Procedure continues on following page

Expected Outcomes

- Arterial sheath removed with hemostasis achieved before the patient leaves the procedure room and during deflation of the radial compression device's air bladder
- Adequate peripheral vascular and neurovascular integrity of the digits distal to the site of sheath removal (positive sensation, movement, capillary refill, color, temperature, radial and ulnar pulse, good pulse oximeter waveform with sensor on the thumb or index finger of the affected extremity)
- No evidence of peripheral vascular or neurovascular complications
- Cardiovascular and hemodynamic stability

Unexpected Outcomes

- Inability to achieve hemostasis during deflation of the radial compression device's air bladder
- Impaired perfusion to the digits distal to the site of sheath removal
- Impaired motor/sensory status of the extremity distal to the site of sheath removal
- Loss of the radial or ulnar pulse
- Development of a hematoma or new bruit
- Development of a pseudoaneurysm or arteriovenous fistula
- Development of a dampened or absent pulse oximeter waveform
- Hemodynamic instability
- Unrelieved pain

Patient Monitoring and Care

Steps	Rationale	Reportable Conditions
		These conditions should be reported if they persist despite nursing interventions.
1. Assess the peripheral vascular and neurovascular status of the affected extremity every 15 minutes while the compression device is in place. After the compression device is removed, assess every 15 minutes × 4, every 30 minutes × 2, and then every 60 minutes × 4.	Changes in peripheral vascular or neurovascular status may indicate radial artery occlusion or other complications.	• Change in strength of radial or ulnar pulse in the affected extremity (diminished or absent) • Coldness or coolness of the distal extremity • Sluggish capillary refill • Paresthesia in the affected extremity • Pallor, cyanosis of the affected extremity • Pain in the affected extremity • Decreased mobility of the affected extremity • Loss of the pulse oximetry waveform
2. Obtain vital signs after removal of the arterial sheath every 15 minutes × 4, every 30 minutes × 2, and then every 60 minutes × 4 (follow institutional protocol).	Determines hemodynamic stability or instability.	• Abnormal vital signs
3. Assess the puncture site every 15 minutes while the radial compression device is in place. Once it is removed, assess every 15 minutes × 4, every 30 minutes × 2, and then every 60 minutes × 4, including assessment of presence or absence of bruit (follow institutional protocol).	Detects presence of bleeding, hematoma, or bruit.	• Bleeding at arterial site • Hematoma development • New bruit

Patient Monitoring and Care —*Continued*

Steps	Rationale	Reportable Conditions
4. Monitor the pulse oximeter waveform (with the sensor on the thumb or forefinger of the affected extremity) after removal of the sheath every 15 minutes × 4, every 30 minutes × 2, and then every 60 minutes × 4 (follow institutional protocol).	Dampening or loss of the waveform may indicate radial artery occlusion.	• Dampening or loss of the pulse oximeter waveform
5. Monitor the electrocardiographic data during and after sheath removal.	Detects the presence of dysrhythmias.	• Dysrhythmias
6. The patient may raise the head of the bed to the desired level and may get out of bed with assistance.	Radial artery access does not require prolonged bed rest; therefore the head of the bed can be raised to a level of comfort and early mobility can be facilitated.	• Occurrence of bleeding • Hematoma development • Abnormal vital signs • New bruit • Changes in peripheral vascular or neurovascular status
7. Follow institutional standards for assessing pain. Administer analgesia as prescribed.	Identifies need for pain interventions.	• Continued pain despite pain interventions
8. Avoid obtaining blood for laboratory tests and avoid taking the patient's blood pressure in the affected extremity for 24 hours.	Avoids unnecessary pressure on the affected radial artery to promote healing and to prevent complications.	

Documentation

Documentation should include the following:
- Date and time of sheath removal and initial hemostasis in the procedure room
- Quality of arterial sheath removed (e.g., intact, cracked)
- Any difficulties with sheath removal
- Patient and family education
- Patient tolerance of the procedure
- Pain assessment, interventions, and effectiveness
- Any medications administered
- Any issues during radial compression device deflation (e.g. uncontrolled bleeding)
- Date and time radial compression device is removed
- Evidence of patent hemostasis
- Site assessment after hemostasis obtained and radial device removed, including presence or absence of a bruit
- Heart rate and rhythm, blood pressure, and respiratory rate
- Peripheral vascular and neurovascular checks to the affected extremity
- Occurrence of unexpected outcomes
- Nursing interventions
- Evaluation of any nursing intervention

References and Additional Readings

For a complete list of references and additional readings for this procedure, scan this QR code with any freely available smartphone code reader app, or visit http://booksite.elsevier.com/9780323376624.

78

Pericardial Catheter Management

Kathleen M. Cox

PURPOSE: Placement of an indwelling pericardial catheter allows for the slow and/or intermittent evacuation of fluid from the pericardial space. An indwelling pericardial catheter also allows for the infusion of medications (e.g., antibiotics or chemotherapeutic agents) into the pericardial space.

PREREQUISITE NURSING KNOWLEDGE

- Knowledge of anatomy and physiology of the cardiovascular system, to include understanding of the principles of cardiac conduction, electrocardiogram (ECG) lead placement, and dysrhythmia interpretation.
- Knowledge and skills related to aseptic technique is necessary.
- Advanced cardiac life support (ACLS) knowledge and skills.
- The pericardial space normally contains 20 to 50 mL of fluid.
- Pericardial fluid has electrolyte and protein profiles similar to plasma.
- Pericardial effusion is generally defined as the accumulation of fluid within the pericardial sac that exceeds the stretch capacity of the pericardium, generally more than 50 to 100 mL.[12]
- Intrapericardial fluid accumulation can be acute or chronic and therefore it varies in presentation of symptoms. Acute effusions are usually a rapid collection of fluid occurring over minutes to hours and may result in hemodynamic compromise with volumes less than 250 mL.[8] Chronically developing effusions occurring over days to weeks allow for hypertrophy and distention of the fibrous pericardial membrane. Patients with chronic effusions may accumulate greater than or equal to 2000 mL of fluid before exhibiting symptoms of hemodynamic compromise.[8]
- Symptoms of cardiac tamponade are nonspecific, so the diagnosis relies on clinical suspicion and associated signs and symptoms. Acute pericardial effusions are usually a result of trauma, myocardial infarction, or iatrogenic injury, whereas chronic effusions can result from conditions such as bacterial or viral pericarditis, cancer, autoimmune disorders, uremia, etc.[2] With a decrease in cardiac output, the patient often develops chest pain, dyspnea, tachycardia, tachypnea, pallor, cyanosis, impaired cerebral and renal function, diaphoresis, hypotension, neck vein distention, distant or faint heart sounds, and pulsus paradoxus.[6]
- Pericardiocentesis is an effective treatment for pericardial effusion (see Procedures 42 and 43). For chronic or rapidly accumulating effusions, an indwelling pericardial catheter may be placed for continuous or intermittent drainage of excess fluid.

- The pericardial catheter may be connected to a closed drainage system (Fig. 78-1).
- The pericardial catheter may also be left in place to facilitate the infusion of medications (e.g., antibiotics, chemotherapeutic agents) depending on the patient's clinical manifestations.
- An indwelling catheter should usually be removed within 48 to 72 hours after placement to avoid risk of infection or iatrogenic pericarditis.[4] Depending on the patient's underlying condition, the catheter may be left in place for longer periods to facilitate resolution of pericardial effusion, cardiac tamponade, or infusion of medication.[8] Pericardial catheters should be removed immediately for any signs of infection or an abrupt rise in white blood cell count.[9]
- Pericardial catheters are generally removed when the pericardial drainage decreases to less than 25 to 30 mL for the preceding 24-hour period.[6]
- Extended catheter drainage is associated with a reduction of the reoccurrence of cardiac tamponade compared with a single pericardiocentesis in patients with pericardial effusion related to malignancy.[10]

EQUIPMENT

- Pericardial catheter
- Sterile drapes: 4 small drapes and a full-body drape
- Sterile and nonsterile gloves, gowns, masks, protective eyewear
- Sterile 0.9% normal saline (NS) solution for irrigation and sterile basin
- Sterile syringes: 3-, 5-, 30-, or 60-mL Luer-Lok
- Sterile 1000-mL vacuum bottle available for the initial procedure
- Antiseptic solution (e.g., 2% chlorhexidine-based preparation)
- Sterile 4 × 4 gauze
- Sterile transparent occlusive dressing
- Adhesive tape
- Sterile three-way Luer-Lok stopcock with nonvented caps and replacement caps
- Drainage tubing
- Pericardial drainage bag

Additional equipment, to have available as needed, includes the following:

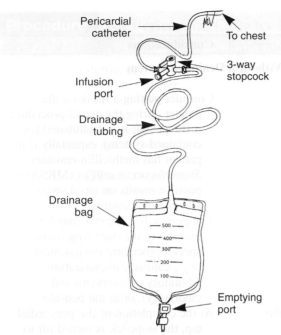

Figure 78-1 Indwelling pericardial catheter system. *(From Hammel WJ: Care of patients with an indwelling pericardial catheter; Crit Care Nurs 18[5]:40–45, 1998.)*

- Anticoagulant flush available for dwell if prescribed (i.e., heparin)
- Cytotoxic disposal receptacle (when chemotherapeutic or cytotoxic agents are prescribed; also used to avoid aerosolization of the medication once disconnected from the patient)
- Emergency cart (defibrillator, emergency respiratory equipment, emergency cardiac medications)

PATIENT AND FAMILY EDUCATION

- Explain to the patient and family the reason necessitating the indwelling pericardial catheter (e.g., relief of pressure on the heart). *Rationale:* Communication of pertinent information helps the patient and family to understand the procedure and the potential risks and benefits, subsequently reducing anxiety and apprehension.[1]
- Discuss potential discomfort the catheter may cause with inspiration and the insertion site. Reassure patient and family that pain medication will be prescribed and administered as necessary. *Rationale:* This explanation prepares and informs the patient of the pain-management plan and reassures the patient that pain management is a priority.
- Instruct the patient and family about the patient's risk for recurrent pericardial effusion, describing the potential

signs and symptoms (e.g., dyspnea, dull ache or pressure within the chest, dysphagia, cough, tachypnea, hoarseness, hiccups, or nausea).[5,6] *Rationale:* Early recognition of signs and symptoms of recurrent pericardial effusion may prompt detection of a potentially life-threatening problem.

PATIENT ASSESSMENT AND PREPARATION

Patient Assessment

- Assess the patient's neurological, cardiovascular, and hemodynamic status including heart rate, cardiac rhythm, heart sounds (S_1, S_2, rubs, murmurs), blood pressure (BP), mean arterial pressure, peripheral pulses, oxygen saturation via pulse oximetry, respiratory status, and if available, pulmonary artery pressures, pulmonary artery occlusion pressure (PAOP), right-atrial pressure (RAP), cardiac output (CO) and cardiac index (CI), and systemic vascular resistance. *Rationale:* Provides baseline data.
- Assess the patient for dyspnea, tachypnea, tachycardia, muffled heart sounds, precordial dullness to percussion, or impaired consciousness; hypotension (systolic BP <100 mm Hg or decreased from patient's baseline); increased jugular venous pressure/jugular distention; pulsus paradoxus (inspiratory decrease in systolic BP amplitude) greater than 12 to 15 mm Hg; equalization of RAP, PAOP, and pulmonary artery diastolic pressure; and decreased CO/CI.[2] *Rationale:* Assessment of these signs and symptoms of possible cardiac tamponade is essential for identification of potential complications and catheter patency.
- Determine the patient's allergy history (e.g., heparin, antiseptic solutions). *Rationale:* This assessment decreases the risk for allergic reactions by avoiding known allergenic products.

Patient Preparation

- Confirm that the patient and family understand preprocedural teaching by having them verbalize understanding. Clarify key points by reinforcing important information and answer all questions. *Rationale:* Preprocedure communication provides a framework of patient expectations, enhances cooperation, and reduces anxiety.[1]
- Verify that the patient is the correct patient using two patient-specific identifiers. *Rationale:* The nurse should always ensure the correct identification of the patient for the intended intervention for patient safety.

Procedure   for Pericardial Catheter Management—*Continued*

Steps	Rationale	Considerations
H. Attach the prescribed medication (either infusion or syringe). With the use of a syringe for delivery, gently instill the medication. If using an infusion pump, set the appropriate medication infusion rate.	Administers the medication as prescribed.	Infusion of the medication may activate signs and symptoms of cardiac tamponade.[11] Monitor vital signs and ECG tracing while infusing the medication to assess response of the patient. If the patient has any abnormal signs or symptoms, stop the infusion and notify the advanced practice nurse or the physician.
I. Turn the stopcock off to the patient when the medication delivery is complete.	Stops the medication administration.	
J. Disconnect the tubing or syringe.	Removes the equipment.	
K. Attach a flush syringe of 0.9% NS.	Prepares the equipment.	
L. Turn the stopcock open to the patient and gently flush the catheter.	Ensures the medication is completely in the pericardium and none remains in the catheter.	
M. Turn the stopcock off to the patient and apply a sterile nonvented cap to the infusion port.	Closes and maintains the integrity of the system.	
N. Allow the medication to dwell for the prescribed time.	Allows time for the medication to act.	
O. When the dwell time is complete, remove the infusion port cap and attach a syringe large enough to retrieve the medication plus the pericardial fluid accumulation.	Prepares the equipment.	
P. Gently withdraw the medication and pericardial drainage.	Removes the medication.	Volume of the retrieved fluid should be equivalent to the volume of medication that was instilled, plus the flush solution and additional pericardial fluid that accumulated during the dwell time.
Q. Turn the stopcock off to the patient and disconnect the syringe.	Removes the equipment.	
R. Attach a flush syringe of 2–5 mL of 0.9% NS with or without heparin as prescribed.[3,8]	Prepares the equipment.	
S. Turn the stopcock open to the patient and instill the 0.9% NS or heparin flush.	Clears the pericardial catheter.	
T. Turn the stopcock off to the patient, remove the flush syringe, and apply a sterile nonvented cap to the infusion port.	Closes the pericardial catheter system and maintains the integrity of the closed system.	

Procedure	**for Pericardial Catheter Management—*Continued***	
Steps	**Rationale**	**Considerations**
U. Remove [PE] and discard used supplies in the appropriate receptacles.		Discard any antineoplastic or cytotoxic agent, tubing, and flush syringes in the designated biohazard receptacle.
V. [HH]		

General Management of the Patient With a Pericardial Catheter Closed Drainage System

1. [HH]		
2. [PE]		
3. Assist the physician or advanced practice nurse with the pericardiocentesis (see Procedures 42 and 43).	Provides assistance as needed.	The pericardial catheter may be inserted in the operating room, in a special procedure environment (e.g., cardiac catheterization laboratory or interventional laboratory), or at the bedside.
4. Determine that the connections between the pericardial catheter and the stopcock are tight.	Ensures the integrity of the system.	At the completion of the pericardial tap, a nonvented sterile cap is placed on the stopcock port and the stopcock is turned off to the patient or open to drainage as prescribed.
5. Position the drainage-collection receptacle lower than the catheter-insertion point to facilitate drainage, and observe the fluid for color, amount, and consistency.	Ensures pericardial catheter patency. The presence of fibrin matrix in the drainage can result in obstruction of the catheter and be problematic for future manual taps.	Pericardial fluid is commonly straw-colored, serous drainage. A 2D or Doppler echocardiogram can be performed after the pericardiocentesis to assess for reaccumulation of pericardial fluid.[8]
6. Perform catheter-site care.	Helps prevent infection.	Observe the site for any evidence of drainage and notify the physician or advanced practice nurse of this finding.
A. [HH]		
B. [PE]		
C. Remove the dressing and discard it in an appropriate receptacle.	Allows for site assessment and prepares for site care.	
D. Assess the catheter and insertion site.	Assesses for signs and symptoms of infection.	
E. Remove and discard the nonsterile gloves in an appropriate receptacle.	Maintains aseptic technique.	
F. [HH]		
G. Apply sterile gloves and establish a sterile field.		
H. Cleanse the skin around the pericardial catheter-insertion site using a back and forth motion while applying friction for 30 seconds with an antiseptic solution (e.g., 2% chlorhexidine-based solution).[3,4] Allow the antiseptic to remain on the insertion site and to air dry completely.[9,11] **(Level D*)**	Reduces the rate of colonization of skin microflora. The Centers for Disease Control and Prevention (CDC) do not have a specific recommendation for care of pericardial catheters or site care.	

*Level D: Peer-reviewed professional and organizational standards with the support of clinical study recommendations.

Procedure continues on following page

Procedure for Pericardial Catheter Management—*Continued*

Steps	Rationale	Considerations
I. Determine whether the catheter and stopcock are securely anchored to the chest.	Ensures a secure system.	
J. Apply a sterile, occlusive dressing over the catheter-insertion site. Label the dressing with the date, time and initials of the person performing the dressing change.	Provides a sterile environment. Identifies the last dressing change.	
K. Remove **PE** and discard used supplies in the appropriate receptacle.		
L. **HH**		
7. *If pericardial fluid removal is desired:* intermittently or continuously drain the pericardial fluid as prescribed by turning the stopcock off to the infusion port and open between the patient and the drainage bag (see Fig. 78-1).	Removes pericardial fluid.	Follow institutional standards regarding personnel permitted to aspirate and flush pericardial catheters (e.g., registered nurses, advanced practice nurses, physicians).
A. *Intermittent drainage:* If intermittent drainage is prescribed, the stopcock is usually off to the patient and opened every 4–6 hours to drainage or as clinically indicated with Doppler scan or 2D echocardiogram and patient presentation until the accumulation of fluid is resolved (follow the prescribed regimen).		
B. *Continuous drainage:* If continuous drainage is prescribed, the stopcock remains open between the patient and the drainage bag and off to the infusion port (follow the prescribed regimen).		
C. Empty the pericardial drainage bag every 8 hours or sooner if prescribed.	Reduces the possibility of colonization in the bag and the potential reflux of fluid to the patient.	Pericardial fluid samples may be collected for selected diagnostic tests.
i. **HH**		
ii. **PE**		
iii. Turn the stopcock off to the patient.	Reduces risk of pneumopericardium.	
iv. Open the emptying port of the drainage bag and drain the pericardial fluid into a receptacle for measurement and waste disposal.	Discard drainage.	

Procedure	for Pericardial Catheter Management—*Continued*	
Steps	**Rationale**	**Considerations**
v. Close the port and secure the drainage bag.	Closes and maintains integrity of the system.	
vi. Resume the prescribed drainage mode.	Continues prescribed treatment.	
D. After completion of intermittent fluid drainage, temporarily turn the stopcock off to the patient for the flush procedure.	Prepares for the procedure.	
i. **HH**		
ii. **PE**		
iii. Remove the infusion port cap and cleanse the infusion port at the top of the stopcock with an antiseptic solution for 15 seconds and allow to dry.[3,4,9,11]	Reduces risk of infection.	
iv. Connect the flush syringe, turn the stopcock open to the syringe and patient, and gently flush the pericardial catheter with 2–5 mL of sterile NS solution or heparinized saline solution as prescribed (use NS if the patient is sensitive to heparin).	Clears the pericardial catheter and maintains catheter patency.	
v. Turn the three-way stopcock off to the patient and disconnect the flush syringe.	Maintains integrity of the closed system and minimizes risk of pneumopericardium.	
vi. Place a new sterile nonvented cap on the infusion port.	Maintains asepsis.	
vii. Remove **PE** and discard used supplies in appropriate receptacles.		
viii. **HH**		
8. *If the pericardial catheter is blocked or obstructed to flow:*		Follow institutional standards regarding personnel permitted to aspirate and flush pericardial catheters (e.g., registered nurses, advanced practice nurses, physicians).
A. **HH**		
B. **PE**		
C. Determine whether the drainage system is lower than the insertion point and reposition if needed.	Facilitates drainage by gravity.	

Procedure continues on following page

Procedure   for Pericardial Catheter Management—*Continued*

Steps	Rationale	Considerations

D. Examine the catheter to determine whether there is an external mechanical cause of the pericardial catheter blockage, and correct if present. Consider the following:
  i. Kinks in tubing.
  ii. Tubing may be compressed underneath patient.
  iii. Turn or reposition patient to facilitate flow.
	Relieves mechanical obstruction to flow.	

E. Assess for loose tubing connections and, if loosened, tighten connections.	Ensures intact drainage system.	
F. Determine correct positioning of the stopcock. If needed, correct the stopcock position.	Facilitates unobstructed fluid drainage.	
G. If the previous steps do not correct the obstruction to flow, do the following: i. Remove the infusion port cap and cleanse the infusion port at the top of the stopcock with an antiseptic solution for 15 seconds and allow to dry.[3,4,9,11]	Decreases the risk of infection.	
ii. Connect the flush syringe, turn the stopcock open to the syringe and patient, and gently flush the pericardial catheter with 2–5 mL of sterile NS solution or heparinized saline solution as prescribed (use NS if patient is sensitive to heparin).	Attempts to improve pericardial catheter patency. Heparinized saline solution may be used for a dwell if the drainage tends to be serous or fibrous in consistency.[7]	Monitor vital signs and ECG tracing while flushing the pericardial catheter to assess patient response. Follow institutional standards for administration of dwell solution, if prescribed.
iii. Turn the stopcock off to the infusion port and allow the fluid to passively drain or turn the stopcock off to the drainage bag and gently attempt to aspirate the flush solution through the attached syringe.	Allows drainage of flush solution and pericardial fluid.	Volume of the drained fluid should be equivalent to the volume of the flush solution and additional accumulated pericardial fluid; deduct the amount of flush used to accurately measure output.
iv. Determine whether the pericardial catheter is draining and patent.	Assesses patency of the system.	
v. If the previous measures are ineffective for drainage but the catheter itself is patent, consider changing the tubing and the drainage-bag system.	Ensures integrity of the system and may facilitate drainage.	Ensure the stopcock is off to the patient at the time of the change.

Procedure for Pericardial Catheter Management—*Continued*		
Steps	**Rationale**	**Considerations**
vi. After the tubing/bag change, assess the patency of the system.	Determines whether the system is functioning.	
vii. If these measures do not remove the catheter blockage, notify the physician or advanced practice nurse immediately.	Additional interventions are necessary.	Accumulation of fluid in the pericardium without the possibility of drainage may result in tamponade.
viii. Remove **PE** and discard used supplies in appropriate receptacles.		
ix. **HH**		
9. *If medications are prescribed for infusion into the pericardium:*		Follow institutional standards for **PE** when administering cytotoxic or antineoplastic medications. Follow institutional standards regarding personnel permitted to instill medications into the pericardial sac.
A. **HH**		
B. **PE**		
C. Review the prescribed medication, dose, method of delivery, amount, and time for dwell. Assemble the medication, tubing, pump or syringe, and two flush syringes of 0.9% NS (2–5 mL each).[3,7]	Ensures the accuracy of medication administration.	
D. Turn the stopcock off to the patient, remove the infusion port cap, and cleanse the infusion port at the top of the stopcock with an antiseptic solution for 15 seconds and allow to dry.[3,4,9,11]	Reduces risk of infection.	
E. Turn the stopcock off to the drainage bag. Attach the prescribed medication (either infusion or syringe).	Prevents inadvertent instillation of medication into the drainage bag.	
F. With the use of a syringe for delivery, gently instill the medication as prescribed. If using an infusion pump, set the appropriate medication-infusion rate. (Patency of the catheter is established by virtue of evident drainage. If there is a question about catheter patency, follow the flush procedure listed in the medication infusion section of General Management of the Patient with a Pericardial Catheter without a Drainage System.)	Administers the medication.	Infusion of the medication may activate signs and symptoms of cardiac tamponade.[11] Monitor vital signs and ECG tracing while infusing the medication to assess patient response. If the patient has abnormal signs and symptoms, stop the infusion and notify the advanced practice nurse or the physician.

Procedure continues on following page

Procedure   for Pericardial Catheter Management—*Continued*

Steps	Rationale	Considerations
G. If the medication is to dwell in the pericardial space before reestablishment of pericardial drainage:		
i. Turn the stopcock off to the patient at the completion of the infusion.		
ii. Disconnect the medication syringe or tubing.		
iii. Attach a syringe with 2–5 mL of 0.9% NS flush and turn the stopcock off to the drainage bag.		
iv. Gently flush the catheter and turn the stopcock off to the patient for the completion of the dwell time as prescribed.	Ensures that the medication is instilled in the pericardial space and does not lie in the catheter.	
v. Disconnect the syringe and close system with a sterile nonvented cap.		
vi. After the dwell time is complete, turn the stopcock off to the infusion port and open to drainage.	Allows pericardial drainage to resume.	The drain time should allow for all of the medication to exit the pericardium.
vii. Measure the amount of the solution infused and the drainage collected.		Volume of the drained fluid should be equivalent to the volume of the medication instilled, the flush solution, and additional accumulated pericardial fluid; deduct the amount of medication infused and flush used to accurately measure output.
viii. Resume the prescribed drainage mode: continuous or intermittent. If intermittent, follow the prescription for the drain time after infusion.		
a. Once the drain time is completed, clean the infusion port of the stopcock with an alcohol swab for 15 seconds.[3,4,9,11]	Reduces the risk for infection.	
b. Connect the flush syringe, turn the stopcock open to the syringe and patient, and gently flush the pericardial catheter with 2–5 mL of sterile NS solution or heparinized saline solution as prescribed (use NS if the patient is sensitive to heparin).	Helps to maintain the pericardial catheter patency.	

Procedure for Pericardial Catheter Management—*Continued*

Steps	Rationale	Considerations
c. Turn the stopcock off to the patient until the next time the patient is due for intermittent drainage. d. Remove **PE** and discard used supplies in appropriate receptacles. e. **HH**	Maintains integrity of the system.	

Expected Outcomes

- Patent pericardial drainage system
- Resolution of pericardial effusion
- Hemodynamic stability
- Patient free of infection
- Patient free of pain and anxiety
- Medications administered as prescribed

Unexpected Outcomes

- Infection
- Pain
- Catheter obstruction
- Reaccumulation of pericardial fluid
- Cardiac tamponade and hemodynamic instability
- Dysrhythmias
- Cardiac arrest

Patient Monitoring and Care

Steps	Rationale	Reportable Conditions
		These conditions must be reported if they persist despite nursing interventions
1. Perform cardiovascular and hemodynamic assessments at least every 60 minutes and as patient condition necessitates, or as prescribed	Assesses for signs of cardiac tamponade and determines hemodynamic stability.	• Signs of cardiac tamponade: dyspnea, tachypnea, tachycardia, hypotension, increased jugular venous pressure, pulsus paradoxus, muffled heart sounds, precordial dullness to percussion, altered level of consciousness. • Equalization of RAP, PAOP • CI <2.5 L/min/m^2 • Dysrhythmias
2. Assess the patency of the pericardial catheter: A. Without a closed drainage system, every 4–6 hours, and as needed or as prescribed. B. With a closed drainage system, every hour, and as needed or as prescribed.	Pericardial catheter blockage may predispose the patient to excessive accumulation of pericardial fluid that may lead to cardiac tamponade and/or hemodynamic instability.	• Inability to obtain pericardial drainage or cessation of pericardial drainage • Signs and symptoms of cardiac tamponade or hemodynamic instability • Evidence of accumulation of pericardial fluid on Doppler or 2D echocardiography
3. Assess the amount and type of fluid draining from the pericardial catheter.	Provides information regarding the continued need for the catheter and potential problems.	• Change in the amount, color, or consistency of pericardial drainage from patient's baseline
4. Change the pericardial catheter dressing every 24 hours.[4]	Provides an opportunity to assess for signs and symptoms of infection. Infective pericarditis is associated with increased mortality and morbidity rates.[10] The CDC recommends replacing dressings on intravascular catheters when the dressing becomes damp, loosened, or soiled or when inspection of the site is necessary.[4]	• Elevated white blood cell counts • Elevated temperature • Signs and symptoms of infection at the insertion site (e.g., pain, erythema, drainage, etc.)

Procedure continues on following page

Patient Monitoring and Care —*Continued*

Steps	Rationale	Reportable Conditions
5. If in use, change the pericardial tubing and drainage bag every 72 hours.[3,8]	Reduces the risk of infection.	
6. Follow institutional standards for assessing pain and administer analgesia as prescribed.	Identifies need for pain interventions. The patient may experience chest pain or pleuritic type pain while the pericardial catheter is in place.	• Continued pain despite interventions
7. Identify parameters that demonstrate clinical readiness for removal of the indwelling pericardial catheter.[8,13]	Facilitates early removal of the pericardial catheter and reduces the risk of infection.	• Pericardial drainage <25–30 mL over the previous 24 hours[12] • Hemodynamic stability as evidenced by systolic BP >100 mm Hg, CI >2.5 L/min/m², absence of pulsus paradoxus, no equalization of RAP, PA diastolic pressure, and PAOP • Absence of pericardial effusion on Doppler or 2D echocardiography[13]
8. Identify situations in which the pericardial effusion cannot be resolved with use of pericardial drainage via tap or closed system.[10]	Additional interventions may be needed.	• Hemodynamic instability • Continued pericardial effusion

Documentation

Documentation should include the following:
- Patient and family education
- Universal Protocol requirements
- Patient tolerance of the indwelling pericardial catheter
- Dressing, tubing, and drainage bag changes
- Amount of pericardial drainage each shift, including net volumes when catheter is flushed or medications are infused
- Volumes of injectate or aspirate
- Characteristics of the pericardial drainage: color, consistency, and/or changes
- Hemodynamic status
- Pain assessment, interventions, and effectiveness
- Occurrence of unexpected outcomes/treatments
- Nursing interventions

References and Additional Readings

For a complete list of references and additional readings for this procedure, scan this QR code with any freely available smartphone code reader app, or visit http://booksite.elsevier.com/9780323376624.

79 Thenar Tissue Oxygen Saturation Monitoring

Kathleen Berns

PURPOSE: Thenar tissue oxygen saturation monitoring is a noninvasive technique to measure an approximated value of percent hemoglobin oxygen saturation in the tissue and is a measure of tissue perfusion status.

PREREQUISITE NURSING KNOWLEDGE

- Tissue oxygen saturation (StO_2) is the measure of hemoglobin oxygen saturation of the microcirculation.
- Oxygen saturation of arterial blood SaO_2 measures and SpO_2 estimates O_2 saturation in the arteries.
- Central venous oxygen saturation ($ScvO_2$) measures O_2 saturation in the superior vena cava.
- Mixed venous oxygen saturation (SvO_2) measures O_2 saturation in the pulmonary artery.
- Tissue oxygenation (StO_2) measures O_2 saturation in the microcirculation, where O_2 diffuses into tissue cells. It is a direct measure of tissue oxygenation and a sensitive indicator of tissue perfusion status (Fig. 79-1).
- StO_2 is measured at the thenar muscle, which is a peripheral muscle. During shock, blood flow to peripheral muscles and core organs (liver, gut, and kidneys) is reduced in order to preserve brain and heart oxygenation. StO_2 measured at the thenar eminence allows noninvasive monitoring of early changes in perfusion status during shock and resuscitation.
- The thenar site is minimally affected by age, gender, edema, and adipose and is not confounded by hypothermia.[1-3]
- Low StO_2 is associated with poor outcomes such as organ dysfunction and mortality; thus further assessment data should be obtained.[4-8]
- Monitoring the StO_2 trend may guide fluid resuscitation (Fig. 79-2).
- Low StO_2 readings can be present even when vital signs are stable.[8,9]
- Patients who may benefit from the use of StO_2 include the following:
  - High-acuity elderly such as those over 65 years old with shortness of breath, chest pain, abdominal pain, weakness, or syncope.[9]
  - Trauma patients of any age in which the mechanism of injury puts them at risk for bleeding.[8,9]
  - Trauma patients who require massive blood transfusion.[10]
  - All patients who are at risk for bleeding or are suspected of having internal bleeding.[8,9]
  - Patients undergoing resuscitation and who are requiring active treatment.[11]
  - Patients being assessed in the prehospital environment where laboratory tests may not be available.[7,12]
- StO_2 monitoring should not be used in the presence of ionizing radiation such as computed tomography (CT) or x-ray. Exposure to ionized radiation will cause cumulative damage to the device resulting in inaccurately low readings. Also, remove the sensor from the patient before magnetic resonance imaging (MRI).

EQUIPMENT

- Tissue oxygenation monitor
- Tissue oxygen disposable sensor or nondisposable clip
- Soap and water or antiseptic solution to cleanse the thenar eminence
- Nonsterile gloves

Additional equipment, to have available as needed, includes the following:

- Batteries

PATIENT AND FAMILY EDUCATION

- Assess patient and family readiness to learn and identify factors that affect learning. *Rationale:* This assessment allows the nurse to individualize teaching.
- Provide information about StO_2 monitoring. *Rationale:* This information helps the patient and family to understand the procedure and why it is needed and may decrease anxiety.
- Explain the displayed values and possible alarms of the monitor. Explain that values may change depending on the sensor positioning and light that may affect the sensor. *Rationale:* This information will help the patient and family know what to expect.

PATIENT ASSESSMENT AND PREPARATION

Patient Assessment

- Assess the patient for signs and symptoms of hypoperfusion, including cyanosis, tachypnea, tachycardia, altered level of consciousness, hypotension, decreased

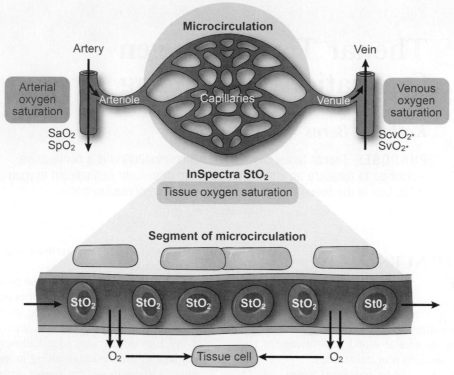

Figure 79-1 Tissue oxygen saturation is measured in the microcirculation where oxygen is exchanged with tissue. *(From Hutchinson Technology pamphlet,* What is InSpectra Sto₂, *2008.)*

urine output, mottling of the lower extremities **Rationale:** Sto₂ monitoring is useful in the early detection of hypoperfusion and can lead to earlier treatment.

- Assess the thenar eminence. **Rationale:** Determines skin integrity.

Patient Preparation

- Verify that the patient is the correct patient using two identifiers. **Rationale:** Before performing a procedure, the

nurse should ensure the correct identification of the patient for the intended intervention.

- Ensure the patient and family understand preprocedural teaching. Answer questions as they arise and reinforce information as needed. **Rationale:** This communication evaluates and reinforces understanding of previously taught information.

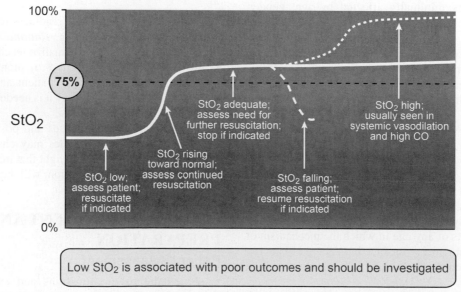

Figure 79-2 It is important to watch the tissue oxygen saturation trend when assessing and treating the patient. *(From Hutchinson Technology website, Education Resources, 2008.)*

Procedure for Thenar Tissue Oxygenation (Sto₂) Monitoring

Steps	Rationale	Special Considerations
1. **HH**		
2. **PE**		
3. Determine whether continuous tissue monitoring will be performed or if a single measurement will be obtained.	A single measurement can be used to quickly assess tissue perfusion. Continuous Sto₂ monitoring is useful in guiding treatments.	The spot-check device has a clip-type cable that is not disposable. The continuous monitor has a sensor cable that attaches firmly to the thenar eminence and is for single patient use. Follow prescribed order for tissue monitoring or institutional standard.
4. Clean and dry the palm and thenar eminence.	The thenar eminence needs to be clean and dry in order for the sensor to adhere to the skin. The sensors also need a clean area so that monitoring is accurate.	Avoid placing the sensor over a hematoma and skin obscured by ink such as tattoos, markers, or pens.
5. Plug the monitor into a grounded wall outlet or ensure that a fully charged battery is installed.	Prepares the equipment.	
6. Attach the optical cable to the Sto₂ monitor.	Prepares the equipment.	Carefully align the pins when connecting the optical cable to the monitor to avoid bending the pins.
7. Press the power button on the monitor.	Prepares the equipment. The start-up time is approximately 30 seconds.	The equipment does not need to be calibrated.
8. Apply the continuous monitoring sensor or clip the nondisposable sensor to the palm and thenar eminence (Fig. 79-3).	Ensure the sensor is attached to the patient to avoid high ambient light conditions that may result in the device not being able to take a measurement or provide inaccurate measurements.	Approximately 20 seconds is needed before determining a value.
9. Observe the tissue hemoglobin index (THI) signal strength on the monitor display.	The THI is an indicator of signal strength based on the measure of the total amount of hemoglobin present in the monitored tissue.	Patient movement can cause changes in measurement values.

Procedure continues on following page

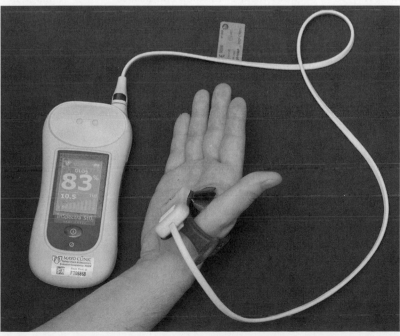

Figure 79-3   Tissue oxygen monitor with nondisposable clip placed on the palm and thenar eminence. *(Photo courtesy of Mayo Clinic.)*

Procedure for Thenar Tissue Oxygenation (Sto₂) Monitoring—*Continued*

Steps	Rationale	Special Considerations
10. If the THI signal is greater than five, observe the Sto₂.	A THI greater than five indicates sufficient hemoglobin to obtain an adequate Sto₂ signal in most circumstances.	
11. Remove PE and discard used supplies in appropriate receptacle.	Reduces the transmission of microorganisms and body secretions; Standard Precautions.	If using the nondisposable sensor cleanse it with a manufacturer's recommended agent.
12. HH		

Expected Outcomes

- Accurate Sto₂ values are obtained.
- Changes in tissue oxygenation are detected and treated.
- The need for invasive techniques for monitoring oxygenation and tissue perfusion is reduced.

Unexpected Outcomes

- Accurate tissue oxygenation is not obtained because of movement or ambient light.
- Sto₂ is not able to be used due to a tattoo on the thenar skin.

Patient Monitoring and Care

Steps	Rationale	Reportable Conditions
		These conditions must be reported if they persist despite nursing interventions.
1. Evaluate the patient's vital signs, level of consciousness, and laboratory values along with the Sto₂ values for evidence of reduced tissue oxygenation and hypoperfusion.	Monitoring Sto₂ is one method for evaluating the patient. A complete assessment of the patient should be done, and reliance on a single measurement should be avoided.	• Trends demonstrating decreasing Sto₂ values • Sto₂ values <75% • Cyanosis • Tachypnea • Tachycardia • Altered level of consciousness • Hypotension • Decreased urine output • Mottling of the lower extremities • Increased lactate level
2. Evaluate the sensor site every 15 minutes if a reusable sensor is used or every 24 hours or per manufacturer's recommendations if a nonreusable sensor is used.	Assessment of the skin and tissues under the sensor identifies skin breakdown or loss of vascular flow.	• Change in skin color • Loss of warmth of tissue • Loss of blood flow to the digits • Evidence of skin breakdown from the sensor • Change in color of the nailbeds • Inability to obtain Sto₂ values
3. Ensure that ambient light does not affect the sensor. • Have the patient rest his or her hand, palm side down, on a flat surface. • A towel or blanket can be placed over the patient's hand/sensor to block out light.	If light gets under the sensor, the values may be inaccurate.	

Documentation

Documentation should include the following:

- Patient and family education
- Indication for use of the StO_2 monitor
- Patient assessment at the time of the StO_2 measurement
- THI level
- StO_2 level

- Other laboratory results such as hemoglobin, lactate, and arterial blood gas
- Skin assessment at sensor site
- Nursing intervention and treatments provided
- Patient response to treatment
- Unexpected outcomes

References and Additional Readings

For a complete list of references and additional readings for this procedure, scan this QR code with any freely available smartphone code reader app, or visit http://booksite.elsevier.com/9780323376624.

80 Transesophageal Echocardiography (Assist)

Janice Y. Dawson and Linda Hoke

PURPOSE: Transesophageal echocardiography (TEE) offers an alternative approach for obtaining high-quality images of the heart structure that are not well visualized with a conventional transthoracic echocardiography (TTE) approach. A TEE obtains images of the heart from a transducer inside the esophagus. The esophagus lies immediately behind the heart, and with this technology clear images of the heart can be obtained.

PREREQUISITE NURSING KNOWLEDGE

- Knowledge of cardiovascular anatomy and physiology is necessary.
- Knowledge of basic arrhythmia recognition and treatment of life-threatening arrhythmias is needed.
- Advanced cardiac life support (ACLS) knowledge and skills are needed.
- A topical anesthetic is used in the oropharyngeal area; thus, the patient's gag reflex may be diminished or absent, putting the patient at risk for aspiration.[4]
- It is essential to know the institution's conscious sedation guidelines.
- Sedation can put the patient at risk for respiratory depression.[9]
- A fiberoptic probe with an ultrasound transducer is inserted through the mouth into the esophagus just behind the heart (Fig. 80-1). The transducer located at the tip of the probe sends high-frequency sound waves toward the heart, which returns as echoes. The echoes are converted, by computer, into moving images of the heart. The image is displayed on a screen and can be recorded on videotape or compact disk (CD), printed on paper, or sent electronically to a picture-archiving communication system. This test is used to visualize structures of the heart and aorta that may not be seen with a standard TTE and to clarify structures that may be otherwise poorly seen. The test may be performed as an outpatient or inpatient procedure or in the operating room.[4]
- Various modes of echocardiography are used to examine the heart, blood vessels, valve function, and blood flow. The three techniques include:
  - Motion-mode (M-mode) echocardiography: This is a one-dimensional echocardiogram that visualizes time, depth, and intensity. It looks like a tracing instead of a picture of the heart and is used to measure the exact size of the heart chambers.
  - Two-dimensional (2D) echocardiography: This shows the actual shape and motion of the different heart

structures. These images represent "slices" of the heart in motion.
  - Three-dimensional (3D) echocardiography provides added dimensions to the 2D echocardiogram. It provides detailed anatomical assessment of cardiac pathology, chamber volume measurement, and views of heart valves, enabling a better appreciation of the severity and mechanisms of valve diseases.
  - Doppler echocardiography: This assesses the flow of blood through the heart. The signals that represent blood flow are displayed as a series of black-and-white tracings or color images on the screen.
- A TEE is considered a safe and relatively noninvasive diagnostic technique. However, severe, even life-threatening complications have been reported.[5]
- General indications for TEE are as follows[1,2,4]:
  - Evaluation of cardiac and aortic structures and function with inadequate TTE images or in whom diagnostic information is not obtainable by TTE
  - Rule out clot prechemical and/or electrical cardioversion
  - Suspected acute thoracic aortic pathology including but not limited to dissection/transection
  - Evaluation of valvular (mitral) structure and function to assess appropriateness for, and to assist with planning of, an intervention
  - Diagnosis of infective endocarditis with a high pretest probability (e.g., staphylococcus bacteremia, fungemia, prosthetic heart valve, or intracardiac device)
  - Evaluation for cardiovascular source of embolus with no identifiable noncardiac source
  - Intraoperative cardiac monitoring
  - Guiding the management of catheter-based intracardiac procedures such as septal defect closure or atrial appendage obliteration and transcatheter valve procedures
  - Prosthetic valve disorders
- Contraindications to TEE can be divided into absolute and relative. Gastrointestinal (GI) evaluation and clearance should be considered before the procedure.

Transesophageal Echocardiogram (TEE)

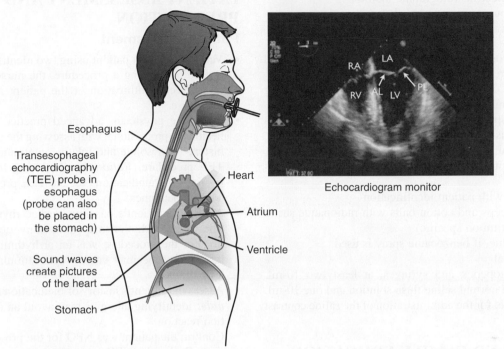

Figure 80-1 Transesophageal echocardiography (TEE) probe inserted through the mouth and into the esophagus just behind the heart.

- Absolute contraindications are as follows[2,5]:
  - Diseases of the throat/esophagus/stomach including, but not limited to, known obstructive esophageal disease, obstruction, stenosis, tumors, fistulae, or varices
  - Esophageal perforation, laceration
  - A history of esophageal radiation or unresolved esophageal dilation
  - Perforated viscus
  - Dysphagia and odynophagia
  - Active upper GI bleeding
  - Patients who ate within 6 to 8 hours of the study, unless emergent as in aortic dissection or trauma
  - Unwilling patients
  - Inability to obtain intravenous access
- Relative contraindications are[2,5]:
  - Upper GI surgery
  - Recent upper GI bleed
  - History of radiation to neck and mediastinum
  - Barrett's esophagus
  - History of dysphagia
  - Restriction of cervical mobility from severe cervical arthritis
  - Esophageal varices
  - Coagulopathy, thrombocytopenia
  - Active esophagitis
  - Active peptic ulcer disease
  - Loose teeth
- A TEE does not pose a risk for infection. Patients with prosthetic values do not need antibiotics prescribed before the procedure.[7]

EQUIPMENT

- Transesophageal ultrasound probe
- Echocardiography machine (compatible with the probe)
- Constant low wall suction with connecting tubing and rigid pharyngeal suction tip catheter
- Protective mask, goggles, nonsterile gloves, and barrier gowns
- Water-soluble lubricant
- Oxygen, with both nasal prongs and mask available
- Topical anesthetic such as lidocaine solution with an administration device (i.e., mucosal atomization device), viscous lidocaine, or benzocaine spray (as prescribed)
- Premedication for sedation and appropriate reversal agents (as prescribed)
- Syringes, blunt needles, and labels for medications
- Antiseptic agents for IV connection cleansing such as alcohol prep pads
- IV insertion kit (if adequate IV access is not in place)
- IV tubing
- One bag (500 mL or 1000 mL) of 0.9% normal saline IV solution
- Syringes of proper size for aspirating and flushing IV access if needed
- Tongue depressor
- Emesis basin
- Flashlight (to assess the oropharyngeal area, especially in the case of trauma)
- Disposable bite guard (may use the type with or without a strap to hold it in place)

- Thermometer
- Continuous electrocardiographic monitor
- Continuous pulse oximetry monitor and equipment
- Continuous capnography monitor and tubing (organization specific)
- Automatic blood pressure machine and cuff (with manual blood pressure cuff available for backup use)
- Two pillows, one supporting the neck and one supporting the back, to maintain the side-lying position
- Bags with respective labels for carrying probe to and from procedure (institution specific)
- ACLS cart, airway equipment, and medications

Additional equipment, to have available as needed, includes the following:

- Denture cup with patient identification
- Tonsillar forceps and cotton balls with radiopaque string attached (institution specific)
- Methylene blue, if benzocaine spray is used
- Ultrasound gel
- Three-way stopcock and syringes, at least two 10-mL syringes with normal saline flush solution and one 10-mL empty syringe, for the administration of the saline contrast agent if used

PATIENT AND FAMILY EDUCATION

- Assess the patient and family's understanding of the procedure and the indication for therapy. *Rationale:* Information about the procedure increases patient cooperation and decreases patient and family anxiety and apprehension.
- Verify that the patient understands the preparation for the procedure, which includes not having food or nonclear liquids for at least 6 hours and nothing by mouth (NPO) for 2 to 3 hours before the procedure as prescribed.[4,8] Before the test, the patient may take daily medications, with a sip of water, as prescribed or according to institution standards. *Rationale:* Undigested material in the stomach increases the risk for aspiration. Prescribed medications may be needed.
- Explain that the local anesthetic may make the patient's tongue and throat feel swollen and that he or she may feel unable to swallow. The gag reflex will be inhibited by the local anesthetic and may last approximately 1 hour after administration. They may experience gagging or retching during the numbing process and during the initial passage of the probe. *Rationale:* The explanation may assist in decreasing patient anxiety during the procedure.
- Explain to the patient he or she will be sedated to decrease anxiety, to increase comfort, and for ease in passing the probe. *Rationale:* This information may decrease patient and family anxiety.
- Describe to the patient he or she will be monitored closely during and after the procedure. *Rationale:* The explanation assists in decreasing patient and family anxiety.
- Explain to the patient he or she will require transportation after the procedure and needs to be accompanied by a responsible adult if it is performed in an ambulatory setting. *Rationale:* Even short acting medications may not be metabolized for a few hours making it unsafe to drive.

PATIENT ASSESSMENT AND PREPARATION

Patient Assessment

- Verify the correct patient using two identifiers. *Rationale:* Before performing a procedure, the nurse should ensure the correct identification of the patient for the intended procedure.
- Assist the physician, advanced practice nurse, or other healthcare professional with assessing the patient's medical history for absolute and relative contraindications for the TEE procedure. *Rationale:* Screening for absolute and relative contraindications for the TEE procedure prevents adverse outcomes.
- Assess the patient's baseline cardiac rhythm. *Rationale:* The patient's rhythm may have converted if the indication for the procedure was an arrhythmia. Passage of a large-bore tube may cause vagal stimulation and brady arrhythmias.
- Assess the patient's history of medication allergies. *Rationale:* Identifying allergies may avoid an adverse medication reaction.
- Confirm the patient was NPO for the prescribed length of time. *Rationale:* NPO status for an appropriate period of time before the procedure allows for gastric emptying and decreases the likelihood of aspiration.
- Assess the patient's medication history.[1] *Rationale:* Frequent use of certain medications (e.g., analgesics and anxiolytics) or illicit drugs and alcohol may affect the patient's response to moderate sedation and the medications.
- Confirm medications the patient has taken within the last 4 hours. *Rationale:* Recent sedative, analgesic, and vasoactive medications may affect the patient's tolerance and response to the medications given during the procedure.
- Assess the patient's height, weight, baseline respiratory, hemodynamic, and neurological status before anesthetizing the posterior pharynx and administering any sedative agents. *Rationale:* Baseline assessment data provide information to use as a comparison for further assessment once medications have been administered.
- Assess the patient's baseline vital signs, oxygen saturation, and if applicable capnography reading. *Rationale:* Close monitoring of vital signs and oxygenation during the procedure and comparison with baseline are essential to assess the patient's tolerance of the procedure.
- Assess the patient's baseline pain characteristic, site, and severity. *Rationale:* Baseline assessment data provide information to use as a comparison during and after the procedure.
- Assess the patient's presedation level of consciousness, using an organization-approved scoring system (e.g., Modified Aldrete Score).[4] *Rationale:* Using a scoring system for conscious sedation may prevent oversedation, and establish a baseline for postprocedure comparison.
- Assess the patient for medical problems that contraindicate or increase the risk of conscious sedation. Consider using the American Association of Anesthesiologists' Physical Status Classification Score per institution policy.

Rationale: Screening the patient preprocedure may find a history or evidence of difficult intubation, sleep apnea, and complications of sedation or anesthesia.[4]

Patient Preparation

- Verify that the patient and family understand preprocedural teaching. Answer questions as they arise, and reinforce information as needed. *Rationale:* Understanding of previously taught information is evaluated and reinforced. Patient and family anxiety may be decreased.
- Verify that informed consent was obtained, including consent for anesthesia and agitated saline contrast injection, if required. *Rationale:* Informed consent is necessary before invasive procedures and the administration of conscious sedation. Informed consent protects the rights of the patient and makes a competent decision possible for the patient; however, in emergency circumstances, time may not allow the form to be signed.
- Instruct the patient to void before the procedure. *Rationale:* Voiding before the procedure minimizes disruption of the examination.
- Perform a preprocedure verification and time out. *Rationale:* Ensures patient safety. Confirms correct patient, procedure, and equipment availability.
- Initiate or continue electrocardiographic monitoring, apply an automatic blood pressure cuff (if arterial blood pressure monitoring is not already in place), and initiate oxygen saturation monitoring and, if prescribed, capnography. *Rationale:* These measures allow for close cardiovascular and respiratory monitoring during the procedure. Follow organizational practice regarding capnography monitoring.
- Ensure the ordered IV access is in place and functional, usually a 20-gauge or larger IV. *Rationale:* IV access is needed to administer premedication and for possible emergency medications. A 20-gauge or larger IV is needed for the injection of contrast if prescribed.

- Maintain the prescribed IV infusion during the procedure. *Rationale:* IV infusion maintenance ensures the IV is functioning and available should an emergency arise.
- Have the patient remove any dentures or dental prostheses. *Rationale:* Dentures may interfere with the safe passage of the transesophageal probe.
- Set up the suction system with the connecting tubing and a rigid pharyngeal suction tip device attached and ready for use. Check for adequate suction vacuum. *Rationale:* This setup is necessary for suctioning the patient's oral secretions during the procedure.
- Prepare the prescribed local anesthetics (e.g., benzocaine, viscous lidocaine); sedatives (e.g., midazolam, diazepam); analgesics (e.g., fentanyl, morphine sulfate); reversal agents (e.g., naloxone, and flumazenil); medications to decrease salivary secretions as needed; and methylene blue (if benzocaine use is planned).[4] *Rationale:* Sedatives and analgesics reduce patient anxiety, promote comfort, facilitate cooperation during the procedure, and decrease myocardial workload. Reversal agents are required for emergencies. Methylene blue is needed to reverse methemoglobinemia if it occurs with the use of benzocaine.[4]
- Have agitated normal saline solution available per organization protocol if prescribed for saline contrast echocardiography (bubble study). *Rationale:* The contrast agent enhances the ability to evaluate cardiac shunt.
- Administer supplemental oxygen as prescribed. *Rationale:* Administration of oxygen may be needed to maintain adequate patient oxygenation during the procedure.
- Have atropine available at the bedside. *Rationale:* Atropine is necessary if a vagal reaction occurs with the insertion and passage of the transesophageal probe.
- Have an ACLS cart, medications, and airway equipment available at the patient's side.[4] *Rationale:* Emergency equipment is necessary to have close by in case an emergency situation should arise.

Procedure | for Transesophageal Echocardiography (Assist)

Steps	Rationale	Special Considerations
1. **HH**		
2. **PE**		
3. Assist if needed as the physician, advanced practice nurse, or other healthcare professional anesthetizes the patient's posterior pharynx with the topical agent.	Decreases discomfort caused by passage of the probe.	If possible, allow the patient to sit up to increase comfort and decrease anxiety or the feeling of choking.
4. Assist the patient to the left-lateral decubitus position. Use pillows to ensure correct alignment of the spine with the head and body.	The left-lateral decubitus position allows secretions to collect in the dependent areas of the mouth for ease of suctioning and to prevent aspiration in case the patient vomits.	Patients may be examined in the supine position if required by anatomy or hemodynamic stability or if the patient is endotracheally intubated.[4]
5. Reassess vital signs, oxygen saturation, capnography, neurological status, cardiac rhythm, respiratory status, and pain before administration of IV medications for moderate sedation.	Closely monitors the patient and determines whether there are any changes in the patient's condition.	

Procedure continues on following page

Procedure	for Transesophageal Echocardiography (Assist)—*Continued*	
Steps	**Rationale**	**Special Considerations**
6. Administer IV medication for moderate sedation as prescribed.[4] **(Level D*)**	Allows the patient to cooperate in facilitating passage of the probe during the procedure.	Confirm the appropriate antagonists are readily available. Continually assess the patient as he or she may need additional medication throughout the procedure. Gag and cough reflexes may be compromised by topical anesthetics, and the patient may vomit as the probe is passed, increasing the risk for aspiration.
7. Assist the physician, advanced practice nurse, or other healthcare professional as needed with the insertion of the probe.		
A. Prepare to insert a bite guard when directed by the physician, advanced practice nurse, or other healthcare professional.	The bite guard prevents the patient from biting the probe or the fingers of the physician, advanced practice nurse, or other healthcare professional and avoids damage to the teeth and mouth.	
B. Assist the physician, advanced practice nurse, or other healthcare professional as requested with lubrication of the probe and oropharynx and applying ultrasound contact gel or viscous lidocaine to the distal end of the probe.	Lubrication of the probe minimizes mucosal injury and irritation, and facilitates the ease of passage of the probe. Contact gel transmits ultrasound signals.	
C. Ask the patient to slightly bend his or her head in a forward flex.	Proper head position eases insertion of the probe into the esophagus.	
D. Alternatively, if needed assist the physician, advanced practice nurse, or other healthcare professional with the jaw-thrust technique if required to guide the probe insertion.		
E. Encourage the patient to simulate swallowing while the probe is passed if requested by the physician, advanced practice nurse, or other healthcare professional.	The swallowing maneuver causes the epiglottis to close the trachea and directs the probe into the esophagus.	Some physicians, advanced practice nurses, and other healthcare professionals may not want to draw attention to the throat and will not ask the patient to swallow, but rather will wait for a natural swallow motion to occur and then insert the probe.
F. Suction the oral secretions as needed to ensure patency of the airway.	Removes secretions. This may be needed due to the patient's diminished gag reflex and the inability of the patient to swallow oral secretions.	Manipulation of the probe may cause stimulation of secretions.
G. Provide the patient with reassurance and encouragement to keep the bite guard in place, maintain the required position, hold still without attempts to speak, and focus on his or her breathing pattern.	May decrease patient anxiety and promote patient cooperation.	Some patients may be able to tolerate the procedure without analgesia or anesthesia when encouragement is provided.[4]

*Level D: Peer-reviewed professional and organizational standards with the support of clinical study recommendations.

Procedure for Transesophageal Echocardiography (Assist)—*Continued*

Steps	Rationale	Special Considerations
8. Provide the physician, advanced practice nurse, or other healthcare professional with updates of the patient status during the TEE procedure.	Keeps the physician, advanced practice nurse, or other healthcare professional informed of the patient's condition and possible need for additional sedation or analgesics.	
9. Assist with the administration of the saline contrast agent as prescribed and per institutional standards.[4,6]	The administration of saline contrast enhances the view of the cardiac structures and function.	Assist with instructing the patient to perform the valsalva maneuver, sniffing, or coughing to enhance right-to-left shunting images, if requested by the physician, advanced practice nurse, or other healthcare professional.[6]
10. Assist if needed with the removal of the probe.	Provides assistance.	Anesthetics may be less effective at the end of the procedure, increasing the gag and cough reflexes, thus increasing the patient's risk of vomiting as the probe is removed. Using a rigid pharyngeal suction tip catheter, suction as necessary as the tube is removed to prevent aspiration.
11. Place the probe in an appropriate receptacle for cleaning.	Reduces the transmission of microorganisms and prepares the equipment for sterilization.	
12. Continue assessment and monitoring until the patient returns to baseline as prescribed; follow institutional standards.	Ensures patient safety.	Keep the patient on the left side with his or her head slightly elevated until the gag, swallow, and cough reflexes are intact.
13. Discard used supplies in appropriate receptacles.	Removes and safely discards used supplies using standard precautions.	
14. 🅷🅷		

Expected Outcomes

- Clear visualization of cardiac structures and function
- Immediate preliminary diagnosis
- Note: Negative study results are helpful in excluding cardiac sources of compromise
- Patent airway
- Acceptable level of comfort with no adverse reactions to sedation or analgesia

Unexpected Outcomes

- Esophageal or gastric perforation
- Esophageal, oropharyngeal, or gastric injury or lacerations
- Oropharyngeal hematoma
- Vasovagal hypotension from esophageal manipulation
- Substernal chest pain
- Temporary dysphagia
- Aspiration
- Respiratory depression
- Hematoma in the oropharynx
- Unresolved hypotension or hypertension
- Arrhythmias, bradycardia, or tachycardia
- Laryngospasm
- Bronchospasm
- Change in neurological status
- Air embolism in patients with right-to-left shunt with use of saline contrast
- Heart failure
- Pain
- Methemoglobinemia

Procedure continues on following page

Patient Monitoring and Care

Steps	Rationale	Reportable Conditions
		These conditions should be reported if they persist despite nursing interventions. Changes in the following: • Neurological status • Oxygenation • Capnography • Heart rate and rhythm • Blood pressure • Respirations • Cardiovascular status
1. Assess and monitor cardiovascular, respiratory, and neurological status at a minimum of 5-minute intervals during the procedure and 15-minute intervals after the TEE procedure, until the patient's condition returns to baseline, the prescribed parameters (e.g., vital signs within 10% of baseline),[4] and as required by institutional standards.	Changes in vital signs; heart rhythm; capnography values; oxygenation; and neurological, respiratory, and cardiovascular status may indicate complications related to the procedure.	
2. Maintain IV access and infusions as prescribed during and after the procedure.	Maintaining IV access and infusions ensures IV patency in case emergency medications are needed.	
3. Monitor the patient's sedation score using a tool (i.e., Modified Aldrete Score)[4] during and after the procedure following institutional standards.	Determines the patient's response to IV moderate sedation and the need for additional sedation.	• Sedation score outside of prescribed parameters • Worsening sedation score after the discontinuation of sedation
4. Assess pain at a minimum of 5-minute intervals during and 15-minute intervals after the TEE procedure until the patient's condition returns to baseline. Administer analgesia as prescribed.	May indicate a complication of the procedure or identify the need for pain interventions. Mild throat discomfort is common as the topical anesthetic wears off.	• New onset of pain • Unresolved discomfort not relieved after the probe is removed • Unusual throat discomfort
5. Monitor for signs and symptoms of esophageal trauma or perforation.[2,3,5]	Identifies complications.	• Dysphagia • Odynophagia • Mackler's triad: vomiting, pain, and subcutaneous emphysema • Fever • Agitation • Tachycardia • Hypotension • Chest pain • Respiratory distress • Tachypnea • Dyspnea • Pneumothorax • Pleural effusions

Patient Monitoring and Care —*Continued*

Steps	Rationale	Reportable Conditions
6. Monitor for intraprocedure complications or reasons to terminate the TEE early.[4]	Determines the patient's response to the procedure and identifies complications.	• Patient becomes agitated and is unable to cooperate with the procedure • Change in neurological status • Dental or oropharyngeal trauma • Apnea • Hypoxemia • Hypercapnia • New arrhythmia • New hypotension or hypertension • Perforation or subcutaneous emphysema • GI or other bleeding • Chest pain • Benzocaine-induced methemoglobinemia
7. Monitor a patient who received benzocaine for symptoms of methemoglobinemia. Prepare to treat methemoglobinemia with supplemental oxygen and methylene blue solution given by slow IV administration as prescribed.[4]	Severe methemoglobinemia is life threatening.	• Dyspnea • Nausea • Tachycardia • Cyanosis • Decreased pulse oximetry levels
8. Assess the patient for the return of normal pharyngeal function. If the patient is not upright, keep the patient on his or her left side with the head of the bed elevated until the gag, swallow, and cough reflexes are intact.	The topical anesthesia decreases the gag, swallow, and cough reflexes and increases the patient's risk of aspiration.	• Prolonged absence of gag, swallowing, or cough reflexes
9. Offer clear liquids and gradually progress to solid food after return of pharyngeal function as prescribed.	Topical anesthesia decreases the gag reflex and increases the risk for aspiration.	• Nausea • Vomiting • Stomach discomfort • Increase in odynophagia or dysphagia after 24 hours, may possibly indicate soft tissue or esophageal injury.[4]
10. Ask the patient to repeat his or her understanding of the postprocedure instructions.	Having patients repeat the postprocedure instructions confirms their understanding of what they should and should not do.	• Patient unable to understand postprocedure instructions

Procedure continues on following page

Patient Monitoring and Care —*Continued*

Steps	Rationale	Reportable Conditions
11. Ensure the safety of the ambulatory patient. Ensure vital signs have returned to 10% of baseline before ambulation.[4] Have a family member or friend explain postprocedure education and sign appropriate documents as needed. Advise the patient to refrain from important decisions and driving while the effects anesthetic remain (i.e., for the remainder of the day). Provide the patient with a copy of the written discharge instructions, per institutional standards. Counsel the patient to call the physician, advanced practice nurse, or other healthcare professional if odynophagia or dysphagia persists for 24 hours.[4] Ensure the patient is accompanied by a responsible adult.	This information is provided to patients who are being discharged.	

Documentation

Documentation should include the following:

- Date and time of procedure
- Initial patient assessment
- Patient and family education
- Preprocedure verifications and timeout
- Completion of informed consent form

- Vital signs, pulse oximetry, capnography, neurological status, respiratory status, and pain evaluation immediately before sedation, and during and after the procedure
- Establishment and assessment of IV patency

References and Additional Readings

For a complete list of references and additional readings for this procedure, scan this QR code with any freely available smartphone code reader app, or visit http://booksite.elsevier.com/9780323376624.

PROCEDURE

81 Arterial Puncture AP

Joel M. Brown II

PURPOSE: Arterial puncture is performed to obtain a sample of blood for arterial blood gas (ABG) analysis.

PREREQUISITE NURSING KNOWLEDGE

- An ABG analysis measures the pH and the partial pressure of oxygen and carbon dioxide. ABG samples are also analyzed for oxygen saturation and for bicarbonate values. These analyses are done primarily to evaluate a patient's oxygenation status, acid-base balance, and ventilation.[5] Additional laboratory tests (e.g., electrolytes, ammonia and lactate levels) can be performed on arterial blood samples.
- Indications for ABGs vary and include patients with chronic and acute respiratory disorders (e.g., chronic obstructive pulmonary disease, pneumonia, adult respiratory lung disease) and acute metabolic or shock disorders (e.g., sepsis, postcardiac arrest, acute kidney injury). ABG analysis frequently is performed on patients in shock, receiving oxygen or mechanical ventilation therapies, or experiencing changes in respiratory therapy or status.[5]
- Knowledge of principles of aseptic technique is necessary.
- Knowledge is needed of the anatomy and physiology of the vasculature and adjacent structures.
- The brachial artery is a continuation of the axillary artery in the upper extremity. It bifurcates just below the elbow (Fig. 81-1). From the bifurcation, the ulnar artery moves down the forearm on the medial side and the radial artery on the lateral side.[18]
- The preferred artery for arterial puncture is the radial artery. Although this artery is smaller than the ulnar artery, it is more superficial and can be stabilized more easily during the procedure.[7] The use of the brachial artery is a safe and reliable alternative site for arterial puncture.[16]
- At times, the femoral artery is used for arterial puncture. The use of this artery can be technically difficult because of the proximity of the artery to the femoral vein (Fig. 81-2).

- Arterial cannulation is considered for patients who need frequent arterial blood samples, continuous arterial pressure monitoring, or evaluation of vasoactive medication therapy (see Procedures 58 and 59).
- The most common complications associated with arterial puncture include pain, vasospasm, hematoma formation, infection, hemorrhage, and neurovascular compromise.[5,9,16]
- Site selection proceeds as follows:
  - Use the radial artery as first choice. The radial artery is small and easily stabilized because it passes over a bony groove located at the wrist (see Fig. 81-1).
  - Use the brachial artery as second choice, except in the presence of poor pulsation from shock, obesity, or sclerotic vessel (e.g., because of previous cardiac catheterization). The brachial artery is larger than the radial artery. There is risk of median nerve injury due to its proximity to the brachial artery. Hemostasis after arterial puncture is enhanced by its proximity to bone if the entry point is approximately 1.5 inches above the antecubital fossa (see Fig. 81-1).
  - Use the femoral artery in the case of cardiopulmonary arrest or altered perfusion to the upper extremities. The femoral artery is a large superficial artery located in the groin (see Fig. 81-2). It is easily palpated and punctured. Complications related to femoral artery puncture include hemorrhage and hematoma because bleeding can be difficult to control; inadvertent puncture of the femoral vein because of the close proximity of the vein to the artery; infection because aseptic technique in the groin area is difficult to maintain; and limb ischemia if the femoral artery is damaged.
- Ultrasound guidance can be used for arterial puncture if the technology is available.[10]

EQUIPMENT

- One prepackaged ABG kit that contains the following:
  - One 20- to 25-gauge, 1- to 1.5-inch hypodermic needle (note: longer needles are needed for brachial and femoral artery puncture)
  - One 1- to 5-mL preheparinized (if available) syringe with a rubber stopper or cap

AP This procedure should be performed only by physicians, advanced practice nurses, and other healthcare professionals (including critical care nurses) with additional knowledge, skills, and demonstrated competence per professional licensure or institutional standard.

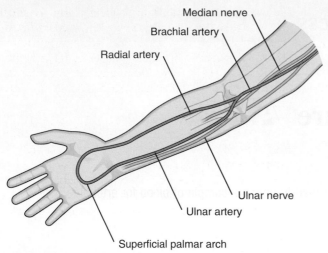

Figure 81-1 Anatomical landmarks for locating the radial and brachial arteries.

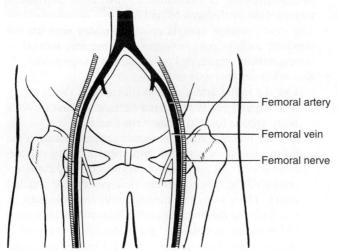

Figure 81-2 Anatomical landmarks for locating the femoral artery.

❖ One 1-mL ampule of sodium heparin, 1 : 1000 concentration (if preheparinized syringe is not available)
❖ Two 2 × 2 gauze pads
❖ 2% chlorhexidine-based antiseptic solution
❖ 70% isopropyl alcohol prep pad
❖ One plastic bag (for transport of sample to the laboratory)
❖ One adhesive bandage
• Appropriate laboratory form and specimen label
• One pair of nonsterile gloves and eye protection
Additional equipment, to have available as needed, includes the following:
• Small, rolled towel (to support the patient's wrist)
• Sterile gloves
• 1-mL syringe with 25-gauge needle (if lidocaine is used)
• 1% lidocaine (without epinephrine), 1-mL, or eutectic mixture of local anesthetics (EMLA) cream
• Bedside ultrasound machine with vascular probe
• Sterile ultrasound probe cover
• Sterile ultrasound gel

PATIENT AND FAMILY EDUCATION

• Explain the reason for the arterial puncture to the patient and family. *Rationale:* Clarification of information is an expressed patient and family need and helps to diminish anxiety, enhance acceptance, and encourage questions.
• Describe the overall steps of the procedure, including the patient's role in the procedure. *Rationale:* This explanation decreases patient anxiety, enhances cooperation, and provides an opportunity for the patient to voice concerns, and prevents accidental movement during the procedure.

PATIENT ASSESSMENT AND PREPARATION

Patient Assessment

• Determine the need for arterial cannulation versus puncture. *Rationale:* Repeated arterial punctures increase patient discomfort and the risk for complications.
• Assess for factors that influence ABG measurements, including anxiety, endotracheal suctioning, nebulizer treatment, change in oxygen therapy/ventilator settings, renal replacement therapy, medications and IV fluid composition, patient positioning, body temperature, metabolic rate, and respiratory status. *Rationale:* These conditions or therapies can alter blood gas analysis results.
• Review the patient's current anticoagulation therapy, known blood dyscrasias, and pertinent laboratory values (e.g., platelets, partial thromboplastin time, prothrombin time, and international normalized ratio) before the procedure. *Rationale:* Anticoagulation therapy, blood dyscrasias, or alterations in coagulation studies could prolong hemostasis at the puncture site and increase the risk for hematoma formation or hemorrhage.
• Review the patient's allergy history (e.g., lidocaine, antiseptic solutions, tape). *Rationale:* Assessment decreases the risk for allergic reactions.
• Review the patient's past surgical history (e.g., use of radial artery for coronary artery bypass surgery, fistulas, or shunts). *Rationale:* Arterial puncture should be avoided in extremities affected by these conditions.
• Ascertain the patient's nondominant hand, if possible. *Rationale:* A complication to the nondominant hand may have fewer consequences.

Patient Preparation

• Verify that the patient is the correct patient using two identifiers. *Rationale:* Before performing a procedure, the nurse should ensure the correct identification of the patient for the intended intervention.
• Ensure that the patient and family understand preprocedural teaching. Answer questions as they arise, and reinforce information as needed. *Rationale:* Understanding of previously taught information is evaluated and reinforced.
• Perform a preprocedure verification and timeout, if nonemergent. *Rationale:* Ensures patient safety.
• If the patient is receiving oxygen or mechanical ventilation, check that the current therapy has been underway for at least 20 to 30 minutes before obtaining ABG.[5] *Rationale:* Ensures that the ABG results reflect the intervention/therapy change.

- Position the patient appropriately. *Rationale:* Positioning enhances the accessibility to the insertion site and promotes patient comfort.
- Radial artery puncture:
  - ❖ Assist the patient to a semirecumbent position. *Rationale:* A position of comfort decreases anxiety and may facilitate respiratory effort.
  - ❖ Elevate and hyperextend the wrist. A small rolled towel may be placed under the wrist for support. *Rationale:* This action moves the artery closer to the skin surface, making the artery easier to palpate.
  - ❖ Palpate for the presence of a strong radial pulse. *Rationale:* Identification and localization of the pulse increases the chance of a successful arterial puncture.
- Brachial artery puncture:
  - ❖ Assist the patient to a semirecumbent position. *Rationale:* A position of comfort decreases anxiety and may facilitate respiratory effort.
  - ❖ Elevate and hyperextend the patient's arm. A small pillow may be placed under the arm for support. *Rationale:* This action increases accessibility for puncture.
  - ❖ Rotate the patient's arm and palpate for the presence of a strong brachial pulse. *Rationale:* Identification and localization of the pulse increase the chance of a successful arterial puncture.
- Femoral artery puncture:
  - ❖ Assist the patient to a supine, straight-leg position. *Rationale:* This position provides the best position for localizing the femoral artery pulse.
  - ❖ Palpate for the presence of a strong femoral pulse. *Rationale:* Identification and localization of the pulse increase the chance of a successful arterial puncture.

Procedure | for Arterial Puncture

Steps	Rationale	Special Considerations
1. **HH**		Ensure that hospital policy permits registered nurses to perform radial, brachial, and femoral arterial punctures.
2. If the radial artery is to be used, perform the modified Allen's test before the puncture (Fig. 81-3). **(Level C*)**	The modified Allen's test has been recommended before a radial artery puncture to assess the patency of the ulnar artery and an intact superficial palmar arch.[5,17]	The modified Allen's test does not always ensure adequate flow through the ulnar artery. A Doppler ultrasound flow indicator can also be used to further verify blood flow.[1-3]
A. With the patient's hand held overhead, instruct the patient to open and close the hand several times.	Forces the blood from the hand.	If the patient is unconscious or unable to perform the procedure, clench the fist passively for the patient.
B. With the patient's fist clenched, apply direct pressure on the radial and ulnar arteries.	Obstructs the flow of blood to the hand.	
C. Instruct the patient to lower and open the hand.	Observe for pallor.	Perform passively if the patient is unconscious or unable to assist.
D. Release the pressure over the ulnar artery and observe the hand for return of color.	Return of color within 7 seconds indicates patency of the ulnar artery and an intact superficial palmar arch, and is interpreted as a normal Allen's test result. If color returns within between 8 and 14 seconds, the test is considered equivocal and the physician, advanced practice nurse, or other healthcare professional must consider the risk and benefits of continuing with performing this procedure. If it takes 15 or more seconds for color to return, the test results are considered abnormal and another site should be considered.	If the test is equivocal or abnormal, the radial artery should not be used and the modified Allen's test should be performed on the opposite hand. A Doppler ultrasound flow indicator can also be used to further verify blood flow.[1-3]

*Level C: Qualitative studies, descriptive or correlational studies, integrative reviews, systematic reviews, or randomized controlled trials with inconsistent results.

Procedure continues on following page

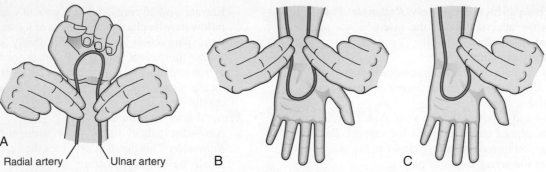

A
Radial artery   Ulnar artery   B   C

Figure 81-3 Modified Allen's test. Elevate the patient's hand and instruct the patient to open and close the fist several times. **A,** With the patient's fist clenched, simultaneously occlude the radial and ulnar arteries. **B,** Instruct the patient to lower and open his or her fist. Observe for pallor in the patient's hand. **C,** Release the pressure over the ulnar artery and observe the hand for the return of color. *(From Bucher L, Melander SD:* Critical care nursing, *Philadelphia, 1999, Saunders.)*

Procedure   for Arterial Puncture—*Continued*

Steps	Rationale	Special Considerations
3. If a preheparinized syringe is not available, heparinize the syringe and needle.	Prevents specimen coagulation.	A small-bore needle is less likely to cause vasospasm of the artery during the procedure.
A. Assemble a 22-gauge needle on the syringe and prime the entire syringe barrel and needle with 1 mL of heparin.	Prepares the syringe.	
B. Expel the heparin from the syringe.	Excess heparin in the syringe can lower the pH and partial pressure of carbon dioxide.	
C. Eliminate any visible air bubbles from the syringe.	Maintains the accuracy of ABG values.	
4. Prepare the site with an antiseptic solution (e.g., 2% chlorhexidine-based preparation).	Limits the introduction of potentially infectious skin flora into the vessel during the puncture.	
A. Cleanse the site with a back-and-forth motion while applying friction for 30 seconds.		
B. Allow the antiseptic solution to dry.		
5. Locally anesthetize the puncture site per institutional standards.[4,7,9,10,13] **(Level C*)**	Provides local anesthesia for arterial puncture.	Most patients report pain during arterial puncture.[6,8] Patients have reported reduced pain when a local, intradermal anesthetic agent is used before the arterial puncture.[8,9]
A. Use a 1-mL syringe with a 25-gauge needle to draw up 0.5 mL of 1% lidocaine without epinephrine.	Minimizes vessel trauma. The absence of epinephrine decreases the risk for peripheral vasoconstriction.	Medications such as lidocaine ointment, amethocaine gel, and EMLA cream may reduce arterial puncture pain.[11–13,15,19] If these medications are used, manufacturer's recommendations should be followed.
B. Aspirate before injecting the local anesthetic.	Determines whether a blood vessel has been inadvertently entered.	
C. Inject intradermally and then with full infiltration around the artery puncture site. Use approximately 0.2–0.3 mL for an adult.	Decreases the incidence of localized pain with injection of all skin layers.	

*Level C: Qualitative studies, descriptive or correlational studies, integrative reviews, systematic reviews, or randomized controlled trials with inconsistent results.

Procedure | for Arterial Puncture—*Continued*

Steps	Rationale	Special Considerations
6. Perform the percutaneous puncture of the selected artery.		Ultrasound technology may be used to assist with insertion.
A. Palpate and stabilize the artery with the index and middle fingers of the nondominant hand.	Increases the likelihood of correctly locating the artery and decreases the chance of vessel rolling.	Use sterile gloves if the site of the artery puncture is palpated after it is antiseptically prepared.
B. With the needle bevel up and the syringe at a 30- to 60-degree angle to the radial or brachial artery, puncture the skin slowly (Figs. 81-4 and 81-5). For a femoral artery puncture, a 60- to 90-degree angle is used (Fig. 81-6).	A slow, gradual thrust promotes entry into the artery without inadvertently passing through the posterior wall.	Enter at an angle that is comfortable; certainty of position is more important than angle entry. If too much force is used, the needle may touch the periosteum of the bone and cause considerable pain.

Procedure continues on following page

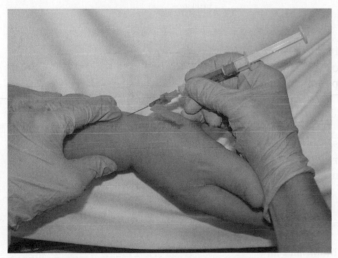

Figure 81-4 Radial artery puncture with the syringe at a 30-degree angle to the artery.

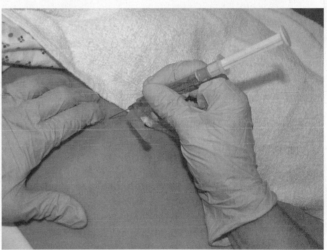

Figure 81-6 Femoral artery puncture with the syringe at a 60-degree angle to the artery.

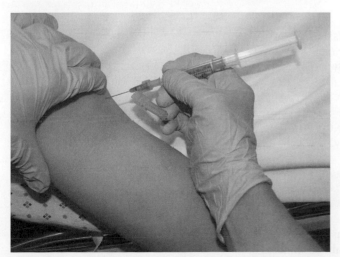

Figure 81-5 Brachial artery puncture with the syringe at a 45-degree angle to the artery.

Procedure for Arterial Puncture—*Continued*

Steps	Rationale	Special Considerations
C. Observe the syringe for a flashback of blood.	Pulsation of blood into the syringe verifies that the artery has been punctured.	Flashback occurs more easily with a glass syringe than a plastic syringe. Gentle aspiration may be necessary with a plastic syringe.
D. If the puncture is unsuccessful, withdraw the needle to the skin level, angle slightly toward the artery, and readvance. Do not withdraw the needle.	Prevents the necessity of a second puncture and changes the needle angle to facilitate the location of the artery.	Excessive probing of the artery may cause vessel or adjacent nerve injury.
7. Obtain 1 mL of blood.	An ABG analysis requires a minimum of 0.2 mL of blood.	Sample volumes may vary with equipment used. Obtain more than 1 mL of blood for additional laboratory tests, as necessary.
8. Withdraw the needle while stabilizing the barrel of the syringe.	Prevents inadvertent aspiration of air during withdrawal.	Equipment may vary. If a safety guard is available, it should be snapped onto the needle with a one-handed technique by gently pressing the device against a hard surface.
9. Press a gauze pad firmly over the puncture site for at least 5 minutes or until hemostasis is established.	Hematomas and hemorrhage can occur if pressure is not applied and maintained correctly. Hematomas can cause circulatory impedance and pain and can predispose to infection.	If the patient is receiving anticoagulation therapy or has a bleeding dyscrasia, pressure may need to be applied for as long as 15 minutes.
10. Cover the puncture site with an adhesive bandage once hemostasis is achieved.	Covers the site until healing occurs.	
11. Check the blood sample in the syringe for air bubbles and express any air bubbles by slowly ejecting the air while covering the syringe tip with a 2 × 2 gauze pad.	Air bubbles can alter the partial pressure of oxygen results.[6,15]	If a safety guard is present, it should be removed and a blood/air filter should be placed on the syringe. Excess air should be evacuated through the blood/air filter.
12. Seal the needle or tip of the syringe immediately with a rubber stopper or cap, respectively. Gently roll the syringe for 30 seconds.	Prevents leakage of blood and air from entering the sample. Mixes blood and heparin, thus preventing clot formation.	
13. Remove gloves and discard used supplies in appropriate receptacles; dispose of needles and other sharp objects in appropriate containers.	Reduces the transmission of microorganisms; Standard Precautions. Safely removes sharp objects.	
14. **HH**		
15. Label the specimen and complete the laboratory form. Note the percentage of oxygen therapy, respiratory rate, and ventilator settings, if appropriate, and the patient's temperature and time the specimen was drawn.	Helps the laboratory to perform the analysis accurately.	Policies may vary regarding the type of patient information required for laboratory analysis.
16. Expedite the delivery of the sample to the laboratory.	Ideally, the blood gas analysis should be performed within 30 minutes of collection to ensure the accuracy of results.[7,14]	

Expected Outcomes

- The ABG sample is collected correctly such that the accuracy of the results is enhanced
- The puncture site remains free of hematoma, hemorrhage, and infection
- The peripheral vascular and neurovascular systems remain intact (free of complications)
- Alterations in the ABG results are identified and treated accordingly

Unexpected Outcomes

- Pain/severe discomfort during the procedure
- Complications during the puncture or vasospasm
- Complications after the puncture: changes in the color, size, temperature, sensation, movement, or pulse of the extremity used for the arterial puncture; hematoma, hemorrhage, or infection at the puncture site

Patient Monitoring and Care

Steps	Rationale	Special Considerations
		These conditions must be reported if they persist despite nursing interventions • Bleeding • Hematoma • Changes in vital signs
1. Observe the puncture site for signs of hemostasis after the procedure.	Postpuncture bleeding can occur in any patient but is more likely to occur in patients with coagulopathies or patients who are receiving anticoagulation therapy.	
2. Assess the puncture site and involved extremity for signs of postpuncture complications.	The arterial puncture can result in peripheral vascular and neurovascular compromise of the extremity distal to the puncture site.	• Changes in color, size, temperature, sensation, movement, or pulse in the extremity used for arterial puncture • Erythema, warmth, hardness, tenderness, or pain at the puncture site • Presence of purulent drainage from the puncture site
3. Assess the puncture site for signs or symptoms of infection.	Determines necessity for further treatment.	
4. Follow institutional standards for assessing pain. Administer analgesia as prescribed.	Identifies need for pain interventions.	• Pain at the puncture site or in the distal extremity

Documentation

Documentation should include the following:
- Patient and family education
- Results of the modified Allen's test or Doppler ultrasound scan
- Preprocedure verification and timeout
- Arterial site accessed
- Number of attempts
- Local anesthetic used
- Patient's tolerance of the procedure
- Pain assessment and interventions
- Appearance of the site
- Appearance of the limb, color, pulse sensation, movement, capillary refill time, and temperature of the extremity
- Occurrence of unexpected outcomes
- Nursing interventions taken
- Laboratory results

References and Additional Readings

For a complete list of references and additional readings for this procedure, scan this QR code with any freely available smartphone code reader app, or visit http://booksite.elsevier.com/9780323376624.

82 Central Venous Catheter AP Insertion (Perform)

Susan Yeager

PURPOSE: Central venous catheters (CVCs) are inserted for measurement of central venous pressure (CVP) with jugular or subclavian catheter placement. Clinically useful information can be obtained about right-ventricular preload, cardiovascular status, and fluid balance in patients who do not need pulmonary artery pressure monitoring. CVCs also are placed for infusion of vasoactive medications and to provide access for pulmonary artery catheters and transvenous pacemakers.

PREREQUISITE NURSING KNOWLEDGE

- Knowledge of the normal anatomy and physiology of the cardiovascular system is needed.
- Knowledge of the anatomy and physiology of the vasculature and adjacent structures of the neck, groin, and chest is needed.
- Knowledge of the principles of sterile technique is essential.
- Clinical and technical competence in central line insertion and suturing is essential.
- Competence in chest radiographic interpretation is necessary.
- Advanced cardiac life support (ACLS) knowledge and skills are needed.
- Knowledge of potential complications and associated interventions/consultations for addressing issues is necessary.
- Follow guidelines regarding institution credentialing.
- Knowledge of ultrasonography technique is needed.
- Indications for CVC placement may include the following:
  - ❖ Severe blood loss
  - ❖ Hemodynamic instability
  - ❖ Administration of vesicant irritant medications
  - ❖ Administration of total parenteral nutrition
  - ❖ Lack of peripheral venous access
  - ❖ Assessment of hypovolemia or hypervolemia
  - ❖ Monitoring of CVPs
  - ❖ Placement of pulmonary artery catheters or placement of transvenous pacemakers
  - ❖ Hemodialysis access
- The normal CVP value is 2 to 8 mm Hg.
- The CVP waveform is identical to the right-atrial waveform.

- Interpretation of right-atrial/CVP waveforms including identification of *a, c,* and *v* waves is important. The *a* wave reflects right-atrial contraction. The *c* wave reflects closure of the tricuspid valve. The v wave reflects passive filling of the right atria during right-ventricular systole.
- The CVP provides information regarding right-heart filling pressures and right-ventricular function and volume.
- The CVP is commonly elevated during or after right-ventricular failure, ischemia, or infarction because of decreased compliance of the right ventricle.
- The CVP can be helpful in the determination of hypovolemia. The CVP value is low if the patient is hypovolemic. Venodilation also decreases the CVP value.
- Electrocardiographic monitoring is essential in the accurate interpretation of the CVP value.
- Some contraindications of CVC insertion include anatomical problems, venous obstructions, and coagulopathies. The subclavian site should be avoided in hemodialysis patients and patients with advanced kidney disease to avoid subclavian vein stenosis.[5]
- It is important to weigh the risks and benefits of placing a CVC against the risk for mechanical complications (e.g., pneumothorax, vein laceration, thrombosis, air embolism, misplacement).[5,6]
- A subclavian site is recommended rather than a jugular or femoral site to minimize the risk of infection.[5]
- The internal jugular site is recommended to minimize catheter cannulation-related risk of injury or trauma.[6]
- Ultrasound guidance is recommended to place CVCs if the technology is available to reduce the number of cannulation attempts and mechanical complications.[4,5,7]
- Regardless of the site selected, complications may occur during or after insertion of a central venous catheter (Table 82-1).

EQUIPMENT

- CVC insertion kit
- CVC of choice (single, dual, or triple lumen) usually supplied with insertion needle, dilator, syringe, and guidewire.
- Full sterile drapes

AP This procedure should be performed only by physicians, advanced practice nurses, and other healthcare professionals (including critical care nurses) with additional knowledge, skills, and demonstrated competence per professional licensure or institutional standard.

TABLE 82-1	**Complications of Central Venous Catheter Insertion**		
Complication	**Clinical Manifestation**	**Treatment**	**Prevention**

Pneumothorax	• Sudden respiratory distress
	• Chest pain
	• Hypoxia/cyanosis
	• Decreased breath sounds
	• Resonance to percussion
		• Confirmation with chest radiograph
		• Symptomatic treatment
		• Small pneumothorax:
		  ❖ Close monitoring
		  ❖ Daily chest radiograph
		  ❖ O_2
		• Large pneumothorax:
		  ❖ Chest tube
		  ❖ Cardiopulmonary support
			• Proper patient preparation
			• Sedation as necessary
			• Proper patient positioning
			• Technique and angle of the needle/catheter on insertion
			• Avoidance of multiple passes with the needle
			• Healthcare provider is skilled and experienced in insertion technique
			• Direct visualization with bedside ultrasonography for internal jugular placement.

Tension pneumothorax	• Most likely to occur in patients on ventilator support
	• Respiratory distress
	• Rapid clinical deterioration:
	  ❖ Cyanosis
	  ❖ Jugular venous distention (may not be present with severe hypovolemia)
	  ❖ Hypotension
	  ❖ Decreased cardiac output
		• Treatment must be rapid and aggressive
		• Immediate air aspiration followed by chest tube
		• Cardiopulmonary support
			• Proper patient preparation
			• Sedation as necessary
			• Proper patient positioning
			• Reduction of positive end-expiratory pressure to ≤5 cm H_2O at the time of venipuncture
			• Technique and angle of the needle/catheter on insertion
			• Avoidance of multiple passes with the needle
			• Healthcare provider is skilled and experienced in insertion technique
			• Use of peripherally inserted central venous catheter

Delayed pneumothorax	• Slow onset of respiratory symptoms • Subcutaneous emphysema • Persistent pleuritic chest or back pain • Insidious increase in peak airway pressures in ventilated patients	• Confirmation with chest radiograph • Chest tube • Cardiopulmonary support	• Proper patient preparation • Sedation as necessary • Proper patient positioning • Technique and angle of the needle/catheter on insertion • Avoidance of multiple passes with the needle • Healthcare provider is skilled and experienced in insertion technique • Use of peripherally inserted central venous catheter
Hydrothorax hydromediastinum	• Dyspnea • Chest pain • Muffled breath sounds • High glucose level of chest drainage • Low-grade fever	• Stop infusion • Confirmation with chest radiograph • Cardiopulmonary support	• Proper patient preparation • Sedation as necessary • Proper patient positioning • Technique and angle of the needle/catheter on insertion • Avoidance of multiple passes with the needle • Healthcare provider is skilled and experienced in insertion technique • Use of peripherally inserted central venous catheter • Placement of catheter tip in lower superior vena cava • Aspiration of blood before catheter use to confirm vascular placement

Continued

TABLE 82-1	Complications of Central Venous Catheter Insertion—cont'd		
Complication	Clinical Manifestation	Treatment	Prevention
Hemothorax	• Respiratory distress • Hypovolemic shock • Hematoma in the neck with jugular insertions	• Confirmation with chest radiograph • Chest tube • Thoracotomy for arterial repair if indicated	• Correction of coagulopathies before insertion • Avoidance of multiple passes with the needle • Evaluation with Doppler scan studies or venogram of suspected thrombosis from prior cannulation before insertion

Arterial puncture/ laceration	• Return of bright red blood in the syringe under high pressure
	• Pulsatile blood flow on disconnection of the syringe
	• Arterial waveform/pressures when the catheter is connected to the transducer system
	• Arterial saturation of sample sent for blood gas analysis
	• Deterioration of clinical status:
	  ❖ Hemorrhagic shock
	  ❖ Respiratory distress
	  ❖ Bleeding from catheter site may or may not be observed
	• Deviation of trachea with large hematoma in the neck
	• Hemothorax may be detected on chest radiograph
		• Application of pressure for 3–5 minutes or as needed to promote hemostasis after removal of the needle
		• Elevate the head of the bed if condition is hemodynamically stable
		• Chest tube as indicated
		• Thoracotomy for arterial repair if indicated
			• Correction of coagulopathies before insertion
			• Avoidance of multiple passes with the needle
			• Evaluation with Doppler scan studies or venogram of suspected thrombosis from prior cannulation before insertion
			• Use of small-gauge needle to first locate the vein
			• Direct visualization with bedside ultrasonography for femoral vein placement.

Bleeding/hematoma; venous or arterial bleeding	• Bleeding from insertion site • Hematoma formation not likely to be seen with subclavian approach • Bleeding may occur internally without visible evidence • Tracheal compression • Respiratory distress • Carotid compression • Pain at insertion site	• Application of pressure to the insertion site • Thoracotomy for arterial repair • Tracheostomy for tracheal deviation from hematoma • With the femoral approach, manual pressure slightly above the inadvertent arterial puncture site (see Procedure 76 for femoral sheath removal) • If retroperitoneal bleeding occurs, external signs may not be apparent except for signs of hypovolemia. Computed tomography (CT) scan of the abdomen may be required for diagnosis.	• Correction of coagulopathies before insertion • Avoidance of multiple passes with the needle at venipuncture • Use of a small-gauge needle to first locate the vein • Immediate control of femoral bleeding may prevent large blood loss or hematoma formation
Cardiac dysrhythmias	• Premature atrial complexes • Atrial fibrillation or flutter • Premature ventricular complexes • Supraventricular tachycardia • Ventricular tachycardia • Sudden cardiovascular collapse	• Withdraw the guidewire or catheter from the heart; dysrhythmias should stop if the cause was mechanical in nature • Pharmacological treatment of persistent dysrhythmias	• Avoidance of entry into the heart with the guidewire • Observation of cardiac monitor; tall, peaked P waves can be identified as the catheter tip enters the right atrium

TABLE 82-1	Complications of Central Venous Catheter Insertion—cont'd		
Complication	**Clinical Manifestation**	**Treatment**	**Prevention**
Air embolism	• Symptoms depend on amount of air drawn in, especially with patients who are spontaneously breathing • Sudden cardiovascular collapse • Tachypnea, apnea, tachycardia • Hypotension, cyanosis, anxiety • Diffuse pulmonary wheezes • "Mill wheel" churning heart murmur • Neurological deficits, paresis, stroke, coma • Cardiac arrest	• Stop airflow • Position patient on left side in the Trendelenburg position • Oxygen administration • Air aspiration; transthoracic needle or intracardiac catheter • Cardiopulmonary support	• Adequate hydration status • Head-down tilt or the Trendelenburg position during catheter insertion • Use of small-bore needle for insertion • Application of thumb over needle or catheter hub during ventilation; needle or hub should not be exposed longer than 1 second • Advancement of catheter during positive-pressure cycle in patients on ventilatory support • Avoidance of nicking of catheter with careful suturing technique • Avoidance of catheter exchange from large-bore catheter (pulmonary artery) to smaller catheter • Use of Luer-Lok connections • Minimal risk with peripherally inserted central venous catheter
Catheter malposition	• Pain in ear or neck • Swishing sound in ear with infusion • Sharp anterior chest pain • Pain in ipsilateral shoulder blade • Cardiac dysrhythmia • Observation on chest radiograph • Signs or symptoms may be absent • No blood return on aspiration	• Ensure that the bevel of the insertion needle is positioned downward (toward feet of patient) before placing guidewire • Repositioning of catheter with guidewire or new venipuncture • Catheter removal	• Proper patient positioning • Avoidance of use of force when advancing the catheter • Use of a guidewire or blunt-tipped stylet
Catheter embolism	• Cardiac dysrhythmias • Chest pain • Dyspnea • Hypotension • Tachycardia • May be clinically silent	• Location of fragment on radiograph • Transvenous retrieval of catheter fragment • Thoracotomy • Interventional radiology retrieval	• Use of "over a guidewire" (Seldinger) insertion technique • Extreme caution with use of through-the-needle catheter designs; never withdraw a catheter through the needle • Use of guidewire or stylet within a catheter that is inserted through a needle
Cardiac tamponade	• Retrosternal or epigastric pain • Dyspnea • Venous engorgement of face and neck • Restlessness, confusion • Hypotension, paradoxical pulse • Muffled heart sounds • Mediastinal widening • Pleural effusion • Cardiac arrest	• Treatment must be rapid and aggressive • Discontinuation of infusions through the central line • Aspiration through the catheter • Emergency pericardiocentesis • Emergency thoracotomy	• Catheter tip position: Parallel to the walls of the superior vena cava 1–2 cm above the junction of the superior vena cava and right atrium • Use of soft, flexible catheters • Minimal risk with peripherally inserted central venous catheter
Tracheal injury	• Subcutaneous emphysema • Pneumomediastinum • Air trapping between the chest wall and the pleura • Respiratory distress with puncture of endotracheal tube cuff	• Emergency reintubation (for punctured endotracheal tube cuff) • Aspiration of air in mediastinum	• Physician, advanced practice nurse, or other healthcare professional is skilled and experienced in insertion technique • Use of peripherally inserted central venous catheter

Continued

TABLE 82-1	Complications of Central Venous Catheter Insertion—cont'd		
Complication	**Clinical Manifestation**	**Treatment**	**Prevention**
Nerve injury	• Patient has tingling/numbness in arm or fingers • Shooting pain down the arm • Paralysis • Diaphragmatic paralysis (phrenic nerve injury)	• Remove catheter if brachial plexus injury is suspected	• Physician, advanced practice nurse, or other healthcare professional is skilled and experienced in insertion technique • Minimal risk with peripherally inserted central venous catheter
Sterile thrombophlebitis	• Potential complication of the peripherally inserted central venous catheter • Redness, tenderness, swelling along the course of the vein • Pain in the upper extremity or shoulder	• Application of heat for 48–72 hours • Removal of catheter	• Strict aseptic technique during catheter insertion • Adequate skin preparation
Pulmonary embolism	• Potential complication of catheter exchange • Often clinically silent • Chest pain, dyspnea, coughing, tachycardia, anxiety, fever	• Spiral chest CT scan • Lung perfusion scan • Cardiopulmonary support with large pulmonary embolism	• Avoidance of catheter exchange in veins with thrombosis

- 1% lidocaine without epinephrine
- One 25-gauge ⅝-inch needle
- Large package of 4 × 4 gauze sponges
- Suture kit (hemostat, scissors, needle holder)
- 3-0 or 4-0 nylon suture with curved needle
- Syringes: one 10- to 12-mL syringe; two 3- to 5-mL syringes; two 22-gauge, 1½-inch needles
- Masks, head coverings, goggles (shield and mask combination may be used), sterile gloves, and sterile gowns
- No. 11 scalpel
- Roll of 2-inch tape
- Dressing supplies
- Waterproof pad
- Chlorhexidine-impregnated sponge
- Antiseptic solution (e.g., 2% chlorhexidine-based preparation)
- Nonsterile gloves
- Normal saline flush syringes or 0.9% sodium chloride vials, 10- to 30-mL
- Bedside ultrasound machine with vascular probe
- Sterile ultrasound probe cover

Additional equipment, to have available as needed, includes the following:

- Hemodynamic monitoring system (see Procedure 75)
- Sutureless catheter securement device
- Intravenous (IV) solution with Luer-Lok administration set for IV infusion
- Luer-Lok extension tubing
- Bedside monitor and oscilloscope with pulse oximetry
- Supplemental oxygen supplies
- Emergency equipment
- Package of alcohol pads or swab sticks
- Package of povidone-iodine pads or swab sticks
- Heparin flushes
- Sterile injectable or noninjectable caps
- Skin protectant pads or swab sticks

PATIENT AND FAMILY EDUCATION

- Explain the need for the CVC insertion and assess patient and family understanding. *Rationale:* Clarification and understanding of information decrease patient and family anxiety levels.
- Explain the procedure and the time involved. *Rationale:* Explanation increases patient cooperation and decreases patient and family anxiety levels.
- Explain the need for sterile technique and patient positioning, and that the patient's face may be covered. *Rationale:* The explanation decreases patient anxiety and elicits cooperation.
- Explain the benefits and potential risks for the procedure. *Rationale:* Information is offered so that the patient and/or family can make an informed decision.

PATIENT ASSESSMENT AND PREPARATION

Patient Assessment

- Determine the patient's medical history including neck, chest, and groin surgeries and previous vascular access devices. *Rationale:* Data obtained will assist with site selection.
- Determine the patient's medical history of pneumothorax or emphysema. *Rationale:* Patients with emphysematous lungs may be at increased risk for puncture and pneumothorax, depending on the approach.
- Determine the patient's medical history of anomalous veins. *Rationale:* Patients may have a history of dextroacardia or transposition of the great vessels, which leads to greater difficulty in catheter placement.
- Assess the intended insertion site. *Rationale:* Scar tissue may impede placement of the catheter. Permanent pacemakers or

implantable cardioverter defibrillators may preclude placement. Previous surgery and previous placement of a CVC may cause a thrombus to be present or there may be stenosis of a vessel.

- Assess the patient's neurological, cardiac, and pulmonary status. **Rationale:** Aids in determining whether the patient can tolerate Trendelenburg position.
- Assess vital signs and pulse oximetry. **Rationale:** Baseline data enable rapid identification of changes.
- Assess electrolyte levels (e.g., potassium, magnesium, calcium). **Rationale:** Electrolyte abnormalities may increase cardiac irritability.
- Assess for a coagulopathic state and determine whether the patient has recently received anticoagulant or thrombolytic therapy. **Rationale:** These patients are more likely to have complications related to bleeding. Therefore site selection and the need/ability to provide interventions before insertion of the CVC can be determined prospectively.[3]

Patient Preparation

- Verify that the patient is the correct patient using two identifiers. **Rationale:** This increases patient safety by ensuring correct identification of the patient for the intended intervention.

- Ensure that the patient and family understand preprocedural teaching. Answer questions as they arise, and reinforce information as needed. **Rationale:** Understanding of previously taught information is evaluated and reinforced.
- Obtain informed consent. **Rationale:** Informed consent protects the rights of the patient and makes a competent decision possible for the patient; however, in emergency circumstances, time may not allow for this form to be signed.
- Perform a preprocedure verification and timeout, if nonemergent. **Rationale:** Ensures patient safety.
- Prescribe sedation or analgesics as needed. **Rationale:** The patient may need sedation or analgesics to promote comfort and to ensure adequate cooperation and appropriate placement.
- Place an order for patient restraints and apply if needed. **Rationale:** In patients with cognitive impairment, restraints may be needed to ensure maintenance of patient positioning and equipment and access site sterility. During the procedure, restlessness and an altered level of consciousness may represent a pneumothorax, hypoxia, or placement in the carotid artery.

Procedure for Performing Central Venous Catheter Insertion

Steps	Rationale	Special Considerations
1. Review indications, contraindications, and potential complications.	Enables appropriate site selection and preprocedural intervention if needed.	
2. Obtain ultrasound equipment if time is available to determine the most appropriate approach.	Prepares equipment.	Assistance may be needed from radiology.
3. **HH**		
4. **PE**		All physicians, advanced practice nurses, and other healthcare professionals in the room should have on protective equipment including head coverings and masks.[5] Persons inserting the catheter or assisting should use face shields or googles.
5. Place a waterproof pad beneath the site to be accessed.	Avoids soiling of bed linens.	
6. Assist the patient to a position that will optimize access to the site selected.	Proper positioning increases vessel access and optimizes comfort of patient and physician, advanced practice nurse, or other healthcare professional throughout the process.	
7. Determine the anatomy of the access site. (**Level E***)	Helps ensure proper placement of the CVC and guides the area to be prepped.[5,6]	Ultrasound guidance to place CVCs (if the technology is available) should be used to reduce the number of attempts and complications.[5,6]

*Level E: Multiple case reports, theory-based evidence from expert opinions, or peer-reviewed professional organizational standards without clinical studies to support recommendations.

Procedure continues on following page

Procedure	**for Performing Central Venous Catheter Insertion—*Continued***	
Steps	**Rationale**	**Special Considerations**

8. Prepare skin with an antiseptic solution (e.g., 2% chlorhexidine-based preparation).[5,6] **(Level A*)**
  A. Subclavian vein: scrub from shoulder to contralateral nipple line and neck to nipple line (Fig. 82-1A).
  B. Internal jugular vein: scrub midclavicle to opposite border of the sternum and from the ear to a few inches above the nipple (Fig. 82-1B).
  C. Femoral vein: scrub the anterior and medial surface of the proximal thigh to the inguinal ligament.
	Limits the introduction of potentially infectious skin flora into the vessel during the puncture.	If there is a contraindication to chlorhexidine, tincture of iodine, an iodophor, or 70% alcohol can be used as alternatives.[5]

9. Discard used supplies, perform hand hygiene, and apply sterile gown and gloves.	Minimizes the risk of infection and maintains standard and sterile precautions.	
10. Place the full drape over the patient with exposure of only the insertion site.	Prepares sterile field.	All physicians, advanced practice nurses, and other healthcare professionals in the room should have on protective equipment including head coverings and masks.[5]

*Level A: Meta-analysis of quantitative studies or metasynthesis of qualitative studies with results that consistently support a specific action, intervention, or treatment (including systematic review of randomized controlled trials).

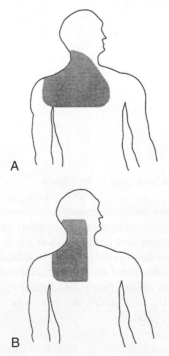

Figure 82-1   Area of skin preparation for central venous catheter insertions. **A,** Subclavian insertion: scrub from shoulder to contralateral nipple line and neck to nipple line. **B,** Jugular insertions: scrub mid clavicle to opposite border of the sternum and from the ear to a few inches above the nipple. *(Courtesy of Suredesign.)*

Procedure	for Performing Central Venous Catheter Insertion—*Continued*	
Steps	**Rationale**	**Special Considerations**
11. Ask critical care nurse or provider assisting to open the CVC insertion kit and drop the sterile items onto the sterile field.	Maintains aseptic technique and prepares the work area.	
12. Check landmarks again for the intended catheter insertion site.	Ensures proper placement of the catheter.	
Site Specific: Internal Jugular Vein (Fig. 82-2) See steps 1–12 above.		
1. Locate the carotid artery.	Helps prevent placing the catheter in the carotid artery.	
2. Identify the jugular vein and mark it if necessary.	Identifies the intended insertion site.	Localization of the vessel may occur with palpation; however, real-time ultrasound should be utilized with the internal jugular approach if equipment and a trained physician, advanced practice nurse, or other healthcare professional are available.[7]
3. Instruct the patient to turn his or her head slightly away from the insertion site.	Helps identify the landmarks.	Ensure that there are no contraindications to neck mobility. If there are no contraindications to neck mobility, the critical care nurse or another physician, advanced practice nurse, or other healthcare professional assisting with the procedure may need to assist the patient to turn his or her head.

Procedure continues on following page

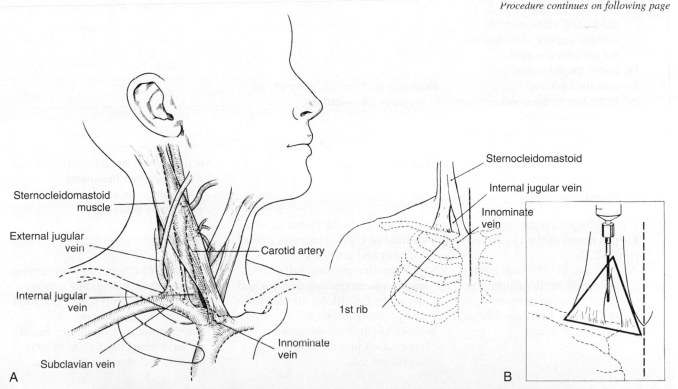

Figure 82-2 Anatomy of the jugular vein. **A,** Anatomy of the internal jugular vein showing its lower location within the triangle formed by the sternocleidomastoid muscle and the clavicle. **B,** Triangle drawn over the clavicle and sternal and clavicular portions of the sternocleidomastoid muscle is centered over the internal jugular vein *(inset). (From Dailey EK, Schroeder JS: Techniques in bedside hemodynamic monitoring. St Louis, 1994, Mosby and redrawn from Daily PO, Griepp RB, Shumway NE: Percutaneous internal jugular vein cannulation,* Arch Surg *101:534–536, 1970. Copyright 1970, American Medical Association.)*

Procedure   for Performing Central Venous Catheter Insertion—*Continued*

Steps	Rationale	Special Considerations
4. Ensure that the patient is in the Trendelenburg position (i.e., 15 to 25 degrees).[1,2] **(Level E*)**	Minimizes the risk for venous air embolus by increasing the pressure in the large veins above atmospheric pressure thus reducing the risk of air aspiration. The patient should be positioned so that the intended puncture site is at or below the level of the heart.[1,2]	Most patients can tolerate Trendelenburg positioning but intracranial, respiratory, or cardiac compromise may occur. Therefore evaluation for the need for alternative sites and close monitoring are necessary.
5. Identify the internal jugular vein from the triangle between the medial aspect of the clavicle, the medial aspect of the sternal head, and the lateral head of the sternocleidomastoid muscle (see Fig. 82-2).	A high entry can be made from a posterior approach, a lateral approach, an anterior approach, or a central approach.	The midanterior approach may be preferred in an obese patient. The posterior approach may present a slightly higher risk. The internal jugular vein is 3–4 cm above the medial clavicle and 1–3 cm within the lateral border of the sternocleidomastoid muscle.
6. Administer an anesthetic: A. Attach a 3- or 5-mL syringe with 2 or 3 mL of 1% lidocaine (without epinephrine) to an 18-gauge needle. B. Align the needle with the syringe parallel to the medial border of the clavicular head of the sternocleidomastoid muscle. C. Aim at a 30-degree angle to the frontal plane over the internal jugular vein, toward the ipsilateral nipple. D. Instill the lidocaine.	Promotes patient comfort during the procedure. Helps to anesthetize below the subcutaneous tissue.	
7. Prepare the catheter: A. Place sterile injectable or noninjectable caps. B. Flush the catheter and ports with normal saline.	Removes air from the catheter and prepares for insertion.	
8. Place the sterile probe over the ultrasound equipment and locate the vessel.	Maintains sterility.	Another physician, advanced practice nurse, or other healthcare professional in sterile attire may assist with this step.
9. Use Seldinger's technique for placement of the catheter (Fig. 82-3). A. Puncture the skin and advance the needle while maintaining slight negative pressure within the syringe until free-flowing blood is obtained.	This technique is the preferred method of CVC placement; it uses a dilator and guidewire. Slight negative pressure helps to ensure placement into the vein and decreases the risk for air embolism and pneumothorax. Without slight negative pressure, penetration into the vein will go unrecognized.	Insert at a 45-degree angle to prevent pneumothorax. Avoiding a too-lateral or too-deep needle insertion can reduce the risk for pneumothorax. Lateral movement of an inserted needle can lacerate vessels and should not be done.

*Level E: Multiple case reports, theory-based evidence from expert opinions, or peer-reviewed professional organizational standards without clinical studies to support recommendations

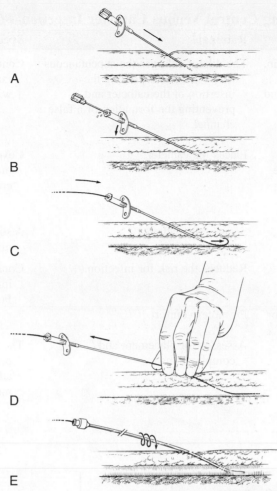

Figure 82-3 Basic procedure for Seldinger's technique. **A,** The vessel is punctured with the needle at a 30- to 40-degree angle. **B,** The stylet is removed, and free blood flow is observed; the angle of the needle is then reduced. **C,** The flexible tip of the guidewire is passed through the needle into the vessel. **D,** The needle is removed over the wire while firm pressure is applied at the site. **E,** The tip of the catheter or sheath is passed over the wire and advanced into the vessel with a rotating motion. *(From Dailey EK, Schroeder JS: Techniques in bedside hemodynamic monitoring. St Louis, 1994, Mosby.)*

Procedure	**for Performing Central Venous Catheter Insertion—*Continued***

Steps	Rationale	Special Considerations
B. After a free flow of blood is returned, turn the bevel to the 3 o'clock position. Once in the vein, have the patient hold his or her breath while the syringe is detached and insert the soft-tipped guidewire 20–25 cm through the needle.	A free flow of blood indicates a vessel has been entered.	When preparing the syringe and needle, line the bevel up with the numbers on the syringe so that you know where the bevel is regardless of how the syringe is manipulated during placement.
C. Remove the needle.		
D. Wipe the guidewire with the sterile 4 × 4 gauze.	Wiping the guidewire dry may ease manipulation.	The guidewire should always pass easily without resistance.
E. Instruct the patient to breathe normally.		
10. With a No. 11 blade, knife edge up, make a small (2–3-mm) stab wound at the insertion site.	Eases the insertion of the dilator through the skin.	

Procedure continues on following page

Procedure	**for Performing Central Venous Catheter Insertion—*Continued***	
Steps	**Rationale**	**Special Considerations**
11. Insert the dilator through the skin, over the guidewire, until 10–15 cm of wire extends beyond the dilator, then remove the dilator while maintaining the position of the guidewire.	The dilator enlarges the subcutaneous tissue and vessel, easing the insertion of the catheter and preventing the formation of a false channel.	Control of the guidewire should be maintained at all times to avoid wire embolization.
12. Advance the catheter over the guidewire until 10–15 cm of the guidewire extends beyond the catheter and then remove the guidewire.	Places the catheter.	Cover the needle hub between manipulations to avoid air embolization.
13. Suture the catheter in place.	Secures the catheter.	A sutureless catheter-securing device may be used to stabilize the CVC.
14. Apply an occlusive, sterile dressing (see Procedure 66).	Reduces the risk for infection.	Consider use of a chlorhexidine-impregnated sponge dressing.[5,6] Follow institutional standards.
15. Return the patient to a neutral, or head-up, position.	Promotes comfort.	
16. Assess lung sounds and peak airway pressures (in ventilated patients), and obtain a chest radiograph.	Assesses for placement and complications.	The radiograph needs to be read before utilization of the catheter for administration of IV fluid and medications.

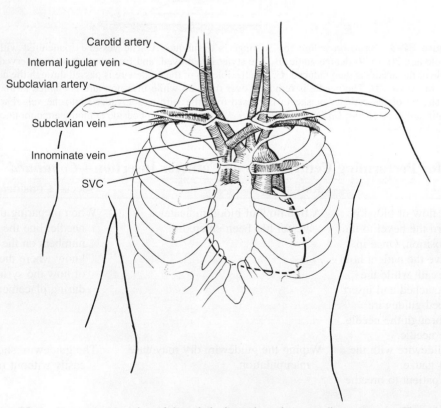

Figure 82-4   Anatomical location of the subclavian vein and surrounding structures. The subclavian vein joins the internal jugular vein to become the innominate vein at about the manubrioclavicular junction. The innominate vein becomes the superior vena cava (SVC) at about the level of the mid manubrium. *(From Dailey EK, Schroeder JS: Techniques in bedside hemodynamic monitoring, St Louis, 1994, Mosby.)*

Procedure | for Performing Central Venous Catheter Insertion—*Continued*

Steps	Rationale	Special Considerations
17. Remove **PE** and discard used supplies in appropriate receptacles.	Reduces the transmission of microorganisms and minimizes exposure to contaminated sharps.	
18. **HH**		

Specific Site: Subclavian Vein (Fig. 82-4)

See steps 1–12 above.

Steps	Rationale	Special Considerations
1. Identify the junction of the middle and medial thirds of the clavicle. The needle insertion should be 1–2 cm laterally.	Identifies the landmarks for catheter placement.	Access from the right side is preferred to avoid inadvertent puncture of the thoracic duct.
2. Depress the area 1–2 cm beneath the junction with the thumb of the nondominant hand and the index finger 2 cm above the sternal notch.	Helps identify the landmarks.	To avoid the subclavian artery, select a puncture site away from the most lateral course of the vein and do not aim too posteriorly.
3. Identify the subclavian vein.	May aid in identifying the intended insertion site.	Utilization of real-time ultrasound should be considered with the subclavian approach if equipment and a trained physician, advanced practice nurse, or other healthcare professional are available.[7]
4. Instruct the patient to turn his or her head away from the insertion site.	Helps identify the landmarks.	Ensure that there are no contraindications to neck mobility. If there are none, the critical care nurse or another physician, advanced practice nurse, or other healthcare professional assisting with the procedure may need to assist the patient to turn his or her head.
5. Position the patient for optimal vein access. A. Ensure that the patient is in the Trendelenburg position (i.e., 15–25 degrees). B. Adduct the patient's arms. C. Consider placing a rolled towel between the patient's shoulder blades.	Minimizes the risk for venous air embolus by increasing the pressure in the large veins above atmospheric pressure thus reducing the risk of air aspiration. The patient should be positioned so that the intended puncture site is at or below the level of the heart.[1,2]	Most patients can tolerate the Trendelenburg positioning but intracranial, respiratory, or cardiac compromise may occur. Therefore evaluation for the need for alternative sites and close monitoring are necessary.
6. Administer a local anesthetic. A. Attach a 3- or 5-mL syringe with 2 or 3 mL of 1% lidocaine (without epinephrine) to an 18-gauge needle. B. Inject the lidocaine into the area surrounding the intended insertion site.	Promotes patient comfort during the procedure. Helps to anesthetize below the subcutaneous tissue.	
7. Prepare the catheter: A. Flush the catheter and ports with normal saline. B. Place sterile injectable or noninjectable caps.	Removes air from the catheter and prepares for insertion.	
8. Place the sterile probe over the ultrasound equipment and locate the vessel.	Maintains sterility.	Another physician, advanced practice nurse, or other healthcare professional in sterile attire may assist with this step.

Procedure continues on following page

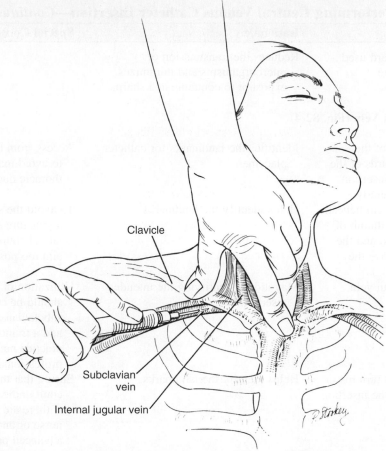

Figure 82-5 Puncture of the subclavian vein with the needle inserted beneath the middle third of the clavicle at a 20- to 30-degree angle aiming medially. *(From Dailey EK, Schroeder JS: Techniques in bedside hemodynamic monitoring. St Louis, 1994, Mosby.)*

Procedure	for Performing Central Venous Catheter Insertion—*Continued*	
Steps	**Rationale**	**Special Considerations**
9. Use Seldinger's technique for placement of the catheter (see Fig. 82-3).	This technique is the preferred method of CVC placement; it uses a dilator and guidewire.	
A. Insert the needle under the clavicle and "walk down" until it slips below the clavicle and enters the vein while maintaining negative pressure within the syringe until free-flowing blood is returned (Fig. 82-5).	Slight negative pressure helps to ensure placement into the vein and decreases the risk for air embolism and pneumothorax. Without slight negative pressure, penetration into the vein will go unrecognized.	Insert at a 45-degree angle to prevent pneumothorax. Avoiding a too-lateral or too-deep needle insertion can reduce the risk for pneumothorax. Lateral movement of an inserted needle can lacerate vessels and should not be done.
B. After a free flow of blood is returned, have the patient hold his or her breath while the syringe is detached and insert the soft-tipped guidewire 20–25 cm through the needle under constant manual control.	A free flow of blood indicates a vessel has been entered.	

In the figure the following labels appear: Clavicle, Subclavian vein, Internal jugular vein.

Procedure	**for Performing Central Venous Catheter Insertion—*Continued***	
Steps	**Rationale**	**Special Considerations**

C. Remove the needle.
  D. Wipe the guidewire with the sterile 4 × 4 gauze.
  E. Instruct the patient to breathe normally.
	Wiping the guidewire dry may ease manipulation.	

10. With a No. 11 blade, knife edge up, make a small (2-mm to 3-mm) stab wound at the insertion site.	Eases the insertion of the dilator through the skin.	
11. Insert the dilator through the skin, over the guidewire, advancing under the clavicle until 20–25 cm of wire extends beyond the dilator, then remove the dilator while maintaining the position of the guidewire.	The dilator enlarges the subcutaneous tissue and vessel, easing the insertion of the catheter and preventing the formation of a false channel.	Control of the guidewire should be maintained at all times to avoid wire embolization.
12. Advance the catheter over the guidewire until 20–25 cm of the guidewire extends beyond the catheter and then remove the guidewire.	Places the catheter.	Cover the needle hub between manipulations to avoid air embolization.
13. Suture the catheter in place.	Secures the catheter.	A sutureless catheter-securing device may be used to stabilize the CVC.
14. Apply an occlusive, sterile dressing to the site (see Procedure 66).	Provides a sterile environment.	Consider use of a chlorhexidine-impregnated sponge dressing.[5,6] Follow institutional standards.
15. Return the patient to a neutral or head up position.	Promotes comfort.	
16. Assess lung sounds and peak airway pressures (in ventilated patients) and obtain a chest radiograph.	Assesses for placement and complications.	The radiograph needs to be read before utilization of the catheter for administration of IV fluid and medications.
17. Remove **PE** and discard used supplies in appropriate receptacles.	Reduces the transmission of microorganisms and minimizes exposure to contaminated sharps.	
18. **HH**		

Specific Site: Femoral Vein (see Fig. 81-2)

See steps 1–12 above.

1. Assist the patient to a supine, flat position with the intended leg extended.	Prepares for the procedure.	
2. Locate the femoral artery and mark it if necessary.	Identifies the intended insertion site.	Localization of the vessel may occur with palpation; however, real-time ultrasound should be utilized with the femoral approach if equipment and a trained physician, advanced practice nurse, or other healthcare professional are available.[5-7]

3. Administer a local anesthetic.
  A. Attach a 3- or 5-mL syringe with 2 or 3 mL of 1% lidocaine (without epinephrine) to an 18-gauge needle.
  B. Inject the lidocaine into the area surrounding the intended insertion site.
	Promotes patient comfort during the procedure. Helps to anesthetize below the subcutaneous tissue.	

Procedure continues on following page

Procedure **for Performing Central Venous Catheter Insertion—*Continued***

Steps	Rationale	Special Considerations
4. Prepare the catheter: A. Flush the catheter and ports with normal saline. B. Place sterile injectable or noninjectable caps.	Removes air from the catheter and prepares for insertion.	
5. Place the sterile probe over the ultrasound equipment and locate the vessel.	Maintains sterility.	Another physician, advanced practice nurse, or other healthcare professional in sterile attire may assist with this step.
6. Use Seldinger's technique for placement of the catheter (see Fig. 82-3).	This technique is the preferred method of CVC placement; it uses a dilator and guidewire.	
A. Insert the needle at a 20–30 degree angle 1–2 cm inferior to the inguinal ligament and just medial to the femoral artery. Maintain slight, continuous, negative pressure during insertion and advance the needle until free-flowing blood is returned.	Slight negative pressure helps to ensure placement into the vein. Without slight negative pressure, penetration into the vein will go unrecognized.	Lateral movement of an inserted needle can lacerate vessels and should not be done.
B. After a free flow of blood is returned, detach the syringe and insert the soft-tipped guidewire 25 cm under constant manual control.	A free flow of blood indicates a vessel has been entered.	
C. Remove the needle.		
D. Wipe the guidewire with the sterile 4 × 4 gauze.	Wiping the guidewire dry may ease manipulation.	
7. With a No. 11 blade, knife edge up, make a small (2-mm to 3-mm) stab wound at the insertion site.	Eases the insertion of the dilator through the skin.	
8. Insert the dilator through the skin, over the guidewire, until 25 cm of wire extends beyond the dilator, then remove the dilator while maintaining the position of the guidewire.	The dilator enlarges the subcutaneous tissue and vessel, easing the insertion of the catheter and preventing the formation of a false channel.	Control of the guidewire should be maintained at all times to avoid wire embolization.
9. Advance the catheter over the guidewire until 25 cm of the guidewire extends beyond the catheter and then remove the guidewire.	Places the catheter.	
10. Suture the catheter in place.	Secures the catheter.	A sutureless catheter-securing device may be used to stabilize the CVC.
11. Apply an occlusive, sterile dressing to the site.	Decreases the risk for infection.	Consider use of a chlorhexidine-impregnated sponge dressing.[5,6] Follow institutional standards.
12. Return the patient to a neutral position with the head of the bed slightly elevated.	Facilitates comfort.	
13. Obtain an x-ray.	Assesses for placement and complications.	The radiograph needs to be read before utilization of the catheter for administration of IV fluid and medications.

Procedure   for Performing Central Venous Catheter Insertion—*Continued*

Steps	Rationale	Special Considerations
14. Remove **PE** and discard used supplies in appropriate receptacles.	Reduces the transmission of microorganisms and minimizes exposure to contaminated sharps.	
15. **HH**		

Expected Outcomes

- Successful placement of the CVC
- If infusing IV solution, the solution infuses without problems
- The *a*, *c*, and *v* waves are identified if hemodynamic monitoring is used
- CVP measurements are obtained

Unexpected Outcomes

- Failure to place catheter
- Arterial puncture
- Catheter embolization
- Vascular injury
- Pain or discomfort during the insertion procedure
- Pneumothorax, tension pneumothorax, hemothorax, or chylothorax
- Nerve injury
- Sterile thrombophlebitis
- Infection
- Cardiac dysrhythmias
- Malposition
- Inadvertent lymphatic or thoracic duct perforation
- Hemorrhage
- Hematoma
- Venous air embolism
- Cardiac tamponade

Patient Monitoring and Care

Steps	Rationale	Reportable Conditions
		These conditions should be reported if they persist despite nursing interventions.
1. Perform respiratory, cardiovascular, peripheral vascular, and hemodynamic assessments immediately before and after the procedure and as the patient's condition necessitates.	Determines whether signs or symptoms of complications are present, for example, an air embolism may present with restlessness.	• Abnormal level of consciousness • Abnormal vital signs • Abnormal waveforms or pressures • Declining oxygen saturation • Increasing peak airway pressures
2. If the catheter was placed for CVP measurement, assess the waveform.	Ensures that the catheter is in the proper location for monitoring. Allows assessment of *a*, *c*, and *v* waves and measurement of pressure.	• Abrupt and sustained changes in CVP • Abnormal waveform
3. Assess the insertion site for presence of a hematoma or hemorrhage.	Determines the presence of complications.	• Bleeding that does not stop • Hematoma or expanding hematoma
4. Assess heart and lung sounds before and after the procedure.	Abnormal heart or lung sounds may indicate cardiac tamponade, pneumothorax, chylothorax, or hemothorax.	• Diminished or muffled heart sounds • Absent or diminished breath sounds unilaterally
5. Assess the results of the chest radiograph.	Ensures accurate placement and may aid in identification of complications.	• Abnormal radiograph results
6. Monitor for signs of complications.	May decrease mortality and morbidity if recognized early.	• Signs and symptoms of complications

Procedure continues on following page

Patient Monitoring and Care —*Continued*

Steps	Rationale	Reportable Conditions
7. Follow institutional standards for assessing pain. Prescribe analgesia as needed.	Identifies need for pain interventions.	• Continued pain despite pain interventions
8. If signs and symptoms of venous air embolus are present, immediately place the patient in the left-lateral Trendelenburg position. (**Level E***)	Venous air embolus is a potentially life-threatening complication. The left-lateral Trendelenburg position prevents air from passing into the left side of the heart and traveling into the arterial circulation.[1,2]	• Respiratory distress • Dyspnea • Coughing • Tachypnea • Altered mental status (agitation, restlessness) • Cyanosis • Gasp reflex • Sucking sound near the site of the catheter insertion/air entrainment • Petechiae • Cardiac dysrhythmias • Chest pain • Hypotension

*Level E: Multiple case reports, theory-based evidence from expert opinions, or peer-reviewed professional organizational standards without clinical studies to support recommendations.

Documentation

Documentation should include the following:
- Patient and family education
- Completion of informed consent
- Preprocedure verifications and timeout
- Insertion of central venous catheter
- Insertion site of central venous catheter
- Date and time of procedure
- Catheter type
- Lumen size

- Right-atrial pressure and CVP waveform in the event of pressure monitoring
- Centimeter marking at the skin
- Patient response to the procedure
- Pain assessment, interventions, and effectiveness
- Confirmation of placement (e.g., chest radiograph)
- Occurrence of unexpected outcomes
- Additional nursing interventions

References and Additional Readings

For a complete list of references and additional readings for this procedure, scan this QR code with any freely available smartphone code reader app, or visit http://booksite.elsevier.com/9780323376624.

83 Central Venous Catheter Insertion (Assist)

Susan Yeager

PURPOSE: Central venous catheters (CVCs) are inserted for measurement of central venous pressure (CVP) with jugular or subclavian catheter placement. Clinically useful information can be obtained about right-ventricular preload, cardiovascular status, and fluid balance in patients who do not need pulmonary artery pressure monitoring. CVCs also are placed for infusion of vasoactive medications and to provide access for pulmonary artery catheters and transvenous pacemakers.

PREREQUISITE NURSING KNOWLEDGE

- Knowledge of the normal anatomy and physiology of the cardiovascular system is needed.
- Knowledge of the anatomy and physiology of the vasculature and adjacent structures of the neck, groin, and chest is needed.
- Knowledge of the principles of sterile technique is essential.
- Advanced cardiac life support (ACLS) knowledge and skills are needed.
- Knowledge of potential complications and associated interventions/consultations for addressing issues is necessary.
- Indications for CVC placement may include the following:
  - ❖ Severe blood loss
  - ❖ Hemodynamic instability
  - ❖ Administration of vesicant irritant medications
  - ❖ Administration of total parenteral nutrition
  - ❖ Lack of peripheral venous access
  - ❖ Assessment of hypovolemia or hypervolemia
  - ❖ Monitoring of central venous pressures
  - ❖ Placement of pulmonary artery catheters or placement of transvenous pacemakers
  - ❖ Hemodialysis access
- The normal CVP value is 2 to 8 mm Hg.
- The CVP waveform is identical to the right-atrial waveform.
- Interpretation of right-atrial/CVP waveforms including identification of a, c, and v waves is important. The a wave reflects right-atrial contraction. The c wave reflects closure of the tricuspid valve. The v wave reflects passive filling of the right atria during right-ventricular systole.
- The CVP provides information regarding right-heart filling pressures and right-ventricular function and volume.
- The CVP is commonly elevated during or after right-ventricular failure, ischemia, or infarction because of decreased compliance of the right ventricle.

- The CVP can be helpful in the determination of hypovolemia. The CVP value is low if the patient is hypovolemic. Venodilation also decreases the CVP value.
- Electrocardiographic monitoring is essential in the accurate interpretation of the CVP value.
- Some contraindications of CVC insertion include anatomical problems, venous obstructions, and coagulopathies. The subclavian site should be avoided in hemodialysis patients and patients with advanced kidney disease to avoid subclavian vein stenosis.[5]
- It is important to weigh the risks and benefits of placing a CVC against the risk for mechanical complications (e.g., pneumothorax, vein laceration, thrombosis, air embolism, misplacement).[5,6]
- A subclavian site is recommended rather than a jugular or femoral site to minimize the risk of infection.[5]
- The internal jugular site is recommended to minimize catheter cannulation-related risk of injury or trauma.[6]
- Ultrasound guidance is recommended to place CVCs if the technology is available to reduce the number of cannulation attempts and mechanical complications.[4,5,7]
- Regardless of the site selected, complications may occur during or after insertion of a central venous catheter (see Table 82-1).

EQUIPMENT

- CVC insertion kit
- CVC of choice (single, dual, or triple lumen) usually supplied with insertion needle, dilator, syringe, and guidewire.
- Full sterile drapes
- 1% lidocaine without epinephrine
- One 25-gauge ⅝-inch needle
- Large package of 4 × 4 gauze sponges
- Suture kit (hemostat, scissors, needle holder)
- 3-0 or 4-0 nylon suture with curved needle
- Syringes: one 10- to 12-mL syringe; two 3- to 5-mL syringes; two 22-gauge, 1½-inch needles
- Masks, head coverings, goggles (shield and mask combination may be used), sterile gloves, and sterile gowns

- No. 11 scalpel
- Roll of 2-inch tape
- Dressing supplies
- Waterproof pad
- Chlorhexidine-impregnated sponge
- Antiseptic solution (e.g., 2% chlorhexidine-based preparation)
- Nonsterile gloves
- Normal saline flush syringes or 0.9% sodium chloride vials, 10- to 30-mL
- Bedside ultrasound machine with vascular probe
- Sterile ultrasound probe cover

Additional equipment, to have available as needed, includes the following:

- Hemodynamic monitoring system (see Procedure 75)
- Sutureless catheter securement device
- Intravenous (IV) solution with Luer-Lok administration set for IV infusion
- Luer-Lok extension tubing
- Bedside monitor and oscilloscope with pulse oximetry
- Supplemental oxygen supplies
- Emergency equipment
- Package of alcohol pads or swab sticks
- Package of povidone-iodine pads or swab sticks
- Heparin flushes
- Sterile injectable or noninjectable caps
- Skin protectant pads or swab sticks

PATIENT AND FAMILY EDUCATION

- Explain the need for the CVC insertion, and assess patient and family understanding. *Rationale:* Clarification and understanding of information decrease patient and family anxiety levels.
- Explain the procedure and the time involved. *Rationale:* Explanation increases patient cooperation and decreases patient and family anxiety levels.
- Explain the need for sterile technique and patient positioning and that the patient's face may be covered. *Rationale:* The explanation decreases patient anxiety and elicits cooperation.
- Explain the benefits and potential risks for the procedure. *Rationale:* Information is offered so that the patient and/or family can make an informed decision.

PATIENT ASSESSMENT AND PREPARATION

Patient Assessment

- Assess the patient's neurological, cardiac, and pulmonary status. *Rationale:* Some patients may not tolerate a supine

or the Trendelenburg position for extended periods of time due to increased intracranial pressure or cardiopulmonary compromise.

- Assess vital signs and pulse oximetry. *Rationale:* Baseline data can be compared with data obtained during and after the procedure.
- Assess electrolyte levels (e.g., potassium, magnesium, calcium). *Rationale:* Electrolyte abnormalities may increase cardiac irritability.
- Assess for a coagulopathic state and determine whether the patient has recently received anticoagulant or thrombolytic therapy. *Rationale:* These patients are more likely to have complications related to bleeding. Therefore, site selection and the need/ability to provide interventions before insertion of the CVC can be determined prospectively.[3]

Patient Preparation

- Verify that the patient is the correct patient using two identifiers. *Rationale:* This increases patient safety by ensuring correct identification of the patient for the intended intervention.
- Ensure that the patient and family understand preprocedural teaching. Answer questions as they arise, and reinforce information as needed. *Rationale:* Understanding of previously taught information is evaluated and reinforced.
- Ensure informed consent has been obtained. *Rationale:* Informed consent protects the rights of the patient and makes a competent decision possible for the patient; however, in emergency circumstances, time may not allow for this form to be signed.
- Assist in performing a preprocedure verification and timeout, if nonemergent. *Rationale:* Ensures patient safety.
- Request and administer sedation or analgesics as prescribed and as needed. *Rationale:* The patient may need sedation or analgesics to promote comfort and to ensure adequate cooperation and appropriate placement.
- Apply patient restraints if ordered and if needed. *Rationale:* In patients with cognitive impairment, restraints may be needed to ensure maintenance of patient positioning and equipment and access site sterility. During the procedure, restlessness and an altered level of consciousness may represent a pneumothorax, hypoxia, or placement in the carotid artery.
- Depending on the site selected and the patient's body habitus, specific positioning may be necessary. Assist with this positioning as needed. (i.e., subclavian vein, assist with placing a towel posteriorly between the shoulder blades.) *Rationale:* Specific positioning techniques for each site assists with optimal vessel access.

Procedure for Assisting with Central Venous Catheter Insertion

Steps	Rationale	Special Considerations
1. **HH**		
2. **PE**		All physicians, advanced practice nurses, and other healthcare professionals in the room should have on protective equipment including head coverings and masks.[5]
3. Prepare the IV solution or flush solution.	Prepares the infusion system.	
4. Prime the IV tubing or flush the entire pressure-transducer system if pressure monitoring is anticipated (see Procedure 75).	Removes air bubbles. Air bubbles introduced into the patient's circulation can cause air embolisms. Air bubbles within the tubing dampen the waveform and can alter pressure results.	
5. Apply and maintain pressure in the pressure bag or device at 300 mm Hg.	Each flush device delivers 1–3 mL/hr to maintain patency of the hemodynamic system.	
6. Place a moisture-proof pad under the patient's back.	Avoids soiling of the bed.	
7. Assist as needed with patient positioning.	Proper positioning increases vessel access and optimizes comfort of the patient and physicians, advanced practice nurses, and other healthcare professionals throughout the process.	
8. If needed remove gloves, wash hands and apply sterile gown and gloves. Then assist as needed with the preparation of the skin with an antiseptic solution (e.g., 2% chlorhexidine-based preparation).[5,6] (**Level A***) A. Subclavian vein: scrub from shoulder to contralateral nipple line and neck to nipple line (see Fig. 82-1, *A*). B. Internal jugular vein: scrub midclavicle to opposite border of the sternum and from the ear to a few inches above the nipple (see Fig. 82-1B). C. Femoral vein: scrub the anterior and medial surface of the proximal thigh to the inguinal ligament.	Limits the introduction of potentially infectious skin flora into the vessel during the puncture.	If there is a contraindication to chlorhexidine, tincture of iodine, an iodophor, or 70% alcohol can be used as alternatives.[5]

*Level A: Meta-analysis of quantitative studies or metasynthesis of qualitative studies with results that consistently support a specific action, intervention, or treatment (including systematic review of randomized controlled trials).

Procedure continues on following page

Procedure   for Assisting with Central Venous Catheter Insertion—*Continued*

Steps	Rationale	Special Considerations
9. While the physician or advanced practice nurse completes the skin preparation, ensure patient comfort by explaining what is happening at the time. A. Application of the antiseptic solution is cold and wet. B. Injection of the local anesthetic may burn or sting as the tissue is infiltrated.	Reduces anxiety and encourages cooperation.	Continue providing support and comfort throughout the procedure.
10. Assist as needed with applying a full drape to the patient with exposure of only the insertion site.	Minimizes the risk of infection; maintains aseptic and sterile precautions.	
11. Assist as needed with placement of the sterile ultrasound probe cover.	Provides help as needed.	
12. Place the bed in the Trendelenburg position (i.e., 15–20 degrees). **(Level E*)**	Minimizes the risk for venous air embolus by increasing the pressure in the large veins above atmospheric pressure, thus reducing the risk of air aspiration. The patient should be positioned so that the intended puncture site is at or below the level of the heart.[1,2]	Most patients can tolerate Trendelenburg positioning but intracranial, respiratory, or cardiac compromise may occur. Therefore evaluation for the need for alternative sites and close monitoring are necessary.
13. Monitor the heart rate, respiratory rate and rhythm, pulse oximetry, intracranial pressure, and any patient response to the procedure.	Assessment may indicate occurrence of complications (see Table 82-1).	Assess patient comfort throughout the procedure.
14. Observe the cardiac monitor while the guidewire and catheter are advanced, and inform the physician or advanced practice nurse immediately if a dysrhythmia occurs.	Advancement of the guidewire or catheter into the heart may induce cardiac dysrhythmias.	Tall, peaked P waves may be observed as the catheter tip enters the right atrium or if the guidewire has been advanced too far into the right atrium. Dysrhythmias may resolve with withdrawal of the guidewire or catheter. If the dysrhythmia continues, antidysrhythmic medications may be necessary.
15. Once the catheter is placed and blood return is ensured, assist if needed with flushing the lumen(s) with normal saline solution.	Maintains aseptic technique and maintains catheter patency.	Ensure a tight connection to prevent accidental disconnection. Luer-Lok devices prevent an accidental disconnection.
16. Assist as needed with applying a sterile, occlusive dressing (see Procedure 66).	Reduces the risk for infection.	A sutureless catheter-securing device may be used to stabilize the CVC. Consider use of a chlorhexidine-impregnated sponge dressing.[5,6] Follow institutional standards.

*Level E: Multiple case reports, theory-based evidence from expert opinions, or peer-reviewed professional organizational standards without clinical studies to support recommendations.

Procedure for Assisting with Central Venous Catheter Insertion—*Continued*

Steps	Rationale	Special Considerations

17. If monitoring:
  A. Connect the hemodynamic monitoring tubing to the catheter.
  B. Level the CVP air-fluid interface (zeroing stopcock) to the phlebostatic axis (see Procedure 75).
  C. Zero the system by turning the stopcock off to the patient, opening it to air, and zeroing the monitoring system (see Procedure 75).
  D. Place a sterile injectable or noninjectable cap on the top port of the stopcock, turn the stopcock open to the patient, and observe the waveform (see Procedure 67).
  E. Obtain a waveform strip.
  F. Measure the pressure.
  G. Set the alarms.
	Prepares the hemodynamic monitoring system and assesses the CVP waveform.	

18. Reposition the patient in a comfortable position.	Promotes comfort.	
19. Assess lung sounds and peak airway pressures (in ventilated patients), and if assistance is needed with obtaining a chest radiograph as prescribed.	Assesses for placement and complications.	The radiograph needs to be read before utilization of the catheter for administration of IV fluid and medications.
20. Remove **PE** and assist as needed with discarding used supplies in appropriate receptacles.	Reduces the transmission of microorganisms and minimizes exposure to contaminated sharps.	The physician or advanced practice nurse who inserted the catheter should dispose of all sharp objects into sharps containers.
21. **HH**		

Expected Outcomes

- Successful placement of the CVC
- If infusing IV solution, the solution infuses without problems
- The *a, c,* and *v* waves are identified if hemodynamic monitoring is used
- CVP measurements are obtained

Unexpected Outcomes

- Failure to place catheter
- Arterial puncture
- Catheter embolization
- Vascular injury
- Pain or discomfort during the insertion procedure
- Pneumothorax, tension pneumothorax, hemothorax, or chylothorax
- Nerve injury
- Sterile thrombophlebitis
- Infection
- Cardiac dysrhythmias
- Malposition
- Inadvertent lymphatic or thoracic duct perforation
- Hemorrhage
- Hematoma
- Venous air embolism
- Cardiac tamponade

Procedure continues on following page

Patient Monitoring and Care

Steps	Rationale	Reportable Conditions
		These conditions should be reported if they persist despite nursing interventions.
1. Assess the patient's vital signs, oxygenation saturation, and level of consciousness before the procedure, after the procedure, and as needed during the procedure.	Identifies signs and symptoms of complications and allows for immediate interventions.	• Abnormal vital signs • Abnormal pulse oximetry value • Changes in level of consciousness
2. If the catheter was placed for CVP measurement, assess the waveform.	Ensures that the catheter is in the proper location for monitoring. Allows assessment of *a*, *c*, and *v* waves and measurement of pressure.	• Abrupt and sustained changes in CVP • Abnormal waveform
3. Observe the catheter site for bleeding or hematoma every 15–30 minutes for the first 2 hours after insertion.	Postinsertion bleeding may occur in a patient with coagulopathies or arterial punctures, with multiple attempts at vein access, or with the use of through-the-needle introducer designs for insertion.	• Bleeding that does not stop • Hematoma or expanding hematoma
4. Assess heart and lung sounds before and after the procedure.	Abnormal heart or lung sounds may indicate cardiac tamponade, pneumothorax, chylothorax, or hemothorax.	• Diminished or muffled heart sounds • Absent or diminished breath sounds unilaterally
5. Follow institutional standards for assessing pain. Administer analgesia as prescribed.	Identifies need for pain interventions.	• Continued pain despite pain interventions
6. If signs and symptoms of venous air embolus are present, immediately place the patient in the left lateral Trendelenburg position. **(Level E*)**	Venous air embolus is a potentially life-threatening complication. The left-lateral Trendelenburg position prevents air from passing into the left side of the heart and traveling into the arterial circulation.[1,2]	• Respiratory distress • Dyspnea • Coughing • Tachypnea • Altered mental status (agitation, restlessness) • Cyanosis • Gasp reflex • Sucking sound near the site of the catheter insertion/air entrainment • Petechiae • Cardiac dysrhythmias • Chest pain • Hypotension

*Level E: Multiple case reports, theory-based evidence from expert opinions, or peer-reviewed professional organizational standards without clinical studies to support recommendations.

Documentation

Documentation should include the following:
- Patient and family education
- Universal Protocol requirements
- Catheter location
- Medications administered
- Right-atrial pressure and CVP waveform if monitored
- Centimeter marking at the skin
- Patient response to the procedure
- Pain assessment, interventions, and effectiveness
- Fluids administered
- Type of dressing applied
- Occurrence of unexpected outcomes
- Additional nursing interventions

References and Additional Readings

For a complete list of references and additional readings for this procedure, scan this QR code with any freely available smartphone code reader app, or visit http://booksite.elsevier.com/9780323376624.

84 Implantable Venous Access AP Device: Access, Deaccess, and Care

Anne Delengowski

PURPOSE: Implantable venous access devices or ports are surgically placed and used for delivery of medications, including cytotoxic agents, parenteral solutions, blood products, and for blood sampling for patients who need long-term venous access.

PREREQUISITE NURSING KNOWLEDGE

- Understanding of the implantable venous access device, including the septum and outer borders, is needed.
- Knowledge of the anatomy of the venous system is needed.
- Understanding is needed of the principles of medication delivery. Intermittent use necessitates flushing with normal saline (NS) solution after each use and instillation of heparin as prescribed when the medication infusion is completed.
- Understanding of the principles of aseptic and sterile techniques is necessary.
- Knowledge of the consequences of infiltration of a vesicant substance is needed.
- There are single- and double-lumen ports. All ports are designed with a portal body and a catheter. The portal body contains a septum and reservoir, which is made of plastic, titanium, polysulfone, or a combination.[4] A slim tube or catheter is connected to the reservoir, which is covered by a disc 2 to 3 cm in width (Figs. 84-1 and 84-2). Provided a noncoring needle is used to access the septum, the septum is capable of resealing when deaccessed. The internal catheter is connected to the patient's venous system and may consist of either silicone or polyurethane.[5,6,13]
- Implanted vascular access ports are accessed using a noncoring safety needle. A noncoring needle allows for repeated access of the venous device without damage to the silicone core.
- The noncoring needle chosen should be of optimal length (0.5–2 inches), with the most commonly used gauge being 19–22.[4] Patients with increased subcutaneous tissue may need a longer needle for access. Too short a needle may cause the flanges to press against the skin surrounding the portal chamber, leading to patient discomfort and possibly resulting in damage to the skin overlying the venous access device. Too long a needle may result in a rocking motion that can cause discomfort, possible migration out of the portal septum, or damage to the integrity of the septum, impairing it for further use.
- Power port implantable ports allow for venous access and the ability for power-injected contrast-enhanced computed tomography (CECT) scans.[1] If the patient has a power-injectable port, the noncoring needle set used must be labeled as power injectable compatible.

EQUIPMENT

- Nonsterile gloves
- Sterile gloves
- Mask
- Noncoring needle, winged with 90-degree angle and extension tubing (ensure that the appropriate size and length of needle is used; also confirm that the port is a power port if being used for power injection and that the correct noncoring needle is being used for access)[4]
- Dressing supplies
- Antiseptic solution (e.g., 2% chlorhexidine–based solution)
- Two 10-mL syringes
- Luer-Lok vial access device
- Needleless injection cap
- Single-use 30-mL vial of NS
- ½-inch Steri-Strips or stabilization device
- Heparin flush, 100 units/mL concentration, if deaccessing
- Central venous catheter dressing change kit

Additional equipment, to have available as needed, includes the following:

- Topical anesthetic if prescribed
- 10% betadine solution and 70% alcohol solution
- Supplies for obtaining blood samples for laboratory analysis
- Needleless blood sampling access device

AP This procedure should be performed only by physicians, advanced practice nurses, and other healthcare professionals (including critical care nurses) with additional knowledge, skills, and demonstrated competence per professional licensure or institutional standard.

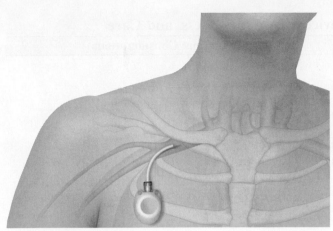

Figure 84-1 Port placement. *(Courtesy of Bard Corporation.)*

PATIENT AND FAMILY EDUCATION

• Assess patient and family readiness to learn, and identify factors that affect learning. *Rationale:* Assessment allows the nurse to individualize teaching and maximize understanding.

• Provide information about the type of implantable venous access device placed and the methods used for accessing and deaccessing it. *Rationale:* Information assists the patient and family in understanding the procedure and decreases patient and family anxiety.

• Encourage the patient to carry a card describing the type of port implanted. *Rationale:* This provides important information that may be needed by other physicians, advanced practice nurses, and other healthcare professionals.

• Explain the patient's role during the procedure and expected outcomes. *Rationale:* The patient is able to participate in care, and cooperation is encouraged.

• Explain the anticipated sensations during the access procedure and infusion of therapies. *Rationale:* Explanation allows the patient to alert the physician, advanced practice nurse, or other healthcare professional to unusual or unexpected sensations.

• Explain site care and signs and symptoms of infection and infiltration. *Rationale:* Explanation enables the patient and family to participate in care and the patient is encouraged to report untoward events to physicians, advanced practice nurses, and other healthcare professionals.

PATIENT ASSESSMENT AND PREPARATION

Patient Assessment

• Review the patient's medical history specifically related to the type of port, problems with device implantation, complications with previous access, and allergies to antiseptic solutions. *Rationale:* Baseline data are provided.

• Obtain the patient's vital signs. *Rationale:* Baseline data are provided.

• Review the patient's current laboratory status, including coagulation results. *Rationale:* Baseline coagulation studies are helpful in determining the risk for bleeding. If results are abnormal, consult with the patient's physician or advanced practice nurse before accessing the device.[2]

• Determine if the patient has a power port by palpating the top of the port to identify three palpations (bumps) on the septum, arranged in a triangle. Also, palpate the sides of the port to identify if the device is in the shape of a triangle.[1] *Rationale:* Determines the type of device in place and guides the use of the correct noncoring needle set.

Patient Preparation

• Verify that the patient is the correct patient using two identifiers. *Rationale:* Before performing a procedure, the nurse should ensure the correct identification of the patient for the intended intervention.

• Ensure that the patient and family understand preprocedural teaching. Answer questions as they arise, and reinforce information as needed. *Rationale:* Understanding of previously taught information is evaluated and reinforced.

• Assist the patient to a supine position with the head of the bed elevated up to a 30-degree angle. *Rationale:* Positioning prepares the patient and allows optimal access to the implanted venous access device.

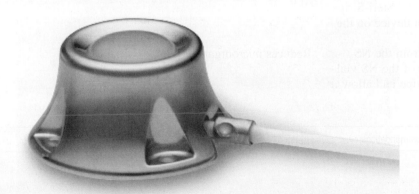

Figure 84-2 PORT-A-CATH reservoir with self-sealing septum and catheter. *(Courtesy of Smiths Medical ASD, Inc., St. Paul, MN.)*

Procedure	for Implantable Venous Access Device: Access, Deaccess, and Care	
Steps	**Rationale**	**Special Considerations**

Accessing an Implantable Venous Access Device

Steps	**Rationale**	**Special Considerations**
1. **HH**		
2. **PE**		
3. Remove the patient's gown away from the venous access device.	Optimizes the viewing area.	
4. Assess the venous access device: A. Palpate the subcutaneous tissue to determine the borders of the access device.[4,6] B. Palpate the venous access device borders and locate the septum and the center of the septum. **(Level M*)**	Allows for identification of the type of port that was implanted and whether the port is single or double lumen.	
5. Assess the site for signs and symptoms of infection or other complications (e.g., erythema, induration, pain, or tenderness at the site).	Minimizes the risk of accessing an infected area.	Before accessing, examine the chest for complications, including evidence of thrombosis (veins of ipsilateral chest and neck), erythema, swelling, or tenderness, which may indicate system leakage. A radiograph is recommended if leakage is suspected.[3,5]
6. Discard gloves in the appropriate receptacle.	Removes and safely discards used supplies.	
7. **HH**		
8. Carefully open the central venous catheter dressing kit with the sterile inner surface of the wrap.	Maintains asepsis and prepares supplies. Creates a sterile field.	Disinfect the table as needed. Venous access devices have the lowest risk for catheter-related blood system infections, provided that aseptic and sterile techniques are used throughout care delivery.[5] The kit should include sterile gloves and masks.
9. Prepare supplies: A. With sterile technique, remove the wrapper from two 10-mL syringes and place them on the sterile field. B. Remove the packaging and place the winged or safety-noncoring needle with extension tubing, needleless injection cap, and Steri-Strips or stabilization device on the sterile field.	Places equipment within reach during the procedure. Maintains the sterility of the procedure.	If prefilled saline syringes are provided in a sterile package, they can be dropped onto the field and **Steps 9-11** can be skipped.
10. Remove the cap from the NS vial; wipe the top of the NS vial with an alcohol wipe and allow it to dry.	Reduces microorganisms.	

*Level M: Manufacturer's recommendations only.

Procedure	for Implantable Venous Access Device: Access, Deaccess, and Care—*Continued*	
Steps	Rationale	Special Considerations
11. Prepare additional supplies: A. Put on face mask. B. Put a sterile glove on your dominant hand. C. With sterile gloved hand, pick up a sterile 10-mL syringe. D. With the nonsterile hand, pick up the NS vial. E. Use the sterile gloved hand to withdraw 10 mL of NS solution, touching only the sterile syringe. F. Repeat the above to fill the second sterile syringe with 10 mL of saline. G. As described previously, use the sterile gloved hand to withdraw 10 mL of NS.	Prepares for the procedure.	
12. Apply the remaining sterile glove.	Maintains asepsis.	
13. With sterile technique: A. Attach the needleless injection cap to the extension tubing on the noncoring needle. B. Attach the 10-mL NS syringe to the needleless cap. C. Prime the tubing with NS solution away from the sterile field.	Prepares the equipment. Removes air from the extension tubing, preventing possible air embolism.	
14. Retain the priming syringe on the needleless cap, and return the primed equipment to the sterile field.		
15. Cleanse the implanted venous access device site or port with a 2% chlorhexidine–based antiseptic solution. Cleanse the site using a back-and-forth motion while applying friction for 30 seconds. Allow the antiseptic to remain on the insertion site and to dry completely before catheter insertion.[4,5,8,9] **(Level D*)**	Reduces the risk of infection.	Administer topical anesthetic if prescribed to reduce discomfort.[4]
16. Pick up the noncoring needle with the NS syringe attached with the dominant hand and remove the protective cap.		
17. Use the nondominant hand to stabilize the borders of the venous access device.		

*Level D: Peer-reviewed professional and organizational standards with the support of clinical study recommendations.

Procedure continues on following page

Procedure   for Implantable Venous Access Device: Access, Deaccess, and Care—*Continued*

Steps	Rationale	Special Considerations
18. Triangulate the venous access device between the thumb and first two fingers of the nondominant hand (Fig. 84-3).	Stabilizes the venous access device within the chest wall and prevents slippage. Protects the physician, advanced practice nurse, or other healthcare professional from a potential needle injury.	
19. With the dominant hand, firmly grasp the protective cap or wings of the noncoring needle and insert it firmly into the center of the port septum using a 90-degree angle perpendicular to the skin surface (Fig. 84-4).		
20. Advance the needle through the skin and septum until reaching the base of the portal reservoir when you feel portal backing (Fig. 84-5).		With use of a noncoring safety needle, grasp the vertical fin between the thumb and middle finger and press downward with the index finger.[4,5,10]
21. Note that resistance is felt as the needle reaches the base of the reservoir.		Once the septum is punctured, avoid tilting or rocking the needle, which may cause fluid leakage or damage to the system.[2]
22. Flush the venous access device with 5 mL of NS solution.	Determines the patency of the venous access device.	Avoid use of syringes with less than a 10-mL volume for flushing or administration of infusate. Smaller syringes exert pressure exceeding 40 psi and may cause catheter rupture or fragmentation with possible embolization.[2,6]
23. Observe the skin surrounding the noncoring needle for leakage of fluid or infiltration at the access site.	Assesses for potential access problems.	

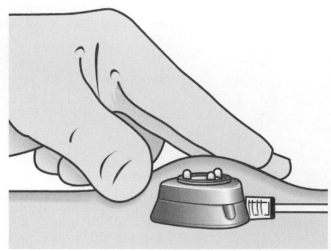

Figure 84-3   Triangulating the PowerPort Implanted Port with the nondominant hand. *(Courtesy of Bard Corporation.)*

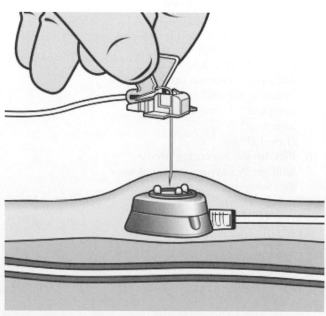

Figure 84-4   Needle access of the PowerPort Implanted Port with a noncoring PowerLoc Needle. *(Courtesy of Bard Corporation.)*

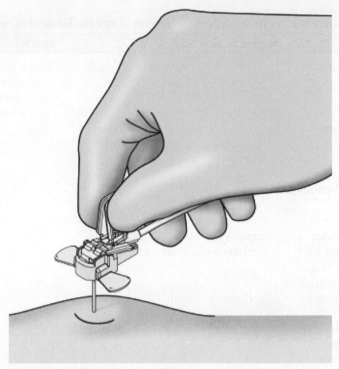

Figure 84-5 The noncoring PowerLoc Needle is inserted until the base of the port reservoir is felt. *(Courtesy of Bard Corporation.)*

Procedure	**for Implantable Venous Access Device: Access, Deaccess, and Care—*Continued***	
Steps	**Rationale**	**Special Considerations**
24. Gently aspirate blood, then flush with the remaining 5 mL of NS.	Verifies placement.	If a blood return is not evident, gently flush with the push-pull method and reposition the patient. If a blood return is still not evident, continue the access procedure and apply a dressing to minimize the risk of infection. Contact the patient's physician or advance practice nurse. Administer a lytic agent and obtain a radiographic or dye shadow study as prescribed.[4,13]
25. Position the wings flush with the patient's skin.	Anchoring minimizes discomfort for the patient.	
26. Stabilize the needle by attaching Steri-Strips in a cross or star pattern over the wings of the noncoring needle or use of the stabilizing device as per protocol.	Stabilizes the needle inserted in the septal core and minimizes rocking of the needle, which can cause damage to the septum and patient discomfort. Also, minimizes needle movement in the septum, thereby ensuring integrity of the septal core for future use.	Follow institutional standards.
27. Apply a sterile, occlusive dressing.	Maintains asepsis.	A gauze dressing is preferred if oozing or blood seepage occurs at the insertion site.
28. Label the dressing with the date, time of cannulation, needle gauge and length, and initial.	Provides important clinical information.	If the accessed device is not to be used immediately, flush it with heparin as prescribed.

Procedure continues on following page

Procedure   for Implantable Venous Access Device: Access, Deaccess, and Care—*Continued*

Steps	Rationale	Special Considerations
29. Initiate continuous or intermittent infusion.	Begins therapy.	Attach intravenous (IV) tubing to the catheter hub for continuous infusion or injection cap for intermittent infusions.
30. Remove **PE** and discard used supplies in appropriate receptacles.	Removes and safely discards used supplies.	
31. **HH**		

Deaccessing an Implantable Venous Access Device

1. **HH**		
2. **PE**		
3. Flush the venous access device with 20 mL of NS, followed by heparin flush as prescribed (e.g., 5 mL of 100 units/mL heparin).[2,4]	Prepares and optimizes catheter patency while not in use.	
4. Loosen the transparent or gauze dressing and Steri-Strips or the stabilization device from the site.	Facilitates removal.	
5. Use the thumb and forefinger of the dominant hand to grasp the dressing and the Steri-Strips or the stabilization device along with the winged flanges of the needle.	Prepares for needle removal.	
6. With the nondominant hand, apply gentle stabilizing pressure to the venous access device while removing the needle by pulling straight up and out in a firm, continuous motion.	Minimizes patient discomfort and ensures controlled withdrawal of a sharp object.	With use of a noncoring safety needle, grasp the horizontal flanges securely, pull up, and squeeze the flanges together. The flanges fold together, forcing the needle inside the locked wings and covering the needle. The wings will lock in place.
7. Assess the site for redness or drainage.	Identifies possible complications.	
8. Discard the noncoring needle in a designated container.	Safely removes sharp objects.	
9. Apply a dressing to the site if oozing occurs.	Provides absorption.	
10. Remove **PE** and discard supplies in appropriate receptacles.	Removes and safely discards used supplies.	
11. **HH**		

Obtaining a Blood Specimen From an Implantable Venous Access Device

1. **HH**		
2. **PE**		
3. If present, shut off the IV infusion and disconnect the IV tubing from the extension tubing on the noncoring needle.	Maintains asepsis.	
4. Place a sterile cap on the end of the IV tubing.	Maintains asepsis.	
5. Thoroughly cleanse the injection cap with an alcohol wipe and allow it to dry. Do not remove the cap.[4,9,11] **(Level D*)**	Minimizes infection and exposure of the physician, advanced practice nurse, or other healthcare professional to blood and body fluids.[6]	

*Level D: Peer-reviewed professional and organizational standards with the support of clinical study recommendations.

Procedure	for Implantable Venous Access Device: Access, Deaccess, and Care—*Continued*	
Steps	Rationale	Special Considerations
6. Attach a 10-mL syringe with NS and flush the venous access device.	Clears the catheter of medication or IV fluid.	
7. Attach a new sterile 10-mL syringe or a needleless blood sampling access device.	Prepares supplies.	
8. Determine the appropriate discard volume. **(Level E*)**	Clears the catheter of solution. The discard volume includes the dead space and the blood diluted by the flush solution. Portal reservoirs average 0.5 mL volume; catheters average 0.6 mL for single-lumen systems.[2] Recommendations are that at least three times the dead space be withdrawn.[7] Discard 5-10 mL of blood.[4,7]	Blood for coagulation tests should not be withdrawn through a heparinized catheter if the results will be used to monitor anticoagulant therapy or to determine whether a patient has a coagulopathy. Blood specimens should be redrawn peripherally when results are abnormal.[8] Follow institutional standards.
9. Gently aspirate the discard volume into the syringe or engage a blood specimen tube into the needleless blood sampling access device to obtain the discard volume and allow the tube to passively fill.[7]	Withdraws the discard.	Minimizes needlestick injury and exposure to blood, and decreases infection risk to the patient by reducing the incidence of opening the catheter system.
10. Remove the discard syringe or the blood specimen tube.	Prepares for blood sampling.	
11. Insert a new syringe into the injection cap or place a new blood specimen tube into the needleless blood sampling access device.	Prepares for removal of the specimen sample.	
12. Slowly and gently aspirate blood or engage the blood specimen tube into the needleless blood sampling access device.	Obtains the blood specimen.	
13. Remove the syringe or the blood specimen tube.	Removes the specimen.	
14. After the blood specimen is obtained, flush the port with 10-20 mL of NS.[4]	Clears blood from the system.	Flush with an additional 10–20 mL of NS if the blood does not clear completely from the extension tubing.
15. Clamp the extension tubing.		
16. Apply a new injection cap with strict aseptic technique.	Reduces infection.	
17. Reconnect the IV and continue the infusion.	Resumes therapy.	If the IV infusion is completed, administer heparin as prescribed.
18. Remove **PE** and discard used supplies in appropriate receptacles.	Removes and safely discards used supplies.	
19. **HH**		
20. Label the specimen(s) and the laboratory form.	Properly identifies the patient and laboratory tests to be performed.	
21. Send the laboratory specimen(s) for analysis.	Expedites determination of laboratory results.	

*Level E: Multiple case reports, theory-based evidence from expert opinions, or peer-reviewed professional organizational standards without clinical studies to support recommendations.

Procedure continues on following page

Expected Outcomes

- Site without redness, pain, or tenderness
- Venous access device stable
- Venous access device is accessed without difficulty
- Venous access device flushes easily without evidence of resistance or infiltration
- No evidence of leakage at the septal site
- Blood specimens are obtained as prescribed
- Venous access device is deaccessed without difficulty

Unexpected Outcomes

- Port reddened, tender, or painful on palpation
- Skin erosion
- Implanted device unstable in chest wall with palpation
- Catheter migration
- Catheter "pinch-off" (compression of catheter between clavicle and first rib)
- Portal body inversion or "twiddler's syndrome"
- Patient describes burning sensation in the subcutaneous tissue with flushing or infusion
- Sluggish or no blood return with aspiration
- Evidence of leakage of flush solution at the septal site
- Patient describes pain at site, chest, ear, or shoulder with flushing
- Signs or symptoms of local or systemic infection
- Swollen neck or arm[14,15]

Patient Monitoring and Care

Steps	Rationale	Reportable Conditions
		These conditions should be reported if they persist despite nursing interventions.
1. During IV infusions, assess the venous access device for patency and signs of infiltration every 4 hours and as needed.	Determines adequate functioning of the venous access device.	• Signs or symptoms of infiltration at the venous access site
2. Replace gauze dressings every 2 days and transparent dressings at least every 7 days.[8,9,12] Follow institutional standards. **(Level D*)**	Decreases the risk for infection at the catheter site. The dressing should be changed if it becomes damp, loosened, or soiled or when inspection of the site is necessary.[4,12]	• Signs or symptoms of infection
3. Follow institutional standards for assessing pain. Administer analgesia as prescribed.	Identifies need for pain interventions.	• Continued pain despite pain interventions
4. Follow-up care for deaccessed device includes reaccessing the device to administer monthly flush with 5 mL of 100 units of heparin as prescribed.[2,4,10,12]	Maintains catheter patency.	
5. Assess for signs and symptoms of infection.	Determines the presence of infection.	• Redness, pain, or drainage at the site; fever, elevated white blood cell count

*Level D: Peer-reviewed professional and organizational standards with the support of clinical study recommendations.

Documentation

Documentation should include the following:

- Assessment of the site before accessing and deaccessing the port
- Location and cannulation of the device
- Needle length and gauge, and rationale for selection including patient's body habitus
- Appearance of blood return before, during, and after infusion
- Date and time of therapy administration

- Specimens obtained and sent for analysis
- Laboratory results
- Pain assessment, interventions, and effectiveness
- Unexpected outcomes
- Additional interventions
- Patient's response to procedure and therapy
- Education of patient and family to procedure and therapies administered

References and Additional Readings

For a complete list of references and additional readings for this procedure, scan this QR code with any freely available smartphone code reader app, or visit http://booksite.elsevier.com/9780323376624.

85 Intraosseous Devices

Michael W. Day

PURPOSE: Intraosseous access is indicated when intravenous (IV) access cannot be obtained or cannot be obtained in a timely manner and access to venous circulation is needed for the administration of medications or fluids.

PREREQUISITE NURSING KNOWLEDGE

- Intraosseous (IO) access is a safe and reliable access point into the noncollapsible marrow cavity that allows direct access to the venous circulation.[6-8] Indications for IO access include status epilepticus, extensive burns, morbid obesity (which may prevent peripheral or central line placement),[6] sepsis, and multiple traumatic injuries.[8]
- IO is significantly faster than central venous placement during actual resuscitation[15] and in simulation.[19]
- Use of IO devices may decrease the use of emergency femoral access, with its attendant complications.[8] "Despite recommendations from a number of specialty societies on the use of IO access when IV access has failed in emergent patients, IO access appears to be an underutilized access tool in the hospital ED (emergency departments)."[21]
- The Volkmann's canals that are located throughout the bone connect with the medullary canal and the blood vessels of the periosteum (Fig. 85-1). When medications and fluids are introduced into the medullary canal, they flow through the vascular plexi directly into the vascular system.[6,7]
- Mechanical insertion devices are available for insertion of IO needles.[6] These devices include the bone injection gun (BIG; Waismed, a Persys Medical Co, Houston, TX; Fig. 85-2), the FASTResponder adult IO infusion system (Pyng Medical Corp, Vancouver, BC, Canada, Fig. 85-3), and the EZ-IO (Teleflex, Shavano Park, TX; Fig. 85-4). These three devices are approved by the US Food and Drug Administration (FDA) for IO access in adult patients. Two of the devices (BIG, Arrow EZ-IO) use a specially designed needle with a stylet or trocar. The third device (FASTResponder) uses a metal-tipped plastic catheter. The attributes of the three devices of this procedure are summarized in Table 85-1.
- In adults, the available IO access sites, depending on the specific device and following each manufacturer's guidelines,[3] include the following:
  - Tibial plateau: 1 to 2 cm distal to the tibial tuberosity
  - Distal tibia: 1 to 2 cm above the medial malleolus
  - Manubrium: 1.5 cm below the sternal notch
  - Greater tubercle of the proximal humerus
- A recent study using the EZ-IO device found that there was a significantly higher success rate with proximal tibial compared with humeral placement.[18]

- IO blood can be used for many laboratory tests, including typing and screening, electrolyte values, chemistries, blood gas values, drug levels, and hemoglobin levels.[7,20]
  - However, specimen samples from the marrow have a lower correlation to serum levels after 30 minutes of resuscitation.[4]
  - IO samples may be used for point-of-care testing.[20]
  - In addition, drawing of blood from an IO device may not be recommended by specific manufacturers and has the potential of occluding the device.[11]
- The onset of action for medications is similar to that of IV medications.[7,8] However, administration via the IO route may result in lower serum concentrations versus the IV route for the following medications: ceftriaxone, chloramphenicol, phenytoin, tobramycin, and vancomycin.[4]
- Marrow-toxic medications should not be infused via the IO route.[13]
- There is some research to support the use of IO devices for IV contrast.[1,12]
- All resuscitation medications, isotonic fluids, and blood products may be given via the IO route[5]; however, myonecrosis has been reported with the infusion of hypertonic saline solution via the IO route.[17]
- Medications administered via the IO route should be followed by a 5- to 10-mL flush of normal saline solution. Resistance to the manual flush will be felt but does NOT indicate incorrect placement. If swelling or infiltration is observed, remove the device and attempt IO access in another bone.[6,7]
- Fluids running into an IO line should be administered with a pressure bag inflated to 300 mm Hg because the pressure needed to push the fluid into the bone marrow may exceed that of volumetric IV pumps. Flow rates can be managed with the IV tubing roller clamp.[6]
- Complications of IO access include compartment syndrome, osteomyelitis, fracture, extravasation,[5] necrosis,[5,10] and infection.[8]
- A syringe should not be attached directly to the hub of the IO needle because it could cause dislodgment, increase the size of the hole, and cause extravasation or loss of the IO site. To extend access to the IO needle, attach extension tubing to the hub of the IO needle and secure it to the skin. Some device insertion kits come with extension tubing.
- Absolute contraindications to attempting an IO access include previous attempts or fractures of the targeted bone.

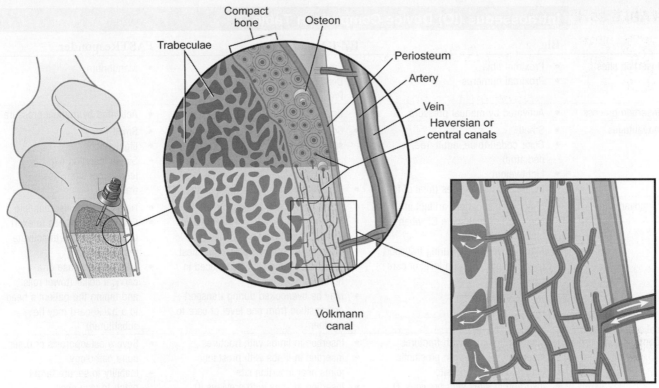

Figure 85-1 Intraosseous circulation. *(From Day MW: Intraosseous devices for intravenous access in adult trauma patients, Crit Care Nurs 31[2]:76–90.)*

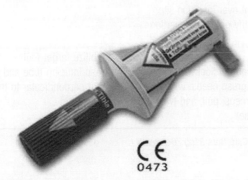

CE 0473

Figure 85-2 Bone injection gun (BIG; adult). *(From Day MW: Intraosseous devices for intravenous access in adult trauma patients, Crit Care Nurs 31[2]:76–90.)*

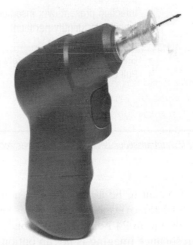

Figure 85-4 EZ-IO power driver. *(From Day MW: Intraosseous devices for intravenous access in adult trauma patients, Crit Care Nurs 31[2]:76–90.)*

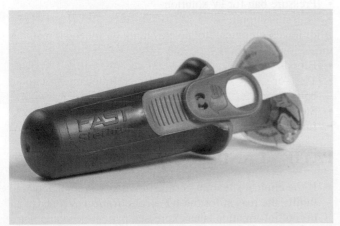

Figure 85-3 The FASTResponder. *(Courtesy Pyng Medical, Richmond, British Columbia.)*

- Relative contraindications to IO access include infection at the access site, artificial joint replacement at the insertion site,[8] fractures above the insertion site, inability to locate landmarks,[5] and bone disorders, such as osteoporosis and osteogenesis imperfecta. Another relative contraindication to the FASTResponder is skin damage at the insertion site, which may preclude the adherence of the target foot patch used to secure the device.
- IO access in obese patients may be more difficult. The Arrow EZ-IO has a needle set specifically designed for the patient with "excessive tissue" at the insertion site.

TABLE 85-1	Intraosseous (IO) Device Comparison Table		
	Big	**EZ-IO**	**FASTResponder**
Insertion sites	• Proximal tibia • Proximal humerus	• Proximal tibia • Distal tibia • Proximal humerus	• Manubrium
Insertion process	• Activated by manual pressure	• Battery-operated power driver	• Activated by manual pressure
Advantages	• Small • Color coded (blue, adult; red, pediatric) • Lightweight • Multiple insertion sites (total of four)	• Color coded, weight-based needle sets (PD, 3–39 kg; AD, >40 kg; LD, >40 kg and "excess tissue" over insertion site) • Multiple insertion sites (total of six)	• Small • Lightweight • Single insertion site (consistent site = less training)
Disadvantages	• May cause "scatter" artifact in chest or cervical spine CT when placed in humerus • May be overlooked during transport or transition from one level of care to another	• Large device and packaging • Requires visualization of needle skin depth before insertion in bone • May cause "scatter" artifact in chest or cervical spine CT when placed in humerus • May be overlooked during transport or transition from one level of care to another	• No alternative insertion site • Requires two hands to exert pressure needed to activate the device • May preclude use of a cervical collar (towel rolls and taping the patient's head to a backboard may be substituted)
Contraindications	• Insertion in limbs with fractures • Insertion in limbs with prosthetic joints near insertion site • Insertion at sites with previous IO attempt • Severe osteoporosis or other bone pathology • Infection present over insertion site • Inability to identify pertinent insertion landmarks	• Insertion in limbs with fractures • Insertion in limbs with prosthetic joints near insertion site • Insertion at sites with previous IO attempt • Severe osteoporosis or other bone pathology • Infection present over insertion site • Inability to identify pertinent insertion landmarks	• Severe osteoporosis or other bone pathology • Inability to secure target patch to skin over manubrium (i.e., burns, wounds, infection)
Removal	• Grasp needle hub with safety latch • Pull and twist	• Attach syringe • Pull and twist counterclockwise (if hub separates, grasp needle with large needle forceps, pull, and twist counterclockwise)	• Stabilize target foot • Grasp infusion tube and pull it out perpendicular to the manubrium

Adapted from Day MW: Intraosseous devices for intravenous access in adult trauma patients, Crit Care Nurs *31(2):76–90, 2011.*

- IO access is meant to be a temporary venous access; IO lines should be removed as soon as other venous access is obtained or within 24 hours of insertion.[8]
- Magnetic resonance imaging is not an option when an IO device is present,[8] whereas an IO humeral placement may interfere with chest, low cervical, or high thoracic computerized tomography (CT).[6]
- Sternal IO devices may interfere with the placement of a cervical collar in trauma patients, requiring alternative methods to maintain cervical stabilization.[6]

EQUIPMENT

- Nonsterile gloves
- Antiseptic solution (e.g., 2% chlorhexidine-based preparation)
- IO insertion device (follow manufacturer's guidelines for information that may be age or weight based)
- Tape
- IV tubing and extension tubing
- Isotonic crystalloid fluid, as prescribed
- Two 5- to 10-mL syringes
- Prescribed medications
- Pressure bag for IV solution
- Dressing supplies

Additional equipment, to have available as needed, includes the following:

- Blood-specimen tubes
- 1% or 2% preservative free lidocaine without epinephrine
- Sterile 2 × 2 gauze pads
- Large needle forceps

PATIENT AND FAMILY EDUCATION

- If the clinical situation permits, explain to the patient and family the reason for the IO access. *Rationale:* Clarification of information is an expressed patient need and helps to diminish anxiety, enhance acceptance, and encourage questions.

- Describe the major steps of the procedure, including the patient's role in the procedure. *Rationale:* Explanation decreases patient anxiety, enhances cooperation, provides an opportunity for the patient to voice concerns, and prevents accidental contamination of the sterile field and equipment.
- Explain the expected outcomes of the procedure. *Rationale:* Explanation reduces anxiety and clarifies the duration and goals of IO access.

PATIENT ASSESSMENT AND PREPARATION

Patient Assessment

- Assess the patient for fractures or infections at the insertion site, for previous bone surgeries at the site, and for a history of osteoporosis or fractures of the target bone. *Rationale:* An alternate site should be accessed to avoid possible complications associated with the previous conditions.

- Obtain the patient's baseline vital signs and cardiac rhythm. *Rationale:* Baseline data facilitate the identification of clinical problems and identify the urgency of obtaining IO access.
- If possible, determine the patient's allergy history (e.g., lidocaine, antiseptic solutions). *Rationale:* This assessment decreases the risk for allergic reactions by avoiding known allergenic products.

Patient Preparation

- Verify that the patient is the correct patient using two identifiers. *Rationale:* Before performing a procedure, the nurse should ensure the correct identification of the patient for the intended intervention.
- Ensure that the patient and family understand preprocedural teaching. Answer questions as they arise, and reinforce information as needed. *Rationale:* Understanding of previously taught information is evaluated and reinforced.
- Perform a preprocedure verification and time out, if nonemergent. *Rationale:* Ensures patient safety.

Procedure for Intraosseous Access

Steps	Rationale	Special Considerations
1. **HH**		
2. **PE**		
3. Assist the patient to a position of comfort for access of the appropriate insertion site.	Prepares the patient for the procedure and allows for optimal visualization.	
4. Palpate the intended insertion site. A. Proximal tibia: 　i. Identify the tibial tuberosity. 　ii. Move 2 cm medially and 1 cm proximally. B. Distal tibia: 　i. Identify the medial malleolus. 　ii. Move two finger widths proximally at the midline of the medial aspect of the leg. C. Manubrium: 　i. Identify the sternal notch. 　ii. Align the target foot with the sternal notch. D. Humerus: 　i. Identify the greater tubercle. 　ii. Move one finger width lateral from the greater tubercle.	Guides IO device placement.	
5. Cleanse the intended site and surrounding area with antiseptic solution (e.g., 2% chlorhexidine-based preparation).	Limits the introduction of potentially infectious skin flora into the insertion site.	

Procedure continues on following page

Procedure   for Intraosseous Access—*Continued*

Steps	Rationale	Special Considerations
6. For those devices placed in extremities, stabilize the insertion site with the nondominant hand.	Prevents movement of the limb during insertion.	Ensure that the nondominant hand is NOT in line with IO placement to prevent inadvertent injury.
7. FASTResponder[9] insertion (see Fig. 85-3):	Inserts the IO device.	Follow manufacturer's guidelines.
A. The FASTResponder is inserted into the manubrium.		It is *critical* that the FASTResponder be held perpendicular to the manubrium and *not* the patient's body.
B. Place the patient in a flat, supine position.		
C. Assume a position at the patient's head.		Attempting to place the FASTResponder device with the patient in a sitting position, from the patient's side, or using one hand is NOT recommended because it may move the physician, advanced practice nurse, or other healthcare professional away from perpendicular to the manubrium.
D. Remove the locking pin and pull away from the device; identify the sternal notch with the thumb of the nondominant hand.		
E. Align the target foot with the sternal notch and press to apply.		
F. Grasp the device with both hands, with the thumbs side by side.		Removing the locking pin exposes the adhesive surface of the target foot and readies the device for insertion.
G. Ensure that the device is perpendicular with the manubrium and NOT the patient's body.		
H. Apply steady pressure until the device is heard and felt to deploy the infusion tube.		
I. Stabilize the target foot with the nondominant hand and slowly withdraw the device with the dominant hand, while remaining perpendicular to the manubrium.		
J. Remove the antibuckle device from the infusion tube.		
K. After correct placement has been confirmed, connect the strain relief hook to the hook on the target foot.		
L. Remove covering from the protective dome and apply over the target foot and infusion tube. **(Level M*)**		

*Level M: Manufacturer's recommendations only.

Procedure for Intraosseous Access—*Continued*

Steps	Rationale	Special Considerations
8. BIG insertion[3] (see Fig. 85-2): A. The BIG can be inserted into the proximal tibia or the humerus. B. Palpate the appropriate landmarks with the dominant hand, and with the nondominant hand place the barrel of the BIG on the skin perpendicular to the intended insertion site. C. With the dominant hand, squeeze and remove the red safety latch. D. Grasp the "shoulders" of the BIG with the fingers of the dominant hand while the palm presses down into the BIG and deploys the needle and trocar. E. Remove the BIG and stabilize the needle. F. Remove the trocar from the needle and secure the needle to the skin by taping the red safety latch around it. **(Level M*)**	Inserts the IO needle.	The BIG device is color coded. The adult device is blue.
9. Arrow EZ-IO[2] insertion (see Fig. 85-4): A. The Arrow EZ-IO can be inserted into the proximal tibia, the distal tibia, or the humerus. B. Connect the appropriately sized needle to the power driver (Fig. 85-5). C. Palpate the appropriate landmark. D. Stabilize the limb and advance the needle at a 90-degree angle through the skin until the bone is felt. E. When the 5-mm mark is visible, apply steady, firm pressure and activate the power driver until the needle hub contacts the skin or a sudden decrease in resistance is noted. F. Stabilize the needle and remove the power driver. G. Remove the stylet from the needle by turning it counterclockwise while withdrawing it. **(Level M*)**	Inserts the IO needle.	Follow manufacturer's guidelines for selection of the size of the needle based on patient weight. If the 5-mm mark is not visible, the needle is withdrawn and a larger size is attached and advanced into the insertion site.

*Level M: Manufacturer's recommendations only.

Procedure continues on following page

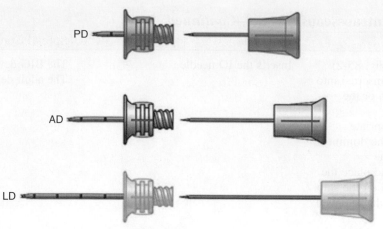

Figure 85-5 EZ-IO needle sets. *(From Day MW: Intraosseous devices for intravenous access in adult trauma patients,* Crit Care Nurs *31[2]:76–90.)*

Procedure	for Intraosseous Access—*Continued*	
Steps	**Rationale**	**Special Considerations**
10. Secure the IO catheter or needle as recommended by the manufacturer. **(Level M*)**	Prevents the needle from moving.	
11. Apply a sterile, occlusive dressing.	Promotes a sterile environment.	
12. Confirm placement by: A. Aspirating blood or marrow. B. Flushing the needle with 10 mL of normal saline solution.	Verifies needle placement in the marrow cavity.	Follow institutional standards. If blood specimens are needed, attach a 5-mL syringe and aspirate bone marrow and blood from the site.[8,14] Aspiration of marrow may occlude the IO device with bone. Lack of marrow aspirate does not indicate improper placement.[8] Resistance to the manual flush will be felt but does NOT indicate incorrect placement. If swelling or infiltration is observed, remove the device and attempt IO access in another bone.[7]
13. Securely attach the tubing and tape it to the patient's skin.	Secures the tubing system.	Care should be taken when positioning and transferring the patient to avoid dislodgment of the IO device.
14. Infuse IV fluids with a pressure bag or manual pressure.	IO lines often need pressure to ensure adequate flow.	The resistance of fluid flow through an IO may exceed the pressure limits on infusion pumps.
15. If the patient is alert, slowly (over 60 seconds)[8] infuse lidocaine (without epinephrine) into the IO device as prescribed.	Promotes comfort.	The infusion of fluids and medications can be painful to the conscious patient.

*Level M: Manufacturer's recommendations only.

Procedure	for Intraosseous Access—*Continued*	
Steps	**Rationale**	**Special Considerations**
16. Administer prescribed medications via the IO device and follow each medication with a 5–10-mL normal saline solution flush as prescribed.[16] **(Level E*)**	Following medications with a saline solution flush ensures delivery of medication into the marrow cavity and blood vessels.	Resistance to the manual flush will be felt but does NOT indicate incorrect placement. If swelling or infiltration is observed, remove the device and attempt IO access in another bone.[7]
17. Remove **PE** and discard used supplies in appropriate receptacles.	Removes and safely discards used supplies.	
18. **HH**		
Procedure for Removal of the Intraosseous Access		
1. **HH**		
2. **PE**		
3. Replace the IO site within 24 hours or as soon as venous access is obtained.	IO access is a temporary access site.	For minimization of the risk of complications, the IO device should be removed as soon as alternate vascular access is obtained or within 24 hours.
4. Follow manufacturer's guidelines for removal: **(Level M*)**	IO device is no longer needed.	Follow manufacturer's guidelines. Be sure to pull *perpendicular* to the patient's manubrium, *not* the patient's body. Inspect the infusion tube upon removal to ensure that the metal tip has been removed. If the metal tip separates from the infusion tube, contact the physician.

A. FASTResponder[9]:
    i. Remove the protective dome and stabilize the target foot with the nondominant hand.
    ii. Grasp the infusion tube as close as possible to the tip and fold it around the finger.
    iii. Pull back in a steady motion until the infusion tube is removed.
  B. BIG removal[3]:
    i. Grasp the IO device hub with the red safety latch.
    ii. Simultaneously rotate and withdraw the IO device.
  C. Arrow EZ-IO removal[2]:
    i. Attach a 5–10-mL syringe to the hub of the IO device.
    ii. Stabilize the limb.
    iii. Simultaneously rotate clockwise and pull the IO device out.
    iv. If the hub separates from the body of the IO device, grasp the body with large (8-inch) needle forceps and simultaneously rotate the body and pull to remove.[6]		

*Level E: Multiple case reports, theory-based evidence from expert opinions, or peer-reviewed professional organizational standards without clinical studies to support recommendations.

*Level M: Manufacturer's recommendations only.

Procedure continues on following page

Procedure for Intraosseous Access—*Continued*

Steps	Rationale	Special Considerations
5. Apply an occlusive, sterile dressing to the site.	Promotes a sterile environment.	
6. Remove **PE** and discard used supplies in appropriate receptacles.	Reduces the transmission of microorganisms; Standard Precautions. Safely remove sharp objects.	
7. **HH**		

Expected Outcomes

- Access to venous circulation for the administration of medications and fluids
- The IO line remains patent
- The tip of the IO needle lies in the marrow cavity
- The insertion site, catheter, and systemic circulation remain free of infection

Unexpected Outcomes

- Inability to infuse medications or fluids
- Infection
- Extravasation
- Complications such as compartment syndrome, fractures, osteomyelitis, and necrosis
- Pain

Patient Monitoring and Care

Steps	Rationale	Reportable Conditions
		These conditions should be reported if they persist despite nursing interventions.
1. Observe for signs and symptoms of infection.	Identifies possible complications.	• Edema around the site • Pain, tenderness, or erythema around the site • Drainage from the site • Increased temperature • Elevated white blood cell count
2. Observe the IO insertion site for signs and symptoms of extravasation or compartment syndrome.	A misplaced device or excessive movement after insertion may lead to a leakage of fluids outside of the marrow cavity and can impair circulation to the extremity.	• Increased circumference of the extremity • Increased pain in the extremity • Change in extremity sensation, temperature, or pulses
3. Follow institutional standards for assessing pain. Administer analgesia as prescribed.	Identifies need for pain interventions.	• Continued pain despite pain interventions

Documentation

Documentation should include the following:
- Patient and family education
- Preprocedure verification and timeout
- Site of insertion
- Number of IO insertion attempts
- Sites of previous IO insertion attempts
- Brand of the IO device inserted and, if appropriate, manufacturer's needle description
- Confirmation of IO needle placement
- Date and time of insertion

- Type and amount of anesthetic used
- Assessment of insertion site
- Method of securing the IO needle in place
- Problems encountered during or after the procedure
- Pain assessment, interventions, and effectiveness
- Vital signs and cardiac rhythm
- Date and time the IO device is removed
- Assessment of site after the IO device is removed

References and Additional Readings

For a complete list of references and additional readings for this procedure, scan this QR code with any freely available smartphone code reader app, or visit http://booksite.elsevier.com/9780323376624.

86 Midline Catheters AP

Debra L. Wiegand

PURPOSE: Midline catheters are peripheral catheters used to provide venous access for patients who have limited peripheral venous access and who require intravenous (IV) therapy for approximately 2 weeks. Midline catheters can be used to administer any infusate that can be administered peripherally such as IV fluid therapy, analgesics, and specific antibiotics.

PREREQUISITE NURSING KNOWLEDGE

- Successful completion of specialized education in ultrasound-guided midline catheter insertion, utilizing a modified Seldinger technique, and demonstrated competency are necessary.[3,4] In addition, opportunities to demonstrate clinical competency on a regular basis (e.g., yearly) may be needed.
- Knowledge of the principles of sterile technique is essential.
- Knowledge is necessary of the anatomy and physiology of the vasculature and adjacent structures in the upper extremity, neck, and chest.
- Knowledge is necessary of assessment of upper extremity venous access using ultrasound.
- Midline catheters do not enter the central vasculature.
- Midline catheters are inserted into the upper arm via the basilic, cephalic, or brachial vein (see Figure 87-1); the catheter tip is located at or near the level of the axilla and below the level of the shoulder.[5]
- The basilic vein is often the larger vessel and is the vein of choice for insertion of a midline catheter.[5]
- Patient indications for the insertion of a midline catheter include administration of IV solutions, analgesic infusions, and specific antibiotics.
- Therapies that should not be administered through a midline catheter include vesicant therapy and parenteral nutrition.[5]
- If IV access is needed for more than 2 weeks, consider placement of a central vascular access device (CVAD).[5]
- Midline catheter placement should be avoided in an extremity on the same side that the patient had a mastectomy with axillary node resection, fistula, shunt, or radial artery surgery.
- Relative contraindications to placement of a midline catheter include upper extremity edema, AV fistulas, and a prolonged bleeding time.[5]

- Midline catheters are available as single-lumen or double-lumen catheters.
- A midline catheter can be inserted with or without the use of the modified Seldinger technique. When a modified Seldinger technique is used, venous access is achieved with a microintroducer needle. A guidewire is introduced and threaded into the microintroducer needle which is then removed and the dilator/introducer is inserted over the guidewire. The dilator and guidewire are removed, leaving the introducer in the vein to allow for passage of the midline catheter into the vein. Once the midline catheter is in place, the introducer is removed.
- There are alternate midline placement techniques and the manufacturer's guidelines should be followed.
- A variety of safety-engineered introducers are available and should be used to reduce the risk for blood exposure and needlestick injury.[4,5,7]
- Ultrasound guidance is recommended to place midline catheters if the technology is available; it is associated with improvement in insertion success rates, reduced number of needle punctures, and decreased insertion complication rates.[4]
- Longitudinal or transverse views can be used when placing the midline catheter with ultrasound. The needle tip should remain in view at all times. If the tip of the needle cannot be visualized, the probe, not the needle, should be moved to reestablish visibility.[4]

EQUIPMENT

- Catheter-insertion kit
- Midline catheter of choice
- Single-use tourniquet
- Sterile and nonsterile measuring tape
- Waterproof underpad/linen saver
- Sterile gown
- Head cover
- Mask
- Goggles or eye protection
- Two pairs of nonpowdered sterile gloves
- Sterile drapes and towels, including one fenestrated full barrier drape
- Antiseptic solution (e.g., 2% chlorhexidine–based preparation)

AP   This procedure should be performed only by physicians, advanced practice nurses, and other healthcare professionals (including critical care nurses) with additional knowledge, skills, and demonstrated competence per professional licensure or institutional standard.

- 10-mL vial of heparin (concentration and use per institutional standard)
- 30-mL vial of normal saline (NS) solution
- Needleless connector with/without short extension tubing
- One to three 10-mL, 20-gauge, 1-inch needle syringes (blunt needles recommended), depending on the number of lumens
- Sterile 4 × 4 gauze pads or sponges
- Sterile 2 × 2 gauze pads or sponges
- Sterile, transparent, semipermeable dressing
- Bedside ultrasound machine with vascular probe
- Sterile ultrasound probe cover
- Sterile ultrasound gel
- Catheter securement device

Additional equipment, to have available as needed, includes the following:
- One 1-mL, 25-gauge, ⅜-inch needle syringe (if intradermal lidocaine is used)
- 1% lidocaine without epinephrine, or 1 to 2 mL of a eutectic mixture of local anesthetics (EMLA) cream

PATIENT AND FAMILY EDUCATION

- Explain the reason for the midline catheter, the benefits and risks associated with the catheter, and the alternatives to midline catheter placement. *Rationale:* Clarification of information is an expressed patient need and helps diminish anxiety, enhance acceptance, and encourage questions.
- Describe the major steps of the procedure, including the patient's role in the procedure. *Rationale:* Explanation decreases patient anxiety, enhances cooperation, provides an opportunity for the patient to voice concerns, and prevents accidental contamination of the sterile field and equipment.
- Instruct the patient and family to refuse injections, venipuncture, and blood pressure measurements on the arm with the midline catheter. *Rationale:* The risk for catheter-related complications and catheter damage is minimized.
- Provide appropriate patient and family discharge education regarding the care and maintenance of the midline catheter if the patient will be discharged with the midline catheter. *Rationale:* Education reduces the risk for catheter-related complications from lack of knowledge and skills needed to care for the midline catheter after discharge.

PATIENT ASSESSMENT AND PREPARATION
Patient Assessment

- Assess the patient's medical history for mastectomy with axillary node dissection, fistula, shunt, or radial artery surgery. *Rationale:* Midline catheter insertion should be avoided in extremities affected by these conditions to preserve veins for future needs and because the risk for complications is increased.
- Obtain the patient's baseline vital signs. *Rationale:* Provides baseline data.
- Assess the vasculature of the antecubital space of both arms, focusing on the basilic and cephalic veins. A tourniquet should be applied on the mid–upper arm for vein assessment and then removed. *Rationale:* Proper vein selection increases the success of insertion and decreases the incidence of postinsertion complications.
- Determine the patient's allergy history (e.g., lidocaine, heparin, EMLA cream, antiseptic solutions, tape, latex). *Rationale:* Assessment decreases the risk for allergic reactions with avoidance of known allergenic products.

Patient Preparation

- Verify that the patient is the correct patient using two identifiers. *Rationale:* Before performing a procedure, the nurse should ensure the correct identification of the patient for the intended intervention.
- Ensure that the patient and family understand preprocedural teaching. Answer questions as they arise, and reinforce information as needed. *Rationale:* Understanding of previously taught information is evaluated and reinforced.
- Ensure that informed consent has been obtained. *Rationale:* Informed consent protects the rights of the patient and allows the patient to make a competent decision.
- Perform a preprocedure verification and timeout. *Rationale:* Ensures patient safety.
- Assist the patient to a supine position with the head of bed elevated. *Rationale:* Promotes a position of comfort.
- Measure the mid–upper arm circumference of the selected extremity. *Rationale:* Measurement provides a baseline for evaluation of suspected catheter-associated venous thrombosis. Post-placement presence of pitting or nonpitting edema may be indicative for venous thrombosis.
- Stabilize the position of the arm with a towel or pillow. *Rationale:* Stabilization increases patient comfort, secures the work area, and facilitates access to the selected vein.

Procedure for Peripherally Inserted Central Catheter

Steps	Rationale	Special Considerations
1. Obtain ultrasound equipment.	Prepares equipment.	Assistance may be needed from radiology.
2. **HH**		
3. **PE**		
4. Place a waterproof pad under the selected arm.	Avoids soiling of bed linens.	
5. Determine the anatomy of the access site. (**Level E***)	Helps ensure proper placement of the midline catheter and guides the area to be prepped.[4,5]	Ultrasound is used to assess veins for vessel size, path, round shape, and compressibility.
6. Wash the insertion area with soap and water.	Prepares insertion site.	
7. Discard used supplies and remove gloves.	Discards used supplies.	
8. **HH**		
9. Don head cover and mask.		
10. Open the midline catheter insertion tray and drop the remaining sterile items onto the sterile field.	Maintains aseptic technique; prepares the work area, including procurement of all necessary equipment; avoids interruption of the procedure and contamination of the work area.	
11. **HH**		
12. Apply sterile gown and sterile gloves.	Midline catheter insertion is a sterile procedure.	Personal protective equipment (e.g., head cover, mask, goggles) is needed as well as sterile equipment. Blood splashing may occur with the use of guidewires, stylets, and breakaway or peel-away introducers.
13. Prepare the catheter according to manufacturer's recommendations.	Each manufacturer recommends a specific preparation protocol for each type of catheter.	
14. Fill the 10-mL syringe with normal saline. Add the needleless connector to the short extension tubing and prime it with normal saline. Leave the syringe attached.	Prepares the equipment.	If inserting a double-lumen catheter, prime the additional lumen of the catheter with normal saline.

15. Prepare the site with a 2% chlorhexidine–based antiseptic solution.[4,5,9]
  A. Cleanse the site with a back-and-forth motion while applying friction for 30 seconds.
  B. Allow the antiseptic to remain on the insertion site and to air-dry completely before catheter insertion.[4,5,9] (**Level D***)
	Limits the introduction of potentially infectious skin flora into the vessel during the puncture.	

16. Discard gloves in the appropriate receptacle.	Removes and safely discards used supplies.	

*Level D: Peer-reviewed professional and organizational standards with the support of clinical study recommendations.
*Level E: Multiple case reports, theory-based evidence from expert opinions, or peer-reviewed professional organizational standards without clinical studies to support recommendations.

Procedure	for Peripherally Inserted Central Catheter—*Continued*	
Steps	**Rationale**	**Special Considerations**
17. 🅷🅷		
18. Apply the tourniquet snugly on the upper arm away from the sterile field.	Provides vasodilation of the vein for venipuncture.	Constriction should effectively cause venous distention without arterial occlusion.
19. 🅷🅷		
20. Apply a new pair of sterile gloves.	Midline catheter insertion is a sterile procedure.	
21. Instruct the patient to lift his or her arm; place a sterile drape underneath and the fenestrated drape over the entire patient, leaving the venipuncture site exposed. Place a sterile 4 × 4 gauze pad over the tourniquet.	Maintains the sterile field and facilitates aseptic technique. Maximal sterile barrier precautions are recommended for midline catheter placement.[5]	Ultrasound scan technology may be used to assist with catheter insertion.
22. Instruct the patient to turn his or her head away from the insertion site.	Prevents contamination of the field by organisms from the patient's respiratory tract.	If the patient is not intubated ensure that the patient has on a mask.
23. Inject a skin weal of approximately 0.5 mL of 1% lidocaine without epinephrine at or adjacent to the venipuncture site. **(Level B*)**	Provides local anesthesia for venipuncture with large-gauge needles and introducers. Local anesthesia should be administered with insertion of a midline catheter.[2-6,8]	Patients report less pain when a local anesthetic agent is used before venipuncture.[2,3] Lidocaine may produce stinging, burning, obscuring the vein, or venospasm. The use of EMLA (a topical anesthetic cream) before venipuncture has been researched.[2,6,8] If it is used, manufacturer's recommendations should be followed.
24. Perform the venipuncture according to catheter design and manufacturer's instructions.	Catheters vary according to design and introducing techniques.	Relocate the intended vein with the ultrasound probe, and use the ultrasound images to guide the insertion process.[4,5]
25. Perform the modified Seldinger technique: A. Insert a microintroducer needle through the skin and into the vein and confirm venous blood return. B. Insert the guidewire at least 10 cm into the microintroducer needle, not to exceed a position beyond the axillary line.[5] C. Remove the IV microintroducer needle and insert the dilator/introducer over the guidewire. D. Gently advance the dilator/introducer, while securing the guidewire, until the tip is well within the vein.	Use of a guidewire enhances the advancement of the dilator/introducer.	Place a finger over the opening of the catheter to limit blood loss and risk for air embolism. If no blood return is found, the procedure should be terminated and an alternate access site selected. A small skin nick may be performed at the venipuncture site to facilitate the advancement of the dilator/introducer. If a scalpel is not provided in the midline catheter insertion kit, a No. 11 blade should be used.

*Level B: Well-designed, controlled studies with results that consistently support a specific action, intervention, or treatment.

Procedure continues on following page

Procedure	for Peripherally Inserted Central Catheter—*Continued*	
Steps	**Rationale**	**Special Considerations**
E. Slowly advance the catheter through the introducer to the measured length.		Place a finger over the opening of the introducer to limit blood loss and the risk for air embolism.
F. Insert the catheter.	Establishes venous access.	
26. Release the tourniquet with sterile technique (e.g., with a sterile 4 × 4 gauze pad).	Continued vasodilation may not be necessary for catheter advancement.	
27. Pull the introducer out of the vein and away from the insertion site and remove.	The introducer sheath is not needed once the catheter is in place.	Methods of removing the introducer vary according to the manufacturer.
28. Measure the length of the catheter remaining outside the skin and reposition, if necessary, to the predetermined length.	Ensures proper catheter tip position.	The ultrasound can guide placement.
29. Attach the primed extension tubing with the needleless connector to the catheter; aspirate for evidence of blood, and flush with normal saline with use of a push/pause technique.	Use of extension tubing provides easier access to the catheter and reduces local trauma at the insertion site. Aspiration affirms patency of the catheter. The push/pause technique during flushing optimizes catheter long-term patency.[4,5]	
30. Inject the recommended amount and concentration of heparin as prescribed into the catheter, clamp the extension tubing, and remove the syringe. Repeat the procedure with use of a double-lumen catheter.	Maintains catheter patency and prevents backflow of blood in the catheter.	Recommendations vary regarding the use, amount, and concentration of heparin to maintain catheter patency.[1,9] Contraindicated in persons with known allergies to heparin. Institutional standards should be followed.
31. Secure the catheter at the insertion site by applying an alternate catheter securement device.	Prevents inward or outward migration of the catheter.	Follow institutional standards.
32. Apply a dressing: A. If bleeding is noted, cover the insertion site with a sterile, 2 × 2 gauze pad and then cover the site with a sterile, transparent, semipermeable dressing.[4] B. If there is no bleeding, omit the gauze and apply a chlorhexidine impregnated gel dressing or sponge to the site and then cover it with a sterile transparent semipermeable membrane dressing.[4]	Decreases catheter-related infections.	A 2 × 2 gauze pad can be folded and placed immediately below the insertion site to act as a "wick" for any drainage in the first 24 hours. If a chlorhexidine impregnated sponge or gel dressing is applied at the insertion site, the dressing can remain for 7 days before changing.
33. Remove **PE** and sterile equipment, and discard used supplies in appropriate receptacles.	Reduces the transmission of microorganisms; Standard Precautions.	Ensure that sharps are safely discarded.
34. **HH**		

Expected Outcomes

- The midline catheter is successfully inserted
- The midline catheter remains patent
- The insertion site and upper extremity remain free of phlebitis and thrombophlebitis
- The insertion site, catheter, and systemic circulation remain free of infection

Unexpected Outcomes

- Pain or discomfort during the procedure
- Complications on insertion, such as catheter embolism, arterial puncture, and nerve (brachial plexus) injury
- Complications after insertion, such as phlebitis, thrombophlebitis, catheter occlusion, infection (e.g., insertion site, catheter, systemic), and infiltration

Patient Monitoring and Care

Steps	Rationale	Reportable Conditions
		These conditions should be reported if they persist despite nursing interventions.
1. Observe the dressing and insertion site every 30 minutes for the first 4 hours after insertion.	Postinsertion bleeding may occur in patients with coagulopathies or with arterial punctures, multiple attempts at venipuncture, or use of the through-the-needle introducer design for insertion.	• Excessive bleeding • Hematoma
2. Assess the insertion site and upper extremity every shift for signs and symptoms of phlebitis, thrombophlebitis, or infiltration.	Mechanical phlebitis is the most common complication within the first 72 hours after insertion. Thrombophlebitis may occur at any time after catheter insertion.	• Pain along the vein • Edema at the puncture site • Erythema • Ipsilateral swelling of the arm, neck, or face • Venous occlusion (changes in arm circumference >2 cm from baseline) • Infiltration

3. Assess the catheter for venous blood return and patency before initiating infusions.
  A. Connect a 10-mL syringe filled with 10 mL of normal saline to the extension tubing.
  B. Release the clamp and aspirate slowly to verify blood return.
  C. Flush with 10 mL of NS (with a push/pause technique) and then administer the infusion.
	Verifies the position of the catheter in the vascular space and patency before initiation of infusions.	• Catheter occlusion (failure to obtain blood return on aspiration or resistance to irrigation)

4. Assess the catheter for dislodgment or migration by measuring the length of the external catheter.	The catheter may no longer be properly positioned if the length of the external catheter is longer or shorter than the length measured at the time of insertion.	• Change in external catheter length • Catheter occlusion • Pain or burning during infusions • Infiltration

Procedure continues on following page

PROCEDURE

87 Peripherally Inserted AP Central Catheter

Debra L. Wiegand

PURPOSE: Peripherally inserted central catheters are used to deliver central venous therapy to provide venous access for patients who require infusates that are not peripherally compatible (e.g., vesicants, irritants). Peripherally inserted central catheters can be used for all types of infusion therapy including chemotherapy, total parenteral nutrition, analgesia, blood products, intermittent inotropic medications, and long-term antibiotics.

PREREQUISITE NURSING KNOWLEDGE

- Successful completion of specialized education in ultrasound-guided peripherally inserted central catheter (PICC) insertion utilizing a modified Seldinger technique and demonstrated competency are necessary.[3,4] In addition, opportunities to demonstrate clinical competency on a regular basis (e.g., yearly) may be needed.
- Knowledge of the principles of sterile technique is essential.
- Knowledge is necessary of the anatomy and physiology of the vasculature and adjacent structures in the upper extremity, neck, and chest.
- Knowledge is necessary of assessment of upper-extremity venous access using ultrasound.
- A patient receiving a PICC should have a peripheral vein that can accommodate a 22-gauge microintroducer needle to perform the modified Seldinger technique. The smallest device in the largest vein allows for maximal hemodilution of the infusate and minimizes the risk of phlebitis and thrombosis.[1] The catheter-vein ratio should be 45% or less.[5]
- The basilic, medial cubital, cephalic, and brachial veins should be considered for cannulation with a PICC (Fig. 87-1). The basilic vein is the larger vessel and is the vein of choice for insertion of a PICC. Brachial veins are a second choice due to close proximity to the brachial artery and nerve structures. The cephalic vein has been associated with an increased risk of thrombosis. Patient preference for arm selection (e.g., nondominant hand, lifestyle, activity restrictions, ability to care for the catheter) should be considered with selection of the insertion site.[2] Once inserted, the PICC is advanced to the lower segment of the superior vena cava at or near the cavoatrial junction.[4,5]

- Patient indications for the insertion of a PICC are not limited to inpatient therapies. A PICC is also placed for patients who require intravenous (IV) therapy in the home setting for chronic heart failure, cancer treatment, chronic pain management, nutritional support, fluid replacement (e.g., hyperemesis gravidarum) and long-term antibiotics.
- PICCs may be preferred over percutaneously inserted central venous catheters for patients with trauma of the chest (e.g., burns) or certain pulmonary disorders (e.g., chronic obstructive pulmonary disease, cystic fibrosis).[7] PICCs eliminate the risks associated with insertion of percutaneously inserted central venous catheters in the neck or chest (e.g., pneumothorax).[1]
- PICCs are contraindicated in patients with sclerotic veins, chronic kidney disease stages 4 and 5, lymphedema, mastectomy with lymph node dissection, arteriovenous graft, fistula, radial artery surgery, or extremities affected by cerebral vascular accident. Other access devices may be a better choice in patients with altered upper extremity skin integrity, or upper extremity fractures where PICC complications could compromise wound healing.
- The most common complications associated with PICCs are phlebitis, thrombosis, and catheter occlusion.[5,9]
- A variety of PICCs are available for use. PICCs are flexible catheters that are made of silicone or polyurethane. Catheter diameters range from 2 Fr to 6 Fr, and the catheter length ranges from 40 cm to 65 cm. For adults, 4 Fr to 5 Fr catheters that are 60 cm in length are typical.
- PICCs are available as single-lumen, double-lumen, and triple-lumen catheters, with and without valves. Some PICCs are designed to handle power injections (e.g., contrast media for computed tomographic scans).
- A PICC can be inserted with or without the use of a modified Seldinger technique. When a modified Seldinger technique is used, venous access is achieved with a small-gauge (20- or 22-gauge) peripheral IV catheter. Once the IV catheter is inserted, the stylet is removed and the guidewire is threaded through the IV catheter. The IV catheter is then removed, and the dilator/introducer is inserted over

---

AP This procedure should be performed only by physicians, advanced practice nurses, and other healthcare professionals (including critical care nurses) with additional knowledge, skills, and demonstrated competence per professional licensure or institutional standard.

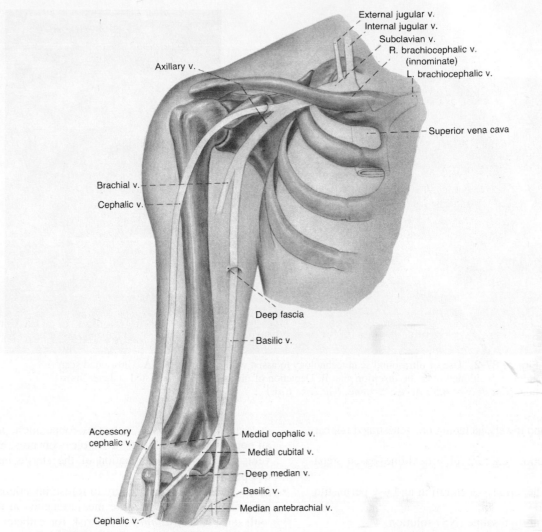

External jugular v.
Internal jugular v.
Subclavian v.
R. brachiocephalic v.
(innominate)
L. brachiocephalic v.

Axillary v.

Superior vena cava

Brachial v.

Cephalic v.

Deep fascia

Basilic v.

Accessory
cephalic v.

Medial cephalic v.

Medial cubital v.

Deep median v.

Basilic v.

Median antebrachial v.

Cephalic v.

Figure 87-1   Location of the veins of the right shoulder and upper arm. *(From Jacob SW, Francone CA: Elements of anatomy and physiology, ed 2. Philadelphia, 1989, Saunders.)*

the guidewire. The dilator and guidewire are removed, leaving the introducer in the vein to allow for passage of the PICC into the vein. Once the PICC is in place, the introducer is removed. Care must be taken with the use of a guidewire. Although advancement of the introducer is enhanced by the firmness provided by the guidewire, the guidewire can inadvertently traumatize the vessel.[5]

- There are alternate PICC placement techniques and the manufacturer's guidelines should be followed.
- A variety of safety-engineered introducers are available and should be used to reduce the risk for blood exposure and needlestick injury.[4,5,7]
- PICCs can be placed at the patient's bedside, in interventional radiology, or in specialized rooms dedicated for PICC insertions.
- Ultrasound guidance is recommended to place PICCs if the technology is available and it is associated with improvement in insertion success rates, reduced number of needle punctures, and decreased insertion complication rates.[4]
- Ultrasound scan technology can be used to assist with vein assessment and PICC insertion (Fig. 87-2). Tip-locating

technology using ECG and Doppler can be utilized to further assist the clinician in confirming tip location in the superior vena cava. This technology can be used in lieu of chest x-ray for verification of tip location.

- Longitudinal or transverse views can be used when placing the PICC with ultrasound. The needle tip should remain in view at all times. If the tip of the needle cannot be visualized, the probe, not the needle, should be moved to reestablish visibility.[4]

EQUIPMENT

- Catheter-insertion kit
- PICC catheter of choice
- Single-use tourniquet
- Sterile and nonsterile measuring tape
- Waterproof underpad/linen saver
- Sterile gown
- Head cover
- Mask
- Goggles or eye protection
- Two pairs of nonpowdered sterile gloves

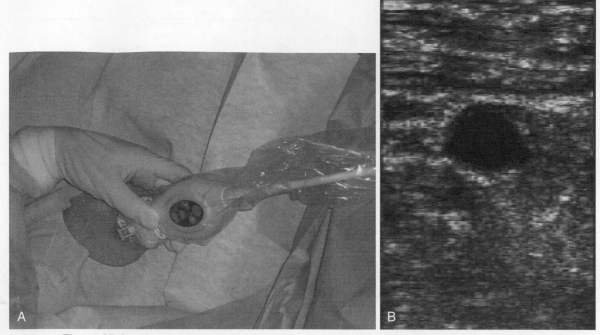

Figure 87-2   Use of ultrasound scan technology to assist with vein location. **A,** Ultrasound scan probe is positioned over the insertion site. **B,** Depiction of ultrasound scan–assisted catheter insertion. *(Courtesy of Bard Access Systems, Salt Lake City.)*

- Sterile drapes and towels, including one fenestrated full barrier drape
- Antiseptic solution (e.g., 2% chlorhexidine–based preparation)
- 10-mL vial of heparin (concentration and use per institutional standard)
- 30-mL vial of normal saline (NS) solution
- Needleless connector with/without short extension tubing
- One to three 10-mL, 20-gauge, 1-inch needle syringes (blunt needles recommended), depending on the number of lumens
- Sterile 4 × 4 gauze pads or sponges
- Sterile 2 × 2 gauze pads or sponges
- Sterile, transparent, semipermeable dressing
- Bedside ultrasound machine with vascular probe
- Sterile ultrasound probe cover
- Sterile ultrasound gel
- Catheter securement device

Additional equipment, to have available as needed, includes the following:

- One 1-mL, 25-gauge, ⅝-inch needle syringe (if intradermal lidocaine is used)
- 1% lidocaine without epinephrine or 1 to 2 mL of eutectic mixture of local anesthetics (EMLA) cream (optional)

PATIENT AND FAMILY EDUCATION

- Explain the reason for the PICC, the benefits and risks associated with the catheter, and the alternatives to PICC placement. *Rationale:* Clarification of information is an expressed patient need and helps to diminish anxiety, enhance acceptance, and encourage questions.
- Describe the major steps of the procedure, including the patient's role in the procedure. *Rationale:* Explanation decreases patient anxiety, enhances cooperation, provides an opportunity for the patient to voice concerns, and prevents accidental contamination of the sterile field and equipment.
- Instruct the patient and family to refuse injections, venipuncture, and blood pressure measurements on the arm with the PICC. *Rationale:* The risk for catheter-related complications and catheter damage is minimized.
- Provide appropriate patient and family discharge education regarding the care and maintenance of the PICC if the patient will be discharged with the PICC in place. *Rationale:* Education reduces the risk for catheter-related complications from lack of knowledge and skills needed to care for the PICC after discharge.

PATIENT ASSESSMENT AND PREPARATION

Patient Assessment

- Assess the patient's medical history for mastectomy, fistula, shunt, CVA, or radial artery surgery. *Rationale:* PICC insertion should be avoided in extremities affected by these conditions to preserve veins for future needs and because the risk for complications is increased.
- Obtain the patient's baseline vital signs and cardiac rhythm. *Rationale:* Cardiac dysrhythmias can occur if the catheter is advanced into the heart. Baseline data facilitate the identification of clinical problems and the efficacy of interventions.
- Assess the vasculature of the proposed extremity for appropriate vessel size, round shape, normal path, and compressibility. These assessments should be performed without a tourniquet to establish the appropriate vein-to-catheter ratio

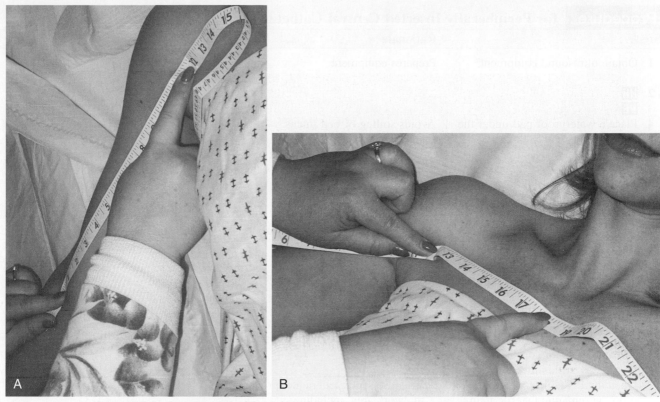

Figure 87-3 Measurement of the catheter length for placement in the superior vena cava. **A,** First, measure the distance from the selected insertion site to the shoulder. **B,** Continue measuring from the shoulder to the sternal notch and add 3 inches (7.5 cm) to this number.

and to ensure there is adequate blood flow around the catheter in situ. *Rationale:* Placing a catheter in a healthy vein with adequate blood flow around the catheter will optimize catheter function and decrease the risk of thrombosis.

- Determine the patient's allergy history (e.g., lidocaine, heparin, EMLA cream, antiseptic solutions, tape, latex). *Rationale:* Assessment decreases the risk for allergic reactions with avoidance of known allergenic products.

Patient Preparation

- Verify that the patient is the correct patient using two identifiers. *Rationale:* Before performing a procedure, the nurse should ensure the correct identification of the patient for the intended intervention.
- Ensure that the patient and family understand preprocedural teaching. Answer questions as they arise, and reinforce information as needed. *Rationale:* Understanding of previously taught information is evaluated and reinforced.
- Ensure that informed consent has been obtained. *Rationale:* Informed consent protects the rights of the patient and allows the patient to make a competent decision.
- Perform a preprocedure verification and timeout. *Rationale:* Ensures patient safety.
- Assist the patient to a supine position with the head of bed elevated. *Rationale:* Ensures patient comfort.
- For catheter placement in the superior vena cava, use the nonsterile measuring tape to measure the distance from

the selected insertion site to the shoulder (Fig. 87-3, *A*) and from the shoulder to the sternal notch (Fig. 87-3, *B*). Add 3 inches (7.5 cm, or the measured distance from the sternal notch to the third intercostal space) to this number for catheter placement in the superior vena cava. *Rationale:* Accurate measurement ensures proper tip position in the distal portion of the superior vena cava at the cavoatrial junction and determines the length of the catheter to be inserted.

- Measure the mid–upper arm circumference of the selected extremity. *Rationale:* Measurement provides a baseline for evaluation of suspected thrombosis after PICC insertion. Increases of greater than 2 cm over baseline may be indicative of venous thrombosis. A diagnostic ultrasound should be obtained.
- Stabilize the position of the arm with a towel or pillow. *Rationale:* Stabilization increases patient comfort, secures the work area, and facilitates access to the selected vein.
- Instruct the patient on proper head positioning. The head is positioned to the contralateral side (away from the insertion site) throughout the procedure, except when the catheter is advanced from the axillary vein to the superior vena cava. At this point, the patient is instructed to position his or her head toward the ipsilateral side (toward the insertion site) with the chin dropped to the shoulder. *Rationale:* Proper positioning limits the risk for the catheter being inadvertently directed into the jugular vein.

Procedure   for Peripherally Inserted Central Catheter

Steps	Rationale	Special Considerations
1. Obtain ultrasound equipment.	Prepares equipment.	Assistance may be needed from radiology.
2. **HH**		
3. **PE**		
4. Place a waterproof pad under the selected arm.	Avoids soiling of bed linens.	
5. Determine the anatomy of the access site. **(Level E*)**	Helps ensure proper placement of the PICC and guides the area to be prepped.[4,5]	
6. Wash the insertion area with soap and water.	Prepares insertion site.	
7. Discard used supplies and remove gloves.	Removes and safely discards used supplies.	
8. **HH**		
9. With the measuring tape, perform the preinsertion anatomical measurements (see Fig. 87-3).	Catheters are provided at various lengths.	This can be guided by ultrasound. Make a note of the required catheter length.
10. Position the tourniquet high on the upper extremity, near the axilla, but do not constrict venous blood flow at this time.	Placement high on the extremity avoids contamination of the sterile field.	
11. Open the PICC insertion tray and drop the remaining sterile items onto the sterile field.	Maintains aseptic technique; prepares the work area, including procurement of all necessary equipment; avoids interruption of the procedure and contamination of the work area.	
12. **HH**		
13. Apply sterile gown and sterile gloves.	PICC insertion is a sterile procedure.	Personnel protective equipment (e.g., head cover, mask, goggles) is needed as well as sterile equipment. Blood splashing may occur with the use of guidewires, stylets, and breakaway or peel-away introducers.
14. Prepare the catheter according to manufacturer's recommendations.	Each manufacturer recommends a specific preparation protocol for each type of catheter.	
15. Fill the 10-mL syringe with normal saline. Add the needleless connector to the short extension tubing and prime it with normal saline. Leave the syringe attached.	Prepares the system.	If inserting a double-lumen or triple-lumen catheter, prime the additional lumen(s) of the catheter with normal saline.

*Level E: Multiple case reports, theory-based evidence from expert opinions, or peer-reviewed professional organizational standards without clinical studies to support recommendations.

Steps	Rationale	Special Considerations
Procedure for Peripherally Inserted Central Catheter—*Continued*		
16. Prepare the site with a 2% chlorhexidine–based antiseptic solution.[4,5,9] A. Cleanse the site with a back-and-forth motion while applying friction for 30 seconds. B. Allow the antiseptic to remain on the insertion site and to air-dry completely before catheter insertion.[4,5,9] **(Level D*)**	Limits the introduction of potentially infectious skin flora into the vessel during the puncture.	
17. Discard gloves in the appropriate receptacle.	Removes and safely discards used supplies.	
18. **HH**		
19. Apply the tourniquet snugly, approximately 6 inches (15 cm) near the axilla well outside of the sterile field.	Provides vasodilation of the vein for venipuncture.	Constriction should effectively cause venous distention without arterial occlusion.
21. **HH**		
20. Apply a new pair of sterile gloves.	PICC insertion is a sterile procedure.	
22. Instruct the patient to lift his or her arm; place a sterile drape underneath and the fenestrated drape over the entire patient, leaving the venipuncture site exposed. Place a sterile 4 × 4 gauze pad over the tourniquet.	Maintains the sterile field and facilitates aseptic technique.	Ultrasound scan technology can be used to assist with catheter insertion (see Fig. 87-2).
23. Instruct the patient to turn his or her head away from the insertion site.	Prevents contamination of the field by organisms from the patient's respiratory tract.	If the patient is not intubated ensure the patient has on a mask.
24. Inject a skin weal of approximately 0.5 mL of 1% lidocaine without epinephrine at or adjacent to the venipuncture site. **(Level B*)**	Provides local anesthesia for venipuncture with large-gauge needles and introducers. Local anesthesia should be administered with insertion of a PICC.[2-6,8]	Patients report less pain when a local anesthetic agent is used before venipuncture.[2,3] Lidocaine may produce stinging, burning, obscuring of the vein, or venospasm. The use of EMLA (a topical anesthetic cream) before venipuncture has been researched.[2,6,8] If it is used, manufacturer's recommendations should be followed.
25. Perform the venipuncture according to catheter design and manufacturer's instructions.	Catheters vary according to design and introducing techniques.	Relocate the intended vein with the ultrasound probe and use the ultrasound images to guide the insertion process.[4,5]

*Level B: Well-designed, controlled studies with results that consistently support a specific action, intervention, or treatment.
*Level D: Peer-reviewed professional and organizational standards with the support of clinical study recommendations.

Procedure continues on following page

Procedure	for Peripherally Inserted Central Catheter—*Continued*		
Steps	**Rationale**		**Special Considerations**
26. Perform the modified Seldinger technique (Fig. 87-4): A. Insert a microintroducer needle or cannula and observe for blood return in the flashback chamber (see Fig. 87-4, *1*). B. Advance the floppy tipped guidewire 2 to 4 inches (5–10 cm) through the needle or cannula (see Fig. 87-4, *2*).[5] C. Remove the needle or cannula back over the guidewire and insert the dilator/introducer over the guidewire (see Fig. 87-4, *4*). D. Gently advance the dilator/introducer until the tip is well within the lumen of the vein (see Fig. 87-4, *5*). E. Remove the guidewire and then the dilator leaving the introducer in place (see Fig. 87-4, *6*). F. Insert the catheter approximately 6–8 inches (15–20 cm).	Use of a guidewire enhances the advancement of the dilator/introducer. Establishes venous access.		Place a finger over the opening of the catheter to limit blood loss and risk for air embolism (see Fig. 87-4, *2*). If unable to access the vein, the procedure should be terminated and an alternate access site selected. A small dermatotomy or nick in the skin using a sterile scalpel adjacent to the guidewire may facilitate the advancement of the dilator/introducer (see Fig. 87-4, *3*). If a scalpel is not provided in the PICC insertion kit, a No. 11 blade should be used. Place a finger over the opening of the introducer to limit blood loss and the risk for air embolism (see Fig. 87-4, *6*). Sterile forceps may be used to insert the catheter into the introducer and advance the catheter into the vein (see Fig. 87-4, *7*).
27. Release the tourniquet with sterile technique (e.g., with a sterile 4 × 4 gauze pad).	The tourniquet may inhibit catheter advancement.		
28. Instruct the patient to turn his or her head toward the cannulated arm and to drop his or her chin to the chest.	Changes the angle of the jugular vein and decreases the potential for malpositioning of the catheter in the jugular vein.		
29. Advance the remainder of the catheter until approximately 4 inches (10 cm) remain while observing the heart rate and rhythm.	Cardiac dysrhythmias may occur if the catheter is advanced into the heart.		Never advance the catheter if resistance is felt. Excessive pushing could lead to perforation of the vein, catheter malposition, or pericardial perforation.
30. Instruct the patient to return his or her head to the contralateral side (away from the insertion site).	Prevents contamination of the field by organisms from the patient's respiratory tract.		
31. Pull the introducer out of the vein and away from the insertion site and remove (see Fig. 87-4, *8* and *9*).	The introducer sheath should remain in place until the catheter is properly positioned.		Methods of removing the introducer vary according to the manufacturer.
32. Measure the length of the catheter remaining outside the skin and reposition, if necessary, to the predetermined length. Approximately 1 inch (2.5 cm) of the catheter should remain externally.	Ensures proper catheter tip position.		The catheter should be advanced to the zero mark. Optimally, no more than 2 cm should remain external to the insertion site.

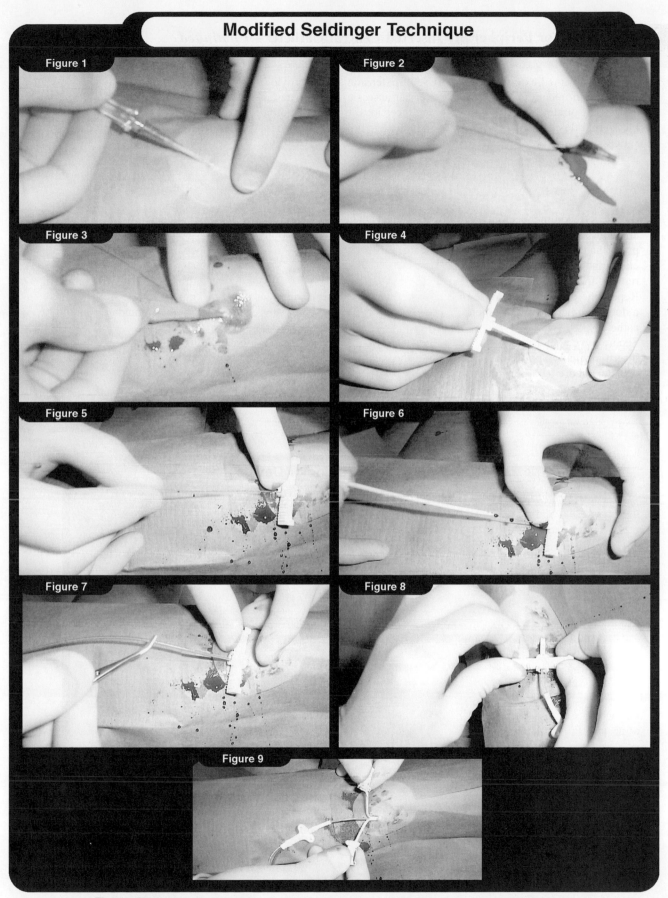

Figure 87-4 Modified Seldinger technique. **1,** Insertion of the peripheral intravenous catheter. **2,** Advancement of the guidewire through the catheter. **3,** Small skin nick to facilitate the advancement of the dilator/introducer. **4,** Insertion of the dilator/introducer over the guidewire. **5,** Advancement of the dilator/introducer. **6,** Removal of the dilator and guidewire. **7,** Insertion of the catheter using sterile forceps. **8,** Removal of the introducer. **9,** Introducer peeled apart and removed. (*Courtesy Bard Access Systems, Salt Lake City, UT.*)

Procedure	for Peripherally Inserted Central Catheter—*Continued*	
Steps	**Rationale**	**Special Considerations**
33. Attach the primed extension tubing (with injection port) to the catheter; aspirate for evidence of blood, and flush with normal saline with use of a push/pause technique.	Use of extension tubing provides easier access to the catheter and reduces local trauma at the insertion site. Aspiration affirms patency of the catheter. The push/pause technique during flushing optimizes catheter long-term patency.[4,5]	Most PICCs have their own extension sets and only require a needleless connector.
34. Inject the recommended amount and concentration of heparin as prescribed into the catheter, clamp the extension tubing, and remove the syringe. Repeat the procedure with use of a double-lumen or triple-lumen catheter.	Maintains catheter patency and prevents backflow of blood in the catheter.	Recommendations vary regarding the use, amount, and concentration of heparin to maintain catheter patency.[1,9] Contraindicated in persons with known allergies to heparin. Institutional standards should be followed.
35. Secure the catheter at the insertion site by applying a catheter securement device (Fig. 87-5).	Prevents inward or outward migration of the catheter.	Follow institutional standards.

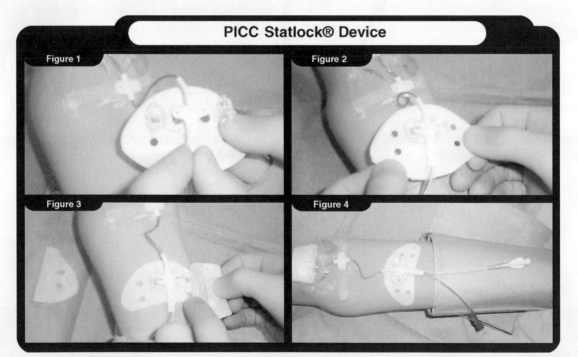

Figure 87-5   PICC Statlock device. **1,** Insertion of the wings of the PICC onto the device. **2,** Placement of the device on the forearm. **3,** Application of the sterile, transparent, semipermeable dressing over the device. **4,** Device properly secured. *(Courtesy Bard Access Systems, Salt Lake City UT.)*

Procedure for Peripherally Inserted Central Catheter—*Continued*

Steps	Rationale	Special Considerations
36. Apply a dressing: A. If bleeding is noted, cover the insertion site with a sterile, 2 × 2 gauze pad and then cover the site with a sterile, transparent, semipermeable dressing.[4] B. If there is no bleeding, omit the gauze and apply a chlorhexidine impregnated gel dressing or sponge to the site and then cover it with a sterile transparent semipermeable membrane dressing.[4]	Decreases catheter-related infections.	A 2 × 2 gauze can be folded and placed immediately below the insertion site to act as a "wick" for any drainage in the first 24 hours. If the chlorhexidine impregnated sponge or gel dressing is applied at the insertion site, the dressing can remain for 7 days before changing.
37. Remove **PE** and sterile equipment and discard used supplies in appropriate receptacles.	Reduces the transmission of microorganisms; Standard Precautions.	Ensure that sharp objects are safely removed.
38. **HH**		
39. Prepare the patient for a chest radiograph to determine tip location if a tip-locating technology was not used.	Confirms placement of the catheter tip and detects any complications.	Some PICCs require contrast media for good visualization. Infusions should not be initiated until the catheter tip placement is confirmed.

Expected Outcomes

- The PICC tip is positioned in the distal portion of the superior vena cava at the cavoatrial junction.
- The PICC remains patent
- The insertion site and upper extremity remain free of phlebitis and thrombophlebitis
- The insertion site, catheter, and systemic circulation remain free of infection

Unexpected Outcomes

- Pain or discomfort during the procedure
- Complications on insertion, such as cardiac dysrhythmias, pericardial tamponade, air embolism, catheter embolism, arterial puncture, and nerve (brachial plexus) injury
- Complications after insertion, such as phlebitis, thrombophlebitis, thrombosis, infection (e.g., insertion site, catheter, systemic), and infiltration

Patient Monitoring and Care

Steps	Rationale	Reportable Conditions
		These conditions should be reported if they persist despite nursing interventions.
1. Observe the patient for signs or symptoms of cardiac dysrhythmias and pericardial tamponade during the procedure. If cardiac dysrhythmias occur, pull the catheter back and reassess the patient.	Cardiac dysrhythmias may occur if the catheter is advanced into the heart. Pericardial tamponade may occur if the catheter penetrates the atrium.	• Cardiac dysrhythmias • Hemodynamic instability (changes in vital signs, level of consciousness, peripheral pulses, narrow pulse pressure, jugular venous distention)
2. Assess the patient and obtain the chest radiographic report confirming proper catheter tip placement before initiating any intravenous solutions.	Ensures accurate catheter tip placement and aids in identification of potentially life-threatening complications.	• Abnormal chest radiographic report • Change in lung sounds • Chest pain • Respiratory distress

Procedure continues on following page

Patient Monitoring and Care —*Continued*

Steps	Rationale	Reportable Conditions
3. Observe the dressing and insertion site every 30 minutes for the first 4 hours after insertion.	Postinsertion bleeding may occur in patients with coagulopathies or with arterial punctures, multiple attempts at venipuncture, or use of the through-the-needle introducer design for insertion.	• Excessive bleeding • Hematoma
4. Assess the insertion site and upper extremity every shift for signs and symptoms of phlebitis, thrombophlebitis, or infiltration.	Mechanical phlebitis is the most common complication within the first 72 hours after insertion. Thrombophlebitis may occur at any time after catheter insertion.	• Pain along the vein • Edema at the puncture site • Erythema • Ipsilateral swelling of the arm, neck, or face • Venous occlusion (changes in arm circumference >2 cm from baseline) • Infiltration

5. Assess the catheter for venous blood return and patency before initiating infusions.
  A. Connect a 10-mL syringe filled with 10 mL of NS to the extension tubing.
  B. Release the clamp and aspirate slowly to verify blood return.
  C. Flush with 10 mL of NS (with a push/pause technique) and then administer the infusion.
	Verifies position of the catheter in the vascular space and patency before initiation of infusions.	• Catheter occlusion (failure to obtain blood return on aspiration or resistance to irrigation)

6. Assess the catheter for dislodgment or migration by measuring the length of the external catheter.	The catheter may no longer be properly positioned if the length of the external catheter is longer or shorter than the length measured at the time of insertion.	• Change in external catheter length • Catheter occlusion • Cardiac dysrhythmias • Pain or burning during infusions • Palpation of the catheter in the internal jugular vein • Palpation of a coiled catheter • Infiltration

7. If there was insertional bleeding, the initial dressing should be left in place for 24 hours.[4] After this:
  A. Assess the insertion site and upper forearm while performing a sterile dressing change.
  B. Transparent, semipermeable dressings should be changed at least weekly.[9]
  C. Sterile gauze dressings should be changed every 48 hours.[4,5]
  D. Dressings should be changed if they become damp, loosened, or visibly soiled.[9]
  (Level D*)
	Policies may vary regarding the type of dressing and frequency of dressing changes after the initial dressing change.	• Redness, warmth, hardness, tenderness, pain, or swelling at the insertion site
		• Presence of purulent drainage from the insertion site
		• Local rash or pustules

*Level D: Peer-reviewed professional and organizational standards with the support of clinical study recommendations.

Patient Monitoring and Care —*Continued*

Steps	Rationale	Reportable Conditions
8. Monitor the insertion site and patient for signs and symptoms of local or systemic infection.	The incidence of infection related to the catheter may result from failure to maintain asepsis during insertion, failure to comply with dressing change protocols, immunosuppression, frequent access to the catheter, and long-term use of a single IV access site.	• Redness, warmth, hardness, tenderness, pain, or swelling at the insertion site • Presence of purulent drainage from the insertion site • Local rash or pustules • Fever, chills, or elevated white blood cell count • Nausea and vomiting
9. Avoid measuring blood pressure, performing venipuncture, or administering injections in the extremity with a PICC. Follow institutional standards regarding placing a sign at the patient bedside regarding avoiding use of the extremity with the PICC.	Minimizes the risk for catheter-related complications and catheter damage.	
10. Follow institutional standards for assessing pain. Administer analgesia as prescribed.	Identifies need for pain interventions.	• Continued pain despite pain interventions

Documentation

Documentation should include the following:
- Patient and family education
- Completion of informed consent
- Preprocedure verification and timeout
- Known allergies
- Mid–upper arm circumference
- Date and time of the procedure
- Catheter type, size, and length, including the length of catheter remaining outside the insertion site
- Type and amount of local anesthetic (if used)

- The location of the PICC insertion site and the vein accessed
- The method of securing the catheter
- Confirmation of the catheter tip placement
- Problems encountered during or after the procedure or nursing interventions
- Patient tolerance of the procedure
- Pain assessment, interventions, and effectiveness
- Vital signs and cardiac rhythm
- Assessment of the insertion site

References and Additional Readings

For a complete list of references and additional readings for this procedure, scan this QR code with any freely available smartphone code reader app, or visit http://booksite.elsevier.com/9780323376624.

PROCEDURE

88

Bispectral Index Monitoring

Richard B. Arbour

PURPOSE: The bispectral index (BIS) is a processed electroencephalogram (EEG)-derived parameter used in critically ill patients for assessing level of consciousness and brain arousal state(s) as well as response to sedative, hypnotic, and anesthetic agents.[4-6,8,9,31] Thorough neurological assessment and judicious interpretation of the single EEG channel and other available parameters may give early indication of progressive brain injury and inform care decisions.[3,4,18,19,22-24,34,38,39,50-52]

PREREQUISITE NURSING KNOWLEDGE

- It is necessary to understand cerebral physiology, including how brain physiology is altered consequent to metabolic and/or structural injury as well as central nervous system (CNS) depressants.[4-6,13,16,29,35]
- Sedative, hypnotic, anesthetic, and analgesic agents produce clinical effects as a result of binding, in a dose-related manner, with specific receptors in the brain modulating cerebral physiology.[16,43,45] Appropriate understanding of these agents is necessary, including side effects and their effects on BIS monitoring parameters.
  - ❖ Opioids may decrease BIS values in a dose-related manner (with the side effect of sedation at higher doses) and decrease BIS values related to attenuation of the arousal response from pain.
  - ❖ Benzodiazepines decrease BIS values in a dose-related manner.
  - ❖ Propofol decreases BIS values in dose-related manner.
  - ❖ Single-agent therapy with ketamine may not result in a dose-related decrease in BIS values. Ketamine results in increased cerebral blood flow and activation of the EEG, specifically in higher frequencies.[43] Higher EEG frequencies are associated with lighter levels of sedation. BIS values may remain elevated in the presence of deeper sedation, as determined with clinical assessment.
- Knowledge of neuromuscular blockade and monitoring issues is necessary.
  - ❖ Differentiation between the monitoring level of sedation and cortical arousal versus the monitoring level of neuromuscular blockade is important.

- ❖ The monitoring level of sedation and cortical arousal is a CNS-mediated phenomenon evaluated by clinical assessment of consciousness and responsiveness. Level of sedation and brain arousal state(s) may also be evaluated by a processed EEG parameter such as the BIS. Medication effects evaluated include CNS depressants, such as propofol, barbiturates, benzodiazepines, and opioids at higher doses.
- ❖ The monitoring level of neuromuscular blockade is a phenomenon mediated by the peripheral nervous system (PNS) and measures the effects of neuromuscular blocking agents at the myoneural junction producing varying degrees of skeletal muscle relaxation. The degree of neuromuscular blockade is evaluated two ways. The primary means include clinical assessment of ventilator synchrony, resolution of life-threatening agitation, and the degree to which clinical goals and end points are met. Secondary means include peripheral nerve stimulation and assessment of the evoked response. Peripheral nerve stimulation is commonly performed at the ulnar nerve in the wrist. After nerve localization and electrode placement, an electrical stimulus is applied and the localized response of the target muscle is assessed (see Procedure 32).
- ❖ Risk of awareness and pain during paralysis should be understood.
- ❖ Clinical goals for aggressive sedation and analgesia during paralysis should be known.
- ❖ Knowledge of monitoring parameters (central versus peripheral nervous system) is needed.
- ❖ Hemodynamic changes (marginal value at best in assessing level of sedation and analgesia and affected by multiple factors) should be understood.
- ❖ Diaphoresis (affected by multiple factors) should be understood.

❖ Knowledge of EEG-based monitoring (BIS) is necessary.

- Indications and contraindications of specific medication classes should be understood.[14,16,31,35,43]
- Knowledge of sedative and analgesic therapy is needed.[14,16]
- Specific medication therapies (e.g., opioids, benzodiazepines, propofol) should be understood.[14,16,31,35,43]
- Understanding of the interrelationship between the electrical activity of the brain and cerebral metabolism is necessary.
- Understanding of factors that affect cerebral metabolism and EEG activity is needed.
  - ❖ Sedation (dose-related): Related to the modulation of the EEG state and level of consciousness from medication administration.[4–8,13,35,41,47]
  - ❖ Analgesic agents (dose-related): Related to attenuation of the arousal response or sedation as a side effect of opioid analgesia in higher doses.[4,5,21]
  - ❖ Anesthetic agents (dose-related).[20,47]
  - ❖ Cerebral injury or hypoperfusion (hemodynamic stability, global neurological injury, severe hypoxemia): Related to direct alterations in cerebral metabolic stability.[4,7,19,24,32]
- Understanding effects of temperature extremes (hypothermia versus hyperthermia) on brain physiology.[4,27]
- EEG tracings are obtained and recorded through the application of scalp electrodes and electrical activity in the brain is displayed and recorded.[4,5,31,32,45,47]
- Evaluation of EEG waveforms provides a complement to CNS evaluation in context with information obtained through clinical neurological assessment.[4,18]
- EEG activity reflects brain physiology and requires successive, energy-using steps. These steps include electrical impulse discharge at the thalamus, impulse transmission to the cerebral cortex, presynaptic neurotransmitter release, and postsynaptic neurotransmitter uptake.[4,6,7,45]
- Any clinical state or drug therapy affecting cerebral metabolism may be reflected in EEG waveforms.[4,5,7,18,29,39]
- See Table 88-1 for terminology associated with BIS technology.
- The close relationship between BIS and EEG activity should be understood.[4,13,32,45,47]
- Goals of care should be known and communicated clearly among all members of the multidisciplinary team.
- Clinical assessment for establishing therapeutic goals and endpoints should be integrated within the plan of care as appropriate.
- BIS monitoring also may indicate an arousal response to painful stimulation.[20–22,28,31,36]
- Information derived from monitoring may be used to guide sedative, hypnotic, and metabolic suppression and analgesic therapies.[4–8,13,31]
- When BIS monitoring is initiated, a sensor is placed across the patient's forehead per manufacturer recommendations to detect one channel of EEG activity across either the right or left frontal-temporal montage (Fig. 88-1).[4,6,9,11,13]
- A single channel of EEG data is then subjected to multiple processing steps.[4,32,45,47]
  - ❖ The EEG signal is filtered and digitized within the digital signal converter (DSC)[4,6,9,11,13] or BISx near the patient's head (Figs. 88-2A and 88-3A).

TABLE 88-1	Bispectral Index Monitoring Terminology
Bispectral index (BIS)	Processed EEG that assesses level of consciousness and response to sedative, hypnotic, and analgesic therapy.
Digital signal converter (DSC)	Amplifies, filters, and digitizes the patient's EEG signals.
Electroencephalogram (EEG)	Measures electrical activity of the brain.
Electromyograph (EMG)	Measures the presence of muscle activity or detects high frequency artifact from patient care devices.
Signal quality index (SQI)	A measure of the signal quality for the EEG channel source and is calculated based on impedance to electronic signal, electrode contact artifact and other variables.
Suppression ratio (SR)	Percentage of EEG suppression (isoelectric EEG) over the past 63 seconds of collected data.

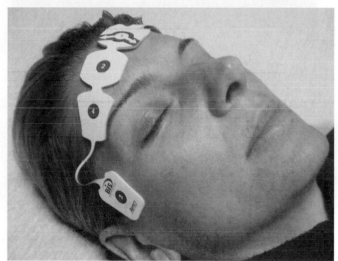

Figure 88-1 BIS sensor in place illustrating anatomical landmarks for optimal sensor placement. BIS Extend sensor in place. Sensor may be placed on right or left side. Circle 1 is positioned at center of forehead approximately 2 inches (5 cm) above nose. Circle 4 is placed directly above and parallel to the eyebrow. Circle 3 is placed on the temple area between the hairline and the outer canthus of the eye. Circle 2 is placed between circles 1 and 4 on the patient's forehead.

- ❖ Artifacts (low-frequency and high-frequency) are eliminated.[4,6,13,32,45,47]
- ❖ Multiple processing steps are applied for the calculation of BIS values based on the EEG state (frequency and amplitude) associated with the level of sedation, brain arousal, or anesthesia.[4,6,13,32,45,47]
- ❖ Levels of EEG suppression versus near suppression are determined.[4,6,13,32,45,47]
- ❖ The BIS value is derived based on the previous 10 to 30 seconds of EEG data (depending on the smoothing

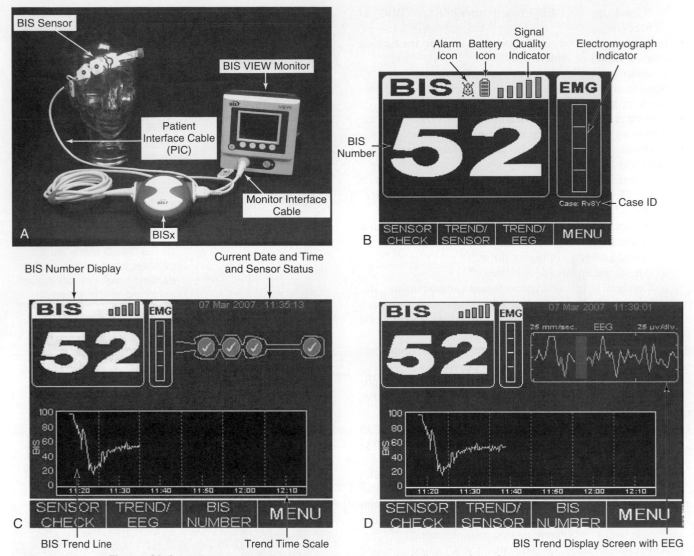

Figure 88-2 BIS View (A and B) monitoring system, including location of menu and power control keys, BISx, (C and D) BIS index/trend, EMG, EEG, and sensor status displays. (*Courtesy Aspect Medical Systems, Norwood, MA.*)

rate setting on the monitoring system) and is updated at intervals. As such, changes in BIS value may lag behind clinical changes.

- BIS monitoring provides a single channel of EEG tracing from the right or left frontal-temporal montage electrode placement (BIS Vista, BIS View; see Figs. 88-2 and 88-3).
- BIS may be utilized for bilateral EEG data acquisition from concurrent right and left frontal-temporal electrode placement (BIS Vista bilateral monitoring system).[10]
- Knowledge is needed to interpret the the BIS display screen, monitor controls, and information array displayed on BIS monitoring system. Information can be on the device (BIS monitor as a stand-alone view) or integrated systems in which data displays are incorporated within critical care monitoring systems (see Figs. 88-2, 88-3, 88-4).[9-11]
- Knowledge of data obtained from BIS monitoring is necessary.

- The BIS value is a single number on a linear (0 to 100) scale that reflects the level of sedation or cerebral arousal. BIS values correspond with specific clinical endpoints, indicating arousal and consciousness. A BIS value at or near 100 typically corresponds with an awake state. A BIS value at or near 0 corresponds with an isoelectric or near-isoelectric EEG reading and a deeply comatose patient, highly suppressed EEG, minimal to no EEG activity.[4-6,8-11,13,32,47] (Description of BIS values and corresponding clinical and EEG states are found in Table 88-2)
- The suppression ratio (SR) is defined as the percentage of suppressed EEG over the previous 63 seconds of collected EEG data. An SR of 15 indicates that the EEG signal was isoelectric over an interval of 15% of the previous 63 seconds of collected data. This parameter may be elevated in patients receiving high-dose propofol, barbiturates or other CNS depressants. The SR may also be elevated in a patient with severe

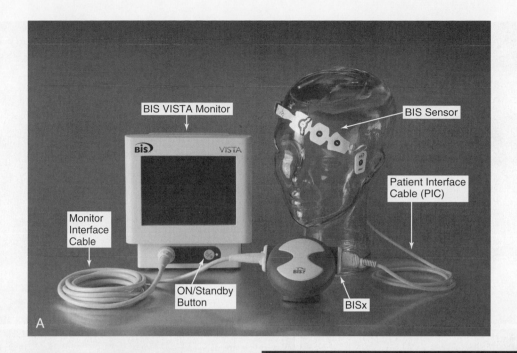

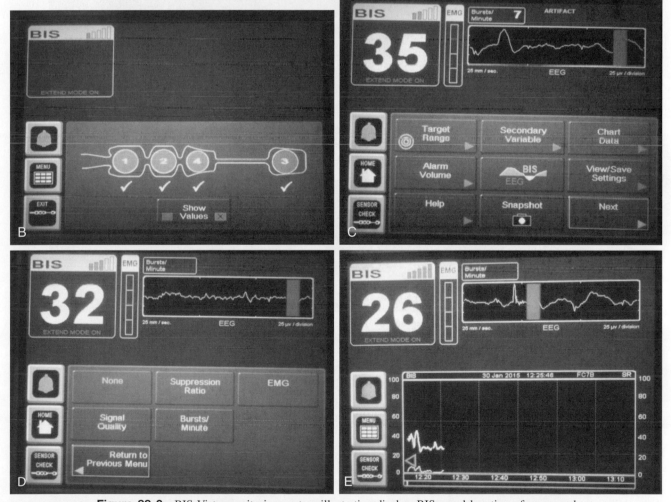

Figure 88-3 BIS Vista monitoring system illustrating display, BISx, and location of menu and power control keys (**A**). **B,** System after activation/patient connection and following successful sensor check. **C,** System initial menu options including choice of secondary variable, frequency of charting data and alarm settings. **D,** Choices for secondary parameter (SR, EMG, burst count, SQI). **E,** BIS monitoring utilizing BIS trend and SR as secondary variable. Single EEG channel visible at top right of image. (*A, Courtesy Aspect Medical Systems, Norwood, MA.*)

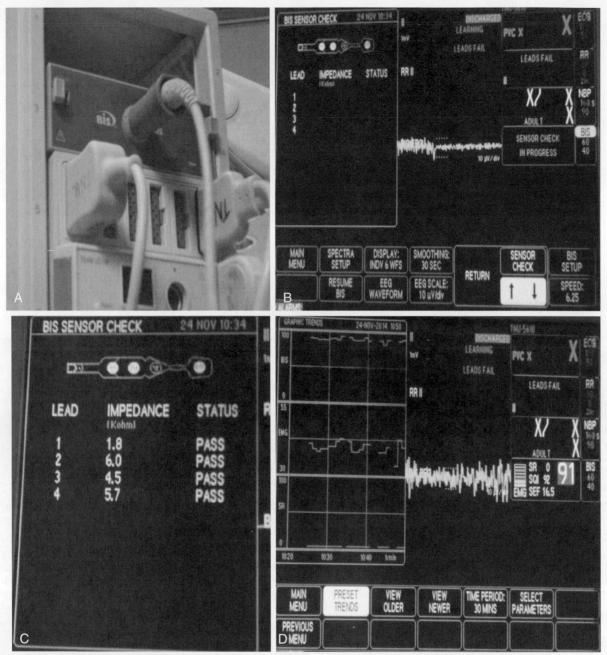

Figure 88-4 Illustration of setup and configuration of BIS monitoring within General Electric (GE) critical care monitoring system. **A,** Placement of BIS module within bedside monitor to establish availability of parameter. **B,** Initial EEG signal and monitor start-up with initial BIS sensor impedance check. In this setup screen, smoothing rate, sensor check, EEG sweep speed and additional options for BIS setup may be determined. **C,** Satisfactory completion of sensor check on all electrodes with impedances within acceptable parameters for acquisition of EEG data. **D,** Completion of sensor check, availability of single-channel EEG tracing (EEG tracing at 6.25 mm/sec sweep speed), SQI indicating adequate signal for BIS determination, EMG and BIS value (91). Graphic trending (BIS, EMG, SR) available by selecting parameters and time indices. This may be utilized for observing data over time and in response to therapies, alterations in clinical state such as shivering during therapeutic hypothermia. BIS technology is licensed to multiple patient monitoring vendors. This illustration using GE monitors is one of multiple options available.

cerebral injury, such as encephalopathy or catastrophic brain trauma, indicating the onset or progression of severe brain injury.[4-6,8-11]

❖ The EMG displays the power (in decibels) within the range of 70 to 110 Hz (cycles per second). This

frequency range includes electrical activity from muscle artifact and patient care devices.[4-6,8-12]

• Initial monitoring and setup of the sensor and equipment includes appropriate setup and configuration of stand-alone BIS monitoring systems (BIS View, BIS Vista) as

TABLE 88-2	BIS Values, Corresponding Level of Sedation, and EEG State[4,6,7,31,32,47]	
BIS Value	**Corresponding Level of Sedation**	**Descriptors**
100	Awake state; patient able to respond appropriately to verbal stimulation	Baseline state before sedation Anxiolysis
80	Patient able to respond to loud verbal, limited tactile stimulation, such as mild prodding/shaking	High-frequency EEG activity (Beta augmentation) Moderate sedation
60	Low probability of explicit recall; patient unresponsive to verbal stimulation	Low-frequency EEG activity Deep sedation
40	Patient unresponsive to verbal stimulation, less responsive to physical stimulation	Deep hypnotic state Drug-induced coma; burst-suppression EEG pattern
20	Minimal responsiveness	
0	No responsiveness mediated by brain function; spinal reflexes may be present	Isoelectric or completely suppressed EEG

Note: Levels of sedation and responsiveness, and corresponding BIS value and EEG state, occur on a continuum.
(Adapted from Arbour R: Continuous nervous system monitoring: EEG, the bispectral index and neuromuscular transmission, AACN Clin Iss 14[2]:192, 2003.)

well as appropriate setup and configuration of BIS modular systems integrated within critical care patient monitoring systems (see Figs. 88-2, 88-3, and 88-4).
* Signal quality index (SQI) is displayed on the monitor screen. The SQI bar that extends to the right side of the SQI bar graph display indicates optimal (100%) EEG signal quality. The BIS value on the numeric region of the monitor display is shown as a solid number. SQI less than 50% (SQI less than the middle range of the display) is indicated by a BIS value shown as an outlined number. If SQI is inadequate for calculation of a BIS value, no data are displayed.
* Potential indications for BIS monitoring include:
  * Use of neuromuscular blockade: BIS monitoring may help in identification of patients at risk for awareness, recall, and pain during paralysis.[2,4,6,31,32,56,57]
  * BIS data may reflect the onset or progression of brain injury not apparent on clinical examination.
  * Use of BIS values to guide sedation and analgesia.[2,4-6,19,21,31,35,36,41,44,48]
  * Titration of sedation or analgesia in patients receiving controlled ventilation.
  * Avoidance of extremes of undersedation and oversedation.
  * Titration of medications for drug-induced coma/metabolic suppression therapies.[4,7,13,46]
  * Procedural sedation.
  * Determination of the dosage of sedation or analgesia during end-of-life care. Using BIS in this setting may be appropriate if concern exists regarding adequacy of sedation and analgesia and clinical assessment is inconclusive on the patient's level of comfort.[4,17]
  * Therapeutic hypothermia
    ○ To titrate sedation and analgesia in real time during hypothermia induction, maintenance and rewarming accounting for temperature-related pharmacokinetics.[14]
    ○ Monitoring BIS value(s)/additional parameters during hypothermia/postcardiopulmonary arrest may give early indications of poor outcome.[19,34,40,49-51,53-55]

  ○ BIS of zero/less than 25, and/or high suppression ratio, may provide early indication of potential poor outcome.[26,34,37,50,51,53-55,58]
  ○ Isoelectric EEG channel or significant ECG artifact indicates significant EEG suppression.[4] Consider reevaluation of hypothermia protocol and neurological evaluation, including diagnostic EEG when clinically appropriate, in determining direction of care.[23]
* Factors that affect the BIS value:
  * Sedation: Decrease in BIS value.[2,4,5,25]
  * BIS value may decrease before impending cardiovascular collapse.[33]
  * Analgesia: Decrease in BIS value from attenuation of cerebral arousal or sedation occurring as a side effect of higher doses of opioids.[2,4,5]
  * Electromyographic (EMG) activity (high-frequency activity from muscle activity across the forehead) may cause increase in BIS value independent of hypnotic state.[1,4,6,12,15,56,57]
  * Neuromuscular blocking agents: If EMG activity is causing false elevation in BIS value due to high-frequency muscle activity across the patient's forehead, neuromuscular blockade administration will decrease BIS value in a dose-related manner.[1,4,6,12,15]
  * Painful (noxious) stimulation: If analgesia is inadequate and CNS/sensory pathways are intact, an arousal response may be produced within the cerebral cortex reflected in the EEG state, resulting in an elevation in BIS value.[20,21]
  * Sleep: BIS range is lower (20 to 70) during deep sleep, and BIS range is higher (75 to 92) during rapid eye movement (REM) sleep.[4,17]
  * Hypothermia: Decrease in BIS value from attenuation of brain metabolism.[4,27]
  * Cerebral ischemia: Decrease in BIS value from deprivation of blood/oxygen supply to affected watershed.[4,7,24,39,52]
  * Neurological injury: Decrease in BIS value depending on location of injury and degree to which overall cerebral metabolism is affected.[4,29]

* Progressive brain injury, including terminal brain herniation/brain death, may produce early indication on BIS monitoring (increased SR, critically low BIS value, possibly isoelectric EEG channel).[22,38]
* Seizure activity can alter/increase BIS value and can be reflected on single EEG channel.[18,40]
* Encephalopathic states: Severe anoxic/ischemic encephalopathy or hepatic encephalopathy (decrease in BIS value).[4,19,30,34,42]
* High-frequency electrical artifact from patient care equipment, such as pacemaker, or muscle activity, such as rapid head or eye movement (increase in BIS value).[1,4,12,59]
* Interpretation of BIS value:
  * BIS is interpreted over time, in response to stimulation and within the context of whether therapeutic endpoints and overall goals of therapy are met.[4,9,11,31]
  * Decisions to increase or decrease titration of sedative or analgesic therapy should be based on the patient's plan of care, clinical assessment, judgment, goals of therapy, and BIS value.
  * Reliance on BIS alone for sedation and analgesia management is not recommended.[9,11,31]
  * Movement such as in response to painful stimulation may occur with low BIS values. This movement may include that produced by spinal reflexes.[20]
  * BIS values should be interpreted with caution and in context with clinical assessment in patients with metabolic or structural brain injury and in those receiving psychoactive medications.[15]
  * BIS monitoring is not intended for regional cerebral ischemia monitoring. With use of BIS in the presence of known CNS injury, a baseline BIS value is recommended before administration of sedative, analgesic, or anesthetic agents.[29]
  * Elevation in BIS value may result from:
    * Sources of noxious stimuli (arousal response and potential increase in EMG activity).
    * Decrease in level of neuromuscular blockade (affecting EMG activity).[1,4]
    * Interruption in sedative therapy (particularly short-acting agents), development of tolerance.
    * Interruption in analgesic therapy, development of tolerance.
    * REM sleep.[4]
    * Seizure activity (potentially).[18]
    * Shivering (particularly in combination with EMG activity).
    * Increased auditory stimulation from environmental noise may cause cerebral arousal and possible BIS elevation.
    * Decrease in BIS value may result from:
    * Attenuation of arousal response or EMG activity after opioid administration.[36]
    * Administration of a neuromuscular blocking agent and attenuation of EMG activity.
    * Excessive sedative dose.
    * Excessive analgesic dosing producing deep sedation as a side effect.
    * Hypothermia (patient cooling).
    * Deeper sleep stages.
    * Hemodynamic instability (compromised blood/oxygen to brain).[33]
    * Onset or progression of neurological injury.

EQUIPMENT

* BIS monitor (or module if using system integrated with the bedside monitor).
* Digital signal converter/BISx
* Patient interface cable
* BIS sensor
* Detachable power cord
* Alcohol pads
* Gauze pads
* Nonsterile gloves

Additional equipment, to have available as needed, includes the following:
* Soap and water
* Emergency equipment

PATIENT AND FAMILY EDUCATION

* Assess factors that affect the patient's (if still awake) and family's readiness to learn. **Rationale:** Teaching is individualized to specific patient and family needs.
* Explain the purpose of BIS monitoring, including content regarding specific information obtained, how it may be used, and an explanation of the equipment. **Rationale:** The patient (if still awake) and family may experience less anxiety and have increased understanding of the patient equipment at the bedside.
* Explain to the patient (if appropriate) and family what will happen with the initiation of BIS monitoring (skin preparation, placement of electrodes, moderate pressure for electrode contact). **Rationale:** The explanation prepares the patient and family for events associated with initiation of BIS monitoring and also provides an opportunity to reinforce preprocedural teaching and assess level of understanding.
* Although rare, some patients may have mild skin irritation develop in the area in contact with the sensor. This irritation typically resolves within 1 hour after sensor removal. **Rationale:** The patient and family are prepared for the possible minor issue with sensor application and the possible need for removal or repositioning of the sensor.
* Explain that BIS monitoring and electrode placement pose no risk to the patient beyond that of mild skin irritation (in rare instances) and that the patient experiences no discomfort as part of monitoring procedure. **Rationale:** Anxiety may be decreased.

PATIENT ASSESSMENT AND PREPARATION
Patient Assessment

* Assess the patient's level of sedation, responsiveness, and arousal. **Rationale:** Baseline data are provided.
* In collaboration with other healthcare physicians, advanced practice nurses, and other healthcare

professionals, establish overall goals and endpoints of sedative and analgesic therapy. ***Rationale:*** A coordinated plan is established with integration of the BIS data into decision making regarding sedation and analgesia.

- Assess the skin at the intended sites for sensor placement. ***Rationale:*** Provides baseline information regarding the patient's skin.
- Assess the patient's neurological status. ***Rationale:*** Baseline data are provided. BIS values may be decreased with significant neurological injury, which needs to be determined before initiation of BIS monitoring. If possible,

obtain a baseline BIS value before initiating therapy with sedative, analgesic, or anesthetic agents.

Patient Preparation

- Verify that the patient is the correct patient using two identifiers. ***Rationale:*** Before performing a procedure, the nurse should ensure the correct identification of the patient for the intended intervention.
- Determine anatomical landmarks for the BIS sensor placement. ***Rationale:*** Landmarks provide for accurate placement of the sensor.

Procedure	for Bispectral Index Monitoring	
Steps	**Rationale**	**Special Considerations**
1. Connect the power cord to the monitor and plug it into the electrical wall outlet.	Prepares the equipment.	Equipment may vary because a stand-alone monitor may be used or a module may be used that is incorporated into the bedside monitoring system.
2. With use of the BIS View or BIS Vista monitoring systems, connect the BISx and related cable to the monitor (see Figs. 88-2A and 88-3A).	Prepares the equipment.	
3. Turn on the monitor and observe as a system check is run. **(Level M*)**	The system initiates a self-test to ensure that the equipment and connections are operating effectively.	If a hardware problem exists, such as DSC failure, a message appears on the display, indicating the need for hardware part replacement or service. If a problem exists, an error message appears. Refer to the operator manual. If needed, remove the device from service and refer to biomedical engineering.
4. Cleanse the intended sensor area with alcohol pads and dry with gauze. **(Level M)**	A thorough skin preparation removes debris and oily residue from the skin and facilitates optimal electrical contact for EEG data acquisition.	Mild soap and water is an acceptable alternative. Ensure that the skin is dry before applying the sensors.
5. **HH**		
6. **PE**		

*Level M: Manufacturer's recommendations only.

Procedure continues on following page

Procedure for Bispectral Index Monitoring—*Continued*

Steps	Rationale	Special Considerations
7. Apply the BIS sensor to the patient's forehead (see Fig. 88-1). A. Position circle 1 electrode at the center of the forehead, approximately 2 inches above the patient's nose. B. Position circle 4 electrode directly above and parallel to the eyebrow. C. Position circle 3 electrode on the temple area between the hairline and the outer canthus of the eye. D. Position circle 2 electrode between the first and fourth sensors on the patient's forehead. E. Press the edges of the sensors to ensure adhesion and seal in the conductive gel. F. Press each of the electrodes with continuous direct pressure for 5 seconds to ensure optimal skin contact. G. With use of the BIS VISTA bilateral monitoring systems, refer to operator's manual. **(Level M*)**	Ensures consistency of the anatomical location for sensor placement and optimizes the electrical contact between the monitoring system and the skin for facilitation of EEG data acquisition. EEG data acquisition begins shortly after optimal connection is established between the patient and the monitoring system.	The conductive parts of the electrodes, sensor, or connectors should not contact other conductive parts of the monitoring system. The patient interface cable should be carefully placed and secured. Data acquisition begins when impedances are acceptable. Electrodes that show high impedance are highlighted on the sensor check display seen at startup. For electrodes identified as having high impedance, repeat pressing of electrodes to optimize electrical contact. If significant artifact is present, the DSC should be moved away from sources of external electrical or mechanical artifact. Sources of artifact include fluid or forced-air warming systems, ventricular assist devices, high-frequency ventilation, suction, pacemakers, and oscillating mattresses. Sensor check is initiated automatically. In the event of an error message, such as high impedance or sensor removal, repreparation, and replacement of the sensor may be necessary.
8. Insert the sensor tab into the patient interface cable until it is engaged.	Connects the BIS sensor and the patient interface cable.	
9. Secure the DSC to an accessible location near the patient's head (e.g., patient's pillow or sheet), avoiding close proximity to sources of mechanical or electrical interference.	The digital signal converter amplifies, filters, and digitizes the patient's EEG signals. It is located close to the patient's head to minimize the vulnerability of the EEG signal to interference from other electronic equipment or patient care devices.	
10. Access the setup menu by pressing "MENU" on the monitor to select the specific monitor settings, including BIS smoothing rate, event markers, and display type (see Figs. 88-2 and 88-3). This also provides access to the advanced setup menu. The touch keys may be used to choose options. **(Level M)**	Settings such as display type and BIS smoothing rate (in seconds) may be chosen.	A 10- or 15-second smoothing rate provides increased sensitivity and expedited feedback to altered hypnotic or arousal states. A 30-second smoothing rate generates a smoother trend with less variability, is less sensitive to artifact, and is often chosen for long-term monitoring; 10-second, 15-second, and 30-second smoothing rate options are available.

*Level M: Manufacturer's recommendations only.

Procedure for Bispectral Index Monitoring—*Continued*

Steps	Rationale	Special Considerations
11. As noted previously, access the advanced setup menu by initially pressing "MENU" and then highlighting "Advanced Setup" by using the up or down arrows. Press select when "Advanced Setup" is highlighted (see Figs. 88-2 and 88-3).	Used to select secondary parameters displayed with BIS trend, such as EMG activity, SR, and SQI, and to alter settings that may be changed less frequently. SQI of 100% indicates an optimal EEG signal. SR is the percentage of suppressed (isoelectric) EEG over the previous 63 seconds within the EEG data sample.	If BIS is used to monitor a patient's sedation level during neuromuscular blockade, selection of EMG as a secondary parameter may provide early information regarding "lightening" of the blockade (EMG activity may increase). If used during deep sedation for controlled ventilation, EMG may indicate a pain/arousal response and indicate the need for analgesia. Increased EMG activity may also indicate a lighter state of sedation or increased muscle activity. If BIS is used to monitor a patient in a drug-induced coma, SR may be monitored as a secondary parameter for continuous evaluation of the degree of EEG suppression.
12. Select additional settings as needed, including: A. Intervals for collection of data in the BIS log. B. "Advanced Setup" as outlined earlier to change the alarm limits, display type, time intervals and secondary parameters.	The settings, such as the interval for recording of the BIS log values, log displays, alarm limits, and alternative displays such as EEG density spectral array, may be changed based on clinical or other needs for data collection.	The density spectral array display shows changes and trends in the power spectrum of the EEG over time. The BIS log display shows BIS numeric values averaged over the previous minute and can be displayed at varying intervals such as 1, 5, 15, or 60 minutes. Approximately 1200 hours of data may be stored in the BISx for later retrieval and review.[9] The EEG display provides a single channel of raw EEG from a frontal montage.
13. When the monitor settings have been adjusted to a specific patient, BIS data collection can begin.	BIS data collection can proceed after all preparatory steps and monitor settings are completed appropriately. This ensures optimal electrical contact between the patient and the monitoring system and optimal electrical safety. In addition, confirmation of display settings and secondary parameters at the outset of monitoring effectively tailors the monitor display and data acquisition to the specific patient.	

Procedure continues on following page

Procedure   for Bispectral Index Monitoring—*Continued*

Steps	Rationale	Special Considerations
14. Observe the monitor display for: A. High impedance alarm (it is highlighted on the sensor check display at start-up): If displayed, press each electrode again to optimize electrical contact. Remove the sensor, cleanse the skin, and place a new sensor if necessary. B. Lead off alarm (it is displayed as "LDOFF"): If present, check whether the sensor has loosened. Remove the sensor, cleanse the skin, and apply another sensor. C. Artifact: If artifact is present, move the digital signal converter away from sources of external electrical or mechanical artifact.	Data acquisition begins when impedances are acceptable. Artifact may result from use of fluid or forced-air warming systems, ventricular assist devices, high-frequency ventilation, suction, pacemakers, and oscillating mattresses.	A sensor check is initiated automatically during the system start-up (see Figs. 88-2, 88-3, and 88-4).
15. For a patient receiving neuromuscular blockade, sedation, or analgesia therapy, the medication should be titrated for a BIS value between 45 and 60. **(Level C*)**	A BIS value <60 is associated with a low probability of explicit recall. A patient with a BIS value <45 is approaching a deep hypnotic state.[4,6]	If the BIS value exceeds 60 in a patient receiving neuromuscular blockade in association with stimulation such as airway suctioning or chest physiotherapy, additional analgesics are indicated. If the BIS value decreases to <40–45, downward titration of sedative therapy may be indicated. In addition, the patient should be evaluated for additional clinical changes such as hypotension, hypothermia, or cerebral ischemia, which may cause a decrease in the BIS value.[4,7,19,24,32]
16. For a patient receiving deep sedation for controlled ventilation, correlate the goal for the BIS value with specific clinical endpoints of therapy.	Correlation of the BIS value with clinical goals of therapy identifies patients who may be progressing to deeper levels of sedation and those who may be at risk for impending breakthrough agitation.	With increased agitation and a BIS value <60, movement may be related to pain or reflex responses to noxious stimulation. Additional analgesia should be considered.
17. Discard used supplies in an appropriate receptacle.	Removes and safely discards used supplies.	
18. 🖐		

*Level C: Qualitative studies, descriptive or correlational studies, integrative reviews, systematic reviews, or randomized controlled trials with inconsistent results.

Expected Outcomes

- Optimal placement of the BIS sensor consistent with anatomical landmarks and manufacturer recommendations
- Skin remaining intact in the area of the BIS sensor placement
- Data acquisition and display after monitor setup and completion of self-test
- SQI of more than 50, indicating optimal EEG data acquisition
- Clear EEG waveform visible on the monitor display
- BIS decrease in response to sedative administration in dose-related manner
- BIS decrease after analgesia administration
- BIS value increase after significant noxious stimulation
- BIS values equal between right and left frontal-temporal montage EEG sensor placement
- BIS data effective in providing feedback on the state of the brain in response to sedative, analgesic, or hypnotic administration that can be used to direct therapy

Unexpected Outcomes

- Skin irritation in the area of the BIS sensor placement
- SQI significantly <50, indicating suboptimal EEG signal acquisition
- A sudden decrease in the BIS value independent of changes in sedative or analgesic therapy (may indicate hemodynamic compromise, cerebral ischemia, or the onset or progression of significant neurological injury)
- A sudden rise in the BIS independent of stimulation, increased EMG activity, or an outward change in the patient's condition (may indicate seizure activity or shivering).
- BIS completely unresponsive to noxious stimulation such as endotracheal suctioning or invasive procedures
- BIS values significantly unequal between the right and left frontal-temporal montage sensor placement (may indicate unilateral cerebral injury or ischemia)
- BIS values that do not correlate with clinical assessment of sedation level and respond inconsistently to administration of sedative, hypnotic, or analgesic agents

Patient Monitoring and Care

Steps	Rationale	Reportable Conditions
		These conditions should be reported if they persist despite nursing interventions.
1. Follow institutional standard for assessing pain. Administer analgesia as prescribed.	Identifies need for pain interventions.	• Continued pain despite pain interventions
2. Assess the skin condition in the area of the sensor placement.	Ensures that the skin is intact.	• Altered skin integrity or irritation after sensor placement
3. Maintain the digital signal converter (DSC or BISx) in close proximity to the patient's head.	Decreases the vulnerability of the EEG signals to electrical interference from other sources.	
4. Monitor the BIS values and secondary parameters, including SQI, EMG, and SR, as determined by goals of care, clinical status, and response to interventions. For example, during rapid administration of sedative or analgesic agents before the anticipated use of neuromuscular blockade therapy, it may be appropriate to monitor and record the BIS value multiple times per hour. As therapy is stabilized, BIS can be monitored hourly.	Identifies trends in BIS and secondary parameters. Decrease in SQI to <50% may indicate suboptimal EEG data acquisition.	• Increase in EMG activity without a change in medication therapy (may indicate increased arousal response [pain] or lightening of neuromuscular blockade and result in increase in BIS independent of hypnotic state or decreasing level of sedation or analgesia) • Significant difference in BIS value between right and left frontal montage EEG (may indicate unilateral cerebral injury) • BIS value absolutely invariant to significant noxious stimulation (may indicate significant cerebral injury) • Increased suppression ratio (may indicate onset or evolution of cerebral injury, hemodynamic compromise, ischemia, or excessively deep hypnotic state)

Procedure continues on following page

Patient Monitoring and Care —*Continued*

Steps	Rationale	Reportable Conditions
5. Identify goals or endpoints of therapy at the beginning of BIS monitoring.	Patient outcomes are improved with an organized, evidence-based approach to care.	• Not progressing toward achievement of goals or endpoint of therapy
6. Observe BIS values at least hourly and in response to titration of medication therapy.	Determines changes in BIS values in response to medication therapy and interventions. Also provides the ability to use "event marker" to closely correlate changes in BIS and secondary parameters for later review.	• Abnormal BIS values or trends: • BIS value not decreasing in response to upward titration of sedative or hypnotic therapy • BIS value not increasing after downward titration of sedative or hypnotic therapy
7. Change the BIS sensor at least every 24 hours or more frequently as needed (e.g., diaphoresis, loose electrodes).	Maintains optimal electrical contact between the patient and the monitoring system.	
8. Observe the EEG channel as determined by the patient's clinical state and therapeutic interventions. Significant decrease in EEG amplitude and/or frequency may become visible and reportable.	The EEG amplitude and frequency change based on the patient's clinical state, evolving injury, and medication therapy. The EEG also (under normal conditions) changes in response to varying levels and types of stimulation. In most conditions, electrocardiographic (ECG) artifact is not visible in an EEG waveform. ECG artifact visible in the EEG channel may indicate significant EEG suppression.	• A decrease in EEG frequency or amplitude (e.g., if this occurs with a decrease in the BIS value, may indicate neurological injury) • A significant decrease in the BIS value that is inconsistent with the medication therapy may indicate critical pathology and warrant further evaluation with neuroimaging diagnostic EEG or clinical examination
9. Observe the BIS value in response to stimulation.	The BIS value should, in most patients, rise in response to stimulation. The EEG, on which the BIS is based, normally responds to external stimulation. An EEG unresponsive to stimulation may indicate significant neurological injury and possibly poor prognosis.	• Significant ECG artifact in the EEG channel • A BIS value that is unresponsive to noxious stimulation • A significant difference in BIS values or suppression ratio (SR) between the right and left frontal-temporal montage (may indicate unilateral cerebral injury)

Documentation

Documentation should include the following:

- Goals and endpoints of sedative or analgesic therapy
- Family education regarding BIS monitoring
- Clinical assessment (if appropriate) of level of sedation
- BIS value at start of monitoring and with changes or titration of therapy
- BIS value recording in patient medical record at least hourly and more frequently as indicated (Fig. 88-5)
- Pain assessment, interventions, and evaluation of interventions
- Occurrence of skin irritation at the site of the BIS sensor placement with action taken
- Unexpected outcomes and interventions
- Sudden changes in BIS value (increase or decrease) independent of obvious clinical changes or alterations of medication therapy
- Suppression ratio (SR) (as appropriate) for BIS use in medication-induced coma or monitoring during therapeutic hypothermia

- SQI and EMG activity (as appropriate)
- Documentation of left versus right frontal montage (location of the BIS sensor on the right or the left side)
- BIS value before and after noxious stimulation and the difference between these two values
- Change in the BIS value in response to noxious or painful stimulation
- For case reviews to track, BIS values or trends and response to stimulation or therapeutic interventions over time may be downloaded from the monitoring system or be tracked by electronic medical record systems. These may require validation by the nurse in order to be permanently entered into the medical record (see Fig. 88-5)

Mode: Expanded View All												1m 5m 10m 15m 30m 1h 2h 4h 8h 24h Based On: 0700 Reset Now
						1/29/15						
	0845	0900	0915	0945	1000	1030	1100	1200	1215	1300	1330	1400	**1440**
Hypothermia Flowsheet												
RASS Score	-5	-5	-5	-5	-5	-5	-5	-5	-5	-5	-5	-5
BIS (Bispectral Index)	98	98	96	93	96	14▪	0	3	36	27	69	49
Temp	91.6 (33...	90.8 (32...	90.2 (32...	90.7 (32...	91.2 (32...	92.1 (33...	92.4 (33...	91.7 (33...	91.6 (33...	91.6 (33...		92 (33.3)
Arctic Sun Goal Temp (degrees)	92	92	92	92	92	92	92	92	92	92		92
Arctic Sun Water Temp (degrees)	80.6	91.9	101.7	101.3	95.4	88.2	78.8	86	88.7	91.6		87.3
QTc Interval (Sec)								0.5▪				
Shivering	N/A	N/A	Mild	Mild	Mild˙	N/A	N/A	N/A	N/A	N/A		N/A

Figure 88-5   Documentation of BIS values in an electronic medical record over time on a patient receiving therapeutic hypothermia. From 0845 to1030 BIS values were significantly elevated and inconsistent with clinical assessment. EMG parameter was also significantly elevated raising suspicion of subclinical shivering. Following collaboration with the clinical nurse specialist, the patient received (per order), a neuromuscular blocking agent at 1030. The patient's BIS value rapidly declined to zero with elimination of EMG interference. BIS was recorded at 15 to 30 minute intervals. BIS data were obtained via a BIS module integrated within the patient monitoring system. Depending on system configuration, BIS data may be entered manually or be transmitted automatically from the monitoring system into the electronic medical record, requiring validation for data to permanently become part of the patient medical record.

References and Additional Readings

For a complete list of references and additional readings for this procedure, scan this QR code with any freely available smartphone code reader app, or visit http://booksite.elsevier.com/9780323376624.

89 Brain Tissue Oxygen Monitoring: Insertion (Assist), Care, and Troubleshooting

Megan T. Moyer and Eileen Maloney Wilensky

PURPOSE: Brain tissue oxygen monitoring is performed in patients with, or at high risk of, cerebral ischemia and/or hypoxia. It is used for measurement and continuous monitoring of regional brain tissue oxygenation for prevention and detection of secondary brain injury. Monitoring of brain tissue oxygen provides important information relative to the delivery of oxygen to cerebral tissue of the injured brain.

PREREQUISITE NURSING KNOWLEDGE

- Incorporated as an adjunct monitor of trends in concert with concurrent neurological multimodality monitoring parameters (intracranial pressure [ICP], cerebral perfusion pressure [CPP], systemic jugular venous oxygen [SjvO$_2$], cerebral microdialysis) brain tissue oxygen monitoring reflects the oxygenation of cerebral tissue local to the sensor placement.[1,7,8,10,14,16,18]
- Each of the devices described in this chapter denotes partial pressure of the brain tissue differently, for example Pbto$_2$, Pbro$_2$, Ptio$_2$, tio$_2$, Pto$_2$. For the remainder of the text in this chapter brain oxygen will be referred to as PbO$_2$. The tables that represent the individual devices will denote the nomenclature adopted by that manufacturer.
- In institutions where SjvO$_2$ is used as a monitoring parameter, the difference between SjvO$_2$ measurements and PbO$_2$ values must be noted. SjvO$_2$ is a measure of the oxygen contained in the blood draining from the cerebral venous sinuses into the jugular bulb (a measure of global brain oxygenation), whereas PbO$_2$ measures regional (local to the catheter placement in the cerebral white matter) brain tissue oxygenation. SjvO$_2$ monitoring accuracy can be influenced by poor sampling technique, positioning, and clot formation on the catheter, making this method of monitoring less reliable than PbO$_2$ monitoring. A normal SjvO$_2$ range is between 55% and 75%, making cerebral ischemia any number less than 55%. The choice of monitoring device depends on the patient's pathology.[1,8]
- Understanding of neuroanatomy and physiology, specifically intracranial dynamics, is needed.
- Cellular death is preceded by a cascade of events following low brain oxygen levels that result in anaerobic metabolism, lactic acid accumulation, and release of excitatory neurotransmitter causing neurotoxicity.[1,7,11]
- Knowledge of sterile and aseptic technique is necessary.
- A brain tissue oxygen probe may be inserted into the brain parenchyma through an intracranial bolt or tunneled.[1]

- PbO$_2$ monitoring provides information that reflects brain tissue oxygen levels associated with cerebral oxygen demand and systemic oxygen delivery, therefore identifying cerebral ischemia.[1,6]
- PbO$_2$ values are relative within an individual and vary depending on a range of factors including precondition, duration, location, tissue condition, and sensor type. Establishing and following the patient's cerebral oxygen trends provides the physicians, advanced practice nurses, and other healthcare professionals with information that will aid in the assessment and treatment of cerebral hypoxia and preventing further secondary brain damage. Brain hypoxia is associated with increased mortality and poor outcome.[1,6,10,13]
- Indications for PbO$_2$ monitoring include patients at risk for secondary injury from cerebral edema. Conditions most likely to cause cerebral edema include severe traumatic brain injury, aneurysmal and traumatic subarachnoid hemorrhage, brain tumor, stroke, and any condition that increases ICP.[6]
- Contraindications for PbO$_2$ monitoring include patients with a coagulopathy, those receiving anticoagulation therapy, and those with an insertion site infection.
- PbO$_2$ probes are safe with computed tomography (CT). Consult manufacturer's guidelines for magnetic resonance imaging specificity by probe.
- Cerebral oxygen data are accurate and reliable when the PbO$_2$ probe is located in the deep white matter of the brain, the location where oxygen availability is most stable.[1]
- Insertion depth affects the cerebral blood flow values obtained due to values differing between the cerebral cortex and subcortical white matter.[1]
- Parameters such as ICP and brain tissue temperature can be measured immediately at the time of probe placement, but may be delayed up to 2 hours because time is needed for the brain tissue to settle after the microtrauma caused by probe placement.[5,17]
- PbO$_2$ monitoring has been demonstrated to be safe and effective in both the clinical and laboratory settings.[6]

TABLE 89-1	Management of Increased or Decreased Pbo$_2$ Values

Decreased Pbo$_2$ Values

Increased oxygen demand	Increased ICP	Treat the increased ICP with osmotic diuretics, cerebrospinal fluid drainage, sedation (e.g., barbiturates, propofol), craniotomy.
	Pain	Administer analgesics.
	Shivering	Rewarm, if needed, or administer agents to stop shivering (e.g., demerol, thorazine, paralytic agents). If a cooling device in use, perform skin counterwarming).
	Agitation	Administer sedation agents.
	Seizures	Administer benzodiazepines and adjunct anticonvulsant agents.
	Fever	Treat the underlying cause of the fever, initiate a cooling device, if needed, and administer antipyretic agents.
Decreased oxygen delivery	Hypotension	Administer isotonic fluids (normal saline or hypertonic saline solution) or vasopressors.
	Hypovolemia	Administer isotonic fluids (normal saline or hypertonic saline solution), blood replacement.
	Anemia	Administer blood-replacement products.
	Hypoxia	Increase Fio$_2$, PEEP, and interventions to mobilize pulmonary secretions and maximize pulmonary function.

Increased Pbo$_2$ values

Increased oxygen delivery	Hyperdynamic (elevated ICP)	Consider sedation agents, temperature management, and/or positioning to treat elevated ICP
Decreased oxygen demand	Hypothermia	Rewarm to achieve normothermia or mild hypothermia as prescribed for management of cerebral metabolism.
	Sedatives	Decrease sedation, anesthesia, or paralysis as prescribed.
	Anesthesia	
	Neuromuscular blockade agents	

Fio$_2$, fraction of inspired oxygen; ICP intracranial pressure; Pbo$_2$, brain oxygen; PEEP, positive end-expiratory pressure.

- The normal range for brain tissue oxygen values is between 20 and 35 mm Hg.[7] Treatment goals usually aim to keep the Pbo$_2$ equal to or greater than 20 mm Hg.
- A Pbo$_2$ of less than 20 mm Hg is when an intervention should be considered due to potentially compromised brain oxygen.[1,3,8–10] A Pbo$_2$ of less than 15 represents impending brain hypoxia.[1,9]
- A Pbo$_2$ of less than 10 mm Hg is directly associated with increased lactate and glutamate, severe disability, poor outcome at discharge, and death.[1]
- A Pbo$_2$ of less than 5 mm Hg is indicative of increased cerebral levels of glutamate, glycerol, or the lactate/pyruvate ratio, indicating a critical level of brain tissue oxygen.[16]
- Brain tissue oxygen values can be used to manage potential cerebral hypoxia. Clinical interventions can be aimed at increasing oxygen delivery or decreasing cerebral oxygen demand, including but not limited to ventilator manipulation, CPP augmentation, sedation, head repositioning, intravenous fluid boluses, airway suctioning, and blood transfusions.[1,2,4] Simultaneously increasing the number of Pbo$_2$ interventions has been shown to worsen the time to correcting Pbo$_2$; instead implementing one intervention at a time may have a better impact.[12]
- Decreases in Pbo$_2$ values occur when cerebral blood flow or cerebral oxygen delivery is inadequate or states of increased metabolic demands exist, indicating the potential for secondary brain injury. Pbo$_2$ can detect subtle changes that can lead to the early identification of cerebral hypoxia and ischemia.[6,8] Table 89-1 outlines interventions for increased or decreased Pbo$_2$.
- Increases in Pbo$_2$ values denote decreased oxygen uptake by cerebral cells that may be caused by states of increased oxygen delivery or decreased oxygen utilization.[8]
- Pbo$_2$ monitoring is accurate and safe, and can provide reliable data for up to 10 days with measured responses to interventions.[8,15] However, both manufacturers' recommendations suggest device placement should not exceed 5 days to continue to receive accurate measurement.
- Pbo$_2$ probe placement: The physician, advanced practice nurse, or other healthcare professional placing the probe device determines the catheter placement location after review of the CT scan and after consideration of the most appropriate monitoring area based on diagnosis, pathology, and technical feasibility, avoiding areas of infarct or hematoma.[3,8] Placement of the probe may be ipsilateral or contralateral to the pathology.
  - ❖ The probe may be placed in the nondominant hemisphere (e.g., right frontal region) to minimize risk of injury from catheter insertion. The right hemisphere is a safer location for probe placement than the left hemisphere because speech function is located in the left hemisphere in most individuals.

- ❖ Placement may be near a lesion when the clinical goal is to monitor oxygen availability to damaged but salvageable tissue.
- ❖ If a patient has a subarachnoid hemorrhage, the probe may be placed in the area of the brain expected to develop vasospasm. Placement is determined by the distribution of subarachnoid blood on CT scan and by aneurysm location.
- When interpreting the PbO_2 data, the clinician should be aware of the catheter probe location.[13]
- Neurological outcome and PbO_2 may be affected by the location of the probe.[7,13]
- Currently, two brain tissue oxygen-monitoring systems are available, the Integra Licox monitor and the RAUMEDIC Neurovent-PTO; both are invasive monitors that provide continuous direct PbO_2 monitoring.[1,15]
- The Licox PtO_2 Monitor (Figs. 89-1, *A–G*) and Licox CMP Monitor (Figs. 89-2, *A–C*)[5]:
  - ❖ Catheter: Two catheters, three parameters (one, ICP; two, oxygen and temperature)
  - ❖ Provides functionality for continuously monitoring PtO_2 in brain tissue. Tissue temperature compensation,

which is required for the calculation of PtO_2 measurements, may also be continuously measured with an accuracy of $\pm 1v$ °C. To measure PtO_2 and temperature tissue compensation continuously, the Integra Licox PtO_2 Monitor supports a series of minimally invasive probes that are inserted directly into the patient.

- ❖ The PtO_2 probe uses an electrochemical (polarographic) microcell for oxygen measurements.
- ❖ The temperature probe uses a thermocouple (type K) for temperature measurements.
- ❖ In place of a temperature probe, the monitor also provides an option for entering tissue temperature compensation values manually for the calculation of PtO_2 measurements.
- ❖ O_2 measurement window
- ❖ Probe storage: temperature, 2 to 10 °C; humidity, 25% to 80%; relative humidity, noncondensing.
- ❖ Contraindications for needle insertion into the body include coagulopathy and/or susceptibility to infections or infected tissue. A platelet count of less than 50,000 per μL is considered a contraindication. This value may differ according to different hospital protocols.

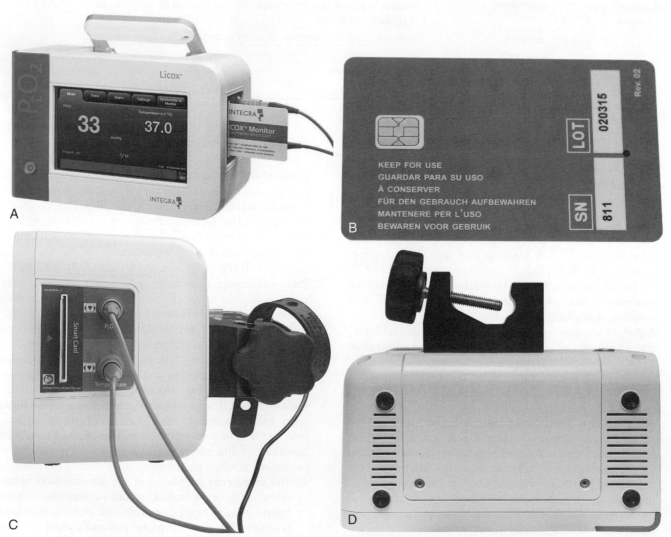

Figure 89-1   **A,** The Integra Licox PtO_2 Monitor with card inserted into slot. **B,** Smart card. **C,** The Integra Licox PtO_2 Monitor right panel. **D,** The Integra Licox PtO_2 Monitor back panel.

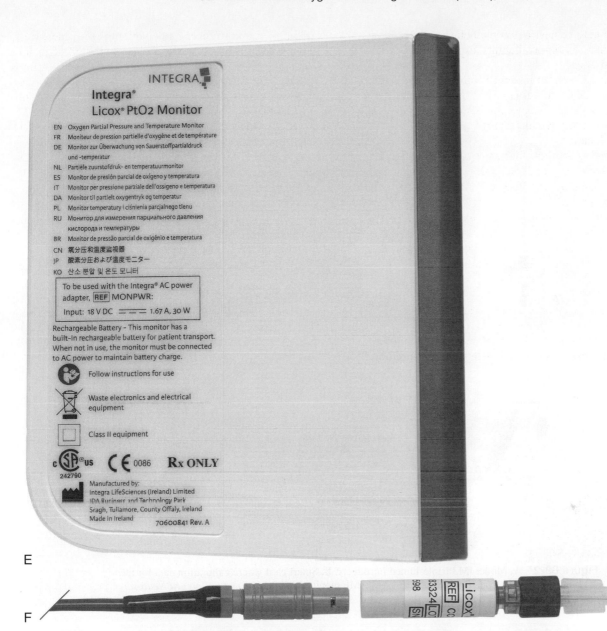

Figure 89-1, cont'd **E,** The Integra Licox Pto$_2$ Monitor left panel. **F and G,** Connecting the Pto$_2$ probe and temperature probe to their probe cables. *(Courtesy Integra Neurosciences, Plainsboro, NJ.)*

- The RAUMEDIC NEUROVENT-PTO Monitor[17]:
  - 5-Fr catheter: one catheter, three parameters (ICP, temperature, and oxygen)
  - Determines the oxygen partial pressure of the available oxygen in the brain tissue. At the same time, the parenchyma pressure and the temperature are measured in one measuring catheter providing information about three parameters: the ICP, the temperature, and the oxygen partial pressure, in one catheter.
  - The NEUROVENT-PTO catheter uses oxygen quenching to measure oxygen partial pressure.
  - The catheter is precalibrated during manufacturing and therefore does not require zeroing.

  - O$_2$ measurement window
  - Temperature accuracy is ±0.1 °C.
  - ICP drift is less than 1 mm Hg during the first 24 hours at 37 °C.
  - Storage is at room temperature and it has a sterility shelf life of 2 years.
  - Contraindications include coagulopathy, those receiving anticoagulation therapy, and those with an insertion site infection. Blood coagulation must be carefully monitored during therapeutic hypothermia, hepatic coma, or other conditions that impair blood coagulation.
  - Monitoring of Pbto$_2$ values may be delayed as long as 2 hours because time is needed for the brain tissue

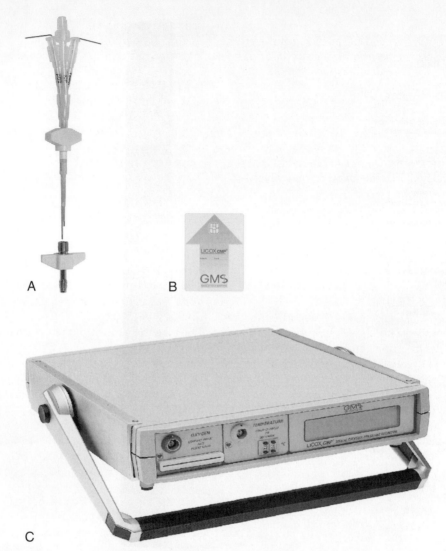

Figure 89-2 **A,** Model IM3 triple-lumen introducer. **B,** Smart card where calibration data for the oxygen probe is electronically stored. **C,** Licox CMP monitor, AC 3.1. *(Courtesy Integra Neurosciences, Plainsboro, NJ.)*

to settle after the microtrauma caused by catheter placement.[7]

PATIENT AND FAMILY EDUCATION

• Assess patient or family understanding of the purpose of Pbo$_2$ monitoring. Most patients who need brain tissue oxygen monitoring have an altered level of consciousness with a score of 8 or less on the Glasgow Coma Scale; education is then directed toward the family. *Rationale:* Understanding may reduce anxiety and stress, stimulates requests for clarification or additional information, and increases awareness of the goals, duration, and expectations of the monitoring system.

• Explain the insertion process, patient monitoring, and care involving the Pbo$_2$ monitoring system. *Rationale:* Explanation may alleviate anxiety and stress and stimulates requests for clarification or additional information.

• Explain the expected outcomes of the Pbo$_2$ system. *Rationale:* Explanation may decrease patient and family anxiety and stress by increasing awareness of Pbto$_2$ monitoring duration and therapy goals.

PATIENT ASSESSMENT AND PREPARATION
Patient Assessment

• Assess the patient's neurological status. *Rationale:* Performing a baseline neurological assessment enables the nurse to identify changes that may occur as a result of the Pbo$_2$ probe insertion.

• Assess the patient for signs or symptoms of local infection at the intended insertion location. *Rationale:* Evidence of local infection is a contraindication to brain tissue oxygen catheter placement.

• Obtain and review coagulation laboratory results (e.g., complete blood count, platelet count, prothrombin time, partial thromboplastin time, bleeding time, international normalized ratio) as prescribed. *Rationale:* Assessment identifies the patient's risk for bleeding.

Patient Preparation

- Verify that the patient is the correct patient using two identifiers. *Rationale:* Before performing a procedure, the nurse should ensure the correct identification of the patient for the intended intervention.
- Ensure that the patient and family understand the procedure teaching. Answer questions as they arise, and reinforce information as needed. Most patients who need brain tissue oxygen monitoring are in an altered level of consciousness with a Glasgow Coma Scale score of 8 or less. *Rationale:* Previously taught information is evaluated and reinforced.
- Ensure that informed consent has been obtained. *Rationale:* Informed consent protects the rights of the patient and makes a competent decision possible for the patient; however, in emergency circumstances, time may not allow for the consent form to be signed.
- Participate in a preprocedure verification and timeout. *Rationale:* Ensures patient safety.
- Administer sedation or analgesia as prescribed before beginning the insertion procedure. *Rationale:* Sedation or analgesia facilitates the insertion process.
- Assist the patient to the semi-Fowler's position with the head in the neutral position and the head of the bed elevated 30 to 45 degrees. *Rationale:* Patients who are candidates for brain tissue oxygen monitoring may have increased ICP. Elevating the head of the bed and placing the head in the neutral position act to decrease ICP by enhancing jugular venous outflow and provides for optimal insertion accessibility.

EQUIPMENT

For the RAUMEDIC Neurovent-PTO Monitoring System

- Sterile gown, sterile drapes, sterile gloves, caps, face masks with eye shield

- Shave preparation kit
- Antiseptic solution
- EASY logO Monitor and connecting fiber optic, yellow, blue, gray, and red cables
- NEUROVENT-PTO catheter (1)
- RAUMEDIC BOLT KIT PTO
- RAUMEDIC DRILL KIT CH5
- Cranial access kit (use the hand drill, not the drill bit)
- 4 × 4 gauze (2)
- Large Tegaderm (2)
- Arm board folded in half (1)
- 2-inch tape

For the Integra Licox Pto$_2$ Monitor

- Sterile gowns, sterile drapes, sterile gloves, nonsterile gloves, caps, goggles, and face masks
- Shave preparation kit
- Antiseptic solution
- Pbto$_2$ monitor (see Fig. 89-1, *A*) or module
- Connecting cables
- Cranial access tray; use the drill, but use the Licox bit in the Licox kit
- Pbto$_2$ probe
- Scalpel
- Dressing supplies, including 4 × 4 gauze and tape
- Sterile dry gauze; may be placed at the insertion site

Additional equipment, to have available as needed, includes the following:

- An intravenous (IV) arm board may be used to stabilize the monitor probe and cable
- Intracranial bolt system
- Extra transparent and soft-cloth adhesive dressing or a dry, sterile occlusive dressing
- A compatible fiber-optic ICP catheter may be inserted through the intracranial bolt system, as well, and will require a separate monitor to measure ICP

Procedure	for Brain Tissue Oxygen Monitoring for the Integra Licox Pto$_2$ Monitor: Insertion (Assist) and Care	
Steps	**Rationale**	**Special Considerations**
1. **HH**		
2. Plug the monitor power cord into an AC power outlet.	Provides the power source.	On the back of the monitor, attach the red connector end of the AC power cord into the red port labeled Input 18V. Insert the plug end of the AC power adapter into an AC wall outlet.
3. Attach the cables (e.g., oxygen cable, temperature cable) to the Pbto$_2$ monitor.	Prepares the equipment.	Refer to manufacturer's guidelines as needed. Monitors and cables may be color coded.

Procedure continues on following page

Procedure	for Brain Tissue Oxygen Monitoring for the Integra Licox Pto₂ Monitor: Insertion (Assist) and Care—*Continued*	
Steps	**Rationale**	**Special Considerations**
4. Turn on the monitor. On the front of the monitor, press the power button. Once the button illuminates, the Integra logo will appear on the touch screen for a few seconds before initiating the setup process.	Prepares the monitor.	
5. After the setup process completes, listen for a 1-second startup tone.	Verifies the audio alarms are functioning correctly; verifies the monitor's screen displays the main panel.	There is a short beep when the monitor is first turned on; this is not the 1-second startup tone.
6. Wash hands and apply goggles or masks with face shields, caps, and gowns, and assist with sterile procedure.	Prepares for sterile procedure.	
7. Assist as needed with site preparation (e.g., shave preparation and cleansing with antiseptic solution).	Prepares for sterile procedure.	Antiseptic solution choice should be determined by institutional policy. Use of povidone-iodine versus chlorhexidine is controversial. The antiseptic solution should be allowed to dry before the initial incision is made.[8] Studies suggest chlorhexidine is neurotoxic.[8]
8. Assist as needed in draping the head, neck, and chest of the patient.	Prepares a sterile environment for the insertion process.	
9. Assist as needed with opening of the sterile trays and probes.	Facilitates efficiency of the insertion process.	
10. Insert the calibration card for calibration of the monitor unique to each Pto₂ probe.[5] **(Level M*)**	The Licox monitor requires insertion of a calibration card referred to as the "smart card," which has numbers on it that match those on the oxygen probe that is being inserted. This card is placed into a card slot located on the right side of the monitor by aligning the arrow on the card with the arrow on the monitor. The calibration card can only be used with the probe that has the same numbers on it and is included in the same packaging (see Fig. 89-1, *A–G*).	Do not discard Pto₂ probe packaging before removing the smart card. Each card contains calibration data specific to that that probe. Inserting a new smart card during the recording of trend data will reset the trend data. Only use the smart card supplied with the Pto₂ probe. If the calibration card is lost, another corresponding Pbto₂ probe and smart card must be used.
11. Assist as needed with insertion of an intracranial bolt (see Procedure 92).	May be inserted before Pto₂ probe insertion.	Use the bit from the Licox kit. It is critical for dural opening to assure accurate parenchymal probe placement.
12. Assist as needed with insertion of the oxygen probe and temperature probe.	Facilitates the insertion process.	The oxygen probe and temperature probe may be separate (triple-lumen bolt system) or may be combined (double-lumen bolt system). The additional lumen is for the ICP probe.

*Level M: Manufacturer's recommendations only.

Procedure	for Brain Tissue Oxygen Monitoring for the Integra Licox Pto$_2$ Monitor: Insertion (Assist) and Care—*Continued*	
Steps	**Rationale**	**Special Considerations**
13. Connect the oxygen and temperature probes to the monitor cables.	Prepares for monitoring.	
14. Observe the temperature and Pto$_2$ values.	Initiates monitoring. The temperature values should be accurate; however, time is needed for the brain tissue to settle after the microtrauma caused by catheter placement.	
15. If possible, use a cable to transfer the values from the Pto$_2$ monitor to the bedside monitor. Set the upper and lower alarm limits.	Allows integration of the monitoring systems. The currently available brain tissue oxygen monitoring system does not have an alarm system. Integrating the monitoring system with the bedside monitor allows (1) a larger display of the numeric values and (2) audible upper and lower alarm limits.[10]	Refer to monitor guidelines for specific information.
16. After the system has been placed, assist with placing a sterile, occlusive dressing at the insertion point.	Prevents contamination of the insertion site by microorganisms and protects the site.	A dressing (formed with dry sterile gauze) provides a base to secure the device to an arm board or other securing method.
17. Secure the Pto$_2$ monitor cables with two points of tension to avoid tension on the Pto$_2$ and ICP probes.		
A. Anchor the cables at the patient's head and at the shoulder.	The monitoring cables need to be secured so that no tension or disruption of the device occurs at the insertion site.	
B. Secure the cables so that they do not get entangled in the side rails and do not touch the floor.	Supports the entire mechanism.	One method to secure the monitor cables is as follows: A. Place an IV arm board or stability anchor to a conical gauze dressing where the device and cables can be secured. B. Anchor the cables from the patient's head to the shoulder in place with a transparent or soft-cloth adhesive dressing. The first tension point is directly on the patient's head where the dressing is anchored to the skin at the point of insertion. The second tension point is at the patient's shoulder. C. Place rolled towels under the secured system.
C. Allow enough slack to accommodate patient movement and turning.	Prevents gravity drag and tension on the cables and the device.	
18. Discard used supplies in appropriate receptacles.	Removes and safely discards used supplies. Safely removes sharp objects.	
19. **HH**		

Procedure continues on following page

Procedure	**for Brain Tissue Oxygen Monitoring for the Integra Licox Pto$_2$ Monitor: Insertion (Assist) and Care—*Continued***	
Steps	**Rationale**	**Special Considerations**

Connecting a Single Pto$_2$ Probe

Steps	Rationale	Special Considerations
1. Connect the Pto$_2$ Probe cable to the monitor.	Allows integration of the monitoring systems.	Refer to monitor guidelines for specific information.
2. Insert the Pbo$_2$ probe's smart card into the monitor.	Prepares the equipment.	Each bedside monitor may have its own unique labels for parameters that are being added (e.g., brain oxygen).
3. Insert the Pto$_2$ probe into the patient and connect the probe to the monitor.	Prepares the equipment.	Depending on hospital protocol, you may either insert the Pbo$_2$ probe into the patient before or after connecting the Pto$_2$ probe to the monitor. The purpose of connecting the Pto$_2$ probe to the monitor before implantation is to verify the functionality of the probe before clinical use.
4. Allow stabilization time for microtrauma.	Prepares the monitor to adjust to measurements obtained on insertion and the continuous monitoring.	This normally applies to the first 20 minutes after insertion and the Pto$_2$ values may not display optimal information about tissue oxygenation due to tissue injury during insertion of the probe.
5. Enter the tissue temperature compensation value manually. A. Enter the tissue temperature compensation that will be used during Pto$_2$ measurements. B. On the temperature manual panel, adjust the manual temperature input arrows to the designated temperature to the nearest whole number.	The calculations for Pto$_2$ measurements require tissue temperature compensation. If you are not measuring the tissue temperature with a probe, the temperature has to be entered manually. Make sure to check the patient's temperature either hourly or before recording the Pto$_2$ value for intervention. If any changes in temperature occur, use the manual temperature input arrows to specify the new temperature value accordingly.	

Connecting a Single Pto$_2$ Probe with a Single Temperature Probe

Steps	Rationale	Special Considerations
1. Connect the Pto$_2$ probe cable to the monitor.	Prepares the monitor.	On the monitor's right side, connect the large plug of the blue Pto$_2$ probe cable into the blue port labeled Pto$_2$.
2. Connect the temperature probe cable to the monitor.	Prepares the equipment/cables connection to the monitor.	On the monitor's right side, connect the green temperature probe cable into the green port labeled "Temperature."
3. Insert the Pto$_2$ probe's smart card into the monitor.	Prepares the monitor.	On the monitor's right side, insert the smart card slot by aligning the arrow on the card with the arrow on the label.
4. Insert the Pto$_2$ and temperature probes into the patient and connect the probes to monitor.	Prepares the equipment/cables connection to the monitor.	Depending on hospital protocol, you may either insert the Pto$_2$ probe and temperature probe into the patient before or after connecting the two probes to the monitor.

Procedure for Brain Tissue Oxygen Monitoring for the Integra Licox Pto₂ Monitor: Insertion (Assist) and Care—*Continued*		
Steps	**Rationale**	**Special Considerations**
5. Allow stabilization time for microtrauma.	Prepares monitor to adjust to measurements obtained on insertion and the continuous monitoring.	This normally applies to the first 20 minutes after insertion and the Pto₂ values may not display optimal information about tissue oxygenation due to tissue injury during insertion of the probe.
6. Check Pto₂ and temperature values.	Initiates monitoring. The temperature values should be accurate.	When using a temperature probe, the temperature measurement being continuously reported by the monitor, with an accuracy of $\pm 1\,°C$, will be applied to the calculation for Pto₂ measurements.

Procedure for Brain Tissue Oxygen Monitoring for the Integra Licox CMP Monitor: Insertion (Assist) and Care		
Steps	**Rationale**	**Special Considerations**
1. ▨		
2. Plug the Pbto₂ monitor power cord into an AC wall outlet.	Provides the power source.	
3. Attach the cables (e.g., oxygen cable, temperature cable) to the Pbto₂ monitor.	Prepares the equipment.	Refer to manufacturer's guidelines as needed. Monitors and cables may be color coded.
4. ▨		
5. Apply goggles or masks with face shields, caps, gowns, and sterile gloves.	Prepares for sterile procedure.	
6. Assist as needed with site preparation (e.g., shave preparation and cleansing with antiseptic solution).	Prepares for sterile procedure.	Antiseptic solution choice should be determined by institutional policy. Use of povidone-iodine versus chlorhexidine is controversial. The antiseptic solution should be allowed to dry before the initial incision. Studies suggest chlorhexidine is neurotoxic.[8]
7. Assist as needed in draping the head, neck, and chest of the patient.	Prepares a sterile environment for the insertion process.	
8. Assist as needed with opening of the sterile trays and probes.	Facilitates efficiency of the insertion process.	
9. Turn on the Pbto₂ monitor.	Prepares the monitor.	
10. Insert the calibration card for calibration of the monitor unique to each Pbto₂ probe.	The Licox monitor requires insertion of a calibration card referred to as the smart card, which has numbers on it that match those on the oxygen probe that is being inserted. This card is placed into a card slot located on the front of the monitor. The calibration card can only be used with the probe that has the same numbers on it and is included in the same packaging (see Fig. 89-1, *A–G*).	If the calibration card is lost, another corresponding Pbto₂ probe and smart card must be used.

Procedure continues on following page

Procedure	for Brain Tissue Oxygen Monitoring for the Integra Licox CMP Monitor: Insertion (Assist) and Care—*Continued*	
Steps	**Rationale**	**Special Considerations**
11. Assist as needed with insertion of an intracranial bolt (see Procedure 92).	May be inserted before Pbto$_2$ probe insertion.	
12. Assist as needed with insertion of the oxygen probe and temperature probe.	Facilitates the insertion process.	The oxygen probe and temperature probe may be separate (triple-lumen bolt system) or may be combined (double-lumen bolt system). The additional lumen is for the ICP probe.
13. Connect the oxygen and temperature probes to the monitor cables.	Prepares for monitoring.	
14. Observe the temperature and Pbto$_2$ values.	Initiates monitoring. The temperature values should be accurate; however, time is needed for the brain tissue to settle after the microtrauma caused by catheter placement.	
15. If possible, use a cable to transfer the values from the Pbto$_2$ monitor to the bedside monitor. Set the upper and lower alarm limits.	Allows integration of the monitoring systems. The currently available brain tissue oxygen monitoring system does not have an alarm system. Integrating the monitoring system with the bedside monitor allows (1) a larger display of the numeric values and (2) audible upper and lower alarm limits.[10]	Refer to monitor guidelines for specific information.
16. After the system has been placed, apply a sterile occlusive dressing at the insertion point.	Prevents contamination of the insertion site by microorganisms and protects the site.	A dressing (formed with dry sterile gauze) provides a base to secure the device to an arm board or other securing method.

17. Secure the Pbto$_2$ monitor cables with two points of tension to avoid tension on the Pbto$_2$ and ICP probes.
  A. Anchor the cables at the patient's head and at the shoulder.
 	
  B. Secure the cables so that they do not get entangled in the side rails and do not touch the floor.
	
	The monitoring cables need to be secured so that no tension or disruption of the device occurs at the insertion site.
	Supports the entire mechanism.
		
		One method to secure the monitor cables is as follows:
		  A. Place an IV arm board or stability anchor to a conical gauze dressing where the device and cables can be secured.
		  B. Anchor the cables from the patient's head to the shoulder in place with a transparent or soft-cloth adhesive dressing. The first tension point is directly on the patient's head where the dressing is anchored to the skin at the point of insertion. The second tension point is at the patient's shoulder.
		  C. Place rolled towels under the secured system.

Procedure	for Brain Tissue Oxygen Monitoring for the Integra Licox CMP Monitor: Insertion (Assist) and Care—*Continued*		
Steps	**Rationale**		**Special Considerations**
C. Allow enough slack to accommodate patient movement and turning.	Prevents gravity drag and tension on the cables and the device.		
18. Discard used supplies in appropriate receptacles.	Removes and safely discards used supplies. Safely removes sharp objects.		
19. **HH**			
Brain Tissue Oxygenation Monitor Setup With the Bedside Monitor			
1. Connect the brain oxygen monitor to the bedside monitor with the attached cable.	Allows integration of the monitoring systems.		Refer to monitor guidelines for specific information.
2. Select a pressure module, and label the parameter. A waveform need not be displayed, only a numeric display.	Prepares the equipment.		Each bedside monitor may have its own unique labels for parameters that are being added (e.g., brain oxygen).
3. Manually adjust the temperature on the front of the monitor to the established number of degrees Celsius determined by the institution.	Prepares the equipment.		Follow institutional guidelines. If a separate brain temperature probe or combined brain tissue oxygen and brain temperature probe is not in use, the temperature on the front of the monitor must be adjusted manually every hour to equal the patient's core temperature for accurate determination of the $Pbto_2$.
4. Disconnect the blue and green cables from the brain oxygen monitor.	Prepares the equipment.		
5. Select the designated pressure module and zero the bedside monitor.	Prepares the equipment.		
6. Plug the blue and green cables back into the front of the brain oxygen monitor.	Allows integration of the monitoring systems.		
7. Note the difference between the brain oxygen monitor reading and the bedside monitor reading.	Confirms that data on the brain oxygen monitor accurately correlate with the bedside monitor.		
8. Readings should be within 1 mm Hg when the blue and green cables are connected to the Licox system at the head of the patient and after the brain tissue has had time to settle (20–120 minutes) after Licox insertion.	Confirms that data on the brain oxygen monitor accurately correlate with the bedside monitor.		Monitoring of Pbo_2 values may be delayed as long as 2 hours because time is needed for the brain tissue to settle after the microtrauma caused by probe placement.

Procedure continues on following page

Procedure	for Brain Tissue Oxygen Monitoring for the RAUMEDIC NEUROVENT-PTO Monitor: Insertion (Assist) and Care	
Procedure	**Rationale**	**Special Considerations**
1. **HH**		
2. Attach the cables to the RAUMEDIC EASY logO (fiber optic cable to Po₂ port, yellow cable P/T port, gray out ICP, blue out Po₂, red power) (Fig. 89-3).	Prepares the equipment.	
3. Plug EASY logO monitor power cord into an AC wall outlet.	Provides the power source.	
4. **HH**	Standard aseptic techniques.	
5. **PE**		
6. Assist as needed with site preparation, opening of sterile trays, draping of head and neck, etc.	Prepares for sterile procedure.	
7. Assist as needed with insertion of the RAUMEDIC bolt (see BOLT Kit PTO IFU) (Fig. 89-4).	Facilitates insertion.	Keep screwing in tool (wrench) for physician, advanced practice nurse, or other healthcare professional to remove bolt when therapy is no longer needed.
8. Assist physician, advanced practice nurse, or other healthcare professional as needed during insertion of the pressure/ temperature/oxygen catheter (see NEUROVENT-PTO catheter IFU) (Fig. 89-5).	Facilitates insertion of catheter by physician, advanced practice nurse, or other healthcare professional.	

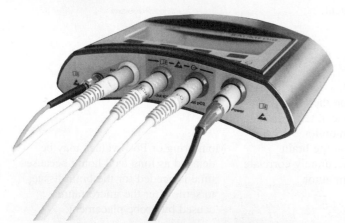

Figure 89-3   *(Courtesy Raumedic Inc., Mills River, NC.)*

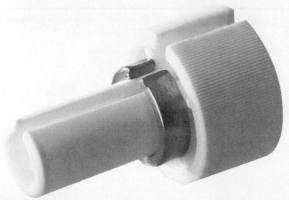

Figure 89-4   *(Courtesy Raumedic Inc., Mills River, NC.)*

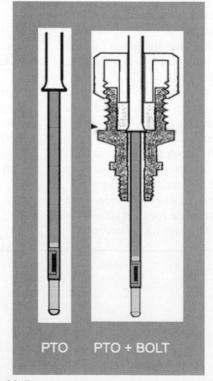

PTO   PTO + BOLT

Figure 89-5   *(Courtesy Raumedic Inc., Mills River, NC.)*

Procedure	**for Brain Tissue Oxygen Monitoring for the RAUMEDIC NEUROVENT-PTO Monitor: Insertion (Assist) and Care—*Continued***	
Procedure	**Rationale**	**Special Considerations**

9. Connect PTO catheter to monitor cables (Fig. 89-7, *A and B*).
  A. Fiber-optic connection on PTO catheter to Cable LWL (fiber optic) (Figs. 89-6 and 89-7, *A and B*).
  B. Blue plug on PTO catheter connects to Cable PTO: gold dot to gold dot (Fig. 89-8).
	Prepares for monitoring.	

10. Observe ICP, temperature, and Pbto$_2$ values.	Initiates monitoring. The temperature and ICP values should be accurate; however, a dwell time is needed (up to 2 hours) for accurate Pbto$_2$ monitoring as it is necessary for the brain tissue to settle after microtrauma caused by catheter placement.	You may document Pbto$_2$ during this time with a comment: "dwell time."
11. After the system has been placed, apply a sterile occlusive dressing at the insertion point.	Maintains sterile environment to prevent infection.	
12. Discard used supplies.		
13. 🅷🅷		
Linking to the Bedside Monitor		
1. Connect the EASY logO to the pressure ports on the bedside monitor using the gray out ICP and blue out Po$_2$ cable.	Allows integration of the monitoring systems.	

Procedure continues on following page

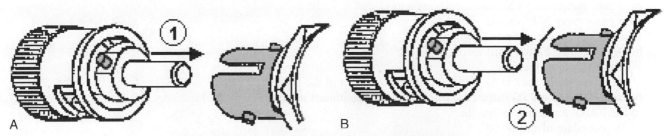

Figure 89-6 *(Courtesy Raumedic Inc., Mills River, NC.)*

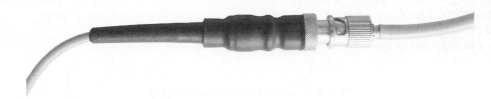

Figure 89-7 A & B *(Courtesy Raumedic Inc., Mills River, NC.)*

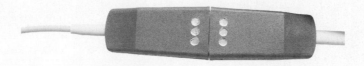

Figure 89-8 *(Courtesy Raumedic Inc., Mills River, NC.)*

Procedure	for Brain Tissue Oxygen Monitoring for the RAUMEDIC NEUROVENT-PTO Monitor: Insertion (Assist) and Care—*Continued*	
Procedure	**Rationale**	**Special Considerations**
2. Select the pressure port labels on the bedside monitor for ICP and Po_2. For Po_2, a waveform does not need to be displayed; only a value needs to be displayed. Set alarm parameter from 20 mm Hg to 40 mm Hg or as prescribed.	Prepares the equipment and establishes alarm parameters for monitoring.	
3. To have ICP and Po_2 values on the bedside monitor, select Menu.	Prepares the equipment to integrate with bedside monitoring systems.	
4. Select "OUT."	Allows integration of the monitoring systems.	
5. Once the cables have been connected to the bedside monitor, press "OK."	Allows integration of the monitoring systems.	
6. Zero the bedside monitor for both ICP and Po_2 pressure ports. When zero appears on the bedside monitor, press "OK."	Prepares the bedside monitor.	
7. Checking the sensitivity: when 20 mm Hg is displayed on the bedside monitor, press "OK."	Allows integration of the monitoring systems.	
8. It is not necessary to rezero the bedside monitor daily. It is only necessary when the EASY logO is disconnected and then reconnected to the bedside monitor.	It is only necessary to rezero after patient transport.	
Preparing RAUMEDIC NEUROVENT-PTO ICP Monitoring for Transport		
1. Disconnect the PTO catheter from the EASY logO, leaving all cables attached to the EASY logO. Attach the catheter (blue plug, gold dot to gold dot) to the transport cable that has the NPS2 (Fig. 89-9).	Oxygen is not monitored during transport.	Do not let cables drag or lay on the floor to prevent accidental removal of the catheter.
2. Plug the NPS2 into the pressure port on the transport monitor.	Provides a connection to the transport monitor.	
3. Press and continue holding the blue zero button on NPS2 and then press "zero ICP" on the transport monitor. Continue holding the blue button until zero is on the transport monitor.	Allows integration of monitoring systems.	
4. Upon return to the patient's bedside, attach the PTO catheter to the EASY logO and follow the OUT procedure of the EASY logO to get ICP and $Pbto_2$ values onto the bedside monitor.	Allows integration of the monitoring systems for continued monitoring.	

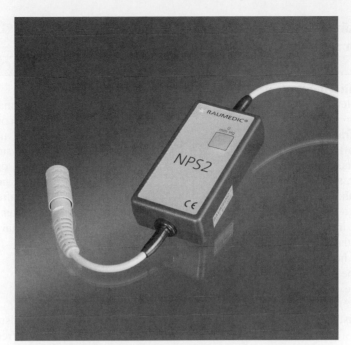

Figure 89-9   *(Courtesy Raumedic Inc., Mills River, NC.)*

Procedure	**for Brain Tissue Oxygen Monitoring for the RAUMEDIC NEUROVENT-PTO Monitor: Insertion (Assist) and Care—*Continued***

Troubleshooting RAUMEDIC NEUROVENT-PTO

Steps	Rationale	Special Considerations
Catheter Implantation Migration 1. Assess for catheter placement. Catheter pulls easily out of the bolt when implanted. The physician, advanced practice nurse, or other healthcare professional will ensure the catheter is fully inserted and tighten the fixing cap (see Fig. 89-5).	Correct catheter insertion and no dislodgement of catheter after placement.	Questionable data or data inconsistent with patient presentation suggest that the catheter may be dislodged.
Catheter Connections to Easy Logo Monitor Disconnections 1. Error: Cable PTO cable not connected to the catheter. Connect Cable PTO blue plug, gold dot to gold dot. Make sure Cable PTO is connected to the yellow socket on EASY logO.	Ensures correct cable connections and that connections are secure.	
2. Error: Cable LWL (fiber optic) not connected/locked to PTO catheter.	Ensures correct cable connection and locking the cable tightly to prevent disconnection.	Avoid forceful locking of cables because it may result in cable breakage.
3. Questionable O_2 value Clean inside Cable LWL (fiber optic) connection to remove dust.	Ensures cable is clean and has a good connection with catheter	Critically assess oxygen values with patient assessment. Evaluate clinical indications for increase/decrease in Po_2.

Procedure continues on following page

Procedure for Brain Tissue Oxygen Monitoring for the RAUMEDIC NEUROVENT-PTO Monitor: Insertion (Assist) and Care—*Continued*		
Procedure	**Rationale**	**Special Considerations**

Troubleshooting Pbo$_2$ Monitoring Systems

Procedure	**Rationale**	**Special Considerations**

1. Perform an oxygen challenge test as prescribed.[7,8]
   A. Place the ventilator fraction of inspired oxygen (Fio$_2$) setting on 100% for 2–5 minutes.
   B. Observe the monitor; an accurate probe will show an increase in Pbto$_2$.
   C. If no response to the increased Fio$_2$ is seen, inform the physician, because a head CT scan may be prescribed to confirm correct probe placement. **(Level D*)**
	After the brain tissue has had time to settle from the initial insertion, an oxygen challenge is performed, particularly if the Pbto$_2$ reading is unexpectedly low or a question of probe accuracy exists.[7,8]	Follow manufacturer guidelines for error codes that are specific to the Pbto$_2$ monitoring system.
		The physician, advanced practice nurse, or other healthcare professional may order a head CT scan after insertion to check catheter placement. Follow hospital-specific guidelines.

2. Assess if an electrical disturbance has occurred.	Strong electromagnetic disturbances can result in Pbto$_2$ measurement errors. Errors can continue for a few seconds after the disturbance.	These disturbances may occur when a high-frequency scalpel or cautery is used or during cardioversion.
3. Assess cable for damage.	If the probe cable or the extension cable is damaged, measured values can be incorrect or the measurement can be interrupted.	Replace damaged cables.
4. Avoid changes in the temperature of the temperature probe connector:	The temperature measurement may be inaccurate if the connector of the temperature probe is subjected to significant changes in temperature or if the temperature of the connector is beyond the defined range of 18° to 30°C.[10]	
A. Avoid holding the temperature probe connector.	If the probe connector is held with a warm hand, the temperature measurement may be inaccurate until it is released.	
B. Protect the temperature probe connector from direct sunlight or warming devices. **(Level M*)**	Warming of the connector can cause inaccurate temperature readings.[10]	

Removal of the Brain Tissue Oxygen Monitoring System

Procedure	**Rationale**	**Special Considerations**
1. **HH**		
2. **PE**		
3. Position the patient in a semi-Fowler's position.	Facilitates the procedure.	
4. Turn off the monitor.	Facilitates the removal process.	
5. Assist with removal of the dressing.	Prepares for removal of the catheter.	
6. Assist the physician, advanced practice nurse, or other healthcare professional as needed with removal of monitoring probes.	The physician, advanced practice nurse, or other healthcare professional will remove catheter and may request assistance.	

*Level D: Peer-reviewed professional and organizational standards with the support of clinical study recommendations.
*Level M: Manufacturer's recommendations only.

Procedure	for Brain Tissue Oxygen Monitoring for the RAUMEDIC NEUROVENT-PTO Monitor: Insertion (Assist) and Care—*Continued*	
Procedure	**Rationale**	**Special Considerations**
7. Apply an occlusive sterile dressing to the site.	Reduces the risk of infection.	Assess for signs of infection, bleeding, and cerebrospinal fluid leakage.
8. Discard used supplies in appropriate receptacles.	Removes and safely discards used supplies.	
9. **HH**		

Expected Outcomes

- Pto$_2$ probe placed in the correct position
- Monitoring is able to begin after brain tissue has had time to settle (20 minutes to 2 hours)
- Pto$_2$ value is between 20 and 35 mm Hg, or as determined by the physician to be an acceptable value for the individual patient
- Accurate and reliable Pbo$_2$ monitoring
- Early detection of cerebral hypoxia
- Immediate intervention and management of compromised cerebral oxygenation hypoxia

Unexpected Outcomes

- Brain tissue oxygen reading low, with no response to oxygen challenge
- Signs and symptoms of infection
- Hematoma from placement
- Worsened neurological assessment

Patient Monitoring and Care

Steps	Rationale	Reportable Conditions
		These conditions should be reported if they persist despite nursing interventions.
1. Assess the patient's baseline neurological status, vital signs, and ICP every 15 minutes and more frequently if necessary during and immediately after the procedure.	Provides assessment of patient status before and during the procedure.	• Changes in neurological status • Changes in vital signs • Changes in ICP and CPP
2. Perform an oxygen challenge test as prescribed. A. Place the ventilator Fio$_2$ setting on 100% for 2–5 minutes. B. An accurate probe shows an increase in Pbo$_2$.[1,6] **(Level C*)**	After the brain tissue has had time to settle from the initial insertion, perform an oxygen challenge, particularly if the Pbo$_2$ reading is unexpectedly low or a question exists of probe accuracy, reliability, or validity.	• Lack of variation response to oxygen challenge • Oxygen challenge tests confirm correct placement of the probe as well as probe functioning
3. Obtain the patient's temperature every 1–2 hours or as prescribed.	Provides a comparison of cerebral and body temperatures. Although the temperature measurements do not correlate exactly, a parallel trend should be seen.	• Abnormal temperatures
4. Maintain the Pto$_2$ value between 20 and 35 mm Hg or as prescribed.[6,8] **(Level D*)**	Represents normal values.	• Elevated Pbo$_2$ values • Decreased Pbo$_2$ values
5. Follow institutional standards for assessing pain. Administer analgesia as prescribed.	Identifies need for pain interventions.	• Continued pain despite pain interventions

*Level C: Qualitative studies, descriptive or correlational studies, integrative reviews, systematic reviews, or randomized controlled trials with inconsistent results.
*Level D: Peer-reviewed professional and organizational standards with the support of clinical study recommendations.

Procedure continues on following page

Documentation

Documentation should include the following:

- After placement of Pbo$_2$ monitor:
  - Patient and family education
  - Preprocedure verifications and time out
  - Completion of informed consent
  - Insertion of the Pbto$_2$ probe
  - Patient tolerance of the procedure
  - Site assessment

- Neurological assessments
- Hourly values, including Pbo$_2$, brain tissue temperature, and neurological multimodality monitoring in use (e.g., ICP, CPP, Sjvo$_2$).
- Occurrence of unexpected outcomes and interventions
- Pain assessment, interventions, and effectiveness

References and Additional Readings

For a complete list of references and additional readings for this procedure, scan this QR code with any freely available smartphone code reader app, or visit http://booksite.elsevier.com/9780323376624.

90 Cerebral Blood Flow Monitoring

Tracey M. Berlin

PURPOSE: Adequate cerebral blood flow (CBF) is essential for the delivery of oxygen and glucose to brain tissue and for maintenance of normal cerebral metabolic processes. CBF monitoring is performed in the patient with acute brain injury for quantitative measurement and continuous monitoring of regional brain perfusion. Monitoring of regional CBF using thermal diffusion flowmetry provides important information related to the delivery of nutrients to brain tissue, autoregulatory status, and cerebral vasoreactivity.

PREREQUISITE NURSING KNOWLEDGE

- Understanding of neuroanatomy and physiology, specifically intracranial dynamics, is needed.
- Knowledge of sterile and aseptic technique is necessary.
- Although representing only 2% of our body tissues, the central nervous system receives 15% of the total cardiac output and uses approximately 20% of the total oxygen consumed by the body.[13]
- The brain depends on a constant supply of oxygen and glucose through CBF to maintain functional and structural integrity.[15]
- If CBF falls below a certain threshold and oxygen extraction has been maximized, certain metabolic and electrical functions may be lost leading to ischemia, infarction and irreversible brain damage.[3,15]
- Used as an adjunct monitor of trends along with other neurological parameters (intracranial pressure [ICP], cerebral perfusion pressure [CPP], and brain tissue oxygen [PbtO$_2$]), CBF monitoring provides a direct measurement of regional cerebral perfusion.
- Direct monitoring of CBF could provide the opportunity to diagnose and to correct insufficient CBF before deficits in tissue oxygenation and metabolism are recognized.[15,17]
- Measurement of CBF is relevant in conditions where alterations in CBF may lead to cerebral ischemia and infarction. Indications for CBF monitoring include patients at risk for secondary brain injury, including severe traumatic brain injury, aneurysmal and traumatic subarachnoid hemorrhage, brain tumor, stroke, and any condition that potentially alters CBF.[3,7]
- Globally, average CBF in adults is considered to be around 50 to 60 mL/100 g/min.[1,13] The normal range for CBF in white matter tissue is 18 to 35 mL/100 g/min.[9] In gray, more metabolically active, cortical tissue, CBF is higher, ranging from 50 to 80 mL/100 g/min.[11] When measured in white matter, treatment goals usually aim to keep CBF between 18 and 50 mL/100 g/min.

- CBF values above 55 to 60 mL/100 g/min may indicate a state of hyperemia.[11] Hyperemia may be a physiological response as the brain attempts to perfuse injured tissue or when the delivery of blood to the brain exceeds demand. Hyperemia may result in increased ICP due to vascular congestion (Table 90-1).
- Globally, failure of electrical activity and neurological dysfunction occur when CBF falls below 18 to 20 mL/100 g/min, indicating a state of ischemia. Although CBF between 10 and 20 mL/100 g/min may be tolerated for minutes to hours before infarction, CBF of less than 10 mL/100 g/min leads rapidly to neuronal death and irreversible brain damage (see Table 90-1).[7,13,19]
- Ischemia is defined as a decrease in blood flow below the level necessary to sustain normal cellular structure and function. Ischemia can be global, as seen in severe hypoperfusion caused by cardiac arrest or intracranial hypertension. Ischemia can also be focal, as seen in occlusion of an intracranial vessel by embolism or thrombus. Focal ischemia does not necessarily lead to irreversible ischemic damage in the entire area of reduced perfusion because of collateral blood flow.[13,19]
- CBF may vary depending on metabolic demands of the brain, factors effecting delivery of blood flow, and factors effecting vasoreactivity, such as carbon dioxide and oxygen levels.[1,13]
- A change of 1 mm Hg PaCO$_2$ results in a 2% to 3% change in CBF between 20 and 80 mm Hg.[11] Hypercapnia, and the resulting decrease in extracellular pH, causes vasodilation and increased CBF, while hypocapnia leads to vasoconstriction and decreased CBF.[8]
- Regional measurements of CBF reflect a local area. Significant variation of CBF occurs in different locations within one hemisphere as well as between hemispheres.[7]
- Thermal diffusion flowmetry (TDF), based on the mathematical separation of the thermal conductive and the perfusion components of thermal diffusion in brain tissue, allows for continuous quantitative measurement of blood flow at the patient's bedside. TDF provides absolute values of CBF expressed as mL/100 g/min and has been validated by comparison with Xenon Flow CT (XeCT) (Table 90-2).[2,3,7,15,17]

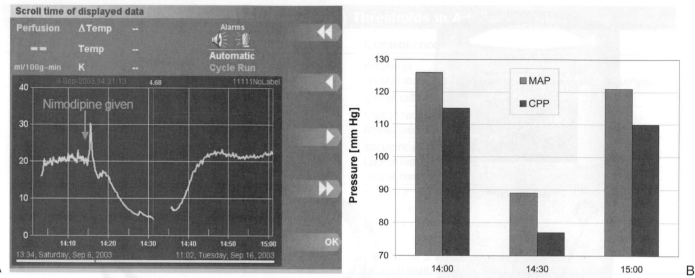

Figure 90-4   A, A screen shot from the Bowman Perfusion Monitor (BPM) showing a graphic trend of the decline and subsequent recovery of cerebral blood flow (CBF) in a patient who received a routine dose of nimodipine. This medication is frequently used as standard of care for prevention of vasospasm after aneurysmal subarachnoid hemorrhage. The sharp increase in CBF just after the time of nimodipine administration represents a motion spike when the patient was repositioned. The gap in data, occurring when CBF was at its lowest, represents a period of recalibration as the BPM verifies the drastic change in perfusion. **B,** The graph shows this patient's mean arterial pressure (MAP) and cerebral perfusion pressure (CPP) in the corresponding timeframes. The decline and recovery of CBF that mirrors the decline and recovery of MAP and CPP indicate a loss of cerebral autoregulation. This screen shot was taken in review mode where data stored on the monitor can be scrolled back and forward at any scale for review. *(Courtesy Hemedex, Inc., Cambridge, MA.)*

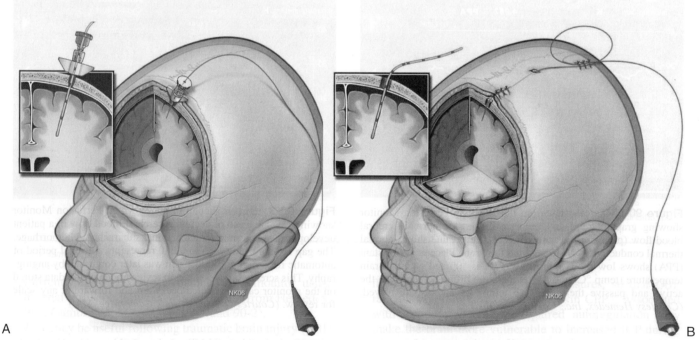

Figure 90-5   **Illustrations of placement options for the thermal diffusion probe. **A, Shows placement of the probe through a single lumen bolt. **B,** Shows tunneling of the probe. Hemedex recommends bolting. One, two, and four lumen bolts are available. *(Courtesy Hemedex, Inc., Cambridge, MA.)*

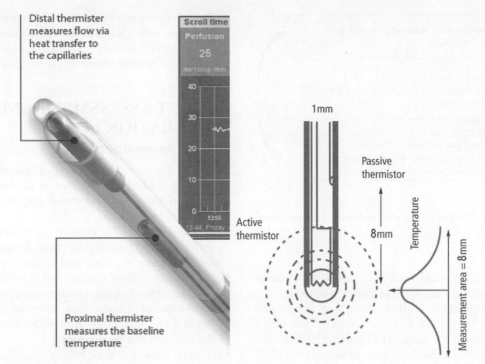

Distal thermister measures flow via heat transfer to the capillaries

Proximal thermister measures the baseline temperature

1mm

Passive thermistor

Active thermistor

8mm

Temperature

Measurement area = 8mm

Scroll time
Perfusion
25
ml/100g-min
40
30
20
10
0
13:55
13:44, Friday

Figure 90-6 Illustrations of the thermal dilution probe showing the active (distal) thermistor that heats brain tissue and measures cerebral blood flow along with the passive (proximal) thermistor that measures baseline tissue temperature.

- Placement of the probe may be ipsilateral or contralateral to the pathology. The physician placing the probe determines the catheter placement location after review of the CT scan and after consideration of the most appropriate monitoring area based on diagnosis and pathology, avoiding areas of infarct or hematoma.[4]
- Contraindications for CBF monitoring include patients with a coagulopathy, those receiving anticoagulation therapy, and those with an insertion site infection.[7]
- Accuracy of the probe is dependent on placement of the probe into white matter. The probe must be positioned in an area not affected by cardiac-induced vessel pulsatility that may introduce artifact. The monitor has a built-in pulse detector (PPA). PPA should be low (between 0 and 2.0) with a green indicator box. As pulsatility rises, values of 2.1 to 5.0 are displayed with a yellow indicator box; and values of 5.1 to 10.0 are displayed with a red indicator box along with a message that the probe should be repositioned away from the pulsating vessel by withdrawing the probe approximately 1 mm. The monitor is programmed to not provide a perfusion measurement if the PPA is red (>5).
- In white matter, tissue thermal conductivity (displayed on the monitor as the K value) is 4.8 to 5.9. If K is abnormally high above this range, it indicates that the probe is in a ventricle. If it is abnormally low, it indicates that the probe temperature sensor is dislodged outside the brain. Thermal conductivity of white matter varies with the amount of water content (edema) in the brain. The K value and PPA function as reliability indicators for the perfusion value displayed.[6]

- A thermistor at the tip of the probe heats surrounding brain tissue ≈2 to 3 °C above baseline tissue temperature (measured by a more proximal thermistor) (Fig. 90-6). The power dissipated by the heated thermistor provides a measure of the tissue's ability to carry heat by thermal conduction in the tissue and by thermal convection due to tissue blood flow.[12,16] Therefore, the greater the blood flow, the higher the thermal dissipation and the greater the power required to maintain the temperature elevation. CBF is measured and displayed on the monitor as a perfusion value of mL/100 g/min.[6,12]
- To prevent thermal injury to brain tissue, the probe tip will not heat above 41 °C. Clinically, perfusion will not be measureable if the patient's brain tissue temperature is ≥39.5 °C.
- The probe is approved for 10 days of single-patient use. The monitor stores 15 days of data. Data can also be downloaded for long-term storage and analysis.[6]
- The monitor has three phases: (1) temperature stabilization—establishes baseline tissue temperature and ensures tissue has returned to baseline since previous measurement (may take 2 to 7 minutes), (2) calibration—calculation of the K value and PPA (10 seconds), and (3) perfusion measurement for a default period of 30 minutes. All phases occur automatically when the probe and cable are connected and also during automatic recalibration periods which occur every 30 minutes (Fig. 90-7).
- Limitations to TDF monitoring include the following: loss of perfusion calculations during periodic recalibration (i.e., reassessment of tissue thermal conductivity and pulsatility), patient movement, or patient fever above 39.5 °C;

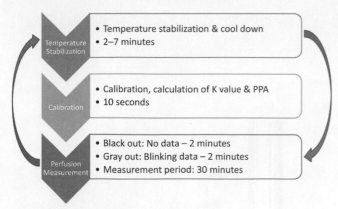

Figure 90-7   Three phases of the perfusion measurement cycle.

probe displacement; and lack of global information because of small volume of tissue being monitored.[3,9]

- Transcranial Doppler (TCD) monitoring may also be performed to measure blood flow velocities of the major vascular branches of the brain. TCD monitoring is a non-invasive ultrasound technology that penetrates the skull providing blood flow velocity measurement to assess vasospasm severity, location of intracranial stenosis, occlusions, or emboli, and monitor hemodynamic changes associated with impaired intracranial perfusion.[7,8] By measuring blood flow velocity, TCD provides an indirect measure of CBF and is best used in conjunction with other parameters for making treatment decisions.[7]

EQUIPMENT

- Cranial access kit
- Cranial bolt kit (if using to secure the probe)
- Thermal diffusion probe
- Bowman perfusion monitor (BPM) with cables
- Sterile gloves and drapes
- Masks, caps, and nonsterile gloves
- Sterile surgical pen
- Sterile dressing supplies

Additional equipment, to have available as needed, includes the following:
- Bedside table
- IV pole

PATIENT AND FAMILY EDUCATION

- Assess patient and family understanding of the purpose of cerebral perfusion monitoring. Most patients who need cerebral perfusion monitoring have an altered level of consciousness with a Glasgow Coma Score of 8 or less, so education is typically directed toward the family. *Rationale:* Understanding may reduce anxiety and stress, stimulate requests for clarification or additional information, and increase awareness of the goals, duration, and expectations of the monitoring system.

- Explain the insertion process, patient monitoring, and care involved with CBF monitoring. *Rationale:* Explanation may alleviate anxiety and stress and stimulates requests for clarification or additional information.

PATIENT ASSESSMENT AND PREPARATION

Patient Assessment

- Assess the patient's neurological status. *Rationale:* Performing a baseline neurological assessment enables the nurse to identify changes that may occur as a result of probe insertion.
- Assess the patient for signs or symptoms of local infection at the intended insertion location. *Rationale:* Evidence of local infection is a contraindication to probe insertion.
- Obtain and review coagulation laboratory results (e.g., complete blood count, platelet count, prothrombin time, partial thromboplastin time, bleeding time, and international normalized ratio). *Rationale:* Assessment identifies the patient's risk for bleeding.
- Assess patient's temperature and institute measures according to orders from the physician, advanced practice nurse, or other healthcare professional to reduce fever. *Rationale:* Thermal diffusion flowmetry technology will not provide perfusion values while the patient's baseline brain temperature exceeds 39.5 °C.

Patient Preparation

- Verify that the patient is the correct patient using two identifiers. *Rationale:* Before performing a procedure, the nurse should ensure the correct identification of the patient for the intended intervention.
- Ensure that the patient and family understand the procedure. Answer questions as they arise, and reinforce information as needed. Most patients who need CBF monitoring have an altered level of consciousness. *Rationale:* Information previously taught is evaluated and reinforced.
- Ensure that informed consent has been obtained. *Rationale:* Informed consent protects the rights of the patient and makes a competent decision possible for the patient. However, in emergency circumstances, time may not allow for the consent form to be signed.
- Perform a preprocedure verification and time out. *Rationale:* Ensures patient safety.
- Administer sedation and/or analgesia as prescribed before beginning the insertion procedure. *Rationale:* Sedation and/or analgesia facilitate the insertion process.
- Assist the patient to the semi-Fowler's position with the head in the neutral position and the head of bed elevated 30 to 45 degrees. *Rationale:* Patients who are candidates for CBF monitoring may have increased ICP. Elevating the head of the bed and placing the head in the neutral position act to decrease intracranial pressure by enhancing jugular venous outflow and provide optimal accessibility for probe insertion.

Procedure	for Cerebral Blood Flow Monitoring: Insertion (Assist), Care, Troubleshooting, and Removal		
Steps	**Rationale**	**Special Considerations**	
1. **HH**			
2. **PE**			
3. Place the perfusion monitor near the head of the bed; either on a flat surface or mounted on a sturdy pole.	Secures the monitor and allows the monitor cable to reach the patient's head.		
4. Plug the power cord into an AC wall outlet.	Provides the power source.		
5. Attach the cable (umbilical cord) to the perfusion monitor.	Prepares the equipment.	The cable connection has a twist collar for proper alignment and connection.	
6. Turn on the perfusion monitor using the toggle switch on the right front of the monitor.	Prepares the monitor.		
7. **HH**			
8. Apply masks, eye protection, caps, sterile gowns, and sterile gloves.	Prepares for sterile procedure.		
9. Assist as needed with site preparation (e.g., shave preparation, cleansing with antiseptic solution).	Prepares for sterile procedure.	Antiseptic solution choice should be determined by institutional policy. Use of povidone-iodine versus chlorhexidine is controversial. The antiseptic solution should be allowed to dry before initial incision. Studies suggest that chlorhexidine is neurotoxic.[5]	
10. Assist as needed with draping the head, neck, and chest of the patient.	Prepares a sterile environment for the insertion process.		
11. Assist as needed with opening of the sterile trays and perfusion probe.	Facilitates efficiency of the insertion process.		
12. Assist as needed with insertion of an intracranial bolt (see Procedure 92).	Bolt system must be inserted before probe.	Physician, advanced practice nurse, or other healthcare professional must use the drill bit provided in the bolt kit (not the one provided with the drill) to assure proper sized hole to accommodate the bolt. Bolt systems may have additional lumens for insertion of other monitoring probes (e.g., ICP, $PbtO_2$ etc.).	
13. Assist as needed with insertion of the perfusion probe.	Facilitates the insertion process.	Physician, advanced practice nurse, or other healthcare professional must be sure to fully incise the dura for correct placement of the probe into brain tissue. Physician, advanced practice nurse, or other healthcare professional should consult the enclosed instructions for use for information on proper depth markings to assure accurate probe placement.	
14. Connect the perfusion probe to the perfusion monitor cable.	Initiates monitoring.	Blue connectors must be completely dry. Moisture in the connectors can cause monitoring to fail.	

Procedure continues on following page

Procedure	for Cerebral Blood Flow Monitoring: Insertion (Assist), Care, Troubleshooting, and Removal—*Continued*		
Steps	**Rationale**	**Special Considerations**	

Steps	Rationale	Special Considerations
15. Observe the message bar on the perfusion monitor screen. If directed to, press the Start button (top soft blue button) to begin monitoring.	Initiates monitoring.	
16. Observe the monitor through the first full cycle of temperature stabilization, calibration, and perfusion calculation. Take note of the initial brain temperature, K value, and PPA. (**Level M***)	Assures adequacy of probe placement if K value is 4.8–5.9 and if PPA is close to zero.	Full cycle takes approximately 6 minutes. The physician should remain at the bedside, in sterile attire until the cycle is complete. This allows the opportunity for repositioning of the probe to achieve better placement if necessary.
17. Assist as needed to mark and secure the probe.	Allows visualization of insertion level and immediate detection if the probe migrates.	A sterile surgical pen should be used to mark the probe where it exits the bolt.
18. Secure the probe and cable with two points of tension: tape the probe to the bolt lumen and anchor the cable to the shoulder.	Secures the cable and probe to prevent tension at the insertion site.	
19. Assist as needed with applying a sterile dressing to the insertion site according to hospital protocol.	Protects the insertion site and prevents contamination.	
20. Secure the cable to the patient's shoulder so that it does not get entangled in the side rails and does not touch the floor.	Supports the entire system and reduces the risk of pulling on the probe.	Use provided cable clip to secure the cable to the patient's gown taking care to avoid contact with or pressure on the patient's skin.
21. Discard used supplies in appropriate receptacles.	Removes and safely discards supplies and sharp objects.	
22. 🄷🄷		
23. Ensure a CT scan is obtained as prescribed.	CT scan is recommended to assess probe placement.	CT scan also helps detect possible complications from insertion (e.g., hemorrhage).

Care of the Perfusion Monitor and Probe

Steps	Rationale	Special Considerations
1. 🄷🄷		
2. 🄿🄴		
3. Visually inspect the probe and insertion site dressing with each neurological assessment. A. Note the probe marking where it exits the bolt. B. Check the security of the probe at the insertion site. C. Assure that the cable remains taped to the patient's shoulder. D. Assess the insertion site for signs of drainage, redness, or swelling.[7]	Alerts caregiver to potential problems with the probe or insertion site.	Notify physician, advanced practice nurse, or other healthcare professional if probe has moved or if there are signs of infection at the insertion site.
4. Assess the perfusion trends on the perfusion monitor screen and correlate the trends with neurological examinations, patient activity, and treatments (e.g., medications), etc.	Allows correlation of perfusion with clinical condition/treatments and helps to individualize care.	If autoregulation is altered, treatments and medications that affect blood pressure (e.g., Nimodipine) may affect cerebral perfusion.

*Level M: Manufacturer's recommendations only.

Procedure	for Cerebral Blood Flow Monitoring: Insertion (Assist), Care, Troubleshooting, and Removal—*Continued*	
Steps	**Rationale**	**Special Considerations**
5. Note regular gaps in data representing probe recalibration.	Probe periodically assesses the tissue environment and characteristics to assure accurate data.	Default recalibration period is every 30 minutes. This can be changed using the Options soft button on the monitor and changing the Perfusion Period.
6. Patient transport: A. Disconnect the probe from the cable. B. Pause monitoring by pushing the Stop button (top blue soft button). C. Resume monitoring upon return by reconnecting the probe and cable, and pressing the same button (now labeled Start).	Pauses monitoring for patient transport.	The probe is CT compatible. The probe is *not* MRI compatible. The monitor is typically left behind for transport. However, some physicians, advanced practice nurses, and other healthcare professionals wish to monitor perfusion during surgery or other procedures, such as angiography.
Troubleshooting the Monitor		
1. **HH**		
2. **PE**		
3. If the screen is blank, check the On/Off switch and the power supply. The perfusion monitor does not have a battery and must be connected to AC outlet for power.	Assures power to the monitor.	
4. Look for paper printout of error code from front of monitor.	Perfusion monitor provides report of monitoring errors.	
5. Check status bar at the top of the monitor screen for message.	Indicates possible reasons for data disruption.	
6. Assess insertion site for security of the probe—the exit mark, tightness of compression cap, etc. Note PPA.	Provides information about possible probe movement and slippage from the bolt.	If the probe has moved, the monitor will have difficulty with temperature stabilization and may display a high PPA. Because sterility cannot be assured, the probe should not be reinserted if it has become dislodged.
7. Assess patient's brain temperature reading on the perfusion monitor screen. The probe is instructed to not operate if brain temperature is ≥39.5 °C.	Assures that active thermistor will not heat brain tissue above 41 °C.	Once brain temperature is below 39.5 °C, the perfusion probe will resume normal operation.
8. Assess patient activity. The probe is sensitive to relative probe-brain tissue motion and may not work well in a patient who is restless without a well-secured probe.	Limited patient movement reduces motion artifact by reducing relative probe-brain tissue motion.	
9. Assess whether the cable is damaged; if so, replace the cable.	If the probe cable is damaged, values can be incorrect or measurement can be interrupted.	Take care when inserting or removing the cable from the monitor—do not pull/push the cable straight in or out. The cable has a twist collar to assure secure connection to the monitor.

Procedure continues on following page

Procedure	for Cerebral Blood Flow Monitoring: Insertion (Assist), Care, Troubleshooting, and Removal—*Continued*	
Steps	Rationale	Special Considerations
Removal of the Probe		
1. **HH**		
2. **PE**		
3. Position the patient in a semi-Fowler's position.	Prepares patient for device removal.	
4. Turn off the monitor.	Facilitates device removal.	If the message bar indicates that data storage is full, notify your supervisor. The perfusion monitor stores 15 days of data. Data will need to be uploaded to the Hemedex web manager or deleted for additional data storage to occur.
5. Assist as needed with removal of the dressing, perfusion probe, and bolt system.	Facilitates device removal.	If multiple probes have been inserted into the bolt system, it is important to remove the probes before removing the bolt to prevent injury to brain tissue with the twisting action of bolt removal.
6. Assist if needed with applying an occlusive sterile dressing to the site.	Reduces risk for infection.	Assess for signs of bleeding, cerebrospinal fluid (CSF) leak, and signs and symptoms of infection.
7. Discard used supplies appropriately.	Removes and safely discards used supplies.	
8. **HH**		
9. Clean monitor, cable, and power cord according to hospital protocol. **PE**	Disinfects equipment and prepares it for use on next patient.	

Expected Outcomes

- Perfusion probe is placed in the correct position as evidenced by:
  - K value is 4.8–5.9
  - PPA box appears "green" with a pulsatility index (PI) of 0–2
  - CT scan verifies proper probe position and no evidence of hemorrhage or hematoma
- Monitoring is able to begin with first perfusion cycle
- Perfusion values are acceptable:
  - Perfusion in white matter is between 18 and 50 mL/100 g/min or as indicated by patient condition
- Detection and monitoring of low perfusion states
- Detection and monitoring of hyperemia
- Assessment of treatment effects (e.g., medications) on perfusion
- Immediate intervention and management of compromised CBF
- Ability to individualize patient care by maintaining adequate perfusion according to cerebral metabolic demand
- No adverse events (e.g., hemorrhage, infection) as a result of monitoring

Unexpected Outcomes

- Perfusion probe not placed correctly as evidenced by poor visualization on CT scan
  - K value <4.8 or >5.9
  - PPA box appears "red" with a PI of 5–10
- Perfusion values in white matter are <15 mL/100 g/min or >50 mL/100 g/min
- Failure to identify low perfusion or high perfusion conditions
- Inability to adequately perfuse the brain according to metabolic demand
- Adverse events such as hemorrhage and infection occur
- Pain

Patient Monitoring and Care

Steps	Rationale	Reportable Conditions
		These conditions should be reported if they persist despite nursing interventions.
1. Assess the patient's baseline neurological status, vital signs, and ICP every 15 minutes and more frequently if necessary during and immediately after the procedure, then hourly or according to institutional standards.	Provides assessment of patient status before, during, and after the procedure.	• Changes in neurological status • Changes in vital signs • Changes in ICP and CPP
2. Maintain perfusion values between 18 and 50 mL/100 g/min or as prescribed.	Represents normal values.	• Decreased perfusion values • Increased perfusion values • Perfusion values that change in response to patient activity or treatment (e.g., a decrease in perfusion following medication administration or adjustment of mechanical ventilator settings)
3. In states of low perfusion, assess for and treat factors that may increase demand for blood flow (pain, fever, agitation, shivering, and seizure) and/or decrease delivery of flow (cardiac issues, bradycardia, hypotension - particularly during loss of cerebral autoregulation, hypovolemia, hypocapnia, and vasoconstriction).[7,10–12] (**Level D***)	Provides assessment of factors that may reduce CBF.	• Uncontrolled pain/agitation • Fever • Shivering • Seizure • Bradycardia • Hypotension • Hypovolemia • Hypocapnia
4. In states of high perfusion, assess for and treat factors that may decrease demand for blood flow (hypothermia, sedation, paralysis, and anesthesia) and/or increase delivery of flow (hypervolemia, hypercapnia/vasodilation).[7,10–12] (**Level D**)	Provides assessment of factors that may increase CBF.	• Hypothermia • Excessive sedation • Hypervolemia • Hypercapnia

*Level D: Peer-reviewed professional and organizational standards with the support of clinical study recommendations.

Documentation

Documentation should include the following:
• Patient and family education
• Preprocedure verifications and time out
• Completion of informed consent
• Insertion of the CBF probe
• Patient tolerance of the procedure
• Insertion site assessment
• Neurological assessments

• Hourly values, including perfusion, K-value, PPA, perfusion temperature, and other hemodynamic parameters (e.g., vital signs, cardiac output [CO], cardiac index [CI], systemic vascular resistance [SVR]), and neurological parameters (e.g., ICP, CPP, $PbtO_2$, $ETCO_2$)
• Occurrence of unexpected outcomes and interventions
• Pain assessment, interventions, and effectiveness

References and Additional Readings

For a complete list of references and additional readings for this procedure, scan this QR code with any freely available smartphone code reader app, or visit http://booksite.elsevier.com/9780323376624.

91 Cerebral Microdialysis

Sandy Cecil

PURPOSE: Cerebral microdialysis is a minimally invasive technique for continuous sampling of the interstitial fluid chemistry of tissues and organs. It is a well-established brain monitoring technology in neurocritical care and can be used in specific regions of the brain to analyze brain tumor substances, neurotransmitters, or other aspects of brain tissue chemistry.[3,7] Microdialysis improves our understanding of energy metabolism in patients with traumatic brain injury or subarachnoid hemorrhage.[3,7] In these patients, microdialysis can provide an early warning sign of impending ischemia by measuring the chemical markers of metabolism and ischemia (glucose, pyruvate, and lactate) as well as markers of cell damage (glutamate and glycerol).[2,6,7]

PREREQUISITE NURSING KNOWLEDGE

- A fundamental understanding of neuroanatomy and physiology is needed.
- A basic understanding of bioenergetics of hypoxia and/or ischemia of the brain is necessary.
- A basic understanding of the ISCUSflex and its use for analyzing microdialysis samples is necessary.
- A basic understanding of catheter positioning within the brain is needed because positioning can influence the sample results.
- A basic understanding of cerebral perfusion pressure (CPP) is important. CPP provides the necessary blood flow for the metabolic needs of the injured brain and for avoiding the exacerbation of ischemic insults.
- A basic understanding of cerebral autoregulation is needed.
- The microdialysis system[3,4] is composed of the microdialysis catheter, perfusion syringe, perfusion pump, microvials, and the tissue chemistry analyzer. The catheter (surrounded by a semipermeable distal end membrane) is placed into brain tissue through a bolt or burr hole or is implanted during an open craniotomy. The catheter is attached to a microdialysis syringe filled with sterile perfusion fluid (artificial cerebrospinal fluid [CSF]). The syringe is placed in a battery-operated pump that is calibrated to pump the perfusion fluid through the catheter at a rate of 0.3 μL/min. The chemical substrates pass from brain tissue through the catheter's semipermeable membrane and are collected with the perfusion fluid in a small vial attached to the catheter (the microvial). The vial is then placed in a point of care (POC) analyzer of the chemical substrates.
- The analyzer can accommodate multiple vials, allowing testing on multiple patients at the same time.
- Normal glucose: 1.7 ± 0.9 mmol/L. The biochemical markers of metabolism and ischemia are reflected in glucose and oxygen as the main components of cell energy.[1-4,7] Glucose is broken down to pyruvate during glycolysis. When oxygen is available, pyruvate goes through the citric acid cycle (aerobic metabolism), generating high production of adenosine triphosphate (ATP). ATP is also produced (minimal amounts) in glycolysis. During ischemia, a lack of oxygen and glucose results in the conversion of pyruvate to lactate during anaerobic metabolism. Glucose is a primary source of energy to the brain and is an important marker of changes in brain metabolism. Cerebral glucose levels account for approximately two thirds of systemic glucose.
- Normal pyruvate: 166 ± 47 μm. Pyruvate and lactate reflect cell metabolism. Pyruvate decreases with inadequate glucose supply.
- Normal lactate: 2.9 ± 0.9 μm. Lactate increases with ischemia. During ischemia, a lack of oxygen and glucose results in anaerobic metabolism, reduced levels of pyruvate, and increased levels of lactate. Lactate alone is insufficient as a marker of brain ischemia.
- Normal lactate/pyruvate ratio (LPR): 23 ± 4 μm. Ischemia is defined by the combined criteria of LPR >40 and glucose <0.2 mmol/L. The LPR reflects anaerobic metabolism and increases with ischemia. The LPR is a good indicator of ischemic and hypoxic conditions as well as possible mitochondrial damage.
- Normal glycerol: 20 to 50 μm. The biochemical markers of cellular damage are reflected in glycerol and glutamate. Glycerol reflects cell injury and lysis and is a marker of cell membrane function. Levels increase when cells do not have sufficient energy to maintain homeostasis.
- Normal glutamate: 10 μm. Glutamate is an early indirect marker of cell damage and reflects cell membrane breakdown. It increases with ischemia.
- Continual assessment of patient's neurological status with continuous sampling of the interstitial fluid chemistry of the brain tissue provides focused information for markers of ischemia and cell damage.

EQUIPMENT

- Sterile gowns, sterile drapes, sterile gloves, nonsterile gloves, caps, gloves, and face masks
- Shave preparation kit
- Antiseptic solution
- The CMA 70 Brain Microdialysis Catheter or CMA 70 Microdialysis Bolt Catheter
- Cranial access tray
- Scalpel
- Dressing supplies, including 4 × 4 gauze
- Sterile dressing supplies
- The ISCUSflex
- The CMA 106 Microdialysis Pump
- Artificial CSF fluid
- Batteries (2 × 3 v)
- Microvials
- Microvial racks
- CMA pump syringe
- Perfusion fluid
- Reagents

Additional equipment, to have available as needed, includes the following:
- Bedside table

PATIENT AND FAMILY EDUCATION

- Assess patient and family understanding of complex brain injuries that require vigilant monitoring of multiple parameters in hopes of preventing secondary brain injuries. *Rationale:* This assessment may help identify patient and family educational needs.
- Explain to the patient and family that the procedure may be performed in the intensive care unit (ICU). *Rationale:* This may reduce patient and family anxiety.
- Explain the basic principles of cerebral metabolites. *Rationale:* This information may answer patient and family questions and reduce anxiety.
- Explain the insertion of the brain microdialysis catheter and the region of the brain where the catheter will be inserted (e.g., at-risk penumbra). *Rationale:* Explain that monitoring areas of the brain may give us crucial information about the biochemistry of the brain and how seriously brain cells are affected by injury to the brain.
- Explain the use of the ISCUSflex equipment. *Rationale:* Explaining how the samples from the brain are transferred to the microdialysis analyzer will allay fears and reduce anxiety regarding the equipment utilized.
- Explain to the patient and family that continual assessment of the patient's neurological status, along with continuous sampling of the interstitial fluid chemistry of the brain tissue, will be completed hourly and as needed. *Rationale:* Use of microdialysis neurointensive care is focused on tissue ischemia and cell damage and requires frequent assessment and sampling.

PATIENT ASSESSMENT AND PREPARATION

Patient Assessment

- Assess the patient's neurological status. *Rationale:* Performing a baseline neurological assessment enables the nurse to identify changes that may occur as a result of the insertion of the microdialysis catheter.
- Assess the patient for signs or symptoms of local infection at the intended insertion location. *Rationale:* Evidence of local infection is a contraindication to microdialysis catheter insertion.

Patient Preparation

- Verify that the patient is the correct patient using two identifiers. *Rationale:* Before performing a procedure, the nurse should ensure the correct identification of the patient for the intended intervention.
- Perform a preprocedure verification and time out. *Rationale:* This ensures patient safety.
- Ensure that informed consent has been obtained. *Rationale:* Informed consent protects the rights of the patient and makes a competent decision possible for the patient; however, in emergency circumstances, time may not allow for the consent form to be signed.
- Administer preprocedural analgesia or sedation as prescribed. *Rationale:* The patient needs to remain still during microdialysis catheter insertion.

Procedure	for Performing Cerebral Microdialysis	
Steps	Rationale	Special Considerations
1. **HH**		
2. **PE**	Sterile procedure in which the physician, advanced practice nurse, or other healthcare professional dons full sterile PE. The critical care nurse assisting will don a surgical hat and mask.	

Procedure | **for Performing Cerebral Microdialysis—*Continued***

Steps	Rationale	Special Considerations
3. The microdialysis catheter may be introduced through an existing intracranial bolt system or be surgically placed. If not using an intracranial bolt system, the physician will insert the microdialysis catheter into brain tissue and secure the catheter to the scalp.	Placing the catheter through an existing intracranial bolt system must be a sterile procedure if performed at the bedside. The patient may also be taken to the operating room for surgery with removal of the bone flap and placement of the catheter under visual inspection.	This is surgical procedure that is most optimally completed in an operating room. Typically a dressing is not required at the catheter insertion site.

4. If using an intracranial bolted catheter, the critical care nurse assists with the procedure.
  A. The physician will place the bolt and secure it to the skull.
  B. The physician, advanced practice nurse, or other healthcare professional will insert the catheter into the intracranial bolt or designated microdialysis port/lumen and fix the catheter at the Luer Lok connector.
	The sterile, single-use CMA 70 Microdialysis Bolt Catheter is designed for implantation in brain tissue through an intracranial access device that is fixed to the skull.
	Tightening the compression screw will help to secure the catheter.
		The intracranial catheters may be inserted in the ICU or the operating room.
		The catheter is location sensitive. Data will differ depending on the proximity of catheter to the area of injury.
		Typically a dressing is not required at the catheter insertion site.

5. Ensure that once the catheter is placed, a brain computed tomography (CT) scan is obtained as prescribed.	Determines the position of the catheter in relation to the tissue pathology.	

6. Fill and connect the syringe. Once the microdialysis catheter is implanted and the wound is closed the critical care nurse will:
  A. Fill the microdialysis syringe with 2.5 mL of artificial CSF perfusion fluid. Ensure there are no air bubbles.
  B. Connect the syringe to the catheter.
	The artificial CSF perfusion fluid (no more than 2.5 mL) primes the tubing/system.	Use only the artificial CSF provided by the manufacturer.

7. Prepare the pump:
  A. Place the syringe in the microdialysis pump tip first and piston second.
  B. Place the battery in the pump.
  C. Close the lid, which will start a flush sequence. A blinking light on the syringe pump indicates the stage in the pump sequence.
  D. Secure the pump near the patient's head.
	Prepares the system.
	The pump is a small battery-driven pump with a flow of 0.3 µL/min.
	Closing the lid starts a flush sequence that removes all air from the tubing and the catheter and initiates the microdialysis process.
	Prevents dislodgement.
		The pump is portable, small, and lightweight and is self-controlled with LED function signals.
		The battery will need to be changed after 5 days of use (or with every new patient).

Procedure continues on following page

Procedure   for Performing Cerebral Microdialysis—*Continued*

Steps	Rationale	Special Considerations
8. Place a microvial in the vial holder of the catheter: A. Discard the first vial after 30–60 minutes. B. Place a new vial in the holder to collect the first sample for analysis.	Discard the first sample because it is diluted by the flush solution. The microvial is the collection vial for the interstitial fluid.	If there is no fluid in the microvial, check the pump's flashing diodes for malfunction. Check the battery, and make sure that the pump lid is closed, there is perfusion fluid in the syringe, and the catheter tubing is not kinked. If the problem persists, open and close the lid of the pump to initiate a flush.
9. Prepare the system. Refer to the user manual of ISCUSflex Microdialysis Analyzer (CMA Microdialysis AB, 2011) for detailed instructions on: A. How to start the ISCUSflex analyzer. B. Loading rinsing fluid. C. Preparing and loading reagents and control samples. D. Registering the patient in the analyzer. E. Adding a new patient: select an empty patient position and add the patient's name. **(Level M*)**	Prepares the system for sample analysis and correct patient identification of samples analyzed.	
10. Prepare the reagents: glucose, lactate, pyruvate, glycerol, and glutamate. A. Mix the solution and powder of each reagent (respectively). B. Mix the solution and powder by first opening the vial with powder. C. Remove and discard the stopper. D. Mix the powder and liquid of each reagent together. E. Set each one aside as you mix the other four reagents. F. Load into the analyzer in the specified position per the user manual.	Prepares the equipment.	Allow up to an hour for the analyzer to calibrate the new reagents and run the controls. Follow all POC and clinical laboratory regulations. Reagents and perfusion fluid must be replaced every 5 days.
11. Analyze the microdialysis samples: A. Change the microvial every 60 minutes or as prescribed.	Results appear in about 8 minutes. Generally samples are run every hour. Samples may be run more frequently as indicated by changes in patient's condition; samples can be run every 10 minutes if necessary.	You do not need to reactivate the pump as you remove microvials.

*Level M: Manufacturer's recommendations only.

Procedure	**for Performing Cerebral Microdialysis—*Continued***	
Steps	Rationale	Special Considerations
B. Remove the microvial from the microvial holder of the catheter and insert a new microvial into the microvial holder of the catheter.	Prepares equipment.	Data are not provided continuously in real time. Clinicians must look for trends.
C. Choose the position of the vial for a specified patient position by adding a catheter name at the preferred vial position in the lower menu of the patient screen.	Prepares equipment.	You may use up to 16 different vial positions for one patient.
12. Discard used supplies.		
13. 🅷🅷		

Expected Outcomes

- Optimal placement of microdialysis catheter confirmed by CT scan; gold catheter tip is visible on CT scan[5]
- Ability to evaluate interventions[4]
- Provides information to assist in delivery of targeted therapy for prevention of secondary ischemic injury
- Identifies changes in chemistry that may develop into secondary damage before clinical signs and symptoms appear[7]
- Ability to see effects of clinical therapies (for example, tight vs. loose glycemic control) on brain metabolism[2,3]

Unexpected Outcomes

- Difficult to interpret if the microdialysis catheter ends up in normal tissue, in penumbra tissue surrounding a contusion, or in dead tissue
- Cerebral hypoglycemia due to increased consumption (hyperglycolysis) and decreased delivery due to lower cerebral blood flow (CBF) after vasospasm or intracranial hypertension
- Infection
- Metabolic crisis as indicated by an elevated lactate-pyruvate ratio (LPR), reduced glucose, and/or the presence of glutamate or glycerol indicating ischemia and cell death

Patient Monitoring and Care

Steps	Rationale	Reportable Conditions
		These conditions should be reported if they persist despite nursing interventions.
1. Assess the patient's neurological status every hour or more frequently if neurological changes are noted.	Provides continual neurological assessment and the ability to note changes.	• Change in level of consciousness (LOC), intracranial pressure (ICP), CPP, pupil response, response to stimuli, blood pressure, and heart rate that suggest compromise in neurological function
2. Monitor the cerebral microdialysis trends (results have [at minimum] a 1-hour lag time).	Provides trending data and allows assessment of changes that may result from procedures, medication adjustments, mobility, and patient care needs. Evaluates changes in CPP, blood glucose levels, and oxygen saturation against changes in tissue chemistry.	• Changes to LPR after medication changes or mobility • Abnormal trends in LPR • Neurological changes such as change in LOC, ICP, CPP, pupil response, response to stimuli, blood pressure, and heart rate that suggest compromise in neurological function • Alert the physician if the chemical condition of the tissue changes, especially when levels and trends are out of normal range

Procedure continues on following page

Patient Monitoring and Care —*Continued*

Steps	Rationale	Reportable Conditions
3. Assess the catheter site every 4 hours or more often if indicated.[1,3] **(Level D*)**	Provides an opportunity to assess the placement of the catheter and for signs and symptoms of infection.	• Redness or swelling at catheter site • Leakage around microdialysis catheter • Catheter dislodgement

*Level D: Peer-reviewed professional and organizational standards with the support of clinical study recommendations.

Documentation

Documentation should include the following:

- Initial documentation (date and time) of catheter insertion, reagent activation, loading of syringe pump, loading of batteries in pump, and registration of patient data into analyzer
- Ensure informed consent was obtained
- Document glucose, lactate, pyruvate, glycerol, and glutamate levels in medical record every hour or as prescribed by the physician
- Patient and family education
- Insertion site assessment
- Hourly vital signs, laboratory values, hemodynamic monitoring
- Assessment of pain and response to pain medication
- Sedation levels
- Neurological assessments
- Patient tolerance of procedure

References and Additional Readings

For a complete list of references and additional readings for this procedure, scan this QR code with any freely available smartphone code reader app, or visit http://booksite.elsevier.com/9780323376624.

92

Intracranial Bolt and Fiberoptic Catheter Insertion (Assist), Intracranial Pressure Monitoring, Care, Troubleshooting, and Removal

Tess Slazinski

PURPOSE: The fiberoptic catheter is a device utilized for continuous measurement of intracranial pressure (ICP). The fiberoptic catheter is placed in the brain parenchyma and reflects pressure exerted by the intracranial contents, brain tissue, blood, and cerebrospinal fluid (CSF) within the skull. The fiberoptic catheter is inserted through a bolt. Unlike a ventricular catheter, which is attached to an external transducer and drainage system, the fiberoptic catheter does not allow for CSF drainage.

PREREQUISITE NURSING KNOWLEDGE

- A fundamental understanding of neuroanatomy and physiology is needed.
- Knowledge of aseptic and sterile technique is necessary.
- Proper equipment assembly and setup specific to the fiberoptic ICP monitoring device must be understood.
- ICP is the pressure exerted by the intracranial contents, brain tissue, blood, and CSF. Increased ICP occurs when the intracranial volume exceeds the brain's ability to compensate for increased volume.[15]
- Normal ICP ranges from 0 to 15 mm Hg; sustained ICPs of greater than 20 mm Hg are generally considered neurological emergencies.[5,6,12]
- ICP is measured via a catheter inserted into the brain parenchyma. The catheter is inserted through an intracranial bolt (Fig. 92-1).
- The normal ICP waveform has three or four peaks with P_1 of greater amplitude than P_2 and P_3. P_1 is thought to reflect arterial pressure; P_2, P_3, and P_4 (when present) have been described as choroid plexus or venous in origin (Fig 92-2).[15] The amplitude of P_2 may exceed P_1 with increased ICP or decreased intracranial compliance (Fig. 92-3).
- ICP waveform trends include a, b, and c waves. The a waves, also referred to as plateau waves, are associated with ICP values of 50 to 100 mm Hg and last 5 to 20 minutes. The a waves (Fig. 92-4) are associated with abrupt neurological deterioration and herniation. The b waves (Fig. 92-5), with ICP values of 20 to 50 mm Hg and lasting 30 seconds to 2 minutes, may become a waves. The c waves (Fig. 92-6) may coincide with ICPs as high as 20 mm Hg but are short lasting and without clinical significance.[1-3,7]

- Cerebral perfusion pressure (CPP) is the pressure at which the brain is perfused. CPP is calculated by subtracting the ICP from the mean arterial pressure. Normal CPP is thought to be approximately 80 mm Hg.[13] In severe traumatic brain injury, the CPP for adults should range between 50 and 70 mm Hg.[4] Patients with other neurological injuries may require individualized CPP parameters reflective of the neuropathology and brain perfusion needs. Research continues regarding the relationship between cerebral blood flow and CPP.
- ICP and CPP must be considered together in management of the patient. Cerebral autoregulation is the intrinsic ability of the cerebral vessels to constrict and dilate as needed to maintain adequate cerebral perfusion. Cerebral autoregulation is impaired with brain injury and the cerebral blood flow becomes passively dependent on the systemic blood pressure. The cerebral blood vessels are no longer able to react to maintain CPP in response to a change in blood pressure.[5,8]
- Sustained ICP elevations of 20 mm Hg or greater necessitate immediate reporting and intervention. ICP waveform changes that indicate loss of cerebral compliance or cerebral autoregulation should be reported immediately.[5,10,12,15]
- ICP monitoring is indicated for the following:
  - ❖ Traumatic brain injury with a Glasgow Coma Scale score of less than or equal to 8 and abnormal computed tomography (CT) scan results or normal CT scan results with two of the following: hypotension, greater than 40 years of age, and motor posturing[4]

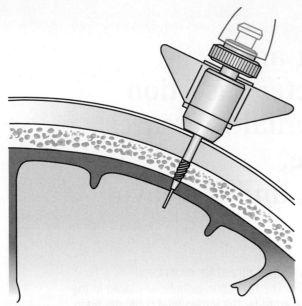

Figure 92-1 Intracranial bolt inserted into the parenchyma. *(From Littlejohns L, Bader MK:* AACN-AANN protocols for practice: Monitoring technologies in critically ill neuroscience patients. *Sudbury, MA, 2009, Jones and Bartlett, p. 35.)*

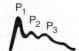

Figure 92-2 Components of the intracranial pressure waveform: P_1, P_2, and P3.

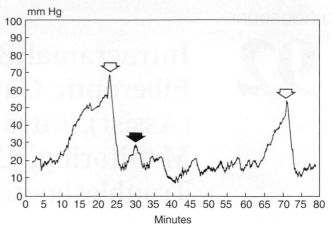

Figure 92-4 *a* or plateau waves. *Open arrows* indicate plateau elevations in intracranial pressure. Note that when intracranial pressure falls, it does not return to baseline preceding the first wave (*closed arrow*). *(From Marshall SB, et al:* Neuroscience critical care: Pathophysiology and patient management. *Philadelphia, 1990, Saunders.)*

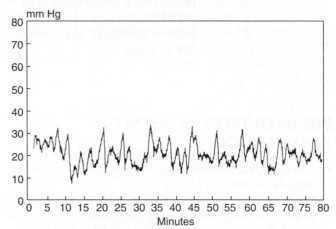

Figure 92-5 Elevations in intracranial pressure represent *b* waves. The intracranial pressure rise is steep and rapid but to heights less than those observed with *a* waves and is also much briefer. *(From Marshall SB, et al:* Neuroscience critical care: Pathophysiology and patient management. *Philadelphia, 1990, Saunders.)*

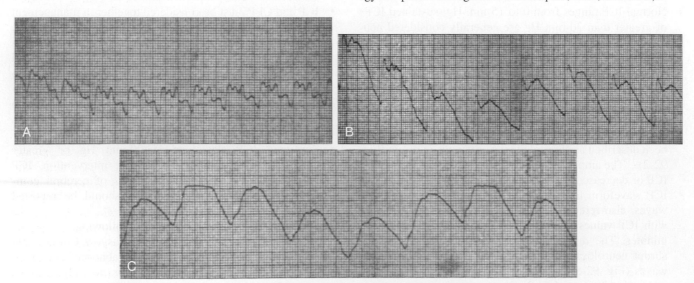

Figure 92-3 Example of intracranial pressure waveforms with P_2 elevation indicating decreased cerebral compliance.

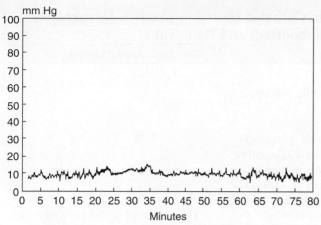

Figure 92-6 *c* waves. The intracranial pressure changes are much less impressive than those in *a* or *b* waves and reflect changes in arterial blood pressure. *(From Marshall SB, et al: Neuroscience critical care: Pathophysiology and patient management. Philadelphia, 1990, Saunders.)*

- ❖ Intracranial hemorrhage[15]
- ❖ Subarachnoid hemorrhage[15]
- ❖ Hydrocephalus[15]
- ❖ Fulminant hepatic failure with encephalopathy[15]
- ❖ Ischemic stroke with massive edema[15]
- ❖ Meningitis[15]
- ❖ Cysts[15]
- Contraindications for inserting ICP monitoring devices include infection and coagulopathies.[17]
- Concerns with accuracy of ICP monitoring values primarily relate to displacement, misplacement, or breakage of the catheter and drift (especially after 5 days).[13,15]
- Management of the patient with increased ICP and decreased CPP is a multitiered approach that includes positioning, maintaining normothermia and normocarbia, administration of pharmacological agents, and surgical procedures.[2,8,11]

EQUIPMENT

- Antiseptic solution
- Sterile gloves, surgical caps, masks, goggles or face shields, and sterile surgical gowns
- Sterile towels, half-sheets, and drapes
- Local anesthetic (lidocaine 1% or 2% without epinephrine), 5-mL or 10-mL Luer-Lok syringe with 18-gauge needle (for drawing up lidocaine), and 23-gauge or 25-gauge needle (for administration of lidocaine)
- Shave preparation kit
- Cranial access tray
  - ❖ Scalpel
  - ❖ Scalpel retractor
  - ❖ Forceps
  - ❖ Needles/needle holders
- Monitoring equipment
  - ❖ Pressure box (bedside monitor)
  - ❖ Pressure cable
  - ❖ Stand-alone monitor (for interpretation of fiberoptic data)
  - ❖ Preamp fiberoptic catheter connector cable
  - ❖ Monitoring cable to connect to bedside monitor
- Sterile dressing supplies

PATIENT AND FAMILY EDUCATION

- Assess patient and family understanding of fiberoptic catheters and management of elevated ICP. *Rationale:* Explanations to patient and family concerning their specific needs may allay fears.
- Explain the fiberoptic catheter–insertion procedure. Review normal parameters and patient care after insertion. Review the family's role in maintenance of an optimal ICP with limitation of patient stimulation. *Rationale:* Explanation of expected interventions may allay patient and family anxieties, encourage questions, and promote therapeutic family interaction.

PATIENT ASSESSMENT AND PREPARATION
Patient Assessment

- Assess the patient's neurological status and vital signs. *Rationale:* Performing a baseline neurological assessment enables the nurse to identify changes that may occur during or as a result of the fiberoptic catheter placement.
- Assess the patient's current laboratory profile, including complete blood count or platelet count, prothrombin time, international normalized ratio, and partial thromboplastin time. *Rationale:* Baseline coagulation study results determine the risk for bleeding during intracranial bolt and catheter insertion.
- Assess for allergies. *Rationale:* Assessment minimizes the risk of allergic reaction.

Patient Preparation

- Verify that the patient is the correct patient using two identifiers. *Rationale:* Before performing a procedure, the nurse should ensure the correct identification of the patient for the intended intervention.
- Perform a preprocedure verification and time out, if nonemergent. *Rationale:* Ensures patient safety.
- Ensure that informed consent has been obtained. *Rationale:* Informed consent protects the rights of the patient and makes a competent decision possible for the patient; however, in emergency circumstances, time may not allow for the consent form to be signed.
- Administer preprocedural analgesia or sedation as prescribed. *Rationale:* The patient needs to remain still during fiberoptic catheter insertion. In an emergency situation, the patient may already be receiving continuous analgesia and sedation.
- Assist the patient to a supine position with the head of the bed at 30 to 45 degrees and the neck in a midline, neutral position. *Rationale:* This position provides access for fiberoptic catheter insertion and enhances jugular venous outflow, contributing to possible reduction in intracranial pressure.

Procedure	**for Intracranial Bolt and Fiberoptic Catheter Insertion (Assist), Intracranial Pressure Monitoring, Care, Troubleshooting, and Removal**	
Steps	**Rationale**	**Special Considerations**
1. **HH**		
2. Apply goggles or masks with face shields, caps, gowns, and sterile gloves.	Prepares for sterile procedure.	
3. Assist as needed with identifying the optimal area for placement of the catheter.	Facilitates catheter placement. Catheters placed adjacent to the intracranial pathology are more likely to identify increased ICP earlier.[15,18,19,21]	
4. Assist as needed with shaving and cleansing the insertion site with an antiseptic solution.	Reduces transmission of microorganisms and minimizes the risk of infection.	The choice of povidone-iodine or chlorhexidine as an antiseptic agent is an unresolved issue.[16] Both should be allowed to dry completely.
5. Assist as needed with covering the patient's head and upper thorax with a sterile half-sheet and drape.	Protects the insertion site from contamination.	
6. Preparation of the fiberoptic system: A. Ensure that the preamp cable connects from the catheter to the stand-alone monitor. B. Follow manufacturer's instructions for zeroing the catheter before insertion. (**Level M***)	The catheter is zeroed before insertion and never rezeroed.[15]	
7. Assist as needed with insertion of the intracranial bolt and fiberoptic catheter.	Facilitates the insertion process.	Manually assisting in maintaining head positioning may be required during cranial drilling while maintaining the sterile field.
8. Assist as needed with applying a sterile occlusive dressing.	Reduces the transmission of microorganisms.	
9. Secure the catheter and preamp cable to the patient in such a way as to prevent accidental removal.	Lessens the likelihood of dislodgment and breakage of the catheter.	
10. After fiberoptic catheter placement, follow the manufacturer's instructions for the "synchronize to monitor" interface. (**Level M**)	Ensures accurate fiberoptic data at the bedside monitor and allows printing of ICP tracing.	
11. Set the appropriate ICP scale for the measured pressure.	Necessary for visualization of the complete ICP waveform and to obtain readings.	
12. Set the monitor alarms.	Goals for ICP management are individualized for each patient based on pathology.	
13. Discard used supplies in an appropriate receptacle.	Removes and safely discards used supplies; safely removes sharp objects.	
14. **HH**		

*Level M: Manufacturer's recommendations only.

Procedure	for Intracranial Bolt and Fiberoptic Catheter Insertion (Assist), Intracranial Pressure Monitoring, Care, Troubleshooting, and Removal—*Continued*	
Steps	**Rationale**	**Special Considerations**

Troubleshooting

1. HH
2. PE
3. Assess the integrity of the fiberoptic device. Note the location and presence of any markers on the fiberoptic catheter system that identify location (depth of the catheter). | Occlusion or dislocation may require manipulation or replacement. | Intracranial device manipulation is not a nursing responsibility in most institutions. Notify the physician if the device is occluded or dislocated.

4. Observe for messages or numeric values that indicate a broken catheter. | Breakage requires replacement. |

5. Correct the ICP monitoring device malfunction. | Fiberoptic catheters may become damaged or dislodged, requiring catheter replacement. | Follow manufacturer's instructions and troubleshooting manuals for identifying and correcting common problems.

6. Change the monitoring system, if needed. | Replaces a malfunctioning system. |

7. Discard used supplies.

8. HH

Fiberoptic Catheter Removal

1. HH
2. Ensure physicians, advanced practice nurses, and other healthcare professionals who are assisting with catheter removal apply sterile gloves and mask with face shield or goggles. | Minimizes the risk of infection; maintains aseptic and sterile precautions. |

3. Assist with the removal of the fiberoptic catheter. | Facilitates the removal process. |

4. Assist as needed with applying a sterile occlusive dressing. | Minimizes contamination by microorganisms. | Observe for any CSF drainage or blood from insertion site.

5. Discard used supplies in an appropriate receptacle. | Removes and safely discards used supplies. |

6. HH

Expected Outcomes

- Accurate and reliable ICP monitoring, CPP calculation, and assessment of cerebral compliance[9,12]
- Maintenance of ICP within the range of 0 to 15 mm Hg or as prescribed[9,12,15]
- Early detection of elevated ICP trends[9,12,15]
- Management of increased ICP and decreased CPP[9,12,15]
- Protection of cerebral perfusion with maintenance of CPP within prescribed parameters[9,12]

Unexpected Outcomes

- CSF infection[14,16,17]
- CSF leakage[15]
- Dislodgment or damage of the fiberoptic catheter[15]
- Dislodgment of the bolt[15]
- Pneumocephalus (rare)[15]
- Cerebral hemorrhage (rare)[4,15]
- Sequelae of sustained increased intracranial pressure and decreased cerebral perfusion pressure: cerebral infarction, herniation, and brain death[8,9,13]

Patient Monitoring and Care

Steps	Rationale	Reportable Conditions
		These conditions should be reported if they persist despite nursing interventions.
1. Assess the patient's neurological status and vital signs during the procedure.	Evaluates the patient's response to the procedure.	• Changes in neurological status • Abnormal vital signs

Procedure continues on following page

Patient Monitoring and Care —*Continued*

Steps	Rationale	Reportable Conditions
2. Note the ICP waveform and numeric values during the insertion procedure.	Provides baseline data.	• P_2 of greater amplitude than P_1
3. Assess the patient's neurological status hourly or more often as indicated.[15]	Provides clinical confirmation of and correlation with the monitored ICP data.	• Changes in neurological status
4. Assess the ICP hourly.	Determines the neurological status.	• Increased ICP • ICP waveform abnormalities • Immediately report sustained ICP elevations of 20 mm Hg or greater[15]
5. Calculate the CPP hourly (or more often as indicated).	A CPP of 50–70 mm Hg should be maintained for adult patients with traumatic brain injury. CPP parameters should be individualized to meet patient perfusion needs.	• Changes in CPP • CPP less than the lowest prescribed parameter may put the patient at risk for cerebral ischemia.[4,6]
6. Set the bedside alarm limits based on the parameter goals.	The ICP limit is usually set to sound an alarm when the ICP is >20 mm Hg; however, this needs to be individualized for each patient.	• Abnormal ICP • Abnormal waveforms
7. Assess the catheter system hourly.	Ensures accuracy and safety of monitoring.	
8. Change the insertion site dressing as needed or based on institutional standards.	Provides an opportunity to assess catheter insertion site and observe for signs and symptoms of infection.[16]	• Significant drainage on ICP insertion site dressing or head dressing • Signs and symptoms of infection
9. Provide a safe environment, preventing inadvertent dislodgment of the fiberoptic catheter through appropriate catheter positioning, sedation, and analgesia as needed and as prescribed.	Catheter dislodgment results in the inability to effectively monitor ICP and may require reinsertion. If intrahospital transportation is required, ICP should be monitored.[20]	• Dislodged device • Abnormal ICP • Abnormal ICP waveform • Increased ICP may occur when patient is lying flat for diagnostic study
10. Follow institutional standard for assessing pain. Administer analgesia as prescribed.	Identifies need for pain interventions.	• Continued pain despite pain interventions

Documentation

Documentation should include the following:
- Insertion time and patient response to procedure
- Completion of informed consent
- Preprocedure verifications and time out
- Procedural and sedation monitoring
- Initial and hourly ICP[1,12,15]
- Initial and hourly CPP calculation[1,12,15]
- Insertion site assessment
- Patient and family education
- Initial ICP tracing (include ICP waveform morphology) and any changes in the waveform[12,15]
- Nursing interventions used to treat ICP or CPP deviations and expected or unexpected outcomes[12,15]
- Pain assessment, interventions, and effectiveness

References and Additional Readings

For a complete list of references and additional readings for this procedure, scan this QR code with any freely available smartphone code reader app, or visit http://booksite.elsevier.com/9780323376624.

93 Intraventricular/Fiberoptic Catheter Insertion (Assist), Monitoring, Nursing Care, Troubleshooting, and Removal

Tess Slazinski

PURPOSE: The combination intraventricular/fiberoptic catheter combines the capability of external ventricular drainage of cerebrospinal fluid with monitoring of intracranial pressure. This hybrid device can be used to monitor intracranial pressure intermittently or continuously and to drain cerebrospinal fluid intermittently or continuously.

PREREQUISITE NURSING KNOWLEDGE

- A fundamental understanding of neuroanatomy and physiology is needed.
- Knowledge of aseptic and sterile technique is necessary.
- Proper equipment assembly and setup specific to fiberoptic intracranial pressure monitoring device should be understood.
- Intracranial pressure (ICP) is the pressure exerted by the intracranial contents, brain tissue, blood, and cerebrospinal fluid (CSF) within the cranium. Increased ICP occurs when the intracranial volume exceeds the brain's ability to compensate for increased volume.[16,18] Increased ICP contributes to secondary neuronal injury.
- The ventricular catheter with external strain gauge transducer is considered the gold standard for ICP monitoring.[3,4] The external ventricular drain is considered the most accurate and reliable method of monitoring ICP and ICP waveform and allows for CSF drainage.[3] However, the fluid-filled system of the external ventricular catheter has the greatest infection rate[1,2,12] and hemorrhage rate, and requires repeated zeroing and leveling with the anatomical reference point for the foramen of Monro.[3]
- The parenchymal fiberoptic catheter provides quality ICP monitoring but cannot be rezeroed once inserted, cannot be used for CSF drainage, and is subject to drift, particularly after 5 days.[3]
- The combination catheter has some of the advantages and disadvantages of both the ventricular catheter with an external strain gauge transducer and the fiberoptic transducer tipped catheter. The combination catheter can only be zeroed before insertion. However, because the transducer is in the tip of the fiberoptic catheter, there is no external strain gauge transducer and therefore no repetitive zeroing and leveling of a transducer with the anatomi-

cal reference point for the foramen of Monro. In addition, the combination catheter allows for CSF drainage but still requires attention to the level of the reference point of the drip chamber to the anatomical reference point for the foramen of Monro and setting of the pressure level at the top of the graduated burette (drip chamber) to prevent underdrainage or overdrainage of CSF.[1]

- The anatomical reference point for the foramen of Monro is the external auditory canal.[1,11]
- Normal ICP ranges from 0 to 15 mm Hg; sustained ICPs of greater than 20 mm Hg are generally considered neurological emergencies.[6,17]
- The normal ICP waveform has three or four peaks, with P_1 being of greater amplitude than P_2, and P_2 of greater amplitude than P_3. P_1 is thought to reflect arterial pressure; P_2, P_3, and P_4 (if present) have been described as choroid plexus or venous in origin (see Fig. 92-2).[18] The amplitude of P_2 may exceed P_1 with increased ICP or decreased intracranial compliance (see Fig. 92-3).
- ICP waveform trends include *a*, *b*, and *c* waves. The *a* waves, also referred to as plateau waves, are associated with ICP values of 50 to 100 mm Hg and last 5 to 20 minutes. The *a* waves (see Fig. 92-4) are associated with abrupt neurological deterioration and herniation. The *b* waves (see Fig. 92-5) with ICP values of 20 to 50 mm Hg, lasting 30 seconds to 2 minutes, may become *a* waves. The *c* waves (see Fig. 92-6) may coincide with ICPs as high as 20 mm Hg but are short lasting and without clinical significance.[3,7,9,18]
- Cerebral perfusion pressure (CPP) is a derived mathematic calculation that indirectly reflects the adequacy of cerebral blood flow. The CPP is calculated by subtracting the ICP from the mean arterial pressure (MAP); thus CPP = MAP − ICP. The normal CPP range for adults is approximately 60 to 100 mm Hg, or a mean of 80 mm Hg. The optimal CPP for a given patient and clinical condition is

not entirely known. ICP and CPP should be managed concomitantly. According to the Brain Trauma Foundation Guides, an acceptable CPP for an adult with a severe traumatic brain injury (Glasgow Coma Scale [GCS] score ≥8) lies between 50 and 70 mm Hg.[4] Patients with aneurysmal subarachnoid hemorrhage vasospasm may need higher CPPs to maintain adequate perfusion through vasospastic cerebral blood vessels. Patients with strokes, aneurysmal subarachnoid hemorrhage, or other neurological injuries may require higher or individualized CPP parameters reflective of the neuropathology and brain perfusion needs. Research continues regarding the relationship between cerebral blood flow and CPP.

- ICP and CPP must be considered together in management of the patient.
- Cerebral autoregulation is the intrinsic ability of the cerebral vessels to constrict and dilate as needed to maintain adequate cerebral perfusion. Cerebral autoregulation is impaired with brain injury, and the cerebral blood flow becomes passively dependent on the systemic blood flow. The cerebral blood vessels are no longer able to react to maintain CPP in response to a change in blood pressure.
- Sustained ICP elevations of 20 mm Hg or greater necessitate immediate reporting and intervention. ICP waveform changes that indicate loss of cerebral compliance or cerebral autoregulation should be reported immediately.[11,16]
- ICP monitoring is indicated for the following[4,18]:
  ❖ Traumatic brain injury with a GCS score less than 8 and abnormal computed tomographic (CT) scan or normal CT scan with two of the following: hypotension, age more than 40 years, and posturing
  ❖ Intracranial hemorrhage
  ❖ Aneurysmal subarachnoid hemorrhage
  ❖ Hydrocephalus
  ❖ Fulminant hepatic failure with encephalopathy
  ❖ Ischemic stroke with massive edema
  ❖ Meningitis
  ❖ Cysts
- CSF drainage is indicated for the following[1]:
  ❖ Acute hydrocephalus
  ❖ Subarachnoid hemorrhage
  ❖ Intracerebral hemorrhage
  ❖ Traumatic brain injury
  ❖ Postoperative craniotomy
  ❖ Meningitis
- Consequences of CSF underdrainage include headache, neurological deterioration, hydrocephalus, increased intracranial pressure, secondary neuronal injury, herniation, and death.
- Consequences of CSF overdrainage include headache, subdural hematoma, pneumocephalus, ventricular collapse, herniation, and death.
- A contraindication for ICP monitoring is coagulopathies.
- Issues regarding accuracy primarily relate to displacement, misplacement, or breakage of the fiberoptic catheter and drift (especially after 5 days).[3,16]
- Management of the patient with increased ICP and decreased CPP is a multitiered approach that includes

nursing interventions (e.g., positioning, maintaining normothermia) and the administration of pharmacological agents and surgical procedures.[4,9,16]
- If intrahospital transportation of the patient is required, ICP should be continuously monitored during transport.[22]

EQUIPMENT

- Antiseptic solution
- Sterile gloves, surgical caps, masks, goggles or face shields, and sterile surgical gowns
- Sterile towels, half-sheets, and drapes
- Local anesthetic (lidocaine 1% or 2% without epinephrine), 5- or 10-mL Luer-Lok syringe with 18-gauge needle (for drawing up of lidocaine), and 23- or 25-gauge needle (for administration of lidocaine)
- Shave preparation kit
- Cranial access tray
  ❖ Scalpel
  ❖ Scalp retractor
  ❖ Forceps
  ❖ Needles/needle holders
  ❖ Intraventricular/fiberoptic catheter
  ❖ Calibration screwdriver (single use)
- Monitoring equipment
  ❖ Pressure module (bedside monitor)
  ❖ Pressure cable
  ❖ Stand-alone monitor (for interpretation of fiberoptic data)
  ❖ Preamp connector cable
  ❖ Monitoring cable to connect to bedside monitor
- External ventricular drainage system
- Sterile dressing supplies

PATIENT AND FAMILY EDUCATION

- Assess patient and family understanding of the purpose of the intraventricular and fiberoptic catheter and management of elevated ICP. *Rationale:* Explaining the purpose of the procedure may decrease patient and family anxiety.
- Explain the intraventricular and fiberoptic catheter insertion procedure. Review normal parameters and patient care after insertion. Review the family's role in maintenance of an optimal ICP with limitation of patient stimulation. *Rationale:* Explanation of expected interventions may allay patient and family anxieties, encourage questions, and promote therapeutic family interaction.

PATIENT ASSESSMENT AND PREPARATION

Patient Assessment

- Assess the patient's neurological status. *Rationale:* A baseline neurological assessment enables the nurse to identify changes that may occur during or as a result of the intraventricular/fiberoptic catheter placement.
- Assess the patient's current laboratory profile, including complete blood count, platelet count, prothrombin time, international normalized ratio, and partial thromboplastin

time. **Rationale:** Baseline coagulation studies determine the risk for bleeding during intraventricular catheter insertion.

- Assess for allergies. **Rationale:** Insertion of the intraventricular fiberoptic catheter may necessitate local anesthetic, an antiseptic to clean the site, and analgesia and sedation. Assessment minimizes the risk of allergic reaction.

Patient Preparation

- Verify that the patient is the correct patient using two identifiers. **Rationale:** Before performing a procedure, the nurse should ensure the correct identification of the patient for the intended intervention.
- Ensure that informed consent has been obtained. **Rationale:** Informed consent protects the rights of the patient

and makes a competent decision possible for the patient; however, in emergency circumstances, time may not allow for the consent form to be signed.

- Perform a preprocedure verification and timeout, if nonemergent. **Rationale:** Ensures patient safety.
- Administer preprocedural analgesia or sedation as prescribed. **Rationale:** The patient needs to remain still during catheter insertion. In an emergency situation, the patient may already be receiving continuous analgesia and sedation.
- Assist the patient to a supine position with the head of the bed at 30 to 45 degrees and the neck in a midline, neutral position. **Rationale:** This position provides access for intraventricular/fiberoptic catheter insertion and enhances jugular venous outflow, contributing to possible reduction in intracranial pressure.

Procedure	for Combination Intraventricular/Fiberoptic Catheter Insertion (Assist), Monitoring, Nursing Care, Troubleshooting, and Removal	
Steps	**Rationale**	**Special Considerations**
1. [HH]		
2. Attach the external drainage system to an intravenous (IV) pole.	Preparation of the external ventricular drainage system allows for stability when priming the tubing.	External ventricular drainage systems are either pole-mount or panel systems. Both systems require attachment to an IV pole for stability.
3. Ensure that all pressure tubing connections on the ventricular drainage system are tightened.	Ensures integrity and sterility of the closed system.	
4. Prime the external ventricular drainage system before patient attachment. Use preservative-free normal saline solution to prevent neuronal damage[8] (see Figs. 94-1 and 94-2).	Air needs to be removed from the pressure tubing.	This system does *not* require an external strain gauge flushless transducer because the fiberoptic portion of this catheter is measuring ICP. Use of a syringe filled with sterile, preservative-free normal saline solution to prime the external ventricular drainage system tubing rather than a bag of flush solution lessens the risk of flush solution being administered through the ventricular catheter into the brain.[13]
5. Apply goggles or masks with face shields, caps, gowns, and sterile gloves.	Ensures aseptic and sterile technique.	
6. Assist as needed with identifying the optimal area for placement of the catheter.	Facilitates catheter placement.	A ventricular catheter is most commonly placed in the nondominant, anterior horn portion of the lateral ventricle.[2]
7. Assist as needed with clipping the hair[12] and cleansing the insertion site with an antiseptic solution.	Reduces the microorganisms and minimizes the risk of infection.	The choice of povidone iodine or chlorhexidine as an antiseptic agent is an unresolved issue.[19] Both should be allowed to dry completely. In addition, the use of prophylactic antibiotics is an unresolved issue.[21]

Procedure continues on following page

Procedure	**for Combination Intraventricular/Fiberoptic Catheter Insertion (Assist), Monitoring, Nursing Care, Troubleshooting, and Removal—*Continued***	
Steps	**Rationale**	**Special Considerations**
8. Assist as needed with covering the patient's head and upper thorax with sterile drapes.	Protects the insertion site from contamination.[4,15,16]	
9. Fiberoptic system: A. Ensure that the preamp cable connects the catheter to the stand-alone monitor. B. Follow manufacturer's instructions for zeroing the catheter before insertion.	Prepares the system. The catheter is zeroed before insertion and is never rezeroed.[17,18]	
10. Assist with the insertion of the intraventricular/fiberoptic catheter.	Facilitates the insertion process.	
11. After intraventricular/fiberoptic catheter placement: A. Follow the manufacturer's instructions for the "synchronize to the monitor" interface. B. Attach the external ventricular drainage device to the proper Y-port. (Refer to Procedure 93.) C. Place the zero reference at the appropriate external anatomical landmark[1] of the external ventricular drainage device (see Fig. 94-2). **(Level D*)**	Ensures accurate fiberoptic data at the bedside monitor and allows printing of ICP tracing. The anatomical reference point for the foramen of Monro is the external auditory canal.[1,4]	Ensure proper CSF drainage amount to prevent ventricular collapse and possible herniation.[1,4]
12. Increase or decrease the height of the graduated burette to the prescribed pressure level.[1]	Ensures proper CSF drainage.	When adjusting the height of the pressure level, the stopcock should be "off" to the patient.[23]
13. The provider will prescribe the desired ICP parameter (see Procedure 93).	If the physician prescribes the ICP to be maintained at <15 mm Hg, drainage of CSF will be initiated if the patient's ICP is >15 mm Hg.	
14. Monitor the ICP and CPP as prescribed.	Assesses ICP waveform and values and CPP value.	
15. Set the appropriate ICP scale for the measured pressure.	Necessary for visualization of the complete ICP waveform.	
16. Set the monitor alarms.	Goals for ICP management are individualized for each patient based on pathology.	
17. Discard used supplies in appropriate receptacles.	Removes and safely discards used supplies; safely removes sharp objects.	
18. ▣▣		

*Level D: Peer-reviewed professional and organizational standards with the support of clinical study recommendations.

Procedure	for Combination Intraventricular/Fiberoptic Catheter Insertion (Assist), Monitoring, Nursing Care, Troubleshooting, and Removal—*Continued*	
Steps	**Rationale**	**Special Considerations**

Troubleshooting

1. HH
2. PE
3. Assess the integrity of the intraventricular/fiberoptic device. | Brain tissue or blood may occlude any of the various intracranial devices, resulting in a dampened waveform. Occlusion may necessitate manipulation or replacement. | Intracranial device manipulation is not a nursing responsibility in most institutions. Notify the provider for assistance as needed.
4. Correct the ICP monitoring device malfunction. | Fiberoptic catheters may become damaged or dislodged, requiring catheter replacement. | Follow manufacturer's instructions and troubleshooting manuals for identifying and correcting common problems.
5. Change the monitoring system, if needed. | Ensures a functional system. |
6. Discard used supplies.
7. HH

Combination Intraventricular/Fiberoptic Catheter Removal

1. HH
2. Ensure physicians, advanced practice nurses, and other healthcare professionals who are assisting with catheter removal don sterile gloves and masks with face shields or goggles.
3. Assist with the removal of the intraventricular/fiberoptic catheter. | Facilitates the removal process. | Culture the tip of the intraventricular catheter as prescribed.
4. Apply a sterile occlusive dressing after the device is removed. | Minimizes contamination by microorganisms. |
5. Dispose of used supplies and the device in the appropriate receptacle. | Removes and safely discards used supplies; safely removes sharp objects. |
6. HH

Expected Outcomes

- Accurate and reliable ICP monitoring, CPP calculation, and assessment of cerebral compliance[1,18]
- Maintenance of ICP within the range of 0–15 mm Hg or as prescribed[1,18]
- Early detection of elevated ICP trends[1,18]
- Management of increased ICP and decreased CPP[1,18]
- Protection of cerebral perfusion with maintenance of CPP within prescribed parameters[1,18]

Unexpected Outcomes

- CSF infection[5,10,12,14,19,20]
- CSF leakage
- Dislodging of the interventricular/fiberoptic catheter[15]
- Dislodging of the fiberoptic bolt[15]
- Pneumocephalus[1]
- Cerebral hemorrhage (rare)[1]
- Sequelae of sustained increased ICP and decreased CPP: cerebral infarction, herniation, and brain death[16,18]

Procedure continues on following page

Patient Monitoring and Care

Steps	Rationale	Reportable Conditions
		These conditions should be reported if they persist despite nursing interventions.
1. Assess the patient's neurological status and vital signs during the procedure.	Evaluates the patient's response to the procedure.	• Changes in neurological status • Abnormal vital signs
2. Note the ICP waveform and numeric values during the insertion procedure.	Provides baseline data.	• P_2 of greater amplitude than P_1
3. Assess the patient's neurological status hourly or more often as indicated.	Provides clinical confirmation of and correlation with the monitored ICP data.	• Changes in neurological status • Changes in vital signs
4. Assess the ICP hourly.	Determines the neurological status.	• Increased ICP • ICP waveform abnormalities • Immediately report sustained ICP elevations of 20 mm Hg or greater
5. Calculate the CPP hourly (or more often as indicated).	A CPP of 50–70 mm Hg should be maintained for adult patients with traumatic brain injuries.[4] CPP parameters should be individualized to meet the patient's perfusion needs.	• Changes in CPP • CPP less than the lowest prescribed parameter may put the patient at risk for cerebral ischemia[4]
6. Set the bedside alarm limits based on the parameter goals.	ICP limit is usually set to alarm when the ICP is >20 mm Hg; however, this needs to be individualized for each patient.	• Abnormal ICP
7. Assess the catheter system hourly.	Ensures accuracy and safety of monitoring.	• Frank blood or clots in the CSF drainage bag may indicate intracranial bleeding • Absence of CSF drainage may indicate an occluded catheter, dislodged catheter, cerebral swelling, or overdrained ventricles • Excessive drainage may lead to infarction and herniation
8. Change the insertion site dressing per institutional policy.[19]	Provides an opportunity to assess insertion site and observe for signs and symptoms of infection.	• Significant drainage on ICP insertion site dressing or head dressing • Signs and symptoms of infection
9. Provide a safe environment, preventing inadvertent dislodgement of the intraventricular/fiberoptic catheter through appropriate catheter positioning, sedation, and analgesia as needed.	Inadvertent dislodgement of the catheter must be avoided because it can result in pneumoencephalopathy or excessive CSF drainage.	• Dislodged device • Abnormal ICP • Abnormal ICP waveform
10. Follow institutional standards for assessing pain. Administer analgesia as prescribed.	Identifies need for pain interventions.	• Continued pain despite pain interventions
11. Change the CSF drainage collection device per institutional policy.	Practices for changing CSF drainage collection devices vary considerably. Maintain closed system.	• Inadvertent disconnection
12. Elevate the head of the patient's bed to 30 degrees or as prescribed.	May decrease ICP.	• Elevated ICP

Documentation

Documentation should include the following:

- Completion of informed consent
- Preprocedure verifications and time out
- Insertion time and patient response to procedure
- Procedural monitoring documentation including vital signs and sedation monitoring
- Initial and hourly ICP reading
- Initial and hourly CPP calculation
- CSF color and clarity

- Insertion site assessment
- Patient and family education
- Initial ICP tracing (include ICP waveform morphology) and any changes in waveform
- Nursing interventions used to treat ICP or CPP deviations and expected or unexpected outcomes
- Hourly amount of CSF drainage
- Pain assessment, interventions, and effectiveness

References and Additional Readings

For a complete list of references and additional readings for this procedure, scan this QR code with any freely available smartphone code reader app, or visit http://booksite.elsevier.com/9780323376624.

94 Intraventricular Catheter with External Transducer for Cerebrospinal Fluid Drainage and Intracranial Pressure Monitoring

Stephanie Cox

PURPOSE: An intraventricular catheter with an external transducer is used to monitor intracranial pressure and, in the presence of pathology, to alleviate increased intracranial pressure by draining cerebrospinal fluid (CSF) from the ventricular system.

PREREQUISITE NURSING KNOWLEDGE

- Knowledge of neuroanatomy and physiology is needed.
- Understanding is needed regarding the assembly and maintenance of the intraventricular catheter with an external transducer and drainage system, care of the insertion site, and drainage techniques.
- Principles of aseptic technique should be understood. Of all the intracranial pressure monitoring devices, external ventricular drains (EVDs) have the greatest risk of infection.[1,4]
- Institutional standards may vary with regard to antiseptic choice—follow your institutional standard. Although the package insert for chlorhexidine warns against use before any neuraxial procedures, a large retrospective study and several anesthesiology societies recommend chlorhexidine as an antiseptic.[14,15,18,33]
- The normal range for intracranial pressure (ICP) is 0 to 15 mm Hg.[1,26,29] This measurement reflects the pressure exerted by the intracranial contents within the skull, including brain, blood, and cerebrospinal fluid.[26]
- Cerebral perfusion pressure (CPP) is a derived mathematic calculation that indirectly reflects the adequacy of cerebral blood flow. The CPP is calculated by subtracting the ICP from the mean arterial pressure (MAP); thus, $CPP = MAP - ICP$.[1,28] The normal CPP range for adults is approximately 60 to 100 mm Hg[22] or a mean of 80 mm Hg.[20,29] The optimal CPP for a given patient and clinical condition is not entirely known. ICP and CPP should be managed concomitantly and recorded. According to the Brain Trauma Foundation Guidelines, an acceptable CPP for an adult with a severe traumatic brain injury (Glasgow Coma Scale [GCS] score of ≤8) lies between 50 and 70 mm Hg.[4] Patients with aneurysmal subarachnoid

hemorrhage vasospasm may need higher CPPs to maintain adequate perfusion through vasospastic cerebral blood vessels.[7] Patients with other neurological injuries require individualized CPP parameters reflective of the neuropathology and brain perfusion needs.

- Elevations in ICP result when one or more intracranial components—blood, CSF, or brain tissue—increase without an accompanying decrease in one or two of the other intracranial components. This is known as the Monro-Kellie doctrine or hypothesis.[1,20]
- Clinical conditions that frequently result in increased intracranial pressure include traumatic brain injury, ischemic stroke,[36] subarachnoid hemorrhage,[7] intraparenchymal hemorrhage,[30] brain tumor, meningitis, and hydrocephalus.[1,27] An EVD may be indicated in the management of intracranial pressure in each of these conditions.[2]
- Fiberoptic catheters and the microsensors that are placed during surgery in the surgical site or through a bolt in the skull are also used to monitor the ICP. They may be placed in the epidural, subdural, subarachnoid, ventricular, and intraparenchymal spaces.[28,29] These catheters are sentinels for increased ICP but may not be designed for treatment of increased ICP with CSF drainage.[28,29] When a ventricular catheter is inserted and transduced at the level of the foramen of Monro, approximately at the level of the external auditory canal, it produces a value and a waveform that reflects the ICP. The EVD is considered the most accurate ICP monitor.[1,4]
- CSF is formed within the lateral ventricles of the cerebral hemispheres by the choroid plexus. From the lateral ventricles, fluid drains into the foramen of Monro, the intraventricular foramina, and into the third ventricle adjacent to the thalamus. Although most of the CSF is made in the choroid plexus of the lateral ventricles, the third ventricle contributes some CSF, which then passes through the

aqueduct of Sylvius into the fourth ventricle at the pons and medulla. The choroid plexus in the roof of the fourth ventricle and the brain parenchyma itself[5] contribute an additional small amount of CSF. The fluid then enters into the subarachnoid space, with the major portion of the fluid moving through the foramen of Magendie, where it is dispersed around the spinal cord and through the foramen of Luschka, where it flows around the brain. CSF is absorbed by the arachnoid villi, also known as arachnoid granulations, where it drains into the venous system to be returned to the heart.[3,6]

- CSF is a clear colorless liquid of low specific gravity with no red blood cells and only 0 to 5 white blood cells (WBCs). Approximately 150 mL of CSF circulates within the CSF pathways in the brain and spinal subarachnoid space. CSF is secreted at the rate of 0.35 mL/min or approximately 20 mL/hr.[3]

- ICP waveform morphology reflects transmission of arterial and venous pressure through the CSF and brain parenchyma. The normal ICP waveform has three or four peaks, with P_1 being of greater amplitude than P_2, and P_2 of greater amplitude than P_3. P_1 is thought to reflect arterial pressure; P_2, P_3, and P_4 (when present) have been described as originating from the choroid plexus or veins (see Fig. 92-2).[1,28] The amplitude of P_2 may exceed P_1 with increased ICP or decreased intracranial compliance (see Fig. 92-3).

- During ICP elevations, pathological (Lundberg) waveform trends include *a, b,* and *c* waves. The *a* waves, also referred to as plateau waves, are associated with ICP values of 50 to 100 mm Hg and last 5 to 20 minutes. The *a* waves are associated with abrupt neurological deterioration and herniation and are the most ominous[1] (see Fig. 92-4). The *b* waves (see Fig. 92-5), with ICP values of 20 to 50 mm Hg, last 30 seconds to 2 minutes and may become *a* waves. The *c* waves (see Fig. 92-6) may coincide with ICPs as high as 20 mm Hg but are short lasting and without clinical significance (see Fig. 92-6).[1]

- Some external ventricular drainage systems may also provide simultaneous drainage and trending of the intracranial pressure.

- Management of acute brain injury is aimed at decreasing secondary brain injury from increased intracranial pressure, decreased cerebral perfusion pressure, impaired autoregulation, hypotension, hypoxemia, cerebral ischemia, hypercarbia, hyperthermia, hypoglycemia, hyperglycemia, seizures or abnormalities in cerebral blood flow. Interventions should include strict blood pressure management, decreased environmental stimuli, elevation of the head of the bed, alignment of the head and neck in a straight position to promote venous drainage, the avoidance of constrictive devices about the neck that might impede arterial flow to the brain and venous drainage from the brain, seizure prophylaxis, glucose control, and attaining and maintaining normothermia without shivering.[1,26]

- In addition to CSF drainage, management of increased ICP frequently requires the use of certain pharmacological agents to lessen intracranial pressure, including sedation and analgesia, osmotic diuretics, hypertonic saline, neuromuscular blockade, and barbiturates. In the case of barbiturate coma, continuous electroencephalographic (EEG)

monitoring (or EEG-based consciousness/sedation monitoring) for burst suppression is necessary to achieve the desired decrease in cerebral oxygen consumption and electrical stimuli.[12] Additional strategies include decompressive craniectomy and hemispherectomy.[1,11,28,35]

- Underdrainage of CSF may result in sustained increased intracranial pressure and herniation.[22,25,28,29]

- Over drainage of CSF may result in headache, subdural hematoma, pneumocephalus, and herniation.[22,25,28,29]

EQUIPMENT

- Cranial access tray with drill
- Ventricular catheter
- Pressure monitor tubing kit, including pressure tubing, transducer, a three-way stopcock, or a flushless transducer with stopcock
- Nonvented sterile caps
- External drainage system, including tubing, collection chamber, and drainage bag
- Preservative-free normal saline solution
- Pressure monitoring cable and module
- Sterile syringes
- Skin/site preparation with antiseptic solution
- Sterile towels, drapes
- Local anesthetic (e.g., lidocaine 1% or 2% without epinephrine)
- Sutures or staples
- Sterile dressing
- Tape
- Laboratory forms and specimen labels (for CSF specimens)
- CSF specimen tubes (for collection of CSF)
- Caps, masks, sterile drapes, gloves, and gowns
- Cautery as required by institutional standard (for bedside insertion)
- Leveling device (e.g., carpenter's, laser, or line level)
- Intravenous (IV) pole

Additional equipment, to have available as needed, includes the following.

- Suction

PATIENT AND FAMILY EDUCATION

- Explain the procedure to the patient/family. This procedure may be performed at the bedside and require the patient to be sedated, paralyzed, and intubated. ***Rationale:*** Patient cooperation during cranial access is of utmost importance. The patient and family should be aware that the patient may need to be intubated to maintain a patent airway, ensure adequate oxygenation, and maintain a normal ICP and an adequate CPP.

- Assess the patient and the family for understanding of ICP pressure monitoring. ***Rationale:*** Knowledge and information may lessen anxiety.

- Explain the potential need for low environmental stimulation, especially during periods of ICP elevations (decreased noise, decreased tactile stimulation, and low lighting). ***Rationale:*** Knowledge and information may lessen anxiety and present expectations of potential events.

- Explain the waveforms on the bedside monitor and how this pressure is continually observed for signs of increased ICP. In the case of increased ICP, the drain is opened to drain CSF continuously or intermittently as prescribed to alleviate the pressure. *Rationale:* This explanation presents to the patient and family a more realistic expectation of the events to come.

PATIENT ASSESSMENT AND PREPARATION

Patient Assessment

- Obtain a baseline assessment to include level of consciousness, mental status, motor capability, sensation, cranial nerves, and vital signs. *Rationale:* This assessment provides baseline data.
- Obtain the patient's medical and surgical history to include use of aspirin, anticoagulants, prior craniotomies, the presence of aneurysm clips, embolic materials, permanent balloon occlusions, detachable coils, or a ventriculoperitoneal shunt. Obtain laboratory results to assess coagulation status as needed. *Rationale:* The information obtained determines and guides future treatment based on the neurological examination results and evidence from radiology and angiography.
- Assess for allergies. *Rationale:* Insertion of an external ventricular catheter requires the use of an antiseptic to

cleanse the site, local anesthetic, and possibly systemic analgesia and sedation. External ventricular catheters may be impregnated with antibiotics (e.g., clindamycin, rifampin, and minocycline), or systemic antibiotics may be given periprocedurally or prophylactically.[4,22,27]

Patient Preparation

- Verify that the patient is the correct patient using two identifiers. *Rationale:* Before performing a procedure, the nurse should ensure the correct identification of the patient for the intended intervention.[34]
- Ensure that the patient and family understand preprocedural information. Answer questions as they arise, and reinforce information as needed. *Rationale:* Understanding of previously taught information is evaluated and reinforced.
- Ensure that informed consent has been obtained. *Rationale:* Informed consent protects the rights of the patient and makes a competent decision possible for the patient. However, in emergency circumstances, time may not allow for the consent form to be signed.
- Initiate IV access or assess the patency of the IV access. *Rationale:* Readily available IV access is necessary if the patient needs to be sedated or paralyzed or needs other medications.
- Perform a preprocedure verification and time out, if nonemergent. *Rationale:* Ensures patient safety.[34]

Procedure	**for Pressure Monitoring and Drainage**	
Steps	Rationale	Special Considerations
External Ventricular Drainage (EVD) System Assembly		
1. 🖐		
2. Open the outer package of the sterile supplies. Apply sterile gloves, gown, and mask with eye shield.[16]	Ensures sterile technique.	
3. With aseptic technique, flush through the pressure tubing and drainage system with preservative-free saline solution, turning the stopcocks as needed to prime the entire system. Remove the syringe and replace with a sterile nonvented cap.	Prepares the drainage system for use; flushes air from the system. If air is left in the tubing, it may alter the numeric value or prevent the flow of CSF.[9,23] The preservative in normal saline may cause cortical necrosis.[15]	Use of a syringe filled with sterile, preservative-free normal saline solution to prime the external ventricular drainage system tubing rather than a bag of flush solution lessens the risk of flush solution being administered through the ventricular catheter into the brain. In addition, the use of a flushless transducer at the zero reference on the drainage system eliminates lengthy tubing that may dampen the waveform (Fig. 94-1).
4. Connect the end of the EVD drainage system tubing to the distal stopcock of the pressure monitor tubing (Fig. 94-2) if not already included in the drainage system. Tighten all the connections.[16,17,24]	Ensures that the system is secure and is a sterile closed system.	

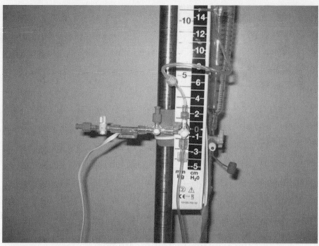

Figure 94-1 External ventricular drainage system with flushless transducer at zero reference level. *(Courtesy of Integra Lifesciences Corporation, Plainsboro, NJ.)*

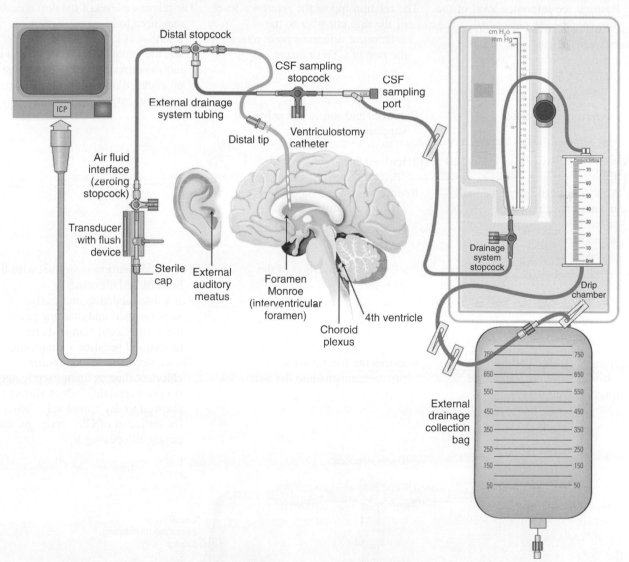

Figure 94-2 External ventricular drainage system. *(Drawing by Paul Schiffmacher, Thomas Jefferson University, Philadelphia, PA.)*

Procedure   for Pressure Monitoring and Drainage—*Continued*

Steps	Rationale	Special Considerations
5. Close the clamp or stopcock between the drip chamber and the external ventricular drainage collection bag (see Fig. 94-2).	Ensures the ability to measure hourly drainage in the drip chamber.	
6. Replace all vented caps with nonvented caps.	Vented caps are used by the manufacturer to permit sterilization of the entire system. These caps need to be replaced with sterile nonvented caps to prevent bacteria and air from entering the system.	
7. After flushing the pressure monitor tubing and the external ventricular drainage system tubing, turn the distal stopcock off to the distal tip of the pressure monitor tubing (Fig. 94-3).	The stopcock in this position readies the entire system for connection to the ventriculostomy catheter.	Prevents the backflow of fluid into the drip chamber.
8. Position the reference level of the drip chamber as prescribed.	The relationship of the reference level of the drip chamber to the anatomical reference point alters the rate of CSF drainage.	The reference level of the drip chamber may need to be adjusted after insertion of the ventricular catheter and the initial ICP is obtained and is individualized for each patient based on etiology, pathophysiology, and management strategies.
9. Discard used supplies.	Removes and safely discards used supplies.	
10. 🔲		

Assisting With Insertion of an Intraventricular Catheter

1. 🔲		
2. Apply nonsterile gloves, gowns, and masks with eye shields. After opening outer packaging, apply sterile gloves to handle sterile supplies.	Reduces transmission of microorganisms and body secretions; Standard Precautions.	
3. Ensure the patient is in position for ventricular catheter placement.	Facilitates the insertion of the catheter.	The usual position is supine, with the head of bed elevated. Administer sedation and analgesia as prescribed and monitor patient per institutional standards for procedural sedation monitoring.
4. Assist as needed with the antiseptic preparation of the insertion site.	Reduces the transmission of microorganisms into the ventricles.	The choice of povidone iodine or chlorhexidine as an antiseptic agent is controversial.[14,18] Both should be allowed to dry completely. Observe for initiation of CSF drainage, and obtain an opening ICP.

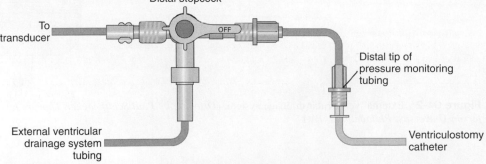

Figure 94-3   Distal stopcock turned off to the distal tip of the pressure monitor tubing. (*Drawing by Paul Schiffmacher, Thomas Jefferson University, Philadelphia, PA.*)

Procedure for Pressure Monitoring and Drainage—*Continued*		
Steps	**Rationale**	**Special Considerations**
5. Connect the drainage/monitoring system to the distal tip of the catheter after it is inserted.	Establishes draining system.	
6. Assist as needed with application of a sterile, occlusive dressing or as per hospital standards. Secure the catheter to minimize manipulation and the risk of inadvertent removal.[16,25] **(Level E*)**	Reduces the risk of infection.	
7. Discard supplies.		
8. **HH**		
Connecting the EVD Transducer with Bedside Monitor		
1. Turn on the bedside monitor.	Prepares the monitor.	
2. Plug a pressure cable into the appropriate pressure module or port in the bedside monitor (see Fig. 94-2).	The signal is transmitted to the bedside monitor so that it may be transmitted to the oscilloscope for display.	
3. Attach the pressure cable to the transducer connection on the pressure tubing of the drainage system.	Prepares the equipment.	
4. Turn on the ICP parameter.	Visualizes correct waveform.	
5. Set the appropriate scale for the measured pressure.[27,29]	It is necessary to visualize the complete waveform and to obtain corresponding numerical values. Waveforms vary in amplitude, depending on the pressure within the system.	The normal ICP for an adult is within the range of 0–15 mm Hg.[8,12]
6. Set the monitor alarm limits for ICP and CPP.	Goals for ICP management are individualized for each patient based on etiology, pathophysiology, and management strategies.	
Leveling the Transducer		
1. Perform hand hygiene.		
2. **PE**		
3. Position the patient in the supine position with the head of the bed elevated as prescribed by the physician, advanced practice nurse, or other healthcare professional.[26,28,31] **(Level E)**	Prepares the patient.	The head of the bed is usually placed at 30 degrees to aid in increasing venous return.[12,27]
4. Place the air-fluid interface (zeroing stopcock) at the level of the external auditory meatus (see Fig. 94-2).[2,31] **(Level B*)**	The external auditory meatus approximates the level of the foramen of Monro (intraventricular foramen).[2,8]	Some institutions use the tragus or a line drawn from the outer canthus of the eye.[2,22] Follow institutional policy.
5. Discard supplies.		
6. **HH**		

*Level B: Well-designed, controlled studies with results that consistently support a specific action, intervention or treatment.

*Level E: Multiple case reports, theory-based evidence from expert opinions, or peer-reviewed professional organizational standards without clinical studies to support recommendations.

Procedure continues on following page

Procedure	for Pressure Monitoring and Drainage—*Continued*

Steps	Rationale	Special Considerations
Zeroing the Transducer		
1. HH		Follow institutional standard.
2. PE		
3. Turn the transducer stopcock off to the patient.	Prepares the system for the zeroing procedure.	
4. If indicated for the drainage/monitoring system in use: remove the nonvented cap from the stopcock, thus opening the stopcock to air. (Some drainage systems may not require removing a cap but simply adjusting the drip chamber to 0 mm Hg, pressing zero on the bedside monitor, and retuning the drip chamber to the level prescribed.)	Allows the monitor to use atmospheric pressure as a reference for zero.	Follow institutional standard.
5. Push and release the zeroing button on the bedside monitor. Observe the digital reading until it displays a value of zero.	The monitor automatically adjusts itself to zero. Zeroing negates the effects of atmospheric pressure.	Some monitors require that the zero be turned and adjusted manually.
6. Place a new, sterile, nonvented cap on the stopcock.	Maintains sterility.	
7. Turn the stopcock so that it is open to the transducer. Observe the ICP waveform and the corresponding numerical value.	Permits pressure monitoring.	
8. Discard used supplies.		
9. HH		
Monitoring Intracranial Pressure		
1. HH		
2. PE		
3. Position the head of the bed as prescribed.	Allows for accurate and consistent monitoring of the ICP.	Ensure that the EVD system is at the prescribed level for ICP measurement (e.g., level with external auditory meatus).
4. Turn the distal stopcock off to the external ventricular drainage system (Fig. 94-4).[22]	Decreases artifact from simultaneous drainage. Allows for accurate monitoring of the ICP.	
5. Record the ICP value and waveform per institutional standard.	Provides a value for ongoing assessment. Allows analysis of the ICP waveform.	The normal ICP waveform has at least three distinct pressure oscillations or peaks. These are referred to as P_1, P_2, and P_3 (see Fig. 92-2).[19,25]

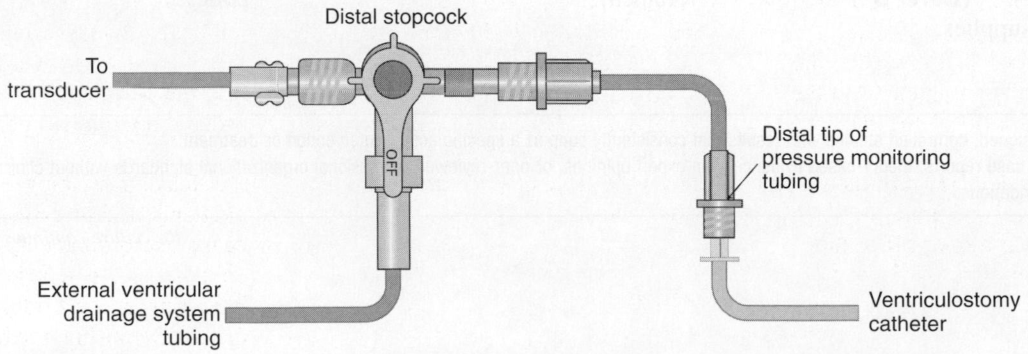

Figure 94-4 Distal stopcock turned off to the external drainage system tubing. (*Drawing by Paul Schiffmacher, Thomas Jefferson University, Philadelphia, PA.*)

Procedure for Pressure Monitoring and Drainage—*Continued*

Steps	Rationale	Special Considerations
6. Monitor and record ICP and CPP as prescribed.	Assesses ICP waveform and values and CPP value.	If continuous drainage is prescribed, the risk of overdrainage is increased. If the drainage system allows, turn the stopcock to simultaneously drain and to trend the ICP. Set alarms. To obtain an accurate ICP, the stopcock must be turned off to the drain with the catheter open to the transducer only and the waveform and numeric value of the ICP given time to stabilize. The waveform and numeric value of the ICP should correspond. Deviations in ICP and CPP may require immediate intervention and should be reported to the physician, advanced practice nurse, or other healthcare professional. If an EVD is in the monitoring position (and off to CSF drainage), special care must be paid to the bedside neurological examination with regard to the potential for deterioration. The catheter may become obstructed with clot, tissue, or protein. Note any changes in CSF flow. Notify the physician, advanced practice nurse, or other healthcare professional who may need to irrigate the catheter to reestablish patency. Other maneuvers may include turning or stimulating a cough. Some institutional policies may allow the critical care nurse to irrigate the catheter with a limited amount of preservative-free saline solution. Follow institutional standard.

7. **PE**
8. **HH**

Draining CSF from the EVD

1. **HH**
2. **PE**

Steps	Rationale	Special Considerations
3. The physician, advanced practice nurse, or other healthcare professional will prescribe the desired ICP parameter and the reference level of the drip chamber.	If the physician, advanced practice nurse, or other healthcare professional prescribes the ICP to be maintained at <15 mm Hg, drainage of CSF will be initiated if the patient's ICP is >15 mm Hg.	Assess patency of the system when applicable by lowering the system briefly to assess for CSF dripping into the burette (then return to ordered anatomical point).[32]
4. To drain the CSF, turn the distal stopcock of the pressure monitoring tubing off to the transducer (Fig. 94-5).[22]	Allows the flow of CSF from the ventricles.	Never leave a draining EVD unattended. Excessive drainage may cause overdrainage and a possible collapse of the ventricles, resulting in tearing of the bridging veins of the brain causing a subdural hematoma.

Procedure continues on following page

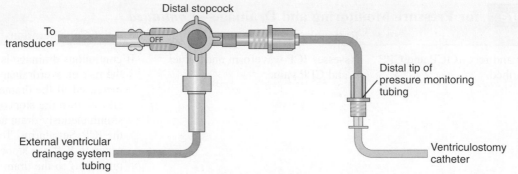

To transducer

Distal stopcock

OFF

Distal tip of pressure monitoring tubing

External ventricular drainage system tubing

Ventriculostomy catheter

Figure 94-5   Distal stopcock turned off to the transducer. *(Drawing by Paul Schiffmacher, Thomas Jefferson University, Philadelphia, PA.)*

Procedure	**for Pressure Monitoring and Drainage—*Continued***	
Steps	**Rationale**	**Special Considerations**
5. Allow 2–5 mL of CSF to enter the drip chamber (see Fig. 94-5).	Prevents overdrainage of CSF.	Never leave a draining EVD unattended.
6. When drainage is completed, turn the distal stopcock off to the external ventricular drainage system (see Fig. 94-4) and record the amount drained and the ICP value.	Check the ICP value to determine whether the parameter is met.	If the patient's CSF is being continuously drained, note and record the amount of drainage every hour. In general, no more than 20 mL, the amount of CSF produced in 1 hour,[3] should be drained each hour.
7. If the goal was not met, repeat **Steps 3–5** until the ICP parameter is met.	Allows gradual draining of CSF.	
CSF Sampling		
1. 🅷🅷		
2. Obtain from a physician, advanced practice nurse, or other healthcare professional an order for a CSF sample, including the frequency.	Prepares for the test.	CSF sampling may include glucose, cell count, protein, culture and sensitivity, and gram stain. If a comparison of serum glucose and CSF glucose is prescribed, a serum glucose sample should be obtained at the same time as the CSF sampling. Normal CSF glucose is two thirds of blood glucose.[3,6]
3. Obtain the supplies for sampling: sterile 3-mL syringes, CSF tubes, antiseptic solution, sterile gloves, mask with face shield, laboratory forms, and specimen labels.	Prepares the equipment.	
4. Apply sterile gloves and mask with face shield.	Reduces the transmission of microorganisms and body fluids; Standard Precautions.	
5. Cleanse the CSF sampling port with an antiseptic solution (Fig. 94-6). Allow solution to dry.	Reduces the transmission of microorganisms into the ventricles.	Follow institutional standard.
6. Turn the distal stopcock of the pressure monitor tubing off to the transducer and turn the drainage system stopcock off to the drop chamber (see Fig. 94-5).	Allows for direct sampling of CSF from the ventriculostomy catheter.	

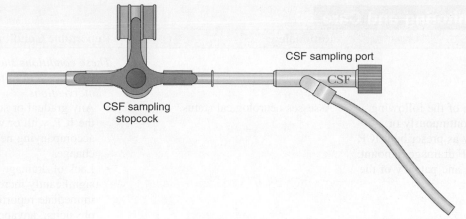

Figure 94-6 CSF sampling port. *(Drawing by Paul Schiffmacher, Thomas Jefferson University, Philadelphia, PA.)*

Procedure for Pressure Monitoring and Drainage—*Continued*

Steps	Rationale	Special Considerations
7. Slowly withdraw two 1- to 2-mL samples from the designated CSF Y-site or sampling port and inject each into a specimen tube. If resistance is met during aspiration, notify physician, advanced practice nurse, or other healthcare professional.	Obtains the prescribed sample.	One sample may be used for laboratory studies, and the other for culture and Gram stain, if prescribed by the physician, advanced practice nurse, or other healthcare professional. Follow institutional standards.
8. Turn the distal stopcock to resume monitoring or open to drainage as prescribed.	Continues monitoring and drainage as prescribed.	
9. Label the CSF specimen tubes and send to the laboratory for analysis.	Prepares the specimen for analysis.	
10. Discard used supplies.	Removes and safely discards used supplies.	
11. HH		

Expected Outcomes

- Aseptic drainage system[21,25,27]
- Air-fluid interface of the transducer is leveled at the foramen of Monro for accurate ICP and CPP monitoring[22,26,28]
- The monitoring system is zeroed
- Drainage chamber at prescribed level
- Intermittent or continuous drainage as prescribed
- Accurate and reliable monitoring of ICP and CPP[22,26,28]
- Continuous flow of CSF when drainage is initiated; appropriate amount of CSF drainage[22,26,28]
- Immediate management of increased ICP and decreased CPP[22,26,28]
- Improvement or stabilization of neurological function[22,28,31]

Unexpected Outcomes

- Loose connections within the external ventricular drainage system
- Stopcocks left open to air without nonvented caps
- Air bubbles within the system[23]
- CSF infection[1,10,30]
- CSF leak
- Lack of CSF flow[6]
- Dislodgment or occlusion of the EVD
- Headache from overdrainage[31]
- Pneumocephalus from overdrainage
- Rebleed from subarachnoid hemorrhage[13,21]
- Subdural hematoma from overdrainage[27]
- EVD-related hemorrhage[27]
- Herniation from underdrainage or overdrainage

Procedure continues on following page

Patient Monitoring and Care

Steps	Rationale	Reportable Conditions
		These conditions should be reported if they persist despite nursing interventions.
1. Monitor each of the following parameters continuously or intermittently as prescribed: ICP, CPP, and CSF drainage, amount, color, clarity, and patency of the system.	Assesses neurological status.	• Any gradual or sudden increase in the ICP, with or without accompanying neurological changes • Lack of drainage in the presence of significantly increased ICP requires immediate reporting to the physician, advanced practice nurse, or other healthcare professional; this may indicate an occlusion of the catheter[21,27] • Lack of drainage in the presence of significantly increased ICP may also indicate occlusion of the drainage system from persistent contact of CSF catheter with the ventricular wall[8] • Persistent large volumes of CSF may indicate the need for a CSF shunt[30]
2. Zero the external ventricular drainage system during the initial setup or before insertion, then after insertion and again if connections between the transducer and the monitoring cable become dislodged, if connections between the monitoring cable and the monitor become dislodged, and when the values do not fit the clinical picture.	Ensures the accuracy of the monitoring process.	
3. During position changes, clamp the EVD. After changing the patient's position, maintain the reference level of the EVD at the external auditory meatus and ensure system is patent.	Minimizes the risk for underdrainage, overdrainage, or erroneous ICP values.	• Increase or decrease in CSF drainage • The inability to obtain CSF drainage • Changes in ICP or neurological assessment
4. Maintain the reference level of the drip chamber as prescribed.	The relationship of the reference for CSF drainage and ICP monitoring level of the drip chamber to the anatomical reference point alters the rate of CSF drainage.	• Underdrainage • Overdrainage
5. Check the system every hour and as needed.	Ensures that all connections are tightly secured and that no cracks occur in the system. Ensures that the system is closed with nonvented caps on all stopcocks. Ensures that the system is free of air bubbles.[23]	

Patient Monitoring and Care —*Continued*

Steps	Rationale	Reportable Conditions
6. Set the alarm parameters relative to the ICP and CPP goals established by the physician, advanced practice nurse, or other healthcare professional.	Provides immediate alarm for high pressures (and an immediate alarm for low pressures associated with inadvertent overdrainage).	• Changes in ICP or neurological assessment
7. All drainage should be measured and recorded as part of the intake and output.	Assesses CSF drainage. Amount, color, and character should be noted.[26]	• Increase or decrease in CSF drainage; change in CSF color, presence of blood or blood-tinged CSF
8. If continuous drainage is used, record and monitor the output every 1–2 hours. Maintain the reference point at the foramen of Monro.	Assesses CSF drainage.	• Increase or decrease in CSF drainage; underdrainage or overdrainage
9. Change the dressing at the insertion site daily or as prescribed with aseptic technique. Follow institutional standard.	Maintains sterility and provides an opportunity for insertion site assessment.[24]	• Signs or symptoms of infection • Loosened sutures
10. Change bag and drainage system as needed by institutional standard.	Practices for changing CSF drainage collection device vary considerably. Maintain closed system.	• Inadvertent disconnection
11. Follow institutional standard for assessing pain. Administer analgesia as prescribed (Fig. 94-7).	Identifies need for pain interventions.	• Continued pain despite pain interventions

Documentation

Documentation should include the following:
- Initial opening ICP and CPP
- Level of the drip chamber and anatomical landmark for zeroing
- Patency of drainage system
- Analysis of waveform[19,26,28,29]
- Description of CSF to include amount, clarity and color
- Insertion site assessment
- Hourly to every 2 hours output or amount drained intermittently[22,29]
- Hourly ICP and CPP[22,29]
- Neurological assessment[22,29]
- Site care and change of drainage system or bag
- Pain assessment, interventions, and evaluation

Monitoring ICP with a Ventricular Drain

To Drain CSF

- *Master System Stopcock* is off to the transducer

- Drainage line is open between the patient and the drip chamber

- When the stopcock is open to drain it is critical that neither the height of the patient nor that of the drainage system be changed to avoid over drainage of CSF

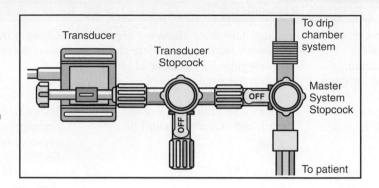

To Zero Transducer

- Requires hand hygiene, sterile gloves and new sterile dead-ender

- Turn the *Transducer Stopcock* off to the *patient* (*off* to the *Master System Stopcock*)

- Remove dead-ender cap from side port of *Transducer Stopcock*

- The Transducer is *OPEN TO AIR* and isolated from any pressures

- Press *ZERO* on the ICP monitor

- Replace dead-ender cap with *NEW STERILE CAP* and turn stopcock back OFF to side port

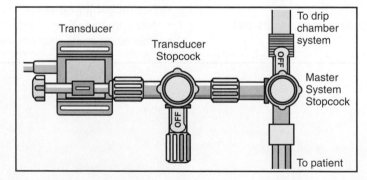

To Monitor ICP

- Turn the *Master System Stopcock* off to the drip chamber

- The drainage line is open between the patient and the transducer

NEVER!

- *NEVER turn the stopcock open three ways to try to drain and monitor at the same time!*

- This gives a false ICP reading – the system is open to drain and therefore also open to air

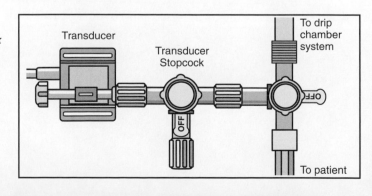

Figure 94-7 Alternate external ventricular drainage monitoring system. *(Drawing by Lorna Prang, Littleton, CO).*

References and Additional Readings

For a complete list of references and additional readings for this procedure, scan this QR code with any freely available smartphone code reader app, or visit http://booksite.elsevier.com/9780323376624.

95

Lumbar Subarachnoid Catheter Insertion (Assist) for Cerebrospinal Fluid Drainage and Pressure Monitoring

Nicolle Schraeder

PURPOSE: Patients with a variety of central nervous system conditions and thoracoabdominal aneurysms may benefit from the monitoring of intraspinal pressure and maintenance of therapeutic levels of cerebrospinal fluid (CSF) drainage. Lumbar subarachnoid catheters may be used for CSF pressure monitoring and drainage.

PREREQUISITE NURSING KNOWLEDGE

- Knowledge of the anatomy and physiology of the vertebral column, spinal meninges, spinal cord, nerve roots, and CSF circulation and intracranial and intraspinal dynamics is needed.
- Knowledge of aseptic techniques is necessary.
- Normal intraspinal pressure in the adult is 0 to 20 cm H_2O (0 to 15 mm Hg or 50 to 150 mm H_2O) and usually corresponds with intracranial pressure.[28] Intraspinal pressure may be influenced by a number of factors including edema and positioning. Further research is needed to ascertain therapeutic levels after various surgical interventions.[25]
- Lumbar subarachnoid catheters, also referred to as lumbar drains or intrathecal catheters, require lumbar puncture (LP) for insertion.[20] Lumbar subarachnoid catheters permit monitoring of CSF pressure. CSF pressure may be monitored intermittently or continuously, and CSF drainage may be performed intermittently or continuously.[11,28,29]
- Lumbar subarachnoid catheters may be used in the prevention or management of spontaneous, traumatic, or surgical CSF fistulas to allow any tears in the dura mater to heal.[5,11,38,40,41] The catheter reduces moisture and pressure at the tear and may be placed before, during, or after surgery.[4,5,10,11,14]
- Lumbar subarachnoid catheters may be used in the diagnostic workup and management of normal pressure hydrocephalus instead of serial lumbar punctures.[16,19]
- Lumbar subarachnoid catheters may be used in the perioperative management of intraspinal pressure during and after thoracoabdominal aortic aneurysmal repair to provide adequate room in the intraspinal space to accommodate spinal cord edema and to improve impaired spinal cord perfusion related to spinal cord edema.

- Lumbar subarachnoid catheters may be used instead of or with an external ventricular drain to decrease intracranial pressure and remove blood from the subarachnoid space, which may lessen aneurysmal subarachnoid hemorrhage vasospasm.[17,20,25–27,35,39] When ventricular and lumbar drainage are used simultaneously, the ventricular drainage output should exceed the lumbar drainage output to lessen the risk of herniation.[11,16,25,39]
- Paraplegia remains the most dreaded neurological complication following thoracoabdominal aortic repair.[2,11,41]
- For patients having thoracic aorta or thoracoabdominal surgery, CSF drainage to maintain pressures less than 10 mm Hg in conjunction with other neuroprotective strategies minimizes the risk of neurological sequelae, allowing for adequate perfusion pressure to the spinal cord.[2–4]
- Lumbar subarachnoid catheters may be use in the management of communicating hydrocephalus related to intraventricular, intracerebral hemorrhage.[11,21,22]
- Complications related to the use of lumbar subarachnoid catheters include infection, headache, nerve root irritation, retained fragments of broken catheters, paraplegia, and neurological deterioration related to overdrainage, including subdural hematomas, pneumocephalus, and herniation.[1,31–34]
- Lumbar subarachnoid catheters have been used, with extreme caution, in the management of patients with meningitis.[24,36,37]
- Lumbar subarachnoid catheter drainage is contraindicated with midline mass effect. A computed tomographic (CT) scan before lumbar subarachnoid catheter insertion to confirm discernible basal cisterns and absence of a mass lesion may lessen the risk of herniation.[1,20,25,26]

- A variety of products are available for lumbar subarachnoid catheter drainage systems, making it essential to follow the manufacturer's guidelines for management of the patient,[28] including the type of pressure measurement unit used for patient monitoring (e.g., monitoring pressures in units mm Hg or cm H_2O).

EQUIPMENT

- Antiseptic solution
- Caps, masks with face shields, sterile gowns, and sterile gloves
- Sterile towels, half-sheets, and drapes
- Local anesthetic (lidocaine 1% or 2% without epinephrine)
- 5- or 10-mL Luer-Lock syringe with 18-gauge needle for drawing of lidocaine and 23-gauge needle for administration of lidocaine
- Sutures (2-0 nylon, 3-0 silk)
- Forceps
- Sterile scissors
- Sterile needle holder
- Preservative-free sterile normal saline solution (vial, bag, or prefilled syringe)
- Lumbar catheter tray containing a sterile catheter and, depending on the tray, additional connection devices
- Lumbar puncture tray
- Sterile occlusive dressing
- Tape (1- and 2-inch rolls)
- External stand-alone transducer with three-way stopcock
- Pressure cable if monitoring pressures is indicated
- External CSF drainage system
- Nonvented sterile caps

Additional equipment, to have available as needed, includes the following:

- Leveling device
- Rolled towels or small pillows to support the patient during positioning

PATIENT AND FAMILY EDUCATION

- Assess the patient and family understanding of the lumbar subarachnoid catheter system. *Rationale:* Any necessary clarification may limit anxiety for the patient and family.
- Explain insertion, monitoring, and care involving the lumbar subarachnoid catheter. *Rationale:* Knowledge of expectations can minimize anxiety and encourage questions regarding goals, duration, and expected outcomes of the lumbar subarachnoid catheter.
- Explain to the patient that the nurse will help with position changes so that the drainage system is protected *Rationale:* Prepares the patient for what to expect. This will also decrease the risk of overdrainage which can result in subdural hematoma or 6th nerve palsy.

PATIENT ASSESSMENT AND PREPARATION

Patient Assessment

- Assess the patient's neurological status, including level of consciousness, cranial nerves, sensory and motor function in the upper and lower extremities, vital signs, and bowel and bladder function. *Rationale:* Baseline data are provided.
- The procedure may be performed on an awake patient. *Rationale:* By having the patient awake, this allows the patient to provide feedback in relation to paresthesis and can assist with placement by adjusting positioning; this further allows for ongoing assessments during the procedure, which allows for detection of changes in patient condition.
- Assess the patient's current laboratory profile, including complete blood count, with platelets, partial thromboplastin time, prothrombin time, and international normalized ratio. *Rationale:* Baseline coagulation study results determine the risk for bleeding during and after lumbar subarachnoid catheter insertion.[20,30,35]
- Assess the patient's medication profile. *Rationale:* Recent anticoagulants or antiplatelet agents may increase the risk of bleeding during and after lumbar subarachnoid catheter insertion.
- Assess known allergies. Notify the physician and/or advance practice nurse of allergies. *Rationale:* Usual medications used during the procedure may be contraindicated by allergy.

Patient Preparation

- Verify that the patient is the correct patient using two identifiers. *Rationale:* Before performing a procedure, the nurse should ensure the correct identification of the patient for the intended intervention.
- Ensure that informed consent is obtained. *Rationale:* Informed consent protects the rights of the patient and makes competent decision-making possible for the patient, however, in emergency circumstances, time may not allow for the consent form to be signed.
- Administer preprocedural analgesia or sedation as prescribed. *Rationale:* The patient must be correctly positioned and immobile during lumbar subarachnoid catheter insertion and therefore may need sedation or analgesia to tolerate the procedure.
- Administer preprocedural antibiotics as prescribed. *Rationale:* Prophylactic intravenous antibiotics may reduce the risk of infection for those patients that are at high risk. Prophylactic antibiotics are not recommended for all patients.
- Perform a preprocedure verification and time out, if nonemergent. *Rationale:* Ensures patient safety; Joint Commission's Universal Protocol for Invasive and Surgical Procedures.

Procedure	**for Lumbar Subarachnoid Catheter Insertion (Assist)**		
Steps	**Rationale**	**Special Considerations**	
1. [HH]		Check latest coagulation laboratory works. Ensure the patient is not on a heparin drip. This will decrease the risk of bleeding and complications.	
2. [PE]		All physicians, advanced practice nurses, and other healthcare professionals involved in the procedure need to apply goggles or masks with face shields, caps, sterile gowns, and sterile gloves.	
3. If pressure monitoring is prescribed, assemble a fluid-filled transducer with stopcock and nonvented cap. Using sterile techniques, flush the external standalone transducer with preservative-free sterile normal saline solution. **(Level E*)**	Facilitates monitoring after catheter insertion. Preservative in normal saline solution may cause cortical necrosis.[28]	Do not attach a pressurized intravenous fluid bag to the transducer.	
4. Using sterile techniques, assemble and flush the sterile CSF drainage system compatible with the lumbar subarachnoid catheter device with preservative-free sterile normal saline solution. Ensure the filter located at the top of the drainage chamber does not get wet during priming because this will affect drainage.[11,25] **(Level E)**	Prepares the equipment.	Allowing the CSF to flush the system after insertion of the catheter may allow air in the fluid-filled system, resulting in a damped waveform, inaccurate intraspinal pressure values, and decreased drainage. Priming the drainage system with preservative-free sterile normal saline solution, not CSF, before connecting the system to the lumbar catheter, is recommended.[11] Follow institutional standards. It is of note that some physicians prefer and are trained to allow CSF to flush the system once the drain is connected to the catheter.[30]	
5. Attach the fluid-filled transducer to the CSF drainage system.	Prepares the equipment.	The transducer may be attached to the CSF drainage system before either is primed, and the transducer may be flushed at the same time the CSF drainage system is primed. Ensure that the tail/cable part of the transducer is facing away from the drainage system.	
6. Connect the fluid-filled transducer to the pressure cable and bedside monitor.	Facilitates insertion and immediate lumbar subarachnoid CSF pressure monitoring on insertion.	Ensure that the waveform chosen for CSF monitoring is read on the "mean" setting.	
7. Set the reference line of the drip chamber at the level of the transducer, which is typically at zero reference (Figs. 95-1 and 95-2).	Prepares the CSF drainage system for use.		
8. Level the transducer and the zero reference to the anatomical reference point of the patient as prescribed or as per institutional standards (see Fig. 95-1). **(Level E)**	Ensures accurate readings on which to base therapy.	The anatomical reference point will be determined by the physician and may be the external auditory meatus, shoulder height, or the level of catheter insertion.[28]	

*Level E: Multiple case reports, theory-based evidence from expert opinions, or peer-reviewed professional organizational standards without clinical studies to support recommendations.

Procedure for Lumbar Subarachnoid Catheter Insertion (Assist)—*Continued*		
Steps	**Rationale**	**Special Considerations**

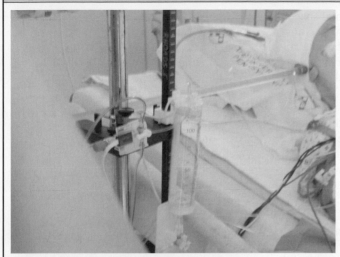

Figure 95-1   Drip chamber at the level of the transducer and the external auditory meatus.

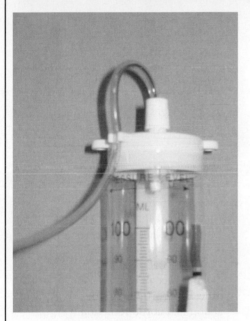

Figure 95-2   Top of the drip chamber with reference line.

9. To zero the system before attaching to the patient, turn the stopcock off to the patient port, remove the nonvented cap on the stopcock, and zero the monitoring system at the anatomical reference point. Replace the sterile nonvented cap. Follow manufacturer's directions.[23] **(Level M*)**	Allows the monitor to use atmospheric pressure as a reference for zero.	The membrane at the top of the drip chamber may allow zeroing without opening the fluid-coupled system to air.
10. Position the reference level of the drip chamber as prescribed.	The relationship of the reference level of the drip chamber to the anatomical reference point alters the rate of CSF drainage.	

*Level M: Manufacturer's recommendations only.

Procedure continues on following page

Procedure	**for Lumbar Subarachnoid Catheter Insertion (Assist)**—*Continued*	
Steps	**Rationale**	**Special Considerations**
11. Assist the patient to a lateral decubitus (side-lying) position with neck, hips, and knees flexed (knees to chest; see Fig. 96-1 and 97-1).[7,8,11,34]	The intervertebral space widens in this position, facilitating the entry of the spinal needle into the subarachnoid space.	The patient may be placed in a sitting position for the procedure, allowing for easier location of midline structures.[8,11,33] In this position the patient can be assessed more readily during the procedure.
12. Assist the physician or advanced practice nurse as needed with cleansing the intended insertion site with antiseptic solution.[10,15,16,31,32] **(Level C*)**	Minimizes the risk for infection and protects the insertion site from recontamination.	The choice of povidone-iodine or chlorhexidine as an antiseptic agent is controversial. Both should be allowed to dry completely. Studies suggest chlorhexidine may be neurotoxic.[18,30,32]
13. Assist as needed with draping the patient with sterile sheets and opening sterile trays.	Prepares for catheter insertion.	
14. Provide supplies as needed during catheter insertion.	Facilitates insertion.	Surgeons may insert the catheter during surgery.
15. Note the opening CSF pressure (initial), color, and clarity.	Provides baseline data.	
16. Assist with the application of an occlusive sterile dressing to the catheter insertion site.	Reduces contamination of the insertion site by microorganisms.	
17. Secure the catheter with tape, with care taken not to alter the catheter position.	Reduces the potential for catheter dislodgment.	Some institutions prefer transparent dressing (e.g., Tegaderm™, Opsite™). This provides visualization of the catheter insertion site.
18. Attach the CSF drainage system to the lumbar drain.		
19. If the intraspinal pressure is to be monitored, turn the stopcock off to the patient and zero the transducer.	Ensures accurate data on which to base therapy.	
20. If intraspinal pressure is to be monitored, observe the waveform morphology, obtain a strip of the waveform, and measure the CSF pressure.	Provides initial baseline data. Confirms correct placement of the catheter.	Lumbar subarachnoid CSF pressure waveform data are similar to traditional intracranial pressure waveform data. Research supports maintenance of an intraspinal pressure of less than 10 mm Hg after thoracic abdominal aortic resection.[2,9,12,25]
21. Position the head of the bed as prescribed. Reassess the level of the transducer, zero reference, and level line of drip chamber. Relevel and rezero as needed. Observe the rate of drainage.	Prevents overdrainage or underdrainage of CSF.	Follow institutional standards and the physician's order (e.g., drain based on volume, level, or specific pressure). Hourly drainage amount is generally 10–20 mL/hr.[34,39] Follow orders regarding when to notify the physician regarding trouble shooting and overdraining.
22. Turn the stopcock to continuously monitor with intermittent drainage or to intermittently monitor with continuous drainage. Set alarm limits. Follow institutional standards and physician orders.	The stopcock must be turned off to the drain to obtain an accurate intraspinal pressure.	Set alarms if continuously monitoring to minimize underdrainage or overdrainage.[10]
23. Discard used supplies in an appropriate receptacle.	Removes and safely discards used supplies; safely removes sharp objects.	
24. 🖐		

---

*Level C: Qualitative studies, descriptive or correlational studies, integrative reviews, systematic reviews, or randomized controlled trials with inconsistent results.

Procedure for Troubleshooting Lumbar Subarachnoid Catheter Insertion (Assist)

Steps	Rationale	Special Considerations
1. **HH**		
2. **PE**		
3. If the CSF waveform is damped:	Damping of the waveform can indicate catheter occlusion or risk for catheter displacement.	Catheter occlusion may result from precipitate in the CSF.
A. Assess the integrity of the lumbar subarachnoid catheter device and correct problems if possible.	Loose connections may cause damped waveforms and increase the risk for infection.	
B. Assess the monitoring system for disconnections and reconnect the system if needed.	Loose cables and connecting devices may contribute to mechanical failure.[28,30]	
C. Assess the level of the transducer, the zero reference point, and the reference line on the drip chamber for the correct position, and readjust the position and rezero if needed (see Figs. 95-1 and 95-2).	The membrane at the top of the drip chamber may allow zeroing without opening the fluid-coupled system to air. However, one-way valves in the drainage system may affect calibration.[23] Also, if the membrane becomes wet, it may no longer permit accurate readings and the drip chamber must be changed.	Changing the drip chamber involves changing the entire CSF drainage system. Responsibility for changing the CSF drainage system varies among institutions and may not be a nursing responsibility in most institutions. Notify the physician or advanced practice nurse for assistance as needed.
D. Assess the lumbar drain site.	The lumbar drain might have migrated or have been pulled accidentally.	Notify physician of a broken, dislodged, or disconnected catheter.
4. Assess for the sudden absence of the pressure waveform or significant changes in pressure measurements without an apparent clinical cause.	Ensures accurate measurement of CSF pressure.[28,39]	Notify the physician or advanced practice nurse if a reversible cause cannot be identified. The CSF drainage system or the catheter may need to be replaced because of catheter dislodgment or blockage.
A. Ensure connections are tight.		
B. Ensure leveling is correct.		
C. Rezero the system.		
5. Assess the flow of CSF through the drainage system by briefly lowering the drip chamber.	Avoids increases in CSF pressure caused by equipment malfunction.[28,39]	Flushing or changing the system may be necessary. Follow institutional standards as to who is responsible for flushing the system.
6. Discard uses supplies.		
7. **HH**		

Procedure for Removal of a Lumbar Subarachnoid Catheter (Assist)

Steps	Rationale	Special Considerations
1. **HH**		Check the latest coagulation laboratory works. Ensure the patient is not on heparin drip.
2. **PE**		Universal personal protection equipment including eye protection should be worn.
3. Assist the physician or advanced practice nurse as needed with removal of the catheter.	Facilitates catheter removal.	Culture the catheter tip as prescribed.

Procedure continues on following page

Procedure | for Removal of a Lumbar Subarachnoid Catheter (Assist)—*Continued*

Steps	Rationale	Special Considerations
4. Apply a sterile occlusive dressing.	Reduces the risk of contamination by microorganisms.	
5. Discard used supplies in an appropriate receptacle.	Removes and safely discards used supplies; safely removes sharp objects.	
6. **HH**		
7. Continue to assess the patient's neurological status and dressing after removal of the catheter for CSF leak.	Removal of the catheter may result in neurological deterioration related to increased CSF pressure. An overt CSF leak may indicate increased CSF pressure.[1,6]	

Expected Outcomes

- Accurate and reliable CSF pressure monitoring
- CSF pressure within the range of 0–15 mm Hg[28] (0–20 cm H_2O)
- Early detection and management of elevated CSF pressure through CSF drainage[1,15,39]
- Resolution of any CSF leak[14,32]
- Resolution of symptoms associated with normal pressure hydrocephalus[5,15]
- Prevention of spinal cord damage or reversal of late-onset symptoms associated with thoracoabdominal aneurysm repair.[2,9,11,12,25]
- Monitor CSF chemistry, cytology physiology
- Drain subarachnoid hematoma blood from CSF; this may decrease risk of vasospasms.[20,26,27]

Unexpected Outcomes

- CSF leak or symptoms associated with excessive drainage[11–13,25]
- CSF infection[16,34]
- Dislodgment or occlusion of the lumbar subarachnoid catheter[32]
- Tension pneumocephalus[1,32]
- Motor function deficits along the myotome distribution of thoracic or lumbar spinal cord[2,9,11,12,25]
- Catheter site pain
- Sensory dysfunction involving dermatome distribution of thoracic or lumbar spinal cord[2,9,11,12,25]
- Bladder or bowel dysfunction[2,9,11,12,25]
- Decreased level of consciousness in association with herniation[1,6]
- Headache
- Subdural hematoma

Patient Monitoring and Care

Steps	Rationale	Reportable Conditions
		These conditions should be reported if they persist despite nursing interventions.
1. Monitor the patient's neurological status and vital signs per physician orders and institutional policy.	Neurological status changes may result from irritation of spinal nerves associated with subarachnoid catheter placement,[3,25,28,39] spinal cord damage related to thoracoabdominal aneurysm repair,[3,6,11,25,28,39] subdural hematoma formation, herniation, or tension pneumocranium resulting from overdrainage of CSF.[1,20,26,32]	• Change in level of consciousness • Change in cranial nerve function • Change in sensation of upper and lower extremities • Change in motor function of upper and lower extremities • Changes in bowel and bladder function • Changes in vital signs
2. Follow institutional standards for assessing pain. Administer analgesia as prescribed.	Identifies need for pain interventions.	• Continued pain despite pain interventions

Patient Monitoring and Care —*Continued*

Steps	Rationale	Reportable Conditions
3. Assess the lumbar subarachnoid CSF waveform and pressure, and the color, clarity, and amount of CSF drainage every hour or as prescribed.	Ensures accurate measurement of CSF pressure and monitoring.[28,39]	• Changes in CSF pressure • Changes in CSF drainage • Changes in the CSF waveform morphology
4. Maintain CSF pressure and drainage as prescribed.	In the management of intraspinal pressure after abdominal aortic aneurysm repair, a CSF pressure of <5 mm Hg is recommended.[2,25,29]	• Abnormal CSF pressure
5. Assess the integrity of the lumbar subarachnoid catheter system at least hourly.	Determines accurate functioning of the system.	• Loose connections or other openings in the catheter system
6. Zero the monitoring system with insertion, disconnection, or position changes; when the values do not fit the clinical picture; and according to institutional standards.	Ensures accuracy of the monitored data.	
7. Assess the insertion site and change the dressing when loose or soiled. Follow institutional standards for dressing changes.	Maintaining an occlusive dressing reduces the risk of infection.	• Signs or symptoms of infection • Significant drainage at the catheter insertion site
8. Continue ongoing assessment of neurological status hourly, as prescribed, or per institutional standards: A. Level of consciousness. B. Cranial nerves. C. Sensation. D. Motor function of lower extremities. E. Bowel and bladder function. F. Comfort level (including headache).	Changes in neurological status or comfort level may indicate dislodgment of the lumbar subarachnoid catheter, spinal cord damage related to thoracoabdominal aneurysm repair, or poorly managed CSF drainage.[28,29,39,41]	• Change in level of consciousness • Change in cranial nerve function • Change in sensation of upper and lower extremities • Change in motor function of upper and lower extremities • Changes in bowel and bladder function • Headache
9. Monitor patient mobility as prescribed to avoid overdrainage or underdrainage.[10,11,20]	Patients may be permitted to sit or ambulate with specific guidelines for placement or clamping of the drainage system.	• Overdrainage or underdrainage with mobility restrictions • Headache
10. Prevent dislodgment of the catheter through ongoing patient education. Ensure that the catheter and drainage system are secured. Provide sedation and analgesia as prescribed.	Catheter dislodgment may result in excessive drainage of CSF.	• Dislodged catheter
11. Change the CSF pressure monitoring and drainage systems aseptically according to institutional standards.	Reduces the risk of infection.	

Procedure continues on following page

Patient Monitoring and Care —*Continued*

Steps	Rationale	Reportable Conditions
12. Obtain or assist with obtaining CSF specimens as prescribed by accessing the sampling port on the CSF drainage system with strict aseptic techniques. Follow institutional standards.	Currently, insufficient data exist to guide or support decisions on the necessary frequency of routine CSF sampling from lumbar subarachnoid catheters.[32]	• Elevated white blood cell (WBC) count • Elevated protein • Decreased glucose in CSF fluid • Positive gram stain • Positive culture and sensitivity • Positive/elevated CSF cytokines (interleukin [IL]–6) may predict bacterial infection earlier than elevated WBC count, elevated protein, and decreased glucose[36,37]
13. Administer antibiotics as prescribed.	Currently, insufficient data are available to guide or support routine prophylactic antibiotic therapy.[10,12,31]	
14. If overdrainage is suspected, clamp the drain, lower the head of the bed,[5,11,16,20,32] and assess neurological status. **(Level E*)** Notify the physician of change of condition and to get any further orders.	The patient may be at increased risk of herniation with overdrainage.	• Change in neurological status and vital signs • Overdrainage

Documentation

Documentation should include the following:
- Completion of informed consent
- Preprocedure verifications and time out
- Insertion site assessment
- Insertion of the lumbar subarachnoid catheter, including opening CSF pressure, any difficulties or abnormalities, and patient tolerance
- CSF description (e.g., clarity, color, characteristics)
- Hourly measurement of CSF pressure and amount of drainage
- Vital signs (intraprocedural) per institutional policy
- Waveform tracing at insertion and with continuous monitoring according to institutional standards
- Description of expected or unexpected outcomes
- Nursing interventions used to treat elevated CSF pressure and expected or unexpected outcomes
- Pain assessment, interventions, and effectiveness

References and Additional Readings

For a complete list of references and additional readings for this procedure, scan this QR code with any freely available smartphone code reader app, or visit http://booksite.elsevier.com/9780323376624.

PROCEDURE

96   Lumbar Puncture (Perform) AP

Susan Chioffi

PURPOSE: A lumbar puncture (LP) is performed for access to the subarachnoid space to obtain a cerebrospinal fluid (CSF) sample, measure CSF pressure, drain CSF, infuse medications or contrast agents, or place a CSF drainage catheter.[1,3,4,7]

PREREQUISITE NURSING KNOWLEDGE

- Knowledge of the anatomy and physiology of the vertebral column, spinal meninges, and CSF circulation, including the location of the lumbar cistern, is needed.
- Technical and clinical competence in performing LPs is necessary.
- Knowledge of sterile technique is needed.
- The presence of meningeal irritation caused by either infectious meningitis or subarachnoid hemorrhage may promote discomfort when the patient is placed in the flexed, lateral decubitus position for the LP.[4-6,18]
- Computed tomography (CT) scan or magnetic resonance imaging supersedes the routine use of LP for many diagnoses.[6,8,19,29]
- Indications for LP include the following[5,6,19,29]:
  - Suspected central nervous system infection
  - Clinical examination results suggestive of subarachnoid hemorrhage accompanied by negative CT scan findings
  - Suspected Guillain-Barré syndrome
  - Suspected multiple sclerosis
  - Intrathecal administration of medications
  - Imaging procedures that require infusion of contrast agents
  - Measurement of CSF pressure
  - CSF drainage in hydrocephalus, pseudotumor cerebri, or CSF fistula
- Contraindications for LP include the following[4,19,29,30]:
  - Increased intracranial pressure (ICP) with mass effect
  - Superficial skin infection localized to the site of entry
  - Bleeding diathesis (relative contraindication)
  - Platelet count less than 50,000/mm[4]
  - International normalized ratio greater than 1.5
  - Anticoagulation therapy (e.g., heparin, warfarin)
- Noncommunicating hydrocephalus
- Infection in the region to be used for LP

- Normal CSF values include the following[19,22,24,29]:
  - Opening pressure, 0 to 15 mm Hg
  - White blood cell count, less than 5/mm
  - Glucose, 60% to 70% of serum blood glucose
  - Protein, 15 to 45 mg/dL
  - Clear colorless appearance
  - Negative culture results
- Recommended CSF tests include the following[19,22,25,29]:
  - Tube #1: Biochemistry:
    - Glucose
    - Protein
    - Protein electrophoresis (if clinically indicated)
  - Tube #2: Bacteriology:
    - Gram stain
    - Bacterial culture
    - Fungal culture (if clinically indicated); requires larger volume
    - Tuberculosis culture (if clinically indicated); requires larger volume
  - Tube #3: Hematology:
    - Cell count
    - Differential
  - Tube #4: Optional studies as indicated:
    - Venereal disease research laboratory test
    - Oligoclonal bands
    - Myelin protein
    - Cytology

EQUIPMENT

- Sterile gloves, caps, masks with eye shields or goggles, and sterile gowns
- Sterile drapes
- Sterile gauze pads
- Antiseptic solution
- Fenestrated drape
- Manometer with three-way stopcock
- Lidocaine, 1% to 2% (without epinephrine)
- 3- to 5-mL syringe
- 20-, 22-, and 25-gauge needles
- 18-, 20-, or 22-gauge spinal needles
- Four numbered capped test tubes
- Adhesive strip or sterile dressing supplies

AP   This procedure should be performed only by physicians, advanced practice nurses, and other healthcare professionals (including critical care nurses) with additional knowledge, skills, and demonstrated competence per professional licensure or institutional standard.

- Specimen labels
- Laboratory forms
- Glucometer/phlebotomy equipment for serum or whole blood glucose
- Lumbar tray (may contain many of the above supplies)

Additional equipment, to have available as needed, includes the following:

- Rolled towels or small pillows to support the patient during positioning
- Alcohol pads or swab sticks
- Two overbed tables (one for the sterile field; one to position the patient, if necessary)

PATIENT AND FAMILY EDUCATION

- Explain the purpose of the LP procedure to the patient and family. *Rationale:* Explanation may decrease patient and family anxiety.
- Explain the need for the patient to remain still and quiet in a lateral decubitus position with the neck, knees, and hips flexed (knees to chest); the axis of the hips vertical; the back close to the edge of the bed; the head of the bed flat; and no more than one pillow under the head (Figs. 96-1 and 97-1). If the LP is not successful in this position, or the patient cannot tolerate this position, explain that the patient may also be positioned leaning over a bedside table or stand.[6,20,23,25] *Rationale:* Patient cooperation during the examination is elicited; the intervertebral space widens in these positions, facilitating entry of the spinal needle into the subarachnoid space.[3,4,6,7]
- Explain that the procedure may produce some discomfort and that local anesthesia will be injected to minimize pain. Also, explain that the patient may receive some mild analgesic and anxiolytic agents as prescribed and needed. *Rationale:* The patient and family are prepared for what to expect.
- Explain that the patient may find it helpful to lie flat for 1 to 4 hours after the LP. *Rationale:* A flat position may promote dural closure; the position was previously thought to reduce the possibility of postprocedure headache, but studies suggest it is not helpful in the prevention of a headache after the procedure.[1,6,13,26]

PATIENT ASSESSMENT AND PREPARATION

Patient Assessment

- Note any pertinent patient history. *Rationale:* An LP is performed to assist with the diagnosis and management of a number of neurological disease processes (see previous indications for LP).
- Obtain a baseline neurological assessment, including assessment for increased ICP, before performing the LP. *Rationale:* Increased ICP during the LP may place the patient at risk for a downward shift in intracranial contents (brain herniation) when the pressure is suddenly released from the lumbar subarachnoid space.[4,19,25,29]
- Assess for coagulopathies, active treatment with heparin or warfarin, local skin infections in close proximity to the site, or pertinent medication allergies. *Rationale:* This assessment identifies potential risks for bleeding, infection, and allergic reactions.[3-6]
- Assess the patient's ability to cooperate with the procedure. *Rationale:* Sudden, uncontrolled movement may result in needle displacement with associated injury or need for reinsertion.
- Identify through history and clinical examination vertebral column deformities or tissue scarring that may interfere with the ability to successfully carry out the procedure. *Rationale:* Scoliosis, lumbar surgery with fusion, and repeated LP procedures may interfere with successful cannulation of the subarachnoid space.[4,23]
- Assess for signs and symptoms of meningeal irritation, which include the following. *Rationale:* A baseline assessment of neurological function is established before the introduction of the needle into the subarachnoid space.
  - ❖ Nuchal rigidity
  - ❖ Photophobia
  - ❖ Brudzinski's or Kernig's sign
  - ❖ Fever
  - ❖ Headache
  - ❖ Nausea or vomiting
  - ❖ Nystagmus

Patient Preparation

- Verify that the patient is the correct patient using two identifiers. *Rationale:* Before performing a procedure, the nurse should ensure the correct identification of the patient for the intended intervention.
- Ensure that the patient and family understand preprocedural teaching. Answer questions as they arise, and reinforce information as needed. *Rationale:* Understanding of previously taught information is evaluated and reinforced.
- Obtain informed consent.[16] *Rationale:* Informed consent protects the rights of the patient and makes competent decision making possible for the patient; however, in emergency circumstances, time may not allow for the consent form to be signed.
- Perform a preprocedure verification and time out, if nonemergent. *Rationale:* Ensures patient safety.
- Obtain the patient's history of allergic reactions. *Rationale:* History can rule out an allergy to lidocaine, the antiseptic solution, and the analgesia or sedation.
- Prescribe an analgesic medication and/or an anxiolytic medication. *Rationale:* These medications may be needed to promote comfort and to decrease anxiety so that positioning can be achieved during the procedure.

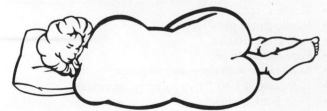

Figure 96-1 The lateral decubitus position appropriate for lumbar puncture. The patient flexes the neck, hips, and knees, and the knees are drawn up tightly to the chest. This increases the intraspinous space for facilitation of needle insertion.

Procedure for Lumbar Puncture (Perform)

Steps	Rationale	Special Considerations
1. **HH**		
2. **PE**		
3. Position or assist the critical care nurse with positioning the patient in the lateral recumbent position near the side of the bed with neck, hips, and knees flexed (knees to chest), head of the bed flat, and no more than one small pillow under the head (see Figs. 96-1 and 97-1). Ask the critical care nurse to assist the patient in attaining and maintaining the position. The critical care nurse should place an arm behind the patient's head and then the other arm around the knees.	The intervertebral space widens in this position, facilitating the entry of the spinal needle into the subarachnoid space.	If the LP is not successful in this position, or the patient cannot tolerate this position, the patient may also be positioned leaning over a bedside table or stand.[4,20,24,26] Also consider performing the LP with fluoroscopy if the patient is morbidly obese or has vertebral column deformities.
4. With the patient in the lateral decubitus position for examination, identify the intervertebral spaces of L3-L4, L4-L5, and L5-S1; the L3-L4 intervertebral space is level with the top of the iliac crests (Fig. 96-2).[4,19] **(Level E*)**	The LP is performed below the level of the conus medullaris, which ends at the L1-L2 in the adult. The most common site used for an LP is the L4-L5 interspace, but the L3-L4 or the L5-S1 interspace may be used when cannulation of the L4-L5 interspace is not possible.[5,6,19,28]	An imaginary vertical line is drawn in the midline through the spinous processes between the two iliac crests. A second line is imagined horizontally at the top of the iliac crests and across the spinous processes by the healthcare provider. These lines should intersect the L3-L4 area, and the puncture can be performed at the L3-L4, L4-L5, or L5-S1 interspace.[4,5]

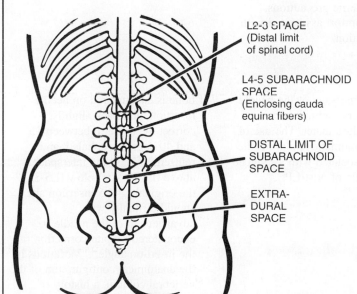

L2-3 SPACE
(Distal limit
of spinal cord)

L4-5 SUBARACHNOID
SPACE
(Enclosing cauda
equina fibers)

DISTAL LIMIT OF
SUBARACHNOID
SPACE

EXTRA-
DURAL
SPACE

Figure 96-2 The body of the spinal cord ends at L2-L3. The region below, L4-L5, encloses the cauda equina (a bundle of lumbar and sacral nerve roots) within the subarachnoid space. It is this area that is appropriate for lumbar puncture.

*Level E: Multiple case reports, theory-based evidence from expert opinions, or peer-reviewed professional organizational standards without clinical studies to support recommendations.

Procedure continues on following page

Procedure for Lumbar Puncture (Perform)—*Continued*

Steps	Rationale	Special Considerations
5. Remove **PE**, wash hands, and apply sterile gowns and gloves.	Minimizes the risk of infection; maintains sterile precautions.	
6. Set up a sterile field on the bedside stand. A. Preassemble the manometer, attaching the three-way stopcock; set it to the side. B. Open the test tubes and place them in order of use in the tray slots. C. Draw approximately 3 mL of 1% lidocaine with a 20-gauge needle. Change to a 25-gauge needle for a superficial injection; change to a 22-gauge, 1.5-inch needle for a deeper injection.[4,6,8,29]	Prepares equipment for use in the procedure.	Have the critical care nurse or assistant prepare the numbered labels for the test tubes; ensure that the tubes are labeled in the order in which they are filled, to facilitate laboratory differentiation of a traumatic tap versus a subarachnoid hemorrhage.[4,21]
7. Cleanse the skin over the L4-L5 puncture site, including one intervertebral space above and below the site with the antiseptic solution.[11,12,17,18] **(Level C*)**	Reduces transmission of microorganisms and minimizes the risk of infection.	The choice of povidone-iodine or chlorhexidine as an antiseptic agent is controversial. Both should be allowed to dry completely. Some physicians, advanced practice nurses, and other healthcare professionals have found chlorhexidine to be safe in practice,[26] although other studies have suggested chlorhexidine is neurotoxic.[11,18]
8. Drape the patient with exposure of the insertion site.	Minimizes the risk of infection; maintains sterile precautions.	
9. Administer a local anesthetic with a 25-gauge needle, raising a wheal in the skin. Inject a small amount into the posterior spinous region with a 22-gauge needle.[6,29]	Reduces discomfort associated with needle insertion.	
10. Insert a 22-, 20-, or 18-gauge spinal needle bevel up[9] through the skin into the intervertebral space of L4-L5, with the needle at an angle of 15 degrees cephalad, aiming toward the umbilicus and level with the sagittal midplane of the body.[4,19] **(Level E*)**	Facilitates the passage of the needle between intervertebral spaces toward the dura mater. The use of a smaller atraumatic spinal needle has been associated with a reduced incidence rate of post-LP headache.[9,10,14,15,30]	If bone is encountered on needle insertion, pull back slightly, correct the angle to between 15 and 40 degrees cephalad, and reinsert.[5,6,29] Use the interspace above (L3-L4) or below (L5-S1) the original L4-L5 insertion site should difficulty with advancement of the needle be encountered despite correction of the insertion angle.[4,5] Variations in the anatomical configuration of the vertebral column, a history of vertebral column surgery, or repeat LPs may necessitate needle insertion at a different level.[4]

*Level C: Qualitative studies, descriptive or correlational studies, integrative reviews, systematic reviews, or randomized controlled trials with inconsistent results.
*Level E: Multiple case reports, theory-based evidence from expert opinions, or peer-reviewed professional organizational standards without clinical studies to support recommendations.

Procedure	**for Lumbar Puncture (Perform)—*Continued***	
Steps	**Rationale**	**Special Considerations**
11. Once the needle has been advanced approximately 3–4 cm, withdraw the stylet, and check the hub for CSF. If CSF is not present, replace the stylet and advance slightly. Once CSF is draining, advance the needle another 1–2 mm.[4,19] **(Level E*)**	In most adults, a 3–4-cm insertion depth is sufficient to enter the subarachnoid space.	A "popping" sensation is often associated with penetration of the dura mater.[4,6,19]
12. Attach the stopcock of the manometer to the needle. Have the patient straighten his or her legs and relax his or her position. Measure the opening pressure, and note the color of the fluid in the manometer.[4,19] **(Level E*)**	Flexing the legs or straining to maintain a position may artificially elevate the CSF pressure.[4,8,19] Opening pressure or normal CSF pressure measurements taken at the lumbar area range from 0–20 cm H_2O (0–15 mm Hg or 50–150 mm H_2O).	If the patient was sitting on the side of the bed leaning over the bedside table for the LP, have the patient lie down on his or her side for the CSF pressure measurement.[5]

13. Consider performing the Queckenstedt test.
  A. Ask the critical care nurse to simultaneously compress the jugular veins for 10 seconds, if not contraindicated and within institutional policy for the critical care nurse to perform.
  B. Watch for a change in subarachnoid CSF pressure on the manometer.[6,18]
	The Queckenstedt test is used if an obstruction in the spinal subarachnoid space is suspected. A normal response indicates that the pathway between the skull and the lumbar needle is patent. This maneuver is contraindicated in patients with known or suspected elevated ICP; a sudden release of CSF pressure distally can result in herniation.[6,19]	Normal findings reflect a sharp increase in spinal subarachnoid CSF pressure on compression of the jugular veins; on release, pressure returns to precompression levels. A lack of change in CSF pressure indicates an obstruction of CSF flow. The Queckenstedt test is contraindicated in patients with increased ICP.[6,19]

14. Obtain laboratory samples:
  A. Position the first test tube over the stopcock port.
  B. Turn the stopcock and drain CSF from the manometer into the first test tube.
  C. Continue filling test tubes from the hub of the spinal needle; a minimum of 1–2 mL CSF should be collected in each of the first three test tubes. The second and fourth test tubes may require up to 8 mL CSF depending on the tests ordered (e.g., fungal or tuberculosis testing).[5,6]
  D. Return the stopcock to the off position and discard the manometer.
	By draining CSF from the manometer into the test tubes, the CSF volume withdrawn is minimized.[4,6] Allows for progressive clearing of CSF blood in the case of a traumatic tap.[5,6,25,29]	In subarachnoid hemorrhage, CSF with the same consistency of blood is drained in all four test tubes. In the case of a traumatic tap, progressive clearing of bloody CSF occurs as drainage continues. Also, the supernatant of centrifuged CSF should be clear if the tap was traumatic and xanthochromic if blood has been present for several hours and has undergone hemolysis.[5,6,25,29]

*Level E: Multiple case reports, theory-based evidence from expert opinions, or peer-reviewed professional organizational standards without clinical studies to support recommendations.

Procedure continues on following page

Procedure for Lumbar Puncture (Perform)—*Continued*		
Steps	**Rationale**	**Special Considerations**
15. Cover the opening of the needle with a sterile gloved finger. Replace the stylet and withdraw the needle.[1,4,8] **(Level E*)**	Covering the opening of the needle with a sterile gloved finger reduces the contamination by microorganisms. Replacing the stylet before withdrawing the needle prevents unnecessary CSF loss and facilitates needle withdrawal without traction on the spinal nerve roots. Reinsertion of the stylet before withdrawal of the spinal needle has also been associated with a reduced incidence rate of post-LP headaches.[7,9,14,30]	Minimizes post procedure headache.[1,3,4] If a lumbar subarachnoid catheter is inserted, refer to Procedure 95.
16. Apply an occlusive sterile dressing to the puncture site.	Decreases the incidence of infection.	
17. Place the patient in a supine or prone position immediately after the procedure.[1,6] **(Level E*)**	In the supine position, the patient's weight acts as site pressure. In the prone position, the increased abdominal pressure transmits pressure to the site.[27] Some physicians, advanced practice nurses, and other healthcare professionals advocate placing the patient in a supine or prone position for 1–4 hours.[1,2,6]	Whether either the prone or supine position facilitates closure of the dura mater after the LP remains unclear. Neither the supine nor prone position has been shown to prevent postdural puncture headaches.[1,4,5,27]
18. Label and send specimens to the laboratory. If there is no same-day serum glucose measurement, consider obtaining a serum glucose sample.	Obtains CSF analysis and assists with the differential diagnosis.[5,19,25,29]	Hyperglycemia or hypoglycemia affects CSF glucose values and can interfere with interpretation of results.[6,19,25,29]
19. Discard used supplies in appropriate receptacles.	Removes and safely discards used supplies; safely removes sharp objects.	
20. **HH**		

*Level E: Multiple case reports, theory-based evidence from expert opinions, or peer-reviewed professional organizational standards without clinical studies to support recommendations.

Expected Outcomes

- Determination of the characteristics of the CSF that supports establishment of the diagnosis
- Recommendation for definitive treatment that promotes restoration of health or optimal functional status
- Postprocedure headache may occur in up to 70% of patients undergoing LP and is usually self-limiting[9,10,14,19]; the incidence of headache may be reduced with the use of smaller-gauge spinal needles and reinsertion of the stylet before the needle is withdrawn[4,7,14,15,19,30]
- No change in neurological status after the procedure

Unexpected Outcomes

- In cases of a supratentorial mass or severely elevated ICP, a shift in intracranial contents (brain herniation) may be promoted by the sudden decrease in pressure incurred with LP[4,6,19,25]
- Injury of the periosteum or spinal ligaments may produce local back pain[6,27]
- Infectious meningitis may result from an improper technique that produces contamination[5,6,18,19]
- Traumatic taps may result from inadvertent puncture of the spinal venous plexuses; usually this is a self-limiting process, but it may result in a hematoma in patients with bleeding disorders[4-6,29]
- Transient lower-extremity pain may occur from irritation of a spinal nerve[6,29]
- Persistent CSF leak from the puncture site associated with nonclosure of the dura[4,13]
- Inability to obtain a CSF specimen because of healthcare provider skill level, patient intolerance of the procedure, pathological blockage of CSF flow, or aberrant anatomy[4]
- Persistent headache despite interventions[4,13-15]

Patient Monitoring and Care

Steps	Rationale	Reportable Conditions
		These conditions should be reported if they persist despite nursing interventions.
1. Monitor the patient's neurological status, including the development of a change in level of consciousness, pupil size and reactivity, new onset of pain, motor weakness, or numbness in the lower extremities, and the patient's procedural tolerance throughout and after the procedure.	Changes in neurological status may be related to sudden intracranial decompression with brain herniation or local irritation of a spinal nerve by the needle or hematoma formation at the puncture site.[3-5,18]	• Deterioration in neurological status • Transient lower-extremity motor or sensory changes associated with spinal nerve irritation or hematoma formation
2. Monitor for postprocedure headache.	Headache occurs in up to 70% of patients after an LP.[9,10,27,29]	• Intractable postprocedure headache
3. Monitor for drainage from the puncture site.	Persistent drainage may indicate an unresolved CSF leak.[1,19,27]	• Drainage from the LP site • Dural tear that necessitates a patch or closure
4. Monitor the patient's neurological status at a minimum of every 4 hours for 24 hours after the LP.	Lower extremity motor or sensory changes may indicate a hematoma at the puncture site.[19]	• Spinal hematoma that necessitates emergent surgical evacuation
5. Monitor the effectiveness of measures taken to prevent or treat postprocedure headache.[14]	Determines level of comfort.	• Unrelieved headache
6. Follow institutional standards for assessing pain. Consider administration of a mild analgesic agent and encourage the patient to remain supine or prone until the headache improves.	Additional treatment measures may be necessary to manage postprocedure headache.[24] Although recent studies do not support either the prone or supine position to prevent postdural puncture headache, lying in one of these positions may relieve the headache once it develops.[1,7,9,13,30]	• Intractable postprocedure headache • Dural tear that necessitates patch[10,12,28] or closure[27]

Procedure continues on following page

Documentation

Documentation Should Include the Following:
- Patient and family education
- Completion of informed consent
- Preprocedure verifications and timeout
- Performance of the procedure, significant findings, CSF appearance, and opening pressure
- Amount of CSF removed
- Patient tolerance of the procedure

- Change in neurological status associated with the procedure
- CSF specimens obtained
- Pain assessment, interventions, and effectiveness
- Unexpected outcomes
- Additional interventions

References and Additional Readings

For a complete list of references and additional readings for this procedure, scan this QR code with any freely available smartphone code reader app, or visit http://booksite.elsevier.com/9780323376624.

PROCEDURE

97

Lumbar Puncture (Assist)

Susan Chioffi

PURPOSE: A lumbar puncture (LP) is performed for access to the subarachnoid space to obtain a cerebrospinal fluid (CSF) sample, measure CSF pressure, drain CSF, infuse medications or contrast agents, or place a CSF drainage catheter.[1,3,4,8]

PREREQUISITE NURSING KNOWLEDGE

- Knowledge of neuroanatomy and physiology is needed.
- LP at L3-L4 or L4-L5 in an adult is usually performed to obtain a CSF sample.[19]
- Indications for LP are as follows:
  - ❖ CSF analysis may be indicated in the differential diagnosis of subarachnoid hemorrhage, central nervous system infection, central nervous system autoimmune processes, and some malignant diseases.[5,6,17,26]
  - ❖ Therapeutically, an LP may be used to treat hydrocephalus, CSF fistulas, and pseudotumor cerebri; to deliver medications or contrast material into the subarachnoid space; or to access the subarachnoid space for placement of a lumbar subarachnoid drain.[5,6,19,27]
- Contraindications for LPs are as follows[5,19,26,27]:
  - ❖ LPs are contraindicated if the patient has a known or suspected intracranial mass or elevated intracranial pressure (ICP), noncommunicating hydrocephalus, or infection in the region to be used for LP, or is coagulopathic or therapeutically anticoagulated. If CSF analysis is necessary, the patient may need pretreatment with fresh frozen plasma, platelets, cryoprecipitate, or the specific factor needed to correct a hematologic abnormality.[6,19,26,27]
  - ❖ LPs are cautioned against in patients suspected of aneurysmal subarachnoid hemorrhage and in patients with complete spinal blocks. In such cases, an LP may be performed if the computed tomographic scan of the patient's head does not indicate signs of increased ICP, such as significant cerebral swelling, hematoma, intracranial tissue shifts, or herniation.[6,19,26,27]
  - ❖ Brain herniation may occur after punctures in the presence of an intracranial mass lesion or increased ICP.[4,19]
- The preferred positioning for an LP is lateral decubitus with the neck, hips, and knees flexed (knees to chest); the axis of the hips vertical; the back close to the edge of the bed; the head of the bed flat; and no more than a small pillow under the head (see Figs. 96-1 and 97-1).[20] If the LP is not successful in this position, or if the patient cannot tolerate this position, the patient may also be positioned sitting on the side of the bed, leaning over a bedside table or stand.[20,22,23,27] This procedure may also be per-

formed with fluoroscopy for patients with marked obesity or spinal deformities. Optimal positioning is necessary to avoid the risk for a "dry tap" or an unsuccessful puncture attempt. Repeated attempts at puncture increase the risk for infection and patient discomfort.[4,19]
- Proper positioning for an LP widens the interspinous process space and facilitates the passage of the needle.[3,4,6,7]

EQUIPMENT

- Sterile gloves, caps, masks with eye shield, and sterile gowns
- Sterile drapes
- Sterile gauze pads
- Antiseptic solution
- Fenestrated drape
- Manometer with a three-way stopcock
- Lidocaine, 1% to 2% (without epinephrine)
- 3- to 5-mL syringe
- 18-, 20-, 22-, and 25-gauge needles
- 18-, 20-, or 22-gauge spinal needles
- Four consecutively numbered, capped test tubes
- Adhesive strip or sterile dressing supplies
- Specimen labels
- Laboratory forms
- Glucometer/phlebotomy supplies for concurrent testing of serum or whole blood glucose
- Lumbar tray (some of the supplies above will be in the tray)

Additional equipment, to have available as needed, includes the following:
- Alcohol pads or swab sticks
- Two overbed tables (one for the sterile field; one to position the patient, if necessary)
- Rolled towels or small pillows to support the patient during positioning

PATIENT AND FAMILY EDUCATION

- Explain the purpose of the procedure to the patient and family. *Rationale:* Understanding of the procedure is reinforced, and anxiety may be decreased.
- Explain positioning requirements for the LP. *Rationale:* Cooperation with positioning requirements facilitates the procedure.

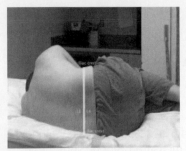

Figure 97-1 Proper positioning of the patient for a lumbar puncture. *(From Ellenby MS, Tegtmeyer K, Lai S, et al: Lumbar puncture, N Engl J Med 355:e12, 2006. Copyright © 2006, Massachusetts Medical Society. All rights reserved.)*

- Explain that the procedure may cause some mild discomfort; the patient will receive local anesthesia and may also receive some mild analgesia and an anxiolytic. ***Rationale:*** This lets the patient know what to expect.

PATIENT ASSESSMENT AND PREPARATION

Patient Assessment

- Obtain vital signs. ***Rationale:*** Baseline values for the patient are established.
- Perform a neurological assessment, including level of consciousness, pupil size and reactivity, and motor and sensory function. ***Rationale:*** Baseline neurological function is established before the insertion of a needle into the proximity of sensitive neurological tissue.
- Assess for signs and symptoms of increased ICP. ***Rationale:*** Increased ICP during the LP may place the patient at risk for a downward shift in intracranial contents (brain herniation) when the pressure is suddenly released from the lumbar subarachnoid space.
- Assess the patient's current laboratory profile, including complete blood cell count, platelets, prothrombin time, partial thromboplastin time, bleeding time, and international

normalized ratio. ***Rationale:*** Baseline values are established, and any coagulopathies that necessitate intervention before the cisternal or LP are identified.
- Assess for signs and symptoms of meningeal irritation, including the following. ***Rationale:*** Baseline neurological function is established before introduction of a needle into the subarachnoid space.
  - ❖ Nuchal rigidity
  - ❖ Photophobia
  - ❖ Brudzinski's sign (flexion of the knee in response to flexion of the neck)
  - ❖ Kernig's sign (pain in the hamstrings on extension of the knee with the hip at 90-degree flexion)
  - ❖ Fever
  - ❖ Headache
  - ❖ Nausea or vomiting
  - ❖ Nystagmus
- Assess for allergies to local anesthetic, antiseptic, and any analgesic or sedative medications. ***Rationale:*** Risk of allergic reaction is decreased.[3-6]

PATIENT PREPARATION

- Verify that the patient is the correct patient using two identifiers. ***Rationale:*** Before performing a procedure, the nurse should ensure the correct identification of the patient for the intended intervention.
- Ensure that the patient and family understand preprocedural teaching. Answer questions as they arise, and reinforce information as needed. ***Rationale:*** Understanding of previously taught information is evaluated and reinforced.
- Ensure that informed consent is obtained.[16] ***Rationale:*** Informed consent protects the rights of the patient and makes competent decision making possible for the patient; however, in emergency circumstances, time may not allow for the consent form to be signed.
- Perform a preprocedure verification and time out, if nonemergent. ***Rationale:*** Ensures patient safety.

Procedure	**for Lumbar Puncture (Assist)**	
Steps	**Rationale**	**Special Considerations**
1. **HH**		
2. **PE**		
3. Ensure that the patient is in the proper lateral decubitus position, near the side of the bed with the neck, hips, and knees flexed (knees to chest). The head of the bed should be flat, and no more than one small pillow should be under the head (see Figs. 96-1 and 97-1). If difficulty is encountered, an alternative position is to have the patient sit on the edge of the bed, leaning over the bed table.[4,20,27]	The intervertebral space widens in this position, facilitating the entry of the spinal needle into the subarachnoid space.	For LPs, to help the patient maintain this position, an arm can be placed behind the patient's head and then the other arm around the knees. If difficulty is encountered, an alternative position is to have the patient sit on the edge of the bed, leaning over the bed table (see Fig. 97-1).[4,20,27]

Procedure for Lumbar Puncture (Assist)—*Continued*

Steps	Rationale	Special Considerations
4. Administer analgesia and/or anxiolytic medications as prescribed.	May be needed to facilitate positioning of the patient and to relieve anxiety.	
5. Apply goggles or masks with face shields, caps, sterile gowns, and sterile gloves.	Minimizes the risk of infection; maintains aseptic and sterile precautions.	
6. Assist as needed with skin preparation with antiseptic solution.[11,12,17,18] **(Level C*)**	Reduces microorganisms and helps prevent infection.	The use of povidone-iodine versus chlorhexidine as an antiseptic solution before LP is controversial. Chlorhexidine may be neurotoxic. Allowing the site to air dry increases the effectiveness of antiseptic solutions and minimizes contact with nervous system tissue.[11,12,17,18]
7. Assist as needed with the application of sterile drapes.	Decreases the risk for contamination and provides a sterile field for the procedure.	
8. Assist if needed in identifying the appropriate anatomical site for puncture.	The LP in an adult is performed below the level of L3 to prevent damage to the spinal cord (the body of the spinal cord ends at L2-L3).	An imaginary line is drawn vertically between the iliac crests, and a second line is imagined horizontally at the top of the spinous processes. These lines should intersect the L3-L4 area, and the puncture can be performed here or one level below at the L4-L5 interspace.[3,4]
9. Assist with the preparation of local anesthesia as needed. Hold medication vials as needed for removal of local anesthetic to assist the provider in maintaining sterile technique.	Prevents or decreases the pain from the needle insertion.	
10. Once the needle is in place, instruct the patient to relax and breathe normally, and to avoid holding his or her breath. Assist the patient to straighten his or her legs when indicated by the provider.[4,8,19] **(Level E*)**	Increased muscle tension or intrathoracic pressure may falsely elevate CSF pressure.[4,8,19]	Patients undergoing LP may also straighten their legs because leg flexion can increase intrathoracic pressure.[4,8,19]
11. With aseptic technique, assist with holding the manometer in place when it is attached to the spinal needle via a three-way stopcock.	Secures the position of the manometer.	

*Level C: Qualitative studies, descriptive or correlational studies, integrative reviews, systematic reviews, or randomized controlled trials with inconsistent results.
*Level E: Multiple case reports, theory-based evidence from expert opinions, or peer-reviewed professional organizational standards without clinical studies to support recommendations.

Procedure continues on following page

Procedure	**for Lumbar Puncture (Assist)—*Continued***	
Steps	**Rationale**	**Special Considerations**
12. Assist with obtaining the CSF pressure measurement.	Opening pressure or normal CSF pressure measurements taken at the lumbar area range from 0–20 cm H_2O (0–15 mm Hg or 50–150 mm H_2O). The opening pressure in a traumatic tap is within normal limits, compared with the opening pressure in patients with subarachnoid hemorrhage and meningitis.	The meniscus should show minimal fluctuation related to pulse and respiration.
13. Assist as needed in performing the Queckenstedt test, if not contraindicated or prohibited by institutional policy, by simultaneously compressing the jugular veins for 10 seconds while observing for a change in subarachnoid CSF pressure on the manometer.[6,19] Follow institutional policy regarding who may perform the Queckenstedt test.	The Queckenstedt test is used if an obstruction in the spinal subarachnoid space is suspected. A normal response indicates that the pathway between the skull and the lumbar needle is patent. This maneuver is contraindicated in patients with known or suspected elevated ICP; a sudden release of CSF pressure distally can result in herniation.[5,18]	Normally, a rapid increase in CSF pressure occurs with resultant decrease when compression is released. If a complete or partial spinal block exists, the level does not rise, or it rises slowly, and remains elevated when the jugular veins are released. No increase in CSF pressure may be caused by improper needle placement.[6,19]
14. Assist with the collection of CSF specimens as needed: A. Assist in stabilizing the manometer with one hand. B. Assist with the handoff of each tube as needed (if not placed upright and in order in the LP tray). Tighten the cap of each tube.	Obtains needed CSF specimens.	
15. Label each tube in order of collection with the type of specimen, patient name, and the order in which the specimen was collected (i.e., "#1 of 3").	Differentiates between subarachnoid hemorrhage and traumatic tap by evaluating each numbered specimen.[5,6,23,26]	Red blood cell (RBC) dissipation through consecutive samples is indicative of a traumatic tap; consistent RBC presence is indicative of a subarachnoid hemorrhage. Also, the supernatant of centrifuged CSF should be clear if the tap was traumatic and xanthochromic if blood has been present for several hours and has undergone hemolysis.[5,6,23,26]
16. Obtain a serum or whole blood glucose value from the patient as prescribed.	Allows for comparison of the serum glucose value and the CSF glucose concentration. A normal CSF glucose value is approximately two thirds of the blood glucose value.[20,21]	Hyperglycemia increases CSF glucose concentration, and hypoglycemia decreases CSF glucose concentration. Either may interfere with the interpretation of the CSF results.[5,6,19,23,26]

Procedure	**for Lumbar Puncture (Assist)—*Continued***	
Steps	Rationale	Special Considerations
17. Assist the patient to a supine or prone position.[1,5] **(Level E*)**	In the supine position, the patient's weight acts as site pressure. In the prone position, the increased abdominal pressure transmits pressure to the site.[24] Some clinicians advocate placing the patient in a supine or prone position for 1–4 hours.[2,9,10,13,15]	Whether either the prone or supine position facilitates closure of the dura mater after the LP remains unclear. Neither the supine or prone position has been shown to prevent postdural puncture headache.[2,4,7,24]
18. Observe the puncture site, dressing, and linen for CSF leakage or bleeding. Reinforce the dressing as needed.	May indicate continued CSF loss after the procedure. Drainage after LP from the insertion site should be minimal.	
19. Discard used supplies in an appropriate receptacle.	Removes and safely discards used supplies; safely removes sharp objects.	
20. **HH**		
21. Send the specimens to the laboratory.	Ensures the specimens are sent for laboratory analysis.	

*Level E: Multiple case reports, theory-based evidence from expert opinions, or peer-reviewed professional organizational standards without clinical studies to support recommendations.

Expected Outcomes

- LP completed
- CSF samples and results obtained
- Patient's vital signs and level of consciousness stable before, during, and after the procedure
- No change or deterioration in neurological examination
- Puncture site clean and dry
- No headache, neck stiffness, local pain at puncture site, leg spasms, or elevated temperature related to the procedure

Unexpected Outcomes

- Significant change in vital signs (respiratory changes, bradycardia, and increased systolic blood pressure)
- Change or deterioration in neurological status (signs of brain herniation, which may include a decrease in the level of consciousness, pupil changes, and motor or sensory impairment)[4,6,19,23]
- Inability to void spontaneously (if able to before procedure)
- Abnormal CSF results
- CSF not obtained or inability to complete procedure
- Prolonged headache, stiff neck, photophobia, and an acute increase in temperature related to the procedure[5,6,18,19]
- Excessive drainage at the puncture site[14,15]
- Persistent headache or low back pain despite interventions
- New and persistent symptoms of pain, numbness, tingling, weakness, or paralysis in the lower extremities[4-6,26]
- Spinal or paraspinal abscess
- Hematoma formation[4-6,26]
- Implantation of epidermal tumors[5]
- Vasovagal syncope
- Seizure
- Pneumocephalus

Procedure continues on following page

Patient Monitoring and Care

Steps	Rationale	Reportable Conditions
		These changes should be reported if they persist despite nursing interventions.
1. Monitor the patient's neurological, respiratory, and cardiovascular status during the procedure.	Pain or abnormal sensation radiating down one or both legs may result from spinal nerve irritation, which may necessitate a change in patient or needle position. Respiratory depression or an altered level of consciousness may result from brain herniation[3-5,20] or analgesia and sedation.	• Respiratory depression • Changes in level of consciousness • Pupil changes • Motor or sensory changes • Change in vital signs • Bowel or bladder dysfunction
2. Assess vital signs and perform systematic neurological assessments every 15 minutes for the first hour, every 30 minutes twice, then every hour for the next 4 hours, and at a minimum of every 4 hours for the following 24 hours after the procedure.	A change in vital signs or neurological assessment could indicate brain herniation, acute hematoma formation at the insertion site, injury to a spinal nerve, or infection.[4,5,19,20]	• Change in vital signs • Changes in level of consciousness • Pupil changes • Motor or sensory changes
3. Monitor the needle puncture site.	Identifies complications at the site.	• Persistent bleeding at the site • Drainage of clear serous fluid
4. Monitor the patient for headache or back or leg pain or discomfort. Follow the institutional standards for assessing pain. Administer analgesia as prescribed.	Identifies traumatic complications of needle placement. Identifies need for management of discomfort.	• Severe, persistent back or leg pain not evident before the procedure • Inability to manage pain • Persistent headache despite interventions[2]
5. Instruct the patient to remain supine or prone in bed for 1–4 hours or for the length of time prescribed.[10,13-15] **(Level E*)**	In the supine position, the patient's weight acts as site pressure. In the prone position, the increased abdominal pressure transmits pressure to the site.[25] Some physicians, advanced practice nurses, and other healthcare professionals advocate placing the patient in a supine or prone position for 1–4 hours.[2,6,7,24]	• Unrelieved headache
6. Ensure adequate oral or intravenous fluid intake.[2,6,24]	May facilitate repletion of CSF.	• Intravascular fluid overload or deficit

*Level E: Multiple case reports, theory-based evidence from expert opinions, or peer-reviewed professional organizational standards without clinical studies to support recommendations.

Documentation

Documentation should include the following:
• Patient and family education
• Completion of informed consent
• Preprocedure verifications and time out
• Date and time of procedure
• Opening pressure
• Status of puncture site
• Specimens sent to the laboratory for analysis
• Amount and character of CSF collected
• CSF laboratory results
• Patient's baseline vital signs and neurological assessment and tolerance of procedure
• Pain assessment, interventions, and effectiveness
• Any unexpected outcomes
• Additional interventions

References and Additional Readings

For a complete list of references and additional readings for this procedure, scan this QR code with any freely available smartphone code reader app, or visit http://booksite.elsevier.com/9780323376624.

98 Pupillometer

DaiWai M. Olson and John C. Bazil

PURPOSE: The pupillometer is a noninvasive, handheld device that is used to provide an objective measurement of the pupils before and after a light stimulus, as well as the pupillary reactivity to light. The pupillometer is capable of providing automated measurement of one pupil at a time and therefore may not be an adequate substitute for evaluating the presence of anisocoria (unequal pupils). However, after completing paired measurements of both pupils within 30 seconds, the device displays data that allow for comparison of pupillary size and reaction.

PREREQUISITE NURSING KNOWLEDGE

- A fundamental understanding of the neuroanatomy and function of the optic cranial nerve (CN II) and the oculomotor cranial nerve (CN III) provides clinical correlates for interpreting the outcome of readings obtained with the pupillometer.[1,2]
  - ❖ The pupil is an opening in the center of the iris of the eye. Light passes through the pupil to the lens where images are reversed before going through the vitreous humor to the rods and cones embedded throughout the retina.
  - ❖ Images are then converted into electrical signals that travel along the optic cranial nerve (CN II) to the optic chiasm, optic tracts, and lateral geniculate nucleus where the images are sorted and then relayed to the visual cortex in the occipital lobe.
  - ❖ The size and shape of the pupil determines the amount of light that can enter the eye. The intrinsic muscles in the iris (sphincter pupillae and dilator pupillae) control the size and shape of the eye. The pupillary light reflex is a brisk, protective mechanism (reflex) that triggers the intrinsic muscles in the iris to contract and thereby decrease the size of the pupil and reduce the amount of light reaching the retina. Testing the pupillary light reflex evaluates components of the second and third cranial nerve (Fig. 98-1).[2] The electrical signal created from light entering the eye travels along CN II (afferent) to the Edinger-Westphal nucleus and triggers an efferent signal to travel along CN III from the Edinger-Westphal nucleus to the intrinsic muscles of both eyes (OU). Thus a normal response to light entering either eye is OU pupil constriction.[3]
  - ❖ The modern pupillometer is a handheld device that uses video recording to analyze the size and reactivity of the pupil to light.[4]
  - ❖ Proper equipment assembly of the pupillometer requires attaching an aseptic SmartGuard to the device with the knowledge that each device is assigned to and linked with a single patient. The neuropupillary index (NPi) is based on a collection of pupil measurements conducted on a healthy control population.[5] All variables representing the pupil dynamics were used to create a multidimensional, normative model. These variables are the maximum size, the latency, the constriction (average and maximum), and the dilation velocity (Fig. 98-2). The NPi quantifies the distance between the single measurement and the model. A normal NPi is >3.0. An index equal to or above 3 indicates that the pupil measurement falls within the boundaries of the NPi model and is defined as normal. A score below 3 means the reflex falls outside the boundaries and is defined as abnormal—that is, weaker than a normal pupil response as defined by the NPi model. The NPi is reported as zero when no constriction is detected. An NPi less than 3 may be reflective of increasing intracranial pressure.[6]
  - ❖ The constriction velocity is measured in mm/sec and calculated as the amount of constriction (size change) divided by the duration (time in seconds) during which the pupil remains constricted. There are medications with known effects on the pupillary response. Alcohol (EtOH) and opioids will generally cause a constriction of the pupil whereas atropine, amphetamines, and many hallucinogens (e.g., psilocybin [mushrooms], LSD) will cause pupillary dilation. It is important to remember that the medication's influence will occur in both pupils. If a patient has had a recent ophthalmological examination, determine whether specific anticholinergic medications such as cyclopentolate (Cyclogyl) have been used to dilate the pupils.[7]
  - ❖ The presence of cataracts, or a history of cataract surgery, may influence pupillary reactivity.

EQUIPMENT

- Nonsterile gloves
- Pupillometer device (Fig. 98-3A)
- Pupillometer docking station (see Fig. 98-3A)
- Pupillometer SmartGuard (see Fig. 98-3B)

Additional equipment to integrate data into an Electronic Medical Record (EMR)
- Pupillometer Scanner
- Pupillometer Reader

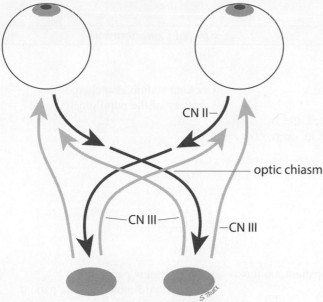

Figure 98-1 CN II and CN III pathways to Edinger-Westphal nuclei.

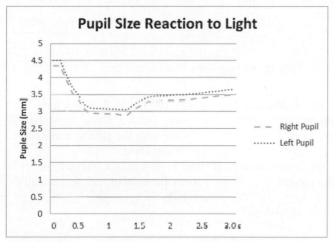

Figure 98-2 Graphic representation of the pupillary light reflex and variables used to calculate the NPi for the left and right pupils.

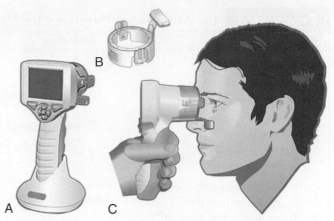

Figure 98-3 NPi-200 Pupillometer shown in docking (**A**) and with SmartGuard (**B**) attached and being held in proper position (**C**) with pad of SmartGuard on zygomatic bone (cheekbone).

- Provide patient and family teaching explaining how the pupillary examination will be completed. *Rationale:* A bright light is used to examine the pupils and may startle or frighten a patient/family if prior instruction is not provided.

PATIENT AND FAMILY EDUCATION

- Explain the purpose of serial neurological assessment to the patient and family. *Rationale:* The pupillary examination is a key assessment element performed during serial neurological examinations.
- Provide education that the pupillometer is an automated assessment device that will be used to track how fast the patient's pupils respond to light. *Rationale:* Assessing pupils is a standard component of the neurological examination. However, patient and family may be unfamiliar with automated pupil assessment.

PATIENT ASSESSMENT AND PREPARATION

Patient Assessment

- Assess patient and family understanding of information. *Rationale:* Provides an opportunity to clarify information, answer questions, and possibly reduce fear and anxiety associated with a device being used near the face and eyes.
- Assess the patient's ability to maintain eye opening. *Rationale:* The patient must maintain eye opening. If the patient is unable to maintain eye opening during the examination, the provider will be required to manually lift the eyelid and keep the eye open during the examination.
- If the patient is conscious, determine whether photophobia is present. *Rationale:* Patients with photophobia will benefit from instructions and warning that a bright light will be used to assess their pupil reactivity.

Patient Preparation

- Verify that the patient is the correct patient using two identifiers. *Rationale:* Before performing a procedure, the nurse should ensure the correct identification of the patient for the intended intervention. The SmartGuard in the pupillometer will automatically upload data to the EMR based on the code entered into the SmartGuard.
- Identify and confirm the correct SmartGuard is available. *Rationale:* To reduce the risk of cross contamination, a separate reusable SmartGuard is used for each patient. The SmartGuard should remain with the patient.

Procedure   for Automated Pupillometer Use

Steps	Rationale	Special Considerations
HH **PE**		
1. Remove pupillometer from docking/charging station If in sleep mode: • NPI 100 model: press and hold the UP arrow to turn device on. • NPI 200 model: touch the screen to turn device on. If the device has been off for more than 30 minutes, press and hold the UP arrow to turn on the device.	Prepares the equipment. If not previously docked, the pupillometer will be in sleep mode.	Docking station also charges the battery of the pupillometer.
2. Obtain correct SmartGuard.	SmartGuard is single-patient multiuse.	If this is a new patient, the SmartGuard must scan the patient ID band.
3. Connect the SmartGuard to the pupillometer as shown in Fig. 98-3A. • For *new* patients, start with Step 6. • For patients with prior examinations done during this admission, start with Step 7.	The pupillometer device must be connected to a SmartGuard to obtain a reading. The device will not operate if the connection is not made or is not secure.	Gently squeeze the SmartGuard slide tabs to position on to the NPI 200 model. You will feel a click as the SmartGuard engages the device.
4. *New* patients: • NPI 100: Obtain and label a SmartGuard • NPI 200: Scan the SmartGuard (see Fig. 98-3 B), and scan the patient ID band using the infrared Pupillometer Scanner	The SmartGuard is single-patient use and scanning the SmartGuard pairs/links the SmartGuard to an individual patient. If using the NPI 200, the SmartGuard must be paired to the patient.	The NPI 100 model does not have the scanning feature. Some units place a sticker with the patient name on the SmartGuard. If there is no barcode scanner, the patient ID number can be manually entered.
5. Confirm that the patient is the correct patient.	Verify the patient's ID (displayed on screen) by selecting "Accept." The screen will display "Ready to scan."	
6. Press the LEFT button on the pupillometer.	This procedure is written to first assess the left eye (OS) and then assess the right eye (OD). However, this is an arbitrary decision and the examiner may start with OD and then assess OS.	If starting with OD, select RIGHT button on pupillometer. Do not hold the button down.
7. Determine whether the patient is able to follow commands. • For awake and cooperative patients, start with Step 10. • For unresponsive patients, start with Step 11.	The patient who is awake and cooperative will be asked to participate in the examination. If the patient is unresponsive or uncooperative, the examiner will need to maintain the patient's eye open throughout the examination (approximately 3–5 seconds).	
8. Awake/cooperative patients: A. Ask patients to open their eyes. B. Ask them to look straight ahead.	Patient should focus on a distant point (at least 6 feet away).	Focusing on nearby objects will cause a reflexive pupillary dilation.

Procedure for Automated Pupillometer Use—*Continued*

Steps	Rationale	Special Considerations

9. Unresponsive patient:
  A. Open the patient's eye by lifting the eyelid gently with your finger or thumb.
  B. Make sure that the eye is open enough to see the entire pupil.
	The entire pupil must be visible or the pupillometer will not provide an accurate reading.	Inability to raise the eyelid is a reportable condition (e.g., periorbital edema).

10. Holding the pupillometer upright, place the pad of the SmartGuard against the patient's left or right zygomatic process (cheek bone) as shown in Fig. 98-3C.	Start with one pupil and then move to the other pupil. The ideal position to hold the pupillometer is perpendicular to the eye.	The choice to start with OS or OD is arbitrary; practitioners should consider asking patients which eye they would prefer to start with.

11. Target the pupil by pressing and holding the LEFT button.
  A. Look at the display screen on the pupilometer.
  B. Ensure that there is a green circle around the pupil.
	This step ensures that the pupillometer has located the pupil.	Novice practitioners may benefit from practice to ensure that the device is pointed directly at the pupil.

12. Provide a light impulse by releasing the LEFT button (when observing the OS). Hold pupillometer in place until the measurement is completed.	The pupillometer will emit a bright light for 0.8 seconds and video-record the change in pupil size in response to the light.	Press LEFT when examining OS and press RIGHT when examining OD.
13. Ensure that reading was obtained.	Device should see the results display on the screen. The device will display the word "Rescan" if a reading was not obtained.	If device reads "Fail" then repeat Steps 12 and 13.
14. Repeat the previous step for the right eye.	Provides systematic evaluation of both eyes.	This procedure is written to first assess the OS and then assess the OD. However, this is an arbitrary decision and the examiner may start with OD and then assess OS. See Step 9 for clarity.
15. Tap the base of the pupillometer against the pupillometer reader.	This step of the procedure uploads readings from the pupillometer directly into the EMR.	Optional step for hospitals/practitioners that document findings in the EMR. Manually input in the document flowsheet NPi readings (for hospitals where interfacing feature is not yet available).
16. Remove and store the SmartGuard	The SmartGuard is a patient-specific device and should not be used with other patients.	Store in a clean (nonsterile) dry location. Clean pupillometer according to hospital policy.
17. Dock the pupillometer in the charging station	The pupillometer charges when docked.	Ensure that the docking station is plugged into an electrical source.
18. Discard used supplies.		
19. **HH**		

Procedure continues on following page

Expected Outcomes

- Accurate and reliable monitoring of the pupil size and the NPi for each pupil (OS and OD)[8]
- The pupils will be of equal size and reactivity[2]
- Early detection of elevated intracranial pressure associated with oculomotor nerve compression[5]

Unexpected Outcomes

- Inability to measure pupil response with pupillometer (e.g., periorbital edema, cataract, prosthetic eye)
- Nonreactive pupil (NPi = 0)
- NPi of <3.0 (indicative of slower than normal pupillary response)[5]
- Unequal pupil size before light stimulus (anisocoria)[7]

Patient Monitoring and Care

Steps	Rationale	Reportable Conditions
		These conditions should be reported if they persist despite nursing interventions.
1. Assess the pupils with each serial neurological examination.[2]	Pupillary examination is considered a normal and vital component of the neurological examination.[9]	• Changes in pupillary reaction noted from pervious examination
2. Note the waveform for each pupil.	Similar shape waveform indicates equal responsiveness of OS and OD pupils.	• Unreactive pupils • Unequal pupils or abnormal waveform
3. Note NPi value.	Normal is >3.0.	• NPi <3.0
4. Upload to the EMR by tapping the base of the NPi-200 against the pupillometer reader.	The NPi-200, links to most EMRs and the results from the pupil examination can be directly uploaded to autopopulate the EMR.	• Fixed pupils • Inability to upload data
5. Report any abnormal values or significant changes of the pupils to the physician, advanced practice nurse, or other healthcare professional.	Changes in pupillary reactivity should be correlated over time.	• Abnormal values (NPi <3)

Documentation

Documentation should include the following:
- Document findings for each eye
- Date and time of examination
- Initial size (rounded to nearest mm)
- NPi
- Inability to obtain examination. If unable to obtain examination, document the reason (e.g., periorbital edema, combative, etc.)

- Comparison of left/right symmetry
- Minimum size
- Constriction velocity
- Note that the pupillometer is programmed to document the findings automatically into the EMR. When using compatible systems, documentation will occur when the upload is completed.

References and Additional Readings

For a complete list of references and additional readings for this procedure, scan this QR code with any freely available smartphone code reader app, or visit http://booksite.elsevier.com/9780323376624.

99 RotoRest Lateral Rotation Surface

Theresa Nino and Mary Beth Flynn Makic

PURPOSE: The purpose of kinetic therapy is to decrease complications associated with immobility. Rotation therapy can aid redistribution of blood flow to pulmonary circulation with the goal of improving oxygenation.[16] Kinetic therapy provides dynamic rotation and benefits pulmonary status by enhancing mobilization and removal of pulmonary secretions, and assisting in preventing and treating physiological complications of immobility. The RotoRest lateral rotation surface is a unique kinetic therapy surface that can be perceived to be technically challenging and requires a coordinated effort for use. This rotation therapy is ideal for patients with traumatic injury, unstable spine, and traction and for patients who need aggressive rotation therapy.

PREREQUISITE NURSING KNOWLEDGE

- Principles of prevention of pressure-induced injury should be understood, including high-risk areas for tissue injury in the critically ill patient.[7,8,16,20,21] Pressure points and locations where moisture or incontinence may occur require special attention to prevent skin breakdown.[1,7,8,13,16,19,20,21] Prolonged external pressure over bony prominences, shear and friction forces, and excessive moisture increase the risk of pressure ulcers.[1,7,8,16,17,20,21]
- Pressure injury may occur while a patient is on a specialty surface. Assess all at-risk areas of the patient's skin, especially the face, ears, occiput, shoulders, and coccyx areas.
- With use of a validated pressure ulcer risk–assessment tool such as the Braden Scale, a patient's risk for a pressure ulcer should be assessed on admission to the intensive care unit and at least every 12 to 24 hours thereafter, or with changes in the patient's condition. Interventions to prevent pressure ulcer development should target characteristics that put the patient at risk.[2,4,7,16,19]
- Knowledge is needed concerning the physiological effects of immobility on body systems, including factors that contribute to impaired circulation. Potential complications in the critically ill patient include the following:
  - Venous stasis and thrombosis[19]
  - Pulmonary and urinary stasis[22]
  - Pressure ulcer formation with potential associated friction, moisture, and shear injury[2,6,13,16,17]
- The RotoRest kinetic therapy bed is based on a platform that provides rotation and pressure relief by continuous rotation. The use of this therapy includes frequent assessments of patient skin, and safety of lines, drains, and tubes.[1,6,11]

- The RotoRest kinetic therapy surface can be used for those patients that require spinal immobilization and the prevention of complications due to immobility.[3,5,10,14,18]
  - Preventive interventions, such as providing skin protectants, monitoring nutrition, containing excessive moisture, and preventing shear and friction, are indicated with the use of the RotoRest surface.
  - Layers of linen placed on the surface should be limited to allow maximal benefit of the surface for the patient's skin.
- The term *kinetic therapy* refers to a 40-degree or greater rotation.[1,9,10,15,18]
- The RotoRest lateral rotation surface is a kinetic therapy surface that does not incorporate low air loss into its technology, but if the patient is in continuous motion (rotation), pressure over bony prominences may be relieved during the continuous turning therapy. However, because of the aggressive degree of the turn, possible shear and friction injuries of the skin can occur during rotation.
- For maximal benefit, the support surface should be in rotation more than 18 hours per day and at optimal rotation.[1,9–12,15,18]
  - The support surface should provide continuous rotation at varying degrees.
  - Serial skin assessments per institutional protocols are required when patients are on rotational therapy surfaces.
  - The clinician should evaluate the patient's tolerance of kinetic therapy and consider sedation and analgesics as appropriate.
- Indications include critically ill patients who are at a higher risk of pulmonary complications such as the following:
  - Patients with increasing ventilatory support requirements

- Patients who have clinical indications for acute lung injury or adult respiratory distress syndrome[3,9,22]
  - ❖ Worsening partial pressure of O_2 in arterial blood to fraction of inspired oxygen ratio
  - ❖ Presence of fluffy infiltrates via chest radiograph concomitant with pulmonary edema
  - ❖ Refractory hypoxemia
- Patients should be placed on a lateral rotation support surface as soon as possible to prevent the negative effects of immobility and possible pulmonary complications.[3,9,15,22]
- When ordering kinetic therapy, the clinician should assess the properties of the pressure redistribution surface and evaluate patient skin/tissue redistribution needs (i.e., moisture control, pressure redistribution).
- Trauma diagnosis and spinal cord injury should be understood. Pressure ulcer–related risks associated with traumatic and spinal cord injury should be understood related to prolonged immobility.[3,9,15,22] Low air-loss surfaces are contraindicated for patients with unstable spine or pelvic injuries until the injury is stabilized. The RotoRest surface may be used with spinal injuries; additional care is necessary to place unstable spinal cord injuries or patients with pelvic instability on a RotoRest surface that has a firm, flat surface. Cervical traction and skeletal traction may be used with a RotoRest therapy surface (see Procedure 100).
- The RotoRest Delta Advanced Kinetic Therapy bed is shown in Figure 99-1.
- Noted principles in caring for a patient receiving kinetic therapy on a RotoRest Delta Advanced Kinetic Therapy bed include technical and clinical competence in the following:
  - ❖ The surface below the patient and the positioning packs consist of pressure-redistributing foam and a pad of nonliquid polymer gel with a low-friction, low-shear nylon fabric with moisture-permeable backing cover that does not absorb body fluids.

- ❖ The gel pads prevent the patient from bottoming out and transfer body heat evenly; they are radiographically transparent.
- ❖ The bed provides continuous, slow, side-to-side turning of the patient by rotating the bed frame. Keeping the patient in maximal rotation assists with prevention of skin breakdown and provides the most effective therapy for pulmonary indications. The bed can turn up to 62 degrees on each side, either intermittently or constantly, providing unilateral or bilateral rotation.
- ❖ The amount of time the patient is held at the rotation limit before rotating in the opposite direction can be adjusted from 7 seconds to 30 minutes.
- ❖ Head and shoulder packs provide cervical stability but should not be used as the primary means of stabilizing cervical spine fractures. Cervical traction, halo, and vest or internal fixation may be required. Lateral arm and leg hatches facilitate range of motion.
- ❖ Hatches underneath the bed (located in the cervical, thoracic, and rectal areas) provide access for skin care, catheter maintenance, and bladder and bowel management. Do not open thoracic and sacral hatches at the same time.
- ❖ The bed has a built-in scale with a maximal patient weight of 300 lbs.[1,7] Overall width of the bed is 34 inches with a height of 94 inches.[1]
- ❖ An optional vibrator pack is available to provide chest physiotherapy to further mobilize pulmonary secretions.

EQUIPMENT

- Nonsterile gloves
- Sheet or slide board to assist with moving the patient onto the surface
- Transparent or foam protective dressings for areas prone to friction or shear

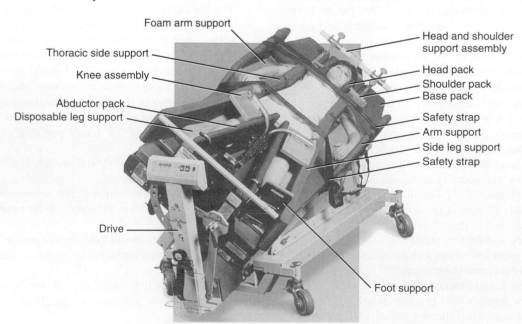

Figure 99-1   Kinetic Concepts Inc. RotoRest Delta Advanced Kinetic Therapy bed. *(Courtesy KCI Licensing, Inc, San Antonio, TX, 2008.)*

- Appropriate support surface and positioning packs for the RotoRest lateral rotation surface

PATIENT AND FAMILY EDUCATION

- Explain to the patient and family the adverse effects of critical illness and immobility, including pulmonary complications, tissue pressure, and excessive moisture of the skin. *Rationale:* Providing an explanation promotes understanding of the need for prevention, interventional strategies and the specialty devices that are utilized based on patient risk assessment. The patient and family are able to share understanding of the plan of care and ask questions
- Describe the goals of RotoRest kinetic therapy and how the therapy can aid in maintaining patient alignment in patients with spinal injuries. *Rationale:* The patient and family are able to share understanding of the plan of care and ask questions
- Explain how the therapy can serve as both a prevention and an interventional care strategy. *Rationale:* Understanding and cooperation are increased.
- Explain to the patient and family the pulmonary benefit of rotation in promoting dynamic movement of pulmonary secretions. *Rationale:* Facilitates the understanding of the role of pulmonary secretion mobility in the critically ill.

PATIENT ASSESSMENT AND PREPARATION

Patient Assessment

- Assess the patient's risk for a pressure ulcer with an evidence-based practice assessment tool (i.e., Braden score).[2,4,16] *Rationale:* Valid assessment tools assist in the identification of patient risk for alterations in skin.
- Assess the patient's skin for evidence of pressure ulcer formation or alterations in skin on admission and throughout care based on institutional policy. *Rationale:* Baseline and ongoing skin status data are provided.
- Assess the patient's wounds: location, size, stage of pressure ulcer, description of tissue in the wound bed, type and amount of drainage, maceration and inflammation in the surrounding skin, and pain on palpation of surrounding skin. *Rationale:* Objective and thorough assessment of wounds on admission and throughout the course of illness is necessary for measuring the effectiveness of therapy and interventions.
- Assess and ensure hemodynamic stability; assess for the presence of edema in lower extremities and the potential for thromboembolism.[22] *Rationale:* Baseline data are provided for serial assessment and if necessary to treat the adverse effects of immobility.
- Assess the patient's pulmonary status to include the quality and presence of adventitious breath sounds, the rate and depth of respirations, cough, cyanosis, dyspnea, nasal flaring, arterial blood gas results, chest radiograph, mental status, and restlessness. *Rationale:* Provides baseline data for additional comparisons. Lateral movement provides postural drainage, mobilizes secretions, and enhances air exchange.[10]
- Assess the patient's bladder for complications associated with urinary stasis from immobility to include the presence of bladder distention, incomplete bladder emptying, or urinary infrequency. *Rationale:* Baseline data are provided before implementation of lateral movement that decreases urinary stasis and associated complications.[22]
- Discuss goals for rotation therapy with the interprofessional team as part of the daily plan of care. *Rationale:* The principles of therapy are evaluated to match patient factors related to type of injury, moisture, and need for redistribution of pressure on skin and wounds.
- Reassess every 12 to 24 hours for the need to continue, change, or discontinue rotational therapy. *Rationale:* Reevaluation of the benefit of the therapy is important in creating an individualized plan of care.

Patient Preparation

- Ensure that the patient and family understand preprocedural teaching. Answer questions as they arise, and reinforce information as needed. *Rationale:* Understanding of previously taught clinical information and rationale is evaluated and reinforced.
- Evaluate the properties of the support surface to meet pulmonary needs, skin factors related to the type of injury, moisture, and need for redistribution of pressure on skin and wounds. Order and inspect the bed functions before the patient is placed on the surface. *Rationale:* Support surface selection should match the clinical indication for patient therapy. Relief of external pressure may decrease the risk of pressure ulcer formation and facilitate wound healing.
- Verify that the patient is the correct patient using two identifiers. *Rationale:* Before performing a procedure, the nurse should ensure the correct identification of the patient for the intended intervention.
- Organize moving the patient to the special surface, ensuring adequate personnel are available. *Rationale:* Transfer of the patient from one bed to another is potentiated.

Procedure for Lateral Rotation Therapy

Steps	Rationale	Special Considerations
Procedure for Kinetic Therapy With the RotoRest Surface		
1. Obtain the bed that will be used for kinetic lateral rotation.	Rental beds may require a physician's order.	These beds are U.S. Food and Drug Administration (FDA) regulated. Ensures the properties of the specialty surface meet the patient's specific needs.
2. Follow manufacturer guidelines for setting up the bed to include patient height, weight, and rotation settings.	Prepares the equipment.	The RotoRest kinetic therapy surface is considered more challenging to use and thus is described in this section.
3. 🔲HH		
4. 🔲PE		
Prepare for Patient Placement		
5. Ensure that the bed is locked in the horizontal position and that the drive is disengaged.	Ensures patient safety.	
6. Check all hatches to be certain they are properly latched; be sure castors are locked.	Prevents unplanned movement of the bed.	
7. Zero the bed scale system.	Prepares bed for patient daily weight.	
8. Prepare the surface: A. Remove all vertical packs. B. Cover support brackets with a wash cloth. C. Slide thoracic and foot packs. to the side and ends of the unit. D. Consider routing for any patient-specific drains/tubes.	Allows for smooth transfer of the patient onto the bed and protects the patient from discomfort. Prepares for safe management of lines, drains, and tubes.	
Prepare for Patient Transfer and Positioning on Kinetic Therapy Surface		
1. Using a draw sheet or slide board, gently move the patient to the center of the surface while maintaining body alignment.[1] **(Level M*)**	Bouncing of the patient can result in skin abrasions and progression of injury.	Pillar bars can be covered with a towel or folded paper sheet to avoid the possibility of abrasion. Assess the security of all lines, drains, and tubes to accommodate a full 62-degree turn.
2. Center the patient on the bed by aligning the nose, umbilicus, and pubis with the center posts.[1] Align both head and shoulder pack posts vertically and horizontally. **(Level M)**	Facilitates proper balance. Rotating to one side indicates that the patient is not centered.	Traction equipment may be installed once the patient is centered.
3. Pack installation for one side of the patient is repeated and mirrored on the opposite side.	Packs are the main supporting apparatus. Packs provide support to prevent lateral movement within the bed, which can lead to skin breakdown.	Packs and supports are labeled for the patient's right and left sides.

*Level M: Manufacturer's recommendations only.

Procedure for Lateral Rotation Therapy—*Continued*

Steps	Rationale	Special Considerations
4. Install shoulder and head pack assemblies by sliding onto head and shoulder posts. Slide head and shoulder packs inward to lightly touch patient head.	Provides support and protects ears from pressure. Proper shoulder and head support help to prevent lateral movement within the bed, which can lead to ear skin breakdown and cervical injury.	Maintain a 1-inch clearance from the shoulder; use passing of hand between the shoulder and pack to verify the clearance. Verify that the pack is not pressing against the ears. If cervical traction causes the patient to slide up on the bed during rotation, place the patient in the reverse Trendelenburg's position.
5. Place thoracic side supports in appropriate holes provided in the frame and ensure that they are tightened securely. Lock cam handles to hold the pack in position.	Provides support to prevent lateral movement within the bed, which may lead to shearing skin injury.	The holes in the frame in which the side supports fit are near the surface of the base packs. Packs are labeled "Right" and "Left." The thicker side of the pack is always against the patient. Maintain a 1-inch clearance between the end of the pack and the axilla.
6. Adjust the knee assembly to a position slightly above the patient's knee. Lock cam handles to hold the pack in position.	Provides support.	
7. Place the disposable leg support under the thigh and calf so that it fits under the ankle and knee but not beneath the heel.	Decreases external pressure on the heels.	Leg supports should be changed with excessive moisture or when soiled.
8. Place the foot supports in the foot bracket assembly. The assembly should be positioned so that the footrest is in anatomical position. Tighten the foot assembly.[1] Lock cam handles to hold the position. **(Level M*)**	Maintains each foot in proper anatomical position and prevents migration.	The foot supports should not be left in place for longer than 2 hours at a time. A schedule of 2 hours on and 2 hours off should be maintained continuously. Side-to-side motion does not relieve pressure on the soles of the feet.
9. Install the abductor packs into the preset metal brackets.	Provides support.	Adjust and lower if extra space is required at the groin.
10. Place the side leg supports snugly against the patient's hips. Lock cam handles to hold the positon.	Provides support.	
11. Install the knee pack by pressing the pin on the support tube while inserting the support tube into the knee pack assembly. Tighten the knob to hold the assembly in position.[1] **(Level M)**	Prevents pressure on the knee.	Maintain a 1-inch clearance between the foam and the skin. Knee packs can be adjusted to allow for variation in abduction and flexion of the patient's legs. They maintain proper posture of the lower limbs in the patient with spasticity, discouraging contracture formation.
12. Install the disposable foam arm supports.[7] **(Level M)**	Ensures that the patient's hands are in a position of function and that the ulnar nerve and elbows are protected.	Disposable arm supports should be changed with excessive moisture or when soiled.
13. Secure the arm supports in the holes provided on the frame.	Provides support and promotes safety.	
14. Place a hand on the patient's shoulder and adjust the shoulder pack to lightly touch your hand.[1] **(Level M)**	Prevents pressure ulcers.	A 1-inch (2.54-cm) clearance should always exist between the patient's shoulders and the shoulder packs.

*Level M: Manufacturer's recommendations only.

Procedure continues on following page

Procedure   for Lateral Rotation Therapy—*Continued*

Steps	Rationale	Special Considerations
15. Verify that all packs are in position, all hatches are closed, all cam handles are locked, and brakes are locked.	Provides support.	Remove any obstructions from the area that may impede the unit rotation cycle.
16. Fasten the restraining straps. Safety straps must be in place at all times. One safety strap is used to hold down the shoulder assembly. Place the other strap across the hip region.	Prevents falls and patient injury.	
17. Initiate therapy.	Determine whether the equipment and positioning works.	Observe the patient through a full rotation cycle; ensure that all packs are appropriately set, pressure points are protected, drains and lines are not pulled or pinched during rotation, and there are no obstructions during the cycle.
18. Monitor patient hemodynamics with rotation therapy.	Determines the patient's response to therapy.	Changes in hemodynamics are expected; monitor the patient's tolerance and hemodynamic goals (e.g., urine output, mentation, mean arterial pressure, intracranial pressure, etc.). The patient may need time to acclimate to kinetic therapy. Interpret vital signs with knowledge of fixed transducer variation caused by degree of rotation (i.e., level may change, providing false data).[10]
19. Remove **PE** and discard used supplies.	Reduces transmission of microorganisms; Standard Precautions.	
20. **HH**		

Expected Outcomes

- Intact skin integrity
- Wound healing
- Absence of friction and shearing
- Absence of excessive skin moisture or dryness
- Improved peripheral circulation
- Improved urinary elimination
- Maximal pulmonary function achieved

Unexpected Outcomes

- Friction, shearing, motion sickness, agitation, disorientation, and falls from lateral movement of the table if the patient is not strapped in properly
- Pressure ulcer formation or further deterioration of existing pressure ulcers
- Desaturation or hemodynamic instability with rotation
- Dislodged invasive lines or tubes
- Development of urinary tract infection
- Development of worsening pulmonary status

Patient Monitoring and Care

Steps	Rationale	Reportable Conditions
		These conditions should be reported if they persist despite nursing interventions.
1. To initiate cardiopulmonary resuscitation (CPR): A. Return the bed to the horizontal position by disengaging rotation and manually rotating. B. Pull the crank arm handle (the clutch) and lock it in place with the lock. C. Follow the manufacturer's guidelines regarding if a back board is needed for CPR.	A flat, firm surface is necessary for CPR.	• Need for emergency care
2. Evaluate the patient's existing pressure areas and ulcers, wounds, flaps, and grafts for evidence of healing according to institutional guidelines. Monitor skin regularly, and provide extra attention to any pressure points and locations where moisture or incontinence may occur.[2,6,7,13,16]	Relief of external pressure facilitates healing.	• New breakdown • Impaired healing
3. Assess the skin for evidence of pressure (especially on the occiput, sacrum, and heels), friction, shearing, or moisture per hospital policy. Consider applying protective dressing to areas prone to friction or shear (i.e., transparent semiocclusive, hydrocolloid, or foam dressings).	Kinetic therapy surface alone does not protect from pressure ulcer formation. Ensure that adequate skin assessment continues throughout therapy.	• Development of pressure ulcers or skin breakdown
4. Evaluate the patient's peripheral vascular circulation. Follow hospital policy for prevention of thromboembolism.	Lateral movement discourages venous stasis.	• Edema • Decreased or absent pulses • Discoloration • Pain
5. Evaluate the patient's pulmonary function.	Lateral movement provides continuous postural drainage and mobilization of secretions.	• Adventitious breath sounds • Decreased respiratory rate and depth • Cough • Cyanosis • Dyspnea • Nasal flaring • Decreased oxygen saturation • Abnormal blood gases • Decreased mental acuity • Restlessness • Abnormal chest radiograph results
6. Evaluate the patient for urinary retention.	Lateral movement decreases urinary stasis.	• Decreased urine output • Bladder distention
7. Evaluate the patient's acceptance of and adaptation to the device (motion sickness, agitation, disorientation).	Increases cooperation and decreases anxiety.	• Intolerance to device

Procedure continues on following page

Patient Monitoring and Care —*Continued*

Steps	Rationale	Reportable Conditions
8. Monitor patient's tolerance and hemodynamic goals (e.g., urine output, mentation, mean arterial pressure, intracranial pressure, etc.). The patient may need time to acclimate to kinetic therapy.	Lateral movement may alter hemodynamics because of the degree of rotation (turn) and changes in transducer positioning.	• Increased or decreased blood pressure • Increased or decreased heartrate • Elevation in intracranial pressure
9. Follow institutional standards for assessing pain. Administer analgesia as prescribed.	Identifies need for pain interventions.	• Continued pain despite pain interventions
10. Maintain bed in motion for 18 hours of every 24-hour period.[5,6] Target rotation on a kinetic therapy surface is 62 degrees.	Provides proper rotation and adequate mobility.	• Inability to rotate as per schedule
11. Maintain safety straps and positioning packs at all times.	Prevents falls and patient injury.	• Falls or injury
12. Maintain schedule for foot supports: 2 hours on and 2 hours off continuously.	Side-to-side movement does not relieve pressure on the soles of the feet.	• Breakdown on the soles of the feet
13. Determine when therapy should be discontinued. Reassess need every 12–24-hour period.	Lateral rotation therapy is no longer required.	• Need for discontinuation of therapy

Documentation

Documentation should include the following:
- Patient and family education
- Date and time therapy is instituted
- Rationale for use of lateral rotation therapy surface
- Number of hours patient is in rotation mode per 24-hour period and degree of rotation achieved
- Patient tolerance of therapy
- Safety straps in place, bed alarms engaged
- Complete skin assessments of pressure areas and wound assessments per institutional standards and as necessary

- Status of wound healing, if applicable
- Patient's response to therapy
- Any unexpected outcomes and interventions taken
- Phone number and name of company representative
- Pain assessment and management according to institutional guidelines

References and Additional Readings

For a complete list of references and additional readings for this procedure, scan this QR code with any freely available smartphone code reader app, or visit http://booksite.elsevier.com/9780323376624.

100 Thermoregulation: External and Intravascular Warming/ Cooling Devices

Karen A. Lovett

PURPOSE: An external surface or hydrogel pad temperature-management device may be used to increase or decrease the body temperature. An intravascular warming and cooling device may be inserted to increase or decrease the body temperature. External surface-cooling devices or intravascular cooling catheters are also used as a therapeutic treatment modality to reduce the body temperature after acute injury (such as global cerebral ischemia, cardiac arrest, or hypoxia) to decrease cellular oxygen consumption and intracranial pressure. Decreasing cerebral blood flow improves the discrepancy between oxygen supply and oxygen demand.[30]

PREREQUISITE NURSING KNOWLEDGE

- The hypothalamus is the primary thermoregulatory center for the body and where the central sensors for the body core temperature are located; it maintains normothermia through internal regulation of heat production or heat loss. Information is sent from the brain, spinal cord, deep abdominal and thoracic tissue, and thermosensors underneath the skin to the hypothalamus.[37,40]
- In the preoptic area of the hypothalamus are thermosensitive neurons that incorporate information from the peripheral and blood receptors and compare it to the body's set point. The body reacts when there is a difference between the set point and the actual temperature.[38]
- Through a negative feedback loop, the warm and cold sensory neurons respond to feedback from the peripheral sensors and balance their signals to maintain a set point of 37.0°C (98.6°F).[21,40]
- When the thermal area of the hypothalamus senses heat gain or a warmer temperature than the set point, the body vasodilates and sweats to assist in lowering the body temperature. Conversely, when the neurons sense a temperature below the set point (heat loss), vasoconstriction and shivering occur to increase catabolism, conserve heat, and raise body temperature.[4,21,28,36,37]
- Thermoregulation is influenced by several factors, such as cellular metabolism, exercise, diurnal variation, and ambient temperature.[36]
- The body has mechanisms to dissipate heat:
  - Conduction occurs when heat is lost by direct transfer from one surface to a second adjacent cooler object.[4,27]
  - Convection is the transfer of heat from a surface to surrounding air.[27]
  - Radiation occurs when heat (thermal energy) is transferred through air or space between separated surfaces without direct contact between the objects.[27]
  - Evaporation occurs when heat loss accompanies water evaporated from the skin and respiratory tract to the surrounding air.[4,27]
- Knowledge of terms associated with temperature is needed (Table 100-1).
- Alteration in thermoregulation can result from a primary central nervous system injury or disease (e.g., subarachnoid hemorrhage, traumatic brain injury, spinal cord injury, or neoplasm) and metabolic conditions (e.g., diabetes mellitus; toxic levels of ethanol alcohol or other drugs, such as barbiturate and phenothiazine agents).
- Body temperature is the measurement of the presence or absence of heat. Body heat is generated, conserved, redistributed, or dissipated during all physiological processes. Factors such as age, circadian rhythm, and hormones influence body temperature.
- Body temperature may be measured with a variety of thermometers and at several body sites. Electronic or digital thermometers are used to obtain rectal, oral, and axillary temperatures. Thermistors within catheters or probes measure rectal, nasopharyngeal, esophageal, bladder, brain, and pulmonary artery temperatures. Infrared thermometers measure tympanic membrane and temporal artery temperatures. Choose the method of temperature monitoring that best meets the patient's clinical condition and obtains results that are reliable, accurate, and safe to support clinical decisions.[23,29,34,37,38]
- When assessing body temperature, some basic aspects have to be considered that influence normal thermoregulation, such as age, gender, and site of measurement.

TABLE 100-1	Terms Associated With Temperature
Term	**Definition**
Normothermia/euthermia	Optimal range of body temperature associated with health.
Hypothermia	Subnormal core body temperature equal to or below 35°C.[20,24]
Induced hypothermia	Intentional reduction of body temperature to decrease the cerebral metabolic rate of oxygen, intracranial pressure, cerebral blood volume, thereby improving the oxygen supply and demand mismatch.[32] This may be accomplished by surface means (transfer of heat from the skin to the cooling device) or central means (circulatory heat exchange in a cardiopulmonary bypass machine or cooling catheter)
Fever	Fever is a response to either endogenous or exogenous pyrogens, or direct effects upon the hypothalamic temperature-control centers.[21]
Hyperthermia	The body temperature is out of control due to failed thermoregulation. The body temperature is high, usually resulting from infection, medication, or head injury.[20]

- The best evaluation of body temperature uses the core temperature; it is the least influenced by environmental and other factors and maintains a stable temperature.[21]
- The most accurate core temperature monitoring methods are intravascular (e.g., pulmonary artery catheter), esophageal, and bladder.[34,40]
- The pulmonary artery catheter is the best representation of core temperature and the "gold standard" for clinical thermometry.[12,16,21,23,33,37,40,42]
- Variations in temperatures normally occur in the body. No accurate conversion table exists that converts the temperature from one site to another. Trying to adjust between sites only contributes to misunderstanding.[38]
- Site choice for temperature monitoring is based on the clinical data needed; the patient's condition, safety, and comfort; environmental factors (e.g., room temperature); the indication for a catheter or a probe (e.g., pulmonary artery catheter); and the availability of equipment.
- Regardless of method and site chosen, the same site and same method should be used repeatedly to trend the serial measurements during the application of warming or cooling therapy.[4,20]
- Trend with two sites, use caution, and question differences in temperature that are >0.3°C, or a temperature difference that would drive a clinical decision to change therapy and/or cause an intervention.[16,21,40]
- An esophageal temperature probe can be inserted into the esophagus. Accurate placement of the temperature probe is necessary to obtain results similar to monitoring the temperature from the pulmonary artery.
- Shivering is an involuntary shaking of the body generated to maintain thermal homeostasis. Shivering causes rhythmic tremors that result in skeletal muscle contraction and is a normal physiological mechanism to generate heat production.[28]
- Early detection of shivering can be accomplished by palpating the mandible and feeling a humming vibration. Electrocardiographic artifacts from skeletal muscle movement is seen on the bedside monitor. If not detected early, shivering can progress from visible twitching of the head or neck to visible twitching of the pectorals or trunk, and then to generalized shaking of the entire body and teeth chattering.

TABLE 100-2	Bedside Shivering Assessment Scale (BSAS)	
Score	**Term**	**Description**
0	None	No shivering noted on palpation of masseter, neck, or chest wall, and no electrophysiological evidence of shivering (using electrocardiographs)
1	Mild	Shivering localized to neck or thorax only
2	Moderate	Shivering involves gross movement of the upper extremities (in addition to neck and thorax)
3	Severe	Shivering involves gross movements of trunk, upper, and lower extremities

- The Bedside Shivering Assessment Scale (BSAS) is a simple and reliable tool for evaluating the metabolic stress of shivering (Table 100-2).[2,25]
- Shivering may be visible on the Bispectral Index Monitor in the form of an increase in electromyogram activity (see Procedure 88).
- Shivering increases the metabolic rate, carbon dioxide (CO_2) production, resting energy expenditure, oxygen consumption, and myocardial work, and lowers brain tissue oxygen levels.[8,15,18,28] The overall metabolic consequences of shivering may eliminate many of the clinical benefits of temperature control.[5,28]
- At a body temperature <35°C, the basal metabolic rate can no longer supply sufficient body heat and an exogenous source of heat is needed.
- Table 100-3 outlines techniques to increase heat gain.
- Hypothermia may be categorized as mild (34 to 35.9°C), moderate (30 to 33.9°C), or severe/deep (<30°C).[10,28] The American Heart Association (AHA) recommends that if ventricular fibrillation or ventricular tachycardia are present with severe hypothermia defibrillation should be attempted. The value of subsequent defibrillations is uncertain; therefore, active rewarming should occur and the AHA suggests that it may be reasonable to further defibrillate, following the basic life support (BLS) algorithm.[10]

TABLE 100-3	Techniques to Increase Heat Gain
Mechanism of Heat Transfer	**Techniques to Increase Heat Gain**
Radiation	Warming lights, warm environment, room temperature, blankets
Conduction	Warm blankets, circulating water blanket, continuous arteriovenous rewarming, cardiopulmonary bypass
Convection	Thermal fans, circulating air blanket
Evaporation	Head and body covers; warm, humidified oxygen

- Hypothermia may be caused by an increase in heat loss, a decrease in heat production, an alteration in thermoregulation, and a variety of clinical conditions.
- An increase in heat loss may occur from the following:
  - Accidental (e.g., cold water drowning)
  - Environmental exposure
  - Induced vasodilation caused by high levels of ethanol alcohol, barbiturates, phenothiazines, or general anesthesia
  - Central nervous system dysfunction (e.g., spinal cord injury)
  - Dermal dysfunction (e.g., burns)
  - Iatrogenic conditions (e.g., administration of cold intravenous fluids, hemodialysis, cardiopulmonary bypass)
  - Trauma
- A decrease in heat production is associated with the following:
  - Endocrine conditions (e.g., hypothyroidism)
  - Malnutrition
  - Diabetic ketoacidosis
  - Neuromuscular insufficiency (e.g., resulting from a pharmacological paralysis caused by a neuromuscular blocking agent or anesthetic agents)
- Clinical conditions associated with hypothermia are sepsis, hepatic coma, prolonged cardiac arrest, and systemic inflammatory response syndrome.
- Severe hypothermia may mimic death; resuscitative efforts should be initiated despite the absence of vital signs.
- Rewarming for cardiac arrest survivors who have undergone therapeutic hypothermia should not occur faster than 0.25 to 0.50°C per hour.[10,22,30,33,35] Rapid rewarming can cause rewarming acidosis, electrolyte shifts, shivering, hypovolemic shock, temperature core afterdrop, and temperature overshoot.[8,41]
- Core afterdrop is a decrease in core temperature after rewarming is discontinued secondary to redistribution of body heat to colder peripheral areas.
- Rapid rewarming could cause an increase in insulin sensitivity and electrolyte disorders caused by shifts from the intracellular to the extracellular compartment.[8,41]
- Rapid rewarming could lead to loss of some or even all of the protective effects of hypothermia.[8,41]

- Overshoot occurs when the thermoregulatory mechanisms rebound or overcompensate.
- Termination of active external rewarming at 36 to 36.5°C may prevent temperature overshoot.
- Rewarming acidosis results from the increase in CO_2 production associated with the temperature increase and from the return of accumulated acids in the peripheral circulation to the heart.
- Rewarming shock occurs when hypothermic vasoconstriction masks hypovolemia. If the patient's circulating volume is insufficient during rewarming vasodilation, sudden decreases in blood pressure, systemic vascular resistance, and preload occur. In cases of severe to profound hypothermia, peripheral rewarming with external devices should be used with extreme caution. Core methods of rewarming should be considered.
- Hyperthermia occurs when the thermoregulatory system of the body absorbs or produces more heat than it is able to dissipate.
- Malignant hyperthermia is a rare, life-threatening hereditary condition of the skeletal muscle that occurs on exposure to a triggering agent or agents.[14] The triggering agents most commonly associated with malignant hyperthermia are volatile anesthetic agents, particularly halogenated inhalation anesthetics and/or the depolarizing muscle relaxant succinylcholine.[31] Malignant hyperthermia involves instability of the muscle cell membrane, which causes a sudden increase in myoplasmic calcium and skeletal muscle contractures.
- The earliest indication of malignant hyperthermia is an increase in end-tidal carbon dioxide level or hyperventilation while breathing spontaneously. Additional symptoms could include tachycardia, supraventricular or ventricular arrhythmia, masseter spasm, or generalized muscular rigidity.[13,31]
- A rapid temperature increase of 1°C every several minutes may occur and that rapid rise is more significant in diagnosing malignant hyperthermia than a peak temperature. The treatment of hyperthermia should be either the use of an internal cooling or specific surface cooling device.[14,31]
- Treatment includes discontinuation of the triggering agent and administration of a muscle relaxant (e.g., dantrolene sodium). The muscle relaxant inhibits the release of calcium from the sarcoplasmic reticulum without affecting calcium uptake.[31] Refer to hospital protocol for storage and administration of muscle relaxant.
- Heat stroke is characterized as a rectal temperature greater than 40.0°C (104°F) and central nervous system dysfunction. It occurs when the outdoor temperature and humidity are excessive and heat is transferred to the body. Increased humidity prevents the body from cooling by evaporation. Other signs of heat stroke include hypotension, tachycardia, tachypnea, mental status changes from confusion to coma, and possibly seizures. The skin is hot and dry, and sweating may occur. Initial interventions include support of airway, breathing, and circulation. Rapid cooling of the patient is the main treatment priority, with a goal of reducing the temperature to 38.9°C (102°F) as soon as possible.

- Fever occurs in response to a pyrogen and is defined as a temperature more than 38.3°C.[24] During fever, the hypothalamus retains its function, and shivering and diaphoresis occur to gain or lose body heat. Fever may be an adaptive response and may be considered beneficial in the absence of neurological disease processes. However, a febrile state increases the heart rate and metabolic rate and may be detrimental to a critically ill patient. The question of whether to reduce or treat a fever still remains unanswered and needs to be based on the patient's physical and hemodynamic stability and provider preference.[21,24]
- Fever worsens neurological outcome and increases mortality in neurological patients.[28,39]
- It is thought that fever occurs in approximately 50% of patients in the intensive care unit and is associated with adverse outcomes, including death with high fever.[21]
- Some external warming or cooling devices transfer warmth or coolness to the patient via conduction. Warmed or cooled fluids circulate through coils or channels in a thermal blanket or pad that is commonly placed under the patient.
- Additional warming and cooling systems are available. Hydrogel pads or external wraps can be placed on the patient's skin in the trunk and upper leg regions. These external systems are controlled through a feedback loop system with a core temperature (e.g., a bladder probe, an esophageal probe) that is attached to a central console and automatically regulates temperature according to programmed temperature target points. The feedback of patient temperature is compared with the set target temperature and the circulating water temperature is adjusted to ensure the target temperature is maintained.
- Other external devices transfer warmth to the patient via convection. A device used for warming blows warm air through microperforations on the underside of a blanket that is placed over the patient. The air is directed through the blanket onto the patient's skin.
- Intravascular cooling and warming devices currently in use include central venous catheters with temperature-controlled saline solution balloons or distal metallic heat-transfer elements that cool and warm the blood as it flows by the catheter. The saline solution is not in direct contact with the systemic circulation. These devices may be inserted in the subclavian, internal jugular, or femoral vein. They are attached to a console with an automatic temperature-control device that adjusts the pressure, temperature, and flow rate of the circulating saline solution based on the patient's continuously monitored temperature (e.g., rectal, bladder, esophageal) and the set points established by the healthcare provider.[8,27]
- Specific information about controls, alarms, troubleshooting, and safety features is available from each manufacturer and must be understood by the nurse before using the equipment.

EQUIPMENT

- Warming or cooling device
- Sheet or bath blanket
- Nonsterile gloves

- Temperature probe, cable, and module to monitor the patient's temperature (varies based on the type of site and thermometer selected and available)
- Hydrogel pads, external wraps or blankets needed by the equipment which is going to be used
- Cardiac monitoring (see Procedure 54)
- Appropriate skin-care products (refer to hospital policy)

Additional equipment, to have available as needed, includes the following:

- Hemodynamic monitoring (see Procedure 72)
- Sterile or distilled water (see manufacturer's recommendations)
- Intravascular cooling/warming central venous catheter
- Startup tubing kit
- Console, including cable for monitoring temperature
- Central venous catheter insertion tray
- Antiseptic solution
- Sterile drape
- Masks with eye shields, hair cover, sterile gloves, and sterile gowns
- Occlusive dressing
- Antimicrobial (e.g., chlorhexidine gluconate)–impregnated disc/dressing
- Normal saline solution
- Water-soluble lubricant

PATIENT AND FAMILY EDUCATION

- Explain the reason for the use of a warming or cooling device and standard of care, including monitoring of the temperature, expected length of therapy, comfort measures, and parameters for discontinuation of the device. ***Rationale:*** Explanation encourages the patient and family to ask questions and verbalize concerns about the procedure.
- Assess the patient and family understanding of the warming or cooling therapy. ***Rationale:*** Clarification and reinforcement of information are needed during times of stress and anxiety.
- Encourage the patient to notify the nurse of any discomfort. If the patient is unable to verbalize discomfort, look for signs and symptoms of discomfort such as grimacing, restlessness, diaphoresis, and etc. ***Rationale:*** Identification of discomfort facilitates early intervention and promotes comfort.

PATIENT ASSESSMENT AND PREPARATION

Patient Assessment

- Assess risk factors, medical history, the cause of the patient's underlying condition, and the type and the length of temperature exposure. ***Rationale:*** Assessment assists in anticipating, recognizing, and responding to the patient's responses and potential side effects to therapy.
- Assess the patient's medication therapy. ***Rationale:*** Medications such as vasopressors and vasodilators may affect heat transfer, increase the potential for skin injury, and contribute to an adverse hemodynamic response.

- Obtain a core temperature (e.g., pulmonary artery, esophageal, bladder). ***Rationale:*** Assessment determines baseline temperature and determines when a warming or cooling device is needed.
- Obtain vital signs and hemodynamic values. ***Rationale:*** Assessment determines baseline cardiovascular data. Initially, tachycardia and hypertension can occur as a result of cutaneous vasoconstriction and shivering with attempts at heat conservation.[32] Rewarming may cause hypotension from vasodilatation.[6]
- Monitor the patient's cardiac rhythm. ***Rationale:*** Monitoring determines the baseline cardiac rhythm. Most common and well-known electrocardiographic changes include presence of J (Osborn) waves, interval prolongation, and atrial and ventricular arrhythmias.[3] Tachycardia and hypertension may occur as a result of cutaneous vasoconstriction and shivering as the patient attempts to conserve heat.[6,27] Once patients begin to cool, bradycardia is the most common arrhythmia, together with PR prolongation, sinus bradycardia, and even junctional or ventricular escape rhythms. Bradycardia should be treated only if it is associated with hypotension. Hypothermia also prolongs the QT interval.[8,28,32] Tachycardia and ventricular dysrhythmias may occur if the patient is hyperthermic.[27]
- Assess the patient's electrolyte, glucose, arterial blood gas, and coagulation study results. ***Rationale:*** Alterations in temperature balance may result in acid-base imbalance, coagulopathy, electrolyte imbalance, glycemic imbalance, and hypoxemia.[1,11,27,28,32] Close monitoring of metabolic parameters with careful consideration of replacement during cooling and warming therapy is necessary.[11,27,28]
- Assess the patient's level of consciousness and neurological function. ***Rationale:*** Assessment determines baseline neurological status. A change in mental status, level of consciousness, or impaired neurological function may occur because of an undesirable high or low temperature or from the condition causing the alteration in mental status. Fatigue, muscle incoordination, poor judgment, weakness, hallucinations, lethargy, and stupor may occur with hypothermia. Seizures may occur with hyperthermia.
- Assess the patient's ventilatory function. ***Rationale:*** Hypoventilation, suppression of cough, and mucociliary reflexes associated with hypothermia may lead to hypoxemia, atelectasis, and pneumonia. Hypothermia shifts the oxygenation-dissociation curve to the left, and less oxygen is released from oxyhemoglobin to the tissues. Because of peripheral vasoconstriction, digit-based pulse oximetry is often unreliable. Hyperthermia shifts the oxygenation dissociation curve to the right, and oxygen is readily released from oxyhemoglobin.[27]
- Assess the patient's bowel sounds, abdomen, and gastrointestinal function. ***Rationale:*** Assessment determines baseline status. Patients with hypothermia may develop an ileus because of decreased intestinal motility. Vomiting and diarrhea may occur with hyperthermia.
- Assess the patient's skin integrity. ***Rationale:*** Assessment provides baseline data. An externally applied warming or cooling device can cause or exacerbate skin injury. Preexisting conditions such as diabetes and peripheral vascular disease increase the patient's risk for skin injury.

Patient Preparation

- Ensure that the patient and family understand preprocedural education. Answer questions as they arise, and reinforce information as needed. ***Rationale:*** Understanding of previously taught information is evaluated and reinforced.
- Verify that the patient is the correct patient using two identifiers. ***Rationale:*** Before performing a procedure, the nurse should ensure the correct identification of the patient for the intended intervention.
- If a warm air device will be used, remove the patient's gown and top sheet. ***Rationale:*** The warm air device works via convection and should be in direct contact with the patient's skin for optimal results.
- If the patient is unintentionally hypothermic, cover the patient's head with a blanket or towel or an aluminum cap. ***Rationale:*** This action minimizes additional heat loss.
- Ensure that informed consent has been obtained for insertion of intravascular catheters. ***Rationale:*** Informed consent protects the rights of the patient and makes a competent decision possible for the patient; however, in emergency circumstances, time may not allow for the consent form to be signed.
- Perform a preprocedure verification and timeout with placement of intravascular catheters, if nonemergent. ***Rationale:*** Ensures patient safety.

Procedure for External Warming/Cooling Devices		
Steps	**Rationale**	**Special Considerations**

Procedure for Obtaining Core Temperatures

1. HH
2. PE
3. Pulmonary artery:

A. Connect the cardiac output temperature cable from the bedside monitor to the pulmonary artery catheter.	Measures the temperature of the blood in the pulmonary artery.	Invasive placement risk for infection or puncture-related complications.[33,40]
B. Observe the temperature display on the bedside monitor.	Provides a temperature value.	

4. Bladder:

A. Connect the bladder temperature cable from the bedside monitor to the bladder probe.	Measures the temperature of the urine in the patient's bladder.	The accuracy of bladder temperatures may be influenced by urine flow rate.[7,28,30,33,34]
B. Observe the temperature display on the bedside monitor.	Provides a temperature value.	Refer to manufacturer's guidelines and follow institutional policy regarding whether the temperature-sensing indwelling urinary catheter is magnetic resonance imaging safe.

5. Esophageal:

A. Assess that the patient does not have any contraindications for placement of an esophageal temperature probe for temperature monitoring.	Ensures that the esophageal temperature probe is inserted safely.	Follow institutional policy regarding whether nurses are able to insert esophageal temperature probes. Contraindications for placement of the esophageal temperature probe include patients with known esophageal strictures or who have a history of esophageal cancer, esophageal perforation, and end-stage liver disease and varicies.[28] If resistance is met, withdraw the probe and gently advance again; this may indicate tracheal intubation of the probe. Never force the probe. If the patient exhibits signs of respiratory distress, such as coughing or gasping, immediately withdraw the temperature probe.
B. Measure from the opening of the patient's mouth to the earlobe and from the earlobe to the upper part of the sternum (manubrium), about two finger widths below the sternal notch for accurate probe placement. Mark the measurement on the tube. Lubricate the tip of the catheter with water-soluble lubricant.	Correct measurement for probe placement is necessary for accurate core temperature monitoring. Eases insertion of the probe.	
C. Insert the esophageal temperature probe into the oral cavity and advance.	Initiates the procedure.	
D. Continue to advance the catheter until the placement marked on the probe reaches the patient's lips.	Positions the probe.	
E. Secure the esophageal temperature sensor to the patient.	Reduces the risk of inadvertent displacement.	
F. Connect the cable from the esophageal probe to the bedside monitor.	Measures the esophageal temperature.	
G. Observe the temperature display on the bedside monitor.	Provides a temperature value.	
H. Placement may be verified with radiograph.[17]	Most catheters have a radiopaque tip visible on radiograph.	

6. Discard used supplies in appropriate receptacles. | Safely discards supplies. |

7. HH

Procedure for External Warming/Cooling Devices—*Continued*		
Steps	**Rationale**	**Special Considerations**

Initiation of a Warming or Cooling Device

1. Plug the device into a grounded outlet.

   Establishes a power source.

2. **HH**

3. **PE**

4. Select a method for continuously monitoring the patient's core temperature.[11,26] (**Level D***)

   Continuous core temperature monitoring is necessary with use of warming or cooling devices.[11,26]

   Some warming or cooling devices have an adapter for connecting a temperature probe from the patient directly to the device.

Use of Traditional Warming or Cooling Fluid Device

1. Place a dry absorbent sheet between the patient and the blanket when using all-vinyl blankets. (**Level M***)

   A dry absorbent sheet placed between the patient and the hypothermia/hyperthermia blanket to provide a sanitary barrier and absorb perspiration. It will also promote more uniform distribution of heat.

   Avoid applying additional sheets or blankets because efficient heating or cooling occurs with maximal contact between the thermal pad and the patient's skin.

2. Vinyl blankets with nonwoven fabric surfaces do not require an absorbent sheet when using the nonwoven side. (**Level M**)

3. Fill the reservoir in the unit to the indicated full level. Follow manufacturer's recommendation on water type.

   The reservoir must contain enough water for the machine to function properly.

4. Attach the hoses to the circulating fluid blanket.

   Allows the flow of warmed or cooled water to the blanket.

   A. Check that the clamps are closed before connecting the hoses from the device to the blanket.

   Prevents water leakage.

   B. After connecting the hoses, ensure that all of the connections are tight before unclamping the hoses.

   C. Check for kinks in the hoses.

5. Press the start switch on.

   Activates the device.

6. Set the controls.

   Follow institutional standards regarding the use of manual or automatic modes.

   A. Manual control of blanket temperature.

      i. Press the manual control switch on.

      ii. Choose the set point for the temperature of the circulating fluid based on the prescribed patient body temperature and the manufacturer's directions.

      The device maintains the circulating fluid in the blanket at the temperature set point.

      The patient's temperature must be continuously monitored.[24]

      iii. Turn the warming or cooling device off when the desired temperature is reached.

      The temperature goal is achieved.

      Closely monitor the patient's temperature for fluctuation.

---

*Level D: Peer-reviewed professional and organizational standards with the support of clinical study recommendations.

*Level M: Manufacturer's recommendations only.

Procedure continues on following page

Procedure for External Warming/Cooling Devices—*Continued*		
Steps	**Rationale**	**Special Considerations**
B. Automatic control of patient temperature.		
i. Connect the patient temperature probe to the unit before pressing a control mode switch.	Prevents triggering of the temperature probe alarm.	Most warming or cooling devices sound an alarm if the probe relays a low temperature; this may be indicative of probe dislodgment.
ii. Select the automatic mode and the set-point based on the prescribed patient body temperature and the manufacturer's directions.	In the automatic mode, the unit warms or cools the circulating fluid in the blanket based on the set-point (desired temperature) for the patient. A temperature probe connected to the unit monitors the patient's temperature.	The unit operates only if the patient's temperature probe is connected to the unit. Lights on the display panel indicate whether the unit is heating or cooling at any given time.
iii. Obtain the patient's temperature from the readout on the display unit.	Indicates the patient's temperature.	
iv. Verify the patient's temperature with another source and compare it with the readout on the device's display unit.	Ensures the warming or cooling device's temperature probe is functioning and correlates with the patient's temperature obtained with another method.	
v. When the desired patient temperature is reached, the warming or cooling device will maintain that set point temperature until the machine is turned off.	The temperature goal is achieved.	May continue to monitor the patient's temperature by pressing on the monitor only switch.

Warming or Cooling Fluid Devices That Use Hydrogel Pads or External Wraps

1. Apply the adhesive hydrogel pads or the external wraps to the body per manufacturer recommendations.	The pads or the wraps should cover approximately 40% of the patient.	Pads and wraps should be placed over clean, dry, intact skin. Inspect and prepare skin according to institutional standards.
2. Connect the hoses from the pads or wraps to the warming or cooling fluid device.	Prepares the system.	
3. Set the patient's target temperature as prescribed.	Sets the desired temperature.	
4. Activate the automatic mode.	The system will automatically adjust to achieve the target temperature.	
5. Set the time to target per institutional standards.	Prepares the system.	
6. Follow provider's prescriptions and follow manufacturer's recommendations for warming/cooling device maintenance.	Ensure safe patient monitoring.	

Use of a Warm Air Device

1. Remove the patient's gown, sheet, and blankets. Then place the circulating air blanket on top of the patient.	Prepares the equipment.	
2. Place a cotton blanket or sheet over the circulating air blanket.	Aids in keeping the air blanket in place.	Maintains privacy.

Procedure for External Warming/Cooling Devices—*Continued*

Steps	Rationale	Special Considerations
3. Connect the air blanket to the hose attached to the device.	The blanket inflates as air flows from the hose into it.	
4. Turn the device on and select the temperature of the air that will flow through the blanket.	The device warms the patient by directing warm airstreams directly onto the patient's skin.	The patient's temperature must be continuously monitored.
After the Warming or Cooling System Is Initiated		
1. Discard used supplies in an appropriate receptacle.	Removes and safely discards used supplies.	
2. **HH**		

Procedure for Intravascular Warming/Cooling Devices

Steps	Rationale	Special Considerations
1. Assist the provider with insertion of the intravascular catheter (see Procedure 82).	Facilitates the insertion process.	The healthcare provider performing the procedure and those assisting with the procedure should use full aseptic technique to include hand washing, sterile gloves, masks, hats, gowns, drapes, and proper use of suitable skin antiseptic. All physicians, advanced practice nurses, and other healthcare professionals in the room during the procedure should have on a mask.
2. Connect the tubing from the warming or cooling fluid device to the intravascular catheter.	Prepares the system.	
3. Set the patient's target temperature as prescribed.	Sets the desired temperature.	
4. Select the treatment mode.	Sets the desired mode of therapy.	
5. Activate the warming or cooling system.	Initiates the system.	
6. If the intravascular catheter device includes lumens for intravenous fluid administration, maintain patency with intravenous fluids or saline solution flush as ordered.	Provides venous access for intravenous fluids and medication administration.	Follow manufacturer's recommendations for warming/cooling device maintenance.
7. Follow provider's orders for desired patient temperature therapy, duration of therapy, and monitoring parameters.	Ensure safe patient monitoring.	
8. Ensure that a postinsertion chest x-ray is obtained if the catheter was placed in the subclavian or internal jugular vein.	Confirms placement.	
9. Discard used supplies in appropriate receptacles.	Removes and safely discards used supplies; safely removes sharp objects.	
10. **HH**		

Procedure continues on following page

Expected Outcomes

- External warming or cooling device applied
- Desirable core body temperature achieved

Unexpected Outcomes

- Inability to achieve desired core body temperature
- Hemodynamic instability
- Cardiac dysrhythmias
- Acid-base, electrolyte, glucose, and coagulation imbalance
- Intolerable discomfort
- Shivering
- Skin injury

Patient Monitoring and Care

Steps	Rationale	Reportable Conditions
		These conditions should be reported if they persist despite nursing interventions.
1. Perform a physical assessment of all systems every 1–2 hours and as needed.	Alterations in temperature affect every system. The condition that caused the change in temperature may worsen or be refractory to treatment.	• Significant changes in assessment
2. Continuously monitor the patient's temperature.[26]	Assesses the patient's response to warming or cooling. Some institutions require two methods of monitoring the patient's temperature when cooling or warming. At least one should have audible alarms for temperatures above and below the desired limit. Follow institutional policy.	• Continued hypothermia or hyperthermia (temperature outside of prescribed target temperature).
3. Measure the patient's blood pressure as frequently as indicated by the patient's condition and according to institutional standards.[9]	Vasodilation occurs with rewarming, and vasoconstriction may occur with cooling. Maintain perfusion and prevent recurrent hypotension	• Hypotension or hypertension
4. Palpate the patient's mandible for humming vibration and observe for shivering.	Aids in the early detection and prompt treatment of shivering. Shivering may contribute to the inability to maintain core temperature goals.	• Shivering • Decreased mixed venous oxygenation saturation • Continued shivering despite prescribed medications
5. Examine the patient's skin condition hourly. Follow manufacturer's recommendations for assessing the patient's skin under hydrogel pads and external wraps (e.g., at least every 4 hours). **(Level M*)**	Detects signs or symptoms of skin irritation so that the temperature of the device can be adjusted or padding can be placed between the skin and the device.	• Signs or symptoms of skin irritation or injury
6. Continuously monitor the patient's cardiac rate and rhythm.	Detects cardiac dysrhythmias associated with warming or cooling therapy.	• Cardiac dysrhythmias

*Level M: Manufacturer's recommendations only.

Patient Monitoring and Care —*Continued*

Steps	Rationale	Reportable Conditions
7. Obtain arterial blood gas results as prescribed and as indicated. Continuously monitor the patient's oxygen saturation and end-tidal carbon dioxide as prescribed.	Detects hypoxemia and acid-base imbalances. Maintains adequate oxygenation and minimizes fraction of inspired oxygen.	• Decreased oxygen saturation • Elevated partial pressure of oxygen in arterial blood • Elevated or decrease partial pressure of CO_2 in arterial blood • Abnormal arterial blood gas results
8. Obtain blood samples as prescribed.	Detects electrolyte shifts associated with warming and cooling therapy.	• Hyper/hypokalemia • Alterations in magnesium and phosphate levels • Hyperglycemia[11] • Coagulation study results[28]
9. Assess for venous thromboembolism (VTE) in vessels that contain intravascular cooling/warming devices.[19] **(Level C*)**	Intravascular cooling devices have been associated with increased risk of VTE.[28]	• VTE or pulmonary emboli
10. Follow institutional standards for assessing pain. Administer analgesia as prescribed.	Identifies need for pain interventions.	• Continued pain despite pain interventions

*Level C: Qualitative studies, descriptive or correlational studies, integrative reviews, systematic reviews, or randomized controlled trials with inconsistent results.

Documentation

Documentation should include the following:

- Patient and family education
- Patient's temperature and site(s) of temperature assessment
- Vital signs, cardiac rhythm, and hemodynamic status
- Physical assessment findings
- Neurological examination findings
- Skin assessment and/or preventative measures
- Mechanical ventilator settings
- Postinsertion chest radiograph (intravascular devices placed in the subclavian or internal jugular veins, confirm secure airway)
- Acid-base, electrolyte, glucose, lactate, and coagulation assessment and interventions
- Type of warming or cooling device used
- Mode of cooling or warming device (automatic or manual), patient's set-point or water temperature (as required by institutional standard)
- Time external warming or cooling is initiated and terminated
- Pain assessment, interventions, and effectiveness of interventions
- Sedation assessment, interventions, and effectiveness of interventions
- Shiver assessment, interventions, and effectiveness of interventions
- Unexpected outcomes
- Additional interventions

References and Additional Readings

For a complete list of references and additional readings for this procedure, scan this QR code with any freely available smartphone code reader app, or visit http://booksite.elsevier.com/9780323376624.

PROCEDURE

101

Cervical Tongs or Halo Ring: Application for Use in Cervical Traction (Assist)

Jennifer Massetti

PURPOSE: Cervical tongs or a halo ring is inserted into the skull so that weighted traction can be applied to the cervical spine. Cervical traction decompresses the spinal cord and immobilizes and realigns the cervical spine. Realignment and immobilization of the cervical spine may decrease the severity of secondary spinal cord injury. Spinal realignment and immobilization allow spinal fractures and supportive structures to heal properly.

PREREQUISITE NURSING KNOWLEDGE

* The nurse must be knowledgeable about the anatomy and physiology of the spinal column, the anatomy of the cervical vertebrae, the spinal cord, the cervical spinal nerves, and the areas of peripheral innervation. In addition, it is important that the nurse understands the pathophysiology and manifestations of spinal cord injury, including ascending edema, spinal shock, and neurogenic shock.
* The nurse should observe the patient for signs of shock, understand the phases of neurogenic and spinal shock, and know the appropriate interventions to implement.
* The nurse needs to continuously monitor the patient for changes in motor and sensory function during and after the procedure.
* The nurse should continuously assess for changes in respiration during the procedure and continue to monitor while the patient is in traction.
* Cervical spine traction is provided to realign, immobilize, and stabilize the cervical spine when it has become unstable as a result of a cervical spine fracture or dislocation caused by trauma or disease, degenerative processes of the cervical vertebrae, or spinal surgery (Fig. 101-1).[3,4] After initial medical stabilization of the patient and assessment and documentation of neurological function, cervical skeletal traction with the tongs or halo ring can be applied to realign the cervical spine. Traction is used to reduce cervical dislocation before the patient undergoes surgery. Occasionally, an unstable cervical spinal injury may necessitate long-term cervical traction for a period of weeks to attain realignment and immobilization to stabilize the spine. The definitive method used to treat cervical

fractures depends on the injury classification and provider or institutional preference.

* Tongs consist of a body with one pin attached at each end (Fig. 101-2). Tong pins are applied to the outer table of the skull on both sides of the skull. Cervical tongs are available in a variety of types, such as Crutchfield, Gardner-Wells, and Vinke tongs.
  * The shape, features, insertion site, and placement vary slightly, but the purpose, principles, and care are the same. Preference of the physician, advanced practice nurse, or other healthcare professional is an important deciding factor in choosing the specific device to be used.[2,11]
  * The insertion of Crutchfield and Vinke tongs necessitates an incision to expose the skull. Two holes are made in the outer table of the skull with a twist drill, and the pins are inserted and tightened until there is a firm fit.[2,11]
  * Gardner-Wells tongs are inserted by placing the razor-sharp pin edges to the prepared areas of the scalp and tightening the screws until the spring-loaded mechanism indicates that the correct pressure has been achieved. To decrease the possibility of tong displacement, all types of pins are well seated into the outer table of the skull and angled inward.[2,6,11]
  * Tongs are made of stainless steel or a graphite body with titanium pins. The graphite body with titanium pins is compatible with magnetic resonance imaging (MRI).
* Traction can be applied with the use of a rope and pulley system or a cable and alignment bracket. Weights are added gradually and followed with radiographic imaging. The physician, advanced practice nurse, or other

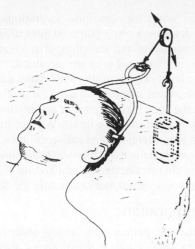

Figure 101-1 Continuous traction provided by weight applied to a cervical external fixation device via a rope and pulley system. *(From McRae R:* Practical fracture treatment, *ed 2, Edinburgh, 1989, Churchill Livingstone.)*

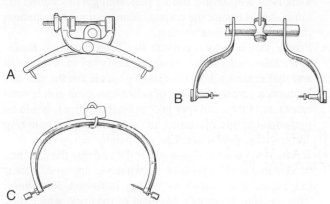

Figure 101-2 All three types of cervical tongs consist of a stainless steel body and a pin with a sharp tip attached to each end. **A,** Crutchfield tongs are placed about 5 inches apart in line with the long axis of the cervical spine. **B,** Vinke tongs are placed on the parietal bones, near the widest transverse diameter of the skull. **C,** Gardner-Wells tongs are inserted slightly above the patient's ears.

healthcare professional uses serial radiographs of the cervical spine to assist in determining the optimal amount of traction (measured in pounds) needed to reduce a fracture and provide optimal alignment. Excessive traction may result in stretching of the spinal cord and subsequent damage.[2-4]

- Cervical traction also may be applied with a halo ring device. This is a stainless steel or graphite ring that is attached to the skull by four stabilizing pins (two anterior and two posterolateral; Fig. 101-3). Skull pins can be made of stainless steel, titanium, or ceramic material.[1,2,5,7] Pins are threaded through holes in the ring, screwed into the outer table of the skull, and locked into place. Traction can be applied to the ring device with the use of a rope and pulley system or a cable and bracket alignment system. Weights are added gradually. After alignment of the cervical spine is achieved, the spine can be immobilized by attaching the ring to a body vest or a custom

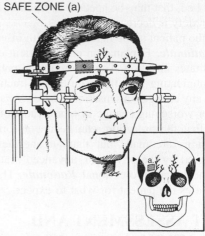

Figure 101-3 Placement of halo pins and ring. The anterior pins are placed anterolaterally 1 cm above the orbital ridge. This "safe zone" avoids the temporalis muscle laterally and an orbital nerve plexus and frontal sinus medially. *(From Batte M, Garfin SR, Byrne TP, et al: The halo skeletal fixator: Principles of applications and maintenance,* Clin Orthop 239:14, 1989.)*

molded body jacket. The patient then is able to move while the head and neck remain immobile.

EQUIPMENT

- Tongs or halo ring
- Insertion tray, including either the specific type of tongs to be used or the halo ring with insertion pins
- Local anesthetic: lidocaine, 1% to 2% (with or without epinephrine, depending on the preference of the physician, advanced practice nurse, or other healthcare professional)
- Needles (18- and 23-gauge)
- Sterile and nonsterile gloves
- Gowns, masks, and eye shields
- Antiseptic solution
- Sterile sponges
- Sterile drill and bits (for insertion of Crutchfield and Vinke tongs)
- Rope and traction assembly for the bed (if a RotoRest Delta Kinetic Therapy™ bed is used, a cable and bracket alignment system is needed; see Procedure 99)
- S and C hooks (to attach to the distal end of the rope for weight application)
- Weights to attach to the traction
- Torque wrench for the halo apparatus as well as the halo vest if this is the definitive treatment

Additional equipment, to have available as needed, includes the following:

- Hair clippers
- Emergency equipment

PATIENT AND FAMILY EDUCATION

- Explain the procedure and the reason for cervical traction. Clarify or reinforce information as needed by the patient or family. Discuss use of any special equipment, such as a special bed, that may be needed. *Rationale:* Patient and family anxiety is decreased.

- Explain the patient's role in assisting with insertion of the tongs. *Rationale:* Explanation elicits patient cooperation and facilitates insertion. The nonintubated patient should be communicating with the team during traction if he or she feels any changes in sensation, new or worsening pain, or new or worsening change in motor function.
- Explain that the procedure can be uncomfortable when the incisions are made but that an anesthetic will be administered by the physician, advanced practice nurse, or other healthcare professional. *Rationale:* This information prepares the patient for what to expect.

PATIENT ASSESSMENT AND PREPARATION

Patient Assessment

- Conduct a complete neurological assessment that includes evaluation of cranial nerve function, motor strength of major muscles, sensation (assessment of light touch, pain, and proprioception, noting highest dermatome level), and deep tendon reflexes (biceps, triceps, patella, and Achilles) and superficial reflexes (abdominal and anal wink). *Rationale:* Baseline data are provided for comparison of postinsertion assessments to determine the presence of neurological compromise or extension of spinal cord injury.
- Assess the patient's vital signs. *Rationale:* Baseline data are provided for comparison with assessments after insertion.
- Assess the patient's respiratory pattern and auscultate lung sounds. Note the use of accessory respiratory muscles and any signs or symptoms of dyspnea. *Rationale:* Baseline data are established to determine any compromise to respiratory function as a result of the procedure.

- Inspect the scalp for abrasions, lacerations, or sites of infection. *Rationale:* Any potential sites of infection that may contraindicate the insertion of a cervical fixation device into the infected area are identified.
- Assess the level of pain or discomfort and anxiety. *Rationale:* Assessment establishes data for decision making regarding the need for analgesia or anxiolytics for comfort and cooperation during the insertion procedure.
- Assess for any allergies to an antiseptic agent, local anesthetic, or analgesia and anxiolytics. *Rationale:* Review of medication allergies before administration of a new medication decreases the chances of an allergic reaction.

Patient Preparation

- Ensure that the patient and family understand preprocedural teaching. Answer questions as they arise, and reinforce information as needed. *Rationale:* Understanding of previously taught information is evaluated and reinforced.
- Verify that the patient is the correct patient using two identifiers. *Rationale:* Before performing a procedure, the nurse should ensure the correct identification of the patient for the intended intervention.
- Ensure that informed consent has been obtained. *Rationale:* Informed consent protects the rights of the patient and makes a competent decision possible for the patient.
- Perform a preprocedure verification and time out, if nonemergent. A time out (per institutional practice) should be performed before placement of cervical tongs or halo ring and traction. *Rationale:* Ensures patient safety.
- Ensure that the head of the bed is flat and that the patient's head is in a neutral position by whatever approved means (e.g., hard/rigid collar) have been instituted. *Rationale:* This measure prevents movement of the neck, which may increase the risk of injury or extension of spinal cord injury.

Procedure	for Assisting With Application of Tongs or Halo Ring for Cervical Traction	
Steps	Rationale	Special Considerations
1. Obtain a bed with an orthopedic traction frame, weights, and rope and pulley system attached to the bed or, if prescribed, obtain a RotoRest Kinetic Therapy™ bed with the wire and bracket alignment device.	Traction must be ready to reduce the potential for movement of the head and neck.	May require assistance from other departments; therefore, plan ahead to coordinate.
2. 🖐		
3. 🛡		All healthcare personnel involved in the procedure need to apply personal protective and sterile attire (e.g., fluid shield masks, eye shields, gowns, and sterile gloves).

Procedure	for Assisting With Application of Tongs or Halo Ring for Cervical Traction—*Continued*	
Steps	**Rationale**	**Special Considerations**
4. Assist the physician, advanced practice nurse, or other healthcare professional with tong or halo ring insertion:	Facilitates the procedure.	Because of the high risk for extension of cervical injury, this procedure usually is performed by a neurosurgeon, who can respond rapidly if neurological deterioration becomes evident.
A. Assist as needed with preparation of the pin sites (clipping a small area of scalp hair if indicated and cleansing with antiseptic solution).	Clipping the hair may prevent it from being trapped when the pins are inserted. Cleansing decreases skin surface bacteria.	
B. Assist if needed with draping the patient, leaving insertion sites exposed.	Aids in maintaining sterility.	
C. Assist as needed with local anesthesia administration.	Decreases patient discomfort during pin insertion.	
D. Stabilize the patient's head and neck during the procedure.	Maintains alignment of the cervical spine and provides support to the injured areas.	Cervical stabilization can be maintained with the use of a rigid collar or other devices that prevent head rotation and neck flexion or extension. A soft collar is not considered a stabilizing device. The head and shoulder packs of the RotoRest Kinetic Therapy™ bed provide some cervical stability but should not be used as the primary means of stabilizing cervical spine fractures before, during, or after tong or halo insertion. Utmost care must be taken to prevent head and neck flexion or extension. Be prepared for the possibility of respiratory insufficiency, respiratory arrest, hypotension, bradycardia or cardiac arrest.
E. Carefully follow institutional policies regarding manual cervical spine immobilization.	Institutional policies may provide strict guidelines for nursing role in manual cervical spine immobilization during traction placement.	Follow institutional policy for confirmatory radiographic studies following the procedure.
5. Monitor the patient for changes in respiratory function, neurogenic shock, spinal shock, changes in motor function, and changes in sensation and pain.	Identifies evidence of untoward effects or complications related to the procedure, and identifies the need for analgesia.	In addition to untoward effects, the patient may need additional reassurance, support, sedation, and analgesia.
6. Follow hospital policy for pin site care (see Procedure 104).	Maintains asepsis.	
7. Assist with application and connection to traction as needed (see Procedure 102).		
A. Maintain the patient's head in a neutral position.	Ensures accurate and safe use of the traction.	

Procedure continues on following page

Procedure	**for Assisting With Application of Tongs or Halo Ring for Cervical Traction—*Continued***

Steps	Rationale	Special Considerations
B. Assist if needed with the application of prescribed weights.	Provides assistance.	
C. Ensure that weights are unobstructed and hanging freely.[2,8–11] **(Level E*)**	Ensures safe use of equipment and maintains principles of traction.	
8. Discard used supplies in an appropriate receptacle.	Removes and safely discards used supplies.	
9. 🖐		

Expected Outcomes

- Tong or halo ring device inserted
- Head and neck immobilized to allow for alignment, stabilization, and healing of fractures
- Prescribed amount of weight applied to tongs or halo
- Traction weights unobstructed and hanging freely
- Improved or stable neurological function (motor and sensory)
- Patient discomfort minimized

Unexpected Outcomes

- Slippage of tongs or halo pins
- Extension or deterioration of neurological deficits or spinal cord injury
- Respiratory compromise or arrest
- Hypotensive episode, bradycardia, cardiac arrest
- Pain
- Bleeding at pin site

Patient Monitoring and Care

Steps	Rationale	Reportable Conditions
		These conditions should be reported if they persist despite nursing interventions.
1. Assess neurological status every 5 minutes during the procedure, including assessment of level of consciousness, movement in arms and legs, sensation, mastication, and eyelid closure.[2,5,7] **(Level E)**	Facilitates early recognition of neurological deterioration. Bitemporal tongs may interfere with mastication and eyelid closure.[2,5,7]	- Any deterioration or extension of baseline neurological function - Increased or new loss of sensation - New or worsening decrease in motor strength
2. Assess respiratory function (respiratory rate, pulse oximetry, lung sounds) before, during, and after the procedure.	Early identification of hypoxia or respiratory distress from neurological deterioration or other potential complications such as aspiration or sedation. Decrease in peripheral oxygen saturation may be an early indicator of respiratory compromise.	- Changes in respiratory function (e.g., decrease in oxygen saturation [Sao_2], increase in end tidal carbon dioxide [$Etco_2$]; increase or decrease in respiratory rate, abnormal lung sounds)
3. Assess for neurogenic shock.	Neurogenic shock can occur rapidly and requires prompt intervention.	- Oversedation - Hypotension - Bradycardia - Decreased vascular tone - Hypoxia - Poikilothermia
4. Provide emotional support and reassurance to the patient during the procedure.	Decreases anxiety and facilitates patient cooperation.	- Unrelieved anxiety

*Level E: Multiple case reports, theory-based evidence from expert opinions, or peer-reviewed professional organizational standards without clinical studies to support recommendations.

Patient Monitoring and Care —*Continued*

Steps	Rationale	Reportable Conditions
5. Monitor pin sites for hemostasis immediately after the procedure, every 15 minutes × four, every 30 minutes × two, and hourly, or as indicated by institutional policy.	The scalp is vascular, and continued bleeding may occur at the pin sites that requires assessment and cleansing.[5,6]	• Unresolved bleeding
6. Check the security of the traction, bed frame, and bed.	The traction frame is attached to the bed and must be secure.	• Break in the integrity of the traction equipment or the bed frame
7. Maintain the patient's head flat on the bed and ensure that the bed is flat. The head of the bed frame may be on shock blocks or placed in reverse Trendelenburg's position to provide countertraction.[8,9]	The head must be flat on the bed to maintain a neutral position. Countertraction is often provided to prevent the patient from being pulled toward the top of the bed.	• Neck or head out of neutral alignment
8. If the knot on the traction rope nears the pulley or the wire band nears the bracket, several physicians, advanced practice nurses, or other healthcare professionals may slowly pull the patient down in bed. The patient should *never* be pulled up in the bed or traction will be released. Do *not* remove the weights to move the patient toward the foot of the bed.[8-11] (**Level E***)	The knot of the traction rope must not be resting against the pulley for effective traction. The cover over the wire and bracket alignment device must not be against the alignment screw (head of the bed) for effective traction.	• Evidence of loss of effective traction
9. If cervical traction is lost for whatever reason (e.g., the loop in traction rope holding the weights slips or the pins dislodge), maintain manual cervical spine immobilization, place the patient in a hard/rigid cervical collar, and notify the physician, advanced practice nurse, or other healthcare professional. Elicit the patient's cooperation to minimize extraneous movement.	Immediate intervention is needed to immobilize the patient's head and neck.	• Changes in motor and/or sensory assessment • Changes in respiratory effort, signs of respiratory distress • Evidence of loss of effective traction
10. Prepare the patient for a bedside confirmatory radiograph of the cervical spine immediately after insertion and application of weights and as prescribed by the physician, advanced practice nurse, or other healthcare professional.	A radiograph is taken to verify alignment of the cervical spine.	• Abnormal radiographic results

*Level E: Multiple case reports, theory-based evidence from expert opinions, or peer-reviewed professional organizational standards without clinical studies to support recommendations.

Procedure continues on following page

Patient Monitoring and Care —*Continued*

Steps	Rationale	Reportable Conditions
11. If additional weights are added or removed by the physician, advanced practice nurse, or other healthcare professional in an attempt to realign the cervical spine, increase the frequency of neurological checks. Expect more frequent cervical radiographs or MRIs to verify alignment.[2,3]	Monitors for possible risk of secondary spinal cord injury.	• Changes in motor and/or sensory assessment • Changes in respiratory effort, signs of respiratory distress
12. Follow institutional standards for assessing pain. Administer analgesia as prescribed.	Identifies need for pain interventions.	• Continued pain despite pain interventions

Documentation

Documentation should include the following:
- Patient and family education
- Completion of informed consent
- Preprocedure verifications and time out
- Type of cervical traction applied
- Date and time traction is applied
- Local anesthetic used
- Sedation and analgesia used
- Amount of weight applied to the traction
- Weights hanging freely
- Pins secure
- Appearance of pin-insertion site and care

- Ongoing comprehensive assessment data and action taken for abnormal response
- Verification of proper functioning and security of traction equipment
- Documentation of radiographic confirmation of alignment
- Occurrence of unexpected outcomes
- Patient response to care
- Additional interventions
- Pain assessment, interventions, and effectiveness

References and Additional Readings

For a complete list of references and additional readings for this procedure, scan this QR code with any freely available smartphone code reader app, or visit http://booksite.elsevier.com/9780323376624.

102 Cervical Traction Maintenance

Jennifer Massetti

PURPOSE: Once cervical traction has been established, the nurse cares for the patient who is immobilized on complete bed rest. Traction must be maintained on a continuous basis until realignment and stabilization with surgical management or orthoses is attained or healing is completed.

PREREQUISITE NURSING KNOWLEDGE

- The nurse must be knowledgeable about the anatomy and physiology of the spinal column, the anatomy of the cervical vertebrae, the spinal cord, the cervical spinal nerves, and the area of peripheral innervation.
- It is important that the nurse understands the pathophysiology and manifestations of spinal cord injury, including ascending edema, spinal shock, and neurogenic shock. Continual assessment of changes in motor, sensory, and respiratory associated with ascending edema, spinal shock, and neurogenic shock is essential in the care of the patient requiring cervical traction.
- After the cervical tongs are inserted, traction is applied by adding weights to a rope and pulley or cable and bracket alignment device attached to the tongs (see Fig. 100-1). Additional weight may be added gradually, followed by radiographic imaging. The physician uses serial radiographs of the cervical spine to assist in determining the optimal amount of traction (measured in pounds) needed to reduce a fracture and provide optimal alignment. Excessive traction may cause stretching of and damage to the spinal cord; the addition of weight to the traction is managed by the physician.[3,5,6,9]
- Once the traction is in place, the patient is maintained on strict bed rest. For facilitation of turning, the patient may be placed on a special bed or turning frame.
- The principles of skeletal traction are the foundation of management of any patient in cervical traction. One must follow key points: (1) never raise/lift the traction weights, (2) never disconnect the traction, (3) never allow the traction weights to rest on the floor, and (4) never allow other objects to compromise freely hanging weights.

EQUIPMENT

- Cervical traction system in place, including rope and pulley system or cable and bracket alignment device and weights for the RotoRest™ Delta Kinetic™ Therapy Bed (see Figs. 99-1, 102-1).
- Pillows

Additional equipment, to have available as needed, includes the following:
- Positioning devices or protective dressings
- Specialty bed

PATIENT AND FAMILY EDUCATION

- Explain the procedure and the reason for the traction. *Rationale:* Patient and family anxiety may be decreased.
- Explain the patient's role in maintaining the traction. *Rationale:* Patient cooperation is elicited. The nonintubated patient should be communicating with the team during traction if he or she feels any changes in sensation, new or worsening pain, or new or worsening change in motor function.[6]
- Explain how the patient's basic needs will be met during the confinement to bed and the maintenance of traction. *Rationale:* The patient and family are reassured that the patient will be cared for and his or her needs met.

PATIENT ASSESSMENT AND PREPARATION

Patient Assessment

- Conduct a complete neurological assessment that includes motor strength of the major muscles and sensory function. (Assess light touch, pain, and proprioception. Note the highest dermatome level with impaired sensation.) Assess deep tendon reflexes (biceps, triceps, patellar, and Achilles), superficial reflexes, and cranial nerves. *Rationale:* Baseline data are established for determination of any change in neurological function.
- Assess the patient's vital signs. *Rationale:* Baseline data are provided for comparison with assessments after insertion.
- Inspect the scalp for abrasions, lacerations, or sites of infection. *Rationale:* Any potential sites of infection that may contraindicate the insertion of a cervical fixation device into the infected area are identified.
- Assess the patient's comfort. *Rationale:* Spinal injuries are often painful. Changes in pain in the head or neck or

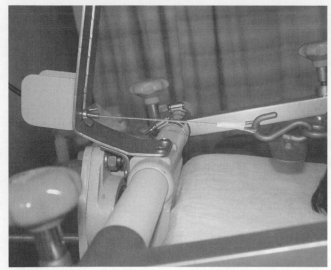

Figure 102-1   Closer view of the tension system for cervical traction.

at the pin sites may suggest misalignment, pin-site infection, or slippage of traction.

• Assess the location and skin around pins. *Rationale:* Pins can slip and pin sites can become irritated and/or infected.[7]

Patient Preparation

• Ensure that the patient and family understand preprocedural teaching. Answer questions as they arise, and reinforce information as needed. *Rationale:* Understanding of previously taught information is evaluated and reinforced.

• Verify that the patient is the correct patient using two identifiers. *Rationale:* Before performing a procedure, the nurse should ensure the correct identification of the patient for the intended intervention.

• Ensure that body alignment is maintained and that the patient is positioned in the middle of the bed. *Rationale:* Positioning facilitates comfort and even distribution of the traction.

• Check the orthopedic traction frame, rope knot, and pulley or cable and bracket alignment device for secure attachment and function. *Rationale:* Ineffective traction or loss of traction may result in loss of realignment and stabilization of the vertebral column, resulting in spinal cord injury.

• Check the ropes and weights to be sure that they are hanging freely. Check the cable and alignment bracket device for patients treated on a kinetic therapy bed. *Rationale:* Assessment maintains function and prevents slippage of the orthopedic equipment.

Procedure | for Traction Maintenance

Steps	Rationale	Special Considerations
1. **HH**		
2. **PE**		
3. Ensure that the orthopedic frame and traction equipment are intact.	Promotes patient safety.	
4. Maintain the weights so that they hang freely at all times.[1,4,8,10] **(Level E*)**	Obstruction to the free hanging of the weights eliminates traction and could precipitate adverse neurological responses in the patient. Do not raise the traction at any time.[4,6,8]	Inform the physician immediately of any interruption of the traction because a cervical radiograph may be necessary to assess cervical alignment.
5. Ensure that the rope is able to slide freely through the pulley and that the knot in the rope is not resting on the pulley. If using the cable and bracket alignment device, ensure that the cable is able to slide freely through the bracket (ensure the band at the end of the cable is not resting on the bracket).[4,8,10] **(Level E)**	The knot resting on the pulley interferes with the adequacy of the weights and traction. The cable must slide freely through the bracket to maintain adequacy of the weights and traction.[4,6,8]	If the knot on the traction rope nears the pulley or the wire band nears the bracket, several healthcare providers may slowly pull the patient down in bed. The patient should *never* be pulled up in the bed or traction will be released.

*Level E: Multiple case reports, theory-based evidence from expert opinions, or peer-reviewed professional organizational standards without clinical studies to support recommendations.

Procedure   for Traction Maintenance—*Continued*

Steps	Rationale	Special Considerations
6. Maintain the patient in a straight line (centered on the bed), in a neutral position and aligned with the pulley and rope or cable and bracket alignment device. Lock the bed controls so the patient and/or visitors cannot accidently move the head of the bed.	Alignment ensures optimal traction that is balanced (does not pull on one side of the body more than on the other side) and prevents traction slippage and pain.	Reposition as necessary; ensure adequate help to prevent extension of a cervical injury.
7. Follow the physician, advanced practice nurse, and other healthcare professionals' prescription regarding turning. When turning manually, logroll with at least three healthcare providers. Follow institutional policy for maintaining cervical spinal alignment during repositioning. When turning automatically with kinetic therapy, increase the angle gradually while assessing how the patient responds to turning.	Maintains alignment.	Begin turning only when prescribed by the physician, advanced practice nurse, or other healthcare professional. Turning or moving the patient in a neutral position with a triple log-rolling technique requires coordination of turning and preplanning.
8. Use pillows and special positioning devices to maintain the patient in body alignment.	Prevents misalignment and possible extension of a cervical injury.	Do not use pillows under the patient's head; maintain the patient flat on the bed; use pillows to support alignment and maintenance of a neutral position.
9. Discard used supplies in an appropriate receptacle.	Removes and safely discards used supplies.	
10. ▦		

Expected Outcomes

- The orthopedic traction frame and all traction equipment are secure and functional
- Proper body alignment of the patient is maintained
- The patient is comfortable and safe
- The patient's neurological function is stable or improved
- The patient tolerates turning

Unexpected Outcomes

- Slippage of tongs, pins, or external fixation device
- Interruption of continuous traction
- Extension or deterioration of neurological deficits or spinal cord injury
- Pain

Patient Monitoring and Care

Steps	Rationale	Reportable Conditions
		These conditions should be reported if they persist despite nursing interventions.
1. Perform a neurological assessment after cervical traction is initiated and then a minimum of every 2–4 hours, as prescribed or according to institution standard.	Determines neurological status and assesses for changes due to edema or spinal shock.	• Any deterioration or extension of baseline neurological function (e.g., loss of more dermatomal sensation, decrease in motor strength, loss of reflexes, difficulty breathing) • Bitemporal tongs may also interfere with eyelid close and mastication[11]

Procedure continues on following page

TABLE 102-1	Acute Physiological Responses to Immobility and Spinal Cord Injury		
Body System	Physiological Response to Immobility	Physiological Response to Spinal Cord Injury	Assessment Parameters
Integumentary	Pressure → ischemia → integumentary disruption	Protective motor and sensory functions lost or impaired below the level of the lesion	Inspect bony prominences. Identify preexisting skin disruptions. Assess specific pressure areas related to traction devices and positioning.
Pulmonary	Decreased chest expansion Secretions pool CO_2 retention → respiratory acidosis	Lost or impaired neuromuscular stimulus to the diaphragm, internal and external intercostals, abdominal muscles, and accessory muscles	Observe the thorax for symmetrical chest expansion. Identify breathing patterns. Auscultate breath sounds. Respiratory parameters (NIF/FVC). Supplemental O_2 ABG/pulse oximetry. Identify associated pulmonary injury.
Cardiovascular	Increased cardiac workload Thrombus formation Orthostasis	Decreased vasomotor tone Loss of sympathetic response Poor venous return Poikilothermia Spinal shock → autonomic dysreflexia	Monitor vital signs, rhythm interpretation, blood pressure, heart rate, and perfusion. Monitor body/skin temperature Organ perfusion assessment: level of consciousness and urine output.
Musculoskeletal	Muscle atrophy Joint immobility → Contractures	Loss/impairment of voluntary motor function Flaccid → spastic paralysis	Identify level of lesion. Serial motor/sensory examinations. Assess joint mobility (flaccidity/spasticity). Confirm that the traction and weights are applied correctly.
Neurological	Increased vasovagal response, bradycardia, hypotension	Neurogenic shock Spinal shock	After spinal shock, assess for autonomic dysreflexia.
Gastrointestinal	Paralytic ileus	Neurogenic bowel	Monitor for absent to hypoactive bowel sounds, inability to tolerate enteral nutrition.
Genitourinary	Bladder atony	Neurogenic bladder Areflexic to eventually reflex voiding	Monitor urine output. Assess for bladder distension.

NIF, negative inspiratory force; *FVC*, forced vital capacity; *ABG*, arterial blood gas.

Patient Monitoring and Care —*Continued*

Steps	Rationale	Reportable Conditions
2. Obtain vital signs after cervical traction is initiated and then a minimum of every 2–4 hours, as prescribed or according to institutional standards. Continue to assess the patient for neurogenic shock.	Determines cardiovascular stability.	• Changes in vital signs (hypotension, bradycardia, respiratory distress), or neurogenic shock will require prompt intervention
3. Assess respiratory status after cervical traction is initiated and then at a minimum of every 2–4 hours, as prescribed or according to institutional standards (Table 102-1).	Provides early identification of atelectasis, pneumonia, respiratory distress, or extension of neurological deterioration.	• Abnormal lung sounds • Abnormal respiratory rate or pattern of breathing • Decreased oxygen saturation • Decreased ventilation parameters (e.g., tidal volume, vital capacity) • Increased sputum • Yellow-green sputum • Elevated temperature • Use of accessory muscles

Patient Monitoring and Care —*Continued*

Steps	Rationale	Reportable Conditions
4. Assess cardiac status after cervical traction is initiated and then at minimum every 2–4 hours, as prescribed or according to institutional standards (see Table 102-1).	Provides early identification of cardiac dysrhythmias or decompensation.	• Dysrhythmias • Abnormal heart sounds • Hemodynamic instability
5. Perform peripheral vascular assessment after cervical traction is initiated and then at a minimum of every 2–4 hours, as prescribed, or according to institutional standards. Consider deep venous thromboembolism (DVT) prophylaxis (e.g., anticoagulation therapy and sequential compression devices).[2,10]	Provides early identification of peripheral vascular insufficiency and DVT.	• Peripheral vascular changes • Signs of DVT
6. Perform gastrointestinal assessment after cervical traction is initiated and then at a minimum of every 2–4 hours, as prescribed, or according to institutional standards; consider gastric prophylaxis.[2,12]	Provides early identification of paralytic ileus and gastric distention; prevention of gastric hemorrhage.	• Abdominal distention • Nausea • Vomiting • Decreased bowel sounds • Constipation
7. Perform genitourinary assessment after cervical traction is initiated and then at a minimum of every 2–4 hours, as prescribed or according to institutional standards.[2,12]	Provides early identification of urinary tract infection and neurogenic bladder.	• Decreased urine output • Increased urine output • Distended bladder • Signs and symptoms of urinary tract infection
8. Perform skin assessment after cervical traction is initiated and then at a minimum of every 2–4 hours, as prescribed or according to institutional standards (see Table 102-1).[2,12]	Provides early recognition of skin breakdown.	• Evidence of skin breakdown
9. Perform musculoskeletal assessment every 8 hours (see Table 102-1).[2,12]	Provides early recognition of musculoskeletal contractures.	• Increased spasticity or malpositioning of an extremity
10. Perform nutritional assessment at least once a day.[1,2]	Determines nutritional status.	• Decreased intake, poor skin turgor, intolerance of nutrition
11. Assess anxiety level, pain, and coping.[1,2]	Provides early recognition of anxiety, depression, agitation, and pain.	• Anxiety, depression, agitation, pain, or other untoward responses
12. Perform pin care (see Procedure 104).	Monitors skin and assesses for infection.	• Evidence of infection
13. Reposition and turn, maintaining neutral body alignment.[1,2] Follow institutional standards.	Maintains skin integrity. Prevents complications of immobility.	• Impaired skin integrity
14. Perform respiratory management (e.g., supplemental oxygen, deep breathing, suctioning, incentive spirometer, quad coughing, chest physical therapy, bronchoscopy, tracheostomy).[2,12]	Supports respiratory function and oxygenation of all body organs.	• Decreased or increased respirations • Abnormal lung sounds • Decreased oxygen saturation • Change in pulmonary secretions • Fever
15. Initiate bladder and bowel programs.[2,12]	Supports adequate emptying of bladder and pattern of bowel activity.	• Bladder distension • Constipation • Decrease in or absence of bowel signs

Procedure continues on following page

Patient Monitoring and Care —*Continued*

Steps	Rationale	Reportable Conditions
16. Perform range of motion every 2 hours and apply splints and other positioners.[1,2]	Maintains intact motor function.	• Evidence of contractures, deformities, functional loss
17. Offer emotional support and other diversional therapy.[1,2]	Supports patient and family through the continuum of care and keeps them actively involved.	
18. Consult support services as needed.[1,2]	Support services can provide items such as prism glasses to help the patient see, read, and increase visual field.	
19. Follow institutional standards for assessing pain. Administer analgesia as prescribed.	Identifies need for pain interventions.	• Continued pain despite pain interventions

Documentation

Documentation should include the following:
- Patient and family education
- Ongoing comprehensive assessment data and interventions for abnormal findings
- Verification of proper functioning and security of traction equipment (e.g., total weight applied, weights hanging freely, traction rope knot not against pulley, band at end of cable, and bracket alignment device not resting on bracket)
- Occurrence of unexpected outcomes
- Patient response to care
- Additional interventions
- Pain assessment, interventions, and effectiveness

References and Additional Readings

For a complete list of references and additional readings for this procedure, scan this QR code with any freely available smartphone code reader app, or visit http://booksite.elsevier.com/9780323376624.

103 Halo Ring and Vest Care

Cara Diaz

PURPOSE: A halo ring attached to a halo vest (commonly referred to as a halo) is designed to immobilize and stabilize the cervical spine. A halo ring and vest may be used alone or in conjunction with surgery for the patient with an unstable cervical spine as a result of spinal fracture or dislocation; degenerative processes, such as C1-C2 changes from rheumatoid arthritis; or spinal surgery. The halo ring and vest stabilizes the vertebral column's movement, reducing subsequent risk of spinal cord injury.[2]

PREREQUISITE NURSING KNOWLEDGE

- Knowledge of neuroanatomy and physiology of the cervical spine—including the spinal column, vertebrae, the spinal cord, and spinal nerves with their areas of innervation—is necessary.
- The nurse must understand the pathophysiology and manifestations of spinal cord trauma, including spinal shock, ascending edema, and related impairment of respiratory function, vasomotor tone, and autonomic nervous system function, including signs and symptoms of autonomic dysreflexia.
- The nurse must be familiar with the components of the halo-vest device, including the halo ring and pins, anterior and posterior posts, vest screws, front and back panels of the vest, and shoulder and side buckles.
- The halo ring and vest may be used as a primary definitive treatment to stabilize the cervical spine, before surgery to reduce spine deformity, or after surgery as an adjunct to interval cervical fixation.
- Although the conventional halo has been used since 1959 and is regarded as a standard of care for external stabilization of the injured cervical spine, new pinless and noninvasive halo options have been introduced to preliminary stages of research, showing promise for future patient options.[13] This procedure focuses on the management of the patient who needs immobilization with a halo ring and vest.
- Basic cardiac life support knowledge and skills are essential.
- The nurse must be knowledgeable about the signs and symptoms of new injury or extension of spinal cord injury and the needed interventions.
- The nurse should have knowledge regarding the indications for halo use in the patient and the risks and signs of halo failure.
- A halo ring device is a graphite ring attached to the skull with four stabilizing pins (two anterior and two posterolateral; see Fig. 101-3). The pins are threaded through holes in the ring, screwed into the outer table of the skull, and locked into place.
- Direct traction may be applied to the halo ring device with a rope and pulley or cable and bracket alignment system and weights (see Procedures 101 and 102). Patients with a halo ring, pins, and traction applied with weights are cared for similarly to patients in cervical traction with tongs (see Procedures 101 and 102).
- When alignment of the cervical spine is achieved, long-term immobilization of the spine can be achieved by attaching the ring to a body vest or a custom-molded body jacket, which allows for mobility of the patient (Fig. 103-1).[2,3]
- With the halo ring and pins in place, traction can be discontinued and a halo vest and struts added for long-term immobilization of the cervical neck (see Fig. 103-1). The advantage of this approach is that the patient can sit upright, mobilize out of bed, and ambulate, if able, while the cervical spine remains stable.
- The nurse should know how to access the patient's anterior chest to administer cardiopulmonary resuscitation (CPR) if cardiac arrest occurs. Refer to information from the manufacturer of the halo vest for specific information on emergency access to the chest. Some vests have a hinged closure; the vest can be lifted up at the hinge to allow quick access to the chest. Other vests are not hinged and require a wrench. The wrench must be available at all times and, depending on institutional policy, may be maintained on the front of the vest for instant access to the chest. If the patient needs defibrillation, avoid touching the bars of the traction with the defibrillator.
- Proper management and monitoring of a patient in a halo-vest device can prevent minor complications that could lead to more serious morbidity and mortality.[9]

EQUIPMENT

- Halo device (in place)
- Soap and a basin of warm water

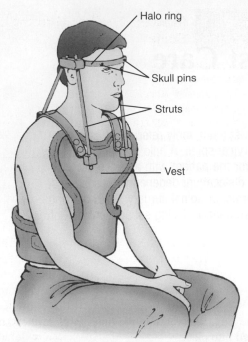

Halo ring

Skull pins

Struts

Vest

Figure 103-1 Halo-vest apparatus. Supportive struts and ring are attached to a plastic vest, applying cervical traction while allowing for patient mobility. *(From Urden LD, Stacy KM, Lough ME: Critical care nursing, ed. 7, St. Louis, 2014, Elsevier.)*

- Washcloth and towel
- Nonsterile gloves
- Flashlight

Additional equipment, to have available as needed, includes the following:
- Sheepskin liner
- Emergency wrench
- Lidocaine for subcutaneous administration at pin site during placement/adjustments

PATIENT AND FAMILY EDUCATION

- Explain that the reason for the halo ring and vest device is to maintain cervical immobilization. *Rationale:* Patient and family anxiety is decreased.
- Describe turning, positioning, and skin care procedures before performing them. *Rationale:* Patient and family anxiety is decreased.
- Explain to the patient and family that the halo vest's side panels should only be opened as prescribed by the physician, advanced practice nurse, or other healthcare professional and according to the manufacturer's guidelines. If the side panels are opened the patient needs to be flat and supine.[2,6,10] *Rationale:* Integrity of the halo-vest device and safety of the patient is maintained. Unbuckling of the halo vest may result in loss of spine alignment and neurological compromise.[10]
- Because the halo vest limits movement of the head, patients must be taught to scan the environment for objects in their path that could lead to falls. *Rationale:* Patient safety and independence are maintained. The halo vest changes the center of gravity and limits movement, thus

requiring adaptations for performing activities of daily living (ADLs).[10]
- If the patient is ambulatory, explain modifications in meeting basic needs such as bathing, toileting, eating, dressing, ambulation precautions, and safety needs. *Rationale:* Self-care skills and awareness of special safety precautions are developed.
- For patients who will be discharged home wearing a halo-vest device, begin a comprehensive teaching program with the patient and family. *Rationale:* The patient and family are prepared for care in the home environment.
- Explain to the patient and family that the patient cannot be turned with the struts (posts) of the halo-vest device. *Rationale:* The patient and family are prepared for care in the home environment.
- Explain that precautions must be used when the ambulatory patient with a halo-vest device gets in and out of a car and walks up and down stairs. *Rationale:* The patient cannot move the head in the halo-vest device to look down.
- Explain that driving, riding a motorcycle or bicycle, and operating machinery are unsafe with a halo-vest device. *Rationale:* Patients recognize that they cannot turn their head.
- Explain that the pins of the halo transmit vibration and cold sensation to the patient's skull. *Rationale:* The patient and family are alerted to possible sensations during ADLs.
- Explain that if the pins in the skull become loose, the patient should contact the physician immediately. Inform the patient and family not to adjust the pins in the skull. Family members may be taught how to tighten the halo washers and bolts with the wrench before discharge as prescribed. *Rationale:* The patient and family are prepared for care in the home and can identify when emergency care may be needed.
- Explain that if the patient has any decline in neurological function (i.e., decreased or abnormal sensory function, decline in motor ability, or increase in pain), the physician should be contacted immediately. *Rationale:* Decline in neurological function may indicate extension of spinal cord injury and the need for immediate interventions.

PATIENT ASSESSMENT AND PREPARATION

Patient Assessment

- Perform a complete neurological assessment (Fig. 103-2; Box 103-1). *Rationale:* This assessment provides baseline data.[5]
- Assess skin integrity along the patient's scalp. *Rationale:* This assessment ensures that there is no skin breakdown near the areas where the screws will be placed.
- Obtain vital signs before halo ring and vest placement. *Rationale:* Baseline data are provided.
- Assess for difficulty swallowing and risk for aspiration.[4,14] *Rationale:* Assessment identifies a patient at high risk and the need to modify oral intake.

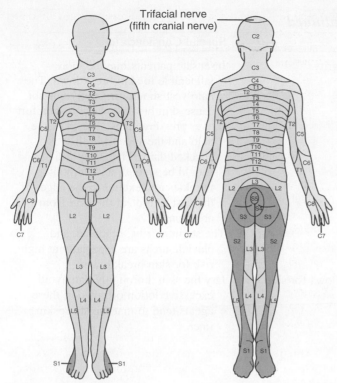

Trifacial nerve
(fifth cranial nerve)

Figure 103-2 Dermatomes. *(From Nagelhout JJ, Plaus KL: Nurse anesthesia, ed 5, St. Louis, 2014, Saunders.)*

BOX 103-1   **Muscle Strength Grading Scale**

0/5—No movement or muscle contraction
1/5—Trace contraction
2/5—Active movement with gravity eliminated
3/5—Active movement against gravity
4/5—Active movement with some resistance
5/5—Active movement with full resistance

(From Urden LD, Stacy KM, Lough ME: Priorities in critical care nursing, ed. 7, St. Louis, 2016, Elsevier.)

- Ensure the emergency wrench is in the packet and attached to the vest after placement. *Rationale:* Allows for emergent removal if necessary.
- Ensure all pins, screws, bolts and washers are intact on the device and no stripping has occurred or pieces are missing. *Rationale:* Tight connections are necessary to ensure stabilization of the device for effective immobilization of the spine.

Patient Preparation

- Ensure that the patient and family understand preprocedural information. Answer questions as they arise, and reinforce information as needed. *Rationale:* Understanding of previously taught information is evaluated and reinforced.
- Verify that the patient is the correct patient using two identifiers *Rationale:* Before performing a procedure, the nurse should ensure the correct identification of the patient for the intended intervention.
- Assist patients, as they lie supine in a neutral position, with proper body alignment for the purpose of halo vest application, liner change, and routine skin care. *Rationale:* Patients are kept safe and accessible for inspection.
- Observe the sides and back of the vest and adjacent skin with the patient standing, if possible. *Rationale:* Observation provides an opportunity to inspect all areas in which the skin and vest come in contact.

- Assess the skin at the edges of the vest and where the vest may overlap for redness or abrasion, especially over bony prominences.[10,14] *Rationale:* Skin irritation related to the halo-vest device is identified.
- Check the fit of the vest for tightness or looseness. *Rationale:* The need for change or modification of the vest is identified. Patient weight loss and position changes (sitting to standing) may contribute to vest looseness.
- Check the halo vest for loose straps or screws, dirt, odor, or evidence of the need to repair the vest. *Rationale:* The vest may need to be repaired or the sheepskin liner changed.

Procedure   for Halo Ring and Vest Care

Steps	Rationale	Special Considerations
1. **HH**		
2. **PE**		
3. If unbuckling is prescribed for vest care, position the patient flat in bed on his or her side; then unbuckle one side of the halo vest while maintaining cervical spinal alignment.[2,10] **(Level E*)**	Gains access to the underlying skin.	Review the manufacturer's recommendations with regard to vest care. Follow institutional policy with regard to vest care.

*Level E: Multiple case reports, theory-based evidence from expert opinions, or peer-reviewed professional organizational standards without clinical studies to support recommendations.

Procedure continues on following page

Procedure   for Halo Ring and Vest Care—*Continued*

Steps	Rationale	Special Considerations
4. Assess the patient's skin. Use a flashlight while pressing the liner toward the vest to facilitate assessment of the skin.	Determines skin integrity.[10,14]	Insensate patients may be more vulnerable to skin breakdown. The halo vest should fit snugly but not cause skin breakdown or discomfort over pressure areas. The fit of the halo and the sheepskin liner is checked daily. The sheepskin should be smooth and without wrinkles and extend to the edges of the vest to protect the skin from abrasions. The sternum, ribs, scapulae, and clavicle areas are especially at high risk for skin breakdown.
5. Bathe the skin with soap and water. Minimize moisture to avoid wetting the liner of the vest. If unbuckling the vest is not recommended by manufacturer or institutional policy, pass a damp thin towel between the skin and sheepskin, reaching all skin surfaces.[10]	Cleanses the skin. Allows for skin assessment.	Dry the skin thoroughly and avoid excessive lotion or powder; these agents tend to mat the sheepskin liner.
6. Auscultate lung sounds.	Identifies adventitious breath sounds.	Lung sounds may be decreased at the bases in patients with poor diaphragm and intercostal muscle function.[1]
7. Perform anterior and posterior chest physiotherapy, if indicated.	May enhance secretion maintenance and facilitate airway clearance.	A slight decrease in vital capacity related to vest placement may be seen.[14]
8. Rebuckle the vest.[8,10] (**Level E***)	Maintains cervical immobilization.	Ensure that the buckle is secured for proper fit.
9. Turn the patient to the opposite side without using the struts of the halo, keep the head of the bed flat, and **repeat Steps 3–8.**[1,2,10,14] (**Level E**)	Facilitates assessment of the opposite side of the patient's body.	
10. If unbuckling is prescribed, change or assist with changing the anterior sheepskin liner as needed:	Provides comfort and cleanliness and protects the skin.	Follow institutional standards for liner change. The anterior portion of the sheepskin liner may require frequent changes because of secretions or drainage from a tracheostomy or from spills during eating.[10] Protect the sheepskin liner during meals and use towels and plastic when washing the hair to minimize the need to change the liner.[10] Follow manufacturer's recommendations and institutional policy regarding washing, reusing, or discarding the liner.
A. Place the patient supine with the head of the bed flat.	Provides support and alignment.	

*Level E: Multiple case reports, theory-based evidence from expert opinions, or peer-reviewed professional organizational standards without clinical studies to support recommendations.

Procedure for Halo Ring and Vest Care—*Continued*

Steps	Rationale	Special Considerations
B. Unbuckle one side strap on the vest while maintaining cervical spine alignment and immobilization.	Provides access to the sheepskin.	
C. Roll the soiled liner on the unbuckled portion of the anterior vest to the center of the vest to facilitate removal of the sheepskin.	Simplifies the liner change.	
D. Match half the clean liner to the corresponding portion of the anterior vest and roll the remainder to the center of the vest.		
E. Buckle the side strap of the vest.	Maintains cervical immobilization.	
F. Unbuckle the other side strap and remove the remainder of the soiled liner.		
G. Unroll the clean liner and match to the corresponding Velcro strips on the vest.		
H. Buckle the side strap.		
11. Change or assist with changing the posterior sheepskin liner as needed:	Promotes comfort and protects the skin.	Follow institutional standards for liner change.
A. Position the patient with the head of the bed flat and the patient turned to the side-lying position. Alternately, the patient can be turned prone, with a pillow under the chest and a pillow under the head, if the patient's respiratory status tolerates this position.	Provides support and protects the skin.	
B. Unbuckle one side strap of the halo vest while maintaining cervical spine alignment and immobilization.	Provides support and alignment.	
C. Roll the soiled liner on the unbuckled portion of the posterior vest to the center of the vest to facilitate removal of sheepskin.	Simplifies the liner change.	
D. Match half the clean liner to the corresponding portion of the posterior vest and roll the remainder to the center of the vest.	Provides comfort and protects the skin.	
E. Buckle the side strap of the vest.	Maintains cervical immobilization.	
F. Roll the patient to the opposite side.	Maintains cervical spine alignment.	
G. Unbuckle the side strap on the vest while maintaining cervical spine alignment and immobilization. Remove the remainder of the soiled liner.	Accesses the opposite side of the liner.	

Procedure continues on following page

Procedure for Halo Ring and Vest Care—*Continued*

Steps	Rationale	Special Considerations
H. Unroll the clean liner and match to the corresponding Velcro strips on the vest.	Secures the liner in place.	
I. Buckle the side strap.	Maintains cervical immobilization.	
12. Discard used supplies in an appropriate receptacle.	Removes and safely discards used supplies.	
13. [HH]		

Expected Outcomes

- Cervical alignment is maintained
- The underlying skin remains intact and free of irritation
- The vest is functional, fits well, and is clean and odorless
- The pin sites are clean
- Mobility and sensation are maintained if the patient is neurologically intact
- The patient's safety is maintained

Unexpected Outcomes

- Loose pins[4,7]
- Pin site infection, osteomyelitis, or intracranial abscess[4,7,12]
- Poor fit (too loose or too tight) of halo vest or body jacket
- Skin breakdown or irritation under or around the vest[4,7]
- Persistent spinal instability and loss of vertebral alignment[4,7]
- New or worsened injury to the spinal cord caused by spine mobility[4,7]
- New or additional loss of neurological function
- Orthostatic hypotension
- Respiratory distress
- Injury from fall during ambulation with a halo vest

Patient Monitoring and Care

Steps	Rationale	Reportable Conditions
		These conditions should be reported if they persist despite nursing interventions.
1. Assess motor and sensory function immediately after application of the halo vest and every 2–4 hours per institutional standard.	Determines neurological status.	- Any deterioration from baseline neurological function (e.g., loss of more dermatomal sensation; decrease in motor strength)
2. Monitor for dyspnea, hypoxia, or decreasing tidal volumes (monitor pulse oximetry, and measure tidal volumes).	Assesses for hypoxia or respiratory distress from extension of neurological dysfunction or compromised respiratory function from vest constriction. A decrease in peripheral oxygen saturation or a decrease in tidal volume may be early indicators of respiratory compromise and risk for pneumonia or mortality.[2,9,12]	- Decreased oxygen saturation - Decreased tidal volumes from baseline - Dyspnea
3. Follow institutional standard for assessing pain. Administer analgesia as prescribed.	Identifies need for pain interventions.	- Continued pain despite pain interventions
4. Monitor for dysphagia.	Dysphagia is a possible side effect of cervical immobilization with a halo vest and can be associated with altered nutritional status and aspiration or risk for pneumonia.[3,4,7,9,12]	- Dysphagia

Patient Monitoring and Care —*Continued*

Steps	Rationale	Reportable Conditions
5. Check the fit of the vest, especially if the patient has lost or gained a significant amount of weight.[2,10]	The vest may be too big if significant weight loss occurs or too small if improperly fitted originally or if the patient gains weight.	• Inability to securely fit the vest
6. At least once each shift, observe the skin at the edges of the vest and where the vest may overlap. Replace the vest liner if it is wet or soiled.[2,10]	Promotes comfort and skin integrity.	• Skin irritation noted; the liner is wet or dirty and needs replacement • Call the physician to replace the liner per institutional standard
7. Wash exposed skin with warm water and soap; rinse well and dry. Be careful not to wet the liner.	Maintains cleanliness of the skin and protects the liner.	• Any assistance needed with the liner replacement
8. Provide pin care (see Procedure 104).[7,11,12]	Monitors pin sites and prevents infection.	• Evidence of infection
9. Check the integrity of the halo, pins, struts, and vest.[10]	Provides for safe use of equipment and appropriate therapy.	• Any break in the integrity of the equipment
10. Move the patient and the halo vest as a unit to avoid pressure that may dislodge the pins. Never use the anterior or posterior struts (posts) that attach the halo to the vest for moving a patient.[11]	Prevents dislodgment of pins and injury.	• Evidence of dislodgment of pins or the halo
11. Support the patient with pillows when positioning the patient in the proper body alignment.	Provides comfort and prevents dislodgment of the halo-vest device. A pillow behind the patient's head decreases the patient's sensation of being suspended.	• Evidence of dislodgment of the pins or halo
12. Discuss possible changes in body image related to the halo-vest device; provide emotional support.[11]	A dramatic change in body image occurs with the wearing of the halo-vest device and needs to be acknowledged.	• Maladaptation to altered body image
13. Discuss safety in ambulation and fall prevention (e.g., scanning with eyes to compensate for inability to move head; walking more slowly).[11] Consider recommendation of a physical therapy consult.	Because of the immobilization of the head and neck, the patient is at risk for falls.	• Patient instability
14. Follow manufacturer's recommendations and institutional policies for obtaining immediate access to the chest in event of an emergency. (Some devices have an anterior vest with a bendable CPR hinge, and some require a wrench for vest removal in emergencies. Keep the wrench readily available at all times.)	Supports basic safety procedures.	• Hemodynamic instability necessitating opening the vest

Procedure continues on following page

Documentation

Documentation should include the following:

- Patient and family education
- Date, time, and name of the physician applying halo vest
- Skin and pin assessment
- Integrity of the vest
- Neurological (motor/sensory assessment) and pulmonary assessment (tidal volume, pulse oximetry)

- Liner changes
- Date and time of chest physiotherapy performed
- Occurrence of unexpected outcomes
- Patient response to care
- Additional interventions
- Pain assessment, interventions, and effectiveness

References and Additional Readings

For a complete list of references and additional readings for this procedure, scan this QR code with any freely available smartphone code reader app, or visit http://booksite.elsevier.com/9780323376624.

104 Pin-Site Care: Cervical Tongs and Halo Pins

Cara Diaz

PURPOSE: Cervical devices (tongs or halo ring) require special care of the skin at the pin-insertion sites (pin-site care) to prevent and monitor for complications. Because the pins are inserted through the skin and into the bone, local infections can develop and proliferate into cranial osteomyelitis. Loosening of the pins may also occur.[3-6]

Pin loosening occurs in 36% to 60% of patients with crown/halo vest, and infection in 20%.[11] Tong and halo pin-site care is provided to cleanse and remove exudate from the sites to minimize the risk of infection and improve patient comfort. In addition, pin-site care allows for better assessment of the pin sites for pin loosening or displacement.

PREREQUISITE NURSING KNOWLEDGE

- The nurse should be knowledgeable about the anatomy and physiology of the spinal column, the cervical vertebrae, the spinal cord, the cervical spinal nerves, and their areas of peripheral innervation. In addition, the nurse must understand the pathophysiology and manifestations of spinal cord injury, including the concepts of primary and secondary spinal cord injury and spinal shock.
- The nurse needs to be able to assess and recognize acute changes in spinal cord examination that may indicate extension of recent spinal cord injury or new injury caused by a complication. This includes changes in motor or sensory function, respiratory function, or autonomic nervous system dysfunction.
- The nurse needs to be knowledgeable about treatment options available to manage cervical injuries with tongs or a halo ring. Tongs (see Fig. 101-2) are applied to the outer table of the cranium on both sides of the skull and attach to a set of weights hanging by a pulley system (amount of weight determined by physician).[3] This places traction along the spine to stabilize various conditions including fractures and trauma. Tongs differ from a halo ring (Procedure 101). A halo ring device can also be used for traction although most often it is used for immobilization. This device is a graphite ring that is attached to the skull with four stabilizing pins (two anterior and two posterolateral). The pins are threaded through holes in the ring, screwed into the outer table of the skull, and locked into place. This device can also be attached to traction equipment or, in cases of external stabilization as definitive treatment, a vest with struts/posts (Procedure 103).
- Various cleansing agents for pin-site care have been used, including, but not limited to, 2% chlorhexidene solution, hydrogen peroxide, sterile normal saline solution, antibac-terial soap and water, alcohol, and povidone-iodine. None have been found superior.[5,8-10,12]
- Definitive guidelines for the frequency of pin-site care, cleansing agents, removal of crust, and the application of dressings have not been established and depend on institutional policies.[8,9]
- The goal is to keep pin sites clean and monitor for loosening, infection, breakage, or other complications.

EQUIPMENT

- Cotton-tipped applicators
- Nonsterile gloves
- Cleansing or antiseptic solution
- Sterile container for cleansing solution
- Rinsing solution (as needed)
- Second sterile container for rinsing solution (as needed)

Additional equipment, to have available as needed, includes the following:

- Hair clippers
- Dressing supplies
- Light source to assist with visualization of posterior pin sites

PATIENT AND FAMILY EDUCATION

- Explain the procedure and the reason for pin care. ***Rationale:*** Patient and family anxiety may be decreased.
- Explain the patient's role in assisting with the procedure. ***Rationale:*** Explanation elicits patient cooperation and facilitates the procedure.
- Teach the family how to perform pin-site care for the patient and monitor for infection (e.g., redness, edema, odor, discharge) after discharge. ***Rationale:*** Education elicits family cooperation and comfort and prevents complications.

- Teach the family to notify the physician, advanced practice nurse, or other healthcare professional if the pins are loose or look infected. *Rationale:* This may lead to informing the physician, advanced practice nurse, or other healthcare professional of a potential problem.
- Teach the family not to adjust the pins. *Rationale:* This helps maintain the stability of the pins.

PATIENT ASSESSMENT AND PREPARATION

Patient Assessment

- Assess the patient's scalp for signs and symptoms of skin irritation; carefully inspect the pin sites for signs and symptoms of infection (e.g., redness, edema, or purulent drainage). *Rationale:* Assessment identifies skin breakdown, irritation, or pin-site infection.
- Assess the pin sites for any signs of dislodged or loose pins including sheering of skin near pin. *Rationale:* Assessment identifies pin loosening.

- Assess the patient's pain and anxiety levels. *Rationale:* Interventions may be needed before the procedure to promote patient comfort and decrease anxiety.

Patient Preparation

- Ensure that the patient and family understand preprocedural teaching. Answer questions as they arise, and reinforce information as needed. *Rationale:* Understanding of previously taught information is evaluated and reinforced.
- Verify that the patient is the correct patient using two identifiers. *Rationale:* Before performing a procedure, the nurse should ensure the correct identification of the patient for the intended intervention.
- Assist the patient to a supine position. The patient in a halo vest may be sitting up in a position of comfort. *Rationale:* Access to the pins is facilitated for care.

Procedure	for Pin-Site Care: Cervical Tong and Halo Pins	
Steps	**Rationale**	**Special Considerations**
1. HH		
2. PE		
3. Prepare the cleansing or antiseptic solution as defined by institutional policy in a sterile container. Recent recommendations include chlorhexidine as a possible antiseptic solution.[7,8] **(Level B*)**	Prepares the cleansing or antiseptic solution for pin care. Recent studies have shown chlorhexidine reduces risk of infection.[7,8]	Solutions may be kept in a covered sterile container for 24 hours. Label with the name of the solution and the date and time the solution was prepared.
4. Cleanse the area around each pin-insertion site with a cotton-tipped swab saturated with cleansing solution. Clean in a single sweeping motion, and then discard the swab. Gently repeat as needed with a new swab each time. Use separate swabs for each site to decrease the chance of cross contamination.[1]	Removes drainage, prevents excessive exudates, and cleanses the area.	Serous drainage may be present the first 2–3 days after insertion. A recent study showed a statistically significant decrease in infection rates dressing the pins with chlorhexidine-soaked gauze for the first 7 days after placement, changing the dressing daily, and cleaning with chlorhexidine each day.[7]
5. Apply a dry dressing if excessive drainage exists and notify the physician. Generally this is not necessary.	Chlorhexidine-soaked gauze dressed around pin sites during the first week has been shown to decrease infection rates.[7]	
6. Discard used supplies in an appropriate receptacle.	Removes and safely discards used supplies.	
7. HH		

*Level B: Well-designed, controlled studies with results that consistently support a specific action, intervention, or treatment.

Expected Outcomes

- Pin or tong sites remain intact
- Pin or tong sites remain free of infection

Unexpected Outcomes

- Infection at pin or tong sites, which may be local or may extend into bone (causing osteomyelitis), through the skull (causing intracranial abscess), or into the bloodstream (causing systemic infection)[4,6,10]
- Loose pins[4,6,10]
- Skin irritation, injury, or scarring[4,6,10]
- Bleeding at the pin site[4,6,10]
- Pain at the pin site[4,6,10]
- Loss of cervical spine immobilization related to loose pins[4,6,10]

Patient Monitoring and Care

Steps	Rationale	Reportable Conditions
		These conditions should be reported if they persist despite nursing interventions.
1. Administer pin care as directed by institution policy. Evidence-based recommendations about the frequency of site care have not been universally developed. Regimens range from daily pin-site care to every other day to weekly.[7,8]	Keeps pin sites clean and provides an opportunity for assessment of pin sites.	• Evidence of infection • Pin dislodgement
2. Examine each pin site for evidence of bleeding, swelling, drainage, redness, or pin loosening.[2,4,7,8,10]	Determines the presence of infection or slippage of pins.	• Evidence of bleeding • Infection • Drainage • Pin dislodgment
3. Obtain a sample of drainage if signs and symptoms of infection are present.[4]	Identifies the presence of infectious organisms for further treatment.	• Culture results from exudate; signs and symptoms of infection
4. Discuss possible changes in body image related to placement of tongs or a halo ring; provide emotional support.	Acknowledges a change in body image that occurs when external traction or immobilization devices are applied.	• Maladaptation to body image
5. Monitor for discomfort at the pin sites. Follow institutional standards for assessing pain. Administer analgesia as prescribed.	Determines evidence of possible infection or slippage of pins.[4,5] Identifies need for pain interventions.	• Continued discomfort or signs of infection • Continued pain despite pain interventions
6. Check pin torque every other day for the first week by using the manufacturer's recommended tools and torque level.[7] **(Level B*)**	Periodically checking pin torque can prevent dislodgement early and avoid irritation or possible pin replacement.	• One study recommends checking torque every other day for week 1, weekly for week 2, and monthly for the remainder of crown wearing[7]

*Level B: Well-designed, controlled studies with results that consistently support a specific action, intervention, or treatment.

Procedure continues on following page

Documentation

Documentation should include the following:

- Patient and family education
- Condition of the skin on the scalp
- Condition of the skin at pin or tong sites
- Evidence of redness or edema and amount and character of drainage at the pin sites
- Loose pins
- Body temperature

- Neurological assessment of sensation and motor function
- Occurrence of unexpected outcomes
- Patient response to care
- Additional interventions
- Pin-site care performed
- Pain assessment, interventions, and effectiveness

References and Additional Readings

For a complete list of references and additional readings for this procedure, scan this QR code with any freely available smartphone code reader app, or visit http://booksite.elsevier.com/9780323376624.

PROCEDURE

105

Epidural Catheters: Assisting with Insertion and Pain Management

Kimberly Williams

PURPOSE: Epidural catheters are used to provide regional anesthesia and analgesia by delivering medications directly into the epidural space surrounding the spinal cord. Medications injected into the epidural space are capable of providing dose-related, site-specific anesthesia and analgesia.

PREREQUISITE NURSING KNOWLEDGE

- State boards of nursing may have detailed guidelines involving the management of epidural analgesia. Each institution that provides this therapy also has policies and/ or guidelines pertaining to epidural therapy. It is important that the nurse is aware of state guidelines and institutional policies.
- The nurse must have an understanding of the principles of aseptic technique.[13,22,23,27]
- The epidural catheter placement and the continuing pain management of the patient should be under the supervision of an anesthesiologist, nurse anesthetist, or acute pain service to ensure positive patient outcomes.[1,13]
- The spinal cord and brain are covered by three membranes, collectively called the meninges. The outer layer is the dura mater. The middle layer is the arachnoid mater, which lies just below the dura mater and, with the dura, forms the dural sac. The innermost layer is the pia mater, which adheres to the surface of the spinal cord and the brain. The cerebrospinal fluid (CSF) circulates in the subarachnoid space, which is also called the intrathecal space.[30]
- The epidural space lies between the dura mater and the bone and ligaments of the spinal canal (Fig. 105-1).
- The epidural space (potential space) contains fat, blood vessels, connective tissue, and spinal nerve roots.
- Epidural catheters can be used effectively for short-term (e.g., acute, obstetrical, postoperative, trauma) or long-term (e.g., chronic, advanced cancer) pain management.[7,20]
- Analgesia via an epidural catheter may be given with a continuous, intermittent, or patient-controlled (PCEA) pump system.[17,30] A variety of medication options are available, including local anesthetics, opiates, mixtures of local anesthetics and opiates, α₂-adrenergic agonists (e.g.,

clonidine), and other agents.[13,17] All medications should be preservative-free for epidural administration.[4,7,13,14]
- Opioids used for neuraxial analgesia include fentanyl, sufentanil, morphine, and hydromorphone.
- All opioids administered via the epidural route can cause respiratory depression, sedation, nausea, vomiting, pruritus, and urinary retention.
- Fentanyl and sufentanil are lipophilic opioids which can have a more rapid onset and a shorter duration than morphine and hydromorphone, which are hydrophilic.[34]
- The lowest efficacious dose of neuraxial opioids should be administered to minimize risk of respiratory depression.[11]
- The pharmacology of agents given for epidural analgesia, including side effects and duration of action, must be understood. Nurses should be familiar with the psychosocial and physiological implications for the appropriate treatment of pain and consequences for undertreatment of acute pain.
- Epidural analgesia provides a number of well-documented advantages in the postoperative period, including attenuation of the surgical/trauma stress response, excellent analgesia, earlier extubation, less sedation, decreased incidence of pulmonary complications, earlier return of bowel function, decreased deep venous thrombosis, earlier ambulation, earlier discharge from high-acuity units,[13,15,20,31] and potentially shorter hospital stays.[1,2,20]

EQUIPMENT

- One epidural catheter kit or the following supplies:
  - One 25-gauge, ⅝-inch (0.5 × 16 mm) injection needle
  - One 23-gauge, 1¼-inch (0.6 × 30 mm) injection needle
  - One 18-gauge, 1½-inch (1.2 × 40 mm) injection needle
  - One 5-mL locking tip syringe
  - One 20-mL locking tip syringe
  - One locking tip loss-of-resistance syringe

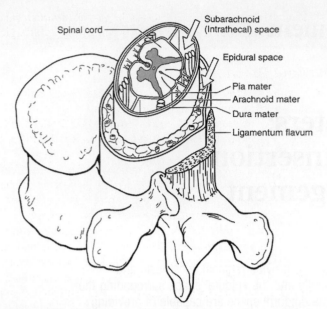

Figure 105-1 Spinal anatomy. The spinal cord is a continuous structure that extends from the foramen magnum to approximately the first or second lumbar vertebral interspace. (*From Lewis SL, Dirksen SR, Heitkemper MM, et al:* Medical-surgical nursing: Assessment and management of clinical problems, *ed 9, St. Louis, 2014, Elsevier.*)

- ❖ One 18-gauge, 3¼-inch (1.3 × 80 mm) epidural needle (pink)
- ❖ One 0.45 × 0.85–inch epidural catheter
- One introducer stabilizing catheter guide
- One screw-cap locking tip catheter
- One 0.2-μm screw-cap locking tip catheter connector
- One epidural flat filter
- Topical skin antiseptic, as prescribed
- Sterile towels
- Sterile forceps
- Sterile gauze, 4 × 4 pads
- Face masks with eye shields
- Sterile gloves and gowns
- 20 mL normal saline solution
- 5 to 10 mL local anesthetic as prescribed (e.g., 1% lidocaine; local infiltration)
- 5 mL local anesthetic as prescribed to establish the block
- Test dose (e.g., 3 mL 2% lidocaine with epinephrine, 1:200,000)
- Gauze or transparent dressing to cover the epidural catheter entry site
- Tape to secure the epidural catheter to the patient's back and over the patient's shoulder
- Labels stating "Epidural only" and "Not for intravenous injection"
- Pump for administering analgesia (e.g., volumetric pump, dedicated for epidural use with rate and volume limited, which has the ability to be locked to prevent tampering and preferably is a color-coded [e.g., yellow] or patient-controlled epidural analgesia pump)
- Dedicated yellow-lined, epidural portless administration set
- Prescribed medication analgesics and local anesthetic medications

- Equipment for monitoring blood pressure, heart rate, and pulse oximetry

Additional equipment, to have available as needed, includes the following:

- Ice or alcohol swabs for demonstrating level of block
- Capnography equipment
- Emergency medications (e.g., naloxone for respiratory depression, intravenous colloids, and a vasoconstrictor such as ephedrine for hypotension and Intralipid, a 20% fat emulsion for local anesthetic toxicity)
- Bag-valve-mask device and oxygen
- Intubation equipment

PATIENT AND FAMILY EDUCATION

- Review the principles of epidural use with the patient and family members. If the patient's pain needs are not met, an assessment of the therapy will be completed and the physician, advanced nurse practitioner, or other healthcare professional may change the dosage or therapy to meet those needs. If available, supply easy-to-read written information. *Rationale:* This information prepares the patient and family for what to expect and may reduce anxiety and preconceptions about epidural use.
- Explain to the patient and family that the insertion procedure can be uncomfortable but that a local anesthetic will be used to facilitate comfort. *Rationale:* Explanation promotes patient cooperation and comfort, facilitates insertion, and decreases anxiety and fear.
- During insertion and therapy, instruct the patient to immediately report adverse side effects, such as ringing in the ears, a metallic taste in the mouth, or numbness or tingling around the mouth, because these are signs indicative of local anesthetic toxicity.[13,30,33] *Rationale:* Immediate reporting identifies side effects and impending serious complications.
- Review an appropriate pain rating scale with the patient. The physician, advanced practice nurse, or other healthcare professional and the patient need to establish a mutually agreeable pain level goal. *Rationale:* Review ensures that the patient understands the pain rating scale and enables the nurse to obtain a baseline assessment. Establishing a pain level goal allows the physician, advanced practice nurse, or other healthcare professional to know an acceptable goal for pain management.
- During insertion and therapy, instruct the patient to report changes in pain management (e.g., suboptimal analgesia), numbness of extremities, loss of motor function of lower extremities, acute onset of back pain, loss of bladder and bowel function, itching, and nausea and vomiting.[4,13,14,17] *Rationale:* Education regarding adverse side effects allows for more rapid assessment and management of potential complications.
- If the epidural infusion is patient-controlled, ensure that patient and family understand that only the patient is to activate the medication release. *Rationale:* The patient should remain alert enough to administer his or her own dose. A safeguard to oversedation is that a patient cannot administer additional medication doses if he or she is sedated.

PATIENT ASSESSMENT AND PREPARATION

Patient Assessment

- Assess the patient for local infection and generalized sepsis. *Rationale:* Assessment decreases the risk for epidural infection (e.g., epidural abscess).[31] Septicemia and bacteremia are contraindications for epidural catheter placement.[4,8,23,27]
- Assess the patient's concurrent anticoagulation therapy. *Rationale:* Heparin (unfractionated) or heparinoids (e.g., low-molecular-weight heparin) administered concurrently during epidural catheter placement increases the risk for epidural hematoma and paralysis. Care must be taken with insertion and removal of the epidural catheter when patients have received anticoagulation therapy. Anticoagulant and fibrinolytic medications may increase the risk for epidural hematoma and spinal cord damage and paralysis. If used, anticoagulants must be withheld before insertion and removal of the epidural catheter.[21,25,26] Removal of the epidural catheter should be directed by the physician. According to Kleinman and Mikhail,[13] aspirin or nonsteroidal antiinflammatory medications (NSAIDs) by themselves do not pose an increased risk for epidural hematoma, assuming the patient's coagulation profile is within normal limits. Therefore aspirin or NSAIDs may be administered while the epidural catheter is in place.[13] However, epidural hematomas have been associated with the concurrent administration of the NSAIDs, ketorolac, and anticoagulants.[12,21] Assessment of sensory and motor function must be regularly performed during epidural analgesia for all patients.
- Obtain the patient's vital signs. *Rationale:* Baseline data are provided.
- Assess the patient's pain. *Rationale:* Baseline data are provided.
- Review the patient's medication allergies. *Rationale:* This information may decrease the possibility of an allergic reaction.

Patient Preparation

- Ensure that the patient and family understand preprocedural information. Answer questions as they arise, and reinforce information as needed. *Rationale:* Understanding of previously taught information is evaluated and reinforced.
- Verify that the patient is the correct patient using two identifiers. *Rationale:* Before performing a procedure, the nurse and team members should ensure the correct identification of the patient for the intended intervention.
- Ensure that informed consent has been obtained. *Rationale:* Informed consent protects the rights of the patient and makes a competent decision possible for the patient.
- Perform a preprocedure verification and time out including all team members. *Rationale:* This action ensures patient safety.
- Wash the patient's back with soap and water and open the gown in the back. *Rationale:* This action cleanses the skin and allows easy access to the patient's back.
- Consider nothing by mouth (NPO), especially if sedation or general anesthesia is to be used. *Rationale:* NPO status decreases the risk for vomiting and aspiration.
- Establish IV access, or ensure the patency of IV catheters, and administer IV fluids as prescribed before epidural catheter insertion. *Rationale:* IV access ensures that medications can be given quickly if needed. The administration of IV fluids may decrease hypotension that may occur during epidural infusions.[4,13]
- Reassure the patient. *Rationale:* Anxiety and fears may be reduced.

Procedure	**for Pain Management: Epidural Catheters (Assisting With Insertion and Initiating Continuous Infusion)**	
Steps	Rationale	Special Considerations
1. **HH**		
2. **PE**		Physicians, advanced practice nurses, and other healthcare professionals should apply personal protective equipment (e.g., face masks with eye shields). All physicians, advanced practice nurses, and other healthcare professionals present during epidural insertion should wear a hat and mask. The individual performing the procedure should wear hat, mask, sterile gown, and gloves.
3. Obtain the prescribed epidural medication infusion from the pharmacy.	The medication should be prepared with aseptic technique by the pharmacy with laminar flow or prepared commercially to decrease the risk for an epidural infection.[23,27,28]	All epidural solutions are preservative-free to avoid neuronal injury.[30]

Procedure continues on following page

Procedure	**for Pain Management: Epidural Catheters (Assisting With Insertion and Initiating Continuous Infusion)**—*Continued*		
Steps	**Rationale**	**Special Considerations**
4. Connect the epidural tubing to the prepared epidural medication infusion and prime the tubing.	Removes air from the infusion system.	
5. Ensure that the patient is in position for catheter placement. Assist with holding the patient in position (lateral decubitus knee-to-chest position or leaning over bedside table) and consider preprocedure analgesia or sedation, if necessary (Fig. 105-2).	Facilitates ease of insertion of the epidural catheter. Both positions open up the interspinous spaces, aiding in epidural catheter insertion (see Fig. 105-2).	Movement of the back may inhibit placement of the catheter.
6. Assist as needed with the antiseptic preparation of the intended insertion site. **(Level C*)**	Reduces the transmission of microorganisms into the epidural space.	The choice of povidone-iodine or chlorhexidine as an antiseptic agent for neurological procedures is controversial. Both should be allowed to dry completely. Studies suggest chlorhexidine is neurotoxic.[10,18,24]
7. Assist if needed with draping the patient with exposure only of the insertion site.	Aids in maintaining sterility.	
8. Assist the physician or advanced practice nurse as needed as the epidural catheter is placed.	Provides needed assistance.	

*Level C: Qualitative studies, descriptive or correlational studies, integrative reviews, systematic reviews, or randomized controlled trials with inconsistent results.

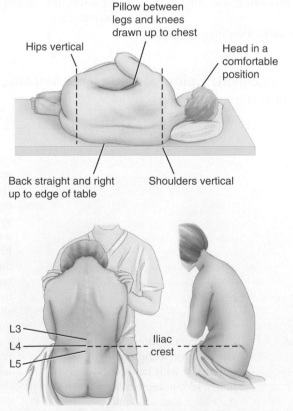

Figure 105-2   Patient positioned for catheter placement. This figure shows two positions patients can assume for the epidural catheter placement procedure. (*From Pasero C, McCaffery M: Pain assessment and pharmacologic management, St. Louis, 2011, Elsevier.*)

Procedure	for Pain Management: Epidural Catheters (Assisting With Insertion and Initiating Continuous Infusion)—*Continued*		
Steps	**Rationale**	**Special Considerations**	
9. Monitor the patient as the physician or advanced practice nurse administers 2–3 mL of 1% lidocaine containing 1:200,000 epinephrine as a test dose.	To confirm proper placement of the epidural catheter	An immediate increase in heart rate indicates the catheter has inadvertently penetrated an epidural vein. If this occurs the physician, advanced practice nurse, or other healthcare professional inserting the catheter should withdraw the catheter slightly or remove it and insert a new catheter.[29]	
10. After the epidural catheter is inserted, assist as needed with application of a sterile, occlusive dressing.	Reduces the incidence of infection.	Use of a transparent dressing allows for ongoing assessment of the insertion site for infection, leakage, or dislodgment.	
11. Secure the epidural filter to the patient's shoulder with gauze padding.	Avoids disconnection between the epidural catheter and filter. Gauze padding prevents discomfort and skin pressure from the filter.		
12. The physician or advanced practice nurse administers a bolus dose of medication.	Facilitates a therapeutic level of analgesia and confirms correct catheter position.[9]	If a local anesthetic is used for the bolus, monitor the blood pressure frequently, with assessment for possible hypotension. Some analgesia medications (e.g., morphine) may take up to 1 hour to be effective.[13,14,30]	
13. Connect the prescribed medication infusion system.	Prepares the infusion system.		
14. Initiate therapy:			
A. Place the system in the epidural pump or PCEA pump and set the rate and volume to be infused.	No other solution or medication (e.g., antibiotic or total parenteral nutrition) should be given through the epidural catheter.[33]	Responses to epidural analgesia vary individually, and epidural analgesia is tailored according to individual responses.	
B. Attach an "Epidural only" label to the epidural tubing. Use a portless system.[4,33] **(Level E*)**	Inadvertent intravenous administration of some epidural solutions can cause serious adverse reactions, including hypotension and cardiovascular collapse.[11,28]		
C. Lock the key pad on the epidural or PCEA pump.	This is an important safety feature.		
15. Assess the effectiveness of the analgesia. Follow institutional standards for assessing pain.	Identifies the need for additional pain medication and interventions.		
A. Determine the pain score.	Tolerable pain scores should be reported at rest, and very little pain should be experienced with deep breathing, coughing, and movement.		
B. Assess the level of the epidural block with ice or an alcohol swab.[6]	The ideal epidural block should be just above and just below the surgical incision or the trauma site (see the dermatomes described in Fig. 105-3).		

*Level E: Multiple case reports, theory-based evidence from expert opinions, or peer-reviewed professional organizational standards without clinical studies to support recommendations.

Procedure continues on following page

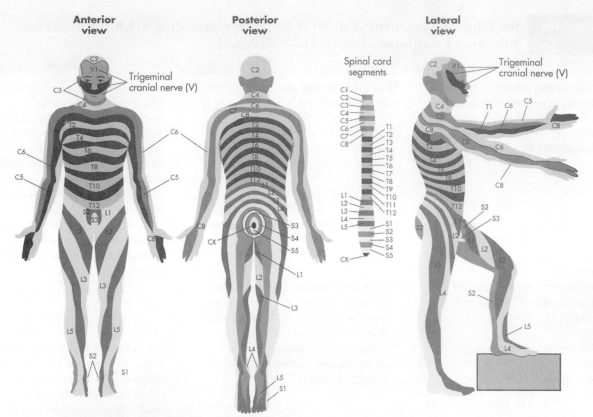

Figure 105-3   Dermatomes. Segmental dermatome distribution of spinal nerves to the front, back, and side of the body. Dermatomes are specific skin surface areas innervated by a single spinal nerve or group of spinal nerves. Dermatome assessment is done to determine the level of spinal anesthesia for surgical procedures and postoperative analgesia when epidural local anesthetics are used. *C,* Cervical segments; *T,* thoracic segments; *L,* lumber segments; *S,* sacral segments; *CX,* coccygeal segment. *(From Patton KT, Thibodeau GA:* Anatomy and physiology, *ed 9, St. Louis, 2016, Elsevier.)*

Procedure	for Pain Management: Epidural Catheters (Assisting With Insertion and Initiating Continuous Infusion)—*Continued*	
Steps	**Rationale**	**Special Considerations**
16. Remove PE and sterile equipment and discard used supplies in an appropriate receptacle.	Removes and safely discards used supplies.	
17. HH		

Procedure	for Epidural Catheter (Bolus Dose Administration) Without a Continuous Infusion	
Steps	**Rationale**	**Special Considerations**
1. HH		
2. PE		
3. Boldly label the epidural catheter used for intermittent bolus dosing (suggest color coding).[4,33] **(Level E*)**	Reduces the risk for administration of medication into intravenous lines.	

*Level E: Multiple case reports, theory-based evidence from expert opinions, or peer-reviewed professional organizational standards without clinical studies to support recommendations.

Procedure	for Epidural Catheter (Bolus Dose Administration) Without a Continuous Infusion—*Continued*	
Steps	**Rationale**	**Special Considerations**
4. Verify the correct medication with the five rights of medication administration.	Before performing a procedure, the nurse should ensure that the correct medication is being administered.	
5. Prepare the bolus dose as prescribed.	Use only preservative-free solution to dilute assuring a decreased risk of neuronal injury.[4,13]	Do not use multidose vials because they increase the risk for contamination and the risk for an epidural infection.[4,14]
6. Prepare and cleanse the epidural port with an antiseptic agent. **(Level C*)**	Do not use an alcohol-based preparation. Use aqueous chlorhexidine or povidone-iodine.	Preparations with alcohol are neurotoxic to the epidural space. The choice of povidone-iodine or chlorhexidine as an antiseptic agent is controversial. Both should be allowed to dry completely. Studies suggest chlorhexidine is neurotoxic.[10,18,14]
7. Use aseptic technique to administer the epidural bolus: A. Connect an empty syringe to the catheter port.	Administers the medication for injection.	Follow state and institutional guidelines as to who is able to provide bolus doses.
B. Aspirate the epidural catheter, limited by the amount allowed by institutional policy. If blood is aspirated, do not reinject the aspirate. Do not inject the medication. Notify the physician or advanced practice nurse. If clear fluid is obtained, it may be CSF. Do not reinject the aspirate. Do not inject the medication. Notify the physician or advanced practice nurse.[6,9,19,30]	If blood is obtained, the epidural catheter may have migrated into an epidural vessel. An amount of only 1–2 mL of blood may be inconclusive because any blood from an epidural vein may have mixed with blood from the trauma of inserting the catheter. If more than 3 mL is aspirated, the catheter is most likely in an epidural vein.[30] If 5 mL or more of CSF is obtained, the catheter may have migrated into the subarachnoid space.[30]	Administration of epidural medications into the epidural vein or into the subarachnoid space may result in increased sedation, respiratory depression, hypotension, and bradycardia.
C. Connect the syringe with the bolus medication to the catheter port.	Prepares for the injection.	
D. Administer the medication slowly. Note: If excessive pressure occurs, assess for kinks in the catheter or reposition the patient.	Some resistance will be felt because the diameter of the epidural space is small and the epidural filter is in place.	Excessive pressure may be more pronounced if the epidural catheter is placed at the lumbar dermatome as opposed to the thoracic dermatome. If resistance continues to impair administration of a bolus dose, contact the physician or advanced practice nurse.
8. Assess the effectiveness of the medication. Follow institutional standards for assessing pain.	Identifies need for pain interventions. Pain should be relieved or decreased.	Report continued pain despite pain interventions.
9. Monitor vital signs.	An epidural bolus may cause hypotension, bradycardia, respiratory depression, or increased sedation.[11,28]	Report untoward decreases in blood pressure, heart rate, respirations, oxygen saturation, and sedation.

*Level C: Qualitative studies, descriptive or correlational studies, integrative reviews, systematic reviews, or randomized controlled trials with inconsistent results.

Procedure continues on following page

Procedure	**for Epidural Catheter (Bolus Dose Administration) Without a Continuous Infusion—***Continued*		
Steps	**Rationale**		**Special Considerations**
10. Monitor for increased motor and or sensory block, and signs and symptoms of local toxicity related to the epidural medications.	Allows for the early identification of signs and symptoms of local anesthetic toxicity which include lightheadedness, tinnitus, metallic taste, visual disturbances, perioral numbness loss of consciousness, seizure, arrhythmia, and asystole.[4]		
11. Remove **PE** and discard used supplies.			
12. **HH**			

Procedure	**for Assisting With Removal of the Epidural Catheter**		
Steps	**Rationale**		**Special Considerations**
1. **HH**			
2. **PE**			Physicians, advanced practice nurses, and other healthcare professionals should apply personal protective gear (e.g., face masks with eye shields), and sterile gloves may be worn by the physician, advanced practice nurse, or other healthcare professional removing the catheter.
3. Assist the physician or advanced practice nurse as needed with removal of the catheter.	Facilitates catheter removal.		
4. Assist if needed with applying a sterile occlusive dressing.	Reduces contamination by microorganisms.		
5. Remove personal protective equipment and discard used supplies in an appropriate receptacle.	Removes and safely discards used supplies.		
6. Assess neurological status, pain, and insertion site after removal of the epidural catheter.	Motor or sensory loss in the extremities may be an early warning sign of an epidural abscess or hematoma or may indicate an excessive dose of a local anesthetic.[26,27] An epidural hematoma is a rare but serious complication; if undetected, it may result in permanent paralysis.[14,16,22,32]		Assess for a change in sensory or motor function in extremities, sudden onset of back pain with increasing motor weakness, and loss in bladder and bowel function.
A. Monitor sensory and motor status of lower extremities and ability to void up to 24 hours after removal of the catheter (see Fig. 105-3).[2,8,14,16]	Identifies potential adverse effects of epidural analgesia.		
B. Monitor insertion site for drainage or infection.	Identifies adverse effects of epidural analgesia such as infection.		
C. Continue to assess pain.	Identifies need for ongoing interventions to manage pain.		
7. **HH**			

Expected Outcomes

- The epidural catheter is inserted into the epidural space
- Pain is decreased and maintained at a tolerable level
- The patient experiences minimal sedation
- The patient experiences minimal numbness and no motor loss in the limbs
- Hemodynamically stable
- No opioid-related respiratory depression or decreased respiratory blockade from local anesthetic affecting the diaphragm or ancillary muscles required for inspiration and expiration

Unexpected Outcomes

- Inability to insert the epidural catheter
- Suboptimal pain relief[13]
- Oversedation or drowsiness[11,28]
- Opioid-induced respiratory depression or hypoxia[11,28]
- Hypotension[14,19,30]
- Motor blockade of limbs; lower extremity weakness[13,19,30]
- Sensory loss in the limbs[13,19,30]
- Patchy block (e.g., uneven pain relief)[13]
- Unilateral block (e.g., pain relief on the contralateral side of the body only)[13]
- Nausea and vomiting[8,14,17,28]
- Pruritus[1,8,14,17,28]
- Urinary retention[1,8,14,16,28]
- Accidental dural puncture into the subarachnoid space[13,33]
- Dural puncture headache[13,33]
- Epidural catheter tip migration into a vessel or adjacent structure[13]
- Redness or signs of skin breakdown at pressure area sites (e.g., sacrum, heels) from decreased sensation
- High epidural block— epidural local anesthetic block above the thoracic fourth vertebrae (T4)[14]
- Total spinal blockade[13]
- Occlusion of epidural catheter[13]
- Accidental epidural catheter dislodgment[13]
- Dressing disruption exposing insertion site
- Leakage from the epidural catheter insertion site[13,33]
- Cracked epidural filter
- Local anesthetic toxicity[13]
- Anaphylaxis[14]
- Epidural hematoma[8,25,26,28]
- Epidural abscess[8,25,27,28]
- Local erythema or drainage at insertion site[32]
- Nerve or spinal cord injury[13]
- Accidental connection of the epidural solution to the intravenous fluids[33]
- Accidental connection of intravenous fluids to the epidural catheter.
- Local anesthetic toxicity[13,14]
- Cardiopulmonary arrest[13]

Patient Monitoring and Care

Steps	Rationale	Reportable Conditions
		These conditions should be reported if they persist despite nursing interventions.
1. Assess the patient's level of pain with use of a pain scale.[9,14,30] The frequency of assessments is determined by institutional standards. Record the patient's subjective level of pain, with use of the institution's standard pain assessment tool.	Describes patient response to pain therapy. A low pain score is expected both at rest and during movement. Analgesic goal is safe, steady pain control at a low level that is acceptable to the patient.	• Moderate to severe pain scores

Procedure continues on following page

Patient Monitoring and Care —*Continued*

Steps	Rationale	Reportable Conditions
2. Assess the patient's level of sedation[9,14,30] with use of the institution's standard assessment scale and frequency standard.	Sedation precedes opioid-related respiratory depression. A sudden change in sedation scale may indicate that the epidural catheter has migrated into an epidural blood vessel or the intrathecal space.[11]	• Increasing sedation and drowsiness or sudden change in sedation scale
3. Assess respiratory rate the first 20 minutes after administration of the epidural medication, and/or bolus then every 1–2 hours and as needed (prn).[11,14,28] **(Level D*)**	Provides data for diagnosis of respiratory depression.	• Increasing respiratory depression or sudden change in respiratory rate combined with increasing somnolence
4. Assess heart rate[14,28] with vital signs every 2 hours, then every 4 hours when stable.	Tachycardia may indicate a condition such as shock. Bradycardia may indicate opioid overmedication and sympathetic blockade by the local anesthetic.[13,19]	• Change in heart rate • Abnormal heart rate • Abnormal cardiac rhythm
5. Assess blood pressure with vital signs every 2 hours, then every 4 hours when stable. If hypotension occurs: A. Turn off the epidural infusion; notify the physician, advanced practice nurse, pain relief service. B. Place the patient in a supine, flat position. C. Administer IV fluids as prescribed or according to protocol. D. Administer vasopressor medications as prescribed.[14,28] E. Use caution when raising patient from lying to sitting or sitting to standing positions.[31]	Epidural solutions that contain a local anesthetic may cause peripheral and venous dilation, providing a "sympathectomy."[14] The hypotensive effect of a local anesthetic is most common when a patient's fluid status is decreased. Epidural analgesia may not be the sole cause of hypotension but may reveal hypovolemia.	• Hypotension
6. Monitor the infusion rate with vital signs. Ensure that the control panel is locked if using the volumetric infuser or ensure that the PCEA program is locked in via key or code access.	Ensures that the medication is administered safely.	
7. Monitor oxygen saturation and end-tidal carbon dioxide if prescribed or continuously as per institutional policy.[11,14] **(Level E*)**	Assesses oxygenation. A decrease in oxygen saturation is a late sign of opioid oversedation and should not be solely relied on to detect oversedation.	• Oxygen saturation <93% or a decreasing trend in oxygenation • Note: Decreased oxygen saturation is a late sign of opioid oversedation and should not be solely relied on to detect oversedation.
8. Obtain the patient's temperature[11,14] every 4 hours; assess more often if febrile. **(Level E*)**	Fever may signify an epidural space infection or systemic infection that is a potential risk when an epidural catheter is in place.[14,17,27,32]	• Temperature >101.3°F (38.5°C)

*Level D: Peer-reviewed professional and organizational standards with the support of clinical study recommendations.

*Level E: Multiple case reports, theory-based evidence from expert opinions, or peer-reviewed professional organizational standards without clinical studies to support recommendations.

Patient Monitoring and Care —*Continued*

Steps	Rationale	Reportable Conditions
9. Assess the epidural catheter site every 4 hours or according to established institutional standards.[14,32]	Identifies site complications and infection. An epidural abscess is a rare but serious complication. Patient recovery without neurological injury depends largely on early recognition.[14,17,27,32]	• Redness • Tenderness or increasing diffuse back pain • Pain or paresthesia during epidural injection induration • Swelling or presence of exudate
10. Monitor ability to void and ability to completely empty bladder.[1,8,14] **(Level E*)**	Provides data regarding urinary retention and possible early signs of epidural abscess or epidural hematoma.[8,14,26,27,32]	• Urinary retention • Change in bladder function • Lack of urination for >6–8 hours
11. Monitor for sensory and or motor loss (e.g., leg numbness or inability to bend knees) at least every 4 hours and prn (see Fig. 105-3).[2,8,14,16] **(Level E*)**	Motor or sensory loss in the extremities may be an early warning sign of an epidural abscess or hematoma or may indicate an excessive dose of a local anesthetic.[26,27] An epidural hematoma is a rare but serious complication; if undetected, it may result in permanent paralysis.[14,16,17,32]	• Change in sensory or motor function in extremities • Sudden onset of back pain with decreasing motor weakness • Loss in bladder and bowel function (e.g., incontinence)
12. Assess for ringing in the ears, tingling around lips, or a metallic taste.[5,13,14] **(Level E*)**	If a local anesthetic is used in the epidural solution, ringing in the ears, tingling around the lips, or a metallic taste may indicate impending local anesthetic toxicity.[5,13,14]	• Ringing in the ears, tingling around the lips, or a metallic taste
13. Monitor and check skin integrity of the sacrum and the heels every 2 hours and as needed. Change the patient's position as needed.	If a local anesthetic is used in the epidural solution, check for pressure points and decubitus ulceration (patient may have sensory loss in lower limbs).[13,19,30]	• Altered skin integrity • Increasing redness or blistering of the skin on the sacrum or heels
14. Change the epidural catheter insertion site dressing as prescribed or if soiled, wet, or loose. Call physician or advanced practice nurse if catheter site is exposed. Follow institutional standards.	Provides an opportunity to cleanse the area around the catheter and to assess for signs and symptoms of infection that may indicate early signs of an epidural abscess.[14,27]	• Swelling • Site pain • Redness • Leakage of epidural solution or drainage
15. Assess for the presence of nausea or vomiting.[8]	Antiemetics may need to be administered; the medication may need adjustment (e.g., opiates may need to be decreased or stopped if nausea and vomiting are not well controlled).	• Unrelieved nausea and vomiting • Note: Nausea and vomiting may be a sign of severe hypotension.

*Level E: Multiple case reports, theory-based evidence from expert opinions, or peer-reviewed professional organizational standards without clinical studies to support recommendations.

Procedure continues on following page

Patient Monitoring and Care —*Continued*

Steps	Rationale	Reportable Conditions
16. Assess for the presence of pruritus.[2,8]	Epidural opiates may cause itching. Medications such as antihistamines may cause sedation and are ineffective for spinally mediated itching. Low-dose opioid antagonists may be necessary to relieve pruritus. Small doses of naloxone (e.g., 0.04 mg) are effective for pruritus without reversing the analgesia.[13,19] Diphenhydramine or hydroxyzine can also be effective for itching associated with dehydration but may cause increased sedation.[13,19]	• Itching • Redness • Rashes
17. Label the epidural pump and tubing[33] and consider placing the epidural pump on one side of the patient's bed and all other pumps on the other side of the bed. Consider the use of a different colored label for the epidural pump and the tubing to differentiate it from pumps and tubing for intravenous fluids and medications.	May aid in minimizing the risk for mistaking the epidural infusion for an IV infusion system. Cardiopulmonary arrest and seizures may occur if the epidural solution is infused intravenously.[13]	• Infusion of IV fluid into the epidural space • Infusion of epidural solution into the IV

Documentation

Documentation should include the following:
- Patient and family education
- Completion of informed consent
- Preprocedure verifications and time out
- Any difficulties associated with insertion
- Type of dressing used
- Confirmation of epidural catheter placement (e.g., decrease in blood pressure, demonstrable block to ice; see Fig. 105-3)
- Site assessment
- Preintervention and serial pain assessment, including levels of motor and sensory blockade (documented on an appropriate flow chart at regular intervals; see Fig. 105-3) and effectiveness of interventions[30]
- Sedation score assessment

- Vital signs and oxygen saturation[11]
- Epidural analgesic medication and medication concentration being infused and infusion rate per hour
- Bolus dose administration and patient response after bolus dose, including effectiveness of pain relief
- Occurrence of unexpected outcomes or side effects
- Nursing interventions taken
- Pump settings when programmed for PCEA
- Medication concentrations, continuous infusion rate, bolus dose, lockout interval, limit for 1 or more hours according to institutional standards
- Pain assessment, interventions, and effectiveness

References and Additional Readings

For a complete list of references and additional readings for this procedure, scan this QR code with any freely available smartphone code reader app, or visit http://booksite.elsevier.com/9780323376624.

PROCEDURE

106 Patient-Controlled Analgesia

Lorie Ann Meek

PURPOSE: Intravenous patient-controlled analgesia empowers patients to manage their pain by allowing them to administer smaller analgesic doses more frequently. Nurses are responsible for ensuring appropriate patient selection, maintaining the intravenous delivery system, and ensuring that patients are able to safely meet their own needs for pain management through frequent assessment and patient education.

PREREQUISITE NURSING KNOWLEDGE

- Pain is defined as an "unpleasant sensory and emotional experience that arises from actual or potential tissue damage" by the International Association for the Study of Pain[20,29] According to the National Institutes of Health, more Americans are affected by pain than by diabetes, heart disease, and cancer combined.[29]
- The most common reason for unrelieved pain in hospitals is the failure of staff to routinely and adequately assess pain and pain relief.[2]
- Additional perceived barriers to adequate pain management are poor pain assessment, patient reluctance to report pain and take analgesics, and physician reluctance to prescribe opioids.[2]
- Tables 106-1 and 106-2 list guidelines for dosing and considerations for selection of opioids.
- Unrelieved postoperative pain may result in clinical and psychological changes, an increase in morbidity and mortality, an increase in costs, and a decrease in quality of life. Negative clinical outcomes related to ineffective pain management for patients after surgery include deep vein thrombosis, pulmonary embolism, coronary ischemia, myocardial infarction, pneumonia, poor wound healing, impairment of the immune system, insomnia, readmissions, and negative emotions.[2,3,32] Unrelieved pain may delay recovery and prolong hospital stays.[2,32,33]
- The Agency for Healthcare Research and Quality (AHRQ) urges healthcare professionals to accept the patient's self-report as "the single most reliable indicator of the existence and intensity" of pain.[2]
- Although pain is prevalent, underdiagnosed and undertreated populations include racial and ethnic minorities, people with lower levels of education and income, women, older adults, military veterans, postsurgical and cancer patients, and patients nearing the end of life.[17]
- Studies and meta-analyses have shown that patients receiving patient-controlled analgesia (PCA) report an increased satisfaction level with pain management and an improvement in pain control.[3,5,8,19,23,35,38] Intravenous (IV)

PCA may be used for both acute and chronic pain,[26,30] although IV administration of opioids is most often used for acute pain.[26]
- IV PCA can be an effective method of pain relief for pediatric and adult patients.[16,27,32,38] Table 106-1 lists dosing guidelines. PCA is not recommended in situations in which oral opioids can readily manage pain (e.g., chronic and relatively stable cancer pain).[26]
- IV PCA can be administered as a continuous (basal) infusion along with patient-initiated boluses or as patient-initiated boluses exclusively. Use caution with continuous infusion because of accumulation of the medication.[1]
- Patient assessment at frequent, regular intervals[7,14] (at least every 4 hours) should include an evaluation of the patient's vital signs, sedation level with a valid and reliable scale, pain level with a valid and reliable scale, and common opioid side effects, such as pruritus, nausea,[6] constipation, and urinary retention.[21] Table 106-2 lists side effects associated with PCA opioids. Patients need more frequent assessments during the first 24 hours after initiation of IV PCA and during the night.[9,10,18,21]
- PCA pump settings should be confirmed at regular intervals.[9,10,18,21] See Box 106-1 for common terms used when administering patient-controlled analgesia. Adverse events during IV PCA may include sedation, respiratory depression, and hypoxemia. Opioid antagonists should be readily available.
- Adjuvant medications can be used to improve pain management,[6,41] such as nonsteroidal antiinflammatory drugs (NSAIDs)[1] and cyclooxygenase (COX-2) inhibitors[1,21,29,40] or to improve opioid side effects.[22,27,28]
- The Joint Commission does not support PCA by proxy (someone other than the patient pushing the PCA button) on the recommendation of the Institute of Safe Medication Practices (ISMP). According to ISMP, patients have experienced oversedation, increased respiratory depression, and death from PCA by proxy.[10,18,37,38] A safety feature of PCA therapy is that an oversedated patient cannot press the button to obtain additional pain medication.
- PCA by an authorized user (typically nurse or designated family member of patient) is a potential alternative to

941

TABLE 106-1	Guidelines for Patient-Controlled Intravenous Opioid Administration for Opioid-Naive Adults and Children With Acute Pain

Adults >50 kg

Drug*	Usual Starting Dose After Loading	Usual Dose Range	Typical Starting Lockout (min)	Usual Lockout Range (min)
Morphine (1 mg/mL)	1.0 mg	0.5–2.5 mg	6	5–10
Hydromorphone (0.2 mg/mL)	0.2 mg	0.05–0.4 mg	6	5–10
Fentanyl (50 mcg/mL)	20 mcg	10–50 mcg	6	5–8

*Typical concentrations are listed in parentheses.

Children <50 kg

Drug	Usual Starting Dose After Loading	Usual Dose Range	Usual Starting Lockout (doses/h)	Usual Lockout Range (min)	Usual Basal Rate
Morphine (1.0 mg/mL)	0.02 mg/kg/dose	0.01–0.03 mg/kg	5	6–8	0.0–0.03 mg/kg/hr
Hydromorphone (0.2 mg/mL)	0.003–0.004 mg/kg/dose	0.003–0.005 mg/kg	5	6–10	0.00–0.004 mg/kg/hr
Fentanyl (50 mcg/mL)	0.5–1.0 mcg/kg/dose	0.5–1.0 mcg/kg/dose	5	6–8	0.0–0.5 mcg/kg/hr

From Miaskowski C, Blair M, Chou R, et al: Principles of analgesic use in the treatment of acute pain and cancer pain, ed 6, Glenview, IL, 2008, American Pain Society.

TABLE 106-2	Patient-Controlled Analgesia: Considerations in Opioid Selection

Opioid	Side Effects	Advantages	Disadvantages	Cautions/Contraindications
Morphine	Nausea Sedation Pruritus Reduced peristalsis Respiratory depression	Vast clinical experience Less expensive than other opioids	Slow onset: 15 min Histamine release Active metabolite (M6G) accumulates in renal patients and causes excessive sedation and other side effects.	Allergy (use fentanyl) Renal dysfunction Hepatic dysfunction Asthma (histamine release)
Hydromorphone (Dilaudid)	Nausea Sedation Pruritus Reduced peristalsis Respiratory depression	Faster onset than morphine Less sedation No active metabolites	More expensive than morphine Less clinical experience than morphine Higher potential for abuse	Allergy (use fentanyl) High doses can result in excitation with impaired renal dysfunction
Fentanyl (Sublimaze)	Nausea Sedation Pruritus Reduced peristalsis Respiratory depression	Rapid onset No active metabolites Less constipation as compared with morphine	More expensive than morphine Less clinical experience than with morphine Short duration of action	Allergy Rapid administration of drug can result in "stiff chest," making ventilation difficult

From Institute for Safe Medication Practices: Patient-controlled analgesia: Making it safer for patients, Horsham, PA, 2006, Institute for Safe Medication Practices.

PCA by proxy. Healthcare institutions that use PCA by an authorized user need to have the following in place before this practice is initiated[10,11,18,37,39]:

- ❖ Policies that guide the practice, including the patient population
- ❖ Definition of PCA by an authorized user
- ❖ Education plan for the authorized user
- ❖ Documentation of the authorized user and education given
- Serious adverse events from errors with opioids include "failure to control pain, oversedation, respiratory depression, seizures and death."[13,14]

- Patients with an increased risk for complications during IV PCA use include those with:
  - ❖ Age more than 61 (greater incidence of desaturation)[21,31,38]
  - ❖ Morbid obesity (greater incidence of desaturation)[21,31,34,35]
  - ❖ Sleep apnea, sleep disorder or asthma, and snoring[10,19,21,34,35,38]
  - ❖ Concurrent medications that potentiate opiates (e.g., sedation)[10,18]
  - ❖ Impaired organ function[25]
  - ❖ No recent opioid use[21]

BOX 106-1	Key Terms for Patient-Controlled Analgesia

- *Basal rate:* The amount of analgesic administered continuously.
- *Breakthrough dose:* A bolus dose administered by the nurse, similar to a loading dose when pain is inadequately managed with the current PCA settings.
- *Cumulative dose limit:* The predetermined maximum drug amount that can be delivered over either 1 or more (usually 4) hours.
- *Demand or PCA dose:* The amount of drug administered each time the patient activates the pump.
- *Loading dose:* A bolus dose given before initiation of PCA therapy, usually higher than the dose administered when the patient activates the pump.
- *Lockout interval:* Predetermined period during which the patient cannot initiate doses.

From Miaskowski C: Patient-controlled modalities for acute postoperative pain management, J Perianesth Nurs 20:255-267, 2005; Miaskowski C, Bair M, Chou R: Principles of analgesic use in the treatment of acute pain and cancer pain, ed 6, Glenview, IL, 2008, American Pain Society; Sharma S, Balireddy RK, Vorenkamp KE, et al: Beyond opioid patient-controlled analgesia: A systematic review of analgesia after major spine surgery, Reg Anesth Pain Med, 37:79-98, 2012.

- ❖ Postsurgery, especially if upper abdominal or thoracic, and longer times receiving anesthesia[21]
- ❖ Increased opioid requirement[21]
- ❖ Preexisting cardiac and pulmonary disease[21]
- Careful patient selection is imperative for effective pain management.[13,14,21]
- Patient assessment for management of pain helps prevent adverse events.[1]
  - ❖ Screen for those with increased risk of complications.
  - ❖ Assess the patient's analgesic use and abuse potential.
- Individualize pain treatment plans, and use multimodal strategies (pharmacology, nonpharmacology, psychosocial support, and complementary and behavioral approaches).[29,38]
- Extra precautions to prevent complications, such as a short-term trial to determine the patient's response and sufficient time for assessment of patient and pain
- Patients who may be poor candidates for PCA include the following:
  - ❖ Anyone with cognitive abilities that prohibit understanding and following directions for IV PCA (e.g., patients with a decreased level of consciousness or developmental disabilities)[10,11,18,22]
  - ❖ Anyone without the physical ability to push the PCA button that controls the dose administration[10,11,18,22]
  - ❖ Anyone with a psychological reason that prohibits using the PCA button for pain management (e.g., psychological disability, refusal to operate the PCA administration button)[10,11,18]
- A number of medication errors have been reported with IV PCA. Factors associated with errors include improper patient selection, inadequate monitoring, inadequate patient education, medication product mix-ups, programming errors, PCA by proxy, inadequate medical and nursing staff education, prescription errors, and PCA pump design flaws.[10,13-15,18]

- PCA is available in various routes, including IV, epidural (patient-controlled epidural analgesia [PCEA]; see Procedure 105), subcutaneous, peripheral nerve catheter (see Procedure 107), oral, intranasal, and transdermal.[24,26] The focus of this procedure is IV PCA.
- An interdisciplinary team approach is beneficial for pain management.[22]

EQUIPMENT

- PCA pump
- PCA tubing with antisiphon valve (may also include a plunger for insertion into PCA medication syringe barrel)
- IV pump
- IV tubing
- Prescribed medication (may be in a syringe, bag, or cassette)
- Antiseptic pad
- Nonsterile gloves
- Electrocardiogram (ECG) and blood pressure monitoring equipment
- Pulse oximetry equipment
- Normal saline solution or other compatible IV fluid

Additional equipment, to have as needed, includes the following:
- Emergency medications, including an opioid reversal agent to reverse oversedation or respiratory depression
- Bag-valve-mask device and oxygen
- End-tidal carbon dioxide monitoring equipment

PATIENT AND FAMILY EDUCATION

- Review an appropriate pain rating scale with the patient. The physician, advanced practice nurse, or other healthcare professional and patient need to establish a mutually agreeable pain level goal. *Rationale:* Review ensures that the patient understands the pain rating scale and enables the nurse to obtain a baseline assessment. Establishing a pain level goal allows the physician, advanced practice nurse, or other healthcare professional to know an acceptable goal for pain management.
- Review the principles of PCA use with the patient and family members.[1,14] If a basal rate has been prescribed, inform the patient that pain medication will be infusing at all times. Explain that if the pain is not relieved with the steady dose, extra medicine can be delivered by pressing the patient bolus button. Be sure the patient understands what the lockout interval is. If the patient's pain needs are not met, an assessment of the therapy will be completed and the physicians, advanced practice nurses, or other healthcare professionals may change the dosage or therapy to meet those needs. *Rationale:* This review may reduce anxiety and preconceptions about PCA use.
- IV PCA is designed for the patient to administer the pain medication. The patient should be the only one to deliver the demand dose. The Institute for Safe Medication Practices (ISMP), the American Society for Pain Management Nursing (ASPMN), and The Joint Commission do not support PCA by proxy because of adverse events, such as oversedation, respiratory depression, cardiopulmonary

arrest, and deaths, that have occurred with PCA by proxy.[10,11,18,19,39] *Rationale:* The patient should remain alert enough to administer his or her own dose. A safeguard to oversedation is that a patient cannot administer additional medication doses if sedated.
- Instruct the patient and family members to report common side effects, such as oversedation, pruritus, nausea or vomiting, constipation, or urinary retention. *Rationale:* Side effects are identified by the patient and family.

PATIENT ASSESSMENT AND PREPARATION

Patient Assessment

- Assess the patient's ability to properly use IV PCA as a method for pain management. *Rationale:* The patient will not achieve adequate pain management if unable to use the PCA.
- Assess the patient's pain and document the intensity, location, and characteristics.[2,28] *Rationale:* A baseline assessment permits an accurate evaluation of the efficacy of the PCA.

- Assess the patient's level of sedation with the use of a sedation scale.[7,21,29] *Rationale:* Sedation generally precedes respiratory depression; a patient who is less alert should be closely monitored if PCA is prescribed.
- Review the patient's medication allergies. *Rationale:* Review of medication allergies before administration of a new medication decreases the chances of an allergic reaction.

Patient Preparation

- Verify that the patient is the correct patient using two identifiers. *Rationale:* Before performing a procedure, the nurse should ensure the correct identification of the patient for the intended intervention.
- Ensure that the patient understands the teaching. Having the patient demonstrate the procedure helps evaluate patient education. Answer questions as they arise, and reinforce information as needed.[1] *Rationale:* Understanding of previously taught information is evaluated and reinforced.
- Obtain IV access and ensure patency of the IV. *Rationale:* Analgesia is delivered intravenously.

Procedure	for Initiating Intravenous Patient-Controlled Analgesia	
Steps	**Rationale**	**Special Considerations**
1. **HH**		
2. **PE**		
3. Review the prescription for the PCA, including the medication, concentration, basal rate, loading dose, demand PCA dose, lockout interval, cumulative dose limit (over 1 or more hours), and basal rate as prescribed.[10,18,33]	Ensures correct PCA prescription is administered to patient.	Ensure coverage for common side effects, such as pruritus, constipation, or nausea. Follow institutional standards. A medication such as naloxone may be prescribed. Naloxone is an opioid reversal agent that is used to reverse oversedation or respiratory depression. Ensure that the patient is physically, psychologically, and cognitively able to use the PCA for pain management. The use of a basal rate is controversial and may result in oversedation in patients who are opioid naive.[26]
4. Check for medication allergies or sensitivities. Check for medications that may potentiate the opioid and for adverse effects of the opioid.[10,19] **(Level E*)**	Prevents allergic or adverse reactions.	
5. Attach the antisiphon valve of the tubing to the medication syringe.	Prepares the equipment.	Many PCA pumps use syringe delivery of the medication. Other PCA pumps use bags and cassettes rather than syringe delivery.

*Level E: Multiple case reports, theory-based evidence from expert opinions, or peer-reviewed professional organizational standards without clinical studies to support recommendations.

Procedure	for Initiating Intravenous Patient-Controlled Analgesia—*Continued*		
Steps	**Rationale**	**Special Considerations**	
6. Purge the PCA tubing of air.	Removes air from the system.	If the injector is the plunger of the syringe, attach the antisiphon valve on the tubing to the syringe and manually purge. The PCA may offer the option of purging via the PCA pump before it is attached to the patient.	
7. Insert the syringe into the PCA pump by first placing the bottom of the syringe in the lower flanges of the cradle and then place the top portion of the syringe in place. If using a cassette system, snap and lock the cassette in place on the infusion pump.	Prepares the PCA system.	Place the syringe barrel into the pump within the area provided by the upper and lower flanges of the cradle. If a cassette system is used unlock the system and place the new cassette into the bottom of the infusion pump where it can be snapped into place and then locked.	
8. Position the medication syringe or cassette so that the name and concentration of the drug and the volume markings are visible.	Ensures ready identification of the medication.		
9. Secure the syringe in the cradle.	Ensures proper positioning of the syringe.		
10. Occlude the PCA tubing with the slide clamp.	Contains the medication until the infusion begins.		
11. Insert the IV tubing of the continuous IV solution into the IV pump.	Prepares the infusion pump.		
12. Connect the IV tubing of the continuous IV solution to the lowest Y-site on the PCA medication tubing, and ensure the tubing from Y-site to the end of the PCA medication tubing is purged with the IV fluid.	Prepares the system and prevents an air bolus.		
13. Program the PCA pump with the medication name and concentration, the loading dose (as prescribed), PCA dose, lockout interval, cumulative dose limit (over 1 or more hours), and basal rate (as prescribed).	Prepares the system.		
14. Independently verify the patient's identification, medication and medication concentration, PCA pump settings, and tubing[4,10,15,18] with another physician, advanced practice nurse, or other healthcare professional. **(Level E*)**	Adverse events can occur as a result of programming errors.	Independent verification of patient identification, medication and concentration, PCA pump settings, and the line attachment before use and before pump refill or programming change may lessen the risk of programming error.[10,15,18]	

*Level E: Multiple case reports, theory-based evidence from expert opinions, or peer-reviewed professional organizational standards without clinical studies to support recommendations.

Procedure continues on following page

Procedure   for Initiating Intravenous Patient-Controlled Analgesia—*Continued*

Steps	Rationale	Special Considerations
15. Program the compatible IV solution at a rate to provide not less than the minimal acceptable rate for a continuous IV solution per institutional standards.	Ensures the delivery of the prescribed medication. Highly concentrated medications, such as hydromorphone, may be administered in bolus doses of <1 mL, but do not reach the patient quickly through most IV tubing without a continuous IV infusion. Some PCA pumps do not use continuous IV solution; however, the PCA tubing is much smaller, increasing the likelihood that the medication will reach the patient although the infused volume is small.	The medication's basal rate combined with any other IV fluids should total the prescribed hourly IV rate. If the PCA is programmed for bolus dosing only, set the IV solution on no less than the minimal rate for the maintenance IV.
16. Cleanse the IV catheter cap with appropriate antiseptic cleanser and connect the PCA tubing directly to the patient's IV line.[36] Release the slide clamp from the PCA tubing. Initiate continuous IV delivery and PCA therapy.	Connects the PCA to the IV access.	Verify patent IV access before connecting or infusing medication. Extension tubing may result in errors in the medication delivery and should not be used.
17. Label the PCA pump and the IV infusion pump.	Ensures quick and clear identification of IV fluids and PCA medications.	
18. Label the IV tubing and the PCA tubing.	Ensures identification of IV fluids and PCA medications infusing via each IV tubing.	
19. Secure the PCA tubing at two points of tension.	Prevents accidental removal of the IV.	
20. Remove **PE** and discard used supplies in an appropriate receptacle.	Removes and safely discards used supplies.	
21. **HH**		

Expected Outcomes

- Pain is minimized or relieved (at an acceptable level for the patient)
- No unmanaged side effects
- Continuous IV access

Unexpected Outcomes

- Extravasation
- Oversedation or respiratory depression
- Loss of IV access and interruption of medication delivery
- Pain not relieved

Patient Monitoring and Care

Steps	Rationale	Reportable Conditions
		These conditions should be reported if they persist despite nursing interventions
1. Ensure that the medication is infusing properly through the IV.	New infusions may precipitate extravasation; an IV catheter may become dislodged through patient movement.	- Extravasation
2. Assess the patient's pain and level of sedation.[7,10] Follow institutional standards.	Monitors effectiveness of therapy; identifies need for adjustment. Institutional assessment policies should take into account the expected.	- Pain is unrelieved - Altered level of sedation

Patient Monitoring and Care —*Continued*

Steps	Rationale	Reportable Conditions
3. Monitor the patient's vital signs, including heart rate, blood pressure, respirations, oxygen saturation (SaO_2), and end-tidal CO_2 (if prescribed) according to institutional standards.[12,14,21]	Determines the presence of potential complications.	• Change in sedation level, respiratory status or other vital signs (e.g., respiratory rate, oxygenation via pulse oximetry, end-tidal CO_2)
4. Verify all PCA prescription changes and pump changes with another registered nurse (independent double-check verification).[10,14,15,18] **(Level E*)**	Decreases the risk of a medication error or programming error.	• Medication dosage and/or programming errors
5. Ensure patient comprehension of PCA use and analgesic goal. Reinforce patient education.	Comprehension can be assessed with patient report, with review of the PCA history for frequency of attempts and through return patient demonstration.	• Patient unable to use PCA • Inability to achieve analgesia goal
6. Assess for the presence of side effects, such as nausea, pruritus, urinary retention, or constipation.	Many side effects from opioid use can be managed.	• Nausea • Pruritus • Constipation • Urinary retention
7. Prevention of constipation by encouraging mobilization and adequate fluid intake, adding fiber to the diet if applicable, and using stool softeners if indicated.	This is a significant complication of opiod use and can lead to other complications.	• Unresolved constipation despite prevention measures
8. Ensure patient continues to be appropriate candidate for IV PCA.	Pain management may be ineffective and patient may be at higher risk for adverse events if patient not an appropriate candidate.	• Patient is cognitively, psychologically, or physically unable to manage IV PCA

*Level E: Multiple case reports, theory-based evidence from expert opinions, or peer-reviewed professional organizational standards without clinical studies to support recommendations.

Documentation

Documentation should include the following:

- Medication, concentration, basal rate, loading dose, any breakthrough dosing, demand dose, lockout interval, and cumulative dose (independent double check verification by another registered nurse after initiation of treatment and with all changes thereafter)[10,14,15,18,33]
- Pain assessment, interventions, and effectiveness of PCA and other adjunctive pain management
- Patient's baseline and follow-up pain scores using a valid and reliable scale
- Patient's baseline and follow-up sedation scores using a valid and reliable scale

- Total dose of medication administered, per institutional standards
- Time the PCA pump was cleared, per institutional policy
- Patient teaching and any reinforcement needed
- Side effects of opioids
- Unexpected outcomes
- Vital signs, oxygen saturation, and if used, end-tidal carbon dioxide level
- Appearance and patency of the IV site
- Additional interventions that were needed

References and Additional Readings

For a complete list of references and additional readings for this procedure, scan this QR code with any freely available smartphone code reader app, or visit http://booksite.elsevier.com/9780323376624.

107 Peripheral Nerve Blocks: Assisting with Insertion and Pain Management

Kimberly Williams

PURPOSE: Peripheral nerve blocks are administered as single local anesthetic injections or continuously through a catheter placed into a precise anatomical area to provide site-specific analgesia or anesthesia.

PREREQUISITE NURSING KNOWLEDGE

- State boards of nursing may have detailed guidelines involving peripheral nerve blockade. Each institution that provides this therapy also has policies and guidelines pertaining to peripheral nerve blockade. It is important that the nurse is aware of state guidelines and institutional policies.[15]
- The nurse must have an understanding of the principles of aseptic technique.[9,12,19,23,39]
- The nurse assisting with the insertion of peripheral nerve blocks requires specific skills and knowledge.[15]
- Catheter placement and management of the patient should be under the direct supervision of an anesthesiologist, nurse anesthetist, or the acute pain service.[24,26,39] Peripheral nerve blocks are used as part of a preemptive and multimodal analgesic technique to provide safe and effective postoperative pain management with minimal side effects.[10,12,14,18,21]
- Peripheral nerve blocks are site specific (e.g., femoral, brachial plexus, axillary, intrapleural, extrapleural, paravertebral, tibial, sciatic, lumbar plexus) and provide prolonged anesthesia or analgesia for postoperative and trauma pain management.[4,26]
- Peripheral nerve blocks in the outpatient setting have facilitated early patient ambulation and discharge by decreasing side effects, such as drowsiness, nausea, and vomiting.[3,11,13,18] In addition, unlike general anesthesia, peripheral nerve blocks do not directly alter the level of consciousness. By preserving the patient's level of consciousness, the patient's protective airway reflexes (e.g., cough and gag) are maintained and the need for airway manipulation and intubation is negated. Furthermore, with the use of peripheral nerve blockade, the complications of general anesthesia are avoided.[3] Continuous peripheral nerve blockade improves postoperative analgesia, patient satisfaction, and rehabilitation compared with intravenous (IV) opioids for upper- and lower-extremity procedures.[11,13,18,26,31]

- The anatomical position of the specific catheter should be clearly defined and documented after insertion by the physician or advanced practice nurse (e.g., femoral, axillary [Figs. 107-1 and 107-2], brachial plexus [Fig. 107-3], intrapleural, extrapleural, paravertebral, tibial, sciatic, lumbar plexus).[5,32] Radiological confirmation[6] of the catheter position may be necessary to avoid suboptimal outcomes (e.g., pneumothorax). Catheters may be placed by the surgeon, anesthesiologist, or certified nurse anesthetist under direct vision, via ultrasound scan–guided techniques or with the use of a peripheral nerve stimulator, either adjacent to or directly into the nerve sheath (e.g., sciatic or tibial nerve during surgery for lower-limb amputation).[16,19,21,23,29,31] Catheters may also be placed after surgery (e.g., intercostal, intrapleural, axillary, brachial plexus, femoral, paravertebral; Table 107-1).
- A three-in-one peripheral nerve block can be used for analgesia after proximal lower-limb orthopedic surgery. A three-in-one peripheral nerve block provides analgesia to block three nerves, including the lateral femoral cutaneous, femoral, and obturator nerves.[4,26] This block is as effective as epidural analgesia, with fewer side effects than epidural analgesia (e.g., urinary retention, nausea, risk for epidural hemorrhage in patients with anticoagulation).[6,7,16,26,27] Some forms of plexus analgesia (e.g., brachial plexus analgesia) in the postoperative setting may serve two purposes: pain relief and sympathetic blockade, the latter of which increases blood flow and may improve outcomes in some cases (i.e., digit reimplantation).[5,16,23,34]
- Analgesia via a catheter may be administered as a continuous infusion with the use of a volumetric pump system, a patient-controlled regional infusion system, or a disposable pump device (e.g., elastomeric). An elastomeric pump is one type of disposable infusion pump designed to provide a constant rate of infusion from a filled reservoir. The infusion rates may or may not be adjustable (Fig. 107-4).[21,30,34] Medication administered is usually a local anesthetic (e.g., bupivacaine, ropivacaine). Other agents have been used on an adjunctive basis as a bolus, including opioids, clonidine, epinephrine,[16,17] and neostigmine.[18]

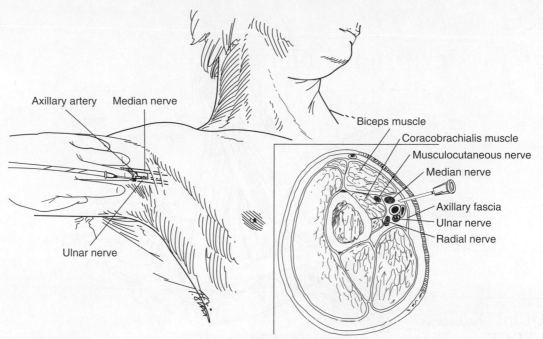

Figure 107-1   Location for needle insertion for an axillary block. *(From Sinatra RS:* Acute pain: Mechanisms & management, *St Louis, 1992, Mosby.)*

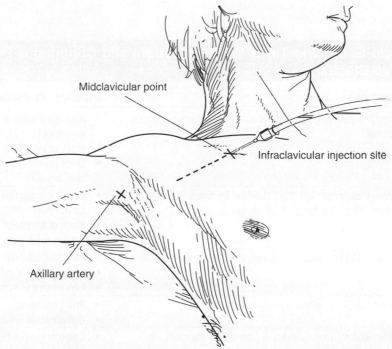

Figure 107-2   Needle insertion for an axillary block. *(From Sinatra RS:* Acute pain: Mechanisms & management, *St Louis, 1992, Mosby.)*

• The pharmacokinetics and pharmacodynamics of local anesthetics and other agents used, including side effects and duration of action, should be clearly understood. Local anesthetic medications used for peripheral nerve blocks provide surgical analgesia (i.e., loss of pain sensation) and anesthesia (i.e., loss of all sensation). The duration of action for each anesthetic medication depends on several factors, including the volume injected, concentration of the medication, site of injection, and absorption. The addition of a vasoconstrictor, such as epinephrine, constricts blood vessels and reduces vascular uptake, which further prolongs the duration of action of the local anesthetic.[16,17] Epinephrine is not recommended with peripheral nerve blocks in areas with end arteries, such as ear lobes, the nose, digits, and the penis.[39] Vasoconstrictor medications may cause spasm of blood vessels,

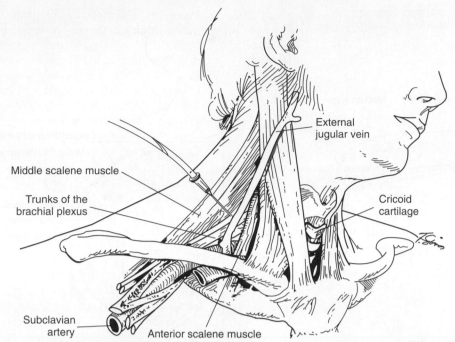

Figure 107-3   Landmarks for interscalene brachial plexus block. (*From Sinatra RS:* Acute pain: Mechanisms & management, *St Louis, 1992, Mosby.*)

TABLE 107-1	Single-Shot (One-Time, Single Injection) and Continuous Peripheral Nerve Blocks	
Block	**Indications**	**Practical Problems**
Interscalene	Shoulder/arm pain (e.g., shoulder dislocation/fractures, humeral fracture)	• Horner's syndrome may obscure neurological assessment • Block of ipsilateral phrenic nerve • Close proximity to tracheostomy and jugular vein line sites
Cervical paravertebral (continuous catheter only)	Shoulder/elbow/wrist pain (e.g., shoulder fractures, humeral fracture, elbow fractures, wrist fractures)	• Horner's syndrome may obscure neurological assessment • Block of ipsilateral phrenic nerve • Patient positioning
Infraclavicular	Arm/hand pain (e.g., elbow fractures, wrist fractures)	• Pneumothorax risk • Steep angle for catheter placement • Interference with subclavian lines
Axillary	Arm/hand pain (e.g., elbow fractures, wrist fractures)	• Arm positioning • Catheter maintenance
Intercostal	Blockade used for management of pain due to traumatic rib fractures. Commonly an elastomeric infusion pump, which is a balloon filled with local anesthetic attached to a catheter placed at the site of injury. This delivery system results in slow infusion of local anesthetic for pain control. This provides pain relief so that patients are able to ventilate more effectively.	• Catheter malposition • Risk of pneumothorax
Paravertebral	Unilateral chest or abdominal pain restricted to a few dermatomes (e.g., rib fractures)	• Patient positioning • Stimulation success sometimes hard to visualize
Combination of femoral and sciatic block	Unilateral leg pain (e.g., femoral neck fracture [femoral], tibial and ankle fractures [sciatic])*	• Patient positioning • Interference of femoral nerve catheters with femoral lines

*Caution: Compartment syndrome.
Modified from Schulz-Stubner S: The critically ill patient and regional anesthesia, Curr Opin Anaesthesiol *19:538–544, 2006.*

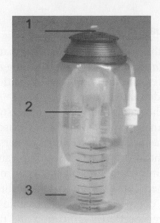

Figure 107-4   An elastomeric infusion pump. Parts include 1, filling port; 2, elastomeric balloon (drug-containing reservoir); and 3, outer protective shell. *(Originally published in Skryabina E, Dunn TS: Disposable infusion pumps,* Am J Health Syst Pharm *63:1260-1268, 2006.)* © *2006, American Society of Health-System Pharmacists, Inc. All rights reserved. Reprinted with permission (R1002).*

resulting in necrosis.[9] Knowledge of signs and symptoms of profound motor and sensory blockade, or overmedication, is essential.[5,9,10,17]

- Sensory and motor blockade may be acceptable or desirable, depending on the goals and preferences of the interdisciplinary team. The loss of sensation at the site is often the primary goal of blocks, and although motor loss is often acceptable, it is not desirable.[3]
- Relative contraindications to peripheral nerve blockade include a history of coagulopathy, preexisting neuropathies, anatomical or pathological deviations at the injection site, and systemic disease or infection.[5,7,10,22,26,27,39]
- Local anesthetic toxicity can result from inadvertent injection of local anesthetic into the vascular system or rapid absorption of the agent from the tissue into the vascular system. Intralipids/20% fat emulsion should be immediately available for IV infusion, to help restore cardiovascular stability.[8]

EQUIPMENT

- One peripheral nerve catheter kit
- Infusion set for continuous plexus anesthesia with or without an adaptor for a nerve stimulator
- Peripheral nerve stimulator
- Topical skin antiseptic, as prescribed
- Sterile towels
- Sterile forceps
- Sterile gauze 4 × 4 pads
- Sterile gloves and gowns
- Fluid shield face masks
- 20-mL normal saline solution
- 5- to 10-mL local anesthetic as prescribed (1% lidocaine) for local infiltration
- Local anesthetic as prescribed (to establish the block)
- Occlusive dressing supplies to cover the catheter entry site
- Gauze and tape to secure the catheter to the patient's body
- Labels stating "Local anesthetic only" and "Not for intravenous injection"

- Pump for administration of analgesia (e.g., volumetric pump, dedicated for peripheral nerve block infusion with rate and volume limited, and preferably a different color from the epidural and IV infusion pumps; patient-controlled analgesic pump or a portable infusion device such as a disposable elastomeric continuous infusion pump
- Specific observation chart for patient monitoring of the peripheral nerve block infusion
- Prescribed analgesics and local anesthetics
- Equipment for monitoring blood pressure, heart rate, and pulse oximetry

Additional equipment, to have available as needed, includes the following:

- Ice or alcohol swabs for demonstrating sensory block
- Emergency medications (e.g., 20% fat emulsion/intralipids for local anesthetic toxicity)
- Bag-valve-mask device and oxygen
- Equipment for end-tidal carbon dioxide monitoring
- Intubation equipment
- Peripheral nerve stimulator and/or ultrasound to facilitate placement

PATIENT AND FAMILY EDUCATION

- Explain the reason and purpose of the catheter. If available, supply easy-to-read patient information. *Rationale:* The patient and the family know what to expect; anxiety may be reduced.
- Explain to the patient and family that the procedure can be uncomfortable but that a local anesthetic will be used to facilitate comfort. *Rationale:* Explanation elicits the patient's cooperation and comfort, and facilitates insertion; anxiety and fear may be decreased.
- During therapy, instruct the patient to report side effects or changes in pain or sensation. Observe for suboptimal analgesia, profound numbness of extremities (beyond the goal of therapy), patient report of lightheadedness, metallic taste, circumoral numbness, dizziness, blurred vision, tinnitus, loss of hearing, and seizures.[5,9,17,23] *Rationale:* Reporting of pain aids the patient's comfort level and identifies side effects. Recognition of early signs and symptoms of local anesthetic toxicity can prevent cardiac arrhythmias, arrest, and death.
- Teach the patient to protect the affected extremity from injury and trauma (e.g., burns).[3,5,23] *Rationale:* Patient safety is increased, and the limb is protected from injury and trauma.
- If a volumetric pump for patient-controlled regional analgesia (PCA) is used, educate the patient and family on its use. Reinforce this education throughout the duration of regional PCA therapy. *Rationale:* This may decrease anxiety and assists the patient in effectively using the infusion system.

PATIENT ASSESSMENT AND PREPARATION
Patient Assessment

- Observe the patient for signs and symptoms of local infection or generalized sepsis. *Rationale:* This decreases the risk for infection at the site of catheter insertion. Septicemia and bacteremia are contraindications for peripheral nerve block catheter placement or continuation of therapy.[10,12]

- Assess the patient's concurrent anticoagulant and fibrinolytic therapy.[6,7,39] *Rationale:* Heparin (unfractionated and low–molecular-weight heparin), heparinoids, and fibrinolytic agents administered concurrently increase the risk for vessel trauma (e.g., hematoma). Care must be taken with insertion and removal of the peripheral nerve block catheter when patients are on anticoagulant and fibrinolytic therapy.[9,27] Special institutional guidelines must be observed.[3,5–7,19,25,27] Insertion and removal of the peripheral nerve catheter should be directed by the physician or advanced practice nurse.[5–7,27]
- Obtain the patient's vital signs. *Rationale:* This provides baseline data.
- Assess the patient's pain and anxiety. *Rationale:* This provides baseline data and helps determine whether premedication is required.
- Reassure the patient. *Rationale:* Anxiety and fears may be reduced.
- Review the patient's medication allergies. *Rationale:* Review of medication allergies before administration of a new medication decreases allergic reactions.
- Consider instructions for nothing by mouth, especially if sedation or general anesthesia is to be used. *Rationale:* The risk for vomiting and aspiration is decreased.

Patient Preparation

- Verify that the patient is the correct patient using two identifiers. *Rationale:* Before performing a procedure, the nurse should ensure the correct identification of the patient for the intended intervention.
- Ensure that the patient and family understand the planned procedure. Answer questions as they arise, and reinforce information as needed. *Rationale:* Understanding of previously taught information is evaluated and reinforced.
- Ensure that informed consent has been obtained. *Rationale:* Informed consent protects the rights of the patient and makes a competent decision possible for the patient.
- Perform a preprocedure verification and time out, if nonemergent. *Rationale:* This ensures patient safety.
- Wash the specific anatomical area of the patient's body with soap and water, and open the gown to expose the site for injection while maintaining the patient's privacy and dignity. *Rationale:* This action cleanses the skin and allows easy access to the specific anatomical area of the patient's body.
- Establish IV access or ensure the patency of IV catheters. *Rationale:* Medications may be needed if side effects occur (i.e., hypotension).
- Position the patient as appropriate, according to which anatomical area of the body is to be blocked. *Rationale:* This prepares the patient for the procedure.

Procedure	for Peripheral Nerve Blocks	
Steps	**Rationale**	**Special Considerations**
1. HH		
2. PE		Physicians, advanced practice nurses, and other healthcare professionals should apply personal protective gear (e.g., face masks with eye shields) and sterile attire (e.g., sterile gowns, sterile gloves).
3. Obtain the prescribed peripheral nerve block medication.	The medication should be prepared with aseptic technique by the pharmacy with laminar flow or prepared commercially.	All peripheral nerve block solutions are preservative free to avoid neuronal injury.[7]
4. Connect the correct tubing to the prepared infusion and prime the tubing.	Removes air from the infusion system.	
5. Ensure that the patient is in position for catheter placement.	Facilitates ease of insertion of the peripheral nerve block catheter.	Assist with holding the patient in position or consider sedation, if necessary.
6. Assist as needed with the antiseptic preparation of the intended insertion site. **(Level C*)**	Reduces the transmission of microorganisms into the nerve sheath or plexus space.[12,23]	The choice of povidone-iodine or chlorhexidine as an antiseptic agent for neurological procedures is controversial. Both should be allowed to dry completely. Chlorhexidine may be neurotoxic.[20]
7. Assist if needed with draping the patient with exposure of the insertion site.	Aids in maintaining sterility.	

*Level C: Qualitative studies, descriptive or correlational studies, integrative reviews, systematic reviews, or randomized controlled trials with inconsistent results.

Procedure	for Peripheral Nerve Blocks—*Continued*	
Steps	**Rationale**	**Special Considerations**
8. Assist the physician or advanced practice nurse as needed with the catheter placement and manipulation of the controls on the peripheral nerve stimulator if used).[3,23] (**Level C***)	Facilitates catheter insertion. Use of a peripheral nerve stimulator assists with identification of the nerve.[23,28]	Ultrasound guidance may be used to place the continuous peripheral nerve block catheter. If ultrasound has print capability, print a reading and include it in the chart for documentation.
9. After the peripheral nerve catheter is inserted, assist as needed with the application of a sterile, occlusive dressing.	Reduces the incidence of infection.[12,23]	
10. Secure the filter to the patient's body with a gauze padding and tape.	Avoids disconnection between the peripheral nerve catheter and the filter. The gauze padding prevents discomfort and skin pressure from the filter.	
11. The physician or advanced practice nurse will administer a bolus dose of medication via the catheter.	Facilitates a therapeutic level of analgesia and ensures correct catheter placement.[39]	An initial test dose of local anesthetic agent with or without epinephrine may be administered, then a bolus dose. Monitor vital signs and symptoms of local anesthetic toxicity and assess the patient's pain. Emergency medications and equipment must be available.[7,25]
12. Connect the prescribed medication infusion system.	Prepares the infusion system.	
13. Initiate therapy:		
A. Place the system in a volumetric pump or elastomeric continuous infusion pump and set the rate and volume to be infused as prescribed.	Prepares the infusion system.	Responses to peripheral nerve block analgesia vary individually, and analgesia is tailored according to individual responses. Note: Peripheral nerve catheters may also be attached to a portable disposable infusion device (e.g., elastomeric pump)[16,21,30,35] that may not have an adjustable rate or volume.[30,35]
B. Attach a label: "Local anesthetic only—Not for intravenous injection" to the tubing and use a portless system.[5] (**Level D***)	Do not give any other solution or medication via this catheter. Inadvertent administration of some IV medications into the peripheral nerve block catheter may cause nerve or tissue damage. Inadvertent administration of local IV anesthetic can cause hypotension and cardiovascular collapse or arrest.[17,21,23]	
C. Lock the key pad on the volumetric pump.	Prevents inadvertent or accidental changes in therapy.	
14. Continue to assess the quality of the analgesia.	Identifies patient comfort level and is an indicator to clinicians regarding the effectiveness of the therapy.	

*Level C: Qualitative studies, descriptive or correlational studies, integrative reviews, systematic reviews, or randomized controlled trials with inconsistent results.
*Level D: Peer-reviewed professional and organizational standards with the support of clinical study recommendations.

Procedure continues on following page

Procedure for Peripheral Nerve Blocks—*Continued*

Steps	Rationale	Special Considerations
A. Determine the patient's pain based on a consistent and reliable pain-assessment tool according to institutional policy.[33]	The amount of pain experienced by the patient should be no more than the amount of what is acceptable to the patient.[1,2,9]	
B. Assist as needed with testing the corresponding dermatome level of the peripheral nerve block with ice or an alcohol swab.	The ideal peripheral nerve block should be just above and just below the (anticipated) surgical incision or the trauma site (see the dermatomes described in Fig. 107-3).[9,23]	
15. Remove **PE** and discard used supplies in an appropriate receptacle.	Removes and safely discards used supplies.	
16. **HH**		

Expected Outcomes

- Regional analgesic catheter inserted; accurate catheter placement confirmed with use of ultrasound scan, nerve stimulator, or radiological imaging when appropriate[5,6,18,22,29,31]
- Pain minimized or relieved[3,31,32]
- No patient oversedation or respiratory depression[5,17,39]
- Reduced need for parenteral opioids, thereby also reducing opioid side effects[18,23]
- Potential for reduction in neuropathic pain states, especially after limb amputation[14]
- Temporary numbness and loss of motor control[23]

Unexpected Outcomes

- Inability to insert the catheter
- Untimely or erroneous medication administration[5,9]
- Suboptimal analgesia
- Adverse medication reactions not recognized
- Altered skin integrity from decreased sensory and motor loss[6,9,16,37,38]
- Accidental dislodgment of the catheter delivery system
- Leakage from the catheter insertion site
- Cracked filter on the delivery system
- Inadvertent injection into a blood vessel[3,5,39]
- Ipsilateral Horner's syndrome—symptoms that arise when a group of nerves known as the sympathetic trunk is damaged or blocked by anesthetic during stellate ganglion block.[26,36] Horner's syndrome may also develop due to inadvertent vascular puncture and hematoma formation in the neck.[4,26] The signs and symptoms occur on the same side as the affected sympathetic trunk (ipsilateral). Miosis (a constricted pupil), ptosis (drooping eyelid), and anhidrosis (decreased sweating) can occur. Enophthalmos (inset eyeball) may also be present, as may hoarseness[5,26,36,39]
- Nerve or vessel trauma[3,5,39]
- Hemorrhage or hematoma[6]
- Respiratory distress related to phrenic nerve paralysis, pneumothorax, or medication effect[3,16,23,32]
- Local infection at the peripheral nerve block catheter insertion site
- Sepsis[12]
- Anaphylaxis[5,17]
- Permanent neurological injuries and damage from insertion[26,39]
- Systemic toxicity from local anesthetics (e.g., tachycardia, hypotension, metallic taste, blurred vision, circumoral numbness, tinnitus, decreased hearing, dizziness, confusion progressing to seizures, cardiac arrest, or even death)[5,17,23]

Patient Monitoring and Care

Steps	Rationale	Reportable Conditions
		These conditions should be reported if they persist despite nursing interventions. • Continued pain despite pain interventions
1. Assess the patient's level of pain with a valid and reliable pain scale. Follow institutional standards for assessing pain. Administer analgesia as prescribed. Continue to assess frequently, especially during the first 12–24 hours of therapy.[2,9,23,33]	Identifies the need for pain interventions. Describes the patient's response to pain therapy. A lower pain score is expected. Assessing and reassessing pain in an objective manner helps determine appropriate treatment measures.	
2. Assess the patient's vital signs, oxygenation and ventilatory status, and level of sedation with a valid and reliable sedation scale.[15,33] Monitoring the patient every 15 minutes has been recommended in the immediate period after initiation of therapy.[23]	Hypotension and sedation may reflect IV infusion, systemic toxicity, or the residual effects of sedation administered for catheter placement.[21,23]	• Change in respiratory status or other vital signs (e.g., respiratory rate, oxygenation via pulse oximetry, blood pressure) • Altered level of consciousness

3. Assess the levels of motor and sensory blockade. Follow institutional standards for these assessments (see Fig. 107-3).[1–3,9,23]	Ensures effectiveness of analgesia and maintenance of the block at the correct level.	• Signs and symptoms of overmedication:
		  • Decreased ability to feel or to move area of the body where the peripheral nerve block is infusing[4]
		  • Excessive sensory or motor blockade in the lower extremities may result in signs of pressure and skin breakdown on the heels[4]

4. Monitor the infusion rate according to institutional policy. Ensure that the control panel is locked if using a volumetric infuser or ensure that the PCA program is locked via a key or code access. Disposable infusion devices (e.g., elastomeric pumps) have been shown to be less accurate than volumetric pumps.[30,35]	Ensures that medication is administered safely and securely.	
5. Monitor oxygen saturation and capnography (if available) continuously, especially if parenteral opioids are administered for pain or mild sedation before, during, or after the procedure.[4,11]	Assesses ventilation and oxygenation.	• Oxygen saturation <93% or decreasing trend in oxygenation
6. Assess temperature regularly; assess more frequently if febrile.	Increasing hyperpyrexia could signify infection.[12]	• Temperature >101.3 °F (38.5 °C)
7. Assess the catheter site every 4–8 hours and as needed.	Identifies site complications.	• A change in the integrity of the peripheral nerve block insertion site (e.g., redness, tenderness, or swelling or the presence of exudate on the dressing)

Procedure continues on following page

Patient Monitoring and Care —*Continued*

Steps	Rationale	Reportable Conditions
8. Observe for signs and symptoms of peripheral nerve catheter migration into a blood vessel.	The catheter is no longer in the correct position.	• Unexpected change in sedation scale • Drowsiness • Dizziness • Blurred vision • Slurred speech • Poor balance • Circumoral numbness • Hypotension • Cardiovascular collapse
9. Monitor sensory or motor loss according to the defined goal of therapy. **(Level D*)**	Motor or sensory loss may result from the local anesthetic infusion. Note: With peripheral nerve blockade, sensory loss is usually acceptable and often desirable. Motor loss is not desirable but often acceptable.[3,5,18,23,39]	• Unexpected change in sensory or motor function beyond the defined goal of therapy • Interference with respiration or excessive spread of local anesthetic beyond the defined area of recommendation
10. Assess for systemic toxicity from the local anesthetic administered through the catheter.	Local anesthetic is used in the solution, and symptoms indicative of systemic toxicity from the agent used to induce anesthesia may occur.	• Metallic taste • Blurred vision • Circumoral numbness • Tinnitus • Decreased hearing • Dizziness • Confusion progressing to seizures
11. Monitor and check the skin integrity of the pressure points relating to the location of the peripheral nerve block (e.g., elbow, sacrum, and heels). Change patient's position as needed. Provide protective positioning.[3,23]	If a local anesthetic is used in the solution, check for pressure ulceration (patient may have sensory loss in areas adjacent to the area of the peripheral nerve block).[3,23]	• Increasing redness or blistering of the skin on pressure points
12. Change the peripheral nerve block catheter insertion site dressing as prescribed or if soiled, wet, or loose.[7] Note: Usually the dressing is left intact for the duration of therapy unless wet or loose.[6]	Provides an opportunity to cleanse the area around the catheter and to assess for signs and symptoms of infection.[12,23]	• Signs of site infection (e.g., swelling, pain, redness, or presence of drainage) • Leakage of the peripheral nerve block solution
13. Label the peripheral nerve block pump and consider placing the pump on one side of the patient's bed and all other pumps on the other side of the bed.[6]	Aids in minimizing the risk for mistaking the local anesthetic infusion for an IV infusion system.[7]	

*Level D: Peer-reviewed professional and organizational standards with the support of clinical study recommendations.

Documentation

Documentation should include the following:

- Patient and family education
- Patient tolerance of procedure
- Completion of informed consent
- Completion of a preprocedure verification and time out
- Catheter location
- Type of dressing used
- Confirmation of peripheral nerve block catheter placement (e.g., radiological confirmation, stimulating peripheral nerve catheter, ultrasound scan)
- Site assessment
- Assessment of pain and levels of motor and sensory blockade documented on an appropriate flow chart (see Fig. 107-3).
- If PCA is used, document medication concentration, PCA bolus dose, continuous infusion, lockout interval, hourly limits, and total dosage

- Regional analgesic medication and the medication concentration being infused and infusion rate; remaining volume of medication in a disposable infusion device
- Bolus dose administration (if appropriate) and patient response after a bolus dose, including quality of pain relief
- Vital signs and oxygenation saturation.
- Occurrence of unexpected outcomes
- Nursing interventions taken
- Date and time of discontinuation of treatment
- Pain assessment, interventions, and effectiveness

References and Additional Readings

For a complete list of references and additional readings for this procedure, scan this QR code with any freely available smartphone code reader app, or visit http://booksite.elsevier.com/9780323376624.

108 Esophagogastric Tamponade Tube

Rosemary Lee

PURPOSE: Esophagogastric tamponade therapy is used to provide temporary control of bleeding from gastric or esophageal varices.

PREREQUISITE NURSING KNOWLEDGE

- Tamponade therapy exerts direct pressure against the varices with the use of a gastric and/or esophageal balloon and may be used for patients who are unresponsive to medical therapy or are too hemodynamically unstable for endoscopy or sclerotherapy.[1,3]

- Esophagogastric tamponade tubes are used to control bleeding from either gastric and/or esophageal varices. The suction lumens allow the evacuation of accumulated blood from the stomach or esophagus. The suction lumens also allow for the intermittent instillation of saline solution to assist with evacuation of blood or clots and provide a means of irrigation if indicated.

- Three types of tubes are available for esophagogastric tamponade therapy. The two most common tubes are the Sengstaken-Blakemore (Bard, Inc., Covington, Georgia) tube (Fig. 108-1) and the Minnesota esophagogastric tamponade tube. The Sengstaken-Blakemore tube has a gastric and esophageal balloon and a gastric aspiration lumen. The four-lumen Minnesota tube (Fig. 108-2) has gastric and esophageal balloons and separate gastric and esophageal aspiration lumens. The third, the Linton or Linton-Nachlas tube, (Mallinckrodt Inc., Tyco Health Care Group, Hampshire, UK) has a gastric balloon and separate gastric and esophageal aspiration lumens and is used only for treatment of bleeding gastric varices. The Minnesota tube is considered the preferred tube for esophagogastric tamponade therapy because it allows for aspiration of drainage above the esophageal balloon and below the gastric balloon.

- Esophagogastric tamponade tubes may be introduced via either the nasogastric or the orogastric route. The tubes are then advanced through the oropharynx and esophagus and into the stomach.

- Contraindications include latex allergy, esophageal strictures, and recent esophageal surgery. Relative contraindications are heart failure, respiratory failure, hiatal hernia, severe pulmonary hypertension, and cardiac dysrhythmias.[4,8,12]

- Because of the risk for aspiration, it is recommended the patient be endotracheally intubated for airway protection before esophagogastric tamponade tube insertion.[13]

- Sedation should be considered, but dosing should be individualized on the assessment of each patient. Sedation should be used with caution in the setting of liver injury and/or failure due to these patients' impaired metabolism of sedating medications. The plan for sedation, if needed, is individualized with the goal to achieve patient comfort.

- Head of bed (HOB) should be at least 30 to 45 degrees at all times to reduce the risk of aspiration.[6]

- The use of esophageal tamponade is decreasing in clinical practice because up to 50% of varices rebleed after the balloons are deflated.[12,13] Additionally, major complications can occur with the use of esophageal balloon tamponade therapy.[13] However, esophagogastric tubes are still used in areas where esophagogastric duodenoscopy is not readily available. The use of esophageal tamponade is designed to be a temporary intervention until more definitive therapy can be carried out. Balloon tamponade is recommended to be used for only 24 to 48 hours.[2,13]

EQUIPMENT

- Tamponade tube (Sengstaken-Blakemore, Minnesota, or Linton-Nachlas)
- Irrigation kit (or catheter-tip, 60-mL syringe and basin)
- Nasogastric (NG) tubes (one for Sengstaken-Blakemore tube)
- Normal saline (NS) solution for irrigation
- Water-soluble lubricant
- Topical anesthetic agent
- Sphygmomanometer or pressure gauge

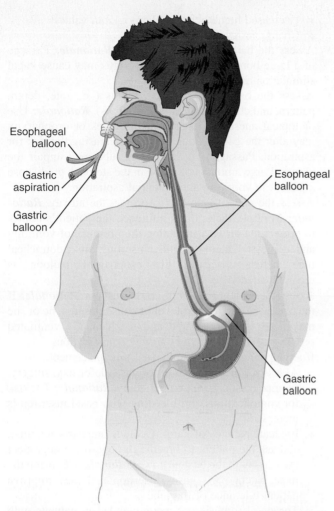

Figure 108-1 Sengstaken-Blakemore tube in place with both the esophageal and gastric balloons inflated. *(From Carlson KK, editor: AACN advanced critical care nursing, Philadelphia, 2009, Saunders.)*

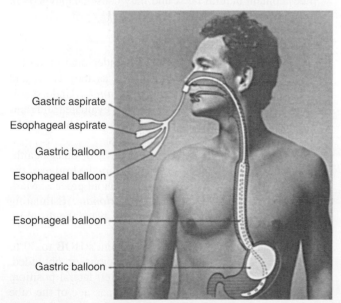

Figure 108-2 Minnesota four-lumen tube. *(From Swearingen PL: Photo atlas of nursing procedures, Reading, MA, 1991, Addison-Wesley.)*

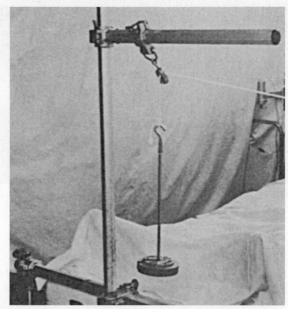

Figure 108-3 Balanced suspension traction securing tamponade tube and placement. *(From DeGroot KD, Damato M: Critical care skills, Norwalk, CT, 1987, Appleton & Lange.)*

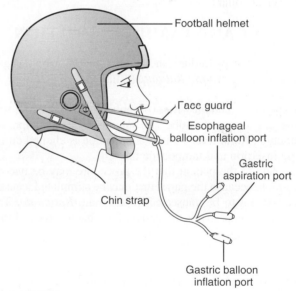

Figure 108-4 Tamponade tube secured in position with helmet.

- Four rubber-shod clamps or plastic plugs that may come with the balloon kit
- Adhesive tape
- Two suction setups and tubing
- Cardiac monitor
- Scissors, must be kept at bedside

Additional equipment, to have available as needed, includes the following:

- Rubber cube sponge (used for nasal tamponade tube placement)—may be used for traction
- Balanced suspension traction apparatus with 1 pound of weights, 500 mL of NS solution (Fig. 108-3), or football helmet with face mask (Fig. 108-4)

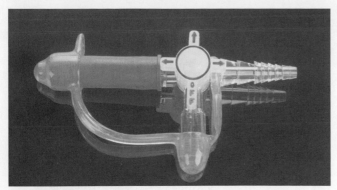

Figure 108-5   Lopez valve. *(Courtesy of ICU Medical, Inc,. San Clemente, CA.)*

- Lopez enteral valve (Fig. 108-5) (ICU Medical, San Clemente, CA), a three-way stopcock used to attach a 60-mL catheter-tip syringe and the handheld manometer to the Minnesota tube
- Emergency medications and equipment, including transcutaneous pacemaker and intubation equipment
- Endotracheal suction equipment
- Marker
- Cervical collar

PATIENT AND FAMILY EDUCATION

- Explain the procedure and reason for the esophagogastric tube insertion. *Rationale:* Patient anxiety may be decreased.
- Explain the patient's role (if applicable) in assisting with the passage of the tube and maintenance of tamponade traction. *Rationale:* Patient cooperation is elicited during the insertion and tamponade therapy.
- Explain to the patient that the procedure may be uncomfortable because the gag reflex may be stimulated, causing the patient to be nauseated or to vomit. *Rationale:* This explanation prepares the patient for what to expect during the procedure.

PATIENT ASSESSMENT AND PREPARATION

Patient Assessment

- Assess signs and symptoms of major blood loss. *Rationale:* Esophageal or gastric varices can cause significant blood loss:
  - Tachycardia
  - Tachypnea
  - Hypotension
  - Decreased urine output
  - Decreased filling pressures (pulmonary artery pressure, pulmonary artery wedge pressure, central venous pressure, stroke volume, stroke volume index)
  - Decreased platelet counts

  - Decreased hematocrit and hemoglobin values
  - Change in level of consciousness
- Assess the baseline cardiac rhythm. *Rationale:* Passage of a large-bore tube into the esophagus may cause vagal stimulation and bradycardia.
- Assess the baseline respiratory status (i.e., rate, depth, pattern, and characteristics of secretions). *Rationale:* Use of topical anesthetic agents in the nares or oropharynx may alter the gag or cough reflex, increasing the risk for aspiration. Passage of a large-bore tube may impair the airway. Large amounts of blood in the stomach predispose a patient to vomiting and potential aspiration.
- Assess the patient's ability to protect the airway. *Rationale:* Multiple factors can influence the patient's ability to protect the airway, including the presence of vomiting and depressed mental status. Inserting an endotracheal tube before inserting the esophageal balloon is recommended.[13]
- Assess the patient's level of consciousness. *Rationale:* If the patient has an altered level of consciousness, he or she may need to be intubated and mechanically ventilated prophylactically to prevent airway complications.
- If anticipating a nasal esophageal tube placement:
  - Assess for medical history of nasal deformity, surgery, trauma, epistaxis, or coagulopathy. *Rationale:* The risk for complications and bleeding with nasal insertion is increased.
  - Evaluate patency of nares. Occlude one naris at a time, and ask the patient to breathe through the nose. Select the naris with the best airflow. *Rationale:* Choosing the most patent naris eases insertion and may improve patient tolerance of the tube.
  - The nasal route is not recommended in patients with coagulopathy. *Rationale:* The risk for bleeding and complications is increased.
- Assess for allergy to latex. *Rationale:* Balloon tamponade tubes contain natural latex and may cause anaphylaxis in patients with a latex allergy.

Patient Preparation

- Ensure that the patient and family understand preprocedural information. Answer questions as they arise, and reinforce information as needed. *Rationale:* Understanding of previously taught information is evaluated and reinforced. Typically this is an emergency procedure and the patient and family will be under stress.
- The physician, advanced practice nurse, or other healthcare professional measures the tube from the bridge of the nose to the earlobe to the tip of the xiphoid process. Mark the length of tube to be inserted. *Rationale:* Estimating the length of tube to be inserted helps place the distal tip in the stomach.
- If the patient is alert, elevate the patient's HOB to 30 to 45 degrees. If the patient is unconscious or obtunded, place the patient's head down in the left lateral position. *Rationale:* Positioning facilitates the passage of the tube into the stomach and reduces the risk for aspiration.

Procedure	**for Inserting Esophagogastric Tamponade Tube**		
Steps	**Rationale**	**Special Considerations**	

Steps	Rationale	Special Considerations
1. **HH**		
2. **PE**	Exposure to blood and gastric fluids is likely.	
3. Assist the physician, advanced practice nurse, or other healthcare professional with assessing gastric balloon integrity before insertion:		The physician, advanced practice nurse, or other healthcare professional performing the procedure may elect to omit this step in the case of a medical emergency.
A. Attach the gastric balloon port to the sphygmomanometer or pressure gauge (Fig. 108-6) before insertion.		
B. Inflate the gastric balloon with 100, 200, 300, 400, and 500 mL of air, noting the pressure reading at each stage of inflation.	Knowing the pressure required at each stage of inflation before insertion may prevent inadvertent perforation of the esophagus after insertion.[1]	
C. If applicable, inflate the esophageal balloon with the volume indicated in the package insert.	Verifies integrity of esophageal balloon.[1]	
D. Hold the air-filled balloon under water to test for air leaks.	Verifies integrity of balloon.[1]	
E. Actively and completely deflate the balloon and clamp. **(Level M*)**	Deflated balloon eases insertion.[1]	
4. Insert a nasogastric tube (see Procedure 113) into the stomach, drain contents, and then remove tube.	Emptying the stomach of blood/gastric contents decreases the risk for aspiration and minimizes occlusion of the tube with blood clots.	There is a risk of lacerating the varices with an NG tube insertion.

*Level M: Manufacturer's recommendations only.

Procedure continues on following page

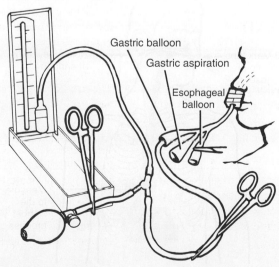

Figure 108-6 Inflation of esophageal balloon. *(Courtesy of Davol, Inc., Warwick, RI)*

Procedure	**for Inserting Esophagogastric Tamponade Tube—***Continued*	
Steps	**Rationale**	**Special Considerations**
5. Lubricate balloons and distal 15 cm of tube with water-soluble lubricant.	Minimizes mucosal injury and irritation during insertion; facilitates insertion.	Use only water-soluble lubricant. Oil-based lubricants, such as petroleum jelly, may cause respiratory complications if inadvertently aspirated. Oil-based lubricants may also damage the latex in the tube and may cause the balloon to rupture.[1]
6. Apply the topical anesthetic agent to the posterior oropharynx as prescribed by the practitioner (apply to nostril if nasally inserted).	Decreases discomfort caused by insertion.	*Caution:* Gag and cough reflexes may be compromised by topical anesthetic, increasing the risk for aspiration. Keep emergency intubation equipment easily available.
7. Position the patient in the supine position with the HOB elevated 30–45 degrees.	Facilitates tube placement and reduces risk of aspiration.	
8. Assist the physician, advanced practice nurse, or other healthcare professional with insertion of the tamponade tube into the mouth or selected nostril. The tube is advanced into the stomach to at least the 50-cm mark on the tube or 10 cm beyond the estimated length needed to reach the stomach. (Fig. 108-7)	Helps placement of entire gastric balloon in the stomach.[1]	Heart rate may decrease as a result of vagal stimulation. Should symptomatic bradycardia occur, atropine may be administered or transcutaneous pacing initiated as prescribed (or per institutional protocol).
9. Lavage the stomach via the gastric aspiration port with NS solution until clear of large blood clots. **(Level E*)**	Ensures patency and prevents clots from blocking the tube.[5,8]	

*Level E: Multiple case reports, theory-based evidence from expert opinions, or peer-reviewed professional organizational standards without clinical studies to support recommendations.

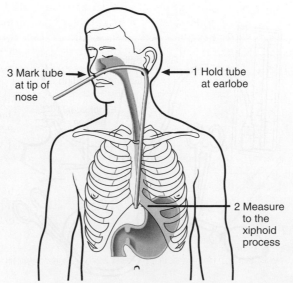

3 Mark tube at tip of nose

1 Hold tube at earlobe

2 Measure to the xiphoid process

Figure 108-7   Measuring nasogastric tube. (*From Luckmann J: Saunders manual of nursing care, Philadelphia, 1997, Saunders.*)

Procedure	**for Inserting Esophagogastric Tamponade Tube—*Continued***	
Steps	**Rationale**	**Special Considerations**
10. Connect the gastric aspiration port to intermittent suction at 60–120 mm Hg.[6] **(Level E*)**	Provides for evacuation of gastric contents and for assessment of continued bleeding.[4,8,11]	
11. Connect the esophageal aspiration port to intermittent suction at 120–200 mm Hg[6] (Minnesota tube only). **(Level E*)**	Provides for evacuation of secretions and for assessment of continued bleeding.[1,4]	
12. Tube placement must be confirmed:		
A. Aspirate drainage from the gastric aspiration port. **(Level M*)**	Prevents gastric balloon from being inflated in the esophagus, causing rupture.[1]	The ability to simply aspirate fluid from the tube is often interpreted as confirmation of gastric intubation. Caution is needed because several reports have shown that fluid can also be aspirated after endotracheal intubation. The gold standard for confirming placement is an abdominal or chest radiograph to ensure proper placement of tamponade tube.[1,7,9,10]
B. The physician, advanced practice nurse, or other healthcare professional slowly inflates the gastric balloon with increments of 100 mL of air, up to a total 500 mL, observing the pressure on the sphygmomanometer or pressure gauge at each increment. (If the pressure exceeds preinflation pressure for a particular volume by more than 15 mm Hg, all of the air is withdrawn and the tube is advanced an additional 10 cm.) **(Level E*)**	A pressure difference of more than 15 mm Hg indicates that the gastric balloon is in the esophagus.[4,8,11]	pH testing of gastric secretions may also be used to assess placement. However, because the patient is actively bleeding this may not be accurate. Auscultation to confirm gastric tube placement by placing a stethoscope over the stomach and instilling 20–50 mL of air via syringe is no longer accepted practice. Alternatively, the gastric balloon can be inflated with 100 mL of air and the position verified by a portable x-ray. Once verified the balloon may be completely inflated.
C. On full inflation of the gastric balloon, clamp the gastric balloon lumen with a rubber-shod clamp or plug with the white plastic plug. An abdominal radiograph is obtained.	The outline of the gastric balloon can be visualized on radiograph. Verifies placement of the entire gastric balloon within the stomach.[4,11,12]	The gastric balloon inflation process may be simplified with the use of a Lopez enteral valve (see Fig. 108-5), which can be connected to one side of the gastric balloon. The catheter-tip syringe goes into the large port, the manometer goes into another, and the tapered end of the valve goes into the Minnesota tube. This alternative may eliminate the need to repeatedly clamp and unclamp the tubing while measuring the volume of air injected through the 60-mL catheter-tip syringe.

*Level E: Multiple case reports, theory-based evidence from expert opinions, or peer-reviewed professional organizational standards without clinical studies to support recommendations.

*Level M: Manufacturer's recommendations only.

Procedure continues on following page

Procedure	for Inserting Esophagogastric Tamponade Tube—*Continued*	
Steps	**Rationale**	**Special Considerations**
13. After radiographic confirmation of placement, the tube is withdrawn until slight resistance is met. Double-clamp the gastric balloon lumen with the rubber-shod clamp, or plug it with the white plug. Disconnect the sphygmomanometer or pressure gauge from the gastric port. **(Level M*)**	Positions the gastric balloon at the gastroesophageal junction where the inflated balloon fills the stomach and creates the tamponade effect.[3,8] The clamp or plug prevents an air leak from the gastric balloon.[1,3,8]	Interval assessment of gastric balloon pressures is not indicated and may result in accidental deflation and loss of tamponade.
14. Use permanent marker or tape to mark the tamponade tube placement at the opening at either the mouth or nose. Place the tape marker around tube as it exits the mouth or nose.	Provides a reference point to assess placement of the tube.	Document the marking, and assess the tube for possible migration.
15. Attach the sphygmomanometer or pressure gauge to the esophageal balloon port. **(Level M*)**	Allows for direct measurement of balloon pressures to prevent excess pressure on esophageal tissue	
16. The physician, advanced practice nurse, or other healthcare professional inserting the tube should inflate the esophageal balloon if bleeding is not controlled with gastric tamponade.	Produces direct pressure on esophageal vessels.[1,3,4]	Maintain esophageal balloon pressures as prescribed or per institutional protocol.
A. The practitioner gradually inflates the esophageal balloon to 25–45 mm Hg. **(Level M*)**	Higher pressures may cause esophageal necrosis or rupture.[1,12,13]	Patient may have chest pain or bradycardia with inflation. Monitor electrocardiographic (ECG) changes during placement, removal, or inflation of the balloon.
B. Double-clamp or plug the esophageal balloon port. **(Level M*)**	Prevents air leaks from esophageal balloon.[1]	

17. Gentle traction is applied to the tube. **(Level E*)**
   A. Apply gentle traction.
     1. Use 1 pound of weight attached to tube with balance suspension traction (see Fig. 108-3).
     2. For alternative traction, use a bag with 500 mL of NS solution. Attach bag to tube with balance system (see Fig. 108-3).
	Positions the gastric balloon and exerts pressure on the varices.[1,8,11–13]	

B. Tape the tube to the sponge cube at the naris, if the tube is passed nasally. *Or*	Prevents excessive pressure on the nares.	

*Level E: Multiple case reports, theory-based evidence from expert opinions, or peer-reviewed professional organizational standards without clinical studies to support recommendations.
*Level M: Manufacturer's recommendations only.

Procedure	for Inserting Esophagogastric Tamponade Tube—*Continued*	
Steps	**Rationale**	**Special Considerations**

C. Apply the football helmet to the patient's head, and tape the tube to the chin or faceguard (see Fig. 108-4). *Or* D. Apply a semirigid cervical collar, and tape the tube to the collar.[5] **(Level E*)**		Pad the inside of the helmet to ensure a snug fit and to prevent pressure ulcer formation on the occipital region of the head. The football helmet makes it difficult to provide oral hygiene and puts the patient at risk for device-related pressure ulcers.
18. Maintain the HOB at 30–45 degrees.	Promotes comfort, minimizes aspiration, and may prevent ventilator-associated pneumonia (if patient is intubated).[7]	
19. Sengstaken-Blakemore tube only: A. Insert an NG tube to just above the esophageal balloon. **(Level E*)**	Reduces secretions and accumulated blood in the esophagus that may result in aspiration into the lungs.[1,8,11,12]	
B. Use permanent marker or tape to mark the tamponade tube placement at the opening of either the mouth or nose.	Creates a reference point to assess migration of the tube.	If the gastric tube migrates upward, it may result in complete blockage of the airway.
C. Connect to intermittent suction 120–200 mm Hg.[6] **(Level E*)**	Reduces secretions and accumulated blood.[1,11,12]	
D. The position of the Sengstaken-Blakemore tube should be checked and documented every hour.		
20. Inflate the gastric balloon: A. The inflated gastric balloon should be kept at the minimal pressure required to control bleeding (approximately 25 mm Hg for at least 48 hours) and deflated for 12–24 hours to assess for any new bleeding. **(Level M*)**	Underinflation can lead to tube displacement into the esophagus. Overinflation can lead to mucosal and submucosal ischemia.[1]	
B. The Sengstaken-Blakemore tube should remain in place for a short period of time. **(Level E*)**	Minimizes the opportunity for mucosal trauma.[2]	
21. Inflation or deflation of the tamponade tube should be performed or prescribed by a physician, advanced practice nurse, or other healthcare professional. A. Connect the sphygmomanometer to the esophageal balloon port.	The esophageal balloon is inflated if the bleeding continues after the inflation of the gastric balloon. Do not inflate the esophageal balloon first.	

*Level E: Multiple case reports, theory-based evidence from expert opinions, or peer-reviewed professional organizational standards without clinical studies to support recommendations.
*Level M: Manufacturer's recommendations only.

Procedure continues on following page

Procedure for Inserting Esophagogastric Tamponade Tube—*Continued*		
Steps	**Rationale**	**Special Considerations**
B. With use of the second access port, gradually inflate the esophageal balloon to 25–45 mm Hg.	High pressures can lead to mucosal and submucosal ischemia or esophageal rupture.	Higher pressures may cause pain with inflation. Monitor ECG for changes during placement, inflation, or removal of the esophageal balloon.
C. Double-clamp the esophageal balloon port with rubber-shod clamps or use the white plug. (**Level M***)	Prevent loss of balloon pressure.	
D. The physician, advanced practice nurse, or other healthcare professional must deflate the esophageal balloon to make any changes to the tube's position. (**Level E***)	Ensures adequate balloon inflation for tamponade. Prevents mucosal ischemia, necrosis, and injury.[1,3,8] Prevents air leaks from the esophageal balloon.[1]	
Discontinuing Tamponade Therapy		
22. Discontinue tamponade therapy in stages. (**Level E***)	Provides for gradual reduction in tamponade to assess cessation of bleeding.[1,11,12]	
A. The physician, advanced practice nurse, or other healthcare professional must deflate the esophageal balloon (if inflation was needed to control bleeding) by unclamping the esophageal balloon port and aspirating to actively deflate the balloon.	Removes the tamponade effect exerted against the esophagus.	Never deflate the gastric balloon while the esophageal balloon remains inflated. A deflated gastric balloon may allow an inflated esophageal balloon to migrate in the airway. If the airway becomes obstructed, immediately cut both balloon ports to deflate the balloons and remove the tube immediately. If a physician, advanced practice nurse, or other healthcare professional is not present, the registered nurse may be able to deflate the balloon and remove the tube to clear the airway; follow institutional standards.
B. Observe for the recurrence of bleeding over 24 hours. If bleeding recurs, notify the physician, advanced practice nurse, or other healthcare professional to reinflate the esophageal balloon.	Bleeding may recur with the release of pressure on the esophageal varices.[1,11–13]	
C. If no further bleeding is noted, the physician, advanced practice nurse, or other healthcare professional deflates the gastric balloon by unclamping the gastric balloon port and aspirating with an irrigation syringe to actively deflate the balloon.		

*Level E: Multiple case reports, theory-based evidence from expert opinions, or peer-reviewed professional organizational standards without clinical studies to support recommendations.
*Level M: Manufacturer's recommendations only.

Procedure for Inserting Esophagogastric Tamponade Tube—*Continued*

Steps	Rationale	Special Considerations
D. Observe for the recurrence of bleeding over 24 hours. If bleeding recurs, notify the physician, advanced practice nurse, or other healthcare professional so he or she can reinflate the gastric balloon.	Bleeding may recur with the release of pressure on esophageal varices.	
E. If bleeding has not recurred in 24 hours, assist with the removal of the tube by cutting the balloon lumens with scissors and slowly withdrawing the tube. **(Level E*)**	Ensures complete balloon deflation before removal.[1,11,12]	
23. Remove **PE** and discard used supplies in appropriate receptacle.	Standard Precautions.	
24. **HH**		

*Level E: Multiple case reports, theory-based evidence from expert opinions, or peer-reviewed professional organizational standards without clinical studies to support recommendations.

Expected Outcomes

- Control of variceal bleeding
- Gastric decompression and evacuation

Unexpected Outcomes

- Rebleeding of varices
- Inappropriate placement of tamponade tube
- Gastric or esophageal necrosis
- Esophageal rupture
- Airway obstruction
- Cardiac dysrhythmias (during insertion or removal)
- Aspiration of gastric or oropharyngeal contents
- Erosion of mucosa around nares, lips, mouth, tongue

Patient Monitoring and Care

Steps	Rationale	Reportable Conditions
		These conditions should be reported if they persist despite nursing interventions.
1. Maintain tamponade therapy as needed: maximum of 24–48 hours for esophageal balloon; 48–72 hours for gastric balloon.	Longer inflation time may cause necrosis or ulceration.[1]	• Continued bleeding
2. Assess and monitor for changes in position of the permanent marker mark or tape mark to ensure the tamponade tube has not slipped out of place.	Allows for rapid identification of proper placement or dislodgement of the tamponade tube.	• Significant changes in tube position
3. Provide care to nares every 2 hours when the tube is inserted nasally. A. Remove dried blood or secretions from the nasal orifice and proximal nares. B. Apply lubricating ointment or lotion to keep the mucosa moist.	Prevents drying and ulcerations of the mucosa.	• Breakdown of tissue around the nares

Procedure continues on following page

Patient Monitoring and Care —*Continued*

Steps	Rationale	Reportable Conditions
4. Provide oral care every 2 hours.	Prevents drying and ulcerations of the mucosa and is also a strategy to thwart the development of ventilator-assisted pneumonia.[7]	• Mouth, tongue, or lip ulcerations
5. Provide frequent oral suctioning. **(Level E*)**	Esophageal balloon prevents the swallowing of secretions and saliva.[7,8]	• Bloody oral secretions
6. Monitor the esophageal balloon pressure hourly or as prescribed. Maintain esophageal balloon pressures at 25–45 mm Hg (pressures vary with respirations and may intermittently reach 70 mm Hg).[12] **(Level E*)**	Prevents excessive pressure on esophageal tissues.[1,8,12] Sudden loss of pressure may indicate rupture of the balloon or esophagus.	• Continued esophageal bleeding • Sudden loss of balloon pressure
7. Decrease the esophageal balloon pressure by 5 mm Hg every 3 hours as prescribed until pressure is 25 mm Hg, without evidence of bleeding. Follow institutional standards. **(Level E*)**	Use of the lowest possible pressure to create tamponade effect reduces the risk of necrosis.[1,8,12]	• Continued esophageal bleeding
8. Assist with the complete deflation of the esophageal balloon for 30 minutes every 8 hours or perform this step as prescribed; follow institutional standards. **(Level E*)**	Intermittent relief of the pressure may prevent necrosis of esophageal tissue.[1]	• Continued esophageal bleeding
9. Evaluate for the recurrence of variceal bleeding.	Bleeding may occur despite tamponade therapy.	• Continued bleeding
10. Monitor for airway patency and respiratory status.	Presence or movement of a large-bore tube may occlude the upper airway.	• Tachypnea • Stridor • Cough • High-pressure alarms on mechanical ventilator
11. Keep scissors at the bedside to immediately deflate the balloons.	Emergency deflation of both balloons may be needed in case of life-threatening complications such as airway occlusion or esophageal rupture.[1] Scissors are used to cut the balloon tubes, resulting in rapid deflation.	• Airway problems such as airway occlusion by migrating balloon • Physiological instability related to displacement of the balloon (i.e., bleeding)
12. Obtain an abdominal radiograph every 24 hours or sooner if there is any indication of displacement of the tamponade tube. **(Level E*)**	Inadvertent deflation of the gastric balloon may cause blockage of the airway by the esophageal balloon.[1,4,8,11,12]	• Balloon deflation • Airway problems (such as occlusion by migrating balloon) • Physiological instability related to displacement of the balloon (i.e., bleeding)
13. Monitor the gastric output. Irrigate the gastric aspiration port with 50 mL of NS solution every 30 minutes, or as needed and prescribed, to keep the lumen patent.	Maintains patency of the gastric lumen.[1]	• Continued gastric bleeding • Change in characteristics of output (e.g., color, quantity)

*Level E: Multiple case reports, theory-based evidence from expert opinions, or peer-reviewed professional organizational standards without clinical studies to support recommendations.

Patient Monitoring and Care —*Continued*

Steps	Rationale	Reportable Conditions
14. Monitor the esophageal output. Irrigate the esophageal aspiration port (or NG with Sengstaken-Blakemore) with 5–10 mL of NS solution every 2–4 hours, or as needed, to maintain patency. **(Level M*)**	Blood clots may occlude the esophageal aspiration lumen (or NG tube).[1]	• Continued esophageal bleeding • Change in characteristics of drainage (e.g., color, quantity)
15. Follow institutional standards for assessing pain. Administer analgesia as prescribed.	Identifies need for pain interventions.	• Continued pain despite pain interventions

*Level M: Manufacturer's recommendations only.

Documentation

Documentation should include the following:

- Patient and family education
- Date and time of the insertion
- Name of the physician, advanced practice nurse, or other healthcare professional inserting tube
- Location of tube placement marker (marker or tape)
- Tube type
- Any difficulties with the insertion
- Patient tolerance of the tube insertion, including pressures with specific balloon volumes
- Confirmation of placement with an abdominal radiograph
- Type and maintenance of the traction device
- Amount and type of suction applied to the various lumens

- Esophageal and gastric balloon pressures as applicable
- Periodic deflation of the esophageal balloon as prescribed
- Appearance and volume of gastric and esophageal drainage, if present
- Nasal or oral care
- Tube site assessments (nasal or oral)
- Unexpected outcomes
- Deflation sequence of the esophageal and gastric balloons
- Medications administered during the tube insertion (if applicable)

References and Additional Readings

For a complete list of references and additional readings for this procedure, scan this QR code with any freely available smartphone code reader app, or visit http://booksite.elsevier.com/9780323376624.

109 Focused Assessment with Sonography in Trauma

Cynthia Blank-Reid and Thomas A. Santora

PURPOSE: The focused assessment with sonography for trauma (FAST) as we know it today is a tool for the rapid assessment of an injured patient that allows reliable bedside identification of internal hemorrhage.

PREREQUISITE NURSING KNOWLEDGE

- When first introduced in the United States,[1] the FAST examination was performed by properly trained individuals and afforded a sensitive bedside evaluation to detect the presence of hemoperitoneum and hemopericardium. As experience and expertise accrued, the FAST examination has now expanded to reliably detect significant hydro- and hemothorax and with advanced training, the presence of pneumothorax.[2,3] Thus ultrasound provides a rapid, noninvasive, accurate, and inexpensive means of diagnosing internal injury of the torso that results in hemorrhage within the chest (pleural or pericardial) or the abdomino-pelvic region.
- The FAST is a "patient-centric" diagnostic intervention performed at the bedside in the resuscitation room while other diagnostic or therapeutic procedures are performed simultaneously. This noninvasive diagnostic intervention can be easily repeated to evaluate either equivocal initial results or clinical deterioration. A traditional or extended FAST may be obtained:
    - Traditional FAST:
        1. Pericardial sac (Fig. 109-1)
        2. Hepatorenal fossa or the right upper quadrant (RUQ) view to include diaphragm-liver interface and Morrison's pouch (liver–right kidney) interface (Fig. 109-2)
        3. Splenorenal fossa or the left upper quadrant (LUQ) view to include the diaphragm-spleen interface and spleen–left kidney interface (Fig. 109-3)
        4. Pelvic or suprapubic view (cul-de-sac of the peritoneum; a.k.a., pouch of Douglas) (Fig. 109-4)
    - Extended FAST (above views, plus the following):
        1. Right supradiaphragmatic or the right lung–diaphragm interface (Fig. 109-5)
        2. Left supradiaphragmatic or the left lung–diaphragm interface

        3. Right pleural slide or the right lung–pleural interface (Fig. 109-6)
        4. Left pleural slide or the left lung–pleural interface (see Fig. 109-6)
- Pertinent Anatomy
    - Solid organs of the abdominal cavity are the spleen, liver, kidneys, and uterus.
    - Hollow organs of the abdominal cavity are the stomach, small and large intestines, and urinary bladder.
- Basic ultrasound physics[4]: Ultrasound (US) involves utilizing a variety of sound frequencies above the 20,000-Hz range (which are above the human hearing range); the usual frequencies used in clinical care are between 2 and 10 MHz (1 MHz = 10,000 Hz). In general, lower-frequency probes provide greater depth penetration but less resolution, whereas higher-frequency probes lack the depth of penetration but give fine resolution of superficial structures. The 3.5-MHz probe is typically used for abdominal study, and the 7.5-MHz probe is used for detection of pneumothorax and evaluation of superficial vascular structures.[1,3,6]
- US waves are produced by electrically charging the piezoelectric crystals within the hand-held probe. The probe acts as both a transmitter of these waves (1%) and a receiver (99%) of waves reflected back from the tissues. As the US wave travels through tissues, it will lose power because of acoustic impedance imposed by the tissues. Different tissues have different acoustic impedance that results in a unique characteristic reflection (similar to an individual's reflection of light in a mirror) called an echo.
- Bone and gases are very dense. As such, US waves cannot permeate them, and they will be reflected. Therefore any structures that are below the bone or gas will not receive any US wave and therefore will not be seen. Fluids, soft tissues, and solid organs will transmit US waves and allow them to pass through.
- The reflected US waves are displayed on a screen as a two-dimensional image with varying echoic appearances. Bone and calcium-containing calculi appear as a white surface with an acoustic shadow beneath. Blood, urine, and water appear black, while solid organs appear in varying shades of gray.

AP This procedure should be performed only by physicians, advanced practice nurses, and other healthcare professionals (including critical care nurses) with additional knowledge, skills, and demonstrated competence per professional licensure or institutional standard.

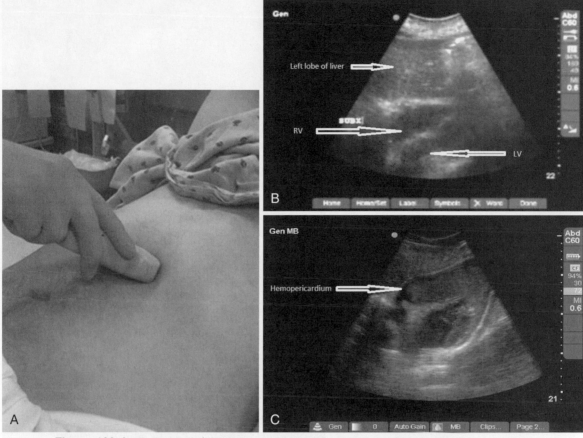

Figure 109-1 Pericardial view. **A,** The 3.5 MHz transducer is positioned below the operator's hand so that with gentle pressure, a satisfactory pericardial view can be obtained. The orientation indicator (on this particular probe, the orange area) is directed to the patient's right. **B,** The resulting pericardial four-chamber view from the subxiphoid orientation. **C,** Subxiphoid pericardial view of a patient after a stab wound to the precordium with evidence of hemopericardium. On dynamic evaluation of this ultrasound, the anterior black stripe seen on this static image resulted in compression of the right ventricular free wall, suggestive of early tamponade physiology. *(From the Temple University Hospital Department of Emergency Medicine Teaching Files.)*

- Tissues are described by their relative echo patterns.
  - *Anechoic* refers to the lack of an echo (e.g., simple fluid, blood). An anechoic finding appears black.
  - *Isoechoic* refers to adjacent tissues/organs with similar echo amplitudes (e.g., solid organs such as liver, spleen, and kidneys). Isoechoic structures appear gray.
  - *Hyperechoic* refers to higher amplitude echoes than adjacent tissues (e.g., diaphragm and liver or spleen). Hyperechoic structures appear white.
  - *Hypoechoic* refers to echoes of lower amplitude than surrounding tissues.
- The US identification of tissues is dependent on the difference in acoustic impedance at the organ interface. The greater the difference in impedance between adjacent structures, the better the US delineation of the structures will be.
- The rate of US wave transmission through a given tissue is constant; therefore the waves returning from the depths of penetration (far field) take longer to return to the probe than those returning from the near field. This understanding is needed to appropriately set up the US machine for optimal visualization.

- A negative FAST does not exclude the possibility of a significant intraabdominal injury producing small volumes of fluid. Although it is difficult to say with certainty, the minimal amount of blood required for US detection has been shown to be 100 mL;[5] however, others have shown in a prospective study done on adults that the average volume needed is 619 mL, with only 10% of the evaluators able to detect volumes less than 400 mL.[6]
- US machines: These machines vary from extremely portable devices about the size of a standard laptop computer to the large machines used in radiology departments. Regardless of the exact machine, there is a minimal amount of technological understanding of particular machines needed to obtain useful US images. The necessary terms to be familiar with are:
  - *Power:* Controls the strength of the US wave. Use the minimal power setting to obtain interpretable images. More power may create distortion and artifact.
  - *Gain:* Amplifies the echo signal returning to the probe. Increasing gain will make the image appear whiter.
  - *Time-gain compensation* (also called near-field, far-field time compensation): Used to compensate for the

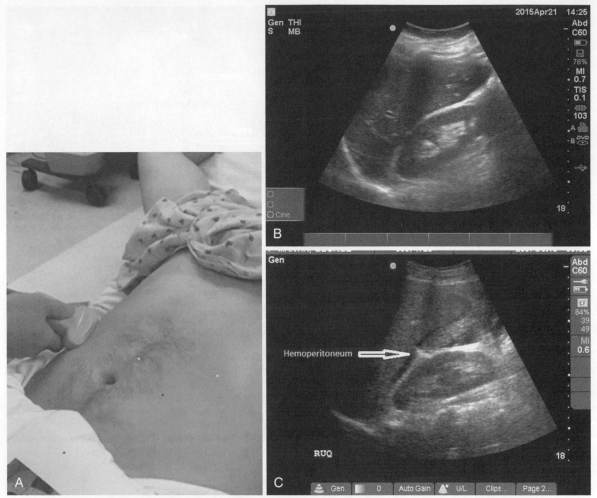

Figure 109-2 Right upper quadrant view. **A,** Note the orientation marker in this case is directed cephalad. If a vertical orientation of the transducer encounters rib artifact, the transducer can be angled diagonally to look between the rib spaces. This maneuver is particularly important to obtain the diaphragm-liver interface in individuals who have high-riding diaphragms. If the patient is able to cooperate, holding a deep breath can facilitate visualization of the diaphragm-liver interface. **B,** In this particular view, the bright interfaces between the diaphragm and liver, as well as the liver and right kidney, are well visualized. **C,** Hemoperitoneum is demonstrated in this image by the black stripe between the liver and kidney. Note that at the right side of the image is a complex fluid collection (just in front of the arrowhead) representing clot in Morison's pouch. *(From the Temple University Hospital Department of Emergency Medicine Teaching Files.)*

time delay from echoes at the depth of penetration. Generally the gain is increased in the far field relative to the near field. Adjustments may be required to create a consistent echogenicity of the organ or structures of interest.

❖ *Depth of penetration:* Should be set to visualize the entire structure of interest.

• Transducers: There are a variety of probe configurations available for clinical use. Most US machines allow rapid exchange of these probes to allow for differing clinical imaging requirements. In general, the following are commonplace probes:

❖ *Annular array:* This probe has a semicircular contact surface and creates a pie-shaped image. This probe configuration is common in the lower frequency probes used to do the abdominal and pericardial portions of the FAST.

❖ Linear array: The probe has a linear patient contact surface and produces a linear image. This arrangement is frequently found in the higher frequency probes used for superficial vascular imaging and is the probe of choice to do the extended portion of the FAST to evaluate potential pneumothorax.

❖ Phased array: This probe has a small profile that allows placement between the ribs to obtain a high-quality cardiac image; it creates a pie-shaped image. It is used primarily for the parasternal cardiac view.

• Regardless of the probe utilized, it is imperative to orient the probe properly. All probes have an indicator for this orientation. This indicator is oriented to the patient's right side when doing the pericardial and pelvic transverse views or toward the head when doing the RUQ, LUQ, pelvic sagittal, and the pleural evaluation for pneumothorax (PTX). When properly oriented, the indicator side of

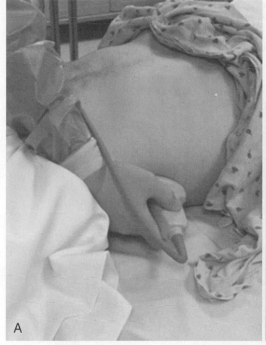
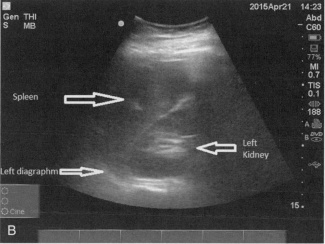

Figure 109-3 Left upper quadrant view. **A,** To obtain this view, the transducer is directed with the orientation marker cephalad (not seen in this image). Because of the posterior position of the spleen, the operator's knuckles frequently need to touch the examining table while directing the transducer slightly anteriorly to obtain the spleen–left kidney interface. As with the right upper quadrant view, a cooperating patient should be asked to take a deep breath and hold it to facilitate visualization of the diaphragm-spleen interface. In the event that rib shadowing occurs, the transducer can be positioned diagonally into the space between the ribs, directing the orientation marker cephalad and posterior. **B,** In this static image, only the most posterior aspect of the diaphragm-spleen interface is visualized. Dynamically, with a slight tilt of the transducer, the entirety of this interface can frequently be visualized. *(From the Temple University Hospital Department of Emergency Medicine Teaching Files.)*

the view will be shown on the left side of the monitoring screen. A trick that many physicians, advanced practice nurses, and other healthcare professionals use if the indicator is no longer recognizable is to apply gel to the probe and gently scratch one edge of the probe; this will create a disturbance of one edge of the image on the screen. The probe should be oriented to have this disturbance on the left side of the monitoring screen.

- FAST is safe in pregnancy and children because it produces no ionizing radiation.
- Indications:
  - *Blunt trauma:* FAST affords rapid bedside evaluation of potential torso cavitary hemorrhage and cardiac tamponade and assists in the clinical diagnosis of pneumothorax.
  - *Penetrating trauma:* Evaluation of the pericardial and upper abdominal views allows for identification of the appropriate body cavity before surgical exploration.
  - *Unexplained hypotension regardless of injury mechanism:* The portability and noninvasive nature of the FAST allows repeated assessments that may detect changes that occasionally occur in the dynamic natural history of traumatic injury. It is helpful when the same operator does repeat FAST examinations because the operator can best evaluate (or assess) any changes. This is especially true if pictures were not taken during previous FAST examinations.

- The FAST is extremely operator dependent and should be performed only by physicians, advanced practice nurses, or other healthcare professionals who have been adequately trained. Training requires an understanding of basic US physics and an understanding of the general operations of the US machine used. Most courses offered include didactic and hands-on experience. Additionally, demonstration of clinical proficiency (usually requiring proctored scans that are correlated with computed tomography [CT] or operative findings) has been debated over the years. In a prospective study, Shackford demonstrated the learning curve for the nonradiologist to detect hemoperitoneum at an acceptable error rate of less than 5% varies based on the prevalence of hemoperitoneum in the study population; if hemoperitoneum occurs in less than 30% of the population, 50 scans are needed, whereas if hemoperitoneum occurs in more than 20% of the population, 30 scans are needed to reach the acceptable error rate of less than 5%.[7]
- The abdominal and pericardial portions of the FAST are typically done with a low-frequency (3.5-MHz) transducer that allows the depth of penetration necessary to obtain the appropriate images.
- Higher-frequency transducers may be appropriate for children who are of average weight for their age and size or extremely thin adults. These probes are used to image superficial vascular structures and to do the pneumothorax

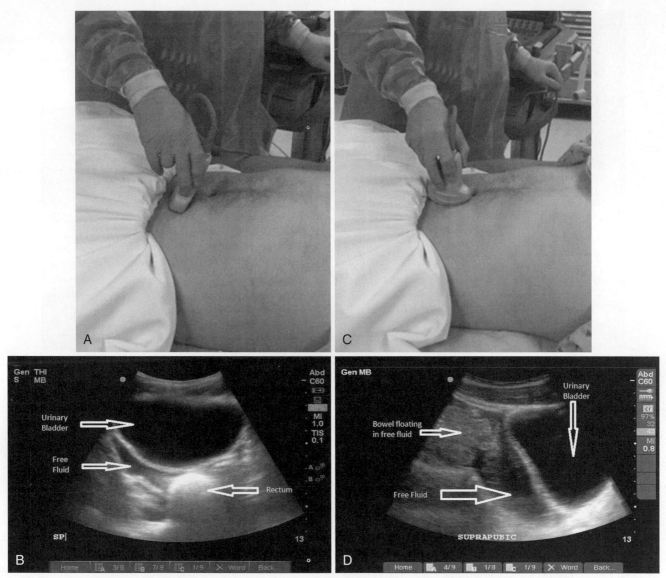

Figure 109-4   Pelvic view. **A,** This view can be obtained in a transverse orientation as depicted in this image; the orientation marker is directed to the patient's right. **B,** Free fluid in the transverse orientation is seen as having a "bowtie" appearance dorsal to (behind) the urinary bladder and anterior to the rectum. **C,** A sagittal image can be obtained by positioning the transducer vertically with the orientation marker directed cephalad. **D,** In this transverse image, free fluid is seen in the rectovesicular pouch of Douglas. The bowel is seen floating in free fluid, which is readily seen at the urinary bladder interface. *(From the Temple University Hospital Department of Emergency Medicine Teaching Files.)*

evaluation in the extended FAST. If the child is an older teenager or is heavy for his or her age, consider other probes.

- Obesity may make it difficult to interpret images; adjusting the gain and frequency (either on the machine or by changing the transducer) may improve the image quality. Lower-frequency transducers may be necessary for adequate penetration in patients who are obese.
- If there is an indication for a laparotomy or immediate surgery, there is no clinical indication for the FAST. However, a FAST may allow the surgeon to know which body cavity to explore initially (i.e., if there is minimal abdominal fluid but a hemopericardium, open the chest first to decompress the hemopericardium and fix the cardiac wound).[8]
- If emergency treatments and therapies are indicated, such as IV fluids, blood transfusions, intubation, pericardiocentesis, or needle decompression of the chest, they should not be delayed for the performance of a FAST. Ideally the FAST and interventions can be conducted simultaneously by multiple physicians, advanced practice nurses, or other health-care professionals.[8]
- Factors that can compromise the utility of US and the accuracy of the FAST are obesity (unable to penetrate for adequate imaging), presence of subcutaneous air (air blocks transmission of US waves), bowel gas, pelvic fractures, and previous abdominal operations (adhesions may not allow blood to pool in the usual dependent portions of the abdominal cavity).
- Clotted blood can generate various degrees of echogenicity and may be mistaken for normal surrounding soft tissue.
- The FAST is not as sensitive with smaller volumes of blood; serial examinations may be required. It will not

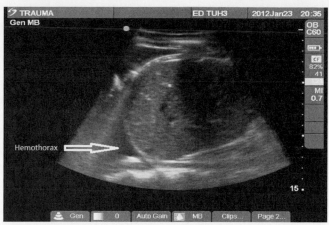

Figure 109-5 Supradiaphragmatic view of the right upper quadrant. This image clearly shows the bright reflectance from the right hemidiaphragm. Just above the diaphragm is a triangular-shaped black area, sometimes called a "sail sign," indicative of free fluid in the pleural space. In this instance a hemothorax was found. *(From the Temple University Hospital Department of Emergency Medicine Teaching Files.)*

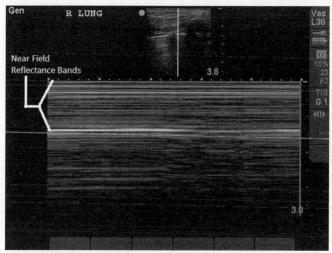

Figure 109-6 Normal M-mode image of the pleura. This evaluation requires a higher-resolution transducer, usually 7.5 to 10 MHz. This static image shows separation of the reflectance of the ultrasound beam off of the pleural surface over time, sometimes referred to as the "beach sign." The separation of these bands in the near field (top of ultrasound image) results from movement of the pleura with normal respiration. This M-mode appearance is seen in patients that have no pneumothorax. Separation of these reflectance bands is much easier to see in real time and is known as a "pleural slide." *(From the Temple University Hospital Department of Emergency Medicine Teaching Files.)*

identify retroperitoneal bleeding. The FAST will not allow for the grading of organ injuries but will show the physician, advanced practice nurse, or other healthcare professional only that fluid is present.

EQUIPMENT

- Ultrasound machine
- Transducer
- Water-based gel
- Gown
- Gloves
- Goggles

PATIENT AND FAMILY EDUCATION

- Explain why the FAST is needed to acquire an accurate diagnosis and to decrease the time to diagnosis. *Rationale:* Explanation may allay anxiety and elicit cooperation to facilitate the procedure.
- Explain that the FAST is noninvasive, performed at the bedside, and can be repeated as needed. *Rationale:* Explanation may allay anxiety.
- Outline the steps of the procedure and the patient's role during the FAST (e.g., positioning). *Rationale:* Patient cooperation may facilitate completion of the procedure.
- Describe the typical sensations experienced during a FAST (the application of cool gel and minor pressure, especially for the subxiphoid view). *Rationale:* Explanation may alleviate anxiety and promote patient cooperation

PATIENT ASSESSMENT AND PREPARATION

Patient Assessment

- Evaluate the patient for hemodynamic stability during the primary survey assessment.[8] *Rationale:* Hemodynamic instability may preclude use of FAST and other diagnostic testing because it may require immediate surgical intervention.
- Obtain baseline pain assessment. *Rationale:* Changes in level of pain during or after the procedure may be an indicator of complications.

Patient Preparation

- Verify that the patient is the correct patient using two identifiers. *Rationale:* Before performing a procedure, the nurse should ensure the correct identification of the patient for the intended intervention.
- Ensure that the patient and family understand preprocedural teaching. Answer questions as they arise, and reinforce information as needed. *Rationale:* Understanding of previously taught information is evaluated and reinforced.
- Obtain informed consent in the nonemergent situation. *Rationale:* This protects the rights of the patient.
- Perform a preprocedure verification and timeout, if nonemergent. *Rationale:* This ensures patient safety.
- The FAST should be performed before Foley catheter insertion to obtain a good pelvic view. *Rationale:* The urine in the bladder provides a way for the US waves to penetrate the depths of the peritoneal cavity surrounding the bladder.
- In those cases in which a Foley catheter has already been placed, if time allows and the patient is not critical, it should be clamped and sufficient time should be allowed for the bladder to fill. *Rationale:* The fuller the bladder, the more urine there is. A normal full bladder will be black in color and triangular in shape. This helps to distinguish it from other abdominal structures.

Procedure	FAST and Extended FAST	
Steps	**Rationale**	**Special Considerations**
1. **HH**		
2. **PE**		
3. Keep the patient as warm as possible using the following: A. Warming lights. B. Warmed IV fluids. C. Warm blankets.	Preservation of body heat; minimizes conductive and convection losses.	Patient needs to be kept warm when exposed for FAST. Keep bare skin area exposure to a minimum.
4. Assist the patient to the supine position with the arms slightly away from the lower torso.	This arm position allows the operator to position the probe at the lower chest to obtain the RUQ and LUQ views.	
5. Evaluate the patient in the supine position and then adjust the patient's position to the Trendelenburg or lateral decubitus position if there are no contraindications (i.e., spinal precautions).	The Trendelenburg position may be required to visualize free fluid during perihepatic and perisplenic examination.	Consider reverse Trendelenburg while evaluating for hemothorax or pelvic free fluid.
6. Place gel on the transducer.	A water-soluble gel between the transducer and the body is necessary to initiate transmission of the ultrasound waves into the body.	Gel is needed to eliminate any air between the surface of the probe and the body contact surface. Air between the probe and the contact surface will block transmission of the US wave, thus preventing visualization.
7. Begin with the cardiac view. A. The heart can be imaged using the subxiphoid or the parasternal view. B. Parasternal approach: the transducer-probe should be placed in the subxiphoid area and directed into the chest toward the left shoulder to view the diaphragm and heart. C. The view may be difficult to obtain if the patient has significant abdominal pain. D. You may need to press the probe into the abdomen and angle the probe so that it is nearly parallel to the sternum. E. You may need to place the palm of your hand over the top of the probe (the surface furthest away from the skin). F. The probe indicator is always to the patient's right side. G. This approach gives a long-axis four-chamber view of the heart (see Fig. 109-1).	Pericardial anechoic or hypoechoic stripes that are circumferential usually represent pericardial fluid. A focal anterior hypoechoic region may be normal pericardial fat. Fluid within the heart should be black. The subxiphoid long-axis is the best view to assess for pericardial effusions and allows the examiner to assess the size of the effusion and collapsibility of the free wall of the right ventricle.	This is particularly important in the unstable patient, especially for those with thoracoabdominal penetrating wounds. It will allow the operator to determine which body cavity requires exploration initially. When using the parasternal approach the curved array transducer or the phased array cardiac transducer can be used. The smaller footprint fits more easily between the ribs. Regardless of the probe used, the indicator is place to the patient's right in the 3rd or 4th intercostal space between the ribs. A focal posterior effusion, seen on the parasternal long axis view, may be a left pleural effusion rather than a pericardial effusion. The hypoechoic stripe of a pericardial effusion usually wraps around the apex of the heart. If the patient is experiencing significant abdominal pain or is obese, consider changing to a parasternal long-axis view.

Procedure **for FAST and Extended FAST—*Continued***

Steps	Rationale	Special Considerations
8. The second view is the RUQ, which is a sagittal view in the midaxillary line at approximately the 10th or 11th rib space (see Fig. 109-2).	Structures to visualize include the diaphragm, liver, and right kidney.	The RUQ is usually the easiest view to obtain due to the large acoustic windowing effect of the liver.
A. The probe is held with the palm upward under the probe.		Not all abdominal injuries produce free fluid.
B. To view Morrison's pouch, the transducer-probe should be placed in the RUQ or laterally along the thoracoabdominal junction.	The entire hepatorenal fossa (Morison's pouch) should be visualized.	Bowel injury and solid organ injury without significant bleeding will not be detected by US.
C. The placement uses the liver as an acoustic window and avoids interference from air-filled bowel.		US will not allow the grading of organ injuries.
D. The probe should be moved toward the inferior margin of the liver to obtain improved images of the right kidney.	Scanning is frequently needed to fully visualize the diaphragm, liver, and right kidney completely.	CT imaging can detect things that US cannot and can grade organ injuries.
		Remember to assess the hepatodiaphragmatic space; blood often accumulates here.
		A common pitfall is to scan only through the hepatorenal spaces.
9. The third view is a sagittal view of the LUQ in the midaxillary line at approximately the 8th or 9th rib space.	Structures to visualize include the diaphragm, spleen, and kidney.	Air artifacts from the stomach and colon, in addition to the smaller acoustic window, make this the most difficult view to obtain.
A. The probe is held with the palm upward under the probe.	The entire splenorenal fossa should be visualized.	It may be necessary to move the transducer posteriorly.
B. To adequately visualize the diaphragm, spleen, and left kidney, the operator's knuckles should be on the patient bed and the probe tilted anteriorly (see Fig. 109-3).	This view allows the spleen to be used as an acoustic window and avoids interference from air-filled bowel.	Free fluid is not always blood; consider ascites, fluid related to a ruptured ovarian cyst, ruptured bladder, or peritoneal dialysis.
C. The probe should then be moved superiorly (toward the thoracoabdominal junction) and inferiorly to assess for the presence of free fluid above the spleen and along the spleen tip.	Scanning is frequently needed to fully visualize the diaphragm, spleen, and left kidney completely.	Remember to assess the splenodiaphragmatic space; blood often accumulates here.
		A common pitfall is to scan only through the splenorenal space.
10. The fourth view is a suprapubic view (see Fig. 109-4).	This view is easier to obtain with a full bladder.	Optimally this should be obtained before placement of a Foley catheter. A distended bladder is helpful in seeing free pelvic fluid.
A. Obtain both a transverse and sagittal view.	It is utilized to view the bladder, lower abdomen, uterus, and pelvic area.	
B. The probe should be placed just above the symphysis and directed inferiorly into the pelvis.	Artifact may be introduced due to posterior enhancement.	Do not look too low; the seminal vesicles are in the retroperitoneum.

Procedure continues on following page

Procedure for FAST and Extended FAST—*Continued*

Steps	Rationale	Special Considerations
C. If areas of fluid disappear with side-to-side movement of the transducer, they are likely artifact.		
11. Extended FAST (see Fig. 109-6).	This technique is used to rule out PTX.	Lack of pleural sliding may indicate PTX, right mainstem intubation, or poor ventilation.
A. If an extended FAST examination is being performed, place a high-frequency linear probe (8–12 MHz) with the indicator toward the patient's head in a long-axis orientation.		Chest US can only detect a PTX that is directly under the probe; consider looking in several sites on the anterior chest.
B. Place the probe high on the patient's chest, just below the clavicles in the midclavicular line.		Comparing one side of the chest to the other is helpful but can be confusing if bilateral PTXs are present.
C. Look for the pleural line sitting at the back of the ribs.		Dimming the lights in the examination room may provide the examiner with an improved display of US findings.
D. The presence of sliding between the visceral and parietal pleura indicates the absence of a PTX in the area being scanned.		
E. The absence of sling implies the presence of a PTX.		
12. Clean the ultrasound gel off of the patient and cover the patient.	Keeps the patient's skin clean.	
13. Reposition the patient.	Promotes comfort.	
14. Remove **PE** and discard used supplies.		
15. **HH**		

Expected Outcomes

- If the patient is experiencing internal bleeding, the source of the bleeding will be determined.
- Rapid bedside detection of potentially life-threatening injuries
- Consider CT as a complementary test, especially when a FAST detects intracavitary fluid in a stable patient. CT can help determine the nature of the fluid and assess the integrity of the solid organs, as well as assess the retroperitoneal structures.

Unexpected Outcomes

- Bowel injury and solid organ injury without significant bleeding will not be detected by FAST
- Patient will continue to deteriorate despite FAST being interpreted correctly

Patient Monitoring and Care

Steps	Rationale	Reportable Conditions
		These conditions should be reported if they persist despite nursing interventions.
1. Monitor vital signs and the patient's electrocardiogram during and after the procedure. Follow institutional standards.	FAST is commonly performed if there is unexplained hypotension.	• Worsening hypotension • Dysrhythmias • Abnormal heart rate
2. Perform serial abdominal examinations as prescribed.	Changes in a patient's abdominal status may be detected before other changes (i.e., alterations in vital signs).	• Guarding • Decreased bowel sounds • Increased girth • Nausea and/or vomiting
3. Monitor pain level.	If the patient continues to have pain or their pain is increasing, it could be a sign of increased internal bleeding. Follow institutional standards for assessing pain. Identifies need for pain interventions.	• Continued pain despite pain interventions, if performed

Documentation

Documentation should include the following:
- Patient and family education
- The date and time the examination is performed
- Documentation of the FAST written report and select photos
- The results of the FAST
- Adequacy of technique to obtain interpretable images in all views

- Interpretation of the study as positive or negative for fluid (in the extended FAST the presence or absence of pneumothorax)
- Unexpected outcomes
- If the FAST is repeated, the above documentation should be undertaken for each procedure
- Pain assessment, interventions, and response to interventions

References and Additional Readings

For a complete list of references and additional readings for this procedure, scan this QR code with any freely available smartphone code reader app, or visit http://booksite.elsevier.com/9780323376624.

110 Gastric Lavage in Hemorrhage and Overdose

Ann Will Poteet

PURPOSE: When gastric hemorrhage is suspected, gastric lavage can be used for the initial assessment of upper gastrointestinal bleeding to potentially identify the severity of bleeding and clear the stomach of blood and clots. Gastric lavage may improve visualization of the gastric fundus in preparation for endoscopy or endoscopic treatments. In overdose, gastric lavage may be used to evacuate drugs or toxins within 1 hour of ingestion, potentially minimizing the consequences of systemic absorption of drugs or toxins.

PREREQUISITE NURSING KNOWLEDGE

- Gastric lavage is not recommended as a routine procedure in the management of hemorrhage and overdose. Current evidence shows limited improvement in patient outcomes after lavage, and the procedure may contribute to additional complications, including gastric or esophageal perforation, aspiration, laryngospasm, dysrhythmias, hypothermia, fluid and electrolyte abnormalities, pain, and hypoxia.[3,6,8,10–13] The risk-benefit ratio of gastric lavage should be considered before the procedure is performed.
- The use of gastric lavage has been found to be of potential benefit in some cases of hemorrhage and overdose. Specific indications for the use of gastric lavage include:
  - ❖ Gastrointestinal (GI) hemorrhage: The patient who has had GI hemorrhage may present with signs and symptoms of volume loss and a decrease in oxygen-carrying capacity. These symptoms include tachypnea, tachycardia, hypotension, orthostatic changes, decreased hemodynamic filling pressures, decreased urine output, pallor, cold and clammy skin, confusion, anxiety, and somnolence. The patient may also show signs of hematemesis, maroon or tarry stools, or hematochezia. Gastric lavage in GI hemorrhage may be helpful in clearing the stomach of blood and clots to facilitate evaluation of the source of bleeding and to improve visualization of the gastric fundus in preparation for endoscopic treatment.[8] The presence of bright red blood in the aspirate could be an indicator for the need for urgent endoscopy.[8,10] Bloody aspirate might also be predictive of higher risk gastric lesions when the patient is hemodynamically stable and has no hematemesis, while clear aspirate might indicate a lower risk lesion.[3,10] In cases of nonvariceal upper gastrointestinal bleeding, placement of a nasogastric tube can be considered for prognostic purposes.[5]
  - ❖ Overdose: The American Academy of Clinical Toxicology and European Association of Poisons Centers and Clinical Toxicologists do not recommend the use of gastric lavage in the routine management of poisoned patients because of the limited evidence of improved patient outcomes and potential risks of the procedure.[6] Supportive care should be considered as the primary treatment before initiating the use of gastric lavage.[2,6] If gastric lavage is utilized for decontamination, it should be performed by individuals specifically trained and skilled in gastric lavage.[6] Lavage may be initiated in symptomatic patients within 1 hour (60 minutes) of ingestion of a potentially life-threatening amount of a highly toxic substance if the substance slows GI motility, if the substance is a sustained-release medication, or in cases where an individual is hypothermic with slowed GI motility.[1,2,9] Gastric lavage is contraindicated in the use of overdose if the patient has consumed strong corrosives or hydrocarbons (e.g., gasoline, strong acids, or alkali) and if the pills or pill fragments are known to be larger than the opening of the orogastric (OG) tube.[9] The administration of activated charcoal (AC) has been used in combination with gastric lavage for specific toxins; however, its use must be approached cautiously because the combination of therapies may result in an increased risk for aspiration. It should be noted that the endpoint of gastric lavage is not clearly defined if particulate cannot be clearly observed; however, the amount of lavage fluid instilled should approximate the amount of fluid returned. Gastric lavage after overdose or toxin ingestion has variable efficacy. The amount of toxin or drug recovered depends on variables such as time from ingestion, whether liquid or pills were ingested, specific agent ingested, and size of lavage tube used. Even if lavage is performed close to the time of ingestion, not all the ingested toxin will be recovered and treatment related to effects of the overdose will still be necessary.[9]
- Nonintubated patients who need gastric lavage must be alert and have adequate pharyngeal and laryngeal reflexes. If the patient has a limited gag reflex or is unable to protect

the airway, the patient should be intubated before gastric lavage is performed.[6,9] All patients undergoing gastric lavage should be positioned in the left lateral decubitus position to assist with passage of the gastric tube.[9]

- Passage of the lavage tube may cause vagal stimulation and precipitate bradydysrhythmias.
- Patients with esophageal varices, coagulopathy, a recent history of upper GI tract surgery, craniofacial abnormalities, head trauma, or an underlying pathology should be carefully evaluated for the risk-benefit ratio before gastric lavage is performed.[6,9]

EQUIPMENT

- Nonsterile gloves
- Eye and face protection
- Barrier gowns and underpads
- Large bore (36–40 Fr for adults) nasogastric or orogastric tube[9]
- 60-mL irrigating syringe
- Water-soluble lubricant
- Lavage fluid (warm normal saline solution or tap water)
- Measurable container for lavage fluid
- Disposable basin or suction canister for aspirate
- Suction source and connecting tubing
- Rigid pharyngeal suction-tip (Yankauer) catheter
- Endotracheal suction equipment
- Tape for securing nasogastric (NG) or OG tube
- Stethoscope
- Cardiac monitor
- Pulse oximeter
- Automatic blood pressure cuff

Additional equipment, to have available as needed, includes the following:
- Specimen container for aspirate (for overdose)
- Absorptive agent for instillation (for overdose, if prescribed)
- Emergency intubation and cardiac equipment
- Bite block or oral airway (if patient needs intubation for procedure)
- Emergency medications (e.g., atropine)

PATIENT AND FAMILY EDUCATION

- Explain the indications and procedure for gastric lavage. *Rationale:* Patient and family anxiety may be decreased.
- Evaluate the patient and family understanding of the risks and benefits of gastric lavage. *Rationale:* The patient and family may be unaware of the risks and benefits of the procedure.
- Explain the patient's role in assisting with passage of the tube and lavage of the stomach. *Rationale:* The patient's cooperation during the procedure is elicited.
- Explain the purpose of the cardiac monitor, automatic blood pressure cuff, and pulse oximeter. *Rationale:* Patient and family anxiety may be decreased.
- Assess the need for family presence during the procedure. *Rationale:* Patient and family anxiety may be decreased and patient cooperation during the procedure could potentially be improved.

- Evaluate patient and family need for information on prevention of accidental ingestion of drugs or toxic agents. *Rationale:* The patient and family may be unaware or uninformed that the agent or drug is potentially toxic.
- Evaluate patient and family need for information on emergency treatment for accidental ingestion of drug or toxic agents. *Rationale:* Emergency first aid measures may be helpful with some ingestions to decrease potential toxicity or systemic absorption.
- Evaluate patient and family need for information regarding monitoring and restrictions postprocedure, including dietary restrictions, and assessment for aspiration and other complications. *Rationale:* The patient and family may be unaware or uninformed about what to expect postprocedure.

PATIENT ASSESSMENT AND PREPARATION
Patient Assessment

- Perform baseline cardiovascular and neurological assessments and assess hemodynamic status, cardiac rhythm, and vital signs. *Rationale:* Passage of the lavage tube may cause heart rate or blood pressure changes or vagal stimulation, which can precipitate bradydysrhythmias or other electrocardiographic (ECG) changes, including ST elevation. In the overdose case, toxic levels of certain classes of drugs can also cause ECG changes.
- Perform baseline respiratory assessment and pulse oximetry. *Rationale:* Gastric lavage has been shown to cause changes in oxygen saturation, leading to hypoxia. Patients who are unable to protect the airway should be intubated before gastric lavage.
- Signs and symptoms of major blood loss are as follows. *Rationale:* Esophageal or gastric varices can cause significant blood loss. The clinical presentation is dependent on amount of blood lost.
  - Tachycardia
  - Tachypnea
  - Decreased urine output
  - Hypotension
  - Decreased hemodynamic filling pressures
  - Pallor, cold and clammy skin
  - Changes in mental status or somnolence
  - Hematemesis
  - Maroon or tarry stools
  - Hematochezia
- Evaluate the patient for a history of esophageal varices, recent GI surgery, coagulopathy, or underlying pathology. *Rationale:* Varices, recent surgery, coagulopathies, or other contraindications may predispose the patient to complications during lavage tube insertion.
- Obtain baseline coagulation studies as prescribed and assess hematocrit and hemoglobin values, basic metabolic panel, renal and liver function tests, and blood type. *Rationale:* Baseline information is provided so that treatment can be determined and progress can be more accurately monitored.
- Obtain as prescribed and assess serum toxicology screen, urinalysis, urine toxicology screen, and anion gap

(overdose case) are other laboratory tests that also may be monitored. *Rationale:* Baseline information for diagnosis is provided so that interventions can be made appropriately and patient progress can be more accurately monitored.

- Obtain as prescribed and assess arterial blood gas (ABG) values. *Rationale:* Overdose victims with hypoventilation and patients with GI hemorrhage with significant blood loss or comorbid disease are at risk for hypoxia, hypercapnea, and acid-base disorders.

- Assess the adequacy of the patient's gag reflex. *Rationale:* Lack of an adequate gag reflex indicates the need for endotracheal intubation before lavage begins.[6,9]

- Assess the type of drugs or toxic substances ingested, quantity ingested, and time since ingestion. Use of common toxidromes (classifications of the signs and symptoms that develop with poisoning) can help to identify unknown ingested substances (for the overdose case). *Rationale:* Certain substances may require neutralization before tube evacuation is attempted. A poison control center should be contacted if the practitioner is unsure that lavage is indicated. Side effects can be anticipated if the drugs or toxins that were swallowed and the quantity are known.

- Perform careful skin assessment (overdose case). *Rationale:* Assessment may give evidence regarding toxin ingested because various drugs can cause cutaneous changes. Changes to look for include diaphoresis, bullae, acneiform rash, flushed appearance, and cyanosis.

- Assess any odors present (overdose case). *Rationale:* Some toxins have a distinctive odor, which can aid in identification of substance ingested.

- As prescribed perform and assess a 12-lead ECG and continuous cardiac monitoring. *Rationale:* In an overdose case, the drug or toxin ingested may be cardiotoxic. For the patient with a GI hemorrhage, comorbid disease states may increase risk for tissue hypoxia and ischemia.

Patient Preparation

- Ensure that the patient understands preprocedural information. Answer questions as they arise and reinforce information as needed. *Rationale:* Understanding of previously taught information is evaluated and reinforced.

- Place the patient on a cardiac monitor, automatic blood pressure cuff, and pulse oximeter. *Rationale:* Allows for close cardiovascular and respiratory system monitoring during the procedure.

- Set up oropharyngeal suction. *Rationale:* Ensures suction is available for the procedure.

- Establish and maintain intravenous (IV) access. For the patient with GI hemorrhage, place a minimum of two large-bore IVs or provide central venous access. *Rationale:* IV access is necessary for emergency IV medication administration and volume resuscitation in the case of GI hemorrhage.[8]

- If not contraindicated, position the patient in the left lateral decubitus position.[9] *Rationale:* This position facilitates passage of the tube into the stomach. The left lateral position is the position of choice to prevent aspiration if the patient should vomit.

- Apply oxygen via nasal prongs or mask as needed. Continue to evaluate the patient for possible need of airway intubation. *Rationale:* Supplemental oxygen may optimize the patient's oxygen saturation.

Procedure	**for Gastric Lavage in Hemorrhage and Overdose**	
Steps	**Rationale**	**Special Considerations**
1. ▨HH		
2. ▨PE		
3. Coat the distal end of the lavage tube with water-soluble lubricant.	Minimizes mucosal injury and irritation during insertion of the tube.	
4. Position the patient (if not contraindicated): A. Assist the patient to the left lateral decubitus position. B. Elevate the head of the bed 10–20 degrees or elevate the bed using a slight (10–20 degree) reverse Trendelenburg's position.	The left lateral decubitus position maximizes access to the stomach and minimizes pyloric emptying. The elevation of the head of the bed or the slight reverse Trendelenburg's position also decreases movement of stomach contents into the duodenum and possibly helps minimize risk of aspiration during procedure.	Ensure adequate ventilation and oxygenation while the patient is positioned for gastric lavage.
5. Prepare suction, lavage fluids, tape, and emergency equipment.	Preprocedure setup facilitates smooth technique, minimizes complications, and prepares for emergency situations.	If the patient does not have an intact gag reflex, endotracheal intubation should be done before the procedure.[6,9]

Procedure	for Gastric Lavage in Hemorrhage and Overdose—*Continued*	
Steps	**Rationale**	**Special Considerations**
6. Insert a large OG or NG tube (36–40 Fr) for adults.[9]	A large-bore OG or NG tube is preferred for the evacuation of blood, clots, undigested pills, or pill fragments. A smaller bore tube may become occluded with solid material.[9]	For overdose situations, an OG or NG tube should be placed that is large enough to capture the pill particulate.[9] A smaller bore nasogastric tube may be used if only known liquid poisons were ingested. Do not cut the end of the tube to create a larger opening because rough edges on the tube can injure the mucosal lining of the GI tract.[9]
A. Measure the distance from the bridge of the patient's nose to the ear (see Fig. 9-2A) and then from the earlobe to the tip of the xiphoid process (Fig. 110-1). Mark this distance on the tube.		
B. Insert an oral airway (see Procedure 9) or bite block if necessary.		Remove patient dentures.
C. Position the tube toward the posterior pharynx over the tongue.	Prevents patient from biting on the lavage tube or harming the practitioner during insertion of the lavage tube.	
D. Pass the tube slowly into the stomach, encouraging the patient to attempt to swallow as the tube is advanced. Continue to advance the tube until the mark previously placed on the tube is reached.	Rapid passage of the tube may lead to perforation or stimulate vomiting, leading to an increased risk of aspiration.	Asking the patient to flex the head forward may facilitate advancement of the tube. Heart rate may decrease as a result of vagal stimulation. Have emergency medication (e.g., atropine) ready for use as necessary. Have oropharyngeal suction available.

Procedure continues on following page

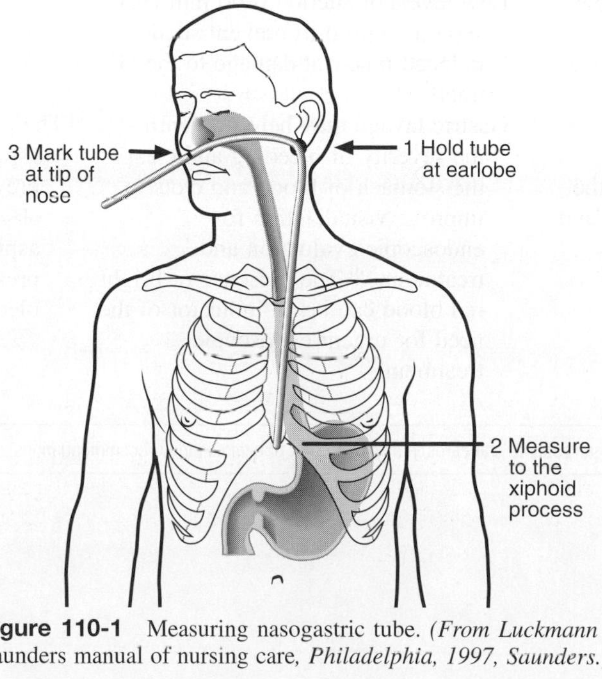

Figure 110-1   Measuring nasogastric tube. (*From Luckmann J, Saunders manual of nursing care, Philadelphia, 1997, Saunders.*)

Procedure for Gastric Lavage in Hemorrhage and Overdose—*Continued*

Steps	Rationale	Special Considerations
7. Utilize a variety of bedside practices to assess tube location during the insertion procedure, including: A. Aspirating with a 60-mL syringe for return of stomach contents.[4] B. Obtain radiographic confirmation of placement.[4] **(Level D*)**	The position of the lavage tube must be confirmed to be in the stomach because of the risk for endotracheal placement of the lavage tube and subsequent pulmonary complications. Radiographic confirmation of lavage tube placement is currently the only definitive way to confirm tube placement.[4]	If not contraindicated, ask the patient to phonate to ensure that the tube has not been placed improperly in the trachea. Be aware that auscultating an air bolus in the stomach is an unreliable method of placement confirmation.[4]
8. After placement is confirmed, secure the tube with tape, and aspirate gastric contents through the lavage tube with a 60-mL syringe.	Manual aspiration withdraws gastric contents and toxic agents or blood and clots out of the stomach.	In cases of overdose, save the aspirate in a specimen container and send to the laboratory for analysis as prescribed.
9. Perform intermittent lavage (with either room-temperature normal saline solution or tap water).[9]	In overdose cases, lavage might aid in removing toxic substances from the stomach before absorption. In GI hemorrhage, lavage might aid in clearing the stomach of blood and clots to help identify the severity of bleeding and improve visualization of the gastric fundus in preparation for endoscopic evaluation or treatment.	
A. Slowly instill lavage fluid into the lavage tube with a 60-mL irrigating syringe (for adults, use 200–300 mL of fluid).[9]	Small amounts of lavage fluid are used to limit fluid from entering the duodenum during lavage.	Lavage fluid should be slightly warmed or at room temperature to prevent hypothermia in the elderly or individuals receiving large amounts of lavage fluids.
B. Aspirate gastric contents through the lavage tube with an irrigating syringe. *or*	Evacuates stomach contents, blood, clots, or ingested toxic agents.	The amount of lavage fluid returned should approximate the amount instilled.
C. Connect lavage tube to low intermittent suction.	Low levels of suction (<60 mm Hg) should be used to prevent suction-induced mucosal damage to the GI tract.	
D. For patients with GI hemorrhage, continue intermittent lavage until the aspirate is clear of blood and clots.[8]	Gastric lavage may help to identify the severity of bleeding and clear the stomach of blood and clots to improve visualization for endoscopic evaluation and treatment.[8,10] The presence of bright red blood can be an indicator of the need for urgent endoscopic treatment.[8,10]	The presence of coffee ground aspirate may indicate a resolving or previous GI bleed. Note that the absence of blood or coffee ground aspirate does not rule out the presence of current or past bleeding.[8]

*Level D: Peer-reviewed professional and organizational standards with the support of clinical study recommendations.

Procedure	**for Gastric Lavage in Hemorrhage and Overdose—*Continued***	
Steps	**Rationale**	**Special Considerations**
E. In the overdose case, continue intermittent lavage until the aspirate is clear of the toxic substance or particulate matter. Once lavage is complete, activated charcoal can be instilled through the tube if indicated.	Gastric lavage may help to remove life-threatening levels of ingested toxic substances from symptomatic patients if performed within 1 hour of ingestion.[2,9] Activated charcoal is used for absorption of the residual substance ingested (unable to be removed with lavage). If the patient is alert and has an intact gag reflex, activated charcoal can be swallowed.	Note that the endpoint of gastric lavage is not clearly defined if particulate cannot be clearly observed and that the lack of poor lavage return does not rule out significant ingestion of the toxic substance.
10. Remove the OG or NG tube.	The OG or NG tube should be for single use only.	
Remove the tape holding the OG or NG tube in place.	Prepares for removal.	If the lavage tube does not remove easily, discontinue removal and evaluate for causes of obstruction.
Pull the OG or NG tube out slowly and steadily.	Minimizes risk for vomiting or complications.	
11. Remove **PE** and dispose of equipment in appropriate receptacle.	Reduces transmission of microorganisms; Standard Precautions.	
12. **HH**		

Expected Outcomes

- Evacuation of blood and clots from the stomach
- Prevention of blood aspiration
- Improved visualization of the gastric fundus for endoscopy
- Identification of the severity of GI hemorrhage
- Prevention or minimization of systemic complications from the absorption of drugs or toxic agents
- Minimization of mucosal damage by toxic agents

Unexpected Outcomes

- Endotracheal intubation rather than gastric intubation with lavage tube
- Esophageal or gastric perforation
- Trauma to the nose, throat, or esophagus
- Epistaxis if NG route is used for lavage
- Hypothermia in the elderly patient
- Bradydysrhythmias or ECG changes
- Vomiting
- Pulmonary aspiration of gastric contents, with risk for aspiration pneumonia
- Movement of gastric contents into the duodenum, potentially increasing the amount of toxin absorbed
- Fluid and electrolyte imbalance
- Laryngospasm
- Hypoxia or hypercapnia
- Intubation as a result of hypoxia, aspiration, or other respiratory compromise
- Prolonged absence of the gag reflex

Procedure continues on following page

Patient Monitoring and Care

Steps	Rationale	Reportable Conditions
		These conditions should be reported if they persist despite nursing interventions.
1. Monitor vital signs every 15 minutes throughout the procedure and every hour after lavage for at least 4 hours or longer, depending on patient condition.	Continued blood loss or side effects of drugs or toxins ingested may cause changes in vital signs. Cold lavage fluid may cause hypothermia in the elderly patient. Complications from the procedure may not present during or immediately after the procedure.	• Increase in heart rate 10–20 beats or more above baseline • Decrease in systolic blood pressure 20–30 mm Hg or more below baseline • Respiratory rate <8 or >24 breaths per minute or rate changes >20% of baseline normal • Temperature <97.5°F (36.5°C) or >101°F (38°C)
2. Monitor the neurological status continuously throughout the procedure and after lavage.	Side effects from toxic agents ingested or significant blood loss may lead to a decrease in level of consciousness.	• Decreasing level of consciousness • Loss of gag reflex
3. Monitor respiratory status continuously throughout the procedure and after lavage.	Determines pulmonary complications.	• Decrease in oximetry below baseline or 92% • Increase in respiratory rate above baseline • Symptoms of shortness of breath • Increasing oxygen requirements
4. Monitor cardiac status continuously throughout the procedure and after the lavage.	Bradydysrhythmias may be caused by passage of the lavage tube or an increase in heart rate may indicate continued blood loss. Toxic effect of drugs ingested may also cause ECG changes, including prolongation of the PR, QRS, and QT intervals.	• Heart rate <60 beats per minute or >100 beats per minute with or without a decrease in blood pressure below baseline • Chest pain, diaphoresis, change in level of consciousness, and shortness of breath • Change in ECG rhythm or length of PR, QRS, and QT intervals from baseline
5. Assess for normal pharyngeal function and laryngospasm. After lavage, keep the patient in the left lateral position with slight head elevation until normal gag reflex returns.	The left lateral position is the position of choice to prevent aspiration should the patient not be able to control secretions or emesis.	• Prolonged absence of gag reflex
6. For the patient with GI hemorrhage:		• Bright red emesis or bleeding from the OG or NG tube • Decrease in hemoglobin or hematocrit below baseline • Decrease in systolic blood pressure 20–30 mm Hg or more below baseline • Increase in pulse 10–20 beats per minute or more above baseline • Urine output <0.5–1 mL/kg/hr • Increasing confusion or decreasing level of consciousness • Continued bleeding • Changes in pulmonary status
A. Measure blood volume loss.	Aids in assessment of fluid balance and volume resuscitation requirements.	

Patient Monitoring and Care —*Continued*

Steps	Rationale	Reportable Conditions
B. Monitor for recurrence of bleeding, color, and consistency of gastric drainage, serial hemoglobin and hematocrit, postural vital signs, urine output, and change in level of consciousness.	Bleeding may recur despite interventions.	
C. Administer crystalloid IV fluids as prescribed for volume resuscitation. Switch to the administration of packed red blood cells and fresh frozen plasma (FFP) or platelets when available for volume replacement and reversal of coagulopathies.	Replaces volume, prevents hemorrhagic shock, and improves oxygen-carrying capacity. Goal hemoglobin level should be 8 g/dL.[7]	
D. Administer proton pump inhibitors (PPIs) as prescribed. Initiation of a PPI should not occur before endoscopic evaluation.[5]	PPIs inhibit the proton pump in the parietal cells of the stomach, suppressing gastric acid secretion.	
E. Prepare for possible administration of intravenous erythromycin (250 mg) before endoscopy as prescribed when a diagnosis of GI hemorrhage is suspected.[11]	Administration of erythromycin may help to accelerate gastric emptying and might decrease the need for repeat endoscopy.[11,12]	
F. Prepare the patient for possible endoscopy.	Endoscopic evaluation is the gold standard in the diagnosis and treatment of GI hemorrhage and should occur within 24 hours of initial presentation.[5,11]	
7. For the patient with drug overdose:		• Patient reporting intent to harm self • Patient reporting that ingestion was a suicide attempt • Deviation of test results outside normal limits
A. Evaluate the patient's need for follow-up psychiatric support for suicide ideation.	The drug or toxin ingestion may be a result of suicidal ideations.	
B. Institute suicide precautions until the patient has been cleared by psychiatric services. Precautions include removal of objects from the patient's room that could be used by the patient to inflict self-harm.		
C. In the hours and days after ingestion, repeat laboratory tests, including electrolytes, glucose, blood urea nitrogen and creatinine, liver function, and drug or toxin levels.	Laboratory tests ordered depend on the drug or toxins ingested. Lavage may cause electrolyte abnormalities. Liver function tests may be necessary if the drug is toxic to the liver. Drug or toxin level tests validate the clearance of the drug or toxin from the patient's system.	

Procedure continues on following page

Documentation

Documentation should include the following:
- Patient and family education
- History of ingestion of drug or toxin or upper GI bleeding
- Date, time, and reason for lavage
- Type and size of lavage tube inserted
- Patient tolerance of tube placement and lavage procedure
- Verification of lavage tube placement (method used)
- Type and amount of lavage fluid used
- Unexpected outcomes
- Nursing interventions

- Amount and characteristics of aspirate
- Assessment of gastric drainage after lavage
- Name and dosage of medications given after the lavage
- Aspirated specimen sent to laboratory for analysis
- Referral to psychiatry if potential for suicide is suspected
- Occurrence of rebleed in the patient with GI hemorrhage
- Blood products given during volume resuscitation

References and Additional Readings

For a complete list of references and additional readings for this procedure, scan this QR code with any freely available smartphone code reader app, or visit http://booksite.elsevier.com/9780323376624.

111 Endoscopic Therapy

Eleanor Fitzpatrick

PURPOSE: Endoscopic therapy is performed to control or prevent bleeding from esophageal or gastric varices, gastric or duodenal ulcer sites, or other selected causes of upper gastrointestinal bleeding.

PREREQUISITE NURSING KNOWLEDGE

- Upper gastrointestinal (GI) hemorrhage is a relatively common, potentially life-threatening emergency that requires rapid assessment and resuscitation.[18,23]
- Esophagogastroduodenoscopy is the diagnostic and therapeutic modality for nonvariceal and variceal upper GI bleeding.[19,20] Endoscopic therapy reduces the occurrence of rebleeding, blood-transfusion requirements, and the need for surgery.[12,18,23]
- Endoscopic therapies are often interventions of choice for upper and lower GI bleeding lesions. Upper endoscopic therapies include injection therapy, ablative therapy, such as heater probe, and mechanical therapy, such as endoclips or endoscopic banding.[11,23]
- For all upper endoscopic interventions, a fiberoptic endoscope is passed through the esophagus and into the stomach and duodenum to identify the source of bleeding. The nurse (or other clinician) assisting the endoscopist typically prepares all of the equipment potentially needed during the procedure. Once the site of bleeding is located, any of the endoscopic techniques identified previously may be used.
- Endoscopic variceal ligation (EVL) is the preferred endoscopic method for control of acute esophageal bleeding and for prevention of rebleeding, unless excess bleeding prevents effective band placement and ligation.[10,15,16,22] Endoscopic sclerotherapy (EST), which involves injection of a sclerosant into or adjacent to a varix, may be used. EST has largely been replaced by the use of EVL, which is a type of mechanical therapy.[15,16,22]
- For gastric varices, a promising intervention is gastric variceal occlusion with tissue adhesives such as N-butyl-cyanoacrylate.[9,15,17] Varied new hemostatic agents, including powders and sprays, which can be delivered via the endoscope have also been developed and promote clotting in the setting of gastrointestinal hemorrhage. Studies are ongoing, but tissue adhesives are not yet approved for this indication in the United States.[5,9]
- Injection therapy is used for hemostasis for bleeding from peptic ulcer disease, Mallory-Weiss tears, other lesions, and postprocedure-related bleeding.[1,20] Epinephrine is the injection agent of choice for these conditions in the United States. Injection therapy alone is not recommended. Additional modalities such as thermal coagulation or endo-

scopic clipping should be employed to achieve or enhance thrombosis.[1,13,20]
- The several proposed mechanisms of action of the various sclerosing agents include vasoconstriction, esophageal or vascular smooth muscle spasm, compression of the bleeding vessel by submucosal edema or by the volume of sclerosing agent used (tamponade effect), and actual coagulation of the vessel. Ultimately, vessel thrombosis occurs.[1,20]
- A variety of sclerosing agents are available (Table 111-1). The physician who performs the endoscopy prescribes the agents to be used during the procedure.
- Endoscopic therapy can combine a number of interventions to promote hemostasis, including esophageal band ligation, endoscopic clipping, injection therapy, laser therapy, and thermal coagulation.[1,2,7,22]
- Ablative therapies, such as the use of a heater probe or bipolar electrocoagulation, are other endoscopic techniques for the management of bleeding from peptic ulcer disease and other nonvariceal causes of upper GI bleeding. These therapies are effective as they result in coagulation of a bleeding vessel.[1,7,13]
- The United States Food and Drug Administration (FDA) has approved a new device for endoscopic clipping. The over-the-scope clip has been approved for achieving hemostasis in the upper and lower gastrointestinal tract and for closure of some luminal perforations. This technique appears to be especially effective after failure of other hemostatic techniques for nonvariceal bleeding episodes.[5]
- Passage of the large-bore therapeutic endoscope may stimulate the vagal response in the patient and precipitate bradydysrhythmias.[19]
- As a result of the sedation and topical anesthetic used, the patient's gag reflex may be diminished or absent, putting the patient at risk for aspiration.[3]
- Moderate sedation is recommended for use during endoscopic procedures. Sedation may increase the risk of respiratory depression, thus appropriate monitoring and emergency equipment should be readily available.

EQUIPMENT

- Therapeutic large-caliber endoscope (rigid or flexible; however, the flexible scope is the usual type used for upper endoscopy)

TABLE 111-1	Sclerosing Agents	
Sclerosants Used for Bleeding Varices	**Sclerosants Used for Other Causes of Upper GI Bleeding**
Sodium morrhuate (5%)	Epinephrine (1 : 10,000–1 : 20,000)
Ethanolamine oleate (5%)	Ethyl alcohol (volumes >1–2 mL can lead to tissue damage)
Sodium tetradecyl sulfate	Thrombin
Ethanolamine acetate	Polidocanol
Polidocanol (0.5–1%)	Sodium tetradecyl sulfate
Ethanol (can cause ulceration)	

From American Society of Gastrointestinal Endoscopy (ASGE): The role of endoscopy in the management of variceal hemorrhage. Gastrointest Endosc 80(2): 221-227, 2014; Bethea ED, Travis AC, Saltzman JR: Initial assessment and management of patients with nonvariceal upper gastrointestinal bleeding. J Clin Gastroenterol 48(10):823-829, 2014.

- Endoscopic injector needle (23- to 26-gauge, 2- to 5-mm needle; as ordered by physician)
- Three 10-mL syringes filled with sclerosing agent, as prescribed by physician
- Additional therapeutic equipment should be available for management of nonvariceal upper GI bleeding (i.e., laser or thermal equipment, endoloops, or endoclips)
- Esophageal bands should be available for management of known or suspected variceal upper GI bleeding
- Suction setup with connecting tubing
- Rigid pharyngeal suction-tip (Yankauer) catheter
- Safety goggles for each healthcare provider and the patient
- Nonsterile gloves
- Barrier gowns
- Nonsterile 4-inch gauze or washcloth
- Water-soluble lubricant
- Topical anesthesia
- Premedications (as prescribed by physician or advanced practitioner)
- Two 30- to 60-mL syringes
- Normal saline solution or tap water for irrigation
- Oral airway or bite block
- Cardiac monitor
- Pulse oximeter
- End-tidal carbon dioxide monitor
- Automatic blood pressure cuff
- Emergency intubation and resuscitation equipment

Additional equipment, to have available as needed, includes the following:

- Nasogastric (NG) tube, Minnesota tube, or Sengstaken-Blakemore tube for esophagogastric tamponade (see Procedure 108)
- Emergency equipment (e.g., intubation)

PATIENT AND FAMILY EDUCATION

- Explain the procedure and indication for endoscopic therapy and the patient's role in the procedure. *Rationale:* Patient and family anxiety may be decreased.
- Explain that sedation will be provided for comfort and ease in passing the endoscope. *Rationale:* Patient and family anxiety may be decreased.
- Explain that the patient will be monitored closely during and after the procedure. *Rationale:* Patient and family anxiety may be decreased.

PATIENT ASSESSMENT AND PREPARATION

Patient Assessment

- Assess for a history of upper GI bleeding, the source of current bleeding, and baseline hematocrit and hemoglobin levels. *Rationale:* This information provides an assessment of risk for bleeding or continued bleeding after endoscopic therapy.
- Assess baseline cardiac rhythm. *Rationale:* Passage of a large-bore tube may cause vagal stimulation and bradydysrhythmias.
- Obtain baseline coagulation study results (i.e., prothrombin time, partial thromboplastin time, platelet count). *Rationale:* Abnormal coagulation values increase the potential for bleeding after endoscopic therapy.
- Review respiratory, hemodynamic, and neurological assessment before the administration of any sedative agents. *Rationale:* Baseline assessment data provide comparison information for further evaluation once medications have been administered.
- Obtain baseline vital signs, pulse oximetry, and end-tidal CO_2 level, if applicable. *Rationale:* Close monitoring of vital signs and pulse oximetry during the procedure and comparison with baseline values are essential to assess patient's tolerance of the procedure.
- Assess sedation using a validated tool (i.e., Aldrete score, Ramsay scale, or the Richmond Agitation/Sedation Score). *Rationale:* Use of a scoring system standardizes assessment of the patient's tolerance of moderate sedation.

Patient Preparation

- Perform a procedural timeout and verify that the patient is the correct patient using two identifiers. *Rationale:* Before performing a procedure, the nurse should ensure the correct identification of the patient for the intended intervention.

- Ensure that the patient understands preprocedural teachings. Answer questions as they arise, and reinforce information as needed. *Rationale:* Understanding of previously taught information is evaluated and reinforced.
- Ensure that informed consent has been obtained. *Rationale:* Informed consent protects the rights of the patient.
- Check that all relevant documents and studies are available before starting the procedure. *Rationale:* Provides information needed before performing the procedure.
- Place the patient on a cardiac monitor and apply a pulse oximeter and automatic blood pressure cuff. *Rationale:* This allows for continuous cardiovascular and respiratory monitoring during the procedure.
- Ensure venous access is in place. *Rationale:* Venous access is needed for procedural and emergency medications.
- Ensure that the patient's status has been nothing-by-mouth for at least 4 hours before the procedure. *Rationale:* Undigested material in the stomach increases the risk for aspiration and decreases visualization of the GI tract.

- Have sedatives and analgesics (common sedatives include midazolam, diazepam, and fentanyl for analgesia) available (as prescribed) and administer when requested by the provider. Naloxone and flumazenil should be available for narcotic or sedative reversal. *Rationale:* Sedation and analgesia provide for patient comfort during the procedure, decrease patient anxiety, and help facilitate cooperation.
- Set up suction with connecting tubing and rigid pharyngeal suction tip attached and ready for use. *Rationale:* This setup is necessary for suctioning the patient's oral secretions during the procedure.
- Have atropine available at the bedside. *Rationale:* Atropine is necessary if a vagal reaction occurs with the insertion and passage of the endoscope.
- Remove the patient's dentures. *Rationale:* Dentures interfere with safe passage of the endoscope.
- Protect the patient's eyes with goggles or a waterproof covering. *Rationale:* Protection is provided against accidental exposure to blood or the sclerosing agents. Sclerosing agents are eye irritants.

Procedure for Assisting With Endoscopic Therapy

Steps	Rationale	Special Considerations
1. **HH**		
2. **PE**		
3. Position the patient in the left-lateral position. **(Level E*)**	The left-lateral position allows predictable views of the stomach as the scope is advanced. This position allows secretions to collect in the dependent areas of the mouth for ease of suctioning and is the position of choice to prevent aspiration should the patient vomit.[1,2,19]	
4. Perform or assist the physician with gastric lavage (see Procedure 110).	Large amounts of blood or clots in the stomach or esophagus can impair visualization of varices and increase the risk for aspiration during the procedure.[14]	
5. Administer analgesic and sedative medications as prescribed. **(Level C*)**	Promotes patient cooperation during the endoscopy, promotes patient comfort, and facilitates the passage of the endoscope.[21]	

*Level C: Qualitative studies, descriptive or correlational studies, integrative reviews, systematic reviews, or randomized controlled trials with inconsistent results.
*Level E: Multiple case reports, theory-based evidence from expert opinions, or peer-reviewed professional organizational standards without clinical studies to support recommendations.

Procedure continues on following page

Procedure   for Assisting With Endoscopic Therapy—*Continued*

Steps	Rationale	Special Considerations
6. Assist the physician if needed with insertion of the endoscope.	Provides assistance.	Gag and cough reflexes may be compromised by topical anesthetics; the patient may vomit as the endoscope is passed, increasing the risk for aspiration. Have emergency intubation equipment available. Monitor heart rate, rhythm, and respiratory status during the endoscopy.
A. Assist as needed in anesthetizing the posterior pharynx with a topical agent as prescribed. **(Level A*)**	Decreases the discomfort caused by passage of the endoscope.[6]	
B. Insert an oral airway (see Procedure 9) or bite block.	Prevents the patient from biting the endoscope or the inserter's fingers.	
C. Lubricate 20–30 cm of the distal end of the endoscope with water-soluble lubricant. (Many physicians prefer to lubricate the scope themselves.)	Minimizes mucosal injury and irritation and facilitates ease of passage of the endoscope.	
D. Encourage the patient to simulate swallowing while the endoscope is passed.	The swallowing maneuver causes the epiglottis to close the trachea and directs the endoscope into the esophagus.	
E. Suction the oral pharynx as needed throughout the procedure.	Because of the diminished gag reflex and the presence of the endoscope in the patient's pharynx, oral secretions may not be able to be swallowed. Blood from the GI tract may be vomited and could be aspirated because of the diminished gag reflex.	
7. The physician performing the esophagogastroduodenoscopy may ask the nurse to assist with preparing equipment for thermal or laser coagulation of a bleeding site.	This technique is frequently used to control bleeding from many upper gastrointestinal sites.	
8. Assist as needed with injecting an irrigant via the endoscope.	Cleanses the area to increase visualization of the tissue.	
9. If a bleeding site is to be sclerosed, manipulate the sclerosing needle as requested (Fig. 111-1). Inject sclerosant if requested.	Ensures that the sclerosing needle is in proper position for injection and does not injure tissue during movement of the endoscope.	The needle must be retracted before manipulation of the endoscope.
10. Endoscopic bands or endoclips may also be requested by the physician performing the intervention (Fig. 111-2).	In EVL, or banding, a rubber band is deployed from the endoscope and contracts around a lesion that has been raised with endoscopic suction into a specially fitted, transparent endoscopic cap (see Fig. 111-2).[7,22]	

*Level A: Meta-analysis of quantitative studies or metasynthesis of qualitative studies with results that consistently support a specific action, intervention, or treatment (including systematic review of randomized controlled trials).

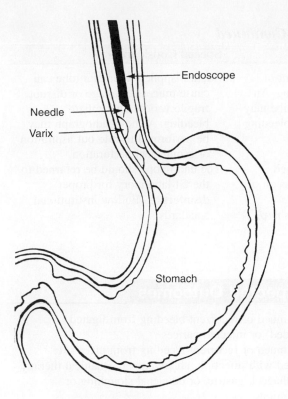

Figure 111-1 Injection of sclerosing agent into engorged varix. *(From Pierce JD, Wilkerson E, Griffiths SA: Acute esophageal bleeding and endoscopic injection therapy,* Crit Care Nurse *10:67–72, 1990.)*

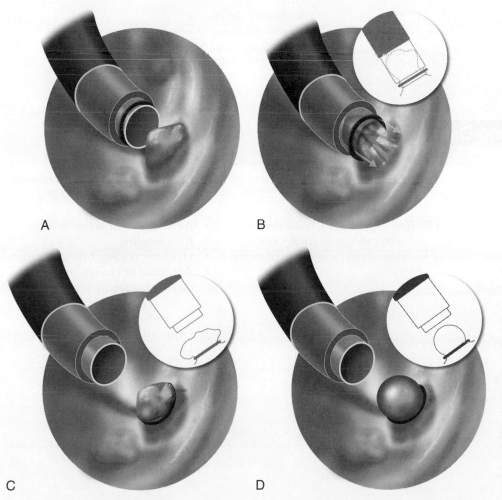

Figure 111-2 Endoscopic variceal ligation. **A,** Endoscope placement over varix. **B,** The varix is drawn into the distal portion of the endoscope. **C,** A rubber band is dropped over the varix. **D,** The rubber band contracts around the varix, causing it to sclerose and eventually slough. *(Drawings by Paul Schiffmacher, Medical Illustrator, Medical Media Services at Thomas Jefferson University Hospital, Philadelphia.)*

Procedure | for Assisting With Endoscopic Therapy—*Continued*

Steps	Rationale	Special Considerations
11. Assist with insertion of an NG tube or esophagogastric tamponade tube (see Procedures 108 or 113) after removal of the endoscope if assistance is needed.	An NG tube provides assessment of continued or recurrent bleeding. An esophagogastric tamponade tube may be used to apply pressure to bleeding varices.	Suction applied to an NG tube can cause mucosal damage or disrupt fragile varices and initiate bleeding. A chest radiograph may be performed to rule out aspiration or esophageal perforation.
12. Remove **PE** and discard used supplies in appropriate receptacles.	Removes and safely discards used supplies, reduces the transmission of microorganisms; Standard Precautions. Safely removes sharp objects.	The endoscope should be returned to the GI laboratory for proper disinfection. Follow institutional standards.
13. **HH**		

Expected Outcomes

- Hemostasis at the site of GI bleeding without recurrent bleeding or prevention of bleeding from esophageal varices
- Stabilization of hematocrit and hemoglobin values

Unexpected Outcomes

- Continued or recurrent bleeding from ligated (banded) or injected varices
- Continued or recurrent bleeding from ulcer site treated with injection, ablative, or mechanical therapy
- Esophageal, gastric, or duodenal sloughing or ulceration
- Esophageal, gastric, or duodenal perforation
- Substernal chest pain
- Fever
- Temporary dysphagia
- Allergic response to sclerosing agent
- Aspiration pneumonia
- Pleural effusion
- Atelectasis
- Bacteremia/sepsis

Patient Monitoring and Care

Steps	Rationale	Reportable Conditions
1. Monitor cardiovascular, respiratory, and neurological status every 5–15 minutes during and after endoscopy until patient condition returns to preprocedure status, then every 30 minutes to 1 hour for 2–4 hours. Includes: A. Level of consciousness. B. Vital signs. C. Oximetry. D. Capnography.[8] (**Level B***) E. Cardiac rhythm.	Changes in vital signs, heart rhythm, oximetry, and capnography may indicate complications related to the procedure.	*These conditions should be reported if they persist despite nursing interventions.* • Altered level of consciousness from baseline • Oximetry reading below baseline • Abnormal or changed end-tidal carbon dioxide from baseline • Pulse rate above or below baseline • Fever >101°F • Decrease in blood pressure 20–30 mm Hg below baseline • Dysrhythmias

*Level B: Well-designed, controlled studies with results that consistently support a specific action, intervention, or treatment.

Patient Monitoring and Care —*Continued*

Steps	Rationale	Reportable Conditions
2. Follow institutional standards for assessing pain.	May indicate continued bleeding or reaction to sclerosant. Identifies need for pain interventions.	• Same pain rating as before procedure • New onset of chest pain • Continued pain despite pain interventions
3. Monitor output from NG tube or any vomitus.	Signs of continued or recurrent bleeding.	• Sudden change in condition, bright red vomitus or NG drainage, or decreased patency of NG tube
4. Monitor serial hematocrit and hemoglobin results as prescribed.	Continued fall in the hematocrit and hemoglobin value indicates continued or recurrent bleeding.	• Decreasing hematocrit and hemoglobin value below baseline
5. Monitor postural vital signs once the patient is able to be out of bed.	Postural changes may indicate volume loss.	• Decrease in blood pressure 20–30 mm Hg below baseline • Increase in pulse 10–20 beats per minute above baseline
6. Assess for return of normal pharyngeal function. A. Keep the patient on left side with slight head elevation until gag, swallow, and cough reflexes are intact. B. Remain with the patient until reflexes return.	Some endoscopic therapies can cause transient dysphagia. Topical anesthesia decreases the gag reflex and increases the risk for aspiration. The left-lateral position is the position of choice to prevent aspiration should the patient not be able to control secretions or vomit.	• Prolonged absence of gag, swallow, or cough reflex
7. Provide clear liquids when prescribed after return of pharyngeal function. Diet should be progressed slowly to solid food.	Food may act as an irritant to the sclerosed ulcer or variceal sites.	• Nausea • Vomiting of bright red blood
8. Administer antacids, histamine (H_2) blockers, sucralfate, proton pump inhibitors, somatostatin, or octreotide as prescribed.[4,7,12,23] **(Level A*)**	Antacids neutralize gastric acid. Histamine blockers decrease gastric acid secretion. Sucralfate reacts with gastric acid, forming a paste that adheres to ulcer sites. Proton pump inhibitors inhibit the proton pump in the parietal cells of the stomach, suppressing gastric acid secretion. Somatostatin and octreotide (synthetic somatostatin) lower portal pressure with splanchnic vasoconstriction.[4,12,16]	
9. Continue patient and family education. A. Explain signs and symptoms to report (fever, chest pain, difficulty swallowing, vomiting bright red blood, and difficulty breathing).	Unexpected outcomes can occur within hours or may be delayed days or weeks after endoscopic therapy.	
B. Explain diet progression.	Decreases the risk for aspiration of liquid or food before the patient is ready for swallowing.	
C. Explain medication therapy.	Knowledge and understanding about the medication regimen promotes safe, effective medication use.	

*Level A: Meta-analysis of quantitative studies or metasynthesis of qualitative studies with results that consistently support a specific action, intervention, or treatment (including systematic review of randomized controlled trials).

Procedure continues on following page

Documentation

Documentation should include the following:

- Completion of informed consent
- Preprocedure verifications and timeout
- Date and time of procedure
- Initial patient assessment
- Preprocedure and postprocedure patient and family education
- Baseline vital signs
- Baseline pulse oximetry
- Baseline capnography
- Premedications administered
- Gastric lavage with results (if performed) and patient's tolerance
- Vital signs, pulse oximetry and capnography during endoscopic therapy
- Type of intervention: injection, ablative or mechanical; sclerosing agents administered and amount or dose; number of bands or clips placed; and location if applicable

- Time of insertion of NG or esophagogastric tamponade tube (if inserted), patient's tolerance, characteristics of any drainage from NG tube, radiographic documentation of placement of NG or tamponade tube, and initial pressure applied
- Postendoscopic therapy vital signs and pulse oximetry
- Position of the patient after the procedure
- Recovery from sedation
- Assessment of gag, swallow, and cough reflexes
- Postprocedure medications administered
- Unexpected outcomes
- Nursing interventions
- Sedation score
- Pain assessment, interventions, and effectiveness

References and Additional Readings

For a complete list of references and additional readings for this procedure, scan this QR code with any freely available smartphone code reader app, or visit http://booksite.elsevier.com/9780323376624.

112 Intraabdominal Pressure Monitoring

Rosemary Lee

PURPOSE: The purpose of this procedure is to present the correct method of measuring intraabdominal pressure via the urinary bladder. Intraabdominal hypertension and abdominal compartment syndrome occur when the abdominal contents expand in excess of the capacity of the abdominal cavity, compromising abdominal organ perfusion and resulting in organ dysfunction or failure and associated mortality. Research has identified that at least 50% of critically ill patients have some degree of intraabdominal hypertension.[2,4,6,9,14,16,18,21,24–26,28,30]

PREREQUISITE NURSING KNOWLEDGE

- Understanding of anatomy and physiology of the abdominal contents is necessary.
- Knowledge of aseptic technique is essential.
- The abdominal cavity should be viewed as a "closed box" with the spine, costal arch, and pelvis as rigid margins and the diaphragm and abdominal wall as flexible margins.[29]
- Intraabdominal hypertension (IAH) and abdominal compartment syndrome (ACS) occur when the abdominal contents expand in excess of the capacity of the abdominal cavity, compromising abdominal organ perfusion and resulting in organ dysfunction or failure and associated mortality.[4–6,9,12,14,18,21,28–30]
- Five major categories of risk are associated with the development of IAH and ACS (Table 112-1). They include[4,18,21]:
  - Diminished abdominal wall compliance
  - Increased intestinal intraluminal contents
  - Increased peritoneal cavity contents
  - Capillary leakage into the bowel wall and mesentery/fluid resuscitation
  - Miscellaneous/other
- IAH is defined as a sustained or repeated pathological elevation of intraabdominal pressure (IAP) greater than or equal to 12 mm Hg.[4,18,21]
- IAH is graded by severity[4,18,21]:
  - Grade I: IAP 12 to 15 mm Hg
  - Grade II: IAP 16 to 20 mm Hg
  - Grade III: IAP 21 to 25 mm Hg
  - Grade IV: IAP greater than 25 mm Hg
- ACS is defined as an IAP greater than or equal to 20 mm Hg that is associated with new organ dysfunction or failure.[1,4,13,18,21,33]
- ACS is categorized into three types. Primary ACS is a condition associated with injury or disease in the abdominopelvic region that frequently requires early surgical or interventional radiological intervention. Secondary ACS refers to conditions that do not originate from the abdominopelvic region. Recurrent ACS refers to the condition in which ACS redevelops following previous surgical or medical treatment of primary or secondary ACS. Primary ACS occurs more frequently, but secondary ACS has a higher mortality rate.
- Both IAH and ACS may compromise perfusion to the visceral organs represented by the parameter abdominal perfusion pressure (APP).[4,18,21,28] APP is derived as follows:

  $$APP = MAP - IAP,$$ where MAP is mean arterial pressure.

- At this time there is not enough evidence to use APP in the management of critically ill patients.[18]
- Measurement of bladder pressure via an indwelling urinary bladder catheter is considered the reference standard for the measurement of IAP and may be performed with equipment readily available in the critical care environment (Fig. 112-1). Bladder pressure monitoring may be performed using a transducer method or manometer method.
- Commercially prepared kits designed for the measurement of IAP are also available and may provide advantages in efficiency, standardization of measurement technique, and data reproducibility.
- Instructions for specific setup and operation of commercially prepared devices are provided by the manufacturer.
- Regardless of the device used, a standardized procedure for measurement should be used to prevent measurement variability between physicians, advanced practice nurses, and other healthcare professionals.[7,10,11,15,17,18,22,23,27,29]
- The bladder acts as a passive reservoir and accurately reflects IAP when intravesicular volumes of 25 mL or less are used. Larger volumes previously suggested (50 to 100 mL) are not necessary and may in fact overdistend the bladder, falsely elevating measured bladder pressure (IAP).[4,11,22]
- Normal IAP is 0 to 5 mm Hg. The typical critically ill patient averages an IAP of 5 to 7 mm Hg.[4,18,21,29]
- Bladder pressure measurement may be contraindicated in certain conditions, such as bladder trauma or bladder surgery. IAP readings are inaccurate in patients with a

TABLE 112-1	Patients at Risk for Development of Intraabdominal Hypertension and Abdominal Compartment Syndrome[2,4,18,21,25,29,31]

Diminished Abdominal Wall Compliance

- Abdominal surgery
- Major trauma
- Major burns
- Prone positioning

Increased Intestinal Intraluminal Contents

- Gastroparesis
- Gastric distention
- Ileus
- Colonic pseudo-obstruction
- Volvulus

Increased Intraabdominal Contents

- Distended abdomen
- Peritoneal dialysis
- Laparoscopy with excessive insufflation pressures
- Acute pancreatitis
- Hemoperitoneum/pneumoperitoneum or intraperitoneal fluid collections
- Intraabdominal infection/abscess
- Intraabdominal or retroperitoneal tumors
- Liver dysfunction/cirrhosis with ascites

Capillary Leak/Fluid Resuscitation

- Metabolic acidosis, pH <7.20
- Hypothermia (core temperature <33°C or <91.4°F)
- Massive fluid resuscitation (>5 L/24 hours) or positive fluid balance
- Polytransfusion (>10 units of blood/24 hours)
- Damage control laparotomy
- Increased severity of disease classification score such as Acute Physiology and Chronic Health Evaluation II (APACHE-II) or Sequential Organ Failure Assessment (SOFA) score

Others/Miscellaneous

- Age (>69 years)
- Coagulopathy (not on anticoagulation)
  - Platelets <55,000/mm³ **OR**
  - A partial thromboplastin time greater than twice normal **OR**
  - International normalized ratio >1.5
- Increased head of bed angle (>20 degrees)
- Large hernia repair
- Mechanical ventilation
- Positive end-expiratory pressure >10 cm H_2O
- Obesity or increased body mass index (BMI >30)
- Diagnosis of:
  - Intraabdominal infections/peritonitis
  - Pneumonia
  - Bacteremia
  - Sepsis
- Shock or hypotension

neurogenic bladder. Risks and benefits of measurement should be discussed with the physician before the procedure is performed in these patients.
- In patients who do not have a urinary catheter in place, the risks and benefits of catheter placement for the purpose of bladder pressure measurement should be considered.

EQUIPMENT

- Nonsterile gloves
- Intravenous (IV) pole
- If using transducer technique:
  - Cardiac monitor and pressure cable for interface with the monitor
  - 500-mL IV bag of normal saline (NS) solution
  - Pressure transducer system, including pressure tubing with flush device, transducer, and two stopcocks
  - 25- to 30-mL Luer-Lok syringe
  - Clamp
  - Chlorhexidine or alcohol swabs
- If using manometer technique:
  - 20 mL of sterile saline
  - 20-mL Luer-Lok syringe
  - Urinary manometer kit

Note: Commercial bladder pressure monitoring system may be substituted for the previous list.

PATIENT/FAMILY EDUCATION

- Explain the procedure of bladder pressure measurement and its purpose to the patient and family. **Rationale:** Patient and family anxiety may be decreased. Understanding of how the procedure is performed may promote the patient's ability to cooperate.
- Inform the patient that fullness may be felt in the bladder when the normal saline solution is injected into the bladder during the procedure. **Rationale:** Patient anxiety may be decreased. Patient is prepared for what to expect.

PATIENT ASSESSMENT AND PREPARATION

Patient Assessment

- Obtain the patient's health history to determine whether risk factors are present that may predispose the patient to IAH or ACS. These conditions are outlined in Table 112-1. **Rationale:** Patients with these conditions may experience an increase in abdominal cavity fluid collection or tissue edema, placing them at risk for IAH and ACS. It is recommended that patients with any one risk factor have their IAPs measured.[18]
- Assess the patient for signs of progression of IAH to ACS. These findings include decreased cardiac output and blood pressure, oliguria and anuria, increased peak inspiratory pressures, hypercarbia and hypoxia, and increased intracranial pressure (ICP) (Table 112-2). **Rationale:** These physical findings indicate pathophysiologic organ system changes associated with the progression of IAH to ACS.

Bladder Pressure Monitoring Setup

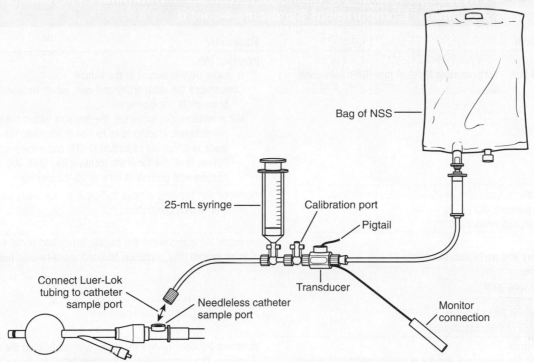

Bag of NSS

25-mL syringe

Calibration port

Pigtail

Connect Luer-Lok tubing to catheter sample port

Needleless catheter sample port

Transducer

Monitor connection

Figure 112-1   Bladder pressure monitoring setup. *(Illustration by John J. Gallagher.)*

TABLE 112-2	Physiological Changes Associated With Intraabdominal Hypertension and Abdominal Compartment Syndrome[1,6,8,9,14,18–21,25,28,29,33]
Organ System	**Rationale**
Cardiovascular ↑ Central venous pressure (CVP), pulmonary artery pressure (PAP), pulmonary capillary wedge pressure (PCWP), systemic vascular resistance (SVR) ↓ Cardiac Output (CO) (more pronounced with hypovolemia) ↓ Venous return from lower extremities (risk for deep vein thrombosis)	Up to 50% of the IAP is reflected into the thoracic cavity. This leads to compression of the heart and decreased venous return (preload reduction), and impedes arterial outflow (increase in afterload). Transmitted backpressure from the abdominal cavity can falsely elevate CVP, PAP, and PCWP. The World Society of the Abdominal Compartment Syndrome recommends using volumetric indices rather than pressure indices for assessment of fluid responsiveness. Indices recommended for use are stroke volume, stroke volume index, global ventricular end-diastolic volume, pulse pressure variation, and stroke volume variation in appropriate situations. Note: The passive leg raise maneuver is not accurate in assessing fluid responsiveness when the IAP is greater than or equal to 12 mm Hg.
Pulmonary ↑ Intrathoracic pressures ↑ Peak inspiratory pressures ↑ Plateau pressures ↓ Functional residual capacity ↑ Dead space shunt ↓ Tidal volume → ↑ hypercarbia + ↓ partial pressure of oxygen in arterial blood ↓ Compliance ↑ Compression atelectasis ↑ Pulmonary infection rate	Increased IAP causes an increase in intrathoracic pressure and limits diaphragm excursion, resulting in hypoventilation and hypoxia. IAH can cause prolonged ventilator time. Patients with primary IAH are at higher risk for developing acute lung injury/acute respiratory distress syndrome.

Continued

TABLE 112-2	Physiological Changes Associated With Intraabdominal Hypertension and Abdominal Compartment Syndrome—cont'd

Organ System	Rationale

Renal
↓ Renal blood flow → ↓glomerular filtration rate (GFR) → ↓urine output
	Increased IAP:
	  Reduces cardiac output to the kidney
	  Compresses the renal artery and vein, which reduces perfusion pressure to the glomerulus.
	  IAP simultaneously increases the pressure within the renal parenchyma, leading to reduction in filtration. The combination leads to a marked reduction in GFR and urine production. Patient is at risk for acute kidney injury (AKI). AKI is known to happen with persistent IAPs of 10–12 mm Hg.

Neurological ↑ Intracranial pressure (ICP) ↓ Cerebral perfusion pressure (CPP)	Increased IAP impedes venous outflow from the brain, increasing cerebral venous congestion.

Hepatic
↓ Hepatic artery and portal vein blood flow
↓ Liver function:
  • Lactate clearance
  • Glucose metabolism
  • Cytochrome P450 function
  • Clearance of toxic metabolites
	Increased IAP compresses the hepatic artery and portal vein, leading to decreased liver perfusion and decreased hepatic function.

Gastrointestinal
↓ Blood flow to the celiac axis and the superior mesenteric artery
↓ Perfusion of the abdominal organs
↑ Compression of mesenteric veins leading to abdominal venous hypertension
↓ Successful enteral nutrition
↑ Ileus
↑ Intestinal edema and permeability
↑ Bacterial translocation
↑ Visceral swelling
↑ Bowel ischemia
↑ Abdominal wound complications:
  • Edema
  • Ischemia
  • Dehiscence
  • Infection
	Increased IAP compresses the major arteries feeding the abdominal organs. The compression of the veins leads to venous congestion. The poor perfusions leads to the gastrointestinal complications listed.

Endocrine ↑ Antidiuretic hormone ↑ Renin, angiotensin, aldosterone	As a result of decreased cardiac output and blood pressure, the baroreceptors stimulate the sympathetic nervous system to maintain homeostasis.

Patient Preparation

• Ensure that the patient and family understand preprocedural teachings. Answer questions as they arise, and reinforce information as needed. *Rationale:* Understanding of previously taught information is evaluated and reinforced.
• Ensure the presence of a conventional (single-lumen) urinary catheter connected to a drainage system. *Rationale:*

A urinary catheter with a drainage system is required to obtain bladder pressure measurements.
• Verify that the patient is the correct patient using two identifiers. *Rationale:* Before performing a procedure, the nurse should ensure the correct identification of the patient for the intended intervention.
• Perform a preprocedure verification and timeout, if nonemergent. *Rationale:* This ensures patient safety.

Procedure	for Intraabdominal Pressure Monitoring	
Steps	**Rationale**	**Special Considerations**
1. **HH**		
2. **PE**		
3. Assemble the entire pressure transducer system as shown (see Fig. 112-1): A. Attach the two stopcocks between the transducer and the pressure tubing. B. Spike the normal saline bag with the pressure transducer system and flush.	Ensures that all air is out of the system.	If the pressure transducer already has a stopcock attached to the transducer, only one stopcock is needed. Note that a pressure bag is not required.
4. Attach the 25- or 30-mL syringe to the distal stopcock (see Fig. 112-1).	The syringe is used to fill the bladder with normal saline solution.	
5. Cleanse the sampling port on the urinary drainage system with an antiseptic solution and aseptically attach the end of the pressure tubing to the sampling port.	Cleansing the sampling port reduces the incidence of hospital-acquired urinary tract infection (UTI) from system contamination.	
6. Connect the system to the pressure module of the monitoring system with the transducer cable. Select a 30 mm Hg scale, and use an IAP label if available or label as "P."	Connects the system for monitoring. The 30–mm Hg scale is sufficient to measure most IAP ranges. Monitors may not have an IAP label; it is best to use the "P" for pressure.	Using the label "CVP" or "ICP" can cause confusion.
7. Level the transducer: A. With the patient in the supine position and the head of the bed (HOB) flat, level the transducer (zeroing stopcock) to the iliac crest at the level of the midaxillary line 9 (Fig. 112-2).[3,11,18,29] **(Level D*)** B. If the patient must remain with the HOB elevated, the transducer must be placed at the level of the bladder (iliac crest; see Fig. 112-2).	The supine position limits the effect of the abdominal cavity contents on the bladder that may falsely elevate bladder pressure measurements. Approximates the level of the bladder and should be used as the reference point.	Marking the position ensures consistent use of the same reference point. The transducer system may be secured to an IV pole beside the patient or can be secured to the patient. If the patient is unable to be placed in the supine position, the degree of HOB elevation should be noted on the medical record, along with the bladder pressure, to allow future measurements to be done in the same position so they may be compared with one another accurately. Note that the phlebostatic axis should not be used to level the transducer for bladder pressure measurement.
8. Zero the IAP monitoring system.	Negates the effect of atmospheric pressure. Ensures accuracy of the system with the established reference point.	
9. Clamp the bladder drainage system just distal to the catheter and drainage bag connection on the drainage bag tubing.	Prevents drainage of the normal saline solution out of the bladder during bladder filling.	

*Level D: Peer-reviewed professional and organizational standards with the support of clinical study recommendations.

Procedure continues on following page

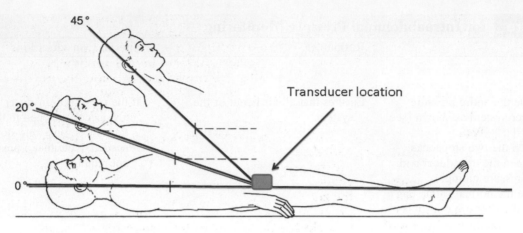

The correct transducer position at the iliac crest in the mid-axillary line in the supine position and with head of bed elevation.

Figure 112-2　Correct position of the transducer for bladder pressure measurement. *(Illustration by John J. Gallagher.)*

Procedure for Intraabdominal Pressure Monitoring—*Continued*

Steps	Rationale	Special Considerations
10. Turn the stopcock attached to the syringe off to the patient and open to the fluid bag and syringe. Activate the fast-flush mechanism while pulling back on the syringe plunger to fill the syringe to 25 mL.[4,15,19,22,27] **(Level D*)**		
11. Turn the stopcock off to the fluid bag and open to the syringe and patient. Inject the 25 mL of saline solution into the bladder.[4,15,19,22,27] **(Level D*)**	The fluid-filled bladder accurately reflects IAP. Use of a volume of 25 mL prevents overdistention of the bladder and false elevation of the bladder pressure.	
12. Expel any air seen between the clamp and the urinary catheter by opening the clamp and allowing the saline solution to flow back past the clamp; then reclamp.	Air in the system may dampen the pressure reading.	
13. Measure the IAP at end expiration with the graphic scale on the monitor display and numeric display of the mean pressure (Fig. 112-3). IAP should be measured with the patient in the supine position. The patient should be relaxed, not coughing or moving.	Measurement at end expiration is most accurate when the effects of pulmonary pressures are minimized. Patient movement and coughing can elevate the IAP	The numeric mean IAP pressure displayed on the monitor may be used in most circumstances. The numeric reading is a mean pressure value, reflecting the average of both inspiratory and expiratory IAP. Consider reading the IAP from the monitor graphic scale or a printed strip if noticeable excursions are found in the waveform with ventilation.

*Level D: Peer-reviewed professional and organizational standards with the support of clinical study recommendations.

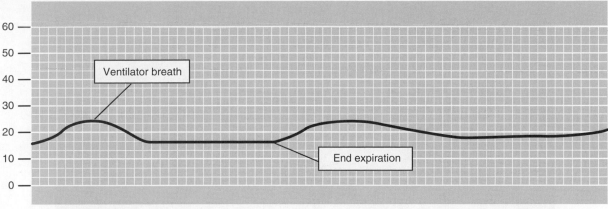

Figure 112-3   Intraabdominal (IAP) waveform. The IAP read at end expiration is 16 mm Hg in this patient on mechanical ventilation.

Procedure for Intraabdominal Pressure Monitoring—*Continued*		
Steps	**Rationale**	**Special Considerations**
14. Once a reading has been obtained, unclamp the urinary drainage system. The pressure monitoring system may be left connected or disconnected and capped to maintain the sterility of the system. Note: The urinary drainage system should be left unclamped between readings.	Unclamping the drainage system discontinues pressure measurement and resumes the normal urinary drainage function of the catheter system. If the monitoring system is maintained connected to the urinary catheter, repeated reentry into the catheter tubing is avoided.	Monitoring requires clamping the drainage system and filling the bladder to obtain a reading. Minimizing entry into the urinary drainage system may reduce the chance of UTI. Specific data to support this practice in IAP measurement do not exist.
15. Record the bladder pressure on the patient flow sheet, and remember to subtract the 25 mL of instilled saline solution from the hourly urine output.	The volume of instilled normal saline solution falsely elevates the calculation of hourly urine output if it is not subtracted.	
16. Discard used supplies and gloves in the appropriate receptacles.		
17. **HH**		

Procedure for Intraabdominal Pressure Monitoring With the AbViser (Convatec) Bladder Pressure Monitoring System With AutoValve (Fig. 112-4)		
Steps	**Rationale**	**Special Considerations**
1. **HH**		
2. **PE**		
3. Hang the bag of normal saline on an IV pole.	Prepares the system for priming.	Note that a pressure bag is not required.
A. Open the AbViser Auto Valve Device packaging.		
B. Remove the protective cap from the saline bag tubing spike and insert the spike into the saline bag (Fig. 112-5, Step 1).		

Procedure continues on following page

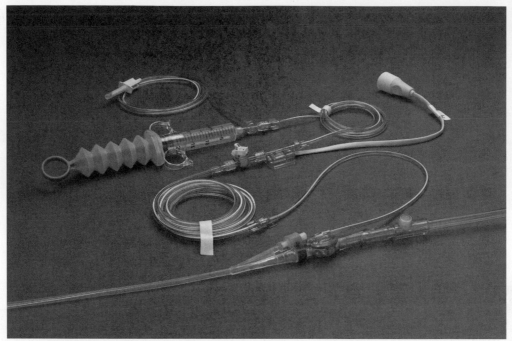

Figure 112-4   Commercially prepared bladder pressure measurement system (AbViser). *(Courtesy Wolfe Tory Medical, Salt Lake City, UT.)*

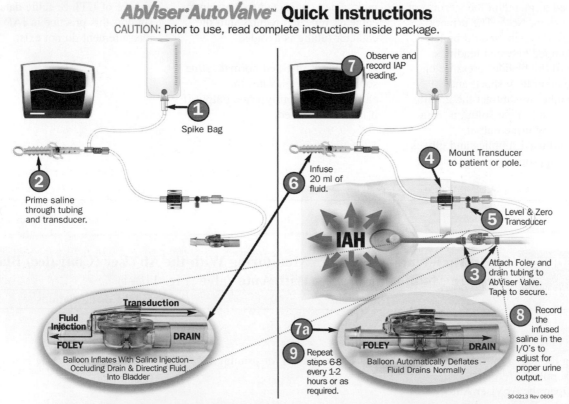

Figure 112-5   AbViser Bladder Pressure Monitoring System. *(From ConvaTec, Bridgewater, NJ.)*

Procedure	for Intraabdominal Pressure Monitoring With the AbViser (Convatec) Bladder Pressure Monitoring System With AutoValve—*Continued*	
Steps	**Rationale**	**Special Considerations**
4. Prime the system with normal saline solution by aspirating and compressing the syringe to remove all air from the tubing. Continue this process until the normal saline solution runs through the AutoValve at the distal end of the system (see Fig. 112-5, Step 2).	Removes all air from the system to establish a fluid column for accurate pressure measurement.	
5. Place the sterile drape under the urinary catheter/drain bag connection and cleanse the connection with the antiseptic solution (see Fig. 112-5, Step 3).	Reduces the chance of bacterial contamination of the urinary drainage system.	
6. With aseptic technique, detach the urinary catheter from the drainage bag (see Fig. 112-5, Step 3).	Reduces the chance of bacterial contamination of the urinary drainage system.	
7. Pick up the AutoValve and tear the perforation on the protective bag, exposing the barbed end of the AutoValve. Slide the urinary catheter over the barbed end of the AutoValve. Connect the other end of the AutoValve to the urinary drainage bag connection. Ensure the connections are dry and wrap the tape strip included with the kit around the catheter/AutoValve connection (see Fig. 112-5, Step 3).	Reduces the risk of contamination; secures the connection to reduce the chance of system component separation.	
8. Place the syringe in a convenient area.	The syringe may be easily hung from an IV pole.	
9. Attach the pressure transducer to the patient or pole mount at the level of the iliac crest in the midaxillary line (see Fig. 112-5, Step 4).	Approximates the level of the bladder and should be used as the reference point.	Marking the position may ensure consistent use of the same reference point. The transducer may be secured to an IV pole beside the patient and leveled in the standard fashion, or it may be secured to the patient at the level described.
10. Connect the AbViser system to the monitor with the pressure transducer cable. Select a 30–mm Hg scale on the monitor and use an IAP label if available or label as "P."	Connects to the system for monitoring. The 30–mm Hg scale is sufficient to measure most IAP ranges. Monitors may not have an IAP label; it is best to use "P" for pressure.	Using the label "CVP" or "ICP" can cause confusion.

Procedure continues on following page

Procedure	for Intraabdominal Pressure Monitoring With the AbViser (Convatec) Bladder Pressure Monitoring System With AutoValve—*Continued*	
Steps	**Rationale**	**Special Considerations**
11. Zero the pressure transducer at the level of the iliac crest (see Fig. 112-2) in the midaxillary line (see Fig. 112-5, Step 5). A. Turn the stopcock (OFF) towards the patient. B. Remove the yellow cap and now "zero" the monitor. C. Reposition the yellow cap. D. Turn the stopcock (OFF) to its original position facing the yellow cap. The transducer is now open to the patient and ready for monitoring.	Negates the effect of atmospheric pressure. Ensures accuracy of the system with the established reference point.	Note that the phlebostatic axis should not be used to level the transducer for bladder pressure measurement.
12. Place the patient in the supine position. The patient should be relaxed, not coughing or moving.	Limits the effect of the abdominal cavity contents on the bladder that may falsely elevate bladder pressure measurements. Patient movement or coughing can elevate the IAP.	If the patient is unable to be placed in the supine position, the degree of HOB elevation should be noted on the medical record, along with the bladder pressure measurement.
13. Retract the plunger of the syringe on the system to aspirate 20 mL of saline solution into the syringe and briskly inject the saline solution into the bladder (for pediatric patients use 1 mL/kg + 2 mL, not to exceed 20 mL total; see Fig. 112-5, Step 6).	This process will inflate the valve, closing off the connection between the urinary catheter and the urine drain tubing allowing a hydrostatic pressure reading.	The AutoValve closes to retain the injected normal saline solution in the bladder for up to 3 minutes.
14. Allow the system to equilibrate and then note the bladder pressure reading on the monitor at end expiration (see Fig. 112-5, Step 7).	Measurement at end expiration is most accurate because the effects of pulmonary pressures are minimized.	The reading lasts for 1–3 minutes until the AutoValve opens, allowing for drainage of the normal saline solution from the bladder. The pressure should drop to zero. Note: If the reading does not go to zero, fluid may remain in the drainage tubing. Drain any remaining fluid into the drainage bag and the reading should decrease to zero. The numeric mean IAP pressure displayed on the monitor may be used in most circumstances. The numeric reading is a mean pressure value, reflecting the average of both inspiratory and expiratory IAP. Consider reading the IAP from the monitor graphic scale or a printed strip if noticeable excursions are found in the waveform with ventilation.

Procedure	for Intraabdominal Pressure Monitoring With the AbViser (Convatec) Bladder Pressure Monitoring System With AutoValve—*Continued*	
Steps	**Rationale**	**Special Considerations**
15. Confirm that the AutoValve has opened and that urine is draining normally (see Fig. 112-5, Step 7, A).	The AutoValve normally opens within 1–3 minutes.	The valve remains open until the next volume of fluid is infused.
16. Discard used supplies and gloves in the appropriate receptacles.		
17. 🄷🄷		
18. Repeat measurement every 4 hours or as clinically indicated (see Fig. 112-5, Step 9).	Measurements should be trended to detect the onset of IAH.	

Procedure	for Intraabdominal Pressure Monitoring With the Foley Manometer LV System	
Steps	**Rationale**	**Special Considerations**

Note: Intended for patients who are at least 10 kg.

Steps	**Rationale**	**Special Considerations**
1. 🄷🄷		
2. 🄿🄴		
3. Open the Foley Manometer LV pouch and close the tube clamp.	The clamp is left open for effective device sterilization. During urine drainage, the filter must be clamped; the clamp is open only when IAP is measured.	
4. Place the urine collection device below the patient's bladder and tape the drainage tube to the bedsheet. **(Level M*)**	This is to prevent dependent loops in the drainage tubing.	
5. Carefully cleanse the catheter connection with an antiseptic before disconnecting the urinary catheter system.	To maintain sterility and prevent a catheter-associated UTI.	
6. Using aseptic technique insert the Foley Manometer LV between the catheter and the drainage device.	To maintain sterility and prevent a catheter-associated UTI.	This step is key in preventing contamination of the urinary drainage system.
7. Prime the Foley Manometer LV with 20 mL of sterile saline solution through its needle-free injection/sampling port. **(Level M*)**	Removes air from the system.	Prime only once, at initial setup or subsequently, to remove any air from the manometer tube. The manometer tube should always be fluid filled. Note: In patients who are anuric, repriming at each pressure determination is not necessary. The fluid returned to the bladder from the manometer tube provides an adequate volume for a reliable pressure determination. Carefully disinfect the needle-free port before urine sampling.

*Level M: Manufacturer's recommendations only.

Procedure continues on following page

Procedure	**for Intraabdominal Pressure Monitoring With the Foley Manometer LV System—***Continued*		
Steps	**Rationale**	**Special Considerations**
8. Place the "0 mm Hg" mark of the manometer tube at the midaxillary line at the iliac crest, and elevate the filter vertically above the patient (Fig. 112-6). Place the patient in the supine position, and ensure the patient is relaxed, not coughing or moving.	Approximates the level of the bladder and should be used as the reference point. Limits the effect of the abdominal cavity contents on the bladder that may falsely elevate bladder pressure measurements. Patient movement or coughing can elevate the IAP.	Note that the phlebostatic axis should not be used to level the transducer for bladder pressure measurement.
9. Open the clamp and read the bladder pressure (end-expiration value) when the fluid meniscus has stabilized (see Fig. 112-6).	Allows for equilibration of the fluid column to accurately represent bladder pressure.	Slow descent (>20–30 seconds) of the meniscus during a bladder pressure determination suggests a blocked or kinked urinary catheter.
10. Close the clamp and place the Foley Manometer LV in its drainage position (Fig. 112-7).	Allows normal flow through the urinary drainage system.	Avoid a U-bend of the large urimeter drainage tube (which will impede urine drainage). Never empty the manometer tube into the urine drainage device during use. The Foley Manometer LV tube should be fluid filled during drainage. Only reprime with sterile normal saline solution to remove any air or bladder debris in the manometer tube. Note: Never use the Foley Manometer LV for more than 7 days. (**Level M***)

*Level M: Manufacturer's recommendations only.

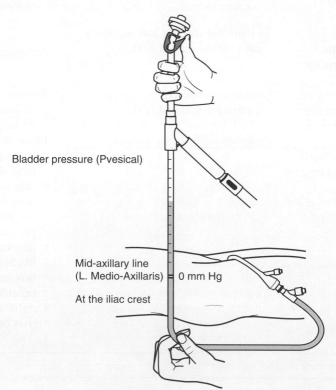

Bladder pressure (Pvesical)

Mid-axillary line
(L. Medio-Axillaris)   0 mm Hg

At the iliac crest

Figure 112-6 Commercially prepared Foley Manometer LV pressure monitoring system. *(Redrawn with permission from Holtech Medical.)*

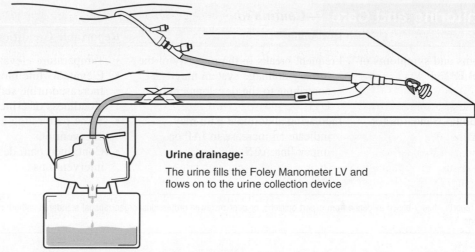

Urine drainage:
The urine fills the Foley Manometer LV and
flows on to the urine collection device

Figure 112-7   The urine fills the Foley Manometer LV and flows on to the urine collection device.
(Redrawn with permission from Holtech Medical.)

Procedure	for Intraabdominal Pressure Monitoring With the Foley Manometer LV System—*Continued*	
Steps	**Rationale**	**Special Considerations**
11. Discard used supplies gloves in the appropriate receptacles. 12. **HH**		

Expected Outcomes

- IAP is monitored in at risk patients.
- IAP is within normal limits.
- Elevated IAP is detected and therapeutic interventions are initiated.

Unexpected Outcomes

- Inability to monitor IAP
- Inaccurate pressure readings obtained
- Development of a hospital-acquired UTI from urinary drainage system manipulation
- Patient discomfort
- Abdominal compartment syndrome develops

Patient Monitoring and Care

Steps	Rationale	Reportable Conditions
		These conditions should be reported if they persist despite nursing interventions.
1. Monitor IAP every 4 hours or more frequently, as prescribed and depending on clinical need.[25,29] **(Level E*)**	Serial measurements detect a trended increase in IAPs, reflecting development of IAH or ACS.	• IAP >12 mm Hg
2. Assess the patient for signs of increasing IAP.[1,6,8,9,12–14,19,25,28,29,31,33]	Patients may have symptoms develop slowly over time. The symptoms may mimic other clinical conditions, such as acute respiratory distress syndrome, acute renal failure, congestive heart failure, and intracranial hypertension.	• Decrease in blood pressure and cardiac output • Oliguria or anuria • Increase in peak inspiratory pressures • Hypoxia and hypercarbia • Elevated ICP

*Level E: Multiple case reports, theory-based evidence from expert opinions, or peer-reviewed professional organizational standards without clinical studies to support recommendations.

Procedure continues on following page

Patient Monitoring and Care —*Continued*

Steps	Rationale	Reportable Conditions
3. Monitor for signs and symptoms of UTI.[23,27] **(Level E*)**	Frequent breaks in the integrity of the urinary drainage system may contribute to the development of UTI.	• Temperature elevation • Elevated white blood cell count • Increased urine sediment or cloudiness of urine
4. Follow institutional standards for assessing pain.	Increasing abdominal pain may indicate an increase in IAP or impending ACS.	• Same pain rating as before interventions • Continued pain despite pain interventions

*Level E: Multiple case reports, theory-based evidence from expert opinions, or peer-reviewed professional organizational standards without clinical studies to support recommendations.

Documentation

Documentation should include the following:
- Patient and family education
- Assessment findings before obtaining IAPs
- Intraabdominal (bladder) pressure value
- Degree of HOB elevation when measurements are not obtained in the supine position.[3,21,32]
- Postprocedure assessment
- Changes in the patient's assessment that indicate onset of IAH or ACS

- The amount of fluid instilled into the bladder to be subtracted from the hourly urine output
- Unexpected outcomes
- Additional interventions
- Pain assessment, interventions, and effectiveness
- Reportable conditions

References and Additional Readings

For a complete list of references and additional readings for this procedure, scan this QR code with any freely available smartphone code reader app, or visit http://booksite.elsevier.com/9780323376624.

PROCEDURE 113

Nasogastric and Orogastric Tube Insertion, Care, and Removal

Carol McGinnis

PURPOSE: Nasogastric (NG) and orogastric (OG) tubes are inserted to facilitate gastric decompression and drainage. This may involve removal of air, retained food materials, secretions, or blood, as well as ingested drugs or toxins. These tubes are also used to deliver fluid and medication and sometimes enteral tube feeding via the gastric route on a short-term basis until a smaller feeding tube or percutaneous tube can be inserted. OG tubes might be inserted when nasal tubes are contraindicated or unable to be placed (e.g., basilar skull or nasal fracture) or sometimes preferentially, as in critical care settings. Consider that the OG tube position may be more difficult to maintain in a conscious, nonintubated patient who might be at risk for tube displacement secondary to tongue movement or difficulty securing the tube.

PREREQUISITE NURSING KNOWLEDGE

- Knowledge of the anatomy and physiology of the gastrointestinal (GI) tract is necessary.
- Knowledge about use and care of the variety of tubes that may be used in clinical practice can help guide practice. Knowing the intended use for the NG tube may help determine the best type and size of the tube.
- Knowledge of means to guide and comfort the patient during a potentially uncomfortable procedure is beneficial.[13,18,20]
- Critical thinking skills are important, especially in terms of determining and monitoring appropriate tube position and assessing that the tube is accomplishing its intended purpose.
- Knowledge of evidence-based measures to verify appropriate tube position is important.
- Knowledge of means to prevent or monitor for adverse effects that could be related to an NG tube, which may include sinus infection, tube misplacement and displacement, tube clogging, pressure ulcers related to tube securement, and patient discomfort.

EQUIPMENT

- NG tube, preferably with numeric markings to help identify depth of insertion and to determine whether the external tube amount has changed
- Water-soluble lubricant
- A 50- or 60-mL syringe with a tip that is appropriate for the tube being inserted and that will meet standards to prevent administration into an inappropriate port.[11]
- Small towel
- Clean gloves
- Stethoscope
- pH strips; follow institutional protocol for quality control and bedside testing

- Emesis bag or basin (keep discretely out of sight) and tissues for eye watering, etc.
- Tape and securement device of choice, which may include transparent dressing or nasal securement device
- Skin prep agent or agent to promote adherence to skin, such as tincture of benzoin; optional (e.g., if skin is oily)
- Indelible marker

Additional equipment, to have available as needed, includes the following:

- Local anesthetic agent (e.g., lidocaine gel) per physician, advanced practice nurse, or other healthcare professional order/institutional protocol. If using lidocaine gel administered via syringe, use tip that meets standards to prevent administration into an inappropriate port.[11]
- Clean cup and supplies if specimens are to be obtained
- Ice chips or a cup of water with a straw if the patient is able to safely swallow fluid

PATIENT AND FAMILY EDUCATION

- Explain the purpose of the NG or OG tube and that efforts will be made to minimize discomfort and provide support. Some patients may appreciate that having an NG is less unpleasant than abdominal distention and vomiting. *Rationale:* Patient and family anxiety may be decreased.
- Explain what the patient might expect as well as the patient's role in assisting with the passage of the tube. *Rationale:* This information may decrease patient anxiety and help during the procedure.

PATIENT ASSESSMENT AND PREPARATION

Patient Assessment

- Obtain history, including recent facial or head injury with basilar skull fracture or transsphenoidal pituitary resection. Determine whether the patient has had prior

1011

nasal or upper GI surgery, esophageal stent, or anatomical anomalies (e.g., deviated nasal septum, esophageal diverticulae or varices, known hiatal hernia). *Rationale:* Contraindications to placing an NG tube include basilar skull fracture and may include nasal or pharyngeal, esophageal, or gastric injury or surgery. Other conditions may require special care or complicate placement.

- If the patient is susceptible to epistaxis or sinusitis, determine which naris is more susceptible. Inquire whether the patient has a preference for which naris should be used for NG intubation. *Rationale:* Preliminary assessment provides an alert to contraindications or potential issues that can be avoided or minimized related to tube placement.
- Assess the nares to determine patency by assessing air exchange and by visual inspection. *Rationale:* The naris with the best airflow may be easiest to access.
- Assess physical status before tube insertion, including assessing for abdominal distention, firmness, tenderness, tympany, and presence or absence, as well as quality, of bowel sounds. *Rationale:* This provides preliminary information that will be useful in monitoring patient status.

Patient Preparation

- Verify that the patient is the correct patient using two identifiers. *Rationale:* Before performing a procedure, the nurse should ensure the correct identification of the patient for the intended intervention.
- Perform a preprocedure verification of patient need for the procedure, and so on, and a timeout, if nonemergent. *Rationale:* This ensures patient safety.
- Ensure that the patient understands what the procedure will involve and how the tube will be helpful. *Rationale:* Patient understanding can reduce anxiety and increase cooperation.
- Assess what helps the patient deal with stressful procedures and offer suggestions for dealing with temporary discomfort (e.g., related to tube insertion, such as distraction, focal point, washcloth or other item to squeeze, breathing techniques). If the patient is restless, having another person present for the patient to have a hand to hold may be helpful. *Rationale:* This maintains the patient's sense of self-control.
- If the patient may safely sip on water, he or she may find this to be helpful during the NG insertion, or it may be overwhelming; assess patient preference. *Rationale:* Following the swallow mechanism may facilitate tube insertion if it is not distracting.

Procedure   for NG or OG Tube Insertion

Steps	Rationale	Special Considerations
1. **HH**		
2. Don **PE** as indicated.		
3. Position the patient in Fowler's or semi-Fowler's position, as possible, providing for patient comfort as well as easy access. If water is to be sipped during the procedure, the head of the bed needs to be appropriately elevated.	Patient and staff comfort, as possible, are important for any procedure. Provide for safety of patient swallow if there is to be sipping of water.	
4. Discuss and provide comfort measures, including administration of lidocaine gel or other agent per physician, advanced practice nurse, or other healthcare professional order via the appropriate naris for NG insertion. If used, follow proper medication administration procedure.	To reduce patient discomfort. Patients may be able to aid in self-comforting means.	A calming nurse presence also provides comfort and a sense of security.
5. Place a clean towel over the patient's upper chest area.	To provide a clean work surface and keep supplies as clean as possible.	Although this is not a sterile procedure, optimal cleanliness is in the patient's best interest.
6. Prepare supplies for easy access (e.g., on clean overbed table).	To aid in organization and avoid unnecessary delays in the procedure.	
7. Perform **HH** again, and don clean gloves.	To aid in cleanliness of procedure.	Repeat if interrupted for nonprocedural-related reasons.

Procedure	for NG or OG Tube Insertion—*Continued*	
Steps	**Rationale**	**Special Considerations**
8. Estimate the length of tube to be inserted: A. The traditional method of measuring insertion distance (from tip of nose to ear or earlobe to xiphoid process or NEX) may underestimate the amount of tube needed to access the gastric fluid pool. Adding the amount of ½ the distance from the tip of the xiphoid process to the umbilicus to this measurement may help ensure that the tube tip opening(s) reach the gastric pool. This method has been called NEMU for nose/ear/midumbilicus.[6–9,12,22] B. Identify the corresponding number on the tube to be inserted or, if without numbers, mark the tube or note identifier at the intended exit point	To help determine the appropriate amount of tube insertion length.	Anatomy differs from patient to patient; know that there is no exact method to determine the best tube insertion length; correlate with clinical condition, aspirated returns, etc.
9. Lubricate the end of the tube with water-soluble lubricant.	To facilitate easier tube passage across potentially dry tissue.	
10. Ensure that the head is in the chin-tuck position if this is not contraindicated.	Aids in accessing the GI tract versus the trachea.	The chin-tuck position has been shown to be more successful in accessing the GI tract than the neutral head position.[3,14] A slight chin-tuck position might be possible if a neck collar is being used.
11. For NG tube insertion: Insert the tube gently through the naris at an angle parallel to the floor of the nasal canal and then with a gentle downward motion as the tube advances through the nasal passage toward the distal pharynx. If resistance is felt, try gentle rotation of the tube tip until it advances beyond the nasal passage. If resistance continues, withdraw the tube and allow the patient to rest, relubricate the tube, and retry or insert the tube via the other naris. **Do not force past resistance.**	To best guide the tube through the opening in the naris toward the nasopharynx.	This may be the most uncomfortable portion of the procedure for the patient. One naris may be more patent that the other.
12. For NG tube insertion: If the patient agrees and is able to swallow safely, sipping on water may enhance NG insertion after the tube is in the oropharynx. If swallowing is not safe, the patient could try dry swallowing to facilitate tube insertion, if desired.	Tube may follow the swallow mechanism and aid insertion. However, this may be distracting to a patient who prefers to have the tube inserted quickly.	Swallowing is not necessary for successful NG insertion, although it may be helpful.

Procedure continues on following page

Procedure for NG or OG Tube Insertion—*Continued*

Steps	Rationale	Special Considerations
13. For OG tube insertion: Insert the tube via the oral cavity, guiding it downward toward the esophagus. If resistance is met, rotate the tube end to guide it toward the esophagus. **Do not force the tube**. If continued resistance is met, stop the procedure and investigate barriers to tube advancement.	To guide the tube into the esophagus, then the stomach.	The tongue might provide a barrier to tube insertion, and gentle guidance over and past it might be helpful.
14. Watch for patient cues (e.g., cough, discomfort) as the tube is advanced.	Patient discomfort could signal potential tube advancement via the respiratory tract or that the tube is kinked or curled in the nasopharyngeal or oral cavity.	Sense of gagging may not be unexpected, but do not advance the tube if the patient is coughing because tube is more likely to enter respiratory tract (pull back to nasopharyngeal area and readvance). Patient cues can be very helpful, although respiratory intubation can occur with no overt signs such as coughing.
15. Continue to advance the tube to the intended distance as previously determined. If there is any resistance, **do not force the tube past resistance.** If the tube is difficult to advance, pull it back to the naso- or oropharyngeal area and gently advance again. Insertion of a small amount of air via syringe can help assess for tube kinking. Gentle resistance may be felt when the tube has been inserted to the distal stomach.	Advance tube to the stomach with sliding motion through the esophagus. Forcing the tube can cause kinking or trauma.	Anatomical anomalies such as hiatal hernias may present challenges to NG insertion. Guide but never force tube insertion.
16. Instill 20–30 mL of air into the tube with a large syringe while listening for the air bolus over the epigastric region.	Although this is unreliable in assessing tube placement alone, it can provide valuable information to add to other information regarding tube placement.	If air is difficult to hear, the tube may not be in the stomach. If the injected air is audible in the mouth area, the tube tip may have curled in the upper GI tract. If unable to instill air, the tube may be kinked.
17. Once the tube has been inserted to the predetermined length, aspirate using a 60-mL syringe to assess for gastric content. The tube may need to be advanced or withdrawn slightly to best obtain gastric content, which may help determine best placement.	Gastric returns can indicate that the hole(s) of the tube are in a pool of gastric fluid.	May need to insert a small volume of air to clear the tube of thick secretions to facilitate aspiration of gastric returns.
18. Observe the quantity, color, and quality of the aspirated returns and store in a clean container to assess pH when the tube has been secured.	Can help differentiate between gastric fluid and returns from the upper small bowel.[15,16] Also provides valuable clinical information (e.g., evidence of recent gastric bleeding or a large volume of dark fluid, which might predispose to reflux or emesis).	Returns from the small bowel might be clear gold in color and perhaps thick and oily as opposed to typical gastric returns.[16] Gastric decompression will be missed if the tube terminates in the upper small bowel.

Procedure for NG or OG Tube Insertion—*Continued*

Steps	Rationale	Special Considerations
19. Cleanse the area for tube securement. Use a skin prep agent as indicated. If using the split-tape method to secure the tube to the nasal area: A. Split the tape lengthwise, leaving 1–2 inches unsplit. B. Clean the top of the nose with alcohol or a skin prep agent and apply an adhesive or tacifier agent (e.g., tincture of benzoin) for adhesiveness as indicated. C. Secure the unsplit tape to the top of the nose and wrap the split ends around the tube in opposite directions, leaving a gap at the tip of the nose to avoid pressure on nasal tissue. Pull up on the tip of the naris during taping to prevent the tube from pressing against the external aspect of the nares *Or* Secure the tube using a nasal securement device, also avoiding pressure on any nasal tissue *Or* If the tube is relatively small and soft, it may be able to secure across the cheek using transparent dressing up to the naris, overlapping two dressings as needed. Secure to the neck area to reduce pressure on the cheek dressings—pinch the tape around the tube, then to the neck for additional security.	Reduces potential for inadvertent tube misplacement. **Avoid pressure from the tube against nasal mucosa with tube securement.** Ensure that there is space between the tube and internal or external aspects of the naris or skin; serious pressure ulcers can and do develop related to NG securement. Using a skin prep agent may aid the adhesiveness of the tape or other dressing material.	If it is possible to adequately secure the tube to the cheek and neck area, the patient may prefer this as opposed to having it hang from the nose.
20. For OG tube securement, the tube might be secured to the endotracheal tube that is often present when this method is used. If the endotracheal tube is not present, secure the tube to the corresponding cheek and neck area, monitoring frequently for potential tube displacement.	The risk of displacement for an orally placed tube is increased when there is difficulty securing it.	Ongoing need for oral gastric access is often considered as endotracheal extubation is planned.
21. Measure the amount of tube that is external (from the naris to the distal tube end) and/or note numerical marking of tube at exit and mark the tube where it exits the naris with an indelible marker.	Provides an objective measure to determine placement; marking aids in quickly determining tube misplacement.	Document in a place that is visible for ongoing monitoring.

Procedure continues on following page

Procedure   for NG or OG Tube Insertion—*Continued*

Steps	Rationale	Special Considerations
22. Assess the pH of aspirated returns.	Gastric returns are typically acidic, with a pH of 1–5.5,[5,10,17] unless affected by medication or feeding. (**Level E***)	Assess the pH before administering proton pump inhibitors (PPI) or histamine (H_2) antagonist to avoid the alkalinizing effect of these agents.
23. Remove gloves, and cleanse hands.	As done with any procedure involving patient contact.	

24. Utilize a variety of bedside practices to assess tube location during the insertion procedure,[2] including:
  A. Obtaining an abdominal x-ray before instillation of fluid or medication into a blindly placed tube (either small or large bore) in the absence of other reliable confirmatory methods of placement verification. [2,4,19,21] (**Level D***)
  B. Aspirating with a 60-mL syringe for gastric returns, assessing quantity, quality, color as well as pH for acidity.
	NG tubes can be misplaced into the esophagus, small intestine, or even lung, and placement must be ascertained before use. Radiographic confirmation of tube placement is currently the only definitive way to confirm tube placement.[2] (**Level D***)	Auscultation of air bolus may be heard in the gastric region, even if the tube terminates in the esophagus, and should not be relied on for verification of placement.

*Level D: Peer-reviewed professional and organizational standards with the support of clinical study recommendations.
*Level E: Multiple case reports, theory-based evidence from expert opinions, or peer-reviewed professional organizational standards without clinical studies to support recommendations.

Procedure   for NG or OG Tube Removal

Steps	Rationale	Special Considerations
1. **HH**		
2. **PE**		
3. Place a clean hand towel on the patient's upper chest area.	Keeps the patient's clothing and linens clean.	There could be fluid splash with this procedure.
4. Verify the order to remove the tube, and identify the patient with two patient identifiers.	Prevents wrong patient or wrong procedure.	Sometimes clamping of the tube is done before discontinuance of the tube to ascertain patient tolerance first.
5. Explain the procedure to the patient and what to expect; reassure the patient that tube removal is less uncomfortable than insertion.	Prevents undue patient anxiety.	
6. Ensure that the patient is comfortably positioned.	For the patient's comfort as well as his or her ability to cooperate with the procedure.	
7. Disconnect from suction if indicated.	Avoids suction and potential trauma to tissues as the tube exits the GI tract.	
8. Have available, or offer the patient, facial tissue.	If indicated for dripping nose or eye watering.	
9. Remove tube securement.	Aids in tube removal.	

Procedure | for NG or OG Tube Removal—*Continued*

Steps	Rationale	Special Considerations
10. Instill small air bolus into the tube to clear secretions from it.	Reduces potential aspiration of gastric fluid with tube removal.	If air is difficult to insert, the tube may have a kink; withdrawing slightly may reduce the kink.
11. Kink or clamp the tubing, ask the patient to hold his or her breath, and then pull out steadily and smoothly into the towel.	Reduces potential aspiration of any fluid and provides a focal point for the patient.	
12. Inspect the tube to ensure that it is intact, and discard it into the appropriate container.	Unlikely that the tube would be damaged, but evidence of tube damage warrants further investigation.	Use caution as one would with any equipment that has been a carrier of bodily fluids.
13. Clean, or assist the patient in cleaning, the naris, and assist with oral care.	Nasal secretions are likely after tube removal; oral care may be very welcome.	Ascertain that damage has not occurred on related body tissue due to the tube or tube securement.

Expected Outcomes

- The NG tube will be inserted safely with no adverse effects or unintended consequences.
- The NG tube will remain appropriately positioned for as long as it is needed, with no adverse effects, including displacement or pressure sores related to the tube and its securement.
- The tube will help accomplish its intended purpose (e.g., the patient will experience relief from gastric distention and emesis, and potential aspiration will be avoided).
- The patient will experience as little discomfort as possible related to the NG tube.

Unexpected Outcomes

- Difficulty is experienced in inserting the tube: If two attempts are unsuccessful, obtain assistance from staff members who are more experienced in this procedure.
- The tube inadvertently intubates the respiratory tract. Immediate recognition of this will reduce other potential adverse events.
- The tube becomes displaced. Monitoring the external amount can help in recognizing this, and tube securement can help with prevention.[2] To determine the amount of tube that is internal, subtract the length of the external tube from the total length of the tube (see manufacturer package insert). Compare with typical measurement assessment, but also consider that the tube could have become coiled in the back of the pharynx or esophagus and monitor for this possibility as well.
- Gastric content is not able to be aspirated manually or via suction. Reassess tube placement; the tube tip may not be deep enough, or the tube may have intubated the upper small intestine. Ensure that the tube is not clogged.
- The patient will develop a pressure ulcer from pressure of the tube against nasal or other tissue. Secure the tube without pressure on surrounding tissue and monitor for pressure frequently.

Patient Monitoring and Care

Steps	Rationale	Reportable Conditions
		These conditions should be reported if they persist despite nursing interventions.
1. Monitor tube securement and amount external before use and every 4 hours or per institutional protocol.	Ensures that the NG or OG tube is secure.	- Report deviations to the physician, advanced practice nurse, or other healthcare professional.

Procedure continues on following page

Patient Monitoring and Care —*Continued*

Steps	Rationale	Reportable Conditions
2. Monitor for signs of pressure on surrounding tissue before use and every 4 hours or per institutional protocol. The tube should be secured in a different manner if there are signs of pressure on surrounding tissue. Report signs of tissue damage to the physician, advanced practice nurse, or other healthcare professional.	Reduces the potential for tissue damage or pressure ulcers.	• Report signs of tissue damage to the physician, advanced practice nurse, or other healthcare professional.
3. Ensure that the tube is connected to low suction, as prescribed. Consider manual aspiration of gastric content if suction is not being used and the patient exhibits nausea or other signs of potential for aspiration.	Avoid a high level of continuous suction. Maintain the sump feature of the tube, if used, to reduce potential tissue damage.	• Nausea • Signs of aspiration
4. Assess and measure output (volume, color, quality) every 4 hours and as indicted. Document output and intake via the tube. Compare overall intake to output daily, as well as trending pattern.	Helps quantify and characterize output for ongoing clinical correlation. Detect potential fluid imbalance. Patients with a large NG output are at risk for fluid, electrolyte and possibly acid-base imbalance. Correlate with laboratory values that might reflect a trend toward dehydration and/or electrolyte imbalance.	• Sudden cessation of output, especially if coupled with increased patient discomfort, may signal tube misplacement or clogging, problem with suction, etc. • Report pattern of output greater than intake.
5. Assess and monitor patient status including abdominal assessment every 4 hours and as indicated.	Provides information about clinical condition as well as effectiveness of NG suction.	• Increased abdominal distress
6. Irrigate the NG or OG tube as needed.	Maintains tube patency. Clean warm water, if used, may be better tolerated than cold fluid.	• Lack of patency despite interventions
7. Unless contraindicated, keep the head of the bed elevated 30 degrees or more.	A patient with an NG tube may not be able to clear secretions well; reduces risk for aspiration.[1,14]	
8. Follow institutional standards for assessing pain. Administer analgesia as prescribed.	Identifies the need for pain interventions. NG use can be associated with patient discomfort.	• Continued pain despite pain interventions
9. Keep equipment used for the NG tube (e.g., syringes) as clean and dry as possible and change per institutional protocol.	Moisture provides media for bacterial growth.	

Documentation

Documentation should include the following:
- Type and size of tube
- Naris of insertion
- Numerical mark at the tube exit and/or external length in an area where it can be monitored on an ongoing basis
- A description and volume of aspirated returns
- How placement was verified
- Use of anesthetic agent if used
- Assessment of change in patient condition (e.g., abdomen more soft, less distended with fluid removal or fluid administration, if used for that purpose)
- Any adverse events related to insertion or indwelling tube
- NG tube removal date and time and any adverse events related to tube removal

References and Additional Readings

For a complete list of references and additional readings for this procedure, scan this QR code with any freely available smartphone code reader app, or visit http://booksite.elsevier.com/9780323376624.

PROCEDURE

114

Molecular Adsorbent Recirculating System (MARS)

Mary D. Still

PURPOSE: Molecular Adsorbent Recirculating System (MARS) therapy is a technology that combines traditional continuous renal replacement therapy (CRRT) technology with the added benefit of the removal of large protein-bound particles via albumin dialysis. The MARS system supports rapid removal of toxic substances that contribute to acute liver injury.

PREREQUISITE NURSING KNOWLEDGE

- The liver is responsible for synthesis of clotting factors, detoxification of toxins, breakdown of hormones and medications, metabolism of essential nutrients, and biotransformation. When the liver fails, the loss of these functions leads to the accumulation of lethal toxins with life-threatening complications.
- Acute liver failure (ALF) is defined as the onset of encephalopathy that occurs within 8 weeks of symptom appearance in the absence of any preexisting liver disease.[1]
- In the United States, the most common cause of ALF is paracetamol (acetaminophen) toxicity and idiosyncratic drug reactions (i.e., antibiotics, antiseizure, and antidepressants). The overall outcome for these patients is dependent on early recognition, and intervention to address the cause of the disease.
- Over the past 10 years, new technology, collaborative medical management, and liver transplantation have improved the outcome for these patients. Regardless of the cause of hepatic failure, frequent clinical manifestations of encephalopathy, altered coagulation, and multiple organ failure can occur.
- Despite advances in critical care therapies, liver failure, acute or chronic, continues to carry a high mortality.[1]
- Extracorporeal albumin liver dialysis was designed for use as support in ALF until effective liver function returns or liver transplantation becomes available. MARS is a two-part dialysis system designed to support the lost detoxification function of the liver.[6] The advantage of this technology is that it uses human albumin to cleanse the protein-bound toxins along with a bicarbonate-based dialysate to clear water-soluble elements. By supporting the injured liver and decreasing the opportunity for encephalopathy, coagulopathy, and multiple organ failure to occur, time to allow for return of function or transplant is provided.
- MARS technology is approved for use in ALF from drug overdoses and acute toxicity of unknown origin by the US Food and Drug Administration (FDA). Substances removed by this combined technology include but are not limited to ammonia, bilirubin, bile acids, aromatic amino acids, nitric oxide, tryptophan, copper, creatinine, protoporphyrin, urea, and diazepam.[6] CRRT is an extracorporeal blood purification therapy by which the kidneys are supported 24 hours per day to remove circulating toxins via a dialysis filter. This process is commonly applied when a patient cannot hemodynamically tolerate conventional hemodialysis.
- CRRT is an integral part of the MARS system. The blood pump in the CRRT machine drives blood through the MARS dialyzer to remove larger protein-bound toxins using albumin as the dialysate. The toxin-filled albumin is then pumped by the MARS.
- Albumin is pumped back to the CRRT machine, where it is cleansed of water-soluble molecules via a standard dialysate solution. CRRT is a critical adjunct in the management of acute liver failure because it removes ammonia, a substrate believed to play a large role in hepatic encephalopathy and subsequent cerebral edema.
- MARS therapy has been approved in the United States for use in the treatment of drug overdose and poisonings resulting in ALF. In the ALF patient with a high expected mortality, MARS treatment is recommended to begin as soon as the diagnosis is made and the patient is transferred to a liver transplant facility.[6] The MARS system is primed with both standard dialysis solution and albumin. The procedure is designed to remove albumin bound toxins in the blood by passing the blood through the MARS Flux filter where it is cleansed via an albumin dialysate. The albumin dialysate is then circulated through the CRRT diaFlux filter where it is passed through an activated charcoal and an anion exchange resin filter to remove the bound toxins from the albumin. This process regenerates the albumin to be circulated back to the dialyzer for additional removal of toxins and bilirubin.
- Setup time may vary, but the recommended mode for treatment is intermittent with treatment lengths of 8 hours per day for 3 consecutive days.

- CRRT may be used between therapy sessions to support renal function and continue the filtration of smaller particles such as ammonia.
- Adverse events such as mild thrombocytopenia, and bleeding have been observed.[10] Disseminated intravascular coagulation (DIC), also described in ALF, has also been observed. Kramer described three patients with DIC that occurred in the intervention group studied, and two experienced fatal outcomes.[4]
- MARS is associated with the same risk as other extracorporeal devices, including air embolus, bleeding, infection, and hypothermia. Patient selection and timing are critical to the success of this treatment. Some of the toxins that MARS can remove are bilirubin, bile acids, phenols, mercaptans, dioxin-like substances, tryptophan, copper, and iron.[1]

EQUIPMENT

- Prismaflex CRRT machine with MARS software enabled.
- MARS kit (contains three filters, Prismaflex filter, and units 1 to 4 to set up the MARS dialysis system)
- Priming solutions:
  - ❖ Three 1-L bags of 0.9% normal saline for priming the system
  - ❖ One 5-L bag of Prismasate for priming the MARS
- Prescribed anticoagulant
- Prescribed replacement solutions.
- Albumin dialysate: 400 mL (100 g 25% albumin in 200 mL of 0.9% normal saline = total volume 600 mL)
- Nonsterile gloves
- Antiseptic solution

Additional equipment, to have available as needed, includes the following:

- Arterial catheter and single-pressure system
- Ultrasound equipment

PATIENT AND FAMILY EDUCATION

- Explain the purpose and anticipated outcome of MARS therapy to the patient (if possible) and family. Review with them what to expect during and after the three treatments. *Rationale:* It is important for patients and families to understand the MARS system and how it works. CRRT has been a standard for treatment of acute kidney injury/failure for many years. The new MARS system is an added tool to CRRT to help in the removal of toxic substances normally removed by a healthy liver. In the absence of a healthy liver, MARS therapy supports liver function. The treatment will last 8 hours each day. The timing of treatments may vary based on transplant candidacy, organ availability, patient's response, and overall goals of care and is evaluated daily. As the blood is cleaned by the albumin, the white resin filter will turn dark, reflecting the absorption of toxic particles.
- Explain all elements of the MARS procedure and setup to the patient (if possible) and family/significant other before initiating treatment. Answer any questions that develop during the process of preparation of the system. *Rationale:* Explanation provides information and may decrease patient and family anxiety.

- Explain to the patient (if possible) and family that once the therapy is initiated, mobility may be limited. Review institutional guidelines and standards for mobility in critical care. *Rationale:* Explanation provides information and may decrease patient and family anxiety. Patients receiving this therapy are often critically ill and remain on bed rest, but those who are more stable at the time of the treatment may not require extreme mobility restrictions.
- Explain the need for careful monitoring of the patient for complications. *Rationale:* Both the underlying disease process and the MARS therapy can result in complications. Explanation provides information and may decrease patient and family anxiety.

PATIENT ASSESSMENT AND PREPARATION

Patient Assessment

- Perform baseline cardiovascular, neurological, respiratory, and integumentary assessments before initiating therapy. *Rationale: Cardiovascular:* Attention should be paid to fluid management and hemodynamic monitoring. Monitor for dysrhythmias related to electrolyte imbalance and fluid shifts. Hypotension may also occur due to decrease of plasma proteins in the liver. *Respiratory:* Assess for the ability to protect the airway. Change in mental status may alter this, and intubation may be required to protect the airway. *Neurological assessment:* Neurological changes can range from simple personality changes to coma. The onset of encephalopathy can also occur quickly with the development of asterixis, delirium, hyperreflexia, seizures, and coma. Signs of increased intracranial pressure should also be monitored such as changes in level of consciousness (LOC) pupillary response and ability to follow commands. Hepatic encephalopathy, arterial ammonia greater than 150 mmol/L, hyponatremia seizure, and pupil changes may indicate a poor prognosis[14,15] *Integumentary:* Special attention should also be given to the patient's skin integrity, not only because of the disease process, but also because of limited mobility. Minimize pressure and maintain function with active and passive range of motion.
- If computed tomography (CT) or magnetic resonance imaging (MRI) are required, these and any other diagnostic testing should be performed before initiation of MARS therapy. Once the therapy is operational, transport of the patient for testing should be avoided to limit discontinuation of the therapy. *Rationale:* CT or MRI of the head provides baseline evidence of cerebral edema. Manufacturer guidelines for MARS, unlike the CRRT system, do not support recirculation via the albumin circuit. The MARS circuit is bathed with albumin, presenting a greater risk of clogging. No studies have been completed to date that validate recirculation, which would allow for temporary disconnection of the patient from the system for transport.
- Obtain laboratory specimens as prescribed, including toxicology screens, ammonia, phosphorus, coagulation studies, hematocrit and hemoglobin values, basic metabolic panel, renal and liver function tests, and blood type.

Rationale: Baseline information is necessary so that appropriate interventions can be implemented before initiation of MARS in order to correct fluid and electrolyte derangements. This will allow the effect of therapy to be more accurately monitored.

Patient Preparation

- Verify that the patient is the correct patient using two identifiers. *Rationale:* Before performing a procedure, the nurse should ensure the correct identification of the patient before the intervention is initiated.
- Ensure that informed consent has been obtained. *Rationale:* Informed consent protects the rights of the patient and makes a competent decision possible for the patient.
- Assist the physician or advanced practice nurse with obtaining necessary vascular access, including a dialysis catheter, 13 Fr or greater in size, and additional central access for monitoring and medication administration.[17] *Rationale:* Patent access is essential to successful dialysis.
- The recommended site for line placement of vascular access for MARS should be the right internal jugular vein and the second choice should be the left internal jugular vein. These (or other) veins are accessed under ultrasound (US) guidance, which is recommended to minimize the risk of arterial puncture. *Rationale:* These vessels allow for successful therapy.
- Ensure there is adequate blood flow in the dialysis catheter, and instill appropriate anticoagulation per institutional guidelines and/or manufacturer recommendations to prevent clotting or occlusion of the lumens. *Rationale:* This enhances the patency of the line.
- The line should be placed and verified by chest radiograph before initiation of CRRT/MARS therapy.[16] *Rationale:* This ensures proper anatomical placement of the access catheter.
- Prophylactic FFP transfusion to improve coagulopathy in patients with ALF is not recommended. *Rationale:* This action does not reduce the risk of significant bleeding or transfusion requirements, and it can mask the trend of international normalized ratio (INR) as a prognostic marker as well as increasing the risk of volume overload and occlusion of the circuit.
- The patient will be in an intensive care unit (ICU) and placed on a cardiac monitor, with an arterial line. *Rationale:* This allows for close physiological monitoring.
- Ensure that the patient understands pre-procedural information. Answer questions as they arise, and reinforce information as needed. *Rationale:* Understanding of previously taught information is evaluated and reinforced.

Procedure	**for Molecular Adsorbent Recirculating System (MARS)**	
Steps	Rationale	Special Considerations
1. **HH**		
2. **PE**		
3. Secure MARS and CRRT machines to bedside.	Place the MARS machine to the right of the Prismaflex. This will allow accurate set up of lines for proper system function.	
4. Verify that MARS/CRRT orders, including therapy management, are completed by the appropriate physicians, advanced nurse practitioners, or other healthcare professionals.	Orders are needed to maintain machine settings for accurate removal of both volume and toxins.	
5. Confirm accurate placement, and size, 13 Fr or greater of hemodialysis catheter and verify blood flow of dialysis catheter to ensure patency.	This size is necessary to provide adequate blood flow to the CRRT and MARS circuits.	
6. Place the MARS machine and the Prismaflex machine side by side with the Prismaflex to the right of the MARS machine.	The MARS is dependent on the Prismaflex blood pump to circulate blood through both machines.	
7. Level the MARS Flux and the diaFLUX filters with one another.	The blood lines connecting the blood flow between the machines require that the machines be aligned appropriately for this to occur.	

Procedure **for Molecular Adsorbent Recirculating System (MARS)—*Continued***

Steps	Rationale	Special Considerations
8. Plug machines into emergency power outlets, and turn on both machines.	Emergency outlets are necessary to prevent interruption of blood pump and continuation of treatment.	There are two power buttons on the MARS machine. One is located in the back and the other on the front of the machine. The Prismaflex machine power button is located on the side of the machine.
9. Open the MARS treatment kit and supplies. Follow directions on the Prismaflex screen to set up the system: A. Follow initial setup screens for entering patient information and MARS/CRRT therapy mode. B. Closely follow each instruction line on the Prismaflex screen, and check off each step as it is completed. C. Install the Prismaflex filter system as directed. D. Install the MARS Flux filters, resin, and charcoal filters on the MARS machine (units 1–4 and accessory kit) as directed. E. Connect the lines as directed by the Prismaflex screen. F. Hang the CRRT solutions as prescribed, and initiate the prime solution when the systems are loaded. (**Level M***)	Step-by-step instructions are located on the Prismaflex screen and should be used for set up. Verify that each step on each screen has been completed before moving to the next screen.	Follow manufacturer's recommendations when initiating set up of the Prismaflex. Any deviation from the directions can result in delays in patient care and the MARS/CRRT system not working properly.
10. After the priming is complete, prepare the anticoagulation if prescribed. A. Medication: i. Unfractionated heparin. *Or* ii. Trisodium citrate. B. If heparin is used, initiate the anticoagulation as you attach to the patient. If citrate is ordered, it is delivered via the pre–blood pump and should be part of the Prismaflex system.	Anticoagulation may be used to prevent clotting of the CRRT circuit. Systemic unfractionated heparin may be prescribed for patients with a lower risk of bleeding and trisodium citrate may be prescribed for patients with a higher risk of bleeding.[10] Regional citrate anticoagulation in patients with liver failure is feasible. **Citrate anticoagulation was identified as providing superior patency of the extracorporeal circuit.**[5,7] Avoidance of anticoagulation during MARS can result in significant loss of treatment time, due to downtime.[5,7]	If trisodium citrate is used, calcium replacement must be initiated based on ionized calcium (iCa) levels and need to be monitored during treatment. Titration of a continuous infusion is based on the level of iCa++.[12] Patients may require additional supplements of calcium during treatment beyond what a continuous infusion can provide. Calcium chloride may be prescribed if difficulty is met maintaining stable calcium levels.[2] Calcium gluconate may also be used for the prevention and/or management of a hypocalcemic state. Goal: Maintain ionized calcium between 1.1 and 1.35 mmol/L.[3]

*Level M: Manufacturer's recommendations only.

Procedure continues on following page

Procedure	for Molecular Adsorbent Recirculating System (MARS)—*Continued*	
Steps	**Rationale**	**Special Considerations**
11. Step 1. Prime the Prismaflex. *Prime Cycle 1:* Three 1-L saline bags are used for the initial Prismaflex prime. *Prime Cycle 2:* A 5-L dialysate bag is hung on the MARS machine; follow the Prismaflex instructions.	Use 3 L of normal saline (NS) to prime the access line, MARS Flux and return line.	
12. Step 2. MARS priming. *Prime Cycle 3:* 600 mL albumin. (**Level M***)	Use a 5-L bag on the MARS machine to prime the albumin circuit, and add 600 mL of albumin to the MARS circuit to complete the final prime of the system.	
13. Set the pump rates as prescribed: A. Blood pump. B. Albumin pump. C. Replacement pump. D. Anticoagulant if prescribed placed on the pre–blood pump. E. Dialysis pump: Fluid removal rates.	Flow rates for the blood pump and albumin pump should be set in the range of 180–220 mL/min. Provides volume and electrolyte solutions that return to the patient and are adjusted based on patient needs. All fluids placed on the pre–blood pump are removed in the effluent and do not interface in any way with the patient, only within the system. This prevents an effect on the patient's coagulation. This pump works through diffusion to correct underlying metabolic problems. The dialysate is dependent on buffering agents, electrolytes and glucose. The dialysate solution ordered should reflect normal plasma values to achieve homeostasis.	The blood and albumin pump rates should be equal during therapy.
14. Remove gloves, and wash hands.		
15. Put on new gloves and a mask.	Prevents contamination of the dialysis catheter when it is opened for access and attachment to the MARS circuit. Remember you must start both the MARS and Prismaflex in order to initiate MARS therapy treatment.	
16. Cleanse the dialysis catheter site connection.	The catheter site connector should be cleansed with alcohol before access to ensure the surface is free of bacteria. Wipe the cap in a brisk motion with an alcohol wipe and allow to dry.	

*Level M: Manufacturer's recommendations only.

Procedure	for Molecular Adsorbent Recirculating System (MARS)—*Continued*	
Steps	**Rationale**	**Special Considerations**

17. Clamp both access and return catheters.
  A. Attach sterile syringe to access line, unclamp patient line, and withdraw blood to ensure access is patent. Clamp the line.
  B. Place the unclamped access line from the Prismaflex machine to the patient access port and open access (unclamp).
  C. Next, attach a syringe to the return access line of the patient, and unclamp and flush to assess patency. Clamp the line.
  D. Attach the return line from the Prismaflex to the patient return line. Unclamp the line.
  E. Initiate blood pumps for both the Prismaflex and MARS machines.
	Provides for a safe and patent access between patient and machine. If any resistance is met when flushing the lines initially, stop and reassess patency of the line.	Before connecting the blood return line to the patient, make sure there is no air in the line between the air detector and the patient end of the line.

18. Initiate treatment, and document initial pressures.	Allows trending of pressures with awareness of the baseline.	

19. During therapy, monitor the system pressures and alarms and troubleshoot:
  A. Albumin pump.
  B. pIN pressure and pOUT pressure.
  C. Transmembrane pressure (TMP) and pressure drop.
  D. Access pressure.
  E. Return pressure.
  F. Effluent (bag change required).
  G. Blood leak (machine will stop if this occurs and will clamp the blood return line).
	The albumin pump will stop if an alarm occurs with this pump. pIN and pOUT alarms are most often related to a line being clamped or kinked.
	TMP: Transmembrane pressure exceeds membrane pressure limit. MARS Flux filter and diaFLUX filter combined transmembrane pressure exceeds membrane pressure limit. Too much fluid is being removed (UFR = patient fluid removal rate + replacement solution rate + pre-blood pump rate).
	Pressure drop filter pressure drop exceeds limit for the filter in use, or both the filter is clotting.
	Access pressure and return pressure alarms are related to kinking of the line or the system beginning to clog or clot.
	Effluent alarms usually indicate the effluent bag is full and needs to be changed.
	Blood leak is a critical alarm that will stop the blood pumps because it indicates that an inappropriate presence of blood in the system has been observed by the blood leak sensor or that tubing was not installed correctly in the detector.
	Follow manufacturer's recommendations for response to alarms if they occur.	

Procedure continues on following page

Procedure   for Molecular Adsorbent Recirculating System (MARS)—*Continued*

Steps	Rationale	Special Considerations
20. Maintain the level of the albumin dialysate in the large drip chamber of unit 2 between the two red LED lights and assess at regular intervals to ensure this remains stable. (**Level M***)	This chamber reflects blood flow and pressure via the albumin pump. Keeping the level in this chamber reflects a stable pressure. As pressure increases, this level with rise and the pIN pressure alarm will sound.	
21. Remove **PE** and discard used supplies.		
22. **HH**		

*Level M: Manufacturer's recommendations only.

Expected Outcomes

- Improvement of severe hepatic encephalopathy
- Improvement in hemodynamic impairment as a result of decompensating liver disease
- Improvement in renal function with patient with renal insufficiency
- Effective removal of larger molecular albumin-bound toxins

Unexpected Outcomes

- Hypocalcemia
- Bleeding secondary to use of anticoagulant
- Clotting and clogging of system or catheter
- Alkalosis secondary to citrate infusion
- Hypophosphatemia
- Hyponatremia
- Progressive cerebral edema, brainstem herniation

Patient Monitoring and Care

Steps	Rationale	Reportable Conditions
		These conditions should be reported if they persist despite nursing interventions.
1. Patients may be maintained on bed rest during the entire therapy. The patient's level of consciousness will determine how interactive and mobile the patient can be. A. The patient should be turned every 2 hours during treatment if hemodynamically stable. B. Passive range-of-motion exercises may be needed to decrease issues related to limited mobility and prevent the complications of immobility.	Acute liver failure results in altered mental status ranging from simple confusion to coma. The pathophysiology of this is not fully understood but may be related to circulating toxins such as ammonia and other substances which cross the blood-brain barrier and affect the neurological status, level of consciousness and level of activity.[7] Interventions can reduce risk of complications of immobility.	• Complications of immobility, such as pressure ulcer formation
2. Avoid conditions and interventions that might increase intracranial pressure (ICP) when possible. These include high positive end-expiratory pressure, frequent movements (agitation), neck vein compression, fever, arterial hypertension, hypoxia, coughing, sneezing, seizures, head-low position, and respiratory suctioning.[10]	Elevated ICP is a dangerous sequela of acute liver failure and is worsened by these conditions and interventions.	

Patient Monitoring and Care —*Continued*

Steps	Rationale	Reportable Conditions
3. If using citrate for anticoagulation, calcium replacement will be necessary: Calcium gluconate infusion may be used. • Monitor ionized calcium level 1 hour after initiation of therapy and then every 2 hours until therapy concludes. • Maintain iCA++ between 1.1–1.3 mmol/L[3]. • Assess for citrate lock, a condition which occurs when the total serum calcium levels rises with a serious decreasing level of ionized calcium, which occurs due to a delivery of citrate which exceeds the capacity of the liver to metabolize or the CRRT to clear.	Adding citrate to the blood will bind the free calcium (ionized) in the blood, thus inhibiting clotting. Regional citrate anticoagulation results in removing calcium from the blood before it enters the CRRT filter. To maintain normal patient blood calcium levels, calcium must be reinfused into the patient's blood after the CRRT filter. A separate access for calcium infusion is recommended.[9] Calcium binds to citrate before the filter to prevent clotting. The post filter return is depleted of calcium, resulting in hypocalcaemia. Alkalosis: "Citrate lock"—Citrate is metabolized by the liver and kidneys to bicarbonate. Therefore patients with liver failure are at greater risk of developing citrate toxicity, resulting in metabolic complications such as alkalosis. However, highly positive citrate balance is prevented in protocols that prescribe much higher hemofiltration/UF rates and thereby provide greater buffer clearance.[8,9,11]	• Hypocalcemia: Report level <1.0 for replacement • Citrate lock • Alkalosis
4. Obtain laboratory specimens as prescribed or per institutional standards. Results to monitor include: A. Complete blood count (CBC). B. Albumin. C. Coagulation panel including international normalized ratio (INR); factors VII, V, and VIII; antithrombin. D. Liver panel. E. Arterial ammonia level. F. Sodium (Na++). G. Phosphorus. H. Glucose. I. Thromboelastogram (TEG) measured every day in the setting of profound coagulopathy.[14]	CBC: address for evidence of bleeding. This may occur as a result of liver failure Albumin: Protein is broken down by the liver. Albumin will be decreased as the liver fails. Albumin maintains oncotic pressure within the vasculature, and vessels become leaky to volume resuscitation when the albumin is low. Monitor changes in clotting. Evidence of improvement related to MARS therapy. Enzymes should be stabilizing, ammonia should be decreasing as evidence of improvement. Ammonia is an important factor related to cerebral edema and encephalopathy. For patients with ALI/ALF, hyponatremia should be strictly avoided, as it may exacerbate cerebral edema. Phosphorus replacement is critical in the liver recovery process; hypophosphatemia should be monitored for and treated aggressively.	• Report hemoglobin <7.5g/dL • Report INR >2.0 • Report elevated ammonia level • Abnormal sodium levels <145 mEq/L or >155 mEq/L • Hypophosphatemia with sodium levels <0.8–1.5 mmol/L • Blood glucose <80 mg/dL • Abnormal TEG measurement

Procedure continues on following page

Patient Monitoring and Care —*Continued*

Steps	Rationale	Reportable Conditions
	Other electrolyte concentrations (phosphate, magnesium, and bicarbonate) should be kept within the normal range.[2] Carbohydrate metabolism is an important function of the liver. As the liver fails, it becomes unable to break down carbohydrates and blood glucose begins to drop. When the INR is >7, TEG confirms marked prolongation in the rate of clot formation; FFP transfusion to maintain INR between 5 and 7 is advised.[14]	
5. Monitor the dialysis access site and lines for kinks, clots, leaking, redness, swelling, or drainage (see Procedure 115).	Access pressure alarms are built into the system of the CRRT machine and will alert staff to any significant risk issues. The greatest risks associated with the catheter are kinking of the line, dislodgement, or infection. Monitor the line carefully with change in position of the patient to ensure it is not accidently kinked or dislodged.	• Accidental catheter dislodgement, clots, leaking • Signs of central line associated bloodstream infection (CLABSI)
6. Monitor vital signs every hour for the duration of therapy and more frequently if needed.	Hemodynamic instability is often associated with acute liver insufficiency as a consequence of endogenous accumulation of vasoactive agents in the blood. This results in systemic vasodilatation, a decrease of systemic vascular resistance, arterial hypotension, and an increase of cardiac output that gives rise to a hyper-dynamic circulation. Bradycardia may occur during the therapy.[13] If cerebral edema is identified on CT scan, mean arterial pressure (MAP) may be required to be ≥70 to maintain cerebral perfusion.	• MAP <70 or below the prescribed level • Increase in heart rate 20% or more above baseline • Decrease in systolic blood pressure 20–30 mm Hg or more below baseline.
7. MAP >70 mm Hg.	Strategy used to maintain cerebral perfusion pressure (CPP) >70 mm Hg. Adequate perfusion pressure is necessary to effectively perfuse the brain.	• MAP <70 • CPP <65 • Worsening encephalopathy/ neurological deterioration
8. Closely monitor respirations, oxygen saturation, and lung sounds.	Alerts the team to respiratory problems that may need further interventions.	• Respiratory rate <10 or >20 • Spo$_2$ <92% • Respiratory decompensation

Patient Monitoring and Care —*Continued*

Steps	Rationale	Reportable Conditions
9. Monitor the neurological status every hour. • Assess for evidence of pain every 4 hours and document. • Hypothermia may be used for neurological protection (see Procedure 100).	Neurological changes may indicate increasing intracranial pressure and the need for intervention.	• Abnormal pupil size and/or reactions • Changes in level of consciousness • Pain rating >4 should be reported
10. Follow institutional standards for assessing pain. Administer analgesia as prescribed.	Identifies need for pain interventions.	• Continued pain despite pain interventions

Documentation

Documentation should include the following:
- Patient and family education
- Patient tolerance of therapy
- CRRT system pressures hourly (access, return pressure, effluent pressure, TMP, and filter pressure)
- From the MARS system: pIN and pOUT, blood flow, and alarm limits, including lower pressure alarm (set 100 mm Hg below pIN pressure)
- Date and time therapy initiated
- Mode of CRRT (CVVHD, CVVHDF, or CVVH)
- Blood flow/albumin pump rates
- Location and condition of insertion site and any signs or symptoms of infection
- Vital signs throughout the treatment
- Unexpected outcomes
- Nursing interventions
- Laboratory assessment data
- iCA++ levels and calcium replacement rate
- Anticoagulation rate (if citrate, pre–blood pump rate, white scale)
- Dialysis fluid and rate (green scale)
- Replacement fluid and rate (purple scale)
- Patient fluid removal rate

References and Additional Readings

For a complete list of references and additional readings for this procedure, scan this QR code with any freely available smartphone code reader app, or visit http://booksite.elsevier.com/9780323376624.

PROCEDURE

115

Paracentesis (Perform) AP

Eleanor Fitzpatrick

PURPOSE: Abdominal paracentesis is performed to remove fluid from the peritoneal cavity for diagnostic or therapeutic purposes.

PREREQUISITE NURSING KNOWLEDGE

- Knowledge of anatomy and physiology of the abdomen is important to avoid unexpected outcomes.
- Intestines and bladder lie immediately beneath the abdominal surface.
- Large volumes of ascitic fluid tend to float in the air-filled bowel toward the midline, where the bowel may be perforated during the procedure.
- The cecum is relatively fixed and is much less mobile than the sigmoid colon; therefore bowel perforations are more frequent in the right lower quadrant than in the left.
- Peritoneal fluid is normally straw-colored serous fluid secreted by the cells of the peritoneum. Grossly bloody fluid in the abdomen is abnormal.
- The peritoneal fluid collected is used in evaluation and diagnosis of ascites, acute abdominal conditions such as peritonitis or pancreatitis, and blunt or penetrating trauma to the abdomen.
- Therapeutic paracentesis is used to reduce intraabdominal and diaphragmatic pressures, to relieve dyspnea and respiratory compromise, and to prevent hernia formation and diaphragmatic rupture.[2,8,11] These complications are seen in patients with tense, refractory ascites and failed medical interventions such as sodium restriction and diuresis.[2,3,5,11,15]
- Cirrhosis is the most common cause of ascites formation. However, ascitic fluid is produced as a result of a variety of other conditions.[2,5,7,10] These conditions may include interference in venous return because of heart failure, constrictive pericarditis, or tricuspid valve insufficiency; obstruction of flow in the vena cava or portal vein; disturbance in electrolyte balance, such as sodium retention; depletion of plasma proteins because of nephrotic syndrome or starvation; lymphoma, leukemia, or neoplasms that involve the liver or mediastinum; ovarian malignant disease; and chronic pancreatitis.
- Analysis of the ascitic fluid can determine the cause of ascites. A serum-to-ascites albumin gradient should be calculated by subtracting the ascitic fluid albumin level from the serum albumin value. This calculation differentiates portal hypertensive from nonportal hypertensive ascites.[2,3,5,9,11]
- Paracentesis is contraindicated in patients with an acute abdomen, who need immediate surgery. Coagulopathy should preclude paracentesis only in the case of clinically evident fibrinolysis or clinically evident disseminated intravascular coagulation.[3,10] Absolute contraindications include an acute abdomen, an uncooperative patient, and disseminated intravascular coagulopathy. Relative contraindications include coagulopathy, abdominal adhesions, infected abdominal wall at the entry site, distended bowel or bladder, and pregnancy.[15]
- Caution should be used when paracentesis is performed in patients with severe bowel distention, previous abdominal surgery (especially pelvic surgery), pregnancy (use open technique after first trimester), distended bladder that cannot be emptied with a Foley catheter, or obvious infection at intended site of insertion (cellulitis or abscess).
- The insertion site should be midline one third the distance from the umbilicus to the symphysis, or 2 to 3 cm below the umbilicus (Fig. 115-1). An alternate position is a point one third the distance from the umbilicus to the anterior iliac crest (left side preferred especially in the obese patient or in those requiring removal of large volumes of fluid).[2,10,11,13]
- Ultrasound scan can be used before paracentesis to locate fluid and during the procedure to guide insertion of catheter.
- If ascitic fluid is difficult to localize with physical examination because of obesity or other conditions, ultrasound is effective in identifying the fluid and critical structures which are to be avoided during the procedure.[10,12] Endoscopic transgastric ultrasound scan has also been used in the diagnosis of malignant ascites.[2,13]
- A semipermanent catheter or a shunt may be an option for patients with rapidly reaccumulating ascites.[2,3,10]
- When large-volume paracentesis (>5 L) is performed in patients with cirrhosis and other disorders, the infusion of albumin, (6 to 8 g/L) of fluid removed, may prevent the onset of circulatory compromise associated with massive fluid shifting.[3,9-11,15] Albumin administration may be effective in preventing paracentesis-induced circulatory dysfunction, the most common complication after the procedure.[13-15] Albumin infusion is recommended with large-volume paracentesis.[1]

AP This procedure should be performed only by physicians, advanced practice nurses, and other healthcare professionals (including critical care nurses) with additional knowledge, skills, and demonstrated competence per professional licensure or institutional standard.

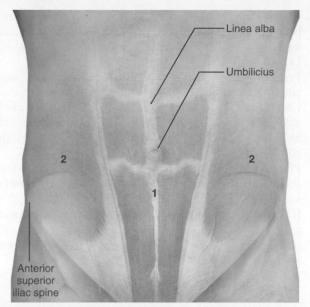

Figure 115-1 Preferred sites for paracentesis: *1,* Primary site is infraumbilical in midline through linea alba. *2,* Preferred alternate (lateral rectus) site is in either lower quadrant, approximately 4 to 5 cm cephalad and medial to the anterior superior iliac spine. *(From Roberts JR:* Roberts and Hedges' clinical procedures in emergency medicine, *ed 6, Philadelphia, 2014, Saunders.)*

EQUIPMENT

- Commercially prepared paracentesis kit if available
- Nonsterile gloves, sterile gloves, mask, gown
- Antiseptic solution (e.g., 2% chlorhexidine-based preparation)
- Sterile marking pen
- Sterile towels or sterile drape
- Local anesthetic for injection: 1% or 2% lidocaine with epinephrine
- 5- or 10-mL syringe with 21- or 25-gauge needle for anesthetic
- Trocar with stylet, needle (16-, 18- or 20-gauge), or angiocatheter, depending on abdominal wall thickness
- 25- or 27-gauge 1½-inch needle
- 20- or 22-gauge spinal needles
- 20-mL syringe for diagnostic tap
- 50-mL syringe if using stopcock technique
- Four sterile tubes for specimens
- Scalpel and No. 11 knife blade
- Three-way stopcock
- Sterile 1-L collection bottles with connecting tubing
- Nylon skin suture material on cutting needle (4-0 or 5-0) and needle holder
- Mayo scissors and straight scissors
- Four to six sterile 4 × 4 gauze pads
- Sterile gauze dressing with tape or adhesive strip

Additional equipment, to have available as needed, includes the following:

- Soft wrist restraints
- Stoma bag
- Ultrasound equipment

PATIENT AND FAMILY EDUCATION

- Explain the indications, procedure, and risks to the patient and family. *Rationale:* Explanation may decrease patient anxiety and encourages patient and family cooperation and understanding of the procedure.
- Explain the patient's role in assisting with the procedure and postprocedure care. *Rationale:* Patient cooperation during and after the procedure is elicited.
- Explain the signs and symptoms to report, such as fever, abdominal pain, decreased urine output, bleeding, and leakage of fluid from surgical wound site. *Rationale:* Unexpected outcomes may not manifest themselves for a period of time after the procedure.

PATIENT ASSESSMENT AND PREPARATION

Patient Assessment

- Obtain the medical history and perform a review of systems for abdominal injury, major gastrointestinal pathology, liver disease, and portal hypertension. *Rationale:* Certain conditions of the gastrointestinal tract may be diagnosed and treated with paracentesis. Contraindications to paracentesis may be identified.
- Identify the presence of any allergies to medication or other substances. *Rationale:* Patients may have allergies to skin preparations or anesthetics used before the invasive procedure is performed. Identification assists the practitioner in choosing the most appropriate skin preparation and anesthetic.
- Assess respiratory status (i.e., rate, depth, excursion, gas exchange, use of accessory muscles, pulse oximetry). *Rationale:* Paracentesis may be indicated to decrease the work of breathing.
- Obtain baseline vital signs. *Rationale:* Hypotension and dysrhythmias may occur with rapid changes in intraabdominal pressure.
- Obtain baseline pain assessment. *Rationale:* Changes in level of pain during or after the procedure may be an indicator of complications.
- Obtain baseline fluid and electrolyte status. *Rationale:* Removal of peritoneal fluid may cause compartment shifting of intravascular volume, electrolytes, and proteins, leading to a decreased circulating volume.
- Assess bowel or bladder distention. *Rationale:* Distension increases the risk for bowel or bladder perforation during the procedure.
- Examine the abdomen, including assessment of abdominal girth, fluid wave, and shifting dullness; mark landmarks as needed. *Rationale:* Knowledge of abdominal landmarks and an understanding of the amount of fluid present are helpful in determining amount to drain as well as where to best insert the catheter.
- Obtain coagulation study results (i.e., prothrombin time, partial thromboplastin time, and platelets). *Rationale:* Abnormal clotting may increase the risk for bleeding during and after the procedure, although this complication is rare.[2,10] Therapy may be necessary to correct clotting

abnormalities before the procedure, particularly if the international normalized ratio is over 2.5.[10,11,13]

Patient Preparation

- Verify that the patient is the correct patient using two identifiers. *Rationale:* Before performing a procedure, the nurse should ensure the correct identification of the patient for the intended intervention.
- Ensure that the patient understands preprocedural information. Answer questions as they arise, and reinforce information as needed. *Rationale:* Understanding of previously taught information is evaluated and reinforced.
- Obtain a written informed consent form. *Rationale:* Paracentesis is an invasive procedure that requires signed informed consent.
- Decompress the bladder either by having the patient void or by inserting a Foley catheter. *Rationale:* A distended bladder increases the risk for bladder perforation during the procedure.

- Obtain plain and upright radiographs of the abdomen before the procedure is performed. *Rationale:* Air is introduced during the procedure and may confuse the diagnosis later.
- Perform a preprocedure verification and time out, if nonemergent. *Rationale:* Ensures patient safety.
- Check that all relevant documents and studies are available before the procedure is started. *Rationale:* This measure ensures that the correct patient receives the correct procedure.
- Place the patient in the supine position (may tilt to side of collection slightly for improved fluid positioning). *Rationale:* Fluid accumulates in the dependent areas.
- If the patient has altered mental status, soft wrist restraints may be needed. *Rationale:* The patient must not move his or her hands into the sterile field once it has been established.

Procedure for Performing Paracentesis

Steps	Rationale	Special Considerations
1. **HH**		
2. **PE**		
3. Prepare equipment and sterile field. Label all medications, medication containers (e.g., syringes, medicine cups, basins), and other solutions that are to be used during the procedure.	Provides a sterile field to decrease risk for infection	Maintain aseptic technique.
4. With the patient in the supine position, determine the site for trocar insertion. Site should be midline one-third the distance from the umbilicus to the symphysis (2–3 cm below the umbilicus; see Fig. 115-1).	Determines correct site for trocar placement. An alternate position, frequently chosen in obese patients or when large volumes of fluid are to be removed, is a point one third the distance from the umbilicus to the anterior iliac crest (left side preferred).	Avoid the rectus muscle because of increased risk for hemorrhage from epigastric vessels; surgical scars because of increased risk for perforation caused by adhesion of bowel to the wall of the peritoneum; and upper quadrants because of the possibility of undetected hepatomegaly.[2,13]
5. Cleanse the insertion site with antiseptic solution (e.g., 2% chlorhexidine-based preparation.[4,6] **(Level C*)**	Reduces risk for infection.	Allergies should be identified before a skin preparation product is chosen. Use sterile technique.
6. Wash hands and apply sterile gloves and sterile gown.	Reduces transmission of microorganisms and body secretions.	
7. Apply sterile drapes to outline the area to be tapped.	Provide sterile field to decrease risk for infection.	

*Level C: Qualitative studies, descriptive or correlational studies, integrative reviews, systematic reviews, or randomized controlled trials with inconsistent results.

Procedure for Performing Paracentesis—*Continued*

Steps	Rationale	Special Considerations
8. Inject the area with local anesthetic (lidocaine with epinephrine preferred). Initially infiltrate the skin and subcutaneous tissues in a circumferential wheel; then direct needle perpendicular to the skin and infiltrate the peritoneum.	Local anesthesia minimizes pain and discomfort. Epinephrine helps eliminate unwanted abdominal wall bleeding and false-positive results.	Usually 1% lidocaine is used, but 0.5% lidocaine with 1:200,000 epinephrine has been shown to provide equivalent anesthetic effect as 1% lidocaine with 1:100,000 epinephrine. The maximum dosage is generally accepted to be 5 mg/kg of 1% plain lidocaine and 7 mg/kg of 1% lidocaine with epinephrine.[16] Assess for anesthesia of the area. Resistance is felt as the needle perforates the peritoneum.
9. With the No. 11 blade and scalpel holder, create a skin incision large enough to allow threading a 3- to 5-mm catheter.	Promotes easier insertion of the catheter.	If lavage is necessary, the opening is large enough to thread the lavage catheter.
10. Insert an 18-gauge needle attached to a 20- or 50-mL syringe through the anesthetized tract into the peritoneum. The needle is inserted through the small stab wound created as noted in Step 9. The stab wound should be made at the midline below the umbilicus. Apply slight suction to the syringe as it is advanced. Grasp the needle close to the skin as it is advanced.	Provides access to peritoneal fluid for evacuation. Slight suction is applied to indicate when the peritoneum is entered and if a blood vessel is entered. Grasping the needle as it is advanced prevents accidental thrusting into the abdomen and possible viscus perforation.	A small pop is felt as the needle advances through the anterior and posterior muscle fascia and enters the peritoneum.
11. Once in the cavity, direct the needle at a 60-degree angle toward the center of the pelvic hollow. When fluid returns, fill the syringe (Fig. 115-2). A flexible catheter/drain can be thread into the abdominal cavity over the needle and left in place if needed.	Removes fluid for laboratory analysis.	Usually, diagnostic tests are ordered dependent on the patient's status and reason for paracentesis.[2] Tests may include the following: tube 1: lactate dehydrogenase, glucose, albumin; tube 2: total protein, specific gravity; tube 3: cell count and differential; tube 4: additional tests as needed. If there is suspicion of infection: gram stain, acid-fast bacillus stain, bacterial and fungal cultures, amylase, and triglyceride tests may be performed.[2,10,13] Also, send a specimen for cytology if malignancy is suspected.[10]
12. Attach syringes or stopcock and tubing and gently aspirate or siphon fluid via gravity or vacuum into the collection device. Drains may be left in and allowed to drain for 6–12 hours.[11,13] **(Level E*)**	Initiates therapy.	Monitor the amount of fluid removed. Removal of large amounts of fluid (>5 L) may cause hypotension.[5,13,15] If large volume paracentesis is performed (>5–6 L) an albumin infusion of 6–8 g/L of fluid removed improves survival and is recommended to prevent circulatory dysfunction.[1,3,5,10,13,15] **(Level A*)**

*Level A: Meta-analysis of quantitative studies or metasynthesis of qualitative studies with results that consistently support a specific action, intervention, or treatment (including systematic review of randomized controlled trials).

*Level E: Multiple case reports, theory-based evidence from expert opinions, or peer-reviewed professional organizational standards without clinical studies to support recommendations.

Procedure continues on following page

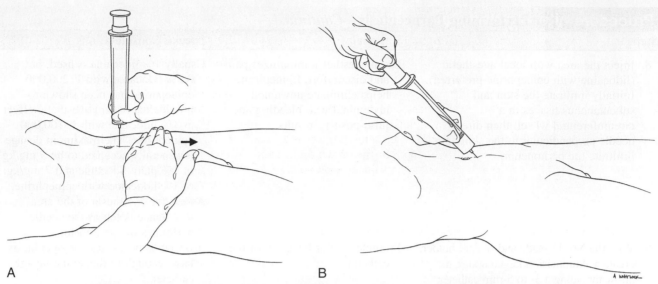

Figure 115-2 **A,** Z-track method of paracentesis. The skin is pulled approximately 2 cm caudal in relation to the deep abdominal wall by the non–needle-bearing hand while the paracentesis needle is slowly being inserted directly perpendicular to the skin. **B,** After the peritoneum is penetrated and fluid return obtained, the skin is released. Note that the needle is angulated caudally. *(From Roberts JR: Roberts and Hedges' clinical procedures in emergency medicine, ed 6, Philadelphia, 2014, Saunders.)*

Procedure for Performing Paracentesis—*Continued*

Steps	Rationale	Special Considerations
13. After the fluid is removed, gently remove the catheter and apply pressure to the wound. If the wound is still leaking fluid after 5 minutes of direct pressure, suture the puncture site with a mattress suture (see Procedure 131) and apply a pressure dressing.	Keeps insertion site clean and dry. Reduces risk for infection.	Inspect catheter to ensure if it intact. If significant leakage is found, apply a stoma bag over the site until drainage becomes minimal.
14. Apply a sterile dressing to the wound site.	Provides a barrier to infection and collects fluid that may leak from wound site.	
15. Remove **PE** and sterile equipment and equipment used during the procedure in appropriate receptacles.	Standard Precautions.	
16. **HH**		

Expected Outcomes

- Evacuation of peritoneal fluid for laboratory analysis
- Decompression of peritoneal cavity
- Relief of respiratory compromise
- Relief of abdominal discomfort

Unexpected Outcomes

- Perforation of bowel, bladder, or stomach
- Lacerations of major vessels (mesenteric, iliac, aorta)
- Abdominal wall hematomas
- Laceration of catheter and loss in peritoneal cavity
- Incisional hernias
- Local or systemic infection
- Hypovolemia, hypotension, shock
- Bleeding from insertion site
- Ascitic fluid leak from insertion site
- Peritonitis

Patient Monitoring and Care

Steps	Rationale	Reportable Conditions
		These conditions should be reported if they persist despite nursing interventions.
1. Evaluate changes in abdominal girth.	Provides evidence of fluid accumulation.	• Increasing abdominal girth
2. Monitor for changes in the respiratory status.	Removal of ascitic fluid should relieve pressure on the diaphragm and the resulting respiratory distress.	• Respiratory rate >24 breaths per minute or significant increase from baseline • Increased depth of breathing • Irregular breathing pattern • Pulse oximetry less than 92%, or significant decrease from baseline
3. Monitor for potential complications, including bowel or bladder perforation, bleeding, and intravascular volume loss.	Paracentesis interrupts the integrity of the skin and underlying peritoneum.	• Hematuria • Hypotension • Tachycardia
4. Monitor vital signs, temperature, and insertion site for drainage or evidence of infection.	Rapid changes in intraabdominal pressure may affect heart rate and blood pressure. Infection is a complication of paracentesis.	• Hypotension • Dysrhythmias • Increased temperature • Purulent drainage from insertion site • Redness, swelling at insertion site • Abnormal laboratory results (e.g., increased white blood cell [WBC] count)
5. Monitor intake and output.	Provides data for evaluation of fluid balance status.	• Inappropriate fluid balance or changes from baseline fluid status
6. Monitor abdominal pain and level of weakness.	Patients often feel weak and have abdominal discomfort for a few hours after the procedure. Follow institutional standard for assessing pain. Identifies need for pain interventions.	• Continued pain despite pain interventions, if performed
7. Evaluate laboratory data when returned.	Provides for evaluation of condition and aids in diagnosis.	• Red blood cell count >100,000/mm^3 • Amylase value greater than 2.5 times normal • Alkaline phosphatase value >5.5 mg/dL • WBC count >100/mm^3 • Positive culture results[10,13]

Documentation

Documentation should include the following:
- Patient and family education
- Date and time of procedure
- Description of procedure step by step
- Patient tolerance of procedure
- Assessment of insertion site after procedure
- Amount and characteristics of fluid removed
- Specimens sent for laboratory analysis
- Postprocedure vital signs, respiratory status
- Postprocedure comfort/pain level
- Abdominal girth
- Unexpected outcomes
- Nursing interventions

References and Additional Readings

For a complete list of references and additional readings for this procedure, scan this QR code with any freely available smartphone code reader app, or visit http://booksite.elsevier.com/9780323376624.

116 Paracentesis (Assist)

Eleanor Fitzpatrick

PURPOSE: Abdominal paracentesis is performed to remove fluid from the peritoneal cavity for diagnostic or therapeutic purposes.

PREREQUISITE NURSING KNOWLEDGE

- Knowledge of anatomy and physiology of the abdomen is important to avoid unexpected outcomes.
- Intestines and bladder lie immediately beneath the abdominal surface.
- Large volumes of ascitic fluid tend to float the air-filled bowel toward the midline, where it may be easily perforated during the procedure.
- The cecum is relatively fixed and is much less mobile than the sigmoid colon; therefore bowel perforations are more frequent in the right lower quadrant than in the left.
- Peritoneal fluid is normally straw-colored, serous fluid secreted by the cells of the peritoneum. Grossly bloody fluid in the abdomen is abnormal.
- The peritoneal fluid collected is used to evaluate and diagnose the cause of ascites, acute abdominal conditions such as peritonitis or pancreatitis, and blunt or penetrating trauma to the abdomen.
- Therapeutic paracentesis is used to reduce intraabdominal and diaphragmatic pressures to relieve dyspnea and respiratory compromise and to prevent hernia formation and diaphragmatic rupture.[2,8,11] These complications are seen in those patients with tense, refractory ascites with failed medical interventions, such as sodium restriction and diuresis.[2,3,5,11,15]
- Cirrhosis is the most common cause of ascites formation. However, ascitic fluid is produced as a result of a variety of other conditions.[2,5,7,10] These conditions may include interference in venous return because of heart failure, constrictive pericarditis, or tricuspid valve insufficiency; obstruction of flow in the vena cava or portal vein; disturbance in electrolyte balance, such as sodium retention; depletion of plasma proteins because of nephrotic syndrome or starvation; lymphoma, leukemia, or neoplasms that involve the liver or mediastinum; ovarian malignant disease; and chronic pancreatitis.
- Analysis of the ascitic fluid can determine the cause of ascites. A serum-to-ascites albumin gradient should be calculated by subtracting the ascitic fluid albumin level from the serum albumin. This calculation differentiates portal hypertensive from nonportal hypertensive ascites.[2,3,5,9,11]

- Paracentesis is contraindicated in patients with an acute abdomen, who need immediate surgery. Coagulopathies and thrombocytopenia are considered relative contraindications. Coagulopathy should preclude paracentesis only in the case of clinically evident fibrinolysis or clinically evident disseminated intravascular coagulation.[3,10] Absolute contraindications include an acute abdomen, an uncooperative patient, and disseminated intravascular coagulopathy. Relative contraindications include coagulopathy, abdominal adhesions, infected abdominal wall at the entry site, distended bowel or bladder, and pregnancy.[15]
- Caution should be used when paracentesis is performed in patients with severe bowel distention, previous abdominal surgery (especially pelvic surgery), pregnancy (use open technique after first trimester), distended bladder that cannot be emptied with a Foley catheter, or obvious infection at intended site of insertion (cellulitis or abscess).
- The insertion site should be midline one third the distance from the umbilicus to the symphysis (2 to 3 cm below the umbilicus; see Fig. 115-1). An alternate position is a point one third the distance from the umbilicus to the anterior iliac crest (left side preferred especially in the obese patient or in those requiring removal of large volumes of fluid).[2,10,11,13]
- Ultrasound scan can be used before paracentesis to locate fluid and during the procedure to guide insertion of the catheter. If ascitic fluid is difficult to localize with physical examination due to obesity or other conditions, ultrasound is effective in identifying the fluid and critical structures which are to be avoided during the procedure.[10,12]
- Endoscopic transgastric ultrasound scan has also been used in the diagnosis of malignant ascites.[2,13]
- A semipermanent catheter or a shunt may be an option for patients with rapidly reaccumulating ascites.[2,3,10]
- When large-volume paracentesis (>5 L) is performed in patients with cirrhosis and other disorders, the infusion of albumin, (6 to 8 g/L) of fluid removed, may prevent the onset of circulatory compromise associated with massive fluid shifting.[3,9,10,11,15] Albumin administration may be effective in preventing paracentesis-induced circulatory dysfunction, the most common complication after the procedure.[13-15] Albumin infusion is recommended with large-volume paracentesis as its use has shown improved survival.[1]

EQUIPMENT

- Commercially prepared paracentesis kit if available
- Nonsterile gloves, sterile gloves, mask, goggles, and gown
- Antiseptic solution (e.g., 2% chlorhexidine-based preparation)
- Sterile marking pen
- Sterile towels or sterile drape
- Local anesthetic for injection: 1% or 2% lidocaine with epinephrine
- 5- or 10-mL syringe with 21- or 25-gauge needle for anesthetic
- Trocar with stylet, needle (16-, 18-, or 20-gauge), or angiocatheter, depending on abdominal wall thickness
- 25- or 27-gauge 1½-inch needle
- 20- or 22-gauge spinal needles
- 20-mL syringe for diagnostic tap
- 50-mL syringe if using stopcock technique
- Four sterile tubes for specimens
- Scalpel and No. 11 knife blade
- Three-way stopcock
- Sterile 1-L collection bottles with connecting tubing
- Nylon skin suture material on cutting needle (4-0 or 5-0) and needle holder
- Mayo scissors and straight scissors
- Four to six sterile 4 × 4 gauze pads
- Sterile gauze dressing with tape or adhesive strip

Additional equipment, to have available as needed, includes the following:

- Soft wrist restraints
- Stoma bag
- Ultrasound equipment

PATIENT AND FAMILY EDUCATION

- Explain the indications, procedure, and risks to the patient and family. *Rationale:* Explanation may decrease patient anxiety and encourages patient and family cooperation and understanding of the procedure.
- Explain the patient's role in assisting with the procedure and postprocedure care. *Rationale:* Patient cooperation during and after the procedure is elicited.
- Explain the signs and symptoms to report, such as fever, abdominal pain, decreased urine output, bleeding, and leakage of fluid from surgical wound site. *Rationale:* Unexpected outcomes may not manifest themselves for a period of time after the procedure.

PATIENT ASSESSMENT AND PREPARATION

Patient Assessment

- Obtain the medical history and a review of systems for abdominal injury, major gastrointestinal pathology, liver disease, and portal hypertension. *Rationale:* Certain conditions of the gastrointestinal tract may be diagnosed and treated with paracentesis. Contraindications to paracentesis may be identified.

- Identify the presence of any allergies to medication or other substances. *Rationale:* Patients may have allergies to skin preparations or anesthetics used before the invasive procedure is performed. Identification assists the practitioner in choosing the most appropriate skin preparation and anesthetic.
- Assess respiratory status (i.e., rate, depth, excursion, gas exchange, use of accessory muscles, and pulse oximetry). *Rationale:* Paracentesis may be indicated to decrease the work of breathing.
- Obtain baseline vital signs. *Rationale:* Hypotension and dysrhythmias may occur with rapid changes in the intraabdominal pressure.
- Obtain a baseline pain assessment. *Rationale:* Changes in the level of pain during or after the procedure may be an indicator of complications.
- Obtain baseline fluid and electrolyte status. *Rationale:* Removal of peritoneal fluid may cause compartment shifting of intravascular volume, electrolytes, and proteins, leading to a decreased circulating volume.
- Assess bowel or bladder distention. *Rationale:* Distension increases the risk for bowel or bladder perforation during the procedure.
- Assess abdominal girth. *Rationale:* Information on changes in fluid accumulation within the peritoneal cavity is provided.
- Obtain coagulation study results (i.e., prothrombin time, partial thromboplastin time, and platelets). *Rationale:* Abnormal clotting may increase the risk for bleeding during and after the procedure, although this complication is rare.[2,10] Therapy may be necessary to correct clotting abnormalities before the procedure, particularly if the international normalized ratio is over 2.5.[10,11,13]

Patient Preparation

- Verify that the patient is the correct patient using two identifiers. *Rationale:* Before performing a procedure, the nurse should ensure the correct identification of the patient for the intended intervention.
- Ensure that the patient understands preprocedural information. Answer questions as they arise, and reinforce information as needed. *Rationale:* Understanding of previously taught information is evaluated and reinforced.
- Ensure that a written informed consent form has been obtained by the practitioner performing the procedure. The assisting practitioner may be a witness to the signing of the consent if needed. *Rationale:* Paracentesis is an invasive procedure and requires a signed informed consent form.
- Decompress the bladder either by having the patient void or by inserting a Foley catheter. *Rationale:* A distended bladder increases the risk for bladder perforation during the procedure.
- The physician or advanced practice nurse orders plain and upright radiographs of the abdomen before the procedure is performed. *Rationale:* Air is introduced during the procedure and may confuse the diagnosis later.
- Perform a preprocedure verification and time out with the physician or advanced practice nurse, if nonemergent. *Rationale:* Ensures patient safety.

- Check that all relevant documents and studies are available before the procedure is started. *Rationale:* This measure ensures that the correct patient receives the correct procedure.
- Place the patient in the supine position (may tilt to side of collection slightly for improved fluid positioning). *Rationale:* Fluid accumulates in the dependent areas.
- The physician or advanced practice nurse will examine the abdomen for areas of shifting dullness, find landmarks, and mark appropriately. *Rationale:* Shifting dullness indicates fluid.
- If the patient has altered mental status, soft wrist restraints may be prescribed. *Rationale:* The patient must not move his or her hands into the sterile field once it has been established.

Procedure   for Assisting With Paracentesis

Steps	Rationale	Special Considerations
1. HH		
2. PE		
3. Assist in preparing the equipment and sterile field. Label all medications, medication containers (e.g., syringes, medicine cups, basins), and other solutions that are to be used during the procedure.	Provides a sterile field to decrease risk for infection.	Maintain aseptic technique.
4. As needed, assist the physician or nurse practitioner to cleanse insertion site with antiseptic solution (e.g., 2% chlorhexidine-based preparation).[4,6] **(Level C*)**	Reduces risk for infection.	Allergies should be identified before a skin preparation product is chosen.
5. As needed, assist the physician or advanced practice nurse with the application of sterile gloves, gown, and mask as well as sterile drapes to outline the area to be tapped.	Provides sterile field to decrease risk for infection.	
6. As needed, assist the physician or advanced practice nurse to draw up local anesthetic (lidocaine with epinephrine preferred).	Local anesthesia minimizes pain and discomfort. Epinephrine helps eliminate unwanted abdominal wall bleeding and false-positive results.	Usually 1% lidocaine is used, but 0.5% lidocaine with 1:200,000 epinephrine has been shown to provide equivalent anesthetic effect as 1% lidocaine with 1:100,000 epinephrine. The maximum dosage is generally accepted to be 5 mg/kg of 1% plain lidocaine and 7 mg/kg of 1% lidocaine with epinephrine.[16] Assess for anesthesia of area.
7. Assist in collection of peritoneal fluid for laboratory analysis.	Assists in collecting fluid for laboratory analysis.	Usually diagnostic tests are ordered depending on patient's status and reason for paracentesis.[2] Tests may include the following: tube 1: lactate dehydrogenase, glucose, albumin; tube 2: total protein, specific gravity; tube 3: cell count and differential; tube 4: additional tests as needed. If there is suspicion of infection: gram stain, acid-fast bacillus stain, bacterial and fungal cultures, amylase, and triglyceride tests may be ordered.[2,10,13] Also, collect a specimen for cytology if malignancy is suspected.[10]

*Level C: Qualitative studies, descriptive or correlational studies, integrative reviews, systematic reviews, or randomized controlled trials with inconsistent results.

Procedure for Assisting With Paracentesis—*Continued*

Steps	Rationale	Special Considerations
8. Assist the physician or advanced practice nurse in attaching syringes or stopcock and tubing and aspirating or siphoning fluid via gravity or vacuum into the collection device. A flexible catheter/drain can be thread into the abdominal cavity over the needle and left in place if needed. Drains may be left in and allowed to drain for 6–12 hours.[11,13] **(Level E*)**	Initiates therapy.	Monitor the amount of fluid removed. Removal of large amounts of fluid (>5 L) may cause hypotension.[5,13,15] If large volume paracentesis is performed (>5–6 L) an albumin infusion of 6–8 g/L of fluid removed improves survival and is recommended to prevent circulatory dysfunction.[1,3,5,10,13,15] **(Level A*)**
9. After the fluid and catheter are removed, apply pressure to the wound. If the wound is still leaking fluid after 5 minutes of direct pressure, the physician or advanced practice nurse may suture the puncture site (see Procedure 124) and apply a pressure dressing.	Keeps the insertion site clean. Reduces the risk for infection.	Inspect catheter to ensure it is intact. If significant leakage is found, apply a stoma bag over the site until drainage becomes minimal.
10. Assist with applying a sterile dressing to the wound site.	Provides a barrier to infection and collects fluid that may leak from wound site.	
11. Remove **PE** and sterile equipment used during the procedure in appropriate receptacles.	Standard Precautions.	
12. **HH**		

*Level A: Meta-analysis of quantitative studies or metasynthesis of qualitative studies with results that consistently support a specific action, intervention, or treatment (including systematic review of randomized controlled trials).

*Level E: Multiple case reports, theory-based evidence from expert opinions, or peer-reviewed professional organizational standards without clinical studies to support recommendations.

Expected Outcomes

- Evacuation of peritoneal fluid for laboratory analysis
- Decompression of peritoneal cavity
- Relief of respiratory compromise
- Relief of abdominal discomfort

Unexpected Outcomes

- Perforation of bowel, bladder, or stomach
- Lacerations of major vessels (mesenteric, iliac, aorta)
- Abdominal wall hematomas
- Laceration of catheter and loss in peritoneal cavity
- Incisional hernias
- Local or systemic infection
- Hypovolemia, hypotension, shock
- Bleeding from insertion site
- Ascitic fluid leak from insertion site
- Peritonitis

Patient Monitoring and Care

Steps	Rationale	Reportable Conditions
		These conditions should be reported if they persist despite nursing interventions.
1. Evaluate changes in abdominal girth.	Provides evidence of fluid reaccumulation.	- Increasing abdominal girth

Procedure continues on following page

Patient Monitoring and Care —*Continued*

Steps	Rationale	Reportable Conditions
2. Monitor for changes in the respiratory status.	Removal of ascitic fluid should relieve pressure on the diaphragm and the resulting respiratory distress.	• Respiratory rate >24 breaths per minute or significant increase from baseline • Increased depth of breathing • Irregular breathing pattern • Pulse oximetry <92%, or significant decrease from baseline
3. Monitor for potential complications, including bowel or bladder perforation, bleeding, and intravascular volume loss.	Paracentesis interrupts the integrity of the skin and underlying peritoneum.	• Hematuria • Hypotension • Tachycardia
4. Monitor vital signs, temperature, and insertion site for drainage or evidence of infection.	Rapid changes in intraabdominal pressure may affect heart rate and blood pressure. Infection is a complication of paracentesis.	• Hypotension • Dysrhythmias • Increased temperature • Purulent drainage from insertion site • Redness, swelling at insertion site • Abnormal laboratory results (increased white blood cell [WBC] count)
5. Monitor intake and output.	Provides data for evaluation of the fluid balance status.	• Inappropriate fluid balance or changes from baseline fluid status
6. Monitor abdominal pain and level of weakness. Follow institutional standards for assessing pain.	Patients often feel weak and have abdominal discomfort for a few hours after the procedure. Identifies need for pain interventions.	• Continued pain despite pain interventions, if performed
7. Evaluate the laboratory data when returned.	Provides for evaluation of the condition and aids in diagnosis.	• Red blood cell count >100,000/mm^3 • Amylase value >2.5 times normal • Alkaline phosphatase value >5.5 mg/dL • WBC count >100/mm^3 • Positive culture results[10,13]

Documentation

Documentation should include the following:
- Patient and family education
- The date and time of the procedure
- Patient tolerance of the procedure
- Assessment of the insertion site after the procedure
- The amount and characteristics of fluid removed
- Specimens sent for laboratory analysis
- Postprocedure vital signs, respiratory status
- Postprocedure comfort/pain level
- Abdominal girth
- Unexpected outcomes
- Nursing interventions

References and Additional Readings

For a complete list of references and additional readings for this procedure, scan this QR code with any freely available smartphone code reader app, or visit http://booksite.elsevier.com/9780323376624.

117 Peritoneal Lavage (Perform) AP

Kate Deis

PURPOSE: Percutaneous peritoneal lavage is performed for both therapeutic and diagnostic purposes. Peritoneal lavage can determine whether surgery is necessary for patients who have experienced blunt or penetrating trauma to the abdomen. Peritoneal lavage can also be used for therapeutic purposes for conditions such as peritonitis and hypothermia.

PREREQUISITE NURSING KNOWLEDGE

- Knowledge of the anatomy and physiology of the abdomen is important to avoid unexpected outcomes.
- Knowledge of the use of sterile technique is needed.
- The intestines and the bladder lie immediately beneath the abdominal surface. In adults, a full bladder is raised out of the pelvis. An indwelling urinary catheter is necessary to decompress the bladder in preparation for peritoneal lavage.
- The cecum is relatively fixed and is much less mobile than the sigmoid colon; therefore bowel perforations are more frequent in the right lower quadrant than in the left.
- A distended stomach can extend to the anterior abdominal wall. A nasogastric or orogastric tube is necessary before peritoneal lavage in order to decompress the stomach.
- Peritoneal fluid is normally straw-colored, serous fluid secreted by the cells of the peritoneum. Grossly bloody fluid, a red blood cell (RBC) count of greater than 100,000/mm,[3,7,11] or the presence of bacteria or bile in the return fluid in the abdomen is abnormal. A white blood cell (WBC) count greater than 500,000/mm and the presence of bile or amylase in the lavage fluid are parameters, in addition to the RBC count, that can lead to operative intervention.[3,7,11]
- Diagnostic peritoneal lavage (DPL) is used less frequently than noninvasive diagnostic testing, such as focused abdominal sonography in trauma (FAST) examinations and multidetector helical computed tomography (CT) scanning in patients with blunt abdominal trauma.[4,6,12]
- DPL can be used after blunt abdominal trauma or in trauma patients who have head injuries, are unconscious, or have preexisting paraplegia to determine the presence of the following[2,3]:
  - Hemoperitoneum (blood in lavage returns)
  - Organ injury (intestinal enzymes or microorganisms in lavage returns)
- DPL is a highly sensitive predictor of blood in the peritoneal cavity.[1,2,10]

- Therapeutic lavage is used to:
  - Irrigate and cleanse purulent exudate in patients with peritonitis or intraabdominal abscess
  - Warm the abdominal cavity in patients with hypothermia
  - Remove unwanted or toxic chemicals through peritoneal dialysis
  - Obtain cytology specimens in patients with cancer
- For trauma patients with stab wounds and gunshot wounds to the lower chest or anterior abdomen, DPL is controversial; most trauma centers operate on patients with gunshot wound injuries to the lower chest or anterior abdomen.[1]
- DPL can be used as a tool in patients with hypotension of uncertain etiology in the presence of trauma.[6]
- DPL is not necessary if abdominal surgery is already indicated.[9,11]
- Because it is an invasive procedure, DPL does have a small risk of visceral injury (0.6%).[7]
- DPL is 95% sensitive and 99% specific for intraperitoneal blood; however, it cannot exclude retroperitoneal hemorrhage, disruption of the diaphragm, or hollow viscus perforation.[2,9,10]
- CT is frequently used as the diagnostic procedure of choice in trauma patients with hemodynamically stable conditions.[7] Also abdominal ultrasound scans and FASTs have been increasingly used to screen cases of blunt abdominal trauma for hemoperitoneum.[11]
- DPL is quick, inexpensive, and safe.[7] Patients with hemodynamically unstable conditions may also go directly to the operating room (OR) for laparotomy.
- Complementary CT scan and DPL decrease nontherapeutic laparotomy rates and allow nonoperative management of those patients with solid-organ injury.[11]
- Peritoneal lavage is absolutely contraindicated in an acute abdomen that needs immediate surgery as indicated by free air on radiography or penetrating abdominal trauma.
- Relative contraindications for DPL include the following[7,8]:
  - Thrombocytopenia
  - Coagulopathy[9]
  - Morbid obesity[9]
  - Severe bowel distention
  - Advanced cirrhosis[9]

AP This procedure should be performed only by physicians, advanced practice nurses, and other healthcare professionals (including critical care nurses) with additional knowledge, skills, and demonstrated competence per professional licensure or institutional standard.

❖ Previous abdominal surgery, especially pelvic surgery
❖ Distended bladder that cannot be emptied with a Foley catheter
❖ Obvious infection at intended site of insertion (cellulitis or abscess)
❖ Pregnancy of greater than 12 weeks' gestation[9]
• Use caution when performing DPL in patients with suspected pelvic fractures (may use a supraumbilical site) because of false-positive results[9]: if DPL is performed in pregnant patients of more than 12 weeks' gestation, use an open technique, superior to the uterus.[9]
• The insertion site should be midline, one-third the distance from the umbilicus to the symphysis, or 2 to 3 cm below the umbilicus (see Fig. 115-1). An alternate position is a point one-third the distance from the umbilicus to the anterior iliac crest (left side preferred).
• An ultrasound scan can be used before peritoneal lavage to locate fluid and during the procedure to guide insertion of the catheter.[11]

EQUIPMENT

• Commercially prepared kit or the following:
  ❖ Personal protective equipment, including sterile gloves, mask, goggles, and gown
  ❖ Antiseptic solution (e.g., 2% chlorhexidine based preparation)
  ❖ Sterile marking pen
  ❖ Sterile towels or sterile drape
  ❖ Local anesthetic for injection: 1% or 2% lidocaine with epinephrine
  ❖ 5- or 10-mL syringe with 25- or 27-gauge needle for anesthetic
  ❖ Scalpel and No. 11 knife blade
  ❖ Trocar with stylet; needle (16-, 18-, or 20-gauge) or angiocatheter; depending on abdominal wall thickness, may use guidewire with floppy tip and 9 to 18 Fr peritoneal lavage catheter
  ❖ 20-mL syringe for diagnostic tap
  ❖ Sterile intravenous (IV) tubing (without valves) with appropriate sterile connectors for lavage catheter and IV bags
  ❖ Sterile tubes for specimens
  ❖ Warmed Ringer's lactate (RL), normal saline (NS), or antibiotic solution for infusion into abdomen
  ❖ Three-way stopcock for therapeutic lavage
  ❖ Nylon skin suture material on cutting needle (4-0 or 5-0) and needle holder
  ❖ Four to six sterile 4 × 4 gauze pads
  ❖ Sterile gauze dressing with tape or adhesive strip
  ❖ Pressure bag
Additional equipment, to have available as needed, includes the following:
• Razor or scissors
• Soft wrist restraints

PATIENT AND FAMILY EDUCATION

• Explain the indication, the procedure, and the risks to the patient and family. *Rationale:* Explanation may decrease patient anxiety and may encourage patient and family cooperation and understanding of the procedure.
• Explain the patient's role in assisting with the procedure and postprocedure care. *Rationale:* Patient cooperation during and after the procedure is elicited.
• Explain the signs and symptoms to report, such as fever, abdominal pain, decreased urine output, bleeding, and leakage of fluid from the wound site. *Rationale:* This alerts the nurse to signs and symptoms of complications.

PATIENT ASSESSMENT AND PREPARATION

Patient Assessment

• Obtain the medical history and a review of systems to identify abdominal injury, peritonitis, intraabdominal abscess, or pregnancy. *Rationale:* Certain conditions of the gastrointestinal tract may be diagnosed and treated with peritoneal lavage. Contraindications to peritoneal lavage may be identified.[8]
• Identify the presence of any allergies to medication or other substances. *Rationale:* Patients may have allergies to skin preparations or anesthetics used before the invasive procedure is performed. This identification assists the physician, advanced practice nurse, or other healthcare professional in choosing the most appropriate skin preparation and anesthetic.
• Assess for bowel or bladder distention. *Rationale:* Distention increases the risk for bowel or bladder perforation during the procedure.[9]
• Review coagulation studies (i.e., prothrombin time [PT], partial thromboplastin time [PTT], and platelets). *Rationale:* Abnormal clotting studies may increase the risk for bleeding during and after the procedure. Therapy may be necessary to correct clotting abnormalities before the procedure is performed.
• Obtain plain radiographs of the abdomen and upright abdominal films if possible (before the procedure). *Rationale:* Air is introduced during the procedure and may confound the diagnosis later.[9]
• Obtain vital signs and assess pain. *Rationale:* This provides baseline data.

Patient Preparation

• Ensure that the patient understands preprocedural teachings. Answer questions as they arise, and reinforce information as needed. *Rationale:* Understanding of previously taught information is evaluated and reinforced.
• Obtain signed informed consent from the patient or decision maker, if possible. In a trauma situation or unresponsive patient, this may be implied consent. *Rationale:* Peritoneal lavage is an invasive procedure that requires signed informed consent.
• Insert or ask for assistance in inserting an indwelling urinary catheter. *Rationale:* A distended bladder increases the risk for bladder perforation during the procedure.[9]
• Insert or ask for assistance in inserting a nasogastric tube unless contraindicated (e.g., in significant facial trauma) and attach to low intermittent suction. *Rationale:* A distended stomach increases the risk for perforation during the procedure.[8]

- Check that all relevant documents and studies are available before starting the procedure. **Rationale:** This measure ensures that the correct patient receives the correct procedure.
- Verify that the patient is the correct patient using two identifiers. **Rationale:** Before performing a procedure, the physician or advanced practice nurse should ensure the correct identification of the patient for the intended intervention.
- Perform a preprocedure verification and timeout, if nonemergent. **Rationale:** Ensures patient safety.

- Place the patient in the supine position (may tilt to the side of collection slightly for improved fluid positioning). **Rationale:** Fluid accumulates in the dependent areas.
- Examine the abdomen for landmarks and mark appropriately. Shave or clip hair from the area, if necessary. **Rationale:** Assists with correct placement of the catheter for peritoneal lavage and minimizes complications.
- Prescribe analgesia and/or sedation as needed. **Rationale:** Promotes comfort and may be needed for patient safety during the procedure. The patient must not move his or her hands into the sterile field once it has been established.

Procedure for Performing Peritoneal Lavage

Steps	Rationale	Special Considerations
1. HH		
2. PE		
3. Set up or ask for assistance in setting up lavage equipment.	Facilitates easy access to needed equipment.	
A. Attach the IV tubing to the lavage fluid and clear the tubing of air.	Provides a closed system for instillation and drainage of lavage fluid.	
B. Attach the IV tubing to one port of the three-way stopcock and attach the drainage collector to the second port of the three-way stopcock.	Priming the tubing prevents instillation of air into the peritoneum.	
C. Use IV tubing with a roller clamp and use the lavage fluid bag as the drainage bag.		
4. Remove gloves, wash hands, prepare the sterile field, and apply sterile gown and gloves.	Maintaining sterile technique throughout procedure minimizes risk for infection.	
5. Cleanse the insertion site with antiseptic solution (e.g., 2% chlorhexidine-based preparation).		
6. Apply sterile drapes to outline the insertion site.	Minimizes risk for infection and aids in site identification.	Avoid the rectus muscle because of increased risk for hemorrhage from epigastric vessels; avoid surgical scars because of the increased risk for perforation caused by adhesion of bowel to the wall of the peritoneum; avoid the upper quadrants because of the possibility of undetected hepatomegaly.[2,3]
A. The site should be in the midline about one third the distance from the umbilicus to the symphysis (usually 2–3 cm below the umbilicus; Fig. 117-1).		
B. An alternate position is a point about one third the distance from the umbilicus to the anterior iliac crest (left side preferred).		
C. Consider marking the site.		
7. Inject the area with local anesthetic (lidocaine with epinephrine preferred).	Promotes comfort during the procedure. Epinephrine helps eliminate unwanted abdominal wall bleeding and false-positive results.[5]	The maximum dose of lidocaine is 30 mL of 1% or 15 mL of 2%. Assess for anesthesia of area. Resistance is felt as the needle perforates the peritoneum.
A. Initially direct the needle perpendicular to the skin.		
B. Infiltrate the peritoneum with the anesthetic.		

Procedure continues on following page

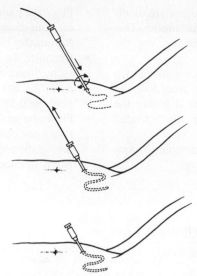

Figure 117-1   The plastic catheter is placed over the guidewire and inserted into the peritoneal cavity by means of a twisting motion at the skin level. After the catheter has been advanced, the guidewire is removed. *(From Pfenninger JL, Fowler GC, eds: Pfenninger and Fowler's procedures for primary care, ed 2, St. Louis, 2003, Mosby.)*

Procedure	for Performing Peritoneal Lavage—*Continued*	
Steps	**Rationale**	**Special Considerations**
8. With the No. 11 blade scalpel: A. Create a vertical skin incision large enough to allow threading of a 3–5-mm lavage catheter. B. Spread the subcutaneous tissue and incise the fascia to expose the peritoneum. C. Nick the peritoneal membrane to pass the catheter.	Creates an opening large enough to thread the lavage catheter.	When the subcutaneous tissue is nicked with the scalpel, a tough, gritty sensation is felt.
9. Insert an 18-gauge needle attached to a 20- or 50-mL syringe perpendicular through the anesthetized tract into the peritoneum. A. Apply slight suction to the syringe as it is advanced. B. Grasp the needle close to the skin as it is advanced.	Provides access to the peritoneal space. Slight suction is applied to indicate when the peritoneum is entered or if a blood vessel is entered. Grasping the needle as it is advanced prevents accidental thrusting into the abdomen and possible viscus perforation.	The needle is inserted through a small incision at midline below the umbilicus. A small pop is felt as the needle advances through the anterior and posterior muscle fascia and enters the peritoneum.
10. Once in the cavity, direct the needle at a 60-degree angle toward the center of the pelvic hollow. If fluid returns, fill the syringe.	Collects fluid for laboratory studies.	A free return of 10 mL of blood is a strong positive finding for a hemoperitoneum.[4] If blood is returned, remove the needle and prepare for immediate surgical intervention.
11. If the tap is dry, perform the lavage technique.	Assesses for hemoperitoneum if the initial aspiration was dry.	

Procedure for Performing Peritoneal Lavage—*Continued*

Steps	Rationale	Special Considerations
12. Introduce the guidewire through the 18-gauge needle.	Provides an access for insertion of the peritoneal lavage catheter.	The wire should insert easily. If any resistance is felt, advance or redirect the needle until the wire advances easily. Difficulty in advancing the catheter may indicate that the stylet is not in the peritoneal cavity or the presence of adhesions.
13. Insert about half of the wire into the pelvis and remove the needle while securely holding the guidewire.	Releasing the guidewire could allow the wire to inadvertently migrate into peritoneum.	
14. Slide the peritoneal lavage catheter over the wire with a gentle twisting motion.	A twisting motion minimizes visceral perforation and displaces the abdominal contents.	Always keep a firm hold on the guidewire to prevent it from slipping into the peritoneal cavity.
15. Remove the guidewire after the catheter is in the peritoneal cavity.	The guidewire is no longer needed.	
16. Attach the lavage catheter to the remaining port of the stopcock and tubing to withdraw the peritoneal fluid.	Fluid may be gently aspirated, siphoned via gravity, or collected into a vacuum device.	Retain the first 100 mL of fluid for laboratory analysis. **Refer to Step 24** for specific laboratory tests.[1,9]
17. Instill the lavage fluid: A. If a drainage collector is used, turn the stopcock off to the drainage collector. B. Open clamp on the IV tubing. C. For adult patients, instill 700–1000 mL of warmed lactated Ringer's solution, 0.9% normal saline solution, or antibacterial fluid.	Directs lavage fluid into the peritoneal space.	Infuse over 10–15 minutes. This may be done with a pressure bag to decrease time.
18. Rotate the patient side to side (if not contraindicated).	Facilitates sampling of fluid that may accumulate in pockets on either side. Mixes the solution with any free material in the abdominal cavity.	
19. Drain the lavage fluid: A. If the drainage collector is used, turn the stopcock off to the IV tubing. B. If the drainage collector is not used, lower the IV bag to a level below the patient. C. Allow the fluid to drain into the drainage collector or the lowered IV bag.	Directs the lavage fluid from the peritoneal space to the drainage collector.	In therapeutic lavage, consider the dwell time of the fluid before drainage (usually 5–10 minutes). When draining fluid, be careful that no tension is put on the tubing.
20. Rotate the patient side to side (if not contraindicated).	Facilitates the drainage of fluid that may accumulate in pockets on either side.	Lavage fluid may be absorbed into the intravascular space, creating a potential fluid volume excess. Twisting the catheter may free the catheter from adhering to peritoneum and facilitate drainage of fluid.

Procedure continues on following page

Procedure for Performing Peritoneal Lavage—*Continued*

Steps	Rationale	Special Considerations
21. **Repeat Steps 17–20** as needed.	Continued lavage may be needed to cleanse the peritoneal space.	
22. If the lavage is positive for blood: A. Prepare the patient for immediate surgery. B. Leave the incision open and cover the area with a sterile, NS solution–soaked dressing.	Immediate repair of the bleeding site is needed.	
23. After the fluid is removed: A. Gently remove the catheter. B. Apply pressure to the wound. C. Suture the puncture site with a mattress suture with 4–0 nylon. D. Apply a sterile dressing.	Keeps the insertion site clean. Reduces the risk for infection. Provides a barrier to infection and collects the fluid that may leak from the wound site.	Inspect the catheter to ensure it is intact.
24. Prepare and send the fluid specimens for laboratory analysis.	Provides information about patient status.	Have the first 100 mL of fluid analyzed for RBCs, WBCs, bilirubin, amylase, lipase, alkaline phosphate, and culture and sensitivity.[1,9]
25. Remove **PE** and discard supplies in appropriate receptacles.		
26. **HH**		

Expected Outcomes

- Lavage fluid is obtained and sent to the laboratory for analysis
- The peritoneum is cleansed of purulent exudate and microorganisms
- Stable vital sign
- No increase in pain level

Unexpected Outcomes

- Perforation of the bowel, bladder, or stomach
- Lacerations of the major vessels (mesenteric, iliac, aorta)
- Laceration of the catheter or guidewire with loss in the peritoneal cavity
- Local or systemic infection
- Hypovolemia or hypotension
- Bleeding from the insertion site
- Inadequate drainage of lavage fluid
- Respiratory compromise
- Unrelieved pain

Patient Monitoring and Care

Steps	Rationale	Reportable Conditions
		These conditions should be reported if they persist despite nursing interventions.
1. During the procedure, monitor the patient's vital signs.	Determines the patient's response to the procedure.	• Abnormal heart rate • Hypotension • Hypertension • Increased or decreased respiratory rate
2. During the procedure, monitor the patient's pulmonary status. Monitor for changes in respiratory status (i.e., rate, depth, and pattern).	Retained lavage fluid increases pressure on the diaphragm and may cause breathing difficulty.	• Respiratory rate significantly (>20%) increased or decreased from baseline • Irregular breathing pattern • Pulse oximetry <93% or significant decrease from baseline

Patient Monitoring and Care —*Continued*

Steps	Rationale	Reportable Conditions
3. Monitor for potential complications, including bowel or bladder perforation, bleeding, and intravascular volume loss.	Determines whether additional interventions are needed.	• Acute abdominal pain, distention, rigidity, and guarding • Decreased bowel sounds • Tachycardia • Hypotentsion • Blood in urine
4. Monitor for evidence of infection.	Infection is a complication of peritoneal lavage.	• Redness at the insertion site • Chills • Increased temperature
5. Monitor intake and output.	Provides data for evaluation of fluid balance status.	• Urine output <30 mL/hr • Symptoms of excess volume losses caused by significant drainage of fluid or blood from the catheter • Signs of overzealous fluid resuscitation in the face of trauma (hypertension, edema, rising peak inspiratory pressures in the intubated and ventilated patient, falling pulse oximetry [SpO_2] levels)
6. Evaluate laboratory data when returned.	Provides for an evaluation of the condition and aids in diagnosis.	• RBC count >100,000/mm^3 • Amylase value >2.5 times normal • Alkaline phosphate value >5.5 mg/dL • Positive bilirubin • Vegetable matter present • WBC count >500,000/mm • Positive culture results
7. Monitor for the presence of pain	Follows institutional standards for assessing pain. Identifies need for pain interventions	• Continued pain despite pain interventions, if performed

Documentation

Documentation should include the following:
- Patient and family education
- Performance of timeout
- Informed consent
- Date and time of the procedure
- Patient tolerance of the procedure
- Assessment of the insertion site after the procedure
- Type and amount of the fluid instilled and the dwell time
- True drainage (total drainage minus lavage fluid input)
- Medications administered

- Amount and characteristics of the fluid removed
- Specimens sent for laboratory analysis
- Vital signs and respiratory status before and after procedure
- Assessment of pain level according to institutional standards and any acute changes
- Unexpected outcomes
- Nursing interventions

References and Additional Readings

For a complete list of references and additional readings for this procedure, scan this QR code with any freely available smartphone code reader app, or visit http://booksite.elsevier.com/9780323376624.

118 Peritoneal Lavage (Assist)

Kate Deis

PURPOSE: Percutaneous peritoneal lavage is performed for both therapeutic and diagnostic purposes. Peritoneal lavage can determine whether surgery is necessary for patients who have experienced blunt or penetrating trauma to the abdomen. Peritoneal lavage can also be used for therapeutic purposes for conditions such as peritonitis and hypothermia.

PREREQUISITE NURSING KNOWLEDGE

- Knowledge of the anatomy and physiology of the abdomen is needed in order to avoid unexpected outcomes.
- Knowledge of the use of sterile technique.
- The intestines and the bladder lie immediately beneath the abdominal surface. In adults, a full bladder is raised out of the pelvis. An indwelling urinary catheter is necessary to decompress the bladder in preparation for peritoneal lavage.
- The cecum is relatively fixed and is much less mobile than the sigmoid colon; therefore, bowel perforations are more frequent in the right lower quadrant than in the left.
- A distended stomach can extend to the anterior abdominal wall. A nasogastric or orogastric tube is necessary before peritoneal lavage in order to decompress the stomach.
- Peritoneal fluid is normally straw-colored, serous fluid secreted by the cells of the peritoneum.
- Grossly bloody fluid, a red blood cell (RBC) count of greater than $100,000/mm^3$,[3,7,11] and the presence of bacteria or bile in the return fluid in the abdomen are abnormal. A white blood cell (WBC) count greater than $500,000/mm^3$ and the presence of bile or amylase in the lavage fluid are parameters, in addition to the RBC count, that can lead to operative intervention.[3,7,11]
- Diagnostic peritoneal lavage (DPL) is used less frequently than noninvasive diagnostic testing such as FAST examination and multidetector helical CT scanning in patients with blunt abdominal trauma.[4,6,12]
- DPL is used after blunt abdominal trauma or in trauma patients with head injuries, those who are unconscious, or those with preexisting paraplegia to determine the presence of the following:[2,3]
  - ❖ Hemoperitoneum (blood in lavage returns)
  - ❖ Organ injury (intestinal enzymes or microorganisms in lavage returns)
- Therapeutic lavage is used to:
  - ❖ Irrigate and cleanse purulent exudate in patients with peritonitis or intraabdominal abscess
  - ❖ Warm the abdominal cavity in patients with hypothermia

- ❖ Remove unwanted or toxic chemicals through peritoneal dialysis
- ❖ Obtain cytology specimens in patients with cancer
- For trauma patients with stab wounds and gunshot wounds to the lower chest or anterior abdomen,[1] DPL is controversial; most trauma centers operate on patients with gunshot wound injuries to the lower chest or anterior abdomen.[1]
- In the presence of trauma DPL can be used as a tool in patients with hypotension of uncertain etiology.[6]
- DPL is not needed if abdominal surgery is already indicated.[9,11]
- Because it is an invasive procedure, DPL does have a small risk of visceral injury (0.6%).[7]
- DPL is 95% sensitive and 99% specific for intraperitoneal blood; however, it cannot exclude retroperitoneal hemorrhage, disruption of the diaphragm, or hollow viscus perforation.[2,9,10]
- Computed tomographic (CT) scans are frequently used in hemodynamically stable trauma cases as the diagnostic procedure of choice.[7] Also, abdominal ultrasound scan and focused abdominal sonography in trauma (FAST) have been increasingly used to screen blunt abdominal trauma cases for hemoperitoneum.[6,11]
- DPL is quick, inexpensive and safe.[7] Hemodynamically unstable cases may also go directly to the operating room for laparotomy.
- Complementary CT and DPL decreases nontherapeutic laparotomy rates and allows nonoperative management of those patients with solid-organ injury.[11]
- Peritoneal lavage is absolutely contraindicated in an acute abdomen that needs immediate surgery as indicated by free air on radiograph or penetrating abdominal trauma.
- Relative contraindications include the following:[7,8]
  - ❖ Thrombocytopenia
  - ❖ Coagulopathy[9]
  - ❖ Morbid obesity[9]
  - ❖ Severe bowel distension
  - ❖ Advanced cirrhosis[9]
  - ❖ Previous abdominal surgery, especially pelvic surgery
  - ❖ Distended bladder that cannot be emptied with a Foley catheter

* Obvious infection at intended site of insertion (cellulitis or abscess)
* Pregnancy of greater than 12 weeks' gestation[9]

* Practitioners should use caution when performing DPL in patients with suspected pelvic fractures (a supraumbilical site may be used) because of false-positive results;[9] if performed in pregnant patients of more than 12 weeks' gestation, an open technique, superior to the uterus, is used.[9]
* The practitioner who performs peritoneal lavage should choose an insertion site midline, one third the distance from the umbilicus to the symphysis, or 2 to 3 cm below the umbilicus (see Fig. 115-1). An alternate position is a point one-third the distance from the umbilicus to the anterior iliac crest (left side preferred).
* The physician or advanced practice nurse can use ultrasound scan before peritoneal lavage to locate fluid and during the procedure to guide insertion of the catheter.[11]

EQUIPMENT

* Commercially prepared kit or the following:
  * Personal protective equipment, including sterile gloves, mask, goggles, and gown
  * Antiseptic solution (e.g., 2% chlorhexidine based preparation)
  * Sterile marking pen
  * Sterile towels or sterile drape
  * Local anesthetic for injection: 1% or 2% lidocaine with epinephrine
  * 5- or 10-mL syringe with 25- or 27-gauge needle for anesthetic
  * Scalpel and no. 11 knife blade
  * Trocar with stylet; needle (16-, 18-, or 20-gauge) or angiocatheter; depending on abdominal wall thickness, may use guidewire with floppy tip and 9 to 18 Fr peritoneal lavage catheter
  * 20-mL syringe for diagnostic tap
  * Sterile intravenous (IV) tubing (without valves) with appropriate sterile connectors for lavage, catheter, and IV bags
  * Sterile tubes for specimens
  * Warmed Ringer's lactate (RL), normal saline (NS), or antibiotic solution for infusion into abdomen
  * Three-way stopcock for therapeutic lavage
  * Nylon skin suture material on cutting needle (4-0 or 5-0) and needle holder
  * Four to six sterile 4 x 4 gauze pads
  * Sterile gauze dressing with tape or adhesive strip
  * Pressure bag

Additional equipment, to have available as needed, includes the following:
* Razor or scissors
* Soft wrist restraints

PATIENT AND FAMILY EDUCATION

* Reinforce the indications, the procedure, and the risks to the patient and family. *Rationale:* Patient anxiety may be decreased, and patient and family cooperation and understanding of procedure are encouraged.

* Explain the patient's role in assisting with the procedure and postprocedure care. *Rationale:* Patient cooperation during and after the procedure is elicited.
* Explain the signs and symptoms to report, such as fever, abdominal pain, decreased urine output, bleeding, and leakage of fluid from wound site. *Rationale:* Alerts the nurse to signs and symptoms of complications.

PATIENT ASSESSMENT AND PREPARATION

Patient Assessment

* Obtain the medical history and perform a review of systems to identify abdominal injury, peritonitis, intraabdominal abscess, or pregnancy. *Rationale:* Certain conditions of the gastrointestinal tract may be diagnosed and treated with peritoneal lavage. Contraindications to peritoneal lavage may be identified.[6]
* Identify the presence of any allergies to medication or other substances. *Rationale:* Patients may have allergies to skin preparations or anesthetics used before the invasive procedure is performed. Identification assists the practitioner in choosing the most appropriate skin preparation and anesthetic.
* Assess for bowel or bladder distention. *Rationale:* Distension increases the risk for bowel or bladder perforation during the procedure.[9] Insertion of a nasogastric or orogastric tube and an indwelling urinary catheter are necessary in order to decompress the bladder and stomach and prevent injury during the procedure.
* Assess coagulation study results (i.e., prothrombin time [PT], partial thromboplastin time [PTT], and platelets). *Rationale:* Abnormal clotting study results may increase the risk for bleeding during and after the procedure. Therapy may be necessary to correct clotting abnormalities before the procedure is performed.
* Obtain vital signs and assess pain. *Rationale:* Provides baseline data.

Patient Preparation

* Ensure that the patient understands preprocedural teachings. Answer questions as they arise, and reinforce information as needed. *Rationale:* Understanding of previously taught information is evaluated and reinforced.
* Ensure that a written informed consent form has been obtained by the physician, advanced practice nurse, or other healthcare professional performing the procedure (if possible). The physician, advanced practice nurse, or other healthcare professional who is assisting may be a witness to the signing of the consent if needed. In a trauma situation or with an unresponsive patient, this consent may be implied. *Rationale:* Peritoneal lavage is an invasive procedure that requires signed informed consent.
* If prescribed, insert a urinary drainage catheter. *Rationale:* A distended bladder increases the risk for bladder perforation during the procedure.[9]
* If prescribed, insert a nasogastric tube unless contraindicated (e.g., in significant facial trauma) and attach to low intermittent suction. *Rationale:* A distended

stomach increases the risk for perforation during the procedure.[8]
- Perform a preprocedure verification and time out, if non-emergent. *Rationale:* Ensures patient safety.
- Verify that the patient is the correct patient with two identifiers. *Rationale:* Before performing a procedure, the physician or advanced practice nurse and the healthcare provider assisting in the procedure should ensure the correct identification of the patient for the intended intervention.

- Place the patient in the supine position (may tilt to side of fluid collection slightly for improved fluid positioning). *Rationale:* Fluid accumulates in the dependent areas.
- Administer analgesia and/or sedation as prescribed. *Rationale:* Analgesia and sedation may promote patient comfort and safety during the procedure.
- If the patient has altered mental status, soft wrist restraints may be needed and prescribed. *Rationale:* The patient must not move the hands into the sterile field once it has been established.

Procedure   for Assisting With Peritoneal Lavage

Steps	Rationale	Special Considerations
1. HH		
2. PE		
3. Assist the physician, advanced practice nurse, or other healthcare provider performing the procedure with applying personal protective and sterile equipment (e.g., head cover, mask, eye protection, sterile gown).	Minimizes the risk of infection. Maintains aseptic and sterile precautions.	
4. Assist as needed with preparing the equipment.	Facilitates easy access to needed equipment.	
5. Assist as needed with setting up the lavage equipment.	Provides a closed system for instillation and drainage of lavage fluid.	
A. Assist with attaching the IV tubing to the lavage fluid and clear the tubing of air.	Priming the tubing prevents instillation of air into the peritoneum	
B. Assist with attaching the IV tubing to one port of the three-way stopcock and drainage collector to the second port of the three-way stopcock.		
C. Use the IV tubing with a roller clamp and use the lavage fluid bag as the drainage bag.		
6. Assist the physician or advanced practice nurse by providing antiseptic solution if needed.	Provides assistance.	
7. Assist the physician or advance practice nurse as needed with preparing the local anesthetic (lidocaine with epinephrine preferred).	Local anesthesia minimizes pain and discomfort. Epinephrine helps eliminate unwanted abdominal wall bleeding and false-positive results.[5]	The maximum dose of lidocaine is 30 mL of 1% or 15 mL of 2%. The physician or advanced practice nurse will need to assess for anesthesia of the area.
8. Assist the physician or advance practice nurse as needed by providing supplies during the catheter insertion.	Provides assistance.	
9. Assist as needed with attaching the lavage catheter to the remaining port of the stopcock and the tubing to withdraw peritoneal fluid.	Fluid may be gently aspirated, siphoned via gravity, or collected into a vacuum device.	Retain the first 100 mL of fluid for laboratory analysis. **Refer to Step 27** for specific laboratory tests.[1,9]

Procedure	for Assisting With Peritoneal Lavage—*Continued*	
Steps	**Rationale**	**Special Considerations**

10. Assist as needed with instilling lavage fluid:
  A. If a drainage collector is used, turn the stopcock off to the drainage collector.
  B. Open the clamp on the IV tubing.
  C. Instill 700 to1000 mL of warmed RL or NS solution or antibacterial fluid.
	Directs lavage fluid into the peritoneal space.	Infuse over 10 to15 minutes. This may be done with a pressure bag to decrease time.

11. Assist as needed with turning the patient side to side (if not contraindicated).	Facilitates sampling of fluid that may accumulate in pockets on either side. Mixes the solution with any free material in the abdominal cavity.	

12. Assist as needed with draining the lavage fluid:
  A. If a drainage collector is used, turn the stopcock off to the IV tubing.
  B. If a drainage collector is not used, lower the IV bag to a level below the patient.
  C. Allow fluid to drain into the drainage collector or the lowered IV bag.
	Directs the lavage fluid from the peritoneal space to the drainage collector.	In therapeutic lavage, consider the dwell time of fluid before drainage (usually 5 to10 minutes).
		When draining fluid, be careful that there is no tension on the tubing.

13. As needed, assist with turning the patient side to side (if not contraindicated).	Facilitates drainage of fluid that may accumulate in pockets on either side.	Lavage fluid may be absorbed into the intravascular space, creating a potential fluid volume excess. Twisting of the catheter may free the catheter from adhering to the peritoneum and facilitate drainage of fluid.
14. **Repeat Steps 10–13** as needed.	Continued lavage may be needed to cleanse the peritoneal space.	
15. If the lavage is positive for blood, assist with preparing the patient for immediate surgery.	Immediate repair of the bleeding site is needed.	The incision may be left open and covered with a sterile NS solution–soaked dressing.

16. After the fluid is removed:
  A. The catheter is gently removed by the physician or advanced practice nurse.
  B. Pressure is applied to the wound.
  C. The puncture site is sutured.
  D. Assist as needed with applying a dry dressing.
	Keeps the insertion site clean.
	Reduces the risk for infection.
	Provides a barrier to infection and collects fluid that may leak from wound site.
		The catheter should be inspected on removal to ensure it is intact.

17. Prepare and send the fluid specimens for laboratory analysis as prescribed.	Provides information about patient status.	Have the first 100 mL of fluid analyzed for RBCs, WBCs, bilirubin, amylase, lipase, alkaline phosphate, and culture and sensitivity.[9]
18. Remove **HH** and discard used supplies in appropriate receptacles.	Standard Precautions.	
19. **HH**		

Procedure continues on following page

Expected Outcomes

- Lavage fluid is obtained and sent to the laboratory for analysis
- The peritoneum cleansed of purulent exudate and microorganisms
- Stable vital signs
- No increase in pain level

Unexpected Outcomes

- Perforation of the bowel, bladder, or stomach
- Lacerations of the major vessels (mesenteric, iliac, aorta)
- Laceration of the catheter or guidewire with loss in the peritoneal cavity
- Local or systemic infection
- Hypovolemia, hypotension
- Bleeding from the insertion site
- Inadequate drainage of lavage fluid
- Respiratory compromise
- Unrelieved pain

Patient Monitoring and Care

Steps	Rationale	Reportable Conditions
		These conditions should be reported if they persist despite nursing interventions.
1. During the procedure monitor the patient's vital signs.	Determines the patient's response to the procedure	• Abnormal heart rate • Hypotension • Hypertension • Increased or decreased respiratory rate
2. During the procedure monitor the patient's pulmonary status. Monitor for changes in respiratory status (i.e., rate, depth, and pattern).	Retained lavage fluid increases pressure on the diaphragm and may cause breathing difficulty.	• Respiratory rate significantly (>20%) increased or decreased from baseline • Irregular breathing pattern • Pulse oximetry <93%, or significant decrease from baseline
3. Monitor for potential complications, including bowel or bladder perforation, bleeding, and intravascular volume loss.	Determines whether additional interventions are needed.	• Acute abdominal pain, distention, rigidity, and guarding • Decreased bowel sounds • Blood in urine • Hypotension • Tachycardia
4. Monitor for evidence of infection.	Infection is a complication of peritoneal lavage.	• Redness at the insertion site • Increased temperature • Chills
5. Monitor intake and output.	Provides data for evaluation of fluid balance status.	• Urine output <30 mL/hr • Symptoms of excess volume losses caused by significant drainage of fluid or blood from catheter • Signs of overzealous fluid resuscitation in the face of trauma (hypertension, edema, rising peak inspiratory pressures in the intubated and ventilated patient, falling pulse oximetry [Spo_2] levels)

Patient Monitoring and Care —*Continued*

Steps	Rationale	Reportable Conditions
6. Evaluate laboratory data when returned.	Provides for an evaluation of the condition and aids in diagnosis.	• RBCs >100,000/mm³ • Amylase value >2.5 times normal • Alkaline phosphate value >5.5 mg/dL • Positive bilirubin results • Vegetable matter present • WBCs >500,000/mm • Positive culture results
7. Monitor for the presence of pain	Follow institutional standards for assessing pain. Identifies need for pain interventions	• Continued pain despite pain interventions, if performed

Documentation

Documentation should include the following:
- Patient and family education
- Performance of time out
- Informed consent
- Date and time of the procedure
- Patient tolerance of the procedure
- Assessment of the insertion site after the procedure
- Type and amount of the fluid instilled and the dwell time
- True drainage (total drainage minus lavage fluid input)

- Medications administered
- Amount and characteristics of the fluid removed
- Specimens sent for laboratory analysis
- Preprocedure and postprocedure vital signs, respiratory status
- Assessment of pain level according to institutional standards and any acute changes
- Unexpected outcomes
- Nursing interventions

References and Additional Readings

For a complete list of references and additional readings for this procedure, scan this QR code with any freely available smartphone code reader app, or visit http://booksite.elsevier.com/9780323376624.

PROCEDURE

119 Continuous Renal Replacement Therapies

Sonia M. Astle

PURPOSE: Continuous renal replacement therapies are used in the critical care unit setting for volume regulation, acid-base control, electrolyte regulation, drug intoxications, management of azotemia, and immune modulation. These methods are most often used in critically ill patients whose hemodynamic status does not tolerate the rapid fluid and electrolyte shifts associated with intermittent hemodialysis or who need continuous removal or regulation of solutes and intravascular volume.

PREREQUISITE NURSING KNOWLEDGE

- Continuous renal replacement therapy (CRRT) is an extracorporeal blood-purification therapy intended to substitute for impaired renal function over an extended period of time for, or attempted for, 24 hours per day.[1]
- CRRT can be accomplished through a variety of methods, with either arteriovenous (AV) access or venovenous (VV) access. The VV access is used almost exclusively because of its less invasive nature. In the past, AV access was used, requiring both arterial and venous cannulation. With AV access, the patient's systemic blood pressure is required for blood to flow into the extracorporeal circuit, making it unreliable for hypotensive patients. The newer-generation CRRT machines have an added extracorporeal blood pump that pulls the patient's blood into the circuit, so it is better suited to treat hemodynamically unstable patients.[10,18]
- The following methods of CRRT are included as listed (details are outlined in Table 119-1):
  - ❖ Slow, continuous ultrafiltration (SCUF)
  - ❖ Continuous venovenous hemofiltration (CVVH)
  - ❖ Continuous venovenous hemodialysis (CVVHD)
  - ❖ Continuous venovenous hemodiafiltration (CVVHDF)
- Basic knowledge is required to understand the principles of diffusion, ultrafiltration (UF), osmosis, oncotic pressure, and hydrostatic pressure and how they pertain to fluid and solute management during dialysis.
  - ❖ *Diffusion:* The passive movement of solutes through a semipermeable membrane from an area of higher to lower concentration until equilibrium is reached.
  - ❖ *Convective transport:* The rapid movement of fluid across a semipermeable membrane from an area of

high pressure to an area of low pressure with transport of solutes. When water moves across a membrane along a pressure gradient, some solutes are carried along with the water and do not require a solute concentration gradient (also called solute drag). Convective transport is most effective for the removal of middle-molecular-weight and large-molecular-weight solutes.

- ❖ *UF:* The bulk movement of solute and solvent through a semipermeable membrane in response to a pressure difference across the membrane. This movement is usually achieved with positive pressure in the blood compartment in the hemofilter and negative pressure in the dialysate compartment. Blood and dialysate run countercurrent. The size of the solute molecules compared with the size of molecules that can move through the semipermeable membrane determines the degree of UF.
- ❖ *Osmosis:* The passive movement of solvent through a semipermeable membrane from an area of higher to lower concentration.
- ❖ *Oncotic pressure:* The pressure exerted by plasma proteins that favor intravascular fluid retention and movement of fluid from the extravascular to the intravascular space.
- ❖ *Hydrostatic pressure:* The force exerted by arterial blood pressure that favors the movement of fluid from the intravascular to the extravascular space.
- ❖ *Absorption:* The process by which drug molecules pass through membranes and fluid barriers and into body fluids.
- ❖ *Adsorption:* The adhesion of molecules (solutes) to the surface of the hemofilter, charcoal, or resin.
- CRRT uses an artificial kidney (i.e., hemofilter, dialyzer) with a semipermeable membrane to create two separate

| TABLE 119-1 | Continuous Renal Replacement Therapies |

Ultrafiltration Mode of Therapies	Principles Involved	Access	Indications	Advantages	Complications/ Disadvantages
SCUF (slow, continuous ultrafiltration)	Ultrafiltration	Venovenous	Patients with diuretic-resistant, volume-overloaded, hemodynamically unstable conditions who cannot tolerate rapid fluid shifts	Continuous, gradual treatment (fewer high and low extremes) Precise fluid control can be done in patient with low mean arterial pressure	Anticoagulation, bleeding Hypotension Hypothermia Access complications (bleeding, clotting, infection) Requires strict monitoring of fluid and electrolyte replacement to avoid deficits or overload Air embolism Critical care setting only Poor control of azotemia; dialysis may be needed Minimal solute clearance Not recommended for emergently treating hyperkalemia or acidosis
CVVH (continuous venovenous hemofiltration)	Ultrafiltration Convection Solute removal	Venovenous	Patient with volume-overloaded, hemodynamically unstable condition with azotemia or uremia	Precise fluid control can be done in patients with low mean arterial pressure Ease of initiation	Anticoagulation, bleeding Hypotension Hypothermia Access complications (bleeding, clotting, infection) Requires strict monitoring of fluid and electrolyte replacement to avoid deficits or overload Air embolism Critical care setting only Recommended 1:1 nurse/ patient ratio Metabolite removal not as efficient as CVVHDF
CVVHD (continuous venovenous hemodialysis)	Ultrafiltration Diffusion Solute removal	Venovenous	Patients with volume-overloaded, hemodynamically unstable conditions with azotemia or uremia	Precise fluid control can be done in patients with low mean arterial pressure Ease of initiation	Same as CVVH Hyperglycemia Hypernatremia Hypophosphatemia
CVVHDF (continuous venovenous hemodiafiltration)	Ultrafiltration Convection Diffusion Solute removal	Venovenous	Patient with volume-overloaded, hemodynamically unstable conditions with azotemia or uremia, catabolic acute renal failure, electrolyte imbalance/ metabolic acidosis	Precise fluid control can be done in patient with low mean arterial pressure Better solute clearance than CVVH/ CVVHD Ease of initiation	Same as CVVH Hyperglycemia Hypernatremia Hypophosphatemia

Adapted from Giuliano K, Pysznik E: Renal replacement therapy in critical care: implementation of a unit-based CVVH program, Crit Care Nurse 18:40–45, 1998.

compartments: the blood compartment and the dialysis solution compartment. The semipermeable membrane allows the movement of small molecules (e.g., electrolytes) and middle-size molecules (e.g., creatinine, vasoactive substances) from the patient's blood into the dialysis solution but is impermeable to larger molecules (e.g., red blood cells, plasma proteins).

• Each dialyzer has four ports: two end ports for blood (blood flows in one end and out the other) and two side ports for dialysis solution ultrafiltrate (dialysate solution flows in one end and out the other). In most cases, the blood and dialysate run through the dialyzer in opposite or countercurrent directions.

- Hollow-fiber dialyzers are used almost exclusively for CRRT. The blood flows through the center of hollow fibers, and the dialysis solution (dialysate) flows around the outside of the hollow fibers. The advantages of hollow-fiber filters include a low priming volume, a low resistance to flow, and a high amount of surface area. The major disadvantage is the potential for clotting as a result of the small fiber size.

- All dialyzers have a UF coefficient; thus, the dialyzer selected varies in different clinical situations.[2–6,8,9] The higher the UF coefficient, the more rapid the fluid removal.[12,16,19] UF coefficients are determined with in vivo measurements done by each dialyzer manufacturer.

- Clearance refers to the ability of the dialyzer to remove metabolic waste products or drugs from the patient's blood. The blood flow rate, the dialysate flow rate, and the solute concentration affect clearance. Clearance occurs by the processes of diffusion, convection, and UF.

- The dialysate (when used during CRRT) is composed of water, a buffer (i.e., lactate or bicarbonate), and various electrolytes. Most solutions also contain glucose. The buffer helps neutralize acids that are generated as a result of normal cellular metabolism. The concentration of electrolytes is usually the normal plasma concentration, which helps to create a concentration gradient for removal of excess electrolytes. The glucose aids in increasing the oncotic pressure in the dialysate (thus aiding in fluid removal) and in caloric replacement. Although glucose comes in various concentrations, it is usually used in normal plasma concentrations to prevent hyperglycemia.

- Heparin or citrate are often used during CRRT to prevent clotting of the extracorporeal circuit during treatment. Saline solution flushes can be used alone or with other anticoagulants to maintain circuit patency.[31,33]

- An anticoagulant may be used to maintain vascular access patency when CRRT is not in use.[4,18,33]

- If the patient is taking angiotensin-converting enzyme (ACE) inhibitors, contact with certain filters or membranes in the CRRT system can cause an anaphylactic reaction and severe hypotension as a result of increased levels of bradykinin, a potent vasodilator.[15] ACE inhibitors are recommended to be withheld for 48 to 72 hours before treatment, if possible.

- Continuous venovenous renal replacement therapy is achieved with a pumped system.

- The patient's volume status and serum electrolyte levels are changed gradually so that patients have fewer problems maintaining hemodynamic stability than with hemodialysis. Specifics of these therapies are outlined in Table 119-1.[1,3,6,10,22–24,28,29]

- SCUF (Fig. 119-1) is a nonpumped system; CVVH (Fig. 119-2), CVVHD (Fig. 119-3), and CVVHDF (Fig. 119-4) use pump-driven systems. These therapies are used to remove both plasma water and solutes and require venous access, most commonly provided with a double-lumen vascular access catheter (VAC). Hemodialysis shunts or surgically created hemodialysis anastomoses have been

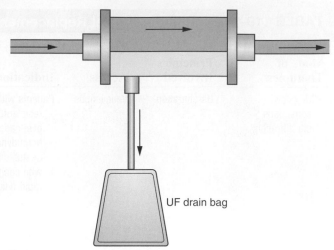

Figure 119-1 Slow continuous ultrafiltration (SCUF). Fluid removal, no fluid replacement. *(Copyright Rhonda K. Martin. All rights reserved. Used with permission.)*

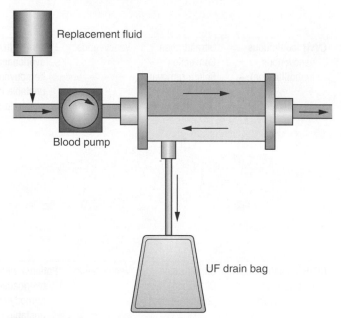

Figure 119-2 Continuous venovenous hemofiltration (CVVH). Fluid removal and fluid replacement. *(Copyright Rhonda K. Martin. All rights reserved. Used with permission.)*

used in the past for CRRT; however, because of increased incidence rates of vascular injury, bleeding, and infection, they are *not* recommended for CRRT access.[1,18] Common sites for the VAC are the internal jugular, subclavian, and femoral veins. The internal jugular approach is the preferred access. Cannulation of the subclavian vein may cause stenosis and prevent placement of upper extremity grafts or fistulas if long-term dialysis is necessary.[4,25,28] Femoral cannulation is associated with increased infection.[4,16,32]

- A blood pump provides the pressure that drives the extracorporeal system; the blood circuit consists of blood lines, a blood pump, and various monitoring devices. The blood lines are connected to the vascular access and carry the blood to and from the patient. The blood pump controls the speed of the blood through the circuit. The monitoring

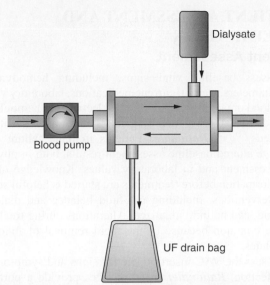

Figure 119-3 Continuous venovenous hemodialysis (CVVHD). Fluid and solute removal with dialysate. *(Copyright Rhonda K. Martin. All rights reserved. Used with permission.)*

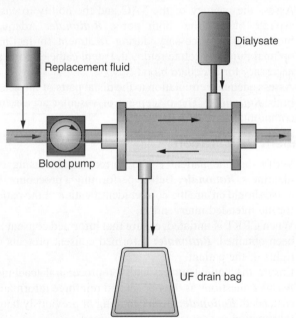

Figure 119-4 Continuous venovenous hemodiafiltration (CVVHDF). Fluid replacement with dialysate. *(Copyright Rhonda K. Martin. All rights reserved. Used with permission.)*

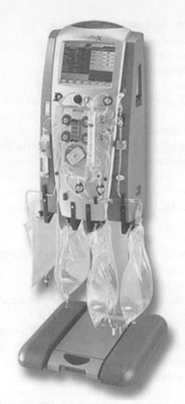

Figure 119-5 Gambro Prismaflex Continuous renal replacement therapy machine. *(Courtesy Gambro USA, Lakewood, Colo.)*

devices include arterial and venous pressure monitors and an air detection monitor to prevent air that may have entered the circuit from being infused to the patient. Anticoagulant, dialysate, and replacement fluids can also be added to the system.

❖ Integrated pump systems have separate pumps for blood, dialysate, ultrafiltrate/effluent, and replacement fluids (Fig. 119-5). The pumps are controlled by a computerized control module. Blood flow rate, dialysate flow rate, anticoagulation rate, and fluid-removal rates are entered by the nurse as prescribed. Dialysate, ultrafiltrate/effluent, and replacement fluids are measured by weight or volumetric scales on the machine.

The module calculates and adjusts pump speeds to achieve the selected fluid goal. The module also records and displays treatment data.

- SCUF (see Fig. 119-1) is used primarily to remove plasma water. A hemofilter with a large surface area, high sieving coefficient, and low resistance is used to facilitate slow continuous fluid removal.
- CVVH (see Fig. 119-2) removes fluids and solutes via convective clearance. Replacement solution is part of the setup; the replacement solution creates a solute drag effect.
- CVVHD (see Fig. 119-3) is used to remove solutes primarily via diffusion. Dialysate solution is part of the setup; flow of the dialysate is countercurrent to the blood flow.
- CVVHDF (see Fig. 119-4) removes fluids and solutes via diffusion and convection. Dialysate runs countercurrent to the blood flow and clears toxins by diffusion. Replacement fluid is infused at a prescribed rate and clears by convection.
- Other extended renal replacement therapy techniques or "hybrid" techniques (sustained low-efficiency dialysis, extended daily dialysis) generally use standard hemodialysis equipment with reduced blood flow and dialysate rates to gradually remove plasma water and solutes. They are used from 4 to 12 hours a day.[26]

EQUIPMENT

- Dedicated vascular access
- Hemofilter/pump system with blood lines

- Replacement fluid as prescribed
- Dialysate fluid as prescribed
- Fluid shield, face masks, or goggles
- Sterile and nonsterile gloves
- Fluid warmer
- Two 10-mL prefilled syringes with normal saline (NS) solution
- Sterile NS solution, 1 to 2 L
- Dressing supplies (alcohol wipes, sterile barrier, gauze pads, transparent dressing, tape)
- Antiseptic solution (e.g., 2% chlorhexidine–based preparation)
- Heparin, 1000 units/mL, or citrate (for priming, as prescribed)
- Drainage bag
- Intravenous (IV) accessory spike to connect NS bag to arterial tubing
- Two dialysis luer caps for the VAC

Additional equipment, to have available as needed, includes the following:

- Two 5-mL syringes and blunt-tip needles (if needed to draw up NS for injection)
- NS for injection (if prefilled NS syringes are not used)
- Plastic hemodialysis clamps

PATIENT AND FAMILY EDUCATION

- Explain the purpose of CRRT—specifically why the treatment is performed and the expected clinical outcomes. *Rationale:* The patient and family should understand that CRRT is necessary to perform the physiological functions of the kidneys if the patient is hemodynamically unstable.
- Explain the procedure, including risks, anticipated length of treatment, and patient positioning, and review any questions the patient may have. *Rationale:* Explanation provides information and may decrease patient anxiety.
- Explain the need for careful sterile technique for the duration of treatment. *Rationale:* The patient and family must know the importance of sterile technique to decrease the likelihood of systemic infection.
- Explain the need for careful monitoring of the patient during the treatment, particularly for fluid and electrolyte imbalance. *Rationale:* The patient and family should understand that careful monitoring is a routine part of CRRT.
- Explain the signs and symptoms of possible complications during CRRT. *Rationale:* Patients and family should be fully prepared if complications occur (e.g., hypotension, hemorrhage, manifestations of fluid/electrolyte/acid-base imbalance).
- Explain the CRRT circuit setup to the patient and family. *Rationale:* It is important that the patient and family know that blood will be removed from the patient's body and will be visible during the CRRT treatment.

PATIENT ASSESSMENT AND PREPARATION

Patient Assessment

- Assess baseline vital signs, including hemodynamic parameters, weight, current medications, laboratory values (blood urea nitrogen, creatinine, electrolytes, hemoglobin, and hematocrit), neurological status, and nutritional needs.[7,11,17,27] *Rationale:* Patients in renal failure often have altered baseline assessment results, both in physical assessment and in laboratory values. Knowledge of this information before treatments are started is helpful so that interventions, including net fluid balance and dialysate fluid, can be individualized. Alterations during treatment are common because of the rapid removal of fluid and solutes.
- Assess the VAC insertion site for signs and symptoms of infection. *Rationale:* Insertion sites provide a portal of entry for organisms, which may result in septicemia if unrecognized or untreated. If the insertion site appears to be infected, further interventions (e.g., site change, culture, antibiotic treatment) may be necessary.
- Assess the patency of the VAC and the ability to easily aspirate blood from both ports. *Rationale:* Adequate blood flow is necessary during treatment to facilitate optimal fluid and solute removal. Patent catheter ports are necessary for adequate blood flow.
- Assess adequate circulation to the distal parts of the access limb. *Rationale:* The placement of vascular access may compromise circulation.

Patient Preparation

- Verify that the patient is the correct patient using two identifiers. *Rationale:* Before performing a procedure, the nurse should ensure the correct identification of the patient for the intended intervention.
- When CRRT is initiated, ensure that informed consent has been obtained. *Rationale:* Informed consent protects the rights of the patient.
- Ensure the patient understands preprocedural teachings. Answer questions as they arise, and reinforce information as needed. *Rationale:* Understanding of previously taught information is evaluated and reinforced.
- Position the patient in a comfortable position (that also facilitates optimal blood flow through the vascular access). *Rationale:* The patient and family must understand that movement may affect blood flow through the system and that a comfortable position is important.
- Following initiation of treatment, continue to reposition the patient at regular intervals. *Rationale:* Critically ill patients are at a high risk for pressure points and skin breakdown.

Procedure	**for Initiation and Termination of Continuous Renal Replacement Therapy**	
Steps	**Rationale**	**Special Considerations**

Systems (SCUF, CVVH, CVVHD, CVVHDF)

1. **HH**
2. **PE**
3. Verify orders, which should include the following:
   - A. Modality
   - B. Vascular access
   - C. Type of hemofilter/dialyzer
   - D. Anticoagulant type, concentration, infusion rate, monitoring parameters
   - E. Replacement fluid and rate (if used)
   - F. Hourly ultrafiltration UF rate
   - G. Hourly net fluid goal
   - H. Dialysate solution and rate (if used)
   - I. Blood pressure/vital sign parameters
   - J. Laboratory testing

   Rationale: Familiarizes the nurse with the individualized patient treatment and reduces the possibility of error.[4,6]

   Special Considerations: Ensure patient weight and laboratory values are assessed and recorded before initiation of therapy. Communicate with the nephrologist/intensivist ordering therapy if questions arise.[14,30]

4. Prepare the system:
   - A. Turn the machine on.
   - B. Load the circuit according to the manufacturer's instructions.
   - C. Attach solutions as prescribed.
   - D. Prepare anticoagulant infusion as prescribed.
   - E. Prepare replacement fluid, dialysate, and flush infusion as prescribed.
   - F. For integrated pump units follow the manufacturer's instructions and prompts from the control screen.
   - G. Automated setup instructions include:
     1. Select therapy/modality.
     2. Calibration (if indicated).
     3. Load set.
     4. Priming.
     5. Anticoagulant.
     6. Dialysate and replacement fluid rates.
     7. Blood flow. rate
     8. Fluid removal rate.
   - H. After priming per manufacturer instructions, **go to Step 5.**

   Rationale: Correct system setup is imperative for safety and optimal functioning. The use of anticoagulants prolongs the function of the hemofilter.[4,6]

   Special Considerations: The pump must be plugged into a generator outlet because some pumps do not have battery power. Heparin, if ordered, is usually administered on a prefilter port; citrate is usually administered at the arterial port of the VAC or infused via the preblood pump. Replacement solutions are administered through the arterial (access) or venous (return) infusion port as ordered (usually arterial) with blood tubing. Connect 1 L NS to arterial infusion port (for flushing system). Dialysate solution (if CVVHD/CVVHDF are used) is connected to the outlet port of the hemofilter near the venous end with blood tubing. Each integrated pump is loaded and primed according to the manufacturer's recommendations, ranging from assembly and priming of all components to "one-touch" circuit loading and priming. Some unit's air detectors are activated after the machine is primed.

5. Leave the priming bag, collection bag, and protective caps in place until the blood lines are attached to the VAC.

   Rationale: Preserves the sterility of the system.

   Special Considerations: Some systems have a collection bag for the priming solution, which stays attached to the venous blood line until it is attached to the VAC.

6. Remove gloves and discard in the appropriate receptacles.

   Rationale: Reduces transmission of microorganisms; Standard Precautions.

Procedure continues on following page

Procedure	for Initiation and Termination of Continuous Renal Replacement Therapy—*Continued*	
Steps	**Rationale**	**Special Considerations**
7. Wash hands.	Reduces transmission of microorganisms on the hands after removal of gloves and before performing a sterile procedure.	
8. Prepare a sterile field with sterile barrier under the VAC.	Prepares material and maintains aseptic technique.	
9. Place 4 × 4 gauze pads onto the sterile field. Open sterile container, syringes, blunt-tip needles, and NS (or prefilled NS syringes) and place on the sterile field.	Prepares material and maintains aseptic technique.	
10. Add antiseptic solution (e.g., 2% chlorhexidine–based preparation) to sterile container or use prepackaged bactericidal agents. **(Level D*)**	Prepares solution used to cleanse VAC ports. Povidone-iodine, hypochlorite, and chlorhexidine solutions are acceptable bactericidal agents.[4,18,31]	
11. Wash hands and apply sterile gloves.	Maintains aseptic technique.	
12. Attach blunt-tip needles to two 10-mL syringes; with help of assistant, fill with NS or use prefilled syringes per institutional standards.	Prepares syringe for VAC flushing.	With Quinton catheters, a 20–30 mL per lumen flush for hemocaths and permacaths is recommended.[1]
13. Saturate four of the 4 × 4 pads in the antiseptic solution. Using two of the soaked pads, perform a 1-minute scrub of the arterial and venous ports of the VAC. Alternatively, perform a 30-second scrub of the ports with antiseptic swabs.	Prevents introduction of pathogens.	Be sure to remove any crust or drainage at the catheter insertion site.
14. Ensure clamps are closed on the arterial and venous ports of the VAC; then remove the cap from the arterial port of the VAC and discard. Alternatively, many facilities are using dialysis-specific luer caps that lock into the VAC.	Provides access to the arterial side of the VAC. The VAC is not opened to air unless caps require changing, reducing the chance of contamination and infection.	Be sure the VAC clamp is closed before removing arterial and venous port caps.
15. Attach an empty 5-mL syringe to the arterial port, open the clamp, and gently aspirate 5 mL of blood and anticoagulant. Close the clamp, remove the syringe, and discard it in an appropriate receptacle.	Verifies the patency of the arterial port. Note any resistance, which may indicate a clotted or kinked port. Prevents bolus of anticoagulant to the patient (if used) and decreases transmission of microorganisms.[4,18]	Do not forward-flush an indwelling port before aspirating. This prevents dislodgment/embolism of clots and prevents a bolus of anticoagulant to the patient. Observe for clots. A clotted or kinked port decreases blood flow and reduces efficacy of the treatment.
16. Attach a 10-mL syringe with NS flush solution to the arterial port. Open the clamp and flush; then close the clamp.	Prevents clotting of blood until dialysis is initiated.	Note any resistance on flushing.

*Level D: Peer-reviewed professional and organizational standards with the support of clinical study recommendations.

Procedure	for Initiation and Termination of Continuous Renal Replacement Therapy—*Continued*	
Steps	**Rationale**	**Special Considerations**
17. **Repeat Steps 15–16** on the venous port.	Provides access to the venous side of the catheter.	
18. Disconnect the access line from the primed circuit and attach it to the arterial port of the VAC; secure the connection.	Loose connections introduce air into the circuit.	
19. Disconnect the return line from the primed circuit and attach it to the venous port of the VAC; secure the connection.	Loose connections introduce air into the circuit.	
20. Open the clamps on the VAC ports and the access and return blood lines.	Opens the circuit in preparation for starting the blood pump.	Perform a final check for air in the circuit.
21. Check that all alarms are on and parameters are set.	Ensures safe delivery of therapy.	
22. Turn the blood pump on and gradually increase the blood flow to the prescribed rate.	Prevents hypotension from rapid blood and fluid shifts.	Observe for blood leaks, air in the system, and pressure alarms. Assess the patient's vital signs, which should remain within 20% of baseline parameters.
23. Note blood pump flow rate, arterial and venous monitor pressures, transmembrane (TMP) filter pressure, the amount and color of UF, and vital signs on initiation and hourly or per institutional standards.	Ensures safe delivery of therapy.	Increased arterial pressure indicates problems with the vascular access or blood inflow. Increased venous pressure indicates clotting of the system. Decreased venous pressure indicates clotting of the hemofilter.
24. Remove **PE** and discard supplies in the appropriate receptacles.	Safely discards used supplies.	
25. **HH**		
26. Prepare a fluid balance flow sheet and calculate the net fluid gain/loss prescribed each hour or document in the electronic health record.	Accurate calculations of hourly fluid balance prevent hypervolemia and hypovolemia and ensure that clinical goals are being met.	Hourly fluid balance is usually calculated by subtracting the total output (including UF removed) from the total intake.
Flushing		
1. **HH**		
2. **PE**		
3. Connect the NS with primed tubing to the arterial port of the VAC and the access line of the circuit via a three-way stopcock.	Prepares port for flushing.	
4. Clamp the arterial port of the VAC by turning the stopcock off to the VAC port.	Prevents any more blood from entering the circuit via the arterial port during flushing.	**Note:** Be sure that the NS flush is running freely to prevent rupture or back filtration. Hemostasis and clot formation in the arterial limb of the tubing are possibilities if the flushing procedure is prolonged.
5. Open the NS flush while the pump continues to run. Note the amount of NS that has infused.	Flushing allows the nurse to assess the patency of the system.[3]	Flushing contributes to the patient's IV intake; the volume of fluid should be documented. When the circuit is flushed of blood, clots may be observed. Flushing does not dissolve existing clots.

Procedure continues on following page

| Procedure | for Initiation and Termination of Continuous Renal Replacement Therapy—*Continued* | | |

Steps	Rationale	Special Considerations
6. If clots are not observed, turn off the NS by moving the stopcock "off" to the NS flush and open to the arterial port of the VAC.	Continues therapy.	If numerous clots are observed, the hemofilter may need to be replaced. Heparin will not dissolve existing clots.
7. Remove **PE** and discard used equipment in appropriate receptacles.	Safely discards used supplies.	
8. **HH**		
Termination		
1. **HH**		
2. **PE**		
3. Turn off all infusions into the circuit.	Prepares for termination of therapy.	
4. With the IV accessory spike, attach the NS flush solution to the arterial infusion line of the circuit. If using NS flushes, this line can be used to flush the circuit when terminating the treatment.	Prepares for flushing blood from the tubing.	
5. Return the blood in the circuit to the patient. When the entire circuit is clear of blood, turn off the pump and clamp off both the arterial and venous lines.	Follow instructions on the pump for termination. The blood should be flushed from the circuit back to the patient to prevent unnecessary blood loss.	If clots are identified beyond the venous bubble trap, stop the pump; do not return blood to the patient.
6. Continue terminating the procedure according to the manufacturer's guidelines.		
7. If the VAC is to be discontinued, remove it per institutional guidelines.	CRRT therapy may no longer be needed.	
8. Record the amount of NS infused.	Ensures accurate fluid balance.	The flush solution infused to the patient must be recorded as intake.
9. If the VAC is not to be removed, prepare the sterile field. Open and place the sterile barrier under the VAC.	Maintains aseptic technique.	
10. Place 4 × 4 gauze pads onto the sterile field. Open the sterile container, syringes, blunt-tip needles, and NS (or prefilled NS syringes) and place them on the sterile field.	Maintains aseptic technique.	
11. Add antiseptic solution (e.g., 2% chlorhexidine–based preparation) to the sterile container (or use prepackaged bacterial solution). **(Level D*)**	Prepares solution used to cleanse VAC ports. Povidone-iodine, hypochlorite and chlorhexidine solutions are acceptable bactericidal agents.[3,10,19]	
12. Remove gloves and discard in appropriate receptacles.	Safely discards used supplies.	
13. Wash hands.		
14. Don sterile gloves.		

*Level D: Peer-reviewed professional and organizational standards with the support of clinical study recommendations.

Procedure	**for Initiation and Termination of Continuous Renal Replacement Therapy—***Continued*		
Steps	**Rationale**		**Special Considerations**
15. Attach blunt-tip needles to two 10-mL syringes; with the help of an assistant, fill the syringes with NS or use prefilled syringes per institutional standards.	Prepares the syringe for VAC flushing.		A 20–30 mL per lumen flush is recommended.[1]
16. Saturate two 4 × 4 gauze pads in antiseptic solution. Perform a 1-minute scrub of the arterial and venous ports of the VAC. Alternatively, perform a 30-second scrub of the ports with chlorhexidine swabs (if approved by the catheter's manufacturer).	Prevents introduction of infection.		Be sure to remove any crust or drainage.
17. Be sure clamps are closed on the arterial and venous ports of the VAC before disconnecting the arterial blood line from the arterial vascular access. Alternatively, if dialysis luer caps are used, the circuit lines can be disconnected without opening the VAC ports.	Opens the system under sterile conditions for system termination.		Be sure the port clamp is closed before removing the arterial line.
18. **Repeat Step 18** on the venous system line.			
19. Attach a 10-mL syringe with NS to the arterial port. Open the clamp and flush, then close the clamp.	Prevents clotting of blood until anticoagulant is instilled.		
20. **Repeat Step 20** on the venous port.			
21. Instill the prescribed anticoagulant into each access port according to institutional standards. Use only the "fill" amount listed on the VAC ports to avoid instilling anticoagulant into the patient. (Many facilities are now using NS instead of heparin and dialysis-specific locking caps to prevent opening the VAC ports to air.)	Maintains patency of the accesses.		Label each port with the date, time, and anticoagulant used, and your initials.
22. Clamp and cap the arterial and venous ports with the sterile needleless luer caps.	Maintains sterility of the VAC.		
23. Change the vascular access dressings according to institutional guidelines.	Prevents infection.		
24. Remove **PE** and discard used equipment in the appropriate receptacle.	Safely discards used supplies.		
25. **HH**			

Procedure continues on following page

Expected Outcomes

- VAC accessed without complications
- Blood easily aspirated from the access site
- Accumulated fluid and waste products removed
- Acid-base balance restored
- Blood urea nitrogen and creatinine values restored to baseline levels
- Electrolyte levels within baseline values
- Hemodynamic stability and maintenance of optimal intravascular volume
- Nutritional status maintained

Unexpected Outcomes

- Clotting/decreased patency of the access sites
- Crack in the VAC or end caps
- Bleeding from the VAC insertion site or access/return lines
- Signs and symptoms of infection at the insertion or access site
- Dislodgment of the VAC
- Decreased circulation in the extremity with the vascular access
- Hematoma formation at the VAC insertion site
- Physiological complications (dysrhythmias, chest pain, fluid or electrolyte imbalance, complications related to anticoagulation, air embolism, hypotension, seizures, nausea and vomiting, headaches, muscle cramping, dyspnea, exsanguination, hemorrhage)
- Introduction of pathogens or air into the circuit
- Technical problems with the blood pump (blood leak, air leak, clotting, disconnection of circuit, hemolysis, hemofilter rupture)
- Hypothermia[21]
- Malnutrition

Patient Monitoring and Care

Steps	Rationale	Reportable Conditions
		These conditions should be reported if they persist despite interventions.
1. Obtain and record predialysis and daily weight.	Predialysis weight is an important factor in deciding how much UF is needed and helps guide ongoing treatment.[4]	• Increase or decrease in weight
2. Perform ongoing assessments, including the following: A. Vital signs B. Jugular vein distention C. Presence of edema D. Intake and output E. Neurological assessment F. Pulmonary assessment G. Cardiac monitoring	Provides information in response to treatment.[1,6,10,13] Monitors for complications.	• Hypotension • Hypertension • Tachycardia/bradycardia • Tachypnea • Fever • Hypothermia[21] • Jugular vein distention • Crackles • Edema • Change in level of consciousness, dizziness • Change in cardiac rhythm • Diminished capillary refill
3. Monitor the circulation to the extremity where the VAC is located.	Assesses for any decrease in perfusion distal to the VAC site.[4,6]	• Diminished or absent peripheral pulses, or pain • Pale, mottled, or cyanotic color • Cool to the touch • Diminished or absent movement or sensation.

Patient Monitoring and Care —*Continued*

Steps	Rationale	Reportable Conditions
4. Monitor electrolytes, glucose, and albumin during treatment as prescribed or per institutional standards.	Must be monitored because of continued fluid and electrolyte shifts during treatment. Amino acids are also lost through the hemofilter.	• Hyperkalemia or hypokalemia • Hypernatremia or hyponatremia • Hypercalcemia or hypocalcemia • Hyperglycemia or hypoglycemia • Hypermagnesemia or hypomagnesemia • Hyperphosphatemia or hypophosphatemia • Hypoalbuminemia
5. Administer medications to correct electrolyte abnormalities as needed during treatment. **(Level D*)**	Patients with renal failure are predisposed to many electrolyte abnormalities. During CRRT, medications or electrolyte replacements may be given as prescribed for individual patients.[6,34] Renal diet with adjusted protein, potassium, phosphorous, carbohydrate, and fluid intake that takes into account the patient's current catabolic state, renal function, adequacy of dialysis, and removal of amino acids via dialysis is required.[4,6,7,11]	• Hyperkalemia or hypokalemia • Hypernatremia or hyponatremia • Hypercalcemia or hypocalcemia • Hyperglycemia or hypoglycemia • Hypermagnesemia or hypomagnesemia • Hyperphosphatemia or hypophosphatemia • Hypoalbuminemia • Unexpected change in weight (loss or gain)
6. Monitor the CRRT circuit (e.g., occlusions; kinks in UF, blood, or vascular access lines; hemofilter).	Disconnections or introduction of air into the circuit are always possible during treatment. Bleeding or exsanguination can also occur.[3,4,7,10] Clotting of the circuit is a potential complication. If the hemofilter needs replacing, the extracorporeal blood volume should be returned to the patient if possible. Blood leaks from the dialyzer into the dialysate may occur and necessitate termination of treatment. In the event of a filter leak, do *not* return circuit blood to the patient. Venous or arterial pressures that are out of range may indicate dialyzer or access malfunction.	• Disconnections, cracks, or leaks • Excessive clotting • Blood leaks/hemofilter rupture • Malfunction of dialyzer or access
7. Monitor UF for rate, clarity, and air bubbles.	A decrease in UF production can occur from clotting of the dialyzer.[4,6,10] Pink or blood-tinged UF is indicative of a filter leak or rupture.	• Decreases in UF production • Change in color or characteristics of UF • Air in UF
8. Administer anticoagulant as prescribed.	Heparin or citrate is often used to prevent clotting of the circuit.[4,6] The heparin/citrate dose varies according to patient condition and laboratory values.	• Suspicion of clotting in the circuit
9. Monitor anticoagulation per institutional standards.	Because heparin or citrate is commonly used to prevent system clotting, coagulation studies should be routinely monitored.	• Abnormal coagulation study results

*Level D: Peer-reviewed professional and organizational standards with the support of clinical study recommendations.

Procedure continues on following page

Patient Monitoring and Care —*Continued*

Steps	Rationale	Reportable Conditions
10. Monitor the vascular access.	Bleeding and/or infection can occur from the access site. Clotting of the access can occur.[4,6,25,32]	• Decrease in access function or patency • Bleeding • Site redness or edema • Warmth • Purulent drainage • Pain or tenderness • Fever
11. Monitor the patient for complications associated with CRRT treatment.	Complications are possible with CRRT.[4,6,9,10,13,20]	• Muscle cramps • Dialysis disequilibrium (headache, nausea and vomiting, hypertension, decreased sensorium, seizures, coma) • Air embolism • Dialyzer reaction (hypotension, pruritus, back pain, angioedema, anaphylaxis) • Hypoxemia • Hypothermia[21]
12. Monitor the blood pump for proper functioning.	Alerts the nurse to problems with the procedure.	• Problems with the blood pump
13. Follow institutional guidelines for assessing pain. Administer analgesia as prescribed.	Identifies need for pain interventions.	• Continued pain despite pain interventions

Documentation

Documentation should include the following:
• Patient and family education
• Date and time of treatment initiation, mode of therapy, filter change
• Condition of vascular access regarding patency, quality of blood flow, ease of access procedure
• Date and time of VAC insertion and dressing change
• Condition of insertion site and any signs or symptoms of infection
• Blood flow rate and arterial and venous monitoring pressures
• Type and content of dialysis and replacement fluids
• Anticoagulation type and dose
• Completion of informed consent
• Vital signs/hemodynamic parameters
• Status of pulse distal to vascular access site
• Hourly fluid balance calculation
• Patient's response to CRRT and daily progress toward treatment goals
• Unexpected outcomes
• Nursing interventions
• Daily weight
• Laboratory assessment data
• Pain assessment, interventions, and effectiveness

References and Additional Readings

For a complete list of references and additional readings for this procedure, scan this QR code with any freely available smartphone code reader app, or visit http://booksite.elsevier.com/9780323376624.

PROCEDURE

120 Hemodialysis

Sonia M. Astle

PURPOSE: Hemodialysis is performed for volume regulation, acid-base control, electrolyte regulation, management of azotemia, and the treatment of drug intoxications.

PREREQUISITE NURSING KNOWLEDGE

- Hemodialysis (Fig. 120-1) may be needed for the onset of acute kidney injury, for maintenance therapy for patients with chronic renal failure, or for patients with acute drug intoxication.[5]
- Knowledge of the principles of diffusion, ultrafiltration (UF), osmosis, oncotic pressure, and hydrostatic pressure as they pertain to fluid and solute management during dialysis is necessary.[1,5,7,8,13]
  - ❖ *Diffusion* is the passive movement of solutes through a semipermeable membrane from an area of higher to lower concentration until equilibrium is reached.
  - ❖ *Ultrafiltration* is the bulk movement of solute and solvent through a semipermeable membrane with a pressure movement. This movement is usually achieved with positive pressure in the blood compartment of the hemodialyzer and negative pressure in the dialysate compartment. Blood and dialysate flow countercurrent to each other. The size of the solute molecules compared with the size of molecules that can move through the semipermeable membrane determines the degree of UF.
  - ❖ *Osmosis* is the passive movement of solvent through a semipermeable membrane from an area of higher to lower concentration.
  - ❖ *Oncotic pressure* is the pressure exerted by plasma proteins that favors intravascular fluid retention and movement of fluid from the extravascular to the intravascular space.
  - ❖ *Hydrostatic pressure* is the force exerted by arterial blood pressure that favors the movement of fluid from the intravascular to the extravascular space.
  - ❖ *Absorption* is the process by which drug molecules pass through membranes and fluid barriers and into body fluids.
  - ❖ *Adsorption* is the adhesion of molecules (solutes) to the surface to the hemodialyzer, charcoal, or resin.
  - ❖ *Convective transport* is the rapid movement of fluid across a semipermeable membrane from an area of high pressure to an area of low pressure with transport of solutes. When water moves across a membrane along a pressure gradient, some solutes are carried along with the water and do not require a solute concentration

gradient (also called solute drag). Convective transport is most effective for the removal of middle molecular weight and large molecular weight solutes.
- Vascular access is needed to perform hemodialysis and can be provided with a double-lumen vascular access catheter (VAC), or a surgically created arteriovenous (AV) anastomosis (e.g., fistula or graft).[4,6,19] The AV fistula or graft is used for long-term dialysis management.[6,19]
- The subclavian vein is not recommended for temporary access because of the increased incidence of vascular stenosis, which makes the vein of the ipsilateral arm unsuitable for chronic dialysis if needed. The internal jugular or leg veins are more commonly used.[6]
- Hemodialysis uses an artificial kidney (hemodialyzer, dialyzer) with a semipermeable membrane to create two separate compartments: the blood compartment and the dialysis solution (dialysate) compartment. The semipermeable membrane allows the movement of small molecules (e.g., electrolytes, urea, drugs) and middle-weight molecules (e.g., creatinine) from the patient's blood into the dialysate but is impermeable to larger molecules (e.g., blood cells, plasma proteins).
- Each dialyzer has four ports: two end ports for blood (in one end and out the other) and two side ports for dialysis solution (also in one end and out the other). In most cases, the blood and dialysate are run through the dialyzer in opposite or countercurrent directions.
- The hollow-fiber dialyzer is the most commonly used dialyzer. With this dialyzer, the blood flows through the center of hollow fibers and the dialysate flows around the outside of the hollow fibers. The advantages of hollow-fiber filters include a low priming volume, low resistance to flow, and high amount of surface area. The major disadvantage is the potential for clotting because of the small fiber size.
- All dialyzers have UF coefficients; thus, the dialyzer selected varies in different clinical situations. The higher the UF coefficient, the more rapid the fluid removal. UF coefficients are determined with in vivo measurements done by each dialyzer manufacturer.[1]
- Clearance refers to the ability of the dialyzer to remove metabolic waste products from the patient's blood. The blood flow rate, the dialysate flow rate, and the solute concentration affect clearance. Clearance occurs by the processes of diffusion, convection, and UF.[7,13]

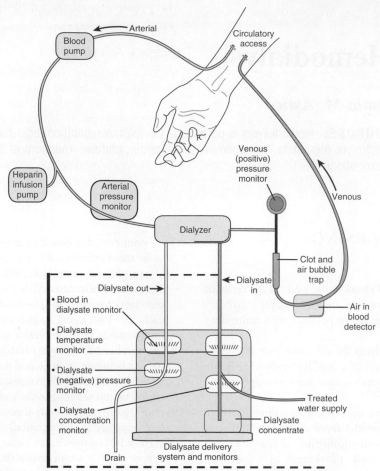

Figure 120-1   Components of a typical hemodialysis system. *(From Thompson JM, et al., editors: Mosby's manual of clinical nursing, St. Louis, 1989, Mosby.)*

- The blood circuit consists of blood lines, a blood pump, and various monitoring devices. The blood lines carry the blood to and from the patient. The blood pump controls the speed of the blood through the circuit. The monitoring devices include arterial and venous pressure monitors and an air detection monitor to prevent air entering the circuit from being returned to the patient.
- The dialysate is composed of water, a buffer (e.g., bicarbonate), and various electrolytes. Most solutions also contain glucose. The buffer helps neutralize acids that are generated as a result of normal cellular metabolism and usually are excreted by the kidney. The concentration of electrolytes is normal plasma concentrations, which help to create a concentration gradient for removal of excess electrolytes. The glucose, available in various concentrations, promotes the removal of plasma water.
- Heparin is usually used during dialysis to prevent clotting of the circuit. In patients with coagulopathies, normal saline (NS) solution flushes can be used to keep the blood circuit patent.[5] Heparin should be avoided in patients with a history of heparin-induced thrombocytopenia (HIT).[1,9,15]
- Because large volumes of water are used during treatments to generate the dialysate, the water must be purified before patient use to prevent patient exposure to

potentially harmful substances present in the water supply (e.g., calcium carbonate, sodium chloride, and iron).[1,5,13]
- Other extended renal replacement therapy techniques or "hybrid" techniques (sustained low-efficiency dialysis [SLED], extended daily dialysis [EDD]) generally use standard hemodialysis equipment and techniques with reduced blood flow and dialysate rates to gradually remove plasma water and solutes in the critically ill patient. They are used from 4 to 12 hours a day.[1,5]
- The adequacy of dialysis and assessment of the patient's residual renal function should be evaluated on a periodic basis. Adequacy of dialysis can be measured with urea kinetic modeling (Kt/V) or urea clearance.[1,7,17,18] Residual renal functioning can be monitored with urine creatinine clearance.[17,18] Collaboration with the nephrology team is necessary to monitor these parameters.[1,10]

EQUIPMENT

- Fluid shield face masks or goggles
- Sterile and nonsterile gloves
- Impermeable gowns
- Sharps container
- Sterile NS solution, 3 L

- Two 10-mL syringes with blunt-tip cannulas (or prefilled NS syringes)
- Two 3-mL syringes
- Dressing supplies (sterile barrier, 4 × 4 gauze pads, transparent dressing, tape, triple-antibiotic ointment or chlorhexidine-impregnated sponge)
- Antiseptic solution (e.g., 2% chlorhexidine-based preparation)
- Heparin (1000 units/mL; for both priming and infusion, if prescribed)
- Sterile container for soaking of 4 × 4 pads with antiseptic solution
- Dialysate fluid as prescribed
- Alcohol wipes
- Dialysis caps for VAC (if used by institution)
- Dialysis machine, tubing, dialyzer, and dialysate solution/water treatment setup
- One 30-mL syringe

Additional equipment, to have available as needed, includes the following:
- Two plastic clamps
- Two fistula needles
- One tourniquet (AV fistula only)
- Equipment for termination of hemodialysis includes the following:
  - ❖ Four hemostats
  - ❖ 2 × 2 gauze pads
  - ❖ NS solution, 1000 mL
  - ❖ Four bandages, tape
  - ❖ Fluid shield face masks or goggles
  - ❖ Nonsterile gloves
  - ❖ Catheter locking solution (VAC) as prescribed

PATIENT AND FAMILY EDUCATION

- Explain the procedure, and review any questions the patient may have. *Rationale:* Explanation provides information and may decrease patient anxiety.
- Explain the purpose of hemodialysis. *Rationale:* This explanation ensures the patient and family know that hemodialysis is necessary to perform the physiological functions of the kidneys when renal failure is present.
- Explain the need for careful monitoring of the patient during the treatment for fluid and electrolyte imbalance. *Rationale:* This explanation prepares the patient for what to expect.
- Explain the importance of input from the patient about how he or she is feeling during the treatment. *Rationale:* Hypotension is a common occurrence during treatment; the patient may experience light-headedness or dizziness if hypotension is present. Patient knowledge of this possibility should help decrease anxiety.
- Explain the hemodialysis circuit setup to the patient. *Rationale:* The patient and family must be aware that blood will be removed from the patient's body and will be visible during the hemodialysis treatment.

PATIENT ASSESSMENT AND PREPARATION
Patient Assessment

- Assess baseline vital signs, weight, and neurological status, and perform a physical assessment of all body systems and fluid and electrolyte status. *Rationale:* Patients in renal failure often have altered baseline assessments, both in physical assessment and in the laboratory values. Having this information before treatments are started is helpful so that interventions, including the dialysate, can be individualized. Alterations during treatment are common because of the rapid removal of fluid and solutes.
- Assess graft, fistula, or VAC site for signs or symptoms of infection. *Rationale:* Because dialysis access sites are used frequently, infection is always a potential risk. Dialysis access sites should only be used for dialysis, and not for other intravenous (IV) access needs, except in an emergency situation. Insertion sites provide a portal of entry for infection, which may result in septicemia if unrecognized or untreated. If the insertion site appears to be infected, further interventions (e.g., site change, culture, and antibiotic treatment) may be necessary.
- Assess VAC patency and the ability to easily aspirate blood from both ports. *Rationale:* Adequate blood flow is necessary during a treatment to facilitate optimal fluid and solute removal. Patent VAC ports are necessary for adequate blood flow.
- With AV fistula use, assess the site for presence of bruit, erythema, swelling, and quality of blood flow. *Rationale:* Physical assessment of the fistula can indicate patency of the graft and the possible presence of infection.
- Assess the circulation to the distal parts of the access limb. *Rationale:* The placement of a vascular access may compromise circulation.

Patient Preparation

- Verify that the patient is the correct patient using two identifiers. *Rationale:* Before performing a procedure, the nurse should ensure the correct identification of the patient for the intended intervention.
- Ensure the patient understands preprocedural instructions. Answer questions as they arise, and reinforce information as needed. *Rationale:* Understanding of previously taught information is evaluated and reinforced.
- Position the patient in a comfortable position (that also facilitates optimal blood flow through the access site and allows for setup of the field). *Rationale:* Facilitation of patient comfort helps to minimize the amount of patient movement during treatment, which can change the amount of blood flow through the access site. Different access sites may require different patient positions to facilitate optimal blood flow. Patient comfort is promoted, and anxiety may be reduced.

Procedure for Hemodialysis

Steps	Rationale	Special Considerations
Cannulation of the AV Fistula or Graft		
1. 🄷🄷		
2. 🄿🄴		
3. Wash access site for 1 full minute with antiseptic solution and a 4 × 4 gauze pad.	Reduces the transmission of microorganisms.	
4. Place arm on a clean barrier.	Maintains aseptic technique.	
5. Starting at the site of insertion and moving out in concentric circles for 2–3 inches, wash access area with bactericidal swabs or soaked 2 × 2 gauze pad. **(Level D*)**	Povidone-iodine, 70% isopropyl alcohol, or chlorhexidine bactericidal solution reduces the transmission of microorganisms. Allow all to air dry.[9,12,15,19] Povidone-iodine solution requires a 2–3-minute scrub for bacteriostatic effect.[9,12,15,19] Isopropyl alcohol is applied using a circular friction motion for 1 minute.[9,12,15,19] Chlorhexidine has a rapid and prolonged antimicrobial effect; apply solution with back-and-forth friction scrub for 30 seconds.[9,12,15,19]	Skin asepsis is crucial to prevent infection.
6. Prepare two 10-mL NS flush syringes: A. Obtain prefilled syringes. or B. Prepare the syringes.	The flush syringes can be used to assess the placement and patency of the fistula/graft.	
7. Attach the flush to the fistula needle tubing and prime through the fistula needle.	Prevents clotting of blood in the fistula needles.	
8. Clamp the tubing.	Prevents loss of solution and backflow of blood.	
9. Apply a tourniquet to the upper portion of the access limb (AV fistula cannulation).	Facilitates site determination for cannulation.	
10. Select the site to be used.	Decreases recirculation of dialyzed blood.	Traditionally, the arterial site is placed at least 3 inches from arterial anastomosis. The venous needle must be in the direction of venous flow and, if possible, 3 inches or more from the arterial needle.[1,5,16,21] However, there is current discussion that needle direction and tip spacing do not influence recirculation of the blood.[6]
11. Grasp the butterfly wings or the hub of the fistula needle between the thumb and index finger of the dominant hand with the needle tip bevel up.	Provides a secure grasp of the needle on cannulation.	
12. Remove the needle guard.	Exposes the fistula needle.	
13. Hold the skin taut with the nondominant hand.	Prevents rolling of the vessel.	

*Level D: Peer-reviewed professional and organizational standards with the support of clinical study recommendations.

Procedure   for Hemodialysis—*Continued*

Steps	Rationale	Special Considerations

14. With the dominant hand:
 	
  A. Insert the needle at a 45-degree angle to the skin.
  B. AV fistula: Advance the bevel up to the hub of the needle.
	Accesses the arterial vascular system.	

15. Remove the tourniquet before infusing NS or the prescribed heparin solution (AV fistula).	Prevents clotting.	
16. Unclamp the tubing and aspirate blood.	Verifies the correct placement and patency of the access.	
17. Infuse the flush solution and then reclamp the tubing.	Prevents clotting and backflow of blood.	
18. Secure the needle with adhesive tape over the insertion site.	Maintains the angle of the needle so that it floats freely in the vessel/graft.	
19. **Repeat Steps 10–18** for insertion of the second needle.	Cannulation of venous site.	Hemodialysis can now be initiated.
20. Remove **PE** and discard used equipment in the appropriate receptacle.		
21. **HH**		
Decannnulation of the AV Fistula or Graft		
1. **HH**		
2. **PE**		
3. Remove both cannulas from the patient's access site, one at a time. With a sterile 2 × 2 gauze pad, apply moderate pressure to each access site until bleeding has stopped.	Discontinues vascular access. Promotes hemostasis at access sites.	Removing the needles one at a time prevents unnecessary loss of blood due to the force of pressure in the access.
4. Apply a sterile dressing to the site.	Provides a protective barrier.	
5. Remove **PE** and discard used equipment in the appropriate receptacle.		
6. **HH**		
Accessing a VAC		
1. **HH**		
2. **PE**		
3. Prepare a sterile field with sterile barrier and 2 × 2 and 4 × 4 gauze pads.	Prepares supplies and maintains aseptic technique.	
4. Open the sterile adaptors and syringes, and place them on the sterile field.	Prepares the equipment and maintains aseptic technique to prevent transmission of microorganisms.	

5. Prepare two 10-mL NS flush syringes:
  A. Obtain prefilled syringes. or
  B. Prepare the syringes.
	Prepares the syringes for VAC flushing.	Refer to manufacturer's recommendations for amount of flush to be used.

6. Remove gloves, wash hands, and apply clean gloves.	Maintains aseptic technique.	
7. Place a sterile barrier beneath the VAC.	Sets up the sterile field.	

Procedure continues on following page

Procedure   for Hemodialysis—*Continued*

Steps	Rationale	Special Considerations
8. Saturate a 4 × 4 gauze pad in antiseptic solution, and perform the appropriate scrub on the arterial port of the VAC. Alternatively, chlorhexidine swabs may be used according to the catheter manufacturer's guidelines; a 30-second scrub is recommended. Allow all bactericidal solutions to dry completely.	Povidone-iodine, 70% isopropyl alcohol, or chlorhexidine bactericidal solution reduces the transmission of microorganisms.[9,19,23] Povidone-iodine solution requires a 2–3-minute scrub for bacteriostatic effect.[9,19,23] Isopropyl alcohol is applied using a circular friction motion for 1 minute.[9,19,23] Chlorhexidine has a rapid and prolonged antimicrobial effect; apply solution with back-and-forth friction scrub for 30 seconds.[9,19,23] Allow all bactericidal solutions to dry completely. (**Level B***)	Be sure to remove any crust or drainage.
9. Remove the cap from the arterial port of the VAC and discard it in the appropriate receptacle.	Provides access to the arterial port of the VAC.	Be sure the slide clamp is closed before removing the arterial cap. Many facilities are now using dialysis caps that lock into the VAC so the catheter is not opened to air unless it requires changing.
10. Clean the connection site with 2 × 2 gauze pads that have been soaked in antiseptic solution or cleanse the site with antiseptic swabs (e.g., 2% chlorhexidine-based preparation).	Minimizes the risk of infection.	Allow the solution to completely dry.
11. Attach an empty 3-mL syringe to the arterial port A. Open the slide clamp. B. Gently aspirate 3 mL of blood. C. Close the slide clamp. D. Remove the syringe	Removes the indwelling heparin from the VAC port and assesses patency.	If difficulty is found in aspirating blood, notify the physician or advanced practice nurse.
12. Attach the flush syringe to the arterial port: A. Open the slide clamp. B. Slowly flush the port. C. Close the slide clamp.	Positive pressure prevents the backup of blood into the port after flushing.	If a dialysis cap is not used, the syringe should be left attached to the VAC port until it is replaced with dialyzer tubing. If a dialysis cap is used, recleanse the access site before connecting the dialyzer tubing.
13. Remove the flush syringe from the arterial and venous ports; attach the arterial line from the dialysis tubing securely to the arterial port of the VAC with a Luer-Lok connector.	Connects the patient to the dialysis machine.	
14. **Repeat Steps 8–13** on the venous port.	Verifies patency of venous port; decreases transmission of microorganisms.	Observe for clots.

*Level B: Well-designed, controlled studies with results that consistently support a specific action, intervention, or treatment.

Procedure for Hemodialysis—*Continued*

Steps	Rationale	Special Considerations
15. Open the clamps on the arterial and venous ports of the VAC and the dialysis tubing, and turn on the blood pump at a slow rate (50–100 mL/min).	Primes the dialysis line with blood.	
16. Assure connections are secure.	Reduces the possibility of accidental disconnection of the lines.	
17. Remove **PE** and discard used equipment in appropriate receptacle.	Safely discards used supplies.	
18. **HH**		
19. Proceed to the initiation of hemodialysis.	Continues treatment.	
Disconnecting From the VAC		
1. **HH**		
2. **PE**		
3. Open the syringes, caps, needles, and 4 × 4 gauze pads; place on the sterile field.	Maintains aseptic technique.	
4. Prepare two 10-mL NS flush syringes: A. Obtain prefilled syringes, or B. Prepare the syringes. C. Place on the sterile field.	Prepares supplies.	
5. Remove gloves, wash hands, and apply clean gloves.		
6. Place a sterile barrier under the VAC ports.	Sets up a sterile field.	
7. Wrap both VAC ports with antiseptic-soaked 4 × 4 pads, and scrub for 1 minute. Alternatively, chlorhexidine swabs may be used according to the catheter manufacturer's guidelines; a 30-second scrub is recommended.	Reduces transmission of microorganisms. Maintains asepsis.[2,3,9]	Allow to dry completely.
8. Remove gloves and wash hands.	Safely discards used supplies.	
9. Apply sterile gloves.	Maintains aseptic technique.	
10. Clamp the arterial and venous ports.	Prevents blood loss from the catheter.	
11. If not using dialysis caps: A. Use the same antiseptic-soaked 4 × 4 gauze pad to handle the dialysis tubing. B. Disconnect the arterial line from the arterial port of the VAC.	Maintains aseptic technique.[23,24]	Many institutions are using specially designed dialysis caps to prevent opening the VAC to air during accessing or deaccessing the dialysis tubing to the VAC.
12. Unclamp the arterial port, and flush with NS, then reclamp the line.	Assures catheter patency.	

Procedure continues on following page

Procedure for Hemodialysis—*Continued*

Steps	Rationale	Special Considerations
13. Attach a 3- or 5-mL syringe with heparin, as prescribed, to the arterial access: A. Unclamp the slide clamp. B. Inject the prescribed amount of heparin or NS per institutional guidelines.	Maintains catheter patency by preventing the clotting of blood.	The heparin dosage varies depending on the type of catheter used and institutional standards. In some cases, the catheter may be flushed with NS solution only. Use only the amount of heparin (or other prescribed solution) listed on the catheter to avoid instilling medication into the patient.[19,22] Label each catheter port with the date, time, anticoagulant used, and nurse's initials.[19]
14. Clamp the line: A. Disconnect the syringe. B. If not using a dialysis cap, cap the arterial port per institutional guidelines.	Prevents the loss of blood and maintains aseptic technique.	
15. **Repeat Steps 10–14** on the venous port.	Maintains patency by preventing clotting of blood.	
16. Assess the dressing to the VAC site at each hemodialysis treatment; change if the dressing becomes damp, loosened, or soiled.	Prevents contamination of the VAC exit site.	An occlusive, transparent dressing should be maintained and changed at least weekly, gauze dressings should be changed every 48 hours, or according to institutional standards. Aseptic technique is followed during dressing changes.[1,2,15,19,24]
17. Apply a chlorhexidine gluconate sponge to the VAC insertion site at each dressing change.	Lowers the incidence of dialysis catheter–related infections.[2,19]	Follow institutional standards regarding use of ointment.
18. Remove **PE** and discard used equipment in appropriate receptacle.	Safely discards used supplies.	
19. **HH**		

Initiation and Termination of Hemodialysis

Steps	Rationale	Special Considerations
1. Verify orders, which should include: A. Vascular access. B. Hours of treatment. C. Type of hemodialyzer/ dialyzer. D. Blood flow rate. E. Anticoagulant type, concentration, infusion rate, monitoring parameters. F. UF goal. G. Dialysate solution and rate. H. Blood pressure and vital sign parameters. I. Laboratory testing.	Familiarizes the nurse with the individualized patient treatment and reduces the possibility of error.[1,5,13]	Ensure that the patient's weight and laboratory values are recorded before initiation of therapy.
2. Set up the dialysis machine according to the manufacturer's instructions.	Ensures safe and proper assembly and allows for testing of all patient alarms and the proper functioning of the machine before the VAC/ graft/fistula is accessed.	

Procedure for Hemodialysis—*Continued*

Steps	Rationale	Special Considerations
3. **HH**		
4. **PE**		
5. Access the VAC, graft, or fistula.	Allows access to the site.	
6. Connect the arterial access to the arterial blood line with a Luer-Lok connector. Repeat the steps with the venous blood line.	Provides a circuit between the patient and the dialyzer.	
7. Remove the clamps from the arterial and venous blood lines.	Permits the flow of blood.	
8. Adjust the blood pump to 50–100 mL/min until blood reaches the venous drip chamber.	The slow rate prevents symptoms of rapid blood loss and allows for assessment of blood flow from the arterial line.	If a heparin loading dose is prescribed it can be given via bolus in the arterial line.
9. Adjust the blood level in the arterial and venous drip chambers to three quarters full.	Prevents accumulation of air in the tubing and dialyzer.	
10. Turn the dialyzer over so that the arterial (red) port is at the top.	Establishes the countercurrent flow.	
11. If the patient is receiving systemic heparinization, set the parameters on the heparin infusion pump as prescribed.	Provides anticoagulation.	
12. Secure the cannula connections.	Additional precaution against accidental disconnection.	
13. Slowly increase the blood pump speed to the prescribed rate while continuing to assess the patient (level of consciousness, symptoms of chest pain, dysrhythmias, and changes in hemodynamic variables).	Prevents complications of rapid removal of blood.	If any question exists as to how well the patient will tolerate hemodialysis, the pump speed should be started at 100 mL/min and gradually increased to goal.
14. Set the arterial and venous alarm parameters.	Sets the safety alarm system.	
15. Observe the patient's transmembrane pressure (TMP) display.	Removes the desired UF.	Most dialysis machines automatically calculate the TMP.
16. Set the TMP alarms.	Allows for UF.	Most machines automatically adjust based on the treatment time and volume removal goal.
17. Remove **PE** and discard used equipment in appropriate receptacle.	Safely discards used supplies.	
18. **HH**		
19. Continuously monitor the patient's status and machine function throughout treatment.	Prevents complications and minimizes the effects of fluid and electrolyte shifts.	Patient assessment should include vital signs and symptoms related to fluid and electrolyte shifts (e.g., cramping, hypotension, nausea, vomiting). Monitor the machine for blood flow rate, arterial and venous pressure readings, dialysate pressure, TMP, and blood circuit for clotting or air.

Procedure continues on following page

Procedure for Hemodialysis—*Continued*

Steps	Rationale	Special Considerations
Termination		
1. **HH**		
2. **PE**		
3. Set the arterial, venous, and dialysate pressure alarms to the maximum low/high limits.	Prevents the machine from alarming when terminating dialysis as pressures drop.	
4. Turn off the TMP or negative pressure.	Removes the negative pressure, thereby stopping UF.	
5. Turn off the heparin infusion pump.	Discontinues heparinization before the end of dialysis, thus allowing clotting times to return to normal shortly after treatment.	May be done 30 minutes to 1 hour before termination of treatment; follow institutional standards.
6. Decrease the blood pump flow rate.	Reduces the blood flow.	
7. Check the amount of NS solution left in the circuit for adequate blood return; hang a new NS solution bag if necessary.	Minimizes the danger of air embolism on return of the blood to the patient.	NS solution (100–300 mL) is used to return blood to the patient.
8. Maintain the blood level in the arterial and venous drip chambers at three quarters full.	Prevents air in the tubing and dialyzer.	
9. Turn off the blood pump.	Stops the blood flow.	
10. Clamp the arterial line:	Prevents the loss of blood.	
A. Disconnect the line from the patient and connect it to the NS flush port on the circuit.		
B. Unclamp the arterial arm of the catheter.		
11. Unclamp the NS:	Promotes the slow return of blood in the tubing back to the patient.	
A. Turn the pump on at a low speed and return the blood to the patient.		
B. Allow the NS flush to infuse until the lines are pink-tinged.		
12. Turn off the blood pump.	Terminates the flow of blood.	
13. Place a sterile 4 × 4 gauze pad under the vascular access and disconnect the dialysis tubing from the vascular access.	Prevents contamination.	
14. Flush the fistula/graft/VAC according to institutional standards.	Prevents clotting.	
15. Sanitize the single-patient machine according to institutional standards.	Reduces transmission of microorganisms and readies it for future use.	
16. Remove **PE** and discard used equipment in appropriate receptacle.	Safely discards used supplies.	
17. **HH**		

Expected Outcomes

- Catheter/fistula/graft accessed without complications
- Blood is easily aspirated from the access site
- Pulsating blood flow occurs in the dialysis tubing set
- Accumulated waste products are removed
- Acid-base balance is restored
- Blood urea nitrogen (BUN) and creatinine values are restored to baseline levels
- Electrolyte values are restored to baseline levels
- Accumulated fluid is removed; dry weight is achieved

Unexpected Outcomes

- Clotting or decreased patency of the AV fistula or catheter lumens
- Poor blood flow
- Bleeding from the insertion site or access site
- Signs or symptoms of infection at the insertion or access site or systemically
- Dislodgment of the catheter
- Decreased circulation in the vascular access limb
- Hematoma formation at the accessed site
- Physiological complications (dysrhythmias, chest pain, fluid-electrolyte imbalance, hypotension, seizures, nausea and vomiting, headaches, muscle cramping, dyspnea)
- Technical problems with the dialysis machine

Patient Monitoring and Care

Steps	Rationale	Reportable Conditions
		These conditions should be reported if they persist despite nursing interventions.
1. Perform and record a predialysis weight.	Predialysis weight is an important factor in deciding how much UF is needed during treatment. It also helps to guide ongoing treatment.[1,5,13]	- Abnormal increase or decrease in weight
2. Perform ongoing assessments, including the following: A. Vital signs B. Jugular vein distention C. Presence of edema D. Intake and output E. Neurological assessment F. Pulmonary assessment	Provides information in response to treatment.[1,5,13] Monitors for complications.	- Hypotension - Hypertension - Tachycardia/bradycardia - Tachypnea - Fever - Hypothermia - Jugular vein distention - Crackles - Edema - Change in level of consciousness, dizziness - Change in cardiac rhythm
3. Monitor the circulation to the extremity where the graft/fistula is located for the following: A. Capillary refill B. Pulses distal to access C. Color/temperature of extremity D. Sensation	Assesses for any decrease in perfusion distal to the graft site.[1,5,13]	- Diminished capillary refill - Diminished or absent peripheral pulses - Pale, mottled, or cyanotic extremity - Cool to touch - Diminished or absent movement - Pain
4. Monitor electrolytes and glucose during treatment as prescribed or per institutional standards.	Must be monitored because of continued fluid and electrolyte shifts during treatment.	- Hyperkalemia or hypokalemia - Hypernatremia or hyponatremia - Hypercalcemia or hypocalcemia - Hyperglycemia or hypoglycemia - Hyperphosphatemia or hypophosphatemia

Procedure continues on following page

Patient Monitoring and Care —*Continued*

Steps	Rationale	Reportable Conditions
5. Administer medications to correct electrolyte abnormalities as prescribed during treatment.	Patients with renal failure are predisposed to many electrolyte abnormalities. During dialysis, several medications/electrolyte replacements may be given, as prescribed for individual patients.[1,20]	<ul><li>Hyperkalemia or hypokalemia</li><li>Hypernatremia or hyponatremia</li><li>Hypercalcemia or hypocalcemia</li><li>Hyperglycemia or hypoglycemia</li><li>Hyperphosphatemia or hypophosphatemia</li></ul>
6. Monitor the dialysis circuit (e.g., occlusions, kinks, or leaks; blood or clots in vascular access lines). **(Level E*)**	Disconnections or introduction of air into the circuit are always possible during treatment. Bleeding or exsanguination can occur.[1,2,11,20] Clotting of the circuit is a potential complication. If the hemodialyzer becomes excessively clotted, the extracorporeal blood volume should be returned to the patient quickly. Blood leaks from dialyzer into the dialysate may occur and necessitate termination of treatment. Venous or arterial pressures, which are out of range, may indicate dialyzer or access malfunction.	<ul><li>Disconnections, cracks, or leaks</li><li>Bleeding</li><li>Excessive clotting</li><li>Blood leaks, hemodialyzer rupture</li><li>Malfunction of dialyzer or access</li></ul>
7. Monitor UF for rate, clarity, and air bubbles.	A decrease in UF production can occur from clotting of the dialyzer.[1,5,13] Pink or blood-tinged UF is indicative of a filter leak or rupture.	<ul><li>Decrease in UF production</li><li>Change in color or characteristic of UF</li><li>Air in UF</li></ul>
8. Administer heparin as prescribed.	Heparin is often used to prevent clotting of the circuit.[2,10,13] Heparin dose varies according to patient condition and laboratory values and type of vascular access.	<ul><li>Suspicion of clotting in the circuit</li></ul>
9. Monitor anticoagulation per institutional standards.	Because heparin is commonly used to prevent system clotting, coagulation studies should be routinely monitored.	<ul><li>Abnormal coagulation studies</li></ul>
10. Monitor the patency of vascular access. A. Gently palpate along the entire length of the graft or over the access for a thrill (feeling of vibration or purring under the fingers). B. Auscultate for the presence of a bruit (sounds like rushing water).	Bleeding can occur from either the venous or arterial catheter or AV fistula. Clotting of the access can occur.[1,2,11,19] Absence of a bruit does not confirm occlusion. Use a Doppler scan if unable to hear a bruit with a stethoscope.	<ul><li>Decrease in access function or patency</li><li>Absence of bruit or thrill</li></ul>

*Level E: Multiple case reports, theory-based evidence from expert opinions, or peer-reviewed professional organizational standards without clinical studies to support recommendations.

Patient Monitoring and Care —*Continued*

Steps	Rationale	Reportable Conditions
11. Monitor the patient for complications associated with dialysis treatment.	Complications are possible with dialysis treatments.[1–3,5,8,14,15,19]	• Muscle cramps • Dialysis disequilibrium (headache, nausea/vomiting, hypertension, decreased sensorium, convulsions, coma)—rare • Air embolism • Dialyzer reaction (hypotension, pruritus, back pain, angioedema, anaphylaxis) • Hypoxemia • Abnormal laboratory values
12. Administer medications to correct metabolic abnormalities as prescribed.	Patients with renal failure are predisposed to many metabolic abnormalities. Common medications administered to patients with renal failure include the following[1,5,8,13]: A. Vitamin D and calcium carbonate to increase the serum calcium level and prevent or treat bone disease. B. Erythropoietin and iron to treat anemia. C. Deferoxamine mesylate to remove excessive iron. D. Phosphate binders to treat hyperphosphatemia.	
13. Reinforce the prescribed renal diet.		
14. Place a sign above patient's bed indicating which limb has the vascular access (AV graft or fistula).	Blood pressures and blood draws should not be done on the access arm.	
15. Follow institutional standards for assessing pain. Administer analgesia as prescribed.	Identifies need for pain interventions.	• Continued pain despite pain interventions

Documentation

Documentation should include the following:
- Patient and family education
- Date and time of treatment initiation
- Condition of catheter or AV fistula regarding patency, quality of blood flow, ease of access procedure
- Condition of insertion site and any signs or symptoms of infection
- Presence of bruit if an AV fistula is used
- Needle gauge size used for cannulation
- Type of machine used for dialysis
- Pain assessment, interventions, and effectiveness
- Arterial and venous pressures during treatment
- Pump speed
- Length of dialysis treatment
- Vital signs throughout the treatments
- Unexpected outcomes
- Any medications/IV fluids given during treatment
- Nursing interventions
- Predialysis and postdialysis weight
- Laboratory assessment data

References and Additional Readings

For a complete list of references and additional readings for this procedure, scan this QR code with any freely available smartphone code reader app, or visit http://booksite.elsevier.com/9780323376624.

121 Peritoneal Dialysis

Sonia M. Astle

PURPOSE: Peritoneal dialysis (PD) is used for the removal of fluid and toxins, the regulation of electrolytes, and the management of azotemia.

PREREQUISITE NURSING KNOWLEDGE

- PD works on the principles of diffusion and osmosis; thus, a basic knowledge of these concepts is necessary.
  - *Diffusion* is the passive movement of solutes through a semipermeable membrane from an area of higher concentration to one of lower concentration. When this concept is applied to PD, diffusion occurs because the patient's blood contains waste products (solute), which gives it a higher osmolarity (concentration) than the dialysate. Therefore waste products in the blood diffuse across the semipermeable membrane into the dialysate solution.
  - *Osmosis* is the passive movement of solvent through a semipermeable membrane from an area of lower concentration to one of higher concentration. The dextrose added to the dialysate gives it a higher osmotic gradient than that of the patient's blood. Therefore excess water in the blood is pulled into the dialysate via osmosis.
- PD uses the peritoneal membrane as the semipermeable membrane for both fluid and solutes.[7,19,23]
- Sterile dialysis fluid (dialysate) is infused into the peritoneal cavity of the abdomen through a flexible catheter (Fig. 121-1).
- A small-framed adult can usually tolerate 2 to 2.5 L of dialysate, whereas a large-framed adult may be able to tolerate up to 3 L in the abdominal cavity. The larger the volume of dialysate, the more effective the removal of blood urea nitrogen (BUN) and creatinine[5,6]; however, peritoneal clearance may be improved with more frequent exchanges rather than an increase in the exchange volume.[1,5,6] The most limiting factor for the volume of dialysate is that it may cause direct pressure on the diaphragm and cause a compromise of respiratory excursion.[7,23,26] The PD dialysate contains higher concentrations of glucose than normal serum levels. These higher concentrations aid in the removal of water via osmosis and small-to-middle-weight molecules (urea, creatinine) via diffusion. Several concentrations of glucose are available in commercially prepared dialysate solutions (1.5%, 2.5%, and 4.25%). The higher the concentration of glucose in the dialysate, the greater the amount of fluid removal. Icodextrin, a relatively new alternative to glucose solutions, may be used as the osmotic agent. It has been shown to enhance ultrafiltration and clearance during the long dwell time in continuous ambulatory PD. This glucose polymer is metabolized to maltose and is not readily absorbed.[6,13,15,18,21] Metabolites may cause erroneously high glucose levels; check with the manufacture's guidelines to assure icodextrin metabolites will not interfere with the glucose analyzer being used for patient testing.
- PD involves repeated fluid exchanges or cycles. Each cycle has three phases: drain, instill, and dwell. If this is the patient's first dialysis cycle, the instillation phase will be first; however, if the patient has been on routine hemodialysis at home, for example, the drain phase will be done first, followed by instillation and dwell.
  - During the drain phase, the dialysate and excess extracellular fluid, wastes, and electrolytes are drained via gravity from the peritoneal cavity via a peritoneal catheter.
  - During the instillation phase, the dialysate is infused via gravity into the patient's peritoneal cavity through a peritoneal catheter.[3,4,21]
  - During the dwell phase, the dialysate remains in the patient's peritoneal cavity, allowing osmosis and diffusion to occur. Dwell time varies based on the patient's clinical need and the delivery method of PD.[1,20]
- PD can be performed either manually with a dialysis administration set (continuous ambulatory PD) or with a cycler machine (continuous cycling PD [CCPD]) (Fig. 121-2). With a cycler machine, multiple exchanges are programmed into the machine and run automatically.[6,24]
- Instillation of dialysate into the peritoneal cavity leads to increased peritoneal pressure. The amount of pressure depends on multiple factors, including the volume of dialysate instilled, patient position, age, body mass index, coughing, lifting, and straining.
- Patients requiring PD may experience complications directly related to increased peritoneal pressure. These may include inguinal and umbilical herniation with potential bowel incarceration, pericatheter and subcutaneous leaks causing abdominal and genital edema, and hydrothorax and hemoperitoneum.
- PD catheters can become clogged with the buildup of fibrin. Heparin or other anticoagulant medications are sometimes added to the dialysate or used as a separate flush to prevent occlusion.[3,5,7,23,26]
- PD dialysate should be warmed in a commercial warmer. *Never* warm the solution in a standard microwave oven, which heats unevenly and does not regulate the fluid temperature.[23,26]

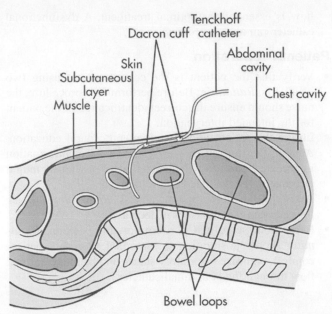

Figure 121-1 Tenckhoff catheter used in peritoneal dialysis. *(From Lewis SM, et al: Medical-surgical nursing: assessment and management of clinical problems, ed 7, St. Louis, 2007, Mosby.)*

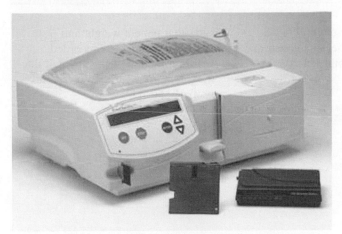

Figure 121-2 Baxter HomeChoice Pro PD Cycler. *(Courtesy Baxter International, Inc, Deerfield, IL.)*

- The adequacy of dialysis and assessment of the patient's residual renal function should be evaluated on a periodic basis. Adequacy of dialysis can be measured with urea kinetic modeling (Kt/V) or urea clearance.[7,10,14] Residual renal functioning can be monitored with urine creatinine clearance. Collaboration with the nephrology team is necessary to monitor these parameters.

EQUIPMENT

- Masks (for anyone in the room)
- Goggles or fluid shield face masks
- Sterile and nonsterile gloves
- 2 to 4 packs of sterile 4 × 4 gauze pads
- Antiseptic solution (follow institutional standards)
- Tape
- Sterile barriers
- Plastic hemostats (or clamps)

- PD administration set (most facilities are using closed delivery systems with attached drainage bag)
- Intravenous (IV) pole
- Warmed dialysate solution (use heating pad or commercial warmer)
- Sterile catheter caps (many facilities are using betadine impregnated caps)
- Labels for catheter
- Scale

Additional equipment, to have available as needed, includes the following:

- Sterile container
- Three clamps (if not included in the PD administration set)
- Cycler with tubing
- Equipment for culture and/or cell count/hematocrit

PATIENT AND FAMILY EDUCATION

- Explain the purpose of PD. *Rationale:* PD is necessary to perform the physiological functions of the kidneys when renal failure is present. PD uses the lining inside the abdomen, called the peritoneal cavity, as a filter to clean the blood and remove excess fluid.
- Explain the procedure, and review any questions. *Rationale:* Explanation provides information and may decrease patient anxiety.
- Explain the need for careful sterile technique when the abdominal catheter is accessed. *Rationale:* Sterile technique is used to decrease the chance of peritoneal infection because pathogens can be introduced into the abdominal cavity via the catheter.[8]
- Explain the three phases of PD. *Rationale:* Because each phase is different, the patient must be informed of all three phases and the purposes, interventions, and possible complications of each.
- Explain the potential for feelings of fullness and possibly shortness of breath during the dwell phase. *Rationale:* The pressure of the dialysate fluid on the diaphragm may cause the patient to have these feelings, which are normal for the dwell phase.

PATIENT ASSESSMENT AND PREPARATION

Patient Assessment

- Obtain baseline vital signs, respiratory status, abdominal assessment, blood glucose level, and pertinent laboratory results (potassium, sodium, calcium, phosphorus, magnesium, renal function tests, complete blood count). *Rationale:* Patients in renal failure often have altered baseline assessments, according to both physical assessment and laboratory values. The availability of this information before treatments are started is helpful so that interventions, including the type and amount of dialysate fluid, can be individualized.
- Assess volume status, as indicated by the following: skin turgor, mucous membranes, edema, lung sounds, weight, intake, and output. *Rationale:* PD is often initiated for the

control of hypervolemia.[17] Knowledge of a patient's pretreatment volume status is essential to allow for the individualization of treatment goals and interventions.

- Assess PD catheter and abdominal exit site for signs and symptoms of infection, leakage or drainage, or peritonitis.[5,10,11,13,16,17,25,26] **Rationale:** The catheter insertion site provides a portal of entry for pathogens that can result in septicemia or peritonitis. If the insertion site or effluent appears to be infected, further interventions (e.g., site change, culture, antibiotics) may be necessary.
  - ❖ Cloudy or bloody dialysate solution
  - ❖ Leakage at the catheter site
  - ❖ Subcutaneous fluid in abdomen, groin, or upper thighs
  - ❖ Abdominal pain
  - ❖ Fever
  - ❖ Chills
  - ❖ Rebound tenderness
- Check the peritoneal catheter and tubing for kinks, puncture sites, and loose connections. **Rationale:** Adequate

flow is essential for optimal treatment. A dysfunctional catheter can alter outcomes.

Patient Preparation

- Verify that the patient is the correct patient using two identifiers. **Rationale:** Before performing a procedure, the nurse should ensure the correct identification of the patient for the intended intervention.
- Ensure the patient understands preprocedural education. Answer questions as they arise and reinforce information as needed. **Rationale:** Understanding of previously taught information is evaluated and reinforced.
- Assist the patient in applying a mask. **Rationale:** The risk for pathogen transmission is decreased.
- Reposition the patient to a comfortable position. **Rationale:** Proper positioning is important to ensure patient comfort, optimize respiratory status, and facilitate optimal flow through the abdominal catheter.

Procedure	for Peritoneal Dialysis		
Steps	**Rationale**		**Special Considerations**
PD Initiation and Discontinuation			
1. Verify PD orders, which should include: A. Manual or automated delivery system B. Dialysis solution type, volume, dextrose/icodextrin and calcium concentrations, and additional medications C. Fill volume/time, dwell time, drain volume/time D. Vital sign parameters E. Laboratory testing	Familiarizes the nurse with the individualized patient treatment and reduces the possibility of error.		Ensure that patient weight and laboratory values are recorded before initiation of therapy and that the patient is wearing a mask and is properly positioned.
2. **HH**			
3. **PE**			
4. Assemble equipment in a clean, draft-free area.	Maintains aseptic technique.		A bathroom is not an appropriate place to prepare supplies or perform PD.
5. Remove the warmed dialysate bag from the protective pouch; check for expiration date, clarity, and leaks.	Assesses for contamination of dialysate.		
6. Hang the PD administration set on the IV pole, and clamp the tubing between the dialysate bag and the patient.	Fills tubing with dialysate; decreases chance of introducing air into the abdominal cavity.		The dialysate solution may have a frangible pin that needs to be broken to allow the solution to flow into the administration tubing.
7. Assure the twist clamp on the catheter adaptor or extension set is in the locked position and the cap is secured.	Prevents inadvertent disconnection.		
8. Don a mask, and assist the patient in applying a mask.	Reduces transmission of pathogens.		
9. Prepare a sterile field. Open a sterile container package or sterile 4 × 4 gauze packs.	Maintains aseptic technique.		

Procedure   for Peritoneal Dialysis—*Continued*

Steps	Rationale	Special Considerations
10. Pour antiseptic solution into a sterile container or onto sterile 4 × 4 gauze pads.	Maintains aseptic technique.	
11. Scrub the area from the catheter cap to the twist/roller clamp.	The effectiveness of the antiseptic is dependent on the scrub time: • Povidone-iodine, 2–3-minute scrub • Hypochlorite, 1-minute scrub • Chlorhexidine, 30-second scrub.	Allow to air dry. Follow the manufacturer's recommendations because chlorhexidine cannot be used for some catheters.[3,11]
12. Remove the cap and connect the catheter to the administration set or to the cycler line.	Ensures a tight connection.	If a cycler is used, follow the manufacturer's instructions for system setup.
13. Remove **PE** and discard used supplies.		
14. **HH**		
Drain Cycle		
1. **HH**		
2. **PE**		
3. Place the drainage bag below the midabdominal area on a clean surface.	Enhances flow by gravity.	
4. Assure the drainage tubing to the empty drainage bag is open.	Allows flow into the drainage bag.	
5. Unclamp the twist clamp on the catheter adaptor or extension set of the catheter.	Allows flow from the peritoneal cavity to the drainage bag.	Allow 15–20 minutes for outflow; observe and record characteristics (e.g., cloudy, bloody, clear, yellow) and amount of outflow. Reposition the patient if flow stops or is sluggish. Notify the physician or advanced practice nurse if drainage is cloudy or bloody.
6. Monitor vital signs as prescribed during outflow.	Assess for hypotension, tachycardia related to hypovolemia, and sudden release of intraperitoneal pressure.	Notify the physician or the advanced practice nurse if the patient becomes hypotensive, has tachycardia, or has abdominal pain.
7. Observe the outflow of the PD cycle.	Turning the patient from side to side ensures that the patient's abdomen is empty of dialysate.	
8. Clamp the catheter when the effluent is completely drained.	Decreases leakage and contamination.	
9. Remove **PE** and discard used supplies.	Safely discards used supplies.	
10. **HH**		
Instillation Cycle		
1. **HH**		
2. **PE**		
3. Assure the tubing to the catheter is clamped and unclamp the tubing between the dialysate and the drainage bag.	Allows flow between the dialysate bag and the drainage bag.	
4. Flush the tubing between the dialysate bag and the drainage bag with approximately 100 mL of dialysate or for approximately 5 seconds.	The "flush before fill" assures the effluent drainage left in the tubing to the drainage bag does not back flow into the peritoneal cavity.[18]	This technique is a key factor in potentially lowering the risk of peritonitis from contamination.
5. Clamp the tubing to the drainage bag.	Allows flow from the dialysate bag to the peritoneal cavity.	

Procedure continues on following page

Procedure for Peritoneal Dialysis—*Continued*

Steps	Rationale	Special Considerations
6. Open the clamp on the catheter.	Allows flow from the dialysate bag to the peritoneal cavity.	
7. Open the clamp from the dialysate bag to the catheter.	Provides open access between the catheter and the PD tubing, allowing inflow of dialysate to the peritoneal cavity.	
8. Set the flow rate as prescribed.	Time for inflow depends on the height of the dialysate bag, the position of the patient, and the patency of the catheter.	Monitor for signs of increased peritoneal volume.
9. Remove **PE** and discard used supplies.	Safely discards used supplies.	
10. **HH**		
Discontinuation of PD		
1. **HH**		
2. **PE**		
3. When inflow is complete, clamp the dialysate tubing and the patient's catheter.	Prepares catheter for disconnection.	
4. Don a mask, and assist the patient in applying a mask.	Maintains aseptic technique.	
5. Open a sterile cap.	Maintains aseptic technique.	Follow institution standard regarding use of a betadine impregnated cap.
6. Disconnect the PD administration set from the patient's catheter.	Preparing to end current dialysis cycle.	
7. With the transfer/extension set tubing pointing in a downward position, apply the sterile cap.	Maintains aseptic technique.	
8. Securely tape the catheter to the patient's abdomen.	Prevents accidental dislodgment.	
9. Obtain and record drainage bag weight.	Accurately assesses intake and output values.	
10. Remove **PE** and discard used supplies.	Safely discards used supplies.	
11. **HH**		
Catheter Exit Site Care		
1. **HH**		
2. **PE**		
3. Don a mask, and assist the patient in applying a mask.		
4. Prepare a sterile field. Open sterile 4 × 4 gauze pads and sterile container.	Maintains aseptic technique.	
5. Pour antiseptic solution into a sterile container.	Reduces transmission of microorganisms.	
6. Remove the old dressing.	Allows for visualization of the catheter site.	Be careful not to tug or dislodge the catheter. Note any odor or drainage on the old dressing.
7. Inspect the catheter exit site and surrounding area for leakage, infection, or trauma.	Provides assessment for complications.	Note any pain, warmth, crusting, bleeding, tenderness, redness, or swelling that may indicate infection.
8. Gently palpate the subcutaneous catheter segments and cuff.	Assesses for pain, erythema, edema, or accumulated drainage.	Obtain a culture if drainage is present and notify the physician or advance practice nurse if the listed signs or symptoms are present.

Procedure   for Peritoneal Dialysis—*Continued*

Steps	Rationale	Special Considerations
9. Remove nonsterile gloves, and wash hands.		
10. Apply sterile gloves.	Maintains aseptic technique.	
11. Use a sterile 4 × 4 gauze pad to hold the catheter off the skin.	Helps prevent contamination of catheter by skin flora.	
12. Cleanse the catheter and exit site with antiseptic solution.	The effectiveness of the antiseptic is dependent on the scrub time:	Allow to dry.
A. Begin at the exit site, and move outward in concentric circles.	• Povidone-iodine, 2–3-minute scrub	
B. Keep cleansing solutions out of the catheter sinus track.[7]	• Hypochlorite, 1-minute scrub • Chlorhexidine, 30-second scrub	
13. Apply a new catheter site dressing with sterile gauze or leave it open to the air. Follow institutional standards.	Gauze wicks drainage away from the site.	Some patients prefer to leave their well-healed catheter sites open to air.
14. Remove **PE** and discard used supplies in appropriate receptacles.	Safely discards used supplies.	
15. **HH**		

Expected Outcomes

- Catheter and exit site maintained without complications
- Instillation and drainage of dialysate without complications
- Respiratory status not compromised during treatment
- BUN and creatinine values restored to baseline levels
- Electrolyte values restored to baseline levels
- Glucose control maintained
- Accumulated fluid removed
- Peritoneum and abdomen intact

Unexpected Outcomes

- Drainage/leakage from the exit site
- Poor dialysate flow during instillation or drainage
- Signs and symptoms of peritonitis
- Inability to drain the total amount of instilled dialysate
- Signs or symptoms of infection at the insertion or access site
- Dislodgment of the abdominal catheter
- Tubing disconnection
- Physiological complications during treatment
- Introduction of pathogens into the abdominal catheter
- Diaphragmatic impingement
- Viscous perforation by PD catheter
- Protein or blood loss from peritonitis
- Increased intraperitoneal volume

Patient Monitoring and Care

Steps	Rationale	Reportable Conditions
		These conditions should be reported if they persist despite nursing interventions.
1. Perform and record predialysis and postdialysis weights. **(Level D*)**	Predialysis weight is an important factor in deciding how much PD is needed during treatment. It also helps to guide ongoing treatment and nutritional status. Postdialysis weight measures the effectiveness of the dialysis treatment.[3–5,7,12,23,26]	• Abnormal increase or decrease in weight.

*Level D: Peer-reviewed professional and organizational standards with the support of clinical study recommendations.

Procedure continues on following page

Patient Monitoring and Care —*Continued*

Steps	Rationale	Reportable Conditions
2. Perform baseline and ongoing assessments, including the following: A. Vital signs B. Jugular vein distention C. Presence or absence of edema D. Skin turgor E. Mucus membranes F. Intake and output G. Pulmonary assessment, including expiratory tidal volume and peak inspiratory pressures on the mechanically ventilated patient H. Abdominal assessment	Important to establish a baseline before initiation of treatment.[7,12,23,26] Monitors for complications.	• Hypotension • Hypertension • Fever • Hypothermia • Jugular vein distention • Dry mucous membranes • Shortness of breath • Crackles • Edema • Abdominal distention or tenderness • Rebound tenderness • Decreased tidal volume • Increased peak inspiratory pressures
3. Monitor BUN, creatinine, and electrolyte levels during treatment at a frequency determined by institutional standards.	Fluids and electrolyte levels shift during treatment.[7]	• Hyperglycemia • BUN or creatinine levels abnormal for the patient • Hyperkalemia or hypokalemia • Hypernatremia or hyponatremia • Hypercalcemia or hypocalcemia
4. Administer medications to correct metabolic abnormalities as prescribed.	Patients with renal failure are predisposed to many metabolic abnormalities. Common medications administered to patients with renal failure include the following[7,23,26]: • Vitamin D and calcium carbonate to increase the serum calcium level and prevent or treat bone disease • Erythropoietin and iron to treat anemia • Deferoxamine mesylate to remove excessive iron • Stool softeners because constipation can impair drainage of PD fluid • Phosphate binders to treat hyperphosphatemia	• Hypercalcemia or hypocalcemia • Abnormal hemoglobin or hematocrit values • Hyperphosphatemia or hypophosphatemia • Decreased albumin or prealbumin levels
5. Monitor serum glucose at the beginning of the treatment and throughout the treatment according to institutional standards. Administer insulin as prescribed to maintain glucose control.	The glucose in the dialysate solution predisposes patients to hyperglycemia, especially patients with diabetes.[1,9]	• Hyperglycemia or hypoglycemia
6. Monitor the integrity of the PD setup.	Disconnections in the setup provide a portal of entry for pathogens that can lead to peritonitis.[3,7,11,17,22]	• Fever • Tachycardia • Cloudy or bloody dialysate • Site redness or edema • Warmth • Bleeding • Purulent drainage • Pain or tenderness • Fever
7. Monitor for signs and symptoms of infection at the catheter exit site.	Identifies the need for intervention.	

Patient Monitoring and Care —*Continued*

Steps	Rationale	Reportable Conditions
8. Monitor the case with which the dialysate is both instilled and drained through the abdominal catheter.	Patients may need repositioning to facilitate flow through the abdominal catheter. Catheters may also become kinked or occluded. Fibrin clots can obstruct outflow; heparin may be added to the dialysate solution if prescribed. Rapid infusion can cause abdominal pain.	• Inability to instill or drain fluid through the abdominal catheter
9. Follow institutional standards for assessing pain. Administer analgesia as prescribed.	Identifies need for pain interventions.	• Continued pain despite pain interventions.
10. Monitor for signs and symptoms related to quality of life.[2]	Patient may require further treatment management. Renal diet may also be prescribed, with adjusted protein, phosphorus, carbohydrate, and fluid intake that takes into account the patient's current catabolic state, residual renal function, adequacy of dialysis, and removal of amino acids by dialysis.[7,12,23,26]	• Fatigue[2] • Depression[2] • Headache[2] • Poor appetite[2] • Pruritis[2] • Constipation.[2]

Documentation

Documentation should include the following:

- Patient and family education
- Date and time of treatment initiation
- Treatment/exchange number
- Condition of the abdominal catheter and exit site at time of treatment
- Date and time of dressing application
- Patient weight before and after treatment
- Pain assessment, interventions, and effectiveness
- Intake and output

- Length and parameters of treatment
- Dialysate solution used
- Total ultrafiltration output
- Vital signs/hemodynamic parameters throughout the treatment
- Unexpected outcomes
- Nursing interventions
- Laboratory assessment data

References and Additional Readings

For a complete list of references and additional readings for this procedure, scan this QR code with any freely available smartphone code reader app, or visit http://booksite.elsevier.com/9780323376624.

PROCEDURE

122 Use of a Massive Infusion Device and a Pressure Infusor Bag

Coleen Dever

PURPOSE: A massive infusion device is used to rapidly replace depleted intravascular volume of a critically ill patient. The infuser can simultaneously warm fluids or blood products and infuse them at rates up to 30,000 mL/hr. The ability to warm the fluids helps prevent and treat hypothermia, which will, in turn, minimize the risk of coagulopathy. Indications to use this device include patients with severe hemorrhage, as seen in trauma, gastrointestinal bleeding, postoperative bleeding, septic shock, and burns. The device utilizes specialized tubing that has the ability to expand during pressure, accommodating the rapid infusion rate and warming ability of the device.

PREREQUISITE NURSING KNOWLEDGE

- Knowledge of aseptic technique and principles of fluid resuscitation and blood transfusion is essential.[14]
- Massive transfusion is the transfusion of plasma to packed red blood cells (PRBCs) in a 1:1 ratio typically consisting of greater than 10 units of PRBCs within a 24-hour period.[5,6,8–10,14]
- Massive transfusion protocols utilizing predetermined ratios are implemented to facilitate the adherence to hemostatic protocols in resuscitation.[2,4,5,9]
- Acute coagulopathy is the result of hypothermia, acidosis, ongoing bleeding, and dilution and decreased activity of clotting factors. Hypothermia, acidosis and coagulopathy are known as the trauma triad of death, occurring in 25% to 30% of trauma patients.[5,7,9–11]
- Acute coagulopathy can be recognized early by laboratory tests such as international normalized ratio (INR), activated partial thromboplastin time (APTT), platelet counts, fibrinogen levels, and thromboelastography (TEG).[2,4,8,10,13]
- Hypothermia is commonly caused by the initial injury and subsequent treatment modalities. Decreased coagulation protease activity and impaired platelet function occur when core temperatures are reduced from 36°C to 33°C.[4,10]
- Measures to prevent and treat hypothermia include solar blankets, heated blankets, warmed blood products and fluids, continuous arteriovenous rewarming, and cardiopulmonary bypass, used in extreme cases of hypothermia (see Procedure 100).
- When large volumes of IV fluids are being infused into patients, the fluids must be warmed to prevent hypothermia. Although institutions vary in what constitutes large volumes, a good rule of thumb is to institute fluid rewarming measures when more than 2 L of fluid are required in less than 1 hour.
- Current resuscitation strategies, known as damage control resuscitation (DCR), focus on rapid hemorrhage control, early recognition and correction of acute coagulopathy, permissive hypotension, minimization of crystalloid, and early initiation of fresh frozen plasma (FFP) in a ratio of 1:1 with PRBCs. DCR is the standard of care and is incorporated into clinical practice guidelines.[2,8-10]
- Uncontrolled hemorrhage and the associated complications account for approximately 40% of trauma-related deaths.[10]
- Goals of therapy are to stop the bleeding, actively rewarm the patient, and administer blood products early to reverse coagulopathy, facilitate clot formation, and restore oxygenated blood carrying capacity to vital organs.[2,4,5,8,10,13,14]
- Ongoing assessment to evaluate for transfusion related complications include: transfusion-related lung injury (TRALI), transfusion-associated circulatory overload (TACO), increased leukocyte adhesion and reperfusion injury acute tubular necrosis, hypothermia, hypokalemia, hypocalcemia, hemolytic and allergic reactions, and air embolism.[2,13]
- Use of a rapid infusion device, such as the one described in this procedure (Fig. 122-1), can warm and infuse fluids at rates from 75 to 30,000 mL/hr (Level 1, Inc., Rockland, MA). The tubing is made of soft plastic that expands to allow rapid infusion of fluids under pressure. Some rapid infusers include automated pressure chambers to compress intravenous (IV) bags. They allow for fast and easy

bag changes and can accommodate both 1-L IV bags and 500-mL blood product bags. Pressure is maintained at a constant 300 mm Hg and is turned on and off via a simple toggle switch at the top of each pressure chamber. Older infusers simply have an IV pole from which to hang fluids, and separate pressure infusor bags must be used.

- IV catheters for aggressive fluid resuscitation should have a large bore and short diameter to facilitate the rapid infusion of large volumes of IV fluids and blood products. Usually, multiple IVs are used, including peripheral and central sites. Venous access may also be obtained surgically via a venous cut-down of the basilic or saphenous veins when peripheral access cannot be obtained.[15]

- Both crystalloid and colloid IV solutions are used for resuscitating patients who are hypovolemic with hemodynamically unstable conditions. Crystalloids directly increase the intravascular volume. Colloids expand plasma volume by pulling interstitial fluid back into the vascular space via osmosis. Numerous crystalloid and colloid preparations are available in isotonic, hypotonic, and hypertonic preparations. Crystalloids most commonly used in aggressive fluid resuscitation are 0.9% normal saline (NS) and lactated Ringer's (LR) solutions.

- The use of colloids such as albumin, dextran, and hetastarch allows the effective restoration of intravascular volume with smaller amounts of fluid; however, these colloids coat red blood cells (RBCs) and platelets, which may result in type and cross-match difficulties and clotting problems. Even slight overresuscitation with colloids increases the risk for fluid overload and pulmonary edema.[1,15]

- Blood and blood products are natural colloids used to replace lost blood and restore coagulation factors. In the patient with significant ongoing hemorrhage, infusion of blood and clotting factors is critical to restoring intravascular volume. Type O-negative blood is the universal donor for all patients and can be given in extreme emergencies before the completion of typing and cross-matching. PRBCs and whole blood are used to replace oxygen-carrying components; FFP, platelets, and cryoprecipitate are used to replace essential clotting factors.[3]

EQUIPMENT

- Rapid infuser (see Fig. 122-1)
- Disposable fluid administration sets (Fig. 122-2)
- Replaceable filter with gas vent (Fig. 122-3)
- Blood administration set

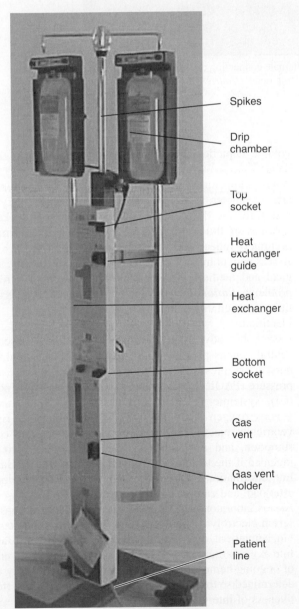

Spikes

Drip chamber

Top socket

Heat exchanger guide

Heat exchanger

Bottom socket

Gas vent

Gas vent holder

Patient line

Figure 122-1 Level 1 rapid infuser. (*Courtesy Level 1, Inc., Rockland, MA.*)

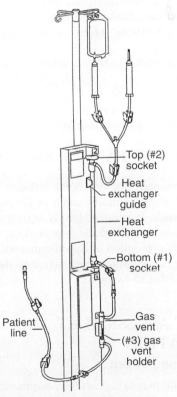

Top (#2) socket

Heat exchanger guide

Heat exchanger

Bottom (#1) socket

Patient line

Gas vent

(#3) gas vent holder

Figure 122-2 Placement of tubing in Level 1 rapid infuser. (*Courtesy Level 1, Inc., Rockland, MA.*)

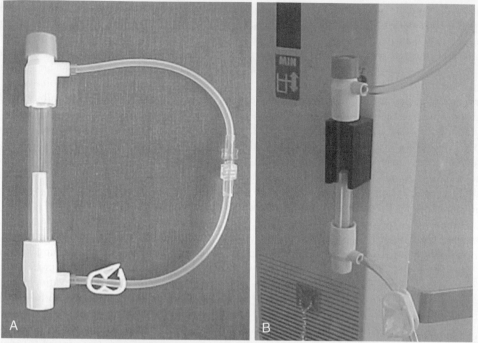

Figure 122-3 **A,** Rapid infuser filter showing male/female connecting ends on the right. **B,** Insertion of the filter in the Level 1 rapid infuser with the clamp open. *(Courtesy Level 1, Inc., Rockland, MA.)*

- Pressure infusor bag
- IV pole
- IV fluids or blood products as prescribed
- Sterile or distilled water for the warmer
- Nonsterile gloves
- Fluid shield face mask or goggles
- Antiseptic solution (e.g., 2% chlorhexidine-based preparation)

Additional equipment, to have available as needed, includes the following:

- Emergency equipment
- Indwelling urinary catheter
- Supplies for blood gas sampling

PATIENT AND FAMILY EDUCATION

- Explain the need for the rapid infusion of fluids, the purpose of warming fluids, and how the equipment operates. *Rationale:* Patient and family anxiety about unfamiliar equipment at the bedside may be decreased.
- Explain that prevention of hypothermia will be a priority. *Rationale:* This explanation prepares the patient and family for what to expect.

PATIENT ASSESSMENT AND PREPARATION

Patient Assessment

- Assess blood pressure, heart rate, respiratory rate, peripheral pulses, and level of consciousness. *Rationale:* Assessment is necessary to determine the severity of the patient's

volume depletion and shock. It also provides baseline data.

- Assess temperature using a bladder probe or pulmonary artery catheter. *Rationale:* Assessment is necessary to assess for the development of hypothermia while large volumes of fluids are infused. Core temperatures most accurately reflect true body temperature.
- Assess patient history, including precipitating events, surgical and medical interventions, and history of cardiac problems. *Rationale:* Potential or actual need for massive fluid resuscitation and risk for fluid overload are identified.
- Assess hemodynamic parameters, including baseline central venous pressure (CVP) and, if available, pulmonary artery pressure (PAP), pulmonary artery occlusion pressure (PAOP), cardiac output (CO) and cardiac index (CI), systemic vascular resistance (SVR), and mixed venous oxygen saturation (Svo_2). Assessment of right ventricular ejection fraction, oxygen delivery and consumption, and oxygen extraction ratio should also be included if the technology is available. *Rationale:* Baseline information is provided about the patient's preload, afterload, and cardiac contractility.
- Assess laboratory values to include arterial blood gases, serum electrolytes, serum lactate, base deficit, hemoglobin, hematocrit, and coagulation studies. *Rationale:* Baseline oxygenation, presence of metabolic acidosis, severity of ongoing hemorrhage, and severity of coagulopathy are determined so that the need for intervention and the effectiveness of interventions can be determined.
- Assess patency of multiple large-bore IV sites. *Rationale:* Multiple sites are often necessary to infuse enough fluids

and blood products to support the patient's vital signs. Extra sites in addition to those used for rapid infusion should be kept patent in case one of the other sites becomes nonfunctional or is accidentally pulled out.

Patient Preparation

- Verify that the patient is the correct patient using two identifiers. *Rationale:* Before performing a procedure, the nurse should ensure the correct identification of the patient for the intended intervention.
- Ensure that informed consent has been obtained. *Rationale:* Informed consent protects the rights of the patient and makes a competent decision possible for the patient.
- Ensure that the patient and family understand the need and purpose for rapid infusion. Answer questions as they arise, and reinforce information as needed. *Rationale:* Understanding of previously taught information is evaluated and reinforced.
- Place additional peripheral IV sites. *Rationale:* Aggressive fluid resuscitation requires additional IV access besides the one site being used with the rapid infuser. Backup IV sites can be used if other sites infiltrate or become pulled out; extra sites may also be used to infuse medications, such as vasopressors, that should be kept separate from rapid infusion lines. Ideal sites for large IV catheter access are the antecubital fossa, saphenous veins, and the veins of the forearm and upper arm.
- Assist the physician or advanced practice nurse with placement of central venous catheter and/or a pulmonary artery catheter. *Rationale:* This placement allows for the assessment of volume status before and after infusion of fluids and blood products. It also allows for assessment of

core temperature with pulmonary artery catheter thermistor and provides central venous access in the event vasoactive medications are needed.

- Place an automatic blood pressure monitor on the patient's arm that is not being infused with the rapid infusion device. Set it to check blood pressure every 5 minutes. *Rationale:* Assessment of patient's hemodynamics and response to fluid replacement is provided. This usually is used temporarily until an arterial catheter is inserted by the physician or advanced practice nurse.
- Assist the physician or advanced practice nurse with placement of an arterial line. *Rationale:* Placement allows for continuous assessment of the blood pressure during resuscitation and provides convenient access for blood sampling.
- Obtain a blood sample for type and cross-match. Two tubes should be sent if a large volume of blood is expected to be transfused. *Rationale:* This action prepares for blood transfusion.
- Obtain baseline hematocrit, chemistry panel, and coagulation studies. Repeat, as prescribed, every 15 to 60 minutes until hemorrhage is controlled. *Rationale:* These studies guide replacement of blood products and essential electrolytes.
- Place an indwelling urinary catheter as prescribed. *Rationale:* Patients who need aggressive fluid resuscitation should have an indwelling urinary catheter placed to determine volume status and end-organ perfusion.
- Cover the patient with warm cotton blankets or a warm-air blanket. Cover the patient's head with a warmed blanket, a towel, or an aluminum cap. *Rationale:* Additional heat loss is minimized.

Procedure for Use of Massive Infusion Device

Steps	Rationale	Special Considerations
1. **HH**		
2. **PE**		
3. Verify the IV fluids and blood products prescribed.	Determines products and amounts to be infused.	The physician or advanced practice nurse will prescribe the volume and type of additional IV fluids and blood products, and laboratory studies. Follow institutional standards for performing pretransfusion blood verification with another physician, advanced practice nurse, or other healthcare professional.
4. Verify that the fluid warmer was prescribed.	Warming fluids helps to prevent hypothermia.[3,4]	
5. Turn on the device.	Allows the system to warm before moving fluid through the warming chamber.	Follow manufacturer's guidelines for setup of each device.
6. Open the Y-set fluid administration package provided by the manufacturer. Close all clamps.	Prevents the accidental spillage of blood or fluid. Prevents the flow of fluid through the circuit before the machine is warmed.	

Procedure continues on following page

Procedure | for Use of Massive Infusion Device—*Continued*

Steps	Rationale	Special Considerations
7. Spike the fluid or blood with both sides of the Y-set.	Allows for a smooth transition from an empty bag to the next bag.	
8. Hang fluid bags on the small hooks inside the rapid infuser pressure chambers, leaving the chamber doors open (see Fig. 122-1) or place the fluid bags in separate pressure infusor bags.	Clearing the tubing of air is easier if the tubing is primed while the bags are still unpressurized.	Autotransfusion bags do not fit into the pressure chambers. Caution needs to be maintained so that air is not pushed through the tubing and into the patient causing an air embolism. Follow institutional standards regarding removal of air from infusion bags.
9. Push the bottom end of the heat exchanger rod firmly into the bottom socket and snap the heat exchanger into the guide (see Fig. 122-2).	The bottom of the heat exchanger must be firmly placed or it will not fit into the top socket.	
10. Slide the top socket up and place the top end of the exchanger into the placement tract.	Locks the warming chamber into place at both the top and the bottom sockets.	
11. Slide the top heat exchanger socket down over the heat exchanger tube until the pole latch clicks into place.	Secures the heat exchanger.	
12. Snap the gas vent filter into the holder on the lower portion of the pole assembly with the orange end up (see Fig. 122-3).	Filters air and blood clots from the tubing.	Only fits into the machine one way because the tubing is not long enough to be placed incorrectly.
13. Squeeze the drip chambers so that they are half full.	Minimizes entrapment of bubbles in the tubing. Allows visualization of the drip chamber so that the drip rate can be assessed.	
14. Open the clamp on one side of the Y-set.	Make sure that only one side of the Y-tubing is open during priming; otherwise, fluid is pumped from one bag to the other and not through the tubing.	
15. Remove the male Luer-Lok cap at the end of the IV tubing; open the clamps.	Does not prime unless the end cap has been removed.	
16. Remove the filter from its holder, and invert it. Prime the tubing; close the roller clamp. Turn the filter back over, and replace it in its holder.	Prevents entrapment of large amounts of air.	
17. Tap the filter or air eliminator against the cabinet several times. Monitor fluid line for bubbles during use.	Releases any residual trapped air.	Never administer fluids if air bubbles are found between the filter chamber and the patient connection. Run IV fluid into the trash container to rid tubing of any residual air. When no more bubbles are observed leaving the gas vent filter, all the air has been vented from the filter or air eliminator.

Procedure for Use of Massive Infusion Device—*Continued*

Steps	Rationale	Special Considerations
18. Open the roller clamp partially, and slowly infuse fluid.	Infusing slowly allows for assessment of any air bubbles. The air filter eliminates bubbles in the tubing.	If unable to clear the line of air and more than $\frac{1}{4}$ inch of air is present at the top of the filter, replace the filter.
19. Replace the male Luer-Lok cap at the end of the tubing; close the clamps.	Maintains asepsis of the tubing.	
20. Close the pressure chamber doors, and latch.	Prepares the fluid bags for pressurization when the machines are turned on and the pressure switch is activated.	Be certain that the latch is secure before the chamber is pressurized.
21. Perform all function and alarm checks as per manufacturer instructions.	Validates proper equipment function.	
22. Wait for the temperature readout to reach the operating temperature of 41°C.	Prevents hypothermia by ensuring the chamber is warm before fluids are run through it and into the patient.	
23. Flip the toggle switch at the top of the pressure chamber to "on/+," or inflate the separate pressure bags.	Pressurizes the chambers.	The pressure automatically inflates to 300 mm Hg. Fluids infuse via gravity flow without being pressurized; however, high flow rates cannot be achieved unless the pressure bags are inflated.
24. Cleanse the injection site with antiseptic solution.[2,12] (Level B*)	Reduces the risk for infection.	Follow institutional standards. Chlorhexidine and povidone-iodine solutions may be more effective than alcohol in reducing external microbial contamination.[2]
25. Connect the distal end of the tubing to the patient's IV.	Prepares for the infusion.	
26. Open the roller clamp to infuse the fluid.	Fluids or blood products now infuse under pressure.	It is best to infuse one side at a time, especially when blood products are infusing, to prevent mixing of fluids and blood products. The pressure system is designed to leave a small volume remaining to prevent air emboli.
27. Set the rate by gradually opening the clamp.	Fluids given via rapid infusers are administered as boluses over short periods; roller clamps are usually left wide open until the bolus is complete.	If a slower bolus is desired, adjust the roller clamp to decrease the flow of fluid.
Changing the Bags		
1. Close the top clamp on the side of the Y-connector with the empty fluid bag.	Prevents air from entering the tubing.	Follow manufacturer's guidelines for changing infusion bags for each device.
2. Open the clamp on the side of the Y-connector with the full fluid bag; infuse the fluid.	Keeping one side of the Y-connector spiked with fluid ready to infuse is helpful when patients have severely unstable conditions and need immediate boluses of fluid.	

*Level B: Well-designed, controlled studies with results that consistently support a specific action, intervention, or treatment.

Procedure continues on following page

Procedure	for Use of Massive Infusion Device—*Continued*	
Steps	**Rationale**	**Special Considerations**
3. Turn the "on/+" switch above the pressure chamber to the "off" position, and remove the empty bag.	Releases pressure from the pressure chamber.	
4. Replace the empty fluid bag with a full one.	The next bag of IV fluid must be ready to infuse to avoid delays in infusion in case the patient's blood pressure falls precipitously.	
5. Close the pressure chamber door and latch; flip the control switch above the pressure chamber to "on/+."	Repressurizes the chamber.	

Replacing the Filter or Air Eliminator

Steps	Rationale	Special Considerations
1. Close the clamps on the disposable fluid administration set just proximal to the filter and between the filter and the patient connection.	The filter should be replaced after 3 hours of use, after 4 units of blood, or if the fluid rate slows because of clotting.	Follow manufacturer's guidelines for replacing the filter or air eliminator for each device.
2. Remove the old filter or air eliminator from the holder, and place the new filter or air eliminator in the holder.	Keep the old filter or air eliminator connected to the disposable fluid administration set until ready to change to new one. Minimizes the potential for contaminating exposed tubing ends.	
3. Disconnect the old filter or air eliminator at the upper Luer-Lok, and connect the tubing to the new filter.	Prepares for placement of new equipment.	
4. Disconnect the patient line Luer-Lok from the old filter or air eliminator, and connect it to the new one.	Prepares for placement of new equipment.	
5. Open the clamp just proximal to the filter or air eliminator to restart fluid. Invert the filter until completely filled with fluid, then turn back to proper position and replace in the holder. Open the clamp between the filter and the patient connection.	Infusion of the fluid resumes.	
6. Remove the filter or air eliminator from the holder, and tap until all bubbles are eliminated; reinsert. Check patient line for bubbles before opening the roller clamp.	Facilitates removal of bubbles.	If air bubbles are present, disconnect the tubing from the patient, and infuse into the trash container until the line is clear of air. Reconnect to the patient, and resume the infusion. If the alarm sounds after setup, check to ensure the filter is properly snapped into place.

Troubleshooting Alarms

Steps	Rationale	Special Considerations
1. If the alarm sounds and the disposable light is illuminated, check to be sure the disposable tubing set is properly placed in the machine.	The system will not run if the disposable tubing is not completely set into the machine.	The tubing set can become inadvertently dislodged. Follow manufacturer's guidelines for troubleshooting alarms for each device.

Procedure   for Use of Massive Infusion Device—*Continued*

Steps	Rationale	Special Considerations
2. If the alarm sounds and the water level light is illuminated, check the water level in the chamber and replace as needed with sterile or distilled water.	The system will not run if the water level is too low.	
3. If the system alarms "overtemp," turn the machine off and use a different rapid infuser.	Fluids inadequately warmed will contribute to hypothermia. Fluids overly warmed will contribute to hemolysis of the RBCs.	Notify biomedical engineering of the problem.

Transporting a Patient With a Rapid Infuser

Steps	Rationale	Special Considerations
1. Turn the rapid infuser off.	If the infuser is still on when the administration set is removed from its holder, water will spurt out of the warming chamber and aluminum tube.	Follow manufacturer's guidelines for each device to transport a patient with a rapid infuser.
2. Remove the disposable administration set from its holder on the infuser, and place it in the bed alongside the patient or hang it on the transport IV pole.	The rapid infusers described here do not operate on a battery. Fluids infuse via gravity, or separate pressure infusor bags can be used.	Fluids run briskly via gravity drainage. If pressure is still necessary to infuse fluids, separate pressure infusor bags need to be used as long as the machine is not plugged in. Interventions to minimize heat loss must be in place while the infuser is not plugged in. An aluminum head covering, warmed cotton blankets, and warm-air blankets help prevent heat loss. Removing the administration set from the machine and transporting the patient separately from the infuser is less awkward and minimizes the risk for pulling out the IV lines during transport.
3. Plug the infuser into an electric outlet once you reach the intended destination.	Establishes power source.	
4. Return the administration set into the infuser. Turn the machine on. Return fluid bags to pressure chambers.	The infuser is now ready to repressurize the chambers and warm the fluid. Any bubbles are eliminated by the filter.	If bubbles are not removed and more than $\frac{1}{4}$ inch of air is at the top of the filter, the filter must be replaced.
5. Remove **PE** and discard used supplies in the appropriate receptacle.	Safely discards used supplies.	
6. **HH**		

Procedure   for Pressure Infusor Bag Use

Steps	Rationale	Special Considerations
1. **HH**		
2. **PE**		
3. Obtain and set up the IV fluid or blood component system.	The infusion system should be assembled before inserting the IV fluid or blood product into the pressure infusor bag.	If administering blood products, follow institution standards for performing pretransfusion blood verification with a physician, advanced practice nurse, or other health care professional.

Procedure continues on following page

Procedure for Pressure Infusor Bag Use—*Continued*

Steps	Rationale	Special Considerations
4. Cleanse the injection site with antiseptic solution.[12] **(Level B*)**	Reduces the risk for infection.	Follow institutional standards. Chlorhexidine and povidone-iodine solutions may be more effective than alcohol in reducing external microbial contamination.[12]
5. If administering a blood component, piggyback the blood tubing into the 0.9% NS solution or connect it directly into the IV line.	Allows the transfusion to proceed.	Follow institutional standard for use of 0.9% NS solution as the primary IV fluid line. FFP and platelets should be given directly into the IV line. Do not piggyback them.
6. Open the roller clamp on the tubing.	Allows infusion to proceed.	The rate of the infusion is dependent on the amount of pressure applied to the unit, not the position of the roller clamp.
7. Place the unit of blood or IV fluid through the mesh or plastic cover of the deflated pressure infusor bag so that the entire bag to be infused remains within the mesh or plastic panel.	Allows pressure to be evenly applied.	Do not allow the top of the bag to be infused appear above the mesh or plastic covering because this interferes with flow.
8. Secure the bag to be infused in place with a Velcro strap or hang on the hook in the pressure infusor bag. Hang the infusor bag on the IV pole.	Prevents the bag to be infused from slipping out of the bag when hung from the IV pole.	A standard sphygmomanometer cuff should never be used to administer large-volume transfusions because it does not exert uniform pressure on all parts of the component container.
9. Inflate the pressure infusor bag to achieve the desired rate of flow.	The pressure of the infusor bag is used to adjust flow, not the position of the roller clamp.	The pressure should not exceed 300 mm Hg to avoid damaging RBCs, rupturing the IV or blood bag, dislodging the IV catheter, or injuring the vein. The patient may have discomfort in an extremity if a peripheral catheter is used; if appropriate, decrease the pressure to maintain patient comfort.
10. When the infusion is complete, deflate the pressure infusor bag.	Slows the infusion.	
11. If infusing blood, close the roller clamp to the blood component and flush the primary infusion tubing with 0.9% NS solution if used as the primary IV line.	Allows the patient to receive blood sequestered in the tubing.	
12. When the infusion is complete, disconnect the IV fluid, NS solution or blood tubing from the IV line.	Completes infusion; Standard Precautions.	
13. Remove gloves and discard used supplies in appropriate receptacle.	Safely discards used supplies.	Blood container and administration set should be handled as hazardous waste.

*Level B: Well-designed, controlled studies with results that consistently support a specific action, intervention, or treatment.

Expected Outcomes

- Patient's blood pressure and heart rate return to baseline
- Patient's core temperature remains above 36°C
- CVP, PAP, PAOP, CO, CI, and SVR reflect return of euvolemia and hemodynamic stability
- IV sites remain patent
- Rapid flow of blood components
- Urine output at least 0.5 mL/kg/hr

Unexpected Outcomes

- Blood pressure remains below baseline despite multiple liters of fluid and blood products
- Core temperature falls below 36°C so that more aggressive rewarming interventions become necessary
- Hypothermia-induced coagulopathy develops as temperature falls below 35°C
- Inability to restore normal intravascular status occurs, as seen by CVP <6, PAOP <6, CO <4 L/min, CI <2 L/min/m^2, or SVR >1500 dynes/sec
- Infiltration of IV site occurs
- Clotting of rapid infuser filter occurs
- Anuria or oliguria with urinary output <0.5 mL/kg/hr
- Patient discomfort

Patient Monitoring and Care

Steps	Rationale	Reportable Conditions
		These conditions should be reported if they persist despite nursing interventions.
1. Monitor the patient's vital signs every 5–15 minutes as indicated. As the patient's condition becomes more stable, assessment of vital signs may be done less frequently (every 15–30 minutes until the blood pressure remains stable for more than 2 hours).	Determines severity of shock, responsiveness to fluids and blood products, and the need for additional fluids.	• Systolic blood pressure below 90 mm Hg despite fluid administration • Abnormal vital signs
2. Assess the patient's core temperature every 15–30 minutes. **(Level E*)**	Patients who are in severe shock have impaired thermogenesis. This, in combination with the infusion of inadequately warmed fluids, leads to hypothermia. Hypothermia-induced coagulopathies begin at a core temperature of 35°C and exacerbate any hemorrhage already occurring. In addition, severe physiological complications from hypothermia, such as cardiovascular instability, electrolyte changes, urine concentration problems, and shifts in the oxygen-hemoglobin dissociation curve, affect the patient's ability to respond to physiological stress. Prevention of hypothermia is a critical goal for patients undergoing massive fluid resuscitation.[1,7]	• Worsening hypothermia or unrelieved hypothermia

*Level E: Multiple case reports, theory-based evidence from expert opinions, or peer-reviewed professional organizational standards without clinical studies to support recommendations.

Procedure continues on following page

Patient Monitoring and Care —*Continued*

Steps	Rationale	Reportable Conditions
3. Assess the integrity of IV sites every 15 minutes.	IV sites under pressure are at higher risk for infiltration. In addition, lines can be inadvertently pulled out during radiographic filming, turning, and other aspects of patient care during a massive resuscitation. Multiple IV sites are recommended to be available at all times in the event an IV infiltrates or is pulled out.	• Infiltrated IV sites • Problems obtaining IV sites
4. Assess hemodynamic parameters every 15–30 minutes.	Determines intravascular volume status and responsiveness to interventions. Patients may still be inadequately resuscitated even though vital signs, urine output, and hemodynamic parameters have returned to normal. A complete clinical picture (including laboratory tests in conjunction with vital signs, urine output, and hemodynamic parameters) is the best way to determine whether a patient has been adequately resuscitated.[11]	• Abnormal hemodynamic parameters • Abnormal trends in hemodynamic monitoring
5. Assess urine output every 30–60 minutes.	Urine output is an assessment of end-organ perfusion. If little or no urine is produced, it is assumed that the kidneys are not being perfused and, therefore, other major viscera are also probably not being adequately perfused. Trauma to the urinary tract may interfere with accurate assessment of urine output because clots may block urine drainage and laceration to ureters may result in extravasation of urine into the peritoneum.	• Urine output <0.5 mL/kg/hr
6. Obtain hemoglobin, hematocrit, and coagulation studies as prescribed. These are usually measured every 30–60 minutes or after transfusion of blood and follow institutional standards.	Determines the presence of ongoing blood loss and coagulopathy.[7]	• Abnormal hemoglobin, hematocrit, and coagulation results
7. Obtain arterial blood gases base deficit and lactic acid as prescribed and indicated.	Determines persistence of metabolic acidosis and identifies the need for additional interventions to improve perfusion to major organs.[11]	• Abnormal laboratory results
8. Obtain electrolytes as prescribed.	Patients undergoing large-volume resuscitation are at risk for hypokalemia, hypomagnesemia, hypocalcemia, and hypophosphatemia.	• Abnormal laboratory results

Patient Monitoring and Care —*Continued*

Steps	Rationale	Reportable Conditions
9. Monitor the patient for signs and symptoms of a transfusion reaction. If a transfusion reaction is suspected, stop the transfusion.	Blood component replacement therapy constitutes the infusion of a foreign substance into the recipient.	• Signs and symptoms of a transfusion reaction.
10. Follow institutional standards for assessing pain. Administer analgesia as prescribed.	Identifies need for pain interventions.	• Continued pain despite pain interventions

Documentation

Documentation should include the following:
- Patient and family education
- Completion of informed consent
- Rationale for use of the rapid infuser
- Blood pressure, heart rate, respiratory rate, lung sounds, and peripheral pulses throughout the resuscitation
- The patient's core temperature while the rapid infusers are used
- Hemodynamic parameters, including CVP, PAP, PAOP, CO, CI, and SVR
- Urine output, estimated blood loss, other measured output
- Laboratory results, including arterial blood gases, hematocrit, hemoglobin, electrolytes base deficit, and lactic acid
- Appearance of IV sites
- IV insertions
- Total IV fluids and blood products in intake and output record
- Unexpected outcomes
- Additional interventions
- Pain assessment, interventions, and effectiveness

References and Additional Readings

For a complete list of references and additional readings for this procedure, scan this QR code with any freely available smartphone code reader app, or visit http://booksite.elsevier.com/9780323376624.

PROCEDURE

123 Apheresis and Therapeutic Plasma Exchange (Assist)

Sonia M. Astle

PURPOSE: Apheresis techniques are used to remove cells, plasma, and other substances from blood. These procedures are used as adjunctive treatments in many diseases, especially in antibody-mediated conditions that produce autoantibodies.

PREREQUISITE NURSING KNOWLEDGE

- Therapeutic apheresis is a technique for selective removal of cells, plasma, and substances from the patient's circulation to promote clinical improvement. The different apheresis techniques vary according to the component of the blood removed or replaced or the substance removed.
  - *Cytapheresis* is the selective removal of the cellular components of blood. Blood is withdrawn from the patient, and a specific cellular component is retained, such as leukocytes (white blood cells); the remainder of the blood components (erythrocytes, platelets, and plasma) are returned to the donor or patient.
  - *Erythrocytapheresis* is the process of removing erythrocytes (red blood cells) from whole blood.
  - *Extracorporeal photopheresis (ECP)* uses apheresis techniques to remove and return blood to the patient. Whole blood is withdrawn into the ECP machine that separates the leukocytes involved in the immune response from the other blood components. The leukocytes remain in the machine and the blood is returned to the patient. While in the machine, the leukocytes are exposed to the photosensitizing medication, methoxsalen, and are then treated with ultraviolet (UV) radiation, which activates the methoxsalen. The leukocytes are then returned to the patient. ECP induces cellular changes that have been shown to be effective in certain diseases such as cutaneous T-cell lymphoma, graft-versus-host disease, post–bone marrow transplant, and solid organ transplant rejection. Apheresis techniques are also used for the procurement of peripheral stem cells for bone marrow transplantation.
  - *Immunoadsorption (IA)* is the removal of an antigen in the blood by a specific antibody lining the surface of a filter or cartridge.
  - *Leukocytapheresis* is the removal of white blood cells from the blood; the remaining blood components are

returned to the patient. It is most commonly used as a therapeutic method for blast cell reduction in leukemias (leukocytosis).
  - *Lymphoplasmapheresis* is the separation and removal of lymphocytes and plasma from the withdrawn blood, with the remainder of the blood retransfused into the donor.
  - *Red blood cell (RBC) exchange* removes the patient's RBCs and replaces them with exogenous normal RBCs.
  - *Rheopheresis* is the process to change the viscosity of blood by filtering out components such as fibrinogen and low-density lipoprotein (LDL) cholesterol.
  - *Plasma adsorption/perfusion* is the removal of plasma with a hollow fiber filter. Blood is returned to the patient, and the plasma is pumped over an adsorptive column that removes certain proteins or pathogens. The treated plasma is then returned to the patient.
  - *Therapeutic plasma exchange (TPE)* is the process of replacing the plasma removed with an equal amount of either plasma or fluid (most commonly a combination of 5% albumin and normal saline solution).
  - *Thrombocytapheresis* is the selective removal of platelets (thrombocytes).
- During plasma exchange procedures, the plasma removed must be replaced; the most common replacement fluids are 5% albumin, fresh frozen plasma (FFP), thawed plasma (derived from thawed FFP and maintained at low temperatures for use within 1 to 5 days), and normal saline.[1] Because clotting factors are transiently reduced by plasma exchange, FFP can also be used as a fluid replacement in patients when bleeding is an issue.
- Plasma volume is an estimate of the patient's total volume based on gender, height, weight, and hematocrit value. Exchange volume is the ratio of the patient's plasma volume to be removed and replaced; this is usually 1:1 or 1.5:1 of the patient's estimated plasma volume.[4]
- In plasma exchange, an average of 3 to 5 L of plasma is removed and replaced.[4]

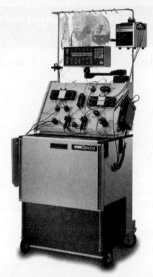

Figure 123-1 COBE Spectra Apheresis System. *(© Caridian-BCT, Inc. 2010. Used with permission.)*

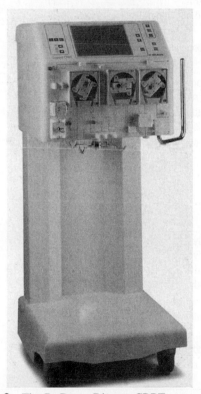

Figure 123-2 The B. Braun Diapact CRRT system can also be used for therapeutic plasma exchange and plasma adsorption/perfusion. *(Photo courtesy B. Braun Medical, Inc.)*

- Treatments can be done with two different systems.[4]
  - *Centrifugal:* Separates plasma and other blood components with use of a centrifuge (Fig. 123-1).
  - *Filtration:* A hollow-fiber cell separator, permeable to plasma proteins, is used to remove the patient's plasma via an apheresis machine or continuous renal replacement machines adapted for apheresis (Fig. 123-2).
- Treatment length and frequency vary according to the disease being treated, rate of production of the substance

being removed, and the patient's response to treatment. Acute conditions, such as thrombotic thrombocytopenia purpura or graft-versus-host disease, usually require daily treatments for 5 to 7 days, depending on the response to the treatment.[6,7] Other conditions usually require plasma exchanges two or three times weekly for up to 6 weeks.[2,5-7] The total amount of plasma to be exchanged is used as a guide for treatment. A single treatment, referred to as a plasma exchange, usually takes 2 to 3 hours with a centrifugal machine and 2 to 6 hours with filtration methods.[4]

- Apheresis procedures are performed by healthcare professionals, such as registered nurses or blood bank personnel, with special knowledge and skills in apheresis. These procedures are commonly performed both in critical care units and on an outpatient basis, depending on the type of disease being treated and on the patient's condition.
- The most commonly used apheresis access systems use either two large-bore peripheral venous catheters, double lumen vascular access catheters (VAC), vortex ports or a dialysis graft/fistula. Peripherally inserted central venous catheters do not provide adequate blood flow and are not acceptable for use.[4]
- The system should be primed with an anticoagulant (e.g., heparin or citrate) to prevent clotting. If citrate is used, the patient must be monitored closely for hypocalcemia. Citrate works as an anticoagulant by binding calcium (Ca^{++}), therefore decreasing the amount of Ca^{++} available for normal clotting.[4]
- Plasma exchange is used to treat antibody-mediated disorders because the pathogenic antibodies are contained in the plasma. Removal of these antibodies through plasma exchange reduces the number of circulating antibodies, temporarily decreasing the patient's symptoms.
- Conditions treated by plasma exchange may include the following[2,5-7]:
  - Myasthenia gravis
  - Guillain-Barré syndrome
  - Various hematologic disorders
  - Nephrologic disorders
  - Rheumatologic disorders
  - Poisoning
  - Drug overdose/drug toxicity
  - Acute liver failure
  - Solid organ transplantation for ABO incompatibility and rejection
  - Cytokine-mediated injury, such as sepsis, burns, and multisystem organ dysfunction syndrome (MODS);
- Current indication categories for therapeutic apheresis, as endorsed by the American Association of Blood Banks (AABB) and the American Society for Apheresis (ASFA), are listed in Table 123-1.
- If the patient is taking angiotensin-converting enzyme (ACE) inhibitors, contact with certain filters or membranes in the apheresis system can cause an anaphylactic reaction and severe hypotension as a result of increased levels of bradykinin, a potent vasodilator. ACE inhibitors are recommended to be withheld for 48 to 72 hours before treatment.
- Invasive procedures should be delayed until the treatment is completed unless FFP is used as a replacement fluid.

TABLE 123-1	American Society for Apheresis (ASFA) 2013 Indication Categories for Therapeutic Apheresis			
Disease Name	**TA Modality**	**Disease Condition**	**Category**	**Grade**
Acute disseminated encephalomyelitis	TPE		II	2C
Acute inflammatory demyelinating polyneurophathy (Guillain-Barré syndrome)	TPE	After IVIG	I	1A
	TPE		III	2C
Acute liver failure	TPE		III	2B
Age-related macular degeneration, dry	Rheopheresis		I	1B
Amyloidosis, systemic	TPE		IV	2C
Amyotrophic lateral sclerosis	TPE		IV	1C
ANCA-associated rapidly progressive glomerulonephritis (Granulomatosis with polyangiitis; Wegener's granulomatosis)	TPE	Dialysis dependence	III	2B
	TPE	DAH	I	1C
	TPE	Dialysis independence	I	1B
Antiglomerular basement membrane disease (Goodpasture's syndrome)	TPE	Dialysis dependence and no DAH	III	2B
	TPE	DAH	I	1C
	TPE	DAH Dialysis independence	I	1B
Aplastic anemia; pure red cell aplasia	TPE	Aplastic anemia	III	2C
	TPE	Pure red cell aplasia	III	2C
Autoimmune hemolytic anemia: WAHA; cold agglutinin disease	TPE	Severe WAHA	III	2C
	TPE	Severe cold agglutinin disease	II	2C
Babesiosis	RBC exchange	Severe	I	1C
	RBC exchange	High-risk population	II	2C
Burn shock resuscitation	TPE		III	2B
Cardiac transplantation	ECP	Refection prophylaxis	II	2A
	ECP	Cellular or recurrent rejection	II	1B
	TPE	Desensitization, positive cross-match due to donor-specific HLA antibody	III	2C
	TPE	Antibody-mediated rejection	III	2C
Catastrophic antiphospholipid syndrome	TPE		II	2C
Chronic focal encephalitis (Rasmussen encephalitis)	TPE		III	2C
	IA		III	2C
Chronic inflammatory demyelinating polyradiculoneuropathy	TPE		I	1B
Coagulation factor inhibitors	TPE	Alloantibody	IV	2C
	IA	Alloantibody	III	2B
	TPE	Autoantibody	III	2C
	IA	Autoantibody	III	1C
Cryoglobulinemia	TPE	Symptomatic/severe	I	2A
	IA	Symptomatic/severe	II	2B
Cutaneous T-cell lymphoma; mycosis fungoides; Sézary syndrome	ECP	Erythrodermic	I	1B
	ECP	Nonerythrodermic	III	2C
Dermatomyositis or polymyositis	TPE		IV	2A
	Leukocytapheresis		IV	2A
Dilated cardiomyopathy, idiopathic	TPE	NYAH II-IV	III	2C
	IA	NYHA II-IV	II	1B
Familial hypercholesterolemia	LDL apheresis	Homozygotes	I	1A
	LDL apheresis	Heterozygotes	II	1A
	TPE	Homozygotes with small blood volume	II	1C
Focal segmental glomerulosclerosis	TPE	Recurrent in transplanted kidney	I	1B
Graft-versus-host disease	ECP	Skin (chronic)	II	1B
	ECP	Skin (acute)	II	1C
	ECP	Nonskin (acute/chronic)	III	2B
HSCT, ABO incompatible	TPE	Major HPC, Marrow	II	1B
	TPE	Major HPC, Apheresis	II	2B
	RBC exchange	Minor HPC, Apheresis	III	2C

| TABLE 123-1 | American Society for Apheresis (ASFA) 2013 Indication Categories for Therapeutic Apheresis—cont'd |

Disease Name	TA Modality	Disease Condition	Category	Grade
Hemolytic uremic syndrome, atypical	TPE	Complement gene mutations	II	2C
	TPE	Factor H antibodies	I	2C
	TPE	MCP mutations	IV	1C
Hemolytic uremic syndrome, infection associated	TPE	Shiga toxin associated	IV	1C
	TPE	*Streptococcus pneumoniae* associated	III	2C
Henoch-Schonlein purpura	TPE	Crescentric	III	2C
	TPE	Severe extrarenal disease	III	2C
Heparin-induced thrombocytopenia	TPE	Precardiopulmonary bypass	III	2C
	TPE	Thrombosis	III	2C
Hereditary hemochromatosis	Erythrocytapheresis		I	1B
Hyperleukocytosis	Leukocytapheresis	Leukostasis	I	1B
	Leukocytapheresis	Prophylaxis	III	2C
Hypertriglyceridemic pancreatitis	TPE		III	2C
Hyperviscosity in monoclonal gammopathies	TPE	Symptomatic	I	1B
	TPE	Prophylaxis for rituximab	I	1C
Immune complex rapidly progressive glomerulonephritis	TPE		III	2B
Immune thrombocytopenia	TPE	Refractory	IV	2C
	IA	Refractory	III	2C
Immunoglobin A nephropathy	TPE	Crescentric	III	2B
	TPE	Chronic progressive	III	2C
Inclusion body myositis	TPE		IV	2C
	Leukocytapheresis		IV	2C
Inflammatory bowel disease	Adsorptive cytapheresis	Ulcerative colitis	III/II	1B/2B
	Adsorptive cytapheresis	Crohn's disease	III	1B
	ECP	Crohn's disease	III	2C
Lambert-Eaton myasthenic syndrome	TPE		II	2C
Lipoprotein (a) hyperlipoproteinemia	LDL apheresis		II	1B
Liver transplantation, ABO incompatible	TPE	Desensitization, live donor	I	1C
	TPE	Desensitization, deceased donor	III	2C
	TPE	Humoral rejection	III	2C
Lung allograft rejection	ECP	Bronchiolitis obliterans syndrome	II	1C
	TPE	Antibody-mediated rejection	III	2C
Multiple sclerosis	TPE	Acute CNS inflammatory demyelinating disease	II	1B
	IA	Acute CNS inflammatory demyelinating disease	III	2C
	TPE	Chronic progressive	III	2B
Myasthenia gravis	TPE	Moderate to severe	I	1B
	TPE	Prethymectomy	I	1C
Myeloma cast nephropathy	TPE		II	2B
Nephrogenic systemic fibrosis	ECP		III	2C
	TPE		III	2C
Neuromyelitis optica (Devic's syndrome)	TPE	Acute	II	1B
	TPE	Maintenance	III	2C
Overdoses, envenomation, and poisoning	TPE	Mushroom poisoning	II	2C
	TPE	Envenomation	III	2C
	TPE	Natalizumab and PML	III	2C
	RBC exchange	Tacrolimus	III	2C
Paraneoplastic neurological syndromes	TPE		III	2C
	IA		III	2C

Continued

TABLE 123-1	American Society for Apheresis (ASFA) 2013 Indication Categories for Therapeutic Apheresis—cont'd			
Disease Name	**TA Modality**	**Disease Condition**	**Category**	**Grade**
Paraproteinemic demyelinating polyneuropathies	TPE	IgG/IgA	I	1B
	TPE	IgM	I	1C
	TPE	Multiple myeloma	III	2C
	IA	IgG/IgA/IgM	III	2C
PANDAS; Sydenham's chorea	TPE	PANDAS exacerbation	I	1B
	TPE	Sydenham's chorea	I	1B
Pemphigus vulgaris	TPE	Severe	III	2C
	ECP	Severe	III	2C
	IA	Severe	III	2C
Peripheral vascular diseases	LDL apheresis		III	2C
Phytanic acid storage disease (Refsum's disease)	TPE		II	2C
	LDL apheresis		II	2C
Polycythemia vera and erythrocytosis	Erythrocytapheresis	Polycythemia vera	I	1B
	Erythrocytapheresis	Secondary erythrocytosis	III	1C
POEMS syndrome	TPE		IV	1C
Post transfusion purpura	TPE		III	2C
Psoriasis	TPE	Disseminated pustular	IV	2C
	Adsorptive cytapheresis		III	2C
	Lymphocytapheresis		III	2C
	ECP		III	2B
Red cell alloimmunization in pregnancy	TPE	Before IUT availability	III	2C
Renal transplantation, ABO compatible	TPE	Antibody-mediated rejection	I	1B
	TPE	Desensitization, living donor, positive cross-match due to donor-specific HLA antibody	I	1B
	TPE	Desensitization, high PRA deceased donor	III	2C
Renal transplantation, ABO incompatible	TPE	Desensitization, live donor	I	1B
	TPE	Humoral rejection	II	1B
	TPE	Group A2/A2B into B, deceased donor	IV	1B
Schizophrenia	TPE		IV	1A
Scleroderma (Progressive systemic sclerosis)	TPE		III	2C
	ECP		III	2B
Sepsis with multiorgan failure	TPE		III	2B
Sickle cell disease, acute	RBC exchange	Acute stroke	I	1C
	RBC exchange	Acute chest syndrome, severe	II	1C
	RBC exchange	Priapism	III	2C
	RBC exchange	Multiorgan failure	III	2C
	RBC exchange	Splenic sequestration; hepatic sequestration; intrahepatic cholestasis	III	2C
Sickle cell disease, nonacute	RBC exchange	Stroke prophylaxis/iron overload prevention	II	1C
	RBC exchange	Vaso-occlusive pain crisis	III	2C
	RBC exchange	Preoperative management	III	2A
Stiff person syndrome	TPE		III	2C
Sudden sensorineural hearing loss	LDL apheresis		III	2A
	Rheopheresis		III	2A
	TPE		III	2C
Systemic lupus erythematosus	TPE	Severe	II	2C
	TPE	Nephritis	IV	1B
Thrombocytosis	Thrombocytapheresis	Symptomatic	II	2C
	Thrombocytapheresis	Prophylactic or secondary	III	2C

TABLE 123-1	American Society for Apheresis (ASFA) 2013 Indication Categories for Therapeutic Apheresis—cont'd				
Disease Name	**TA Modality**		**Disease Condition**	**Category**	**Grade**
Thrombotic microangiopathy, drug associated	TPE		Ticlopidine	I	1B
	TPE		Clopidogrel	III	2B
	TPE		Cyclosporine/Tacrolimus	III	2C
	TPE		Gemcitabine	IV	2C
	TPE		Quinine	IV	2C
Thrombotic microangiopathy, HSCT associated	TPE		Refractory	III	2C
Thrombotic thrombocytopenic purpura	TPE			I	1A
Thyroid storm	TPE			III	2C
Toxic epidermal necrolysis	TPE		Refractory	III	2B
Voltaged gated potassium channel antibodies	TPE			II	1C
Wilson's disease	TPE		Fulminant	I	1C

ANCA, antineutrophil cytoplasmic antibody; *CNS*, central nervous system; *ECP*, extracorporeal photopheresis; *DAH*, diffuse alveolar hemorrhage; *HLA*, human leukocyte antigen; *HSCT*, hematopoietic stem cell transplant; *IA*, immunoadsorption; *IgA*, immunoglobulin A; *IgG*, immunoglobulin G; *IgM*, immunoglobulin M; *IUT*, intrauterine transfusion; *IVIG*, intravenous immunoglobulin; *LDL*, low-density lipoprotein; *MCP*, membrane cofactor protein; *NYHA*, New York Heart Association; *PANDAS*, pediatric autoimmune neuropsychiatric disorders associated with streptococcal infections; *POEMS*, polyneuropathy, organomegaly, endocrinopathy, M protein, and skin changes; *PML*, progressive multifocal leukoencephalopathy; *RBC*, red blood cell; *TPE*, therapeutic plasma exchange; *WAHA*, warm autoimmune hemolytic anemia.

Categories:

I   Disorders for which apheresis is accepted as first-line therapy, either as a primary standalone treatment or in conjunction with other modes of treatment.

II   Disorders for which apheresis is accepted as second line therapy, either as a standalone treatment or in conjunction with other modes of treatment.

III   Optimum role of apheresis therapy is not established. Decision making should be individualized.

IV   Disorders in which published evidence demonstrates or suggests apheresis to be ineffective or harmful. Institutional review board approval is desirable if apheresis treatment is undertaken in these circumstances.

Grades:

Grade 1A: Strong recommendation, high-quality evidence

Grade 1B: Strong recommendation, moderate-quality evidence

Grade 1C: Strong recommendation, low-quality or very low-quality evidence

Grade 2A: Weak recommendation, high-quality evidence

Grade 2B: Weak recommendation, moderate-quality evidence

Grade 2C: Weak recommendation, low-quality or very low-quality evidence

From Schwartz J, et al: Guidelines on the use of therapeutic apheresis in clinical practice-evidence-based approach from the Writing Committee of the American Society for Apheresis; the sixth special issue, J Clin Apherisis *28(3):145–284, 2013.*

- Potential complications of apheresis techniques include the following:
  ❖ Bleeding
  ❖ Thrombocytopenia
  ❖ RBC lysis/hemolysis
  ❖ Air embolism
  ❖ Blood leak
  ❖ Circuit clotting
  ❖ Hypovolemia
  ❖ Hypotension
  ❖ Hypothermia
  ❖ Vascular access complications
  ❖ Fever/chills
  ❖ Shock
  ❖ Anaphylaxis
  ❖ Allergic reactions
  ❖ Transfusion reactions
  ❖ Electrolyte imbalances
  ❖ Dysrhythmias
  ❖ Citrate toxicity
  ❖ Infection

EQUIPMENT

- Blood cell separator or filter machine
- Blood cell separator or filter tubing set
- Replacement intravenous (IV) fluids
- Hemostats
- Vascular access dressings and flushes
- Nonsterile gloves
- Fluid shield face masks or goggles
- Caps

Additional equipment, to have available as needed, includes the following:

- Laboratory specimen tubes
- Sterile gloves if accessing central lines such as VAC or vortex ports

PATIENT AND FAMILY EDUCATION

- Explain the procedure, including risks, length of treatment, and patient positioning, and answer any questions the patient may have. ***Rationale:*** Explanation provides information and may decrease patient anxiety.

- Explain the purpose of the apheresis procedure, why this treatment is being performed, and the expected clinical outcomes. ***Rationale:*** Knowledge about the procedure helps the patient to understand the treatment plan and will decrease anxiety.
- Explain the need for careful sterile technique for the duration of treatment. ***Rationale:*** Sterile technique is important to decrease the chance of systemic infection because pathogens can be transported throughout the entire body via the circulation.
- Explain the need for careful monitoring of the patient for complications. ***Rationale:*** Hypocalcemia, hypotension, bleeding, and hypothermia are all potential complications of apheresis.
- Explain the importance of the patient informing the nurse how he or she is feeling during the treatment. ***Rationale:*** Patient symptoms can be important signs of complications related to the procedure. Examples include lightheadedness as a sign of hypotension and numbness and tingling as a sign of hypocalcemia.
- Explain the importance of preventing bleeding complications: pressure dressings at vascular sites, avoiding shaving, and care of the access catheter. ***Rationale:*** Alterations in blood composition and anticoagulation can put the patient at risk for bleeding.
- Explain the apheresis circuit setup to the patient and family. ***Rationale:*** Blood will be removed from the patient's body and will be visible during apheresis treatment.

PATIENT ASSESSMENT AND PREPARATION

Patient Assessment

- Obtain baseline vital signs, body system assessment, hemodynamic parameters (if appropriate), weight, and pretreatment fluid balance. ***Rationale:*** Total body assessment should be based specifically on the patient's diagnosis and reason for treatment. Pretreatment assessment provides a baseline for comparison once the treatment is started, allowing for appropriate modification of the intervention as needed. Changes in weight during and after treatment are an indicator of fluid balance.

- Review prescribed medications, and ensure that the patient has not taken an ACE inhibitor within 48 hours. ***Rationale:*** Contact with certain fibers or membranes in the apheresis system can cause an anaphylactic reaction and severe hypotension.
- Assess pretreatment laboratory values. ***Rationale:*** Baseline values are needed of the complete blood count (CBC) with differential, platelet count, and electrolytes before these are altered by treatment. Coagulation parameters are particularly important: fibrinogen, prothrombin time (PT), activated clotting time (ACT), and partial thromboplastin time (PTT) if heparin is used, and ACT and ionized Ca^{++} if citrate is used. Serum sodium and serum bicarbonate levels/pH also should be evaluated in patients when citrate is used as the anticoagulant. Disease-specific tests should also be obtained pretreatment as needed.
- Obtain vascular access. ***Rationale:*** A properly functioning vascular access is necessary to perform plasmapheresis.

Patient Preparation

- Verify That the patient is the correct patient using two identifiers. ***Rationale:*** Before performing a procedure, the nurse should ensure the correct identification of the patient for the intended intervention.
- Ensure that informed consent has been obtained. ***Rationale:*** Informed consent protects the rights of the patient and makes a competent decision possible for the patient.
- Ensure that patient understands preprocedural instructions. Answer questions as they arise, and reinforce information as needed. ***Rationale:*** Understanding of previously taught information is evaluated and reinforced.
- Assist the patient to a position of comfort that also facilitates optimal blood flow through the vascular access. ***Rationale:*** Facilitating patient comfort helps to minimize the amount of patient movement during treatment. Movement can change the blood flow through the access site. Different access sites may require different patient positions to facilitate optimal blood flow.

Procedure for Assisting With Apheresis/Plasmapheresis

Steps	Rationale	Special Considerations
1. Verify apheresis orders.	Familiarizes nurse with the individualized patient treatment and reduces the possibility of error.	
2. **HH**		
3. **PE**		
4. Confirm access placement.	Validates line is in correct placement.	

5. Review the following with the apheresis nurse:
A. Exchange volume
B. Anticoagulant
C. Replacement fluids
D. Baseline patient assessment, including
  i. Vital signs
  ii. Jugular vein distention
  iii. Presence of edema
  iv. Intake and output
  v. Neurological assessment
  vi. Pulmonary assessment
  vii. Renal assessment
  viii. Parameters/treatment for heart rate and blood pressure
  ix. Laboratory monitoring
  x. Procedure for emergency resuscitation
	Sets joint goals and actions to provide for patient safety and optimize the patient's outcome.[4]	

6. Gather supplies for vascular access.	Prepares for the procedure.	The process of vascular access depends on whether the site is central or peripheral.
7. Assist in gathering the supplies for apheresis procedure.	Prepares for the procedure.	Obtaining and sending laboratory specimens may be part of the apheresis setup as the vascular system is accessed.
8. Ensure that appropriate replacement fluid is available. Warm replacement fluids as prescribed.	Maintains correct electrolyte balance; avoids hypothermia.[4]	Replacement fluids should be slightly warmed before infusion unless contraindicated (e.g., blood products should be maintained at a specific temperature before infusion to maintain viability of the product). Never use a microwave to warm fluids. Some patients also may need an increase in the ambient room temperature or ventilator cascade and warming blankets to avoid hypothermia. Most apheresis systems have inline blood warmers.
9. Infuse fluid boluses as needed before initiation.	Maintains hemodynamic stability.	
10. Assist with setup and priming of the apheresis circuit as needed.	Ensures safe and proper assembly and complete removal of air from the circuit.	
11. Secure all connections.	Prevents inadvertent disconnection of the system.	
12. Remove gloves and discard used supplies.		
13. **HH**		

Procedure continues on following page

Expected Outcomes

- Therapeutic goals achieved
- Optimal fluid balance is maintained
- Laboratory values are maintained within expected range
- Properly functioning access site
- Patient remains pain free or has pain controlled to an acceptable goal
- Therapeutic medication levels will be maintained
- Patient/family will verbalize understanding of the procedure

Unexpected Outcomes

- Complications related to the treatment (e.g., hypotension, hypocalcemia, hypothermia, hypokalemia, hypernatremia, metabolic alkalosis, air embolism, blood leak, bleeding, infection)
- Poor blood flow through the vascular access
- Bleeding from the access site
- Dislodgment of the access catheter
- Hematoma formation at the access site
- Technical problems with apheresis circuit
- Hemolysis

Patient Monitoring and Care

Steps	Rationale	Reportable Conditions
		These conditions should be reported if they persist despite nursing interventions.
1. Monitor the patient during and after the apheresis treatment: A. Vital signs B. Hemodynamic parameters C. Jugular vein distention D. Presence of edema E. Intake and output F. Neurological assessment G. Pulmonary assessment H. Renal assessment I. Apheresis circuit J. Laboratory values as prescribed (if plasma is removed, include prothrombin time/international normalized ratio [INR], fibrinogen, platelet count)	Patients can experience complications, such as hypotension, hypothermia, blood leak, air embolism, transfusion reactions, hypocalcemia, RBC hemolysis, thrombocytopenia, citrate toxicity, and bleeding, that may need intervention.[1,3,4]	• Hypotension • Hypertension • Tachycardia/bradycardia • Tachypnea/bradypnea • Fever • Hypothermia • Jugular vein distention • Crackles • Edema • Change in level of consciousness • Dizziness • Change in cardiac rhythm • Blood leak • Hemolysis • Thrombocytopenia • Dysrhythmias • Coagulopathies • Allergic reaction • Transfusion reaction
2. Monitor serum ionized Ca^{++}, magnesium, serum sodium, and serum bicarbonate levels/pH (if citrate is used as an anticoagulant).	Citrate binds with Ca^{++} and can cause hypocalcemia. It also metabolizes to sodium and bicarbonate, which may cause hypernatremia, metabolic alkalosis, and citrate toxicity.[4]	• Hypocalcemia • Hypernatremia • Metabolic alkalosis • Increased anion gap
3. Monitor ACT/PTT (if heparin is used as an anticoagulant).	These values primarily reflect the activity of the intrinsic clotting pathway.	• Prolonged ACT/PTT
4. Administer replacement fluid as prescribed and needed.	Replacement fluids are important during the treatment to maintain adequate intravascular volume.	• Hypotension • Tachycardia • Decreased central venous and pulmonary artery pressures • Decreased urine output

Patient Monitoring and Care —*Continued*

Steps	Rationale	Reportable Conditions
5. Hold medication administration as prescribed.	Many medications are withheld during treatment, including vasopressors and pain medications, especially those that are protein-bound.[8] Some medications, such as antihypertensive agents, anticholinergic agents, and Ca^{++} supplements, may be withheld during treatment.[4] Analgesics and antipyretics may be indicated during a treatment, although these medications may mask the symptoms of a transfusion reaction.[8]	• Medications needed (e.g., analgesics, antipyretics) • Transfusion reaction
6. Monitor the access and dressing sites after the termination of the apheresis procedure.	Bleeding or signs or symptoms of infection can be complications of the vascular access.[9]	• Bleeding • Redness, tenderness, pain, or warmth at the access insertion site • Generalized bleeding or fever
7. Appropriately label VACs that contain indwelling anticoagulant.	Prevents the infusion of anticoagulant into the patient.	• Bleeding • Bruising • Oozing
8. Review the following with the apheresis nurse, including: A. Amount and type of fluids removed	For proper patient evaluation and documentation.	• Unexpected volume
B. Amount and type of fluids given		• Unexpected volume
C. Exchange volume and fluid balance		• Unexpected volume
D. Patient reactions during treatment		• Flushing • Dysrhythmias • Tachypnea
E. Medications given during treatment		• Unexpected side effects
9. Follow institutional standards for assessing pain. Administer analgesia as prescribed.	Identifies need for pain interventions.	• Continued pain despite pain interventions

Documentation

Documentation should include the following:

- Patient and family education
- Completion of informed consent
- Date and time of treatment initiation
- Condition of vascular access
- Intake/output/fluid balance
- Vital signs throughout the apheresis treatment
- Daily weight

- Patient's response to apheresis and daily progress toward treatment goals
- Unexpected outcomes
- Nursing interventions
- Laboratory assessment data
- Pain assessment, interventions, and effectiveness.

References and Additional Readings

For a complete list of references and additional readings for this procedure, scan this QR code with any freely available smartphone code reader app, or visit http://booksite.elsevier.com/9780323376624.

124 Bone Marrow Biopsy and AP Aspiration (Perform)

Glen Peterson and Carrie Marvill

PURPOSE: The bone marrow aspiration and biopsy is performed to obtain information on initial diagnosis, staging, or treatment response for hematology/oncology patients.

PREREQUISITE NURSING KNOWLEDGE

- The bone marrow aspiration and biopsy is a common procedure performed on patients with a hematologic disorder or a suspected or previously diagnosed hematological malignancy. It is performed during the initial diagnosis and/or staging and used to determine treatment response in patients with leukemia, lymphoma, multiple myeloma, and other hematologic disorders.
- The procedure is performed by physicians, advanced practice nurses, physician assistants, and other healthcare professionals with special training and experience. It is typically completed at the bedside with local anesthetic and minimal requirement for sedation, however moderate sedation may be performed in patients intolerant to the procedure.
- The procedure is performed at the preferred location of the superior, posterior iliac crest, usually while the patient is positioned in the prone or lateral (side-lying) position. Routinely, an aspirate is obtained from the cancellous (soft, spongy) portion of the bone after a needle is used to penetrate through the outer, firm cortical bone. Similarly, a core biopsy is obtained with the use of a trephine coring needle either manually or with a power drill device. The sternum and anterior iliac crest may also be used in rare situations; however, this is discouraged because of the excessive risk of trauma to underlying tissues including the heart.
- The bone marrow biopsy is generally a safe procedure; however, infection, bleeding, and nerve damage (usually due to nerve compressive hematoma) may occur. Care should be taken to prevent such complications by maintaining strict sterile technique, assuring coagulation laboratory parameters are met, anticoagulation therapy is managed appropriately, and local hemostasis is maintained.
- Multiple tests are required depending on the diagnosis. Common diagnostic tests include morphology, flow cytometry, cytogenetics, fluorescence in situ hybridization (FISH), and molecular studies. Much less commonly, infectious disease testing may be requested, including culture and gram stain, fungal culture, viral culture, polymerase chain reaction (PCR), acid-fast bacillus (AFB), or gomori methenamine silver (GMS) stain.
- A thorough understanding is needed of the anatomy and physiology of the posterior and anterior iliac crest and the sternum. The preferred site for a bone marrow aspirate and biopsy is the posterior iliac crest.[1] The sternum may be used to aspirate marrow; however, a core biopsy cannot be obtained from the sternum because of risk of damage to underlying organs, most significantly the heart.[7,9]
- Clinical and technical competence in performing a bone marrow aspirate and biopsy is necessary.
- Essential knowledge of sterile technique is necessary.
- An understanding is needed of institutional policies and procedures for administration of intravenous (IV) pharmacological agents, including moderate sedation (if indicated) and intradermal and epicortical local anesthesia (lidocaine in most cases; procaine may be used in cases of lidocaine allergy) and procedural care of the patient receiving moderate sedation (if used).
- Procedural care of the patient receiving IV moderate sedation or oral antianxiolytics or pain medication should be understood.
- Knowledge is needed of information to be gained from a bone marrow aspirate sample (i.e., identification of normal and abnormal hematopoietic elements, identification of malignant clones with flow cytometry, immunohistochemistry and other pathological analysis techniques, identification of chromosomal abnormalities that occur in hematologic malignant diseases, identification of molecular diagnostic studies that show gene rearrangements and translocations, and the performance of chimerism studies in patients after allogeneic transplant).
- A bone marrow biopsy is used for morphological analysis of hematopoietic cells and for assessment of the architecture of the bone marrow that may be abnormal in certain disease states.
- Indications for bone marrow aspiration and biopsy include the following:
  - To diagnose a hematologic abnormality or malignancy
  - To monitor a hematologic disease state after initial diagnosis or therapy

---

AP This procedure should be performed only by physicians, advanced practice nurses, and other healthcare professionals (including critical care nurses) with additional knowledge, skills, and demonstrated competence per professional licensure or institutional standard.

○ To diagnose bone marrow involvement before stem cell collection and for staging of various malignant states

○ To assess the status of disease after autologous bone marrow or hematopoietic stem cell transplant

○ To assess chimerism disease status and immune reconstitution after an allogeneic bone marrow or hematopoietic stem cell transplant

○ To evaluate immunodeficiency syndromes or to confirm an infectious disease process in the marrow

❖ Contraindications to bone marrow biopsy and aspirate are the presence of hemophilia, severe disseminated intravascular coagulopathy, or other related severe bleeding disorders. Thrombocytopenia alone is not a contraindication to bone marrow examination,[4,5] although a platelet transfusion may be indicated if the patient is severely thrombocytopenic or if bleeding develops or persists after the procedure.[2] The use of anticoagulant medications may pose a serious bleeding risk; therefore, coagulation studies should be obtained in these patients. The decision on whether anticoagulation can be safely withheld before and restarted after the procedure is patient dependent and may require specialty consultation.

EQUIPMENT

- Bone marrow aspiration and biopsy kit, which includes the following:
  - ❖ Antiseptic solution (e.g., 2% chlorhexidine based preparation)
  - ❖ Two sterile fenestrated drapes
  - ❖ One to two vial(s) of lidocaine (1% or 2%; 5 to 10 mL. Follow institutional standards; administration should not exceed 4.5 mg/kg or 300 mg[12])
  - ❖ 5- or 10-mL syringe for drawing up lidocaine
  - ❖ Filter needle (if lidocaine drawn from glass vial)
  - ❖ Needles of appropriate lengths to anesthetize both skin and periosteum
  - ❖ Sterile 4 × 4 and 2 × 2 gauze pads
  - ❖ Small scalpel blade
  - ❖ Bacitracin or Bactroban ointment (optional; for incision site post procedure)
- Biopsy needle options:
  - ❖ Illinois needle (16 gauge for bone marrow aspirate only)
  - ❖ Jamshidi bone biopsy needle (for aspirate and core biopsy, 8 or 11 gauge, 4 inches or longer)
  - ❖ TrapLok bone marrow biopsy needle (for aspirate and core biopsy, 8 or 11 gauge, 4 inches or longer)
  - ❖ SNARECOIL bone marrow biopsy needle (for aspirate and core biopsy, 8 or 11 gauge, 4 inches or longer)
  - ❖ Powered bone marrow biopsy system (for aspirate and core biopsy, 8 or 11 gauge, 4 inches or longer)
  - ❖ Extra long bone marrow biopsy needle may be required for obese patients
- Two or three 20-mL syringes for bone marrow aspirate
- Blunt tip needles for drawing up ethylenediaminetetraacetic acid (EDTA), heparin
- Adhesive bandage

- Nonadhering dressing (for core biopsy placement and touch preps)
- One-roll paper microporc or Medipore tape
- Sterile gloves
- Sterile gowns
- Fluid shield, face mask, or goggles
- Specimen bags and labels
- Required tubes for specimen processing (variable based on required tests; follow institutional standards): two edetate disodium (liquid EDTA and/or EDTA lavender top) and two sodium heparin (green top) tubes, edetate disodium (EDTA) sterile solution (15 mg/mL; 2 mL total) or prefilled EDTA tube
- Eight glass slides and cover plate
- 3½- to 6-inch spinal needle (may be required for anesthetizing periosteum in the obese patient)
- Container for bone core biopsy specimen, including appropriate fixative (10% formalin)

Additional equipment, to have available as needed, includes the following:

- Power drill
- One vial of 100 units/mL heparin (follow institutional standards)
- One vial of buffered lidocaine (optional: The addition of sodium bicarbonate may minimize pain during lidocaine administration.[7])
- Equipment for patients receiving moderate sedation:
  - ❖ Pulse oximeter with telemetry
  - ❖ Automated blood pressure monitor
  - ❖ Oxygen
  - ❖ Suction
  - ❖ Ambu bag
  - ❖ IV pharmacological agents for sedation (i.e., midazolam, 1 to 4 mg; lorazepam, 1 to 2 mg; fentanyl, 25 to 100 μg; morphine 2 to 4 mg; hydromorphone 0.5 to 2 mg)
  - ❖ IV opiate and benzodiazepine antagonist agents (i.e., naloxone and flumazenil)
  - ❖ Emergency equipment

PATIENT AND FAMILY EDUCATION

- Assess patient and family understanding of the bone marrow aspiration and biopsy procedure and the reason for it. *Rationale:* Clarification of the procedure and reinforcement of information may reduce patient and family anxiety and stress.
- Inform the patient and family (if permitted by patient) that the results will be shared with them as soon as they are available. *Rationale:* The patient and family are usually anxious about the results.
- Explain the actual procedure to the patient and family. *Rationale:* The patient and family are prepared for what to expect and anxiety may be decreased.
- Review safety requirements for patients who will receive pharmacological agents for sedation (i.e., must have transportation and escort home and may not drive until the next day). *Rationale:* Review ensures patient safety and accountability of the physician, advanced practice nurse, or other healthcare professional for patients receiving sedation.

• Encourage the patient to verbalize any pain experienced during the procedure. ***Rationale:*** Additional lidocaine, pain medication, or sedation medication can be administered. The patient becomes a participant in care. Poor relaxation can cause the large gluteal muscles to spasm, making the procedure more difficult for all involved.

PATIENT ASSESSMENT AND PREPARATION

Patient Assessment

• Assess the patient's allergies and home medications, including over-the-counter medications that can increase the risk of bleeding. Anticoagulant medications may need to be held. Specialty consultation may be required to clarify risks and benefits related to anticoagulation. ***Rationale:*** Assessment can decrease the risk of bleeding, hematoma, and allergic reaction.

• Assess the need for antianxiety or analgesic medication or moderate sedation. ***Rationale:*** If the patient is very anxious before the procedure or has had severe pain with previous bone marrow procedures, small doses of analgesia or sedation promote patient comfort. Tense muscles can create a technically difficult procedure and add to pain and anxiety.

• Assess coagulation studies (PT/INR, PTT) in patients who are taking anticoagulant medications. No recommendations exist regarding minimal requirements for coagulation studies before bone marrow biopsy; however, based on clinical guidelines for similar procedures and expert opinion, a PTT goal of less than 1.5 times the control and INR less than 2 (≤1.5 if platelet count <20) are recommended.[10] ***Rationale:*** Patients at risk for bleeding complications are identified and anticoagulant medications may need to be held.

• Assess current cell blood count (CBC) for severe thrombocytopenia requiring pre- or intraprocedure transfusion. No recommendations exist regarding minimal requirements for coagulation studies before the bone marrow biopsy; however, based on clinical guidelines for similar procedures and expert opinion, a platelet count of greater than or equal to 20 is recommended. If the procedure needs to be performed emergently and the platelet count is greater than or equal to 10 but not greater than or equal to 20, platelet transfusion during and possibly after the procedure is recommended.[10] ***Rationale:*** Patients at risk for bleeding complications are identified and interventions for bleeding prevention are completed.

• Assess the ability of the patient to lie in the prone or lateral position, with the head of the bed at no greater than a 25-degree elevation. ***Rationale:*** Access to and control of the posterior iliac crest are best obtained with the patient lying flat, or with the head of the bed only slightly raised, in a side-lying or prone position.

• Assess vital signs and oxygenation status. ***Rationale:*** Baseline data are provided. Assessment ensures that the blood pressure and oxygenation status can be maintained if the patient is placed on his or her side or prone.

• Assess the posterior iliac crest with palpation. In select cases, the anterior iliac crest may be used as a result of positioning limitations or excessive tissue surrounding the posterior iliac crest. However, an increased risk of injury to the surrounding nerves and blood vessels makes this procedure more complicated. The sternum is used for aspiration only in very select cases because of potential fatal complications with this procedure. It should only be performed in the absence of lower-risk techniques and with special equipment and close cardiac monitoring by an experienced physician. ***Rationale:*** Assessment identifies the most suitable area for obtaining optimal samples with a minimum of risk of discomfort and danger to the patient.

• Assess for recent bone marrow aspiration and biopsy sites. ***Rationale:*** The patient may have a painful experience if an additional biopsy is performed at a site that has not yet healed from a previous procedure. Penetration of scar tissue from previous bone marrow biopsy sites may also be difficult and yield inadequate results

Patient Preparation

• Ensure that the patient and family understand information taught. Answer questions as they arise, and reinforce information as needed. ***Rationale:*** Understanding of previously taught information is evaluated and reinforced.

• Verify that the patient is the correct patient using two identifiers. ***Rationale:*** Before performing a procedure, the nurse should ensure the correct identification of the patient for the intended intervention.

• Obtain informed consent for bone marrow aspiration and biopsy and, if indicated, conscious sedation. ***Rationale:*** Informed consent protects the rights of the patient and makes a competent decision possible for the patient.

• Perform a preprocedure verification and timeout. ***Rationale:*** This ensures patient safety.

• Prescribe analgesia or sedation, if needed. ***Rationale:*** Patient may need analgesia or sedation to ensure adequate cooperation and minimize discomfort during the procedure.

• Follow institutional standards for a patient receiving moderate sedation. ***Rationale:*** Preparation ensures that appropriate emergency equipment and medical staff are available.

• Obtain IV access for patients receiving sedation. ***Rationale:*** A secure patent IV line is necessary for administration of IV pharmacological agents and, if necessary, emergency antagonist agents.

• Obtain a complete blood count and differential. ***Rationale:*** Many pathologists prefer to review a peripheral blood sample in conjunction with the marrow to make a complete and accurate diagnostic evaluation.

• Place the patient on a cardiac monitor. ***Rationale:*** This allows for assessment of patient status during procedure.

• Assist the patient to an appropriate position depending on the patient's comfort and the preference of the physician, advanced practice nurse, or other healthcare professional. ***Rationale:*** Positioning ensures good visualization and control of the posterior iliac crest.

• Ensure site markings have been made where appropriate. ***Rationale:*** Procedure site is identified.

Procedure for Performing Bone Marrow Aspiration and Biopsy

Steps	Rationale	Special Considerations
Bone Marrow Aspiration		
1. Confirm availability of personnel who will assist with the procedure.	Slide preparation, specimen processing, and additional supplies require an appropriately trained assistant for the procedure if available.	If the procedure is to be performed without assistance, prepare all equipment and walk through the procedure for concise and accurate specimen acquisition.
2. **HH**		
3. **PE**	Minimizes possible contamination of procedure site.	Apply mask.
4. Open the bone marrow procedure tray; add any additional supplies in a manner that preserves sterility.	Maintains sterility of the procedure.	An extra overbed table works well as a procedure table. Clean before and after each use.
5. **HH**		
6. Apply sterile gown and gloves.	Maintains sterility of the procedure.	
7. Prepare all necessary syringes, including lidocaine syringe and those requiring anticoagulant.	Ensures adequate preparation for the procedure and reduces distraction once the procedure is started.	
8. Prepare the intended site with the antiseptic swabs (e.g., chlorhexidine-based preparation), and place sterile drape.	Minimizes risk for infection.	
9. With a 25–30-gauge needle, inject the skin with lidocaine, creating a wheal.[6]	A small-gauge needle lessens the discomfort associated with administration of local anesthesia.	The use of buffered lidocaine may minimize the pain associated with administration compared with lidocaine alone.[7]
10. With a 21-gauge 1½-inch needle (or spinal needle if necessary), infiltrate the periosteum with lidocaine in a "peppering" fashion with 5–15 mL of lidocaine (1–2%) with 1–2 mL bicarbonate buffer solution, if available. Downward pressure on the tissue and stabilization of the needle with the thumb and forefinger of the opposite hand are helpful.	If the periosteum is not anesthetized the patient may have extreme discomfort. Also, assessing the area of the posterior iliac crest in an obese patient is often difficult. Use of the spinal needle helps the practitioner locate an appropriate site. Buffered lidocaine reduces pain.[7]	If additional lidocaine is needed, ask the critical care nurse or person assisting to invert the extra vial. If the 1½-inch needle does not reach the bone, use the 3½-inch spinal needle to reach it. The spinal needle can also be used to assess the geography of the posterior iliac crest and allows the practitioner to assess the depth of the bone. It is helpful to anesthetize an area of about a quarter to half dollar size so that adjustments can be made in needle placement.
11. Make an incision over the biopsy site with a small scalpel. Advance the aspirate needle (may also use biopsy needle or power drill device needle for aspirate) through the incision (with stabilization of the needle with the thumb and forefinger of the opposite hand) to the periosteum with firm pressure and slight rotation; penetrate the cortex. If a power drill device is used, DO NOT hold the needle. A slight sensation of "giving" is often noticed as the marrow cavity or medulla is reached.	Slight rotation of the needle allows for smooth entry into the marrow cavity. Attempting to stabilize drill needle by holding will tear sterile gloves.	If the patient experiences pain, it is recommended that the needle be placed in another section of bone or additional lidocaine be applied to the outer surface of the bone. Repositioning the needle even 2–3 mm from the site of pain may reduce or eliminate the pain sensation. Follow institutional training guidelines for use of the power drill device.

Procedure continues on following page

Procedure　for Performing Bone Marrow Aspiration and Biopsy—*Continued*

Steps	Rationale	Special Considerations
12. Remove the stylet, attach the 20-mL syringe primed with EDTA, and aspirate 3–5 mL of marrow. Immediately hand this syringe to the critical care nurse or person assisting or place a small portion of aspirate onto a glass slide or petri dish to verify the presence of spicules (small pieces of bone) in the sample if performing the procedure alone. Brisk rotation of the aspirate in the syringe may also reveal spicules.	The syringe is inverted to mix the EDTA and marrow specimen. The first aspirate sample is used to make the slides and to place in the lavender-top EDTA tubes for clot sections or molecular studies.	A volume of spicules is most often found toward the end of the syringe; therefore, place marrow in lavender-top tubes first after spicules have been identified. Follow institutional guidelines for using EDTA in syringes and tubes.
13. If aspirate is not obtained or is raparticulate, replace the stylet, reposition the needle, and attempt to aspirate again. With each pull, rotate the needle slightly.[6] **(Level C*)**	If marrow cannot be obtained after several attempts, another needle may be needed because of blunting.	At times, it is difficult to obtain a bone marrow aspirate. Difficulty can occur if a patient is aplastic, fibrosed, or if the marrow space is packed by disease. This is known as a "dry tap." In these cases, the practitioner should try to obtain an additional core biopsy specimen for pathology analysis that may include flow cytometry and cytogenetics/FISH analysis. The specimen should be placed in RPMI tissue transport medium. The touch preparation in this case also becomes a crucial step in providing the pathologist with material suitable for morphological examination.[6]
14. Obtain additional samples as needed in the 20-mL syringe containing heparin. Place in the green-top sodium heparin tubes (with the help of the person assisting if available).	Heparinized aspirate is used for flow cytometry, chromosome analysis, FISH, and chimerism studies (chimerism may also be performed on EDTA tubes).	Invert syringe to mix heparin and marrow. Follow institutional standards for use of heparinized and nonheparinized tubes for obtaining samples.
15. Have the person assisting help by inverting all of the tubes several times.	Aspirate samples can clot quickly if not thoroughly mixed with anticoagulant.	
16. Remove the aspiration needle from the site with a gentle twisting and pulling motion. Apply firm pressure with sterile gauze. If obtaining a bone biopsy, **proceed to Step 1 (next section).**	Ensures adequate hemostasis and reduces chance of hemorrhage, hematoma, and infection.	Replacing the stylet decreases discomfort with removal of the aspirate needle.

*Level C: Qualitative studies, descriptive or correlational studies, integrative reviews, systematic reviews, or randomized controlled trials with inconsistent results.

Procedure	for Performing Bone Marrow Aspiration and Biopsy—*Continued*	
Steps	**Rationale**	**Special Considerations**

17. If a bone marrow biopsy is not being obtained:
  A. Hold very firm pressure for 5 minutes or until bleeding has stopped.
  B. Cleanse site with antiseptic swab (e.g., chlorhexidine-based preparation).
  C. Apply bacitracin or Bactroban ointment, adhesive bandage, 4 × 4 pressure dressing with paper or Medipore tape. (Follow institutional standards).
  D. Reposition patient into supine position for 10–15 minutes to maintain pressure at the biopsy site.
	Ensures adequate hemostasis and reduces chance of hemorrhage, hematoma, and infection.	Very firm pressure is key.
		If the patient is at high risk for bleeding (severely thrombocytopenic, other coagulopathy, anticoagulation therapy, etc.), have the patient lie on a firm surface (e.g., book, sandbag, firmly rolled towel, etc.) or a large ice pack may be helpful.

18. Label samples in presence of the patient and send for laboratory analysis.	Ensures accuracy of results and timeliness of laboratory analyses.	Ensure that paperwork for specimens is correctly completed to avoid delays in processing.
19. If a biopsy is not being obtained, remove **PE** and discard used supplies in appropriate receptacle.	Safely discards used supplies.	Never allow another individual to clear biopsy tray of sharps. *Always clear your own tray.*
20. **HH**		
Bone Marrow Biopsy		
1. Make a small (3-mm) skin incision with a scalpel, pass the preferred biopsy needle (Jamshidi, TrapLok, SNARECOIL, power drill device, etc.) through the incision, and advance the needle until the periosteum is reached.	Allows smooth entry of the marrow needle into the skin.	Some sections of bone are extremely hard, making placement of the Jamshidi needle difficult. If hard bone is encountered, another section of bone should be used. If a section of bone is extremely soft, it is often difficult to obtain an adequate biopsy, and another section of bone should be chosen. Be sure all of periosteum is anesthetized. Follow institutional training guidelines for use of the power drill device if indicated.
2. Rotate the needle slightly until it is firmly seated in the bone.	Requires constant smooth pressure.	
3. Remove the stylet, replace the cap on the needle, and advance the needle approximately 2 cm with a firm and slightly rotating motion.	Removing the stylet allows the core section of bone to fill the needle. Replacing the cap provides suction to keep the specimen in the needle.	
4. Verify the length of the biopsy sample, with the stylet used as a guide.	Gently insert the stylet so as not to push the core back or damage it.	Optimal length of biopsy sample should be between 1.5 and 2.0 cm.

Procedure continues on following page

Procedure for Performing Bone Marrow Aspiration and Biopsy—*Continued*

Steps	Rationale	Special Considerations
5. Before removal, the manual biopsy needle should be rotated 360 degrees in each direction three to five times. Place the cap back on the hub and gently back the needle out of the bone, skin, and muscle while applying firm gentle pressure.	Giving the manual needle a few 360-degree turns and creating a vacuum by placing the cap over the top of the needle during removal increases the likelihood that the bone core will be retained within the needle.	If no cap is available for the needle, place thumb over the needle to create a vacuum.
6. If available, attach a guide to the distal end of the biopsy needle. With the blunt obturator supplied, remove the core sample by passing the obturator through the guide and pushing the sample out through the needle hub (large end).	Removing the core sample this way prevents damage to the bone by not forcing it through the narrower "drill" end of the needle.	
7. Apply firm pressure to the site for 5 minutes or until bleeding has stopped. A. Cleanse site with antiseptic swab (chlorhexidine-based preparation). B. Apply bacitracin or Bactroban ointment, adhesive bandage, 4 × 4 pressure dressing with paper or Medipore tape. C. Reposition patient into supine position for 10–15 minutes to maintain pressure at the biopsy site.	Reduces chance of bleeding at the site. Prevents hemorrhage, hematoma, and infection.	Very firm pressure is key. If the patient is at high risk for bleeding (severely thrombocytopenic, other coagulopathy, anticoagulation therapy, etc.), have the patient lie on a firm surface (i.e., book, sandbag, firmly rolled towel, etc.) or a large ice pack may be helpful.
8. With the help of the critical care nurse or person assisting: A. Place the bone core sample on a glass slide or nonadherent dressing. B. With six additional glass slides, gently touch each slide against the length of the biopsy sample to make five to six imprints. C. Place the core sample in specimen container with the appropriate solution for processing (i.e., 10% formalin or sterile 2 × 2 gauze soaked with sterile saline solution).	A touch preparation can be useful for a complete pathology analysis.	The core specimen should be kept moist to prevent decay before processing. If aspirate was not obtained, but a second core biopsy was obtained, place the core biopsy in RPMI tissue transport medium.
9. Label samples in presence of the patient and send for laboratory analysis.	Specimens require staining and decalcification for studies.	
10. Remove 🅿🅴 and discard used supplies in appropriate receptacle.	Safely discards used supplies.	Never allow another individual to clear biopsy tray of sharps. *Always* clear your own tray.
11. 🅷🅷		

Expected Outcomes

- Adequate bone marrow aspirate and core biopsy specimens obtained
- Spicules in the aspirate (unless the patient is aplastic, fibrosed, or packed); aspirate not clotted
- Minimal bleeding and discomfort (patient may feel a dull ache for a few days after the procedure)
- Absence of additional complications

Unexpected Outcomes

- Difficulty obtaining a bone marrow aspirate or core biopsy
- Excessive pain
- Inability to perform procedure because of patient fear or intolerance
- Hematoma
- Retroperitoneal bleed
- Local infection
- Nerve damage

Patient Monitoring and Care

Steps	Rationale	Reportable Conditions
		These conditions should be reported if they persist despite nursing interventions.
1. Follow institutional standards for assessing pain. Administer analgesia as prescribed. **(Level B*)**	Identifies the need for pain interventions. Promotes patient comfort.[3,8,11]	- Continued pain despite pain interventions
2. Assess vital signs, oxygenation, level of consciousness, and cardiac rhythm during the procedure and until the patient is completely recovered from sedation medications.	Monitors patient response to positioning, the procedure, and medications.	- Changes in vital signs - Decreases in oxygen saturation (Sao_2) - Changes in cardiac rhythm - Changes in level of consciousness
3. Assess the site at regular intervals with consideration of patient-specific risk factors for bleeding.	Monitors for signs and symptoms of complications.	- Bleeding - Hematoma - Pain - Nerve damage - Infection
4. Instruct the patient and family to keep pressure dressing clean, dry, and in place for 24 hours after the procedure. Ask the patient or family to assess for bruising or hematoma.	Proper dressing care reduces the chance of bleeding and minimizes the chance of infection at the site.	
5. Advise the patient and family to apply a wrapped ice bag to the site over clothing if experiencing discomfort. This will also reduce the risk of bleeding. The ice should never be applied directly to the skin.	Ice reduces swelling, decreases the chance of hematoma, and adds comfort.	
6. Instruct the patient and family to notify the physician, advanced practice nurse, or other healthcare professional immediately if the patient develops fever, increasing pain, erythema, excessive warmth, bruising, and/or bleeding at the biopsy site. Also report numbness, tingling, and/or loss of strength in the extremity of the corresponding biopsy site.	Increasing pain (especially radiating down the leg), numbness, tingling, and/or loss of strength may be signs of a compressive hematoma. Fever, pain, excessive warmth, and erythema may be signs of infection requiring immediate intervention.	

*Level B: Well-designed, controlled studies with results that consistently support a specific action, intervention, or treatment.

Procedure continues on following page

Patient Monitoring and Care —*Continued*

Steps	Rationale	Reportable Conditions
7. Avoid applying heat to the procedure site.	Heat may exacerbate bleeding.	
8. Advise against nonsteroidal antiinflammatory drugs or aspirin for 24 hours after biopsy.	This measure reduces the chance of bleeding or hematoma at site.	
9. Advise the use of acetaminophen for pain relief, if not contraindicated.	Acetaminophen relieves pain and does not promote bleeding.	
10. If the patient has been on prophylactic or treatment-dose anticoagulation, instruct the patient and family on the appropriate time frame to restart anticoagulation if being held.	Clear instruction is required to prevent bleeding complications related to anticoagulation and/or thromboembolism related to a lapse in anticoagulation.	

Documentation

Documentation should include the following:

- Patient and family education
- Completion of informed consent
- Procedure verification and timeout
- Date and time of the procedure
- Indication for the procedure
- Preparation for the procedure
- Any complications that occurred
- Any medications used
- Specimens obtained
- Additional interventions
- For patients receiving moderate sedation, documentation that institution-approved discharge criteria have been met
- Pain assessment, interventions, and effectiveness

References and Additional Readings

For a complete list of references and additional readings for this procedure, scan this QR code with any freely available smartphone code reader app, or visit http://booksite.elsevier.com/9780323376624.

125 Bone Marrow Biopsy and Aspiration (Assist)

Glen Peterson and Carrie Marvill

PURPOSE: The bone marrow aspiration and biopsy is performed to obtain information on initial diagnosis, staging, or treatment response for hematology/oncology patients. Assistance may be required in preparing supplies and the patient before and during the procedure.

PREREQUISITE NURSING KNOWLEDGE

- The bone marrow aspiration and biopsy is a common procedure performed on patients with a hematologic disorder or a suspected or previously diagnosed hematological malignancy. It is performed during the initial diagnosis and/or staging and used to determine treatment response in patients with leukemia, lymphoma, multiple myeloma, and other hematologic disorders.
- The procedure is performed by physicians, advanced practice nurses, physician assistants, and other healthcare professionals with special training and experience. It is typically completed at the bedside with local anesthetic and minimal requirement for sedation; however, moderate sedation may be performed in patients intolerant to the procedure.
- The procedure is performed at the preferred location of the superior, posterior iliac crest, usually with the patient positioned in the prone or lateral (side-lying) position. Routinely, an aspirate is obtained from the cancellous (soft, spongy) portion of the bone after a needle is used to penetrate through the outer, firm cortical bone. Similarly, a core biopsy is obtained with the use of a trephine coring needle, either manually or with a power drill device. The sternum and anterior iliac crest may also be used in rare situations; however, this is discouraged because of the excessive risk of trauma to underlying tissues including the heart.
- The bone marrow biopsy is generally a safe procedure; however, infection, bleeding, and nerve damage (usually due to nerve compressive hematoma) may occur. Care should be taken to prevent such complications by maintaining strict sterile technique, assuring coagulation laboratory parameters are met, anticoagulation therapy is managed appropriately and local hemostasis is maintained.
- Multiple tests are required depending on the diagnosis. Common diagnostic tests include morphology, flow cytometry, cytogenetics, fluorescence in situ hybridization (FISH), and molecular studies. Much less commonly, infectious disease testing may be requested, including culture and gram stain, fungal culture, viral culture, polymerase chain reaction (PCR), acid-fast bacillus (AFB), and gomori methenamine silver (GMS) stain.
- A thorough understanding is needed of the anatomy and physiology of the posterior and anterior iliac crest and the sternum. The preferred site for a bone marrow aspirate and biopsy is the posterior iliac crest.[1] The sternum may be used to aspirate marrow; however, a core biopsy cannot be obtained from the sternum because of risk of damage to underlying organs, most significantly the heart.[7,9]
- Clinical and technical competence in assisting with a bone marrow aspirate and biopsy is necessary.
- Clinical and technical competence in preparing slides and caring for a core biopsy is needed.
- Knowledge of sterile technique is necessary.
- An understanding is needed of institutional policies and procedures for administration of intravenous (IV) pharmacological agents, including moderate sedation (if indicated), intradermal and epicortical local anesthesia (lidocaine in most cases; procaine may be used in cases of lidocaine allergy), and procedural care of the patient receiving moderate sedation (if used).
- Knowledge is needed of information to be gained from a bone marrow aspirate sample (i.e., identification of normal and abnormal hematopoietic elements, identification of malignant clones with flow cytometry, immunohistochemistry and other pathological analysis techniques, identification of chromosomal abnormalities that occur in hematologic malignant diseases, identification of molecular diagnostic studies that show gene rearrangements and translocations, and the performance of chimerism studies in patients after allogeneic transplant).
- A bone marrow biopsy is used for morphological analysis of hematopoietic cells and for assessment of the architecture of the bone marrow that may be abnormal in certain disease states.
- Indications for bone marrow aspiration and biopsy include the following:
  - ❖ To diagnose a hematologic abnormality or malignancy
  - ❖ To monitor a hematologic disease state after initial diagnosis or therapy

- To diagnose bone marrow involvement before stem cell collection and for staging of various malignant states
- To assess the status of disease after autologous bone marrow or hematopoietic stem cell transplant
- To assess chimerism disease status and immune reconstitution after an allogeneic bone marrow or hematopoietic stem cell transplant
- To evaluate immunodeficiency syndromes or to confirm an infectious disease process in the marrow
- Contraindications to bone marrow biopsy and aspirate are the presence of hemophilia, severe disseminated intravascular coagulopathy, or other related severe bleeding disorders. Thrombocytopenia alone is not a contraindication to bone marrow examination,[4,5] although a platelet transfusion may be indicated if the patient is severely thrombocytopenic or if bleeding develops or persists after the procedure.[2] The use of anticoagulant medications may pose a serious bleeding risk; therefore, coagulation studies should be obtained in these patients. The decision on whether anticoagulation can be safely withheld before and restarted after the procedure is patient dependent and may require specialty consultation.

EQUIPMENT

- Bone marrow aspiration and biopsy kit, which includes the following:
  - Antiseptic solution (e.g., 2% chlorhexidine–based preparation)
  - Two sterile fenestrated drapes
  - One to two vial(s) lidocaine (1% or 2%; 5 to 10 mL; follow institutional standards; administration should not exceed 4.5 mg/kg or 300 mg[12])
  - 5- or 10-mL syringe for drawing up lidocaine
  - Filter needle (if lidocaine drawn from glass vial)
  - Needles of appropriate lengths to anesthetize both skin and periosteum
  - Sterile 4×4 and 2×2 gauze pads
  - Small scalpel blade
  - Bacitracin or Bactroban ointment (optional for incision site after procedure)
- Biopsy needle options:
  - Illinois needle (16 gauge for bone marrow aspirate only)
  - Jamshidi bone biopsy needle (for aspirate and core biopsy, 8 or 11 gauge, 4 inches or longer)
  - TrapLok bone marrow biopsy needle (for aspirate and core biopsy, 8 or 11 gauge, 4 inches or longer)
  - SNARECOIL bone marrow biopsy needle (for aspirate and core biopsy, 8 or 11 gauge, 4 inches or longer)
  - Powered bone marrow biopsy system (for aspirate and core biopsy, 8 or 11 gauge, 4 inches or longer)
  - Extra long bone marrow biopsy needle may be required for obese patients
- Two to three 20-mL syringes for bone marrow aspirate
- Blunt tip needles for drawing up ethylenediaminetetraacetic acid (EDTA), heparin
- Adhesive bandage
- Nonadhering dressing (for core biopsy placement and touch preps)

- One roll paper Micropore or Medipore tape
- Sterile gloves
- Sterile gowns
- Fluid shield, face mask, or goggles
- Specimen bags and labels
- Required tubes for specimen processing (variable based on required tests; follow institutional standards): two edetate disodium (liquid EDTA and/or EDTA lavender top) and two sodium heparin (green top) tubes, edetate disodium (EDTA) sterile solution (15 mg/mL; 2 mL total) or prefilled EDTA tube
- Eight glass slides and cover plate
- $3\frac{1}{2}$ - to 6-inch spinal needle (may be required for anesthetizing periosteum in the obese patient)
- Container for bone core biopsy specimen, including appropriate fixative (10% formalin)

Additional equipment, to have available as needed, includes the following:

- Power drill
- One vial of 100 units/mL heparin (follow institutional standards)
- One vial of buffered lidocaine (optional: The addition of sodium bicarbonate may minimize pain during lidocaine administration.[7])
- Equipment for patients receiving moderate sedation:
  - Pulse oximeter with telemetry
  - Automated blood pressure monitor
  - Oxygen
  - Suction
  - Ambu bag
  - IV pharmacological agents for sedation (i.e., midazolam, 1 to 4 mg; lorazepam, 1 to 2 mg; fentanyl, 25 to 100 μg; morphine 2 to 4 mg; hydromorphone 0.5 to 2 mg)
  - IV opiate and benzodiazepine antagonist agents (i.e., naloxone and flumazenil)
  - Emergency equipment

PATIENT AND FAMILY EDUCATION

- Assess patient and family understanding of the bone marrow aspiration and biopsy procedure and the reason for it. *Rationale:* Clarification of the procedure and reinforcement of information may reduce patient and family anxiety and stress.
- Inform the patient and family (if permitted by patient) that the results will be shared with them as soon as they are available. *Rationale:* The patient and family are usually anxious about the results.
- Explain the actual procedure to the patient and family. *Rationale:* The patient and family are prepared for what to expect and may decrease anxiety.
- Review safety requirements for patients who will receive pharmacological agents for sedation (i.e., must have transportation and escort home and may not drive until the following day). *Rationale:* Review ensures patient safety and accountability of the physician, advanced practice nurse, or other healthcare professional for patients receiving sedation.
- Encourage the patient to verbalize any pain experienced during the procedure. *Rationale:* Additional lidocaine,

pain medication, or sedation medication can be administered. Patient becomes a participant in care. Poor relaxation can cause the large gluteal muscles to spasm, making the procedure more difficult for all involved.

PATIENT ASSESSMENT AND PREPARATION

Patient Assessment

- Assess patient's allergies and home medications, including over-the-counter medications that can increase the risk of bleeding. Anticoagulant medications may need to be held. Specialty consultation may be required to clarify risks and benefits related to anticoagulation. *Rationale:* Assessment can decrease the risk of bleeding, hematoma, and allergic reaction.
- Assess the need for antianxiety or analgesic medication or moderate sedation. *Rationale:* If the patient is very anxious before the procedure or has had severe pain with previous bone marrow procedures, small doses of analgesia or sedation promote patient comfort. Tense muscles can create a technically difficult procedure and add to pain and anxiety.
- Assess coagulation studies (PT/INR, PTT) in patients who are taking anticoagulant medications. No recommendations exist regarding minimal requirements for coagulation studies before bone marrow biopsy; however, based on clinical guidelines for similar procedures and expert opinion, a PTT goal of less than 1.5 times control and INR less than 2 (≤1.5 if platelet count <20) are recommended.[10] *Rationale:* Patients at risk for bleeding complications are identified and anticoagulant medications may need to be held.
- Assess current cell blood count (CBC) for severe thrombocytopenia requiring pre- or intraprocedure transfusion. No recommendations exist regarding minimal requirements for coagulation studies before the bone marrow biopsy; however, based on clinical guidelines for similar procedures and expert opinion, a platelet count of greater than or equal to 20 is recommended. If the procedure needs to be performed emergently and the platelet count is greater than or equal to 10 but not greater than or equal to 20, platelet transfusion during and after the procedure is recommended.[10] *Rationale:* Patients at risk for bleeding complications are identified and interventions for bleeding prevention are completed.
- Assess the ability of the patient to lie in the prone or lateral position, with the head of the bed at no greater than a 25-degree elevation. *Rationale:* Access to and control of the posterior iliac crest are best obtained with the patient lying flat, or with the head of the bed only slightly raised, in a side-lying or prone position.
- Assess vital signs and oxygenation status. *Rationale:* Baseline data are provided. Assessment ensures that the blood pressure and oxygenation status can be maintained if the patient is placed on his or her side or prone.
- Assess the posterior iliac crest with palpation. In select cases, the anterior iliac crest may be used as a result of positioning limitations or excessive tissue surrounding the posterior iliac crest. However, an increased risk of injury to the surrounding nerves and blood vessels makes this procedure more complicated. The sternum is used for aspiration only in very select cases because of potential fatal complications with this procedure. It should only be performed in the absence of lower risk techniques and with special equipment and close cardiac monitoring by an experienced physician. *Rationale:* Assessment identifies the most suitable area for obtaining optimal samples with a minimum of risk of discomfort and danger to the patient.
- Assess for recent bone marrow aspiration and biopsy sites. *Rationale:* The patient may have a painful experience if an additional biopsy is performed at a site that has not yet healed from a previous procedure. Penetration of scar tissue from previous bone marrow biopsy sites may also be difficult and yield inadequate results

Patient Preparation

- Ensure that the patient and family understand education. Answer questions as they arise, and reinforce information as needed. *Rationale:* Understanding of previously taught information is evaluated and reinforced.
- Verify that the patient is the correct patient using two identifiers. *Rationale:* Before performing a procedure, the nurse should ensure the correct identification of the patient for the intended intervention.
- Ensure that informed consent has been obtained for bone marrow aspiration and biopsy and, if indicated, moderate sedation. *Rationale:* Informed consent protects the rights of the patient and makes a competent decision possible for the patient.
- Participate in preprocedure verification and timeout. *Rationale:* This ensures patient safety.
- Administer preprocedure medications, as prescribed. *Rationale:* Patient may need analgesia or sedation to ensure adequate cooperation and minimize discomfort during the procedure. Ensures patient has therapeutic effect before procedure.
- Follow institutional standards for a patient receiving moderate sedation. *Rationale:* Preparation ensures that appropriate emergency equipment and medical staff are available.
- Obtain IV access for patients receiving sedation. *Rationale:* A secure patent IV line is necessary for administration of IV pharmacological agents and, if necessary, emergency antagonist agents.
- Obtain a complete blood count and differential as prescribed. *Rationale:* Many pathologists prefer to review a peripheral blood sample in conjunction with the marrow to make a complete and accurate diagnostic evaluation.
- Place the patient on a cardiac monitor. *Rationale:* This allows for assessment of patient status during procedure
- Assist the patient to an appropriate position depending on the patient's comfort and the preference of the physician, advanced practice nurse, or other healthcare professional. *Rationale:* Positioning ensures good visualization and control of the posterior iliac crest.
- Ensure site markings have been made where appropriate. *Rationale:* Procedure site is identified.

Procedure   for Assisting With Bone Marrow Aspiration and Biopsy

Steps	Rationale	Special Considerations
1. **HH**		
2. **PE**		Apply mask.
3. Assist the physician, advanced practice nurse, or other healthcare professional performing the procedure with patient positioning as needed.	Prepares for the procedure.	
4. Assist the physician, advanced practice nurse, or other healthcare professional performing the procedure if needed with opening and assembling necessary supplies.	Prepares supplies. Maintains sterile technique.	
5. Assist the physician, advanced practice nurse, or other healthcare professional performing the procedure with applying personal protective and sterile equipment (sterile gown, sterile gloves, mask, goggles).	Maintains sterile technique.	Gowns may be required in some settings, such as the blood and marrow transplant unit. Follow institutional standards.
6. Assist with or draw up 2 mL of EDTA into one of sterile syringes (10–20 mL) depending on number of specimens needed.	Ensures adequate slide preparation because EDTA is used to preserve spicules (small pieces of bone).	EDTA tubes usually have a lavender top. Follow institutional guidelines for using EDTA in syringes and tubes.
7. Assist with or draw up of heparin into one of syringes (10-mL or 20-mL) depending on number if specimens needed.	Heparinized aspirate is used for flow cytometry, chromosome analysis, FISH, and chimerism studies (chimerism may also be performed on EDTA tubes).	Heparinized tubes usually have a green top. Follow institutional standards for use of heparinized and nonheparinized tubes for obtaining samples.
8. Follow institutional standards for administration of prescribed IV pharmacological agents, including moderate sedation. (**Level B***)	Promotes patient comfort and reduces anxiety.[3,8,11]	Ensure emergency equipment available and functional.
9. Assist with processing the aspirate obtained in the nonheparinized (EDTA) syringe first. A. The aspirate in the 20-mL nonheparinized (EDTA) syringe should be placed in lavender-top tubes and can be used for slide preparation, clot analysis, and polymerase chain reaction (PCR) studies. B. The aspirate in the heparinized syringes should be placed into green-top sodium heparin tubes.	Nonheparinized (EDTA) bone marrow aspirate can clot if it is not placed in the appropriate tubes soon after it is obtained.	If no spicules are visible in the aspirate syringe, there will be no hematopoietic elements for morphological analysis. It may be necessary to attempt aspiration after repositioning the aspirate needle to an alternate site, or the patient may have an "empty marrow." If no blood can be aspirated at all, the procedure may be documented as a "dry tap."
10. Assist as needed with performing the touch preparation with the bone biopsy core sample, and place the sample in 10% formalin fixative or sterile saline solution–soaked sterile gauze in a container.	A touch preparation can be useful for a complete pathology analysis, especially if the aspirate is a particulate or a "dry tap."[6]	

*Level B: Well-designed, controlled studies with results that consistently support a specific action, intervention, or treatment.

Procedure for Assisting With Bone Marrow Aspiration and Biopsy—*Continued*

Steps	Rationale	Special Considerations
11. Assist with holding pressure for 5 minutes or until bleeding has stopped (use sterile technique). Once bleeding stops, assist as needed with applying a sterile pressure dressing.	Ensures adequate hemostasis and reduces hemorrhage, hematoma, and infection.	Very firm pressure is key. If the patient is at high risk for bleeding (severely thrombocytopenic, other coagulopathy, anticoagulation therapy, etc.), have the patient lie on a firm surface (e.g., book, sandbag, firmly rolled towel, etc.) or use of a large ice pack may be helpful.
12. Follow institutional standards for recovering a patient who has received IV moderate sedation.	Ensures recovery parameters have been met.	
13. Label samples in the presence of the patient and send for laboratory analysis.	Ensures accuracy of results and timeliness of laboratory analyses.	Ensure that the paperwork for specimens is correctly completed to avoid delays in processing.
14. Remove **PE** and discard used supplies in appropriate receptacle.	Safely discards used supplies.	Never clear tray of sharps. This will be done by the practitioner.
15. **HH**		

Expected Outcomes

- Adequate bone marrow aspirate and core biopsy specimens obtained
- Spicules in the aspirate (unless the patient is aplastic, fibrosed, or packed); aspirate not clotted
- Minimal bleeding and discomfort (patient may feel a dull ache for a few days after the procedure)
- Absence of additional complications

- Difficulty obtaining a bone marrow aspirate or core biopsy
- Excessive pain
- Inability to perform procedure because of patient fear or intolerance
- Hematoma
- Retroperitoneal bleed
- Local infection
- Nerve damage

Patient Monitoring and Care

Steps	Rationale	Reportable Conditions
		These conditions should be reported if they persist despite nursing interventions.
1. Follow institutional standards for assessing pain. Administer analgesia as prescribed. (**Level B***)	Identifies the need for pain interventions. Promotes patient comfort.[3,8,11]	- Continued pain despite pain interventions
2. Monitor vital signs, level of consciousness, oxygenation, and cardiac rhythm during the procedure and until the patient is completely recovered from sedation medications.	Determines the patient response to positioning and the procedure.	- Changes in vital signs or level of consciousness - Decreased oxygen saturation (Sao_2) - Cardiac dysrhythmias
3. Assess the site at regular intervals with consideration of patient-specific risk factors for bleeding.	Monitors for signs and symptoms of complications.	- Bleeding - Hematoma - Infection

*Level B: Well-designed, controlled studies with results that consistently support a specific action, intervention, or treatment.

Procedure continues on following page

Patient Monitoring and Care —*Continued*

Steps	Rationale	Reportable Conditions
4. Instruct the patient and family to keep pressure dressing clean, dry, and in place for 24 hours after the procedure. Ask the patient or family to assess for bruising or hematoma.	Proper dressing care reduces chance of bleeding and minimizes chance of infection at the site.	
5. Advise the patient and family to apply a wrapped ice bag to the site over clothing if experiencing discomfort. This will also reduce the risk of bleeding. The ice should never be applied directly to the skin.	Ice reduces swelling, decreases the chance of hematoma, and adds comfort.	
6. Instruct the patient and family to notify the physician, advanced practice nurse, or other healthcare professional immediately if the patient develops fever, increasing pain, erythema, excessive warmth, bruising, and/or bleeding at the biopsy site. Also report numbness, tingling, and/or loss of strength in the extremity of the corresponding biopsy site.	Increasing pain (especially radiating down the leg), numbness, tingling, and/or loss of strength may be signs of a compressive hematoma. Fever, pain, excessive warmth, and erythema may be signs of infection requiring immediate intervention.	
7. Avoid applying heat to the procedure site.	Heat may exacerbate bleeding.	
8. Advise against nonsteroidal antiinflammatory drugs or aspirin for 24 hours after biopsy.	This measure reduces the chance of bleeding or hematoma at site.	
9. Advise the use of acetaminophen for pain relief, if not contraindicated.	Acetaminophen relieves pain and does not promote bleeding.	
10. If the patient has been on prophylactic or treatment-dose anticoagulation, instruct the patient and family on the appropriate time frame to restart anticoagulation if being held.	Clear instruction is required to prevent bleeding complications related to anticoagulation and/or thromboembolism related to a lapse in anticoagulation.	

Documentation

Documentation should include the following:
- Patient and family education
- Completion of informed consent
- Procedure verification and timeout
- Indication for the procedure
- Date and time of the procedure
- Practitioner performing the procedure
- Person assisting with procedure
- Any complications that occurred
- Any medications used
- Specimens obtained
- Additional interventions
- Pain assessment, interventions, and effectiveness

References and Additional Readings

For a complete list of references and additional readings for this procedure, scan this QR code with any freely available smartphone code reader app, or visit http://booksite.elsevier.com/9780323376624.

PROCEDURE

126 Burn Wound Care

Cameron Bell

PURPOSE: Burn wound care is performed to promote healing, maintain function, and prevent infection and burn wound sepsis. A major focus during burn wound care also incorporates strategies to effectively manage pain.

PREREQUISITE NURSING KNOWLEDGE

- Burns destroy the structural integrity of the skin, disrupting its normal functions of regulating temperature, maintaining fluid status, protecting against infection, covering nerve endings, and establishing identity.[11] The skin is composed of two layers, the epidermis and the dermis, and is supported by a subcutaneous layer that is rich in blood vessels (Fig. 126-1).
  - The *epidermis* is the outermost layer. It is capable of rapid regeneration through division of cells closest to the dermis; older epidermal cells are pushed outward as the epidermis is regenerated. The epidermis provides a barrier to the environment, containing melanocytes (protection from the sun) and Langerhans cells (protection against foreign organisms).
  - The *dermis* contains blood vessels, sensory fibers (for pain, touch, pressure, and temperature), collagen, sebaceous glands, and sweat glands. Epidermal cells line deep dermal structures (hair follicles and sweat glands); these epidermal elements provide the ability for the skin to regenerate (the more epidermal cells remaining in the wound bed, the faster the healing).
- The depth of burns has historically been classified as first degree (into epidermis), second degree (into dermis), or third degree (through skin into subcutaneous tissue; Table 126-1).[1,11]
- *First-degree,* or superficial, *burns* extend only partially through the epidermis, thereby maintaining the barrier function of the skin. Burns involving only the epidermis are very painful, but do not form blisters. The epidermis is usually regenerated in 3 to 4 days.[11] These burns are not included when estimating the percentage of total body surface area burned (%TBSA) because they do not result in an open wound.
- *Second-degree burns* extend into the dermis and can be superficial (loss of the epidermis and part of the dermis) or deep (destruction of most of the dermis). They are also referred to as *partial-thickness burns* because they extend partially through the skin (Fig. 126-2). These wounds heal by epithelialization from epidermal cells remaining in the dermis. Shallow wounds are associated with rapid healing and less scarring. Deep wounds may result in slow healing (more than 21 days) and are fragile wounds prone to hypertrophic scarring. For that reason, surgical excision of partial-thickness wounds that affect functional and cosmetic areas and application of skin grafts may be preferable.
- A *third-degree,* or *full-thickness, burn* involves complete destruction of the dermis and extends into the subcutaneous tissue. Because the skin is unable to regenerate, the dead tissue is removed and the wound is grafted with skin from another part of the patient's own body (autograft).[11] The grafted wound loses epidermal appendages and is unable to sweat, maintain lubrication, or protect from sun exposure after healing (Fig. 126-3).
- The depth of a burn wound is directly related to the temperature intensity and the duration of contact with the burning agent. The burning agent can be thermal (i.e., flame, contact, or scald), chemical, or electrical. An inhalation injury should always be suspected if the patient was in an enclosed space with a fire; mortality rate is significantly increased when burns are compounded by smoke inhalation.[6]
- The burn injury produces three zones of injury: the zone of coagulation (cellular death), the zone of stasis (vascular impairment, potentially reversible tissue injury), and the zone of hyperemia (increased blood flow and inflammatory response). Decreased perfusion of the burn wound can cause the zone of stasis to deteriorate, deepening the initial wound. This progressive destruction can be minimized by providing adequate oxygenation and fluid resuscitation, alleviating pressure on the injured tissue, maintaining local and systemic warmth, and decreasing edema by elevating the burned area.[1]
- Assess for areas where full-thickness eschar is circumferential. Because of the inelastic nature of eschar, it may act

TABLE 126-1   Depth Characteristics of Burn Wounds

Type	Physical Characteristics	Healing
Superficial burn (first degree): destruction of epidermis, usually caused by overexposure to sun or brief exposure to hot liquid. This type of injury is not included in calculations of burn size.	Red; hypersensitive; no blisters.	Injured layers peel away from totally healed skin at 5–7 days without residual scarring.
Superficial partial-thickness burn (superficial second degree): destruction of epidermis and upper dermis. Usually results from scalding or brief contact with hot objects.	Blistered; very moist; red or pink in color; exquisitely painful; capillary refill intact.	Reepithelializes from epidermal appendages in 7–14 days. Usually has minimal scarring but variable repigmentation.
Deep partial-thickness burn (deep second degree): destruction of epidermis through to lower dermis. May result from grease or longer contact with hot objects.	Mottled pink to white; drier than superficial burns; less sensitive to pinprick; does not blanch to pressure; hair follicles and sweat glands intact.	Slower regeneration from epidermal elements: 14–21+ days in absence of grafting. Prone to hypertrophic scars and contracture formation. May require grafting to reduce healing time and complications.
Full-thickness burn (third degree): destruction of epidermis and all of the dermis. Results from exposure to flames, chemicals that are not immediately washed, electrical injury, or prolonged contact with heat source.	Dry; leathery and firm to touch; pearly white, brown, or charred in appearance; no blanching to pressure; no pain; may see thrombosed vessels.	Incapable of self-regeneration. Preferred treatment is early excision and autografting.

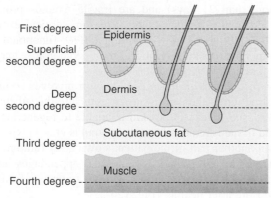

Figure 126-1   Depth of burn wound injury. *(From Townsend CM, et al, editors:* Sabiston textbook of surgery, *ed 19. Philadelphia, 2012, Saunders.)*

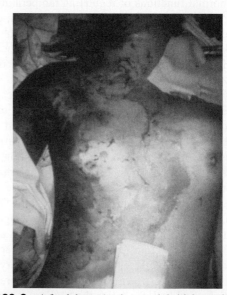

Figure 126-3   A fresh burn that is a partial-thickness burn toward the patient's left side and progresses to a full-thickness burn on the patient's right side.

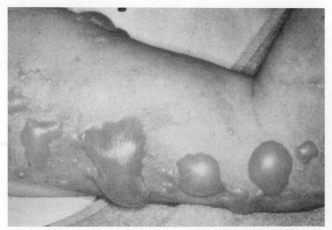

Figure 126-2   Blisters of a partial-thickness burn wound on the arm.

like a tourniquet as edema develops, requiring surgical release (escharotomy) to prevent circulatory or respiratory compromise (Fig. 126-4).

- Monitor pulses, capillary refill, and sensation distal to circumferential eschar. Signs and symptoms that indicate a need for escharotomy include cyanosis of distal unburned skin, unrelenting deep tissue pain, progressive paresthesias, and progressive decrease or absence of pulse.[1]
- Circumferential eschar of the trunk can lead to decreased tidal volume and agitation (Fig. 126-5)[1]; therefore, adequacy of respiratory excursion must be assessed.

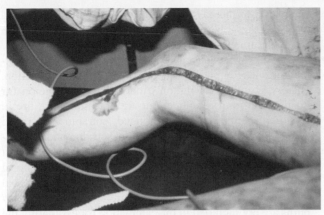

Figure 126-4 Escharotomy of the leg to improve circulation.

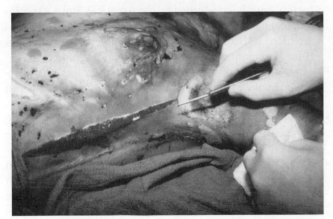

Figure 126-5 Full-thickness burn with chest escharotomy to improve chest expansion.

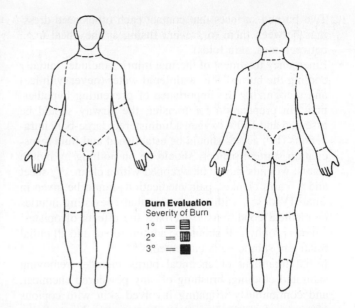

Burn Evaluation
Severity of Burn

1° = 🔲
2° = 🔳
3° = ⬛

- Escharotomy is performed at the bedside by a physician, with a scalpel or electrocautery used to cut the eschar longitudinally. Bleeding should be minimal because only dead tissue is cut; any bleeding can be controlled with sutures, silver nitrate sticks, collagen packing, or electrocautery.[1] Pain is usually managed with small intravenous doses of opiates and benzodiazepines.
- Burn size may be determined with several methods.[19]
  ❖ The *rule of nines* may be used to quickly calculate burn size. In an adult, the head and neck and each upper extremity represent 9% of the patient's body surface area. The anterior trunk, posterior trunk, and each leg represent 18% of the patient's body surface area. This rule only applies to adults; infants and young children have much larger heads in proportion to body size.[1]
  ❖ The *Lund and Browder chart* (Fig. 126-6) breaks the body into smaller areas and takes into consideration the proportional differences of persons of different ages.[14]
  ❖ The *rule of the palm* notes that the patient's hand may be used as a template to represent roughly 1% of the TBSA.[1]
- The inflammatory response causes a massive fluid shift to the interstitial space during the first 24 hours, with mobilization of fluid starting after 72 hours. Fluid resuscitation with a balanced salt solution is based on the patient's weight and burn size (partial-thickness and full-thickness

Lund and Browder chart

AREA	AGE—YEARS					% 2°	% 3°	% TOTAL
	0–1	1–4	5–9	10–15	ADULT			
Head	19	17	13	10	7			
Neck	2	2	2	2	2			
Ant. Trunk	13	17	13	13	13			
Post. Trunk	13	13	13	13	13			
R. Buttock	2½	2½	2½	2½	2½			
L. Buttock	2½	2½	2½	2½	2½			
Genitalia	1	1	1	1	1			
R.U. Arm	4	4	4	4	4			
L. U. Arm	4	4	4	4	4			
R.L. Arm	3	3	3	3	3			
L.L. Arm	3	3	3	3	3			
R. Hand	2½	2½	2½	2½	2½			
L. Hand	2½	2½	2½	2½	2½			
R. Thigh	5½	6½	8½	8½	9½			
L. Thigh	5½	6½	8½	8½	9½			
R. Leg	5	5	5½	6	7			
L. Leg	5	5	5 ½	6	7			
R. Foot	3½	3½	3½	3½	3½			
L. Foot	3½	3½	3½	3½	3½			
					Total			

Figure 126-6 The Lund and Browder chart is used to assess and graphically document size and depth of the burn wound.

wounds).[10] Large wounds are prone to huge evaporative water losses that require close monitoring of volume status.[1,11]

- Effective resuscitation results in adequate urinary output (0.5 mL/kg/hr) as a surrogate marker of end-organ perfusion.[1]
- Burns of specific anatomical areas need special consideration. Assess eyes for injury and treat chemical exposure with copious normal saline solution irrigation; treat burned ears with a topical antimicrobial cream and protect from pressure by eliminating use of pillows or dressings about the head; elevate burned extremities; consider the need for an indwelling urinary catheter in the patient with perineal burns; and clip hair growing through the burn wounds.

Two burned surfaces that contact each other need dressings between them to prevent fusing as they heal (e.g., between toes, skin folds).

- Emergency treatment of thermal injuries includes initially cooling the burned skin with tepid water (never with ice) and recognizing the importance of preventing hypothermia.[1] In preparation for transfer, the airway should be assessed and 100% oxygen administered; large-bore intravenous (IV) access should be established and fluid resuscitation started; patients should be on nothing by mouth status; wounds should be wrapped with a clean, dry sheet and a warm blanket; pain medication should be given in small IV doses, with recognition that coexisting injuries or medical conditions exacerbate the effects of opiates; tetanus prophylaxis should be administered; and all initial treatment should be documented.[1,4,8]
- Initial treatment of chemical burns includes removing saturated clothing, brushing off any powdered chemical, and continuously irrigating involved skin with copious amounts of water for 20 to 30 minutes. Neutralizing chemical burns with another chemical is contraindicated because the procedure generates heat. Burned eyes must be irrigated with large volumes of normal saline solution followed by an eye examination.[1] Some chemicals are absorbed systemically through burn wounds; contact the local poison control center to determine whether further treatment is indicated.[11] Ensure all physicians, advanced practice nurses, and other healthcare professionals wear appropriate personal protective equipment to prevent unintentional chemical exposure.
- Initial treatment of tar burn consists of cooling the tar with cold water until the product is completely cooled.
  - ❖ After cooling, adherent tar should be covered with a petrolatum-based ointment (such as white petrolatum jelly) and dressed to promote emulsification of the tar.[1] Electrical injuries (Fig. 126-7) result when the body becomes part of the pathway for the electrical current. Deep burns may occur from tissue resistance where the patient contacted the electrical source and where the patient was grounded. Initially of greater concern than the burns is the high incidence of cardiac dysrhythmias, myoglobinuria resulting in acute tubular necrosis, and neurological sequelae. Monitoring electrocardiographic (ECG) results, increasing urine output to 1 to 1.5 mL/kg/hr in the presence of dark port-colored urine, assessing for associated trauma, and establishing baseline neurological status are vital in the treatment of the electrical injury patient.[1,19]

- Inhalation of smoke may cause localized airway inflammation and edema that can lead to airway obstruction. History, signs and symptoms that increase suspicion for inhalational injury include, but are not limited to, fire in a closed compartment, prolonged entrapment, singed nares, cough, carbonaceous sputum, stridor and hoarseness. Naso-endoscopy on admission when these are present assists in the assessment for airway edema and mucosal injury. Significant findings may necessitate endotracheal intubation as a precautionary measure. Inhalational injury/burns are not included in the calculation for estimating the percentage of total body surface area burned.[21]
- Criteria for transferring patients to a specialized burn-care facility have been adopted by the American Burn Association and the American College of Surgeons. These criteria are listed in Box 126-1 and are available at the American Burn Association website at www.ameriburn.org.
- Care of the burn wound and associated healing are determined by the extent and depth of the injury and the overall condition of the patient.
- Most burn centers use clean technique for dressing removal and wound cleansing, with sterile technique for sterile dressing application only.[5]
- Wound care should be done in a warm area. Many burn units have replaced traditional hydrotherapy tanks with shower tables for large wound care procedures to allow water runoff, thus decreasing leaching of electrolytes and minimizing wound exposure to perineal-contaminated water. Emergency equipment must always be immediately available during hydrotherapy procedures. As

---

BOX 126-1   Criteria for Patient Transfer to a Specialized Burn-Care Facility

- Partial-thickness burns on more than 10% total body surface area
- Burns that involve the face, hands, feet, genitalia, perineum, or major joints
- Third-degree burns in any age group
- Electrical burns, including lightning injury
- Chemical burns
- Inhalation injury
- Burn injury in patients with preexisting medical disorders that could complicate management, prolong recovery, or affect mortality
- Any patient with burns and concomitant trauma (such as fractures) in which the burn injury poses the greatest risk for morbidity or mortality
- Burned children in hospitals without qualified personnel or equipment to care for children
- Burn injury in patients who will need special social, emotional, or long-term rehabilitative intervention

From Committee on Trauma, American College of Surgeons: Guidelines for the operation of burn centers resources for optimal care of the injured patient. *Chicago, 2006, American College of Surgeons, pp. 79–86.*

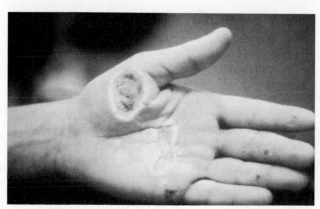

Figure 126-7 Entry site of an electrical burn.

wounds decrease in size and patients approach discharge, bathtubs and showers offer reasonable options for wound cleansing.

- Initial wound cleansing requires thorough débridement of all devitalized tissue. Blisters are generally unroofed.[5,17] Use of a moistened washcloth is effective to gently remove burned tissue, with use of a slow and deliberate wiping motion. Wash the wounds with gentle pH-neutral liquid soap solution or wound cleanser and pat dry with clean towels.
- Topical antimicrobial agents limit bacterial proliferation and fungal colonization in burn wounds. There are numerous dressings used to limit bacterial burden in the wound, including antimicrobial ointments and creams and silver-based long-wear dressings.[23] Systemic antibiotics are not routinely administered to burn patients because of the high risk for development of antibiotic resistance[3] (Table 126-2).
- The wound should be assessed daily for cellulitis and the wound care plan tailored to the needs of the patient. Moist healing may speed the time of burn wound healing.

- An autograft (skin graft taken from the patient) is the only treatment that can heal a full-thickness burn wound.[11] A debrided full-thickness wound may be protected from infection and drying through the use of biologic or biosynthetic dressings when donor sites are not available for autografting. Allograft, or homograft, refers to the use of "nonself" human skin grafts; such a graft becomes vascularized by the patient and risks rejection if it stays in place too long. A xenograft, or heterograft, is nonhuman skin obtained from commercial pigskin (porcine)–processing companies; it forms a collagen bond with the wound and protects it for a period of time until donor sites are available for autografting. Porcine xenografts may be placed over clean partial-thickness wounds to protect the wound while it heals beneath the xenograft.[11,12]
- Negative-pressure wound therapy may be used to maintain fresh-graft placement, improve wound bed vascularization, and reduce microbial activity.[19]
- The burn patient's condition is hypermetabolic until burn wounds are closed and healing is complete, and up to 12 months after the injury.[20,24] Increased caloric and protein

TABLE 126-2 Topical Antimicrobial Agents

Agent	Activity	Advantages	Disadvantages
Silver sulfadiazine 1% cream (Silvadine).	Bactericidal effect on cell membrane and wall; excellent against *Pseudomonas aeruginosa*, *Staphylococcus aureus*, other burn flora, and yeast	Broad-spectrum antimicrobial coverage; low toxicity; no discomfort on application; easy to remove; rare hypersensitivity to sulfa component; may increase neovascularization	Poor eschar penetration; infrequent hypersensitivity; macerates surrounding tissues; contraindicated in pregnant women and newborns (risk for kernicterus); early transient neutropenia when applied to large burns
Mafenide acetate 10% cream (Sulfamylon)	Broad-spectrum against gram-positive and gram-negative organisms; not effective against yeast; diffuses through devascularized areas; is absorbed, metabolized, and excreted by kidneys	Highly soluble and penetrates eschar well; persistent activity against *Pseudomonas*	Pain on application of cream; systemically absorbed; may cause metabolic acidosis (through carbonic anhydrase inhibition); cutaneous hypersensitivity reactions occur; may see yeast overgrowth
Mafenide acetate (Sulfamylon) 5% solution	Broad-spectrum against gram-positive and gram-negative organisms; not effective against yeast	Moist dressings may be used over wounds, such as a new graft, when a liquid soak antibiotic is desired	Expensive; the wet dressings are often uncomfortable and may result in hypothermia
Silver nitrate, 0.5% in water (if dressing is allowed to dry, concentration of silver nitrate increases and becomes caustic at 2%)	Bacteriostatic against many organisms; does not penetrate drainage or debris	Painless application; few organisms are resistant to silver	Must be kept wet; poor penetration of eschar; stains unburned tissue and environment brown-black; hypotonicity of dressing may lead to hyponatremia and hypochloremia; requires thick dressings and resoaking every 4 hours to prevent drying
Silver nylon (a nonadherent nanocrystalline silver-coated dressing with sustained silver release for several days)	Lower minimal inhibitory concentration; a lower minimal bactericidal concentration; faster bacterial killing than other topicals	Decreases dressing changes by being left in place 3 days	Decreases ability to visualize wound

requirements for wound healing are usually met through nasogastric or nasojejunal tube feeding to maintain mucosal integrity in large burns. Dietician consultation is imperative and adjunctive supplemental therapies may be recommended to optimize wound healing.[9,15,20,22] Burn patients should be encouraged to consume a high-protein diet. Supplementation with high-calorie nutritional drinks facilitates meeting energy needs. Large quantities of free water should be discouraged because risk for hyponatremia is high after a large burn.[20]

- An individualized plan for pain control should be in place for both background pain (pain that is continuously present), breakthrough pain (associated with activities of daily living), and procedural pain (intermittent pain related to procedures).[16,25] Unrelieved pain can lead to stress-related immunosuppression, an increased potential for infection, delayed wound healing, and depression.[13] Subcutaneous and intramuscular injections should be avoided because absorption is poor and unreliable as a result of edema.[1] As the wound heals, the patient has more discomfort from itchiness and less discomfort from pain.[16] A moisturizing lotion prevents drying and reduces pruritus. Nonpharmacological techniques can be learned to assist with the management of pain and itch.[2,16]
- Burn wounds contract during the healing phase. Self-care and range-of-motion exercises are encouraged. Stretching exercises and proper positioning are vital to prevent contractures and loss of function.[7] Static splinting is sometimes added to maintain sustained stretch.[7] Hypertrophic scar formation is countered through the use of topical silicone gel sheeting and pressure garments worn 24 hours a day until the scars mature and soften (6–18 months).[18] Keloids, if they form, may require surgery, steroid injections, and pressure treatment.[18]
- Grafts and donor sites on the lower extremities require support during healing when the patient is out of bed. Application of elastic bandages to extremities may prevent pooling of venous blood, permanent discoloration, or skin breakdown.
- The burn wound should not be exposed to the sun for a year because new scars sunburn easily.
- Patients should be instructed to select clothing that blocks sun and to use sunscreen on exposed grafts, generally for life.

EQUIPMENT

- Personal protective equipment as needed (e.g., gown, mask, goggles)
- Nonsterile gloves
- Sterile gloves
- Warm water
- Mild pH-neutral liquid cleansing agent
- Normal saline solution
- Washcloths
- Towels
- Scissors and forceps (clean and sterile)
- Topical agents, as ordered
- Tongue depressors

- Sterile dressings as needed (e.g., gauze, Exu-dry [Smith & Nephew, St. Petersburgh, FL])
- Rolled dressing, gentle tape, or netting to secure dressings
- Pillows to elevate extremities
- Pain and sedation medication (as prescribed)

Additional equipment, to have available as needed, includes the following:

- Emergent intubation and advance airway equipment
- Nasolaryngoscope

PATIENT AND FAMILY EDUCATION

- Provide detailed wound care instructions electronically or in writing. Demonstrate wound care, and have patient and family return the demonstration before the planned discharge. Continue to involve patient and family in wound care for the remainder of the admission, and encourage them to ask questions. Provide positive feedback. Arrange for home care or clinic visits to follow up on wound care. *Rationale:* Education validates patient and family understanding and ability to perform wound care, and allows time for them to develop a level of comfort. The opportunity to reinforce important points is provided.
- Explore resources the patient will have for wound care at home (e.g., availability of running water, shower versus tub). *Rationale:* This measure ensures that the patient is knowledgeable about care based on what adjustments need to be made at home.
- Simplify wound care and assess the family's ability to provide care at home. *Rationale:* Continued care of the wound may be necessary after discharge.
- Teach patient and family about signs and symptoms of infection and the importance of reporting these in a timely manner. *Rationale:* The patient and family can recognize problems early so that appropriate measures can be instituted by the physician, advanced practice nurse, and other healthcare professionals.
- Teach patient and family about pain control; assess the patient's personal acceptable level of pain. *Rationale:* Education and assessment decrease concerns about pain, facilitate an individualized pain-relief plan, and foster cooperation with care.
- Teach patient and family about pain management, including types of medications prescribed, timing of medications in relation to wound care, and nonpharmacological pain strategies.[5] *Rationale:* Comfort at home is supported.
- Provide instruction to the patient and family about the normal changes seen in the wound, including epithelial islands, healing margins, dryness on epithelialization, epidermal fragility on shearing, hypervascularization of the healed wound, and venous congestion in the dependent wound. *Rationale:* Anxiety about appearance is reduced.
- Teach the patient and family about care of healed burns, including medications to reduce itching,[3,14] use of nonperfumed moisturizers, protection from shear, and protection from sun exposure for a minimum of a year. *Rationale:*

Education reduces complications and promotes patient satisfaction.

- Explain the rationale to the patient and family for the wearing and care of pressure garments. *Rationale:* Pressure garments need to fit properly to reduce scar formation, and they can be difficult to apply.[19]
- Discuss the importance of mobility and proper positioning (e.g., splinting) on function. Self-care (activities of daily living) and range-of-motion exercises should be encouraged during the healing phase. *Rationale:* Contractures associated with healing skin, improper positioning, and immobility are prevented.
- Identify caloric needs for healing and suggest appropriate nutritional supplements. *Rationale:* Metabolic needs are increased for months after discharge, and a balanced diet facilitates gain of muscle mass versus adipose tissue.
- Inform patient and family that nightmares, alterations in body image, and psychological disturbances are experienced by many burned patients.[19] Provide resources, including someone to follow up with, if desired. *Rationale:* Information increases awareness of these problems and reassures patient and family that these experiences, although unpleasant, are not abnormal.
- Provide patient and family with follow-up appointments and someone to call with any problems. *Rationale:* Necessary information for further care and follow-up is provided.

PATIENT ASSESSMENT AND PREPARATION

Patient Assessment

- Assess vital signs, including temperature. *Rationale:* Baseline vital signs allow for comparison during and after the procedure to evaluate patient tolerance, normothermia, and adequacy of pain medication.
- Evaluate for signs of healing, including the following. *Rationale:* Healing should occur within a predictable time frame determined by the depth of burns, unless complications occur.
  - ❖ Decreased pain
  - ❖ Reepithelialization from epithelial islands within the wound
  - ❖ Decreasing wound size
  - ❖ Decreased edema
  - ❖ Compare the patient's level of healing with the expected level of healing for the number of days after burn.
- Evaluate for the following signs and symptoms of infection.[19] *Rationale:* Infection can result in delayed wound healing, prolonged hospitalization, and death.
  - ❖ Foul odor
  - ❖ Purulent drainage
  - ❖ Increased pain
  - ❖ Increasing edema
  - ❖ Cellulitis
  - ❖ Fever
  - ❖ Development of eschar or early eschar separation

- ❖ Wound discoloration
- ❖ Increase in burn size or depth
- ❖ Blurring of wound edges
- Monitor for distal circulation (pulses, pain, color, sensation, movement, and capillary refill) to areas with circumferential burns and increased edema. *Rationale:* Edema and circumferential burns impede distal circulation and cause worsening tissue perfusion and cell death.
- Determine patient's understanding of pain-management strategies. Assess patient's pain level on a standardized pain scale (such as the 0 to 10 scale) before, during, and after the procedure. Explore discrepancies between the patient's level of pain and desired level of pain. *Rationale:* An individualized plan for pain control should be in place for background, breakthrough, and procedural pain.[16,23] In addition to the traditional use of pain and anxiety medications, alternative therapies should be included (e.g., relaxation techniques, distraction, massage therapy, music therapy). The patient's needs change based on changes in the wound (e.g., healing, débridement, conversion to a deeper wound).
- Evaluate patient's general level of function, particularly in burned areas. *Rationale:* An individualized plan for range-of-motion exercises, positioning, and splinting should be made to optimize the patient's level of function. Burns contract during the healing phase, and immobility enhances loss of function.

Patient Preparation

- Ensure the patient understands procedural teaching. Answer questions as they arise and reinforce information as needed. *Rationale:* Understanding of previously taught information is evaluated and reinforced.
- Verify that the patient is the correct patient using two identifiers. *Rationale:* Before performing a procedure, the nurse should ensure the correct identification of the patient for the intended intervention.
- Notify other appropriate healthcare providers who need to assess the burn wound (e.g., the physician) or perform a task (e.g., quantitative wound biopsies, range-of-motion exercises by physical therapist) at the time of dressing changes. *Rationale:* Organization of care allows important assessment and intervention to take place without causing extra pain and stress to the patient.
- After checking previous requirements for patient comfort during the dressing change, premedicate the patient with pain medication and any sedative as prescribed, allowing an appropriate amount of time before starting wound care. *Rationale:* Premedication allows time for medication to take effect and promotes optimal comfort for the patient.
- Consider synergistic effects of opioids, sedatives, and drugs that affect the central nervous system. Closely monitor the patient for 30 to 60 minutes after the wound care procedure is completed or until there is a return to baseline. *Rationale:* Stimulatory effects that counteract central nervous system depression are reduced after wounds are covered; decreased noxious stimuli and respiratory depression may occur.

Procedure for Care of Burn Wounds

Steps	Rationale	Special Considerations
1. Prepare all necessary equipment and supplies. The treatment area should be warmed.	Preparation facilitates efficient wound care and prevents needless delays. Warming the room decreases the risk for hypothermia.	Other physicians, advanced practice nurses, and other healthcare professionals who need to observe the wound should be notified ahead of time so that they can be present while the wound is uncovered.
2. **HH**		
3. **PE**		For larger dressing changes, all physicians, advanced practice nurses, and other healthcare professionals participating in the wound care should apply caps, masks, and gowns. Smaller graft changes may require less personal protective equipment.
4. Remove old dressings and discard them in infectious waste containers. Place towel or pad under exposed extremity.	Old dressings can contain large amounts of body secretions and blood. A clean field under the extremity allows the patient a place to rest the extremity during care.	Remove dressings only from areas that can be redressed within 20–30 minutes at one time. Finish wound care to these areas before moving to new areas (decreases heat loss and pain related to nerve endings being exposed to air).
5. Remove and discard gloves and HH, and apply a pair of clean gloves.	Used gloves are contaminated by handling of the burn dressing. Aseptic techniques are necessary for wound care.	
6. Wash the wound with mild pH-balanced soap solution or wound cleanser, rinse with warm tap water, and pat dry.	Cleanses wound of debris with mechanical débridement and reduces microorganisms.	Cleanse beyond wound to reduce microbial count on surrounding tissue. Patient tolerance may improve if allowed to cleanse one's own wounds.
7. Use scissors and forceps to remove loose necrotic tissue and any broken blister tissue.	Bacteria proliferate in necrotic tissue.	Typically, physicians perform this function in hospitals that do not specialize in burn wound care.
8. Assess the burn wound for color, size, odor, depth, drainage, bleeding, edema, cellulitis, epithelial budding, eschar separation, sensation, movement, peripheral pulses, and any signs of pressure areas from splints. For wet dressings, **proceed to Step 9.**	Validates the healing process and identifies complications.	
9. *Creams:* use sterile tongue depressor to remove the required amount of topical agent from the container. *Ointments:* apply a thin layer to the wound as prescribed; apply dressing as needed.	Use of a sterile tongue depressor and removal of only what is needed from the container prevent contamination of the topical agent. Dry dressings protect the topical agent from premature removal.	If the area to be covered has folds and crevices, or if the wound consists of scattered areas, topical agents should be placed directly on the wound, rather than on the burn dressing (ensures good coverage without applying unnecessary amounts of an absorbable topical agent to uninjured areas).
10. *Soaks:* pour the prescribed solution onto sterile gauze pads. Squeeze out excess fluid and apply to the wound.	Ideal moisture is when the dressing is similar to a damp sponge. Excess fluid may macerate tissue.	

Procedure | for Care of Burn Wounds—*Continued*

Steps	Rationale	Special Considerations
11. Loosely wrap extremities with gauze rolls. Secure dressings with elastic net.	Holds dressings in place.	Wrap extremities from distal to proximal. Check pulses and capillary refill after wrapping to ensure circulation is not compromised.
12. Assess need for additional pain medication before continuing.	Patients have a right to good pain control. The success or failure of pain control for the current dressing change affects the way the patient responds to future dressing changes.	
13. **Repeat steps, starting at Step 4,** until all burn wounds have been cared for.	Isolating areas for dressing changes prevents unnecessary temperature loss, pain from increased nerve ending exposure to air movement, and cross contamination of wounds.	The size of the team doing the dressing and the amount of débridement time required determine how much of the wound should reasonably be exposed at any given time.
14. Apply splints as needed and elevate burned extremities with pillows or elastic net sling or both; elevate the head of the bed.	Maintains position of function, prevents contractures and pressure ulcers, and reduces edema. Elevation of donor sites and exposure to air facilitates healing.[8,19]	Do not bend knees if popliteal space is burned. Do not put pillows under the patient's head if neck or ears are burned. Do not inhibit movement with splints if the patient is awake and able to use the involved extremity.
15. Remove gloves and discard used supplies.		
16. 🔲		

Expected Outcomes

- Wounds heal as expected without infectious complications
- Patient maintains a self-identified acceptable level of pain relief
- Patient attains comfort from measures taken for anxiety and itching
- Patient and family verbalize knowledge of patient condition and plan of care
- An optimal level of function is maintained or attained
- Patient and family response and interactions demonstrate adaptation to injury
- Patient and family collaborate in management of care
- At the time of discharge, patient and family verbalize and demonstrate an understanding of posthospital care

Unexpected Outcomes

- Wound converts to deeper injury
- Loss of allograft
- Wound infection or systemic sepsis occurs
- Wound heals with unnecessary loss of function

Procedure continues on following page

Patient Monitoring and Care

Steps	Rationale	Reportable Conditions
		These conditions should be reported if they persist despite nursing interventions.
1. Follow institutional standards for assessing pain. Administer analgesia as prescribed. Evaluate and treat the patient for pain. Ask the patient to rate the pain on a scale of 0–10; check the orders for pain and sedation for dressing changes; check patient's medication requirements with previous dressing changes and have that amount of medication available in the room before starting the procedure; assess the need for more medication throughout the dressing change. Incorporate alternative pain relief techniques (e.g., relaxation techniques, massage therapy, distraction, music, visual imaging).	Identifies need for pain interventions. The burn patient has baseline pain that requires analgesia and increased pain-medication requirements, and possibly sedation requirements for the pain involved in dressing changes. Attention to the patient's pain fosters the patient's trust in healthcare personnel to control pain and promotes cooperation with future burn wound care. The goal of pain management is an alert patient who is able to cooperate, follow commands, and respond to verbal stimuli.	• Continued pain despite pain interventions • Nonverbal indications of pain (restlessness, grimacing, teeth clenching) • Increased respiratory rate • Verbalization of pain • Inability to cooperate with dressing change • Increased heart rate • Increased or decreased blood pressure • Oversedation, depression of respiratory rate, not being arousable
2. Obtain baseline vital signs before the procedure, monitor throughout the procedure, and check for 30 minutes after the procedure is complete.	Changes in vital signs can be an indication that the patient is experiencing pain or anxiety. Decreasing blood pressure, heart rate, and respiratory rate can be complications of pain medication (especially after the dressing change is complete and stimulation has stopped).	• Increased or decreased heart rate • Increased or decreased blood pressure • Increased or decreased respiratory rate; increased need for higher oxygen supplementation • High peak pressures on ventilator
3. Check patient's temperature before dressing changes. Ensure the patient's environment is warm; cover the portions of the patient's body that are not involved in dressing changes. Check the patient's temperature at the end of dressing changes.	Heat is lost through burn wounds. Hypermetabolism and shivering increase caloric demand.	• Hypothermia • Shivering
4. Monitor peripheral pulses and circulation in the burned extremity during the dressing change, within 1 hour after applying the dressing, and every 2 hours thereafter. Keep extremities elevated and assess for increased edema.	Circumferential burns can decrease or prevent blood flow to the involved extremity. The dressing can be too tight, especially if edema increases.	• Increased peripheral edema • Pain or numbness in the extremity • Prolonged or absent capillary refill in the extremity • Decreased or absent pulses • Conversion to deeper burn wound
5. Assess the burn wound for color, size, odor, depth, drainage, bleeding, pain, early eschar separation, healing, and cellulitis in the surrounding tissue. Obtain a wound biopsy as needed for suspected infection.	Observes for usual progression of wound healing versus complications of infection, progression of burn to deeper wound, and bleeding. Wound colonization is common. Histological determination of the level of organism invasion in the presence of systemic symptoms is diagnostic for burn wound infection.	• Foul odor • Purulent or increased amounts of drainage • Elevated body temperatures • Cellulitis • Healthy granulation tissue developing eschar • Increasing necrosis, loss of graft • Blurring of burn wound edges • Discoloration of the wound or the presence of fungal elements • Early eschar separation • Bleeding

Patient Monitoring and Care —*Continued*

Steps	Rationale	Reportable Conditions
6. Encourage exercise and activities of daily living; perform range-of-motion exercises during dressing changes; place patient in a position of optimal function, with splints used as needed, to maintain maximal function.[8,19] Use pain medication as needed to facilitate mobility.[14] **(Level C*)**	Burns and grafts contract during the healing phase if not correctly splinted and exercised; loss of function is a complication of immobility. Pain inhibits patients from moving.	• Contractures • Loss of function
7. Monitor the patient's tolerance of tube feedings or ingestion of a high-calorie and high-protein diet with supplements; encourage a nutritious diet and discourage empty calories.[13,21] Limit free water intake. **(Level D*)**	Nutrition is necessary for wound healing; burn patients are hypermetabolic. Protein-rich fluids promote healing; free water decreases intake of nutritional supplements and can lead to hyponatremia.	• Refusal to eat or inability to ingest adequate amounts of nutrition • Poor wound healing

*Level C: Qualitative studies, descriptive or correlational studies, integrative reviews, systematic reviews, or randomized controlled trials with inconsistent results.
*Level D: Peer-reviewed professional and organizational standards with the support of clinical study recommendations.

Documentation

Documentation should include the following:

- Patient and family education
- Date, time, and duration of wound care
- Areas of burn, other wounds, and pressure ulcers; weekly diagrams (or digital photographs) of unhealed wounds to monitor healing and wound changes
- Appearance of the wound (color, size, odor, depth, drainage, bleeding)
- Assessment of wound areas for level of pain (appropriate for depth and level of healing)
- Progression toward healing (e.g., presence of epithelial budding)
- Evidence of cellulitis around the wound (red, warm, tender)
- Assessment of peripheral pulses; color, movement, sensation, and capillary refill distal to a circumferential wound or an extremity wrapped in dressings
- Pain assessment, interventions, and effectiveness
- Medications given for pain, anxiety, and sedation
- Other comfort measures used
- Dressings and topical agents applied
- Patient's tolerance of the procedure
- Unexpected outcomes
- Nursing interventions

References and Additional Readings

For a complete list of references and additional readings for this procedure, scan this QR code with any freely available smartphone code reader app, or visit http://booksite.elsevier.com/9780323376624.

127 Donor-Site Care

Cameron Bell

PURPOSE: Care of the donor site is performed to promote wound healing and maintain function. A major focus during donor-site care incorporates strategies to effectively manage pain.

PREREQUISITE NURSING KNOWLEDGE

- Across the United States, diversity is found among burn units concerning policy, practice, and procedure in the care of thermal injuries and donor-site care. This procedure in no way reproduces that diversity in practice but strives to provide common tenets that may be used for donor-site care.
- A partial-thickness wound is surgically created when a donor site (Fig. 127-1) is harvested to obtain skin for a full-thickness defect. The more dermis moved with the skin graft, the less the graft shrinks with healing; therefore, deeper donor sites may be created to obtain skin for cosmetically significant areas such as the face or hands. Creation of donor sites adds new wounds that can create significant pain. Depending on the percentage of dermis moved for the graft, donor sites created may be superficial or deep partial-thickness wounds that heal in 10 to 20 days (typically, 10 to 14 days; Fig. 127-2).[6]
- Factors that can disrupt or prolong healing include infection, desiccation, edema, adherent dressing changes, poor nutrition, hemodynamic instability, and a variety of pre-existing medical conditions.[2]
- The longer a partial-thickness wound takes to heal, the more significant the scarring; therefore, donor sites can produce minimal or hypertrophic scars.[2] Donor sites retain deep epidermal appendages, so they are generally capable of sweating and bearing hair after they heal. The site may be procured again once healing is complete, but skin from the first procurement of a donor site is always of higher quality than that of repeat procurements.
- Because the dermis is richly supplied with capillaries and nerve endings, donor sites are at risk for bleeding in the first 24 hours and are exquisitely tender to touch. They produce large volumes of serous exudate.
- Donor-site treatment goals include minimizing bleeding, supporting reepithelialization, managing exudate, preventing infection, controlling pain, and minimizing scarring.[9] Epinephrine-soaked dressings, thrombin spray, or compression dressings may be applied in the operating room to attain stasis.[9] A compression dressing is usually used for the first 12 to 24 hours to ensure stasis.[8] After this initial period, compression may be applied for comfort.

- Wounds epithelialize most rapidly in a moist environment. If donor sites are small enough, use of a thin-film polyurethane or hydrocolloid dressing has been shown to promote rapid healing while providing comfort through dressing flexibility and occlusive coverage of nerve endings.[6] Occlusive dressings (sealed on all sides) can be difficult to maintain on larger donor sites because of the substantial volume of exudate.[6] Calcium alginates can be used under occlusive dressings to manage exudate.[6]
- One of the oldest and most cost-effective methods for treatment of donor sites is to apply xeroform (McKesson Brand, San Francisco, CA), wrap with an outer wrap for 12 to 24 hours, and then remove the outer wrap and allow the inner dressing (Xeroform) to remain exposed and dry until the wound heals beneath. The technique is only effective if the dressing dries well and becomes impermeable to bacteria, essentially acting as a scab.[11] Positioning the patient for maximal exposure of the donor sites, preventing prolonged donor-site contact with sheets and clothing, and increasing airflow across the wound are important for this technique to work.[5] If the donor site is large, this procedure creates a rather stiff and uncomfortable protective layer.
- Antimicrobial creams or ointments have also been used on donor sites, essentially treating the wounds in the same way as partial-thickness burns are treated. The disadvantage to this approach is that it requires daily washing of the wound and reapplication of cream and dressings.[11]
- Slow-release silver dressings are gaining popularity for donor-site use. These dressings release silver for 3 or more days; ideally, they are placed on the donor site in the operating room, and the wound is allowed to heal beneath with infrequent or no dressing changes.[6,11]
- Donor sites need to be assessed daily for signs of infection, including periwound warmth and erythema, increased pain, and purulent drainage. Bacteria can delay healing and increase scarring or convert a partial-thickness donor site to a full-thickness wound.[2] Erythema should be outlined to monitor progression, with consideration of either removing the donor-site dressing or applying a topical antimicrobial to penetrate the donor-site dressing. Reopening or "melting" of epithelium in previously healed donor sites is often the result of colonization with gram-positive organisms and may require antibacterial intervention.[4] Heavy hair-bearing donor sites such as the scalp provide

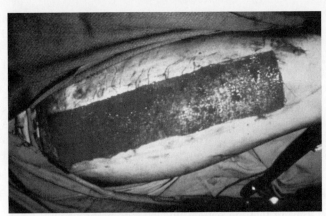

Figure 127-1 Fresh donor site.

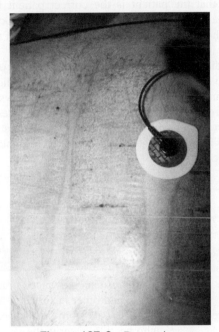

Figure 127-2 Donor sites.

special challenges. Heavy hair growth can lead to matting of hair in the exudate, which can lead to accumulation of protein, proliferation of bacteria, and ingrowth of hair, a condition referred to as chronic folliculitis.[8] This problem can lead to chronic, nonhealing, inflamed wounds or conversion of partial-thickness donor sites to full-thickness wounds. Dressings that prevent drying and wick away the exudate work well.

- Donor sites are often very painful, with the amount of pain variable depending on the dressing technique used. Patients with donor sites usually need scheduled around-the-clock pain medication.[3,7]
- The donor site should not be exposed to the sun for a year after the burn. Apply full-spectrum sunblock to donor sites any time exposure to the sun is anticipated.[10]
- Protect fresh donor sites from dependent edema by wrapping with elastic bandages before sitting or ambulating.

EQUIPMENT

- Personal protective equipment (gown, mask, goggles as needed)
- Nonsterile gloves
- Scissors
- Replacement dressing as needed
- Pain and sedation medication (as prescribed)

Additional equipment, to have available as needed, includes the following:

- Staple remover
- Marking pen

PATIENT AND FAMILY EDUCATION

- Teach the patient and family that donor sites generally heal in 10 to 12 days with variable scarring. *Rationale:* Realistic expectations about healing and scarring are provided.
- Provide donor-site care instructions, and review them with the patient and family. Demonstrate how to assess and manage the donor-site dressing, and have the patient and family return the demonstration. Encourage the patient and family to ask questions. Provide positive feedback. Arrange for home care or clinic visits to follow up on dressings and wound care. *Rationale:* The patient's and family's understanding and ability to perform wound care are validated.
- Patients should be encouraged to avoid smoking. *Rationale:* Smoking causes vasoconstriction, inhibits epithelialization, and decreases tissue oxygenation, all of which delay healing.[2]
- Explain to the patient about the pain and itching sensations associated with donor-site healing.[1,7] *Rationale:* Patients need to know that donor-site pain and itching, although unpleasant, are normal and do not cause concern.
- Teach the patient and family about appropriate use of medications and nonpharmacologic interventions to manage pain and itching.[1] Encourage application of a topical moisturizer after healing.[7] *Rationale:* Comfort is enhanced.
- Teach the patient and family about signs and symptoms of infection and the importance of reporting these in a timely manner.[4] *Rationale:* The patient and family can recognize problems early so that appropriate measures can be instituted by the physician, advanced practice nurse, and other healthcare professionals.
- Provide the patient and family with follow-up appointments and a contact to call with any problems. *Rationale:* This information is necessary for further care and follow-up.
- Assess the family's ability to provide care at home at each follow-up visit. *Rationale:* Continued care of the wound is necessary after discharge.
- Stress the importance of wearing pressure garments if they are indicated. *Rationale:* Pressure garments reduce scarring.[10]
- Inform the patient and family that the donor site should not be exposed to the sun for a year after the burn. Patients should wear clothing that covers wounds or a sunscreen

with sun protection factor (SPF) higher than 15.[10] *Rationale:* The patient and family are prepared for changes that occur after healing.

PATIENT ASSESSMENT AND PREPARATION

Patient Assessment

- Evaluate for the following signs of healing. *Rationale:* Healing should occur within 10 to 12 days unless complications occur.
  - ❖ Decreased pain
  - ❖ Decreased edema
  - ❖ Dressing separation at wound edges with reepithelialization beneath it
  - ❖ Compare degree of healing with expected rate of healing based on number of days since skin procured.
- Evaluate for the following signs and symptoms of infection. *Rationale:* Donor site infection may necessitate antimicrobial intervention.[2]
  - ❖ Foul odor
  - ❖ Purulent drainage
  - ❖ Discoloration
  - ❖ Increased pain
  - ❖ Increasing edema
  - ❖ Cellulitis
  - ❖ Delayed healing
  - ❖ Fever or increasing white blood cell (WBC) count[4]
- Evaluate the adequacy of the pain control by asking the patient to rate the pain on a scale of 0 to 10, both before

and during wound care. *Rationale:* An individualized plan for pain control should be in place for background and procedural pain.[3,7]

- Evaluate the patient's range of motion in the vicinity of the donor site. Physical and occupational therapists may be consulted to assist the patient with maintaining range of motion and with scar management. *Rationale:* Wounds contract during healing; pain and tightness can decrease range of motion. The patient should be encouraged to continue normal movement and range-of-motion exercises.

Patient Preparation

- Ensure that the patient understands preprocedural teaching. Answer questions, and reinforce information as needed. *Rationale:* Understanding of previously taught information is evaluated and reinforced.
- Verify that the patient is the correct patient using two identifiers. *Rationale:* Before performing a procedure, the nurse should ensure the correct identification of the patient for the intended intervention.
- Premedicate the patient for pain and anxiety, as prescribed. Wait to perform the procedure until the medication has had time to work. *Rationale:* Waiting allows time for the medication to take effect and promotes optimal comfort for the patient. Medication reduces pain and anxiety and encourages patient trust and compliance with the procedure.

Procedure for Care of Donor Sites

Steps	Rationale	Special Considerations
1. Prepare all necessary equipment and supplies. Treatment area should be warmed.	Preparation facilitates efficient wound care and prevents needless delays. Warming the room decreases risk for hypothermia.	Notify physician, advanced practice nurse, and other healthcare professionals from other disciplines who need to observe the wound ahead of time so that they can be present while the wound is uncovered.
2. **HH**		
3. **PE**		For larger graft dressing changes, all physicians, advanced practice nurses, and other healthcare professionals participating in the wound care should wear caps, masks, and gowns. Smaller graft changes may require less personal protective equipment.
4. Remove gauze roll and any padding covering inner dressing.	Inner dressing is left in place until the wound heals, unless a problem with infection occurs.	Gauze roll or outer dressing is usually removed after 24 hours if the goal is for inner dressing layer to be exposed to air and dry.
5. Assess the donor site for signs of healing and complications; assess whether the inner dressing needs to be changed. **Proceed to Step 9** if inner donor dressing needs to be changed.	Validates the healing process and identifies complications. Avoid changing inner dressing to facilitate healing.	If inner dressing was stapled in place, staples need to be removed when inner dressing is fully adherent (generally between postoperative days 4 and 7).

Procedure for Care of Donor Sites—*Continued*

Steps	Rationale	Special Considerations
6. Remove and discard gloves; perform HH and apply a pair of clean gloves.	Handling the burn dressing contaminates examination gloves, and clean gloves are needed for wound care.	
7. Gently wash exudate from wound edges with warm tap water and pat dry.	Clears exudate that can harbor microorganisms from area of donor site. Keep covered donor site dry to improve healing.	
8. Use scissors to trim loose edges of donor site dressing. If inner dressing does not need to be changed, **proceed to Step 12 to** complete donor site care.	Because dry inner dressing is not covered, loose edges of dressing can snag and displace inner dressing.	Assess need for outer dressing and apply as needed.
Inner Dressing Change		
1. Remove inner dressing and discard it.		If dressing is adherent, soak with warm tap water to loosen. Do not attempt to remove adherent dressings.
2. Remove and discard gloves; perform HH and apply a pair of clean gloves.	Handling the burn dressing contaminates examination gloves, and clean gloves are needed for wound care.	
3. Gently wash wound with mild pH-neutral soap, rinse with warm tap water, and pat dry.	Cleanses donor site.	Cleanse beyond donor site to reduce microbial count on surrounding tissue. Patients may do better if allowed to cleanse their own wounds.
4. Assess the donor site for progression of healing and complications; outline any inflammation with a marking pen.	Validates the healing process and identifies complications.	
5. Remove and discard gloves; perform HH, and apply a pair of sterile or clean gloves.	Clean gloves are applied after washing a wound.	Sterile gloves may be used when applying dressings to large burn wounds.
6. Cut dressing to the size of the donor site with sterile scissors, apply, and secure in place. Reapply bulky outer dressing if indicated.	Ensures correct fit and adherence. Donor sites may be covered with bulky dressing to maintain moisture barrier, maintain a moist wound surface, or apply a topical antimicrobial soak.	Dressing may be secured with tubular netting or cloth tape applied to the dressing margins.
7. Remove and discard gloves and used supplies.	Reduces transmission of microorganisms.	
8. **HH**		

Procedure continues on following page

Expected Outcomes

- Donor site heals within 2 weeks without complications
- Patient maintains a self-identified, acceptable level of pain relief
- Patient maintains comfort from measures taken for anxiety and itching
- Patient and family verbalize knowledge of patient condition and plan of care
- An optimal level of function is maintained or attained
- Patient and family response and interactions demonstrate adaptation to injury
- Patient and family collaborate in management of care
- At the time of discharge, patient and family verbalize and demonstrate an understanding of posthospital care

Unexpected Outcomes

- Bleeding
- Infection
- Conversion of donor site to deep partial-thickness or full-thickness wound

Patient Monitoring and Care

Steps	Rationale	Reportable Conditions
		These conditions should be reported if they persist despite nursing interventions.
1. Follow institutional standards for assessing pain. Administer analgesia as prescribed. Have the patient rate pain on a validated pain scale; check pain medication orders; and review patient's previous response to pain medication and assess the need to increase the dose. Incorporate nonpharmacologic pain-relief techniques (e.g., relaxation techniques, massage therapy, music, visual imaging).	Identifies need for pain interventions. The donor site pain is minimized by an intact dressing that does not require a dressing change; the patient will have increased pain medication requirements if the dressing needs to be changed. Attention to the patient's pain fosters the patient's trust in the physician, advanced practice nurse, and other healthcare professionals.	- Continued pain despite pain interventions - Nonverbal indications of pain (e.g., restlessness, grimacing, teeth clenching) - Inability to cooperate with wound care - Increased respiratory rate - Verbalization of pain - Increased heart rate - Increased or decreased blood pressure
2. Obtain baseline vital signs before the procedure, monitor them throughout the procedure, and check them for 30 minutes after the procedure is complete.	Changes in vital signs can be a sign that the patient is experiencing pain or anxiety. Decreasing blood pressure, heart rate, and respiratory rate can be complications of pain medication (especially after dressing change is complete and stimulation has stopped).	- Oversedation - Increased or decreased heart rate - Increased or decreased blood pressure - Increased or decreased respiratory rate
3. Assess the donor site for appearance (e.g., dressing wet or dry, dressing adherent, presence of drainage or bleeding, redness at edges) and progression toward healing (e.g., reepithelialization at wound edges).	Observe for usual progression of wound healing versus complications of infection, progression of donor site to deeper wound, and bleeding.	- Foul odor - Purulent or increased amounts of drainage - Cellulitis or edema - Healing tissue developing eschar - Discoloration of wound - Bleeding

Patient Monitoring and Care —*Continued*

Steps	Rationale	Reportable Conditions
4. Encourage exercise and activities of daily living; place patient in a position of optimal function and assess the need for pain medication to facilitate movement. Physical therapy may be necessary to maintain range of motion.[3,10] **(Level D*)**	Donor-site wounds contract during the healing phase. Pain also inhibits movement.	

*Level D: Peer-reviewed professional and organizational standards with the support of clinical study recommendations.

Documentation

Documentation should include the following:
- Patient and family education
- Date and time of wound care
- Appearance (e.g., dressing wet or dry, dressing adherence, presence of drainage or bleeding, redness at edges)
- Progression toward healing (e.g., reepithelialization at wound edges)
- Application of topical agents

- Type of dressing applied
- Pain assessment, interventions, and effectiveness
- Medications given for pain and sedation
- Patient's response to analgesic and sedatives
- Other comfort measures used
- Patient's tolerance of the procedure
- Unexpected outcomes
- Nursing interventions

References and Additional Readings

For a complete list of references and additional readings for this procedure, scan this QR code with any freely available smartphone code reader app, or visit http://booksite.elsevier.com/9780323376624.

128 Skin-Graft Care

Dawn Sculco

PURPOSE: Skin-graft care is performed to promote perfusion to the graft and to prevent infection. Successful graft transplant and care result in maximal function.

PREREQUISITE NURSING KNOWLEDGE

- Skin grafts are used to replace skin on a patient's body that is unable to heal due to the size or thickness of the wound. The original wounds may be from a variety of causes (burns, infections, traumatic injury, etc). An autograft is the only permanent treatment that can heal a large, full-thickness wound, and may also be used to heal partial-thickness wounds with faster closure of the wound. An autograft is a type of skin graft that is created by taking a graft from one site of a patient's body (the donor site) and transplanting it to a different site of the same patient's body (the recipient site). The graft is applied over a clean, surgically excised wound that has been débrided of all nonviable tissue.[1]

- Autografts can be split-thickness skin grafts (STSG), containing the epidermis and part of the dermis, or full-thickness skin grafts (FTSG), containing the epidermis and all of the dermis. The donor site of an STSG is a new exposed wound area that will heal by reepithelization. The FTSG donor site is a full-thickness wound that heals by primary intention due to the harvest of the entire dermis, which will leave a scar.[1,2] The FTSG offers more functionality and a better cosmetic appearance, but is limited by size due to the full-thickness donor site.[3] Therefore, use of the STSG is more common.

- The STSG is procured from an appropriate donor site on the patient's body with a dermatome, a surgical instrument that shaves layers of skin at different depths to be grafted over the wound bed. The STSG is commonly meshed (Fig. 128-1) so that it can be stretched to cover approximately 1.5 to 9 times more surface area than the original donor site. The ability to stretch the donor graft is important when there is limited availability of suitable donor sites or when the wound area that requires grafting is extensive. Meshing the donor skin creates spaces, or interstices, that allow for fluid to escape, which can assist with graft adherence.

- Nonmeshed grafts, called sheet grafts, are used on the face, hands, and some joints because of cosmetic and functional concerns related to appearance and increased shrinkage. A sheet graft covers the same amount of surface area as the donor site. Sheet grafts on the face, neck, and hands are generally inspected within the first 12 to 24 hours to look for fluid collections or graft dislodgement.

- Pockets of serous fluid or blood can accumulate under these grafts and separate the graft from the wound bed, resulting in failure of the graft to adhere or "take" to the wound bed. Therefore evacuation of this fluid is imperative. If the sheet graft has been in place for less than 48 hours and the fluid is near the edge of the sheet graft, the fluid can be rolled to the edge and out (Fig. 128-2).[2]

- Caution should be used when evacuating fluid after vascularization of the graft begins, to avoid disruption of the graft attachment endangering graft take. Another option for fluid removal is to make a small nick in the sheet graft directly over the area of fluid accumulation and gently expressing the fluid through the hole. In either case, the fluid should be gently dabbed away with gauze dampened with sterile normal saline solution or sterile water.[5] Seromas and hematomas tend to redevelop in the same areas, so careful charting should reflect location of any fluid pockets (blebs). Close monitoring of these areas should occur at least every 8 hours until bleb formation is no longer noted.

- Cultured epidermal autografts (CEA) are grown from a sample of the patient's own epidermal cells in a laboratory. CEAs, most frequently used with burn injuries, are an option when the patient does not have enough unburned tissue for donor sites to cover the burn in a reasonable period of time. The use of CEAs has been found to be a successful adjunct to the use of STSG. However, due to cost, CEA use is very limited. In addition, the grafts are fragile, and successful take of the graft is dependent on experience of the burn team with this treatment.[1,10]

- The use of artificial skin and other options for wound coverage has expanded in recent years. Currently, the use of these wound coverings is limited to providing temporary wound coverage or allowing for dermal regeneration while waiting for suitable donor sites for definitive wound closure with autografting.

- Allografts, also called homografts, are fresh or cyropreserved grafts from human donors. Allografts are considered the gold standard for temporary coverage of wounds. Allograft benefits include prevention of wound desiccation, promotion of granulation tissue, and decreased water and heat loss.[1]

- The care for temporary grafts is different than permanent skin grafts and generally unique to the type and manufacturer.

- In the operating room, all nonviable tissue is surgically excised to create a wound bed able to support a skin graft (Fig. 128-3); therefore, the grafted area should be observed for bleeding for the first 24 hours.
- The goals after a graft placement are to protect the wound bed from infection and desiccation and to ensure that no movement (shearing) of the graft occurs while it is

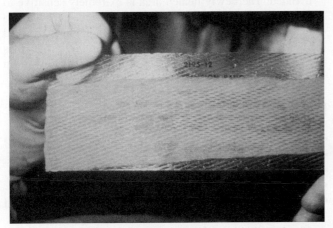

Figure 128-1 Meshed split-thickness skin graft.

becoming vascularized. Neovascularization begins within the first 24 hours of surgery as capillaries grow up into the graft, securing the graft permanently to its new site. The newly grafted tissue must be well protected from shearing forces for 5 to 7 days to allow for graft adherence to the wound bed. With meshed skin grafts, the interstices of the autograft fill with granulation tissue and the epidermis of the autograft migrates over the granulation tissues. Successful grafting is often expressed as a percentage of graft "take," or adherence and vascularization of the graft to the new site.[1] A barrier dressing (e.g., Biobrane allograft [UDL Laboratories, Rockford, IL]) protects the wound (with or without a bulky dressing added), or a minimal nonadherent dressing (e.g., Xeroform [McKesson Brand, San Francisco]) is used with a bulky dressing over the grafted tissue to act as the barrier to infection, prevent drying and shearing. The first dressing change is usually done after 3 to 5 days. Most centers use clean techniques for dressing removal and donor-site cleansing and use sterile techniques for dressing application only.[5]

- Negative-pressure wound therapy (NPWT) may also be used as a dressing on the STSG to enhance the take of the graft, by providing fluid removal, bolstering, and protection of the graft. NPWT is a mechanical wound-care

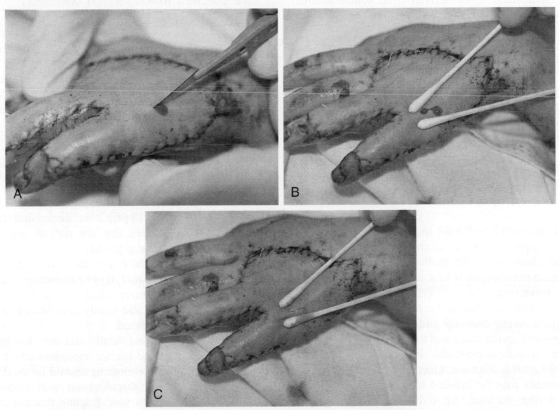

Figure 128-2 **A,** A No. 11 surgical blade and cotton-tipped applicator are used to blade a new sheet graft. Note that the blade is held so that the tip of the cutting surface comes into contact with only the graft. **B,** Cotton-tipped applicators are rolled gently over the graft toward the slit to express fluid that has collected between the graft and the wound bed surface. When deblebbing thick grafts, adequate-sized slits are important to avoid recurring buildup of fluid, which may jeopardize graft survivability and result in scarring. **C,** Blebs tend to recur in the same place. Vigilance about deblebbing at least once every 8 hours until bleb formation ceases is advisable. Documentation of bleb formation and location ensures that the next caregiver is aware of graft sites in need of close monitoring. *(From Carrougher GJ:* Burn care and therapy, *St Louis, 1998, Mosby.)*

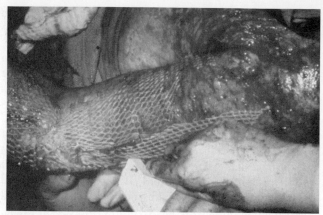

Figure 128-3 Meshed split-thickness skin graft covering the arm, with the remainder of the wound bed ready to be grafted.

treatment that uses controlled negative pressure (via a machine, tubing, foam, and sealed dressing) to accelerate wound healing. A nonadherent dressing is placed on the graft before the NPWT dressing during surgery. The NPWT dressing is usually changed every 3 to 7 days.[6,11] (See Procedure 136 for more information on NPWT.)

- The graft is usually stapled or sutured in place before covering with the dressings or NPWT. Fibrin sealants, a surgical hemostatic agent derived from human plasma, may also be used in place of staples for adherence of sheet grafts.[4]

- Initial healing of the grafted area should occur in 7 to 10 days. The graft area is immobilized for 4 to 5 days to prevent dislocation and shearing. Splints and immobilizers are used during this time to prevent disruption of grafts and to provide therapeutic positioning of extremities.[5]

- If a patient is allowed to mobilize after surgery, leg grafts must be supported with Ace wraps or other compressive dressings when the patient's legs are dependent for the first 3 to 5 days after surgery. This prevents capillary engorgement and hematoma formation beneath the graft.[7,8] Grafted extremities should be elevated when the patient is supine.

- Signs of successful graft take include vascularization of the graft, reepithelialization of the interstices, decreased pain, and adherence of the graft. Signs of complications include graft necrosis, graft loss, cellulitis, purulent drainage, and fever.

- Skin grafts contract during the healing and remodeling phases. Continuing mobility and proper positioning are vital to prevent contractures and loss of function. Self-care and range-of-motion exercises should be encouraged as soon as the graft is adherent. Once the wounds heal, pressure garments may be ordered to be worn at all times, except during bathing, to reduce hypertrophic scar formation.

- Pain related to care of wounds is complicated by several components: background pain (pain that is continuously present), procedural pain (intermittent pain related to procedures and routine care), and anxiety. Unrelieved pain can lead to stress-related immunosuppression, increased potential for infection, delayed wound healing, and depression. The management of pain should use a multi-dimensional approach, including pharmacological and nonpharmacologic methods, tailored to individual patient needs.[3,9]

- Wound healing is dependent on energy production from nutrition. Nutrition that includes protein, carbohydrates, fat, amino acids, and micronutrients is paramount for energy production.[12]

- Exposure of the healed skin graft to the sun should be avoided. The newly healed area is extremely sensitive to sunlight, and permanent discoloration can occur. To prevent discoloration, the patient should protect grafted areas with clothing or sunscreen. During the first year, as the patient's graft matures, the risk for skin discoloration slowly decreases.

EQUIPMENT

- Personal protective equipment (i.e., gowns, mask, goggles)
- Nonsterile gloves
- Sterile gloves
- Scissors and forceps
- Warm tap water (sometimes sterile water or sterile normal saline solution is used for the first dressing change)
- Clean washcloths
- Nonadherent dressing/gauze (e.g., Adaptic [Johnson and Johnson, New Brunswick, NJ], Xeroform)
- Secondary dressings, as needed
- Pain and antianxiolytic medication (as prescribed)

Additional equipment, to have available as needed, includes the following:

- Splints (to be secured with gauze roll, hook and loop closure [e.g., Velcro]), elastic bandage such as ace wraps, or self-adherent wrap (e.g., Coban, 3M, St. Paul, MN)
- Towels or waterproof pads
- Staple remover

PATIENT AND FAMILY EDUCATION

- Explain the procedure for skin-graft care to the patient and family. *Rationale:* Explanation diminishes fear of the unknown and ensures that the patient and family are knowledgeable about graft care.

- Inform the patient and family that the grafted area needs to be protected for 5 to 7 days to encourage graft take and reduce the risk of mechanical trauma to the graft site. *Rationale:* Patient's and family's assistance in protecting the graft site is increased.

- Inform the patient and family that the skin graft should not be exposed to the sun for approximately 1 year. Sunscreen and protective clothing should be used thereafter; some scarring and discoloration will occur but will improve over the first year. Explain that the grafted area will not grow hair or be able to sweat because of permanent loss of these dermal appendages. *Rationale:* The patient and family are prepared for changes that will be present after hospital discharge, and anxieties about body image are addressed.

- Discuss the importance of proper positioning. Explain the need for continuing mobility through self-care and range-of-motion exercises as soon as the graft is adherent and throughout the healing phase. *Rationale:* Education prevents contractures and loss of function associated with healing skin grafts.

- Assess the family's ability to provide care at home. *Rationale:* Continued care of the wound is necessary after discharge.
- As appropriate, provide detailed wound-care instructions in writing and review them with the patient and family. Demonstrate exactly what to do, and have the patient and family return demonstrations before the planned discharge. Continue to involve the patient and family in wound care for the remainder of the admission, and encourage them to ask questions. Provide positive feedback. Arrange for home care or clinic visits to follow up on dressings and wound care. *Rationale:* Education validates patient and family understanding and ability to perform wound care independently and allows time for them to develop a level of comfort. The opportunity to reinforce important points is provided.
- Teach the patient and family about pain and pruritus medications as prescribed. Provide the name of a water-based lotion to apply to healed areas. *Rationale:* Comfort at home is supported.
- Teach patient and family about signs and symptoms of infection and the importance of reporting these in a timely manner. *Rationale:* The patient and family can recognize problems early so that appropriate measures can be instituted by the healthcare team.
- Emphasize the importance of wearing pressure garments and splints. *Rationale:* Scar formation and contractures are reduced.
- Schedule follow-up appointments and provide the name of someone to call with any problems. *Rationale:* This information is necessary for further care and follow-up.
- Work with a vocational rehabilitation counselor to formulate plan for the patient's return to work. *Rationale:* Depending on the severity of the patient's injuries, the patient may be physically unable to return to former employment or may need assistance with job modifications and accommodations. Developing a back-to-work plan based on any new limitations increases the patient's chance of successfully returning to work.

PATIENT ASSESSMENT AND PREPARATION

Patient Assessment

- Assess vital signs, including temperature. *Rationale:* Baseline vital signs allow for comparison during and after the procedure to evaluate patient tolerance and need for pain medication.
- Evaluate the success of graft take: vascularization of the graft; reepithelialization of the interstices; decreased pain;

and adherence of the graft. *Rationale:* Graft success or adherence to the wound is assessed with each episode of care to evaluate healing.

- Monitor for signs of complications: fever, elevated white blood cell count, cellulitis, increased purulent drainage, or saturation of the secondary dressing. *Rationale:* Baseline and ongoing assessment for signs of graft failure to include possible infection are important for early identification of complications to minimize graft loss.
- Compare the patient's rate of healing with the expected rate of wound healing for the number of days after the skin graft. *Rationale:* Initial healing of grafted area should occur in 7 to 10 days.
- Determine adequacy of the pain-control regimen by asking the patient to rate the pain on a scale of 0 to 10 (or other scale as appropriate), both before wound care (background pain) and during the dressing change. *Rationale:* An individualized plan for pain control should be in place for background and procedural pain. In addition to the traditional use of pain and anxiety medications, alternative therapies should be included (e.g., relaxation techniques, distraction, massage therapy, music therapy). The patient's medication requirements should decrease as the grafted area heals.
- Assess the patient's level of function in the grafted area. *Rationale:* Skin grafts contract during the healing phase, and immobility enhances loss of function. The patient should be encouraged to continue normal movement and range-of-motion exercises after graft take has been established.[5]

Patient Preparation

- Ensure that patient understands preprocedural teachings. Answer questions as they arise, and reinforce information as needed. *Rationale:* Understanding of previously taught information is evaluated and reinforced.
- Verify that the patient is the correct patient using two identifiers. *Rationale:* Before performing a procedure, the nurse should ensure the correct identification for the patient for the intended intervention.
- Notify other appropriate physicians, advanced practice nurses, and other healthcare professionals who need to assess the graft (e.g., a physician) or perform a task (e.g., range-of-motion exercises by a physical therapist) at the time of dressing change. *Rationale:* Organization of care allows important assessment and interventions to take place without causing extra pain and stress to the patient.
- Premedicate the patient with pain medication and any sedation and anxiolytic medications as prescribed. Allow an appropriate amount of time for medications to begin to take effect before starting wound care. *Rationale:* Premedication reduces pain and anxiety and allows time for medication to take effect and promote optimal comfort for the patient. Patient trust and compliance with the procedure are encouraged.

Procedure | for Care of Skin Grafts

Steps	Rationale	Special Considerations
1. Prepare all necessary equipment and supplies.	Preparation facilitates efficient wound care and prevents needless delays.	
2. **HH**		
3. **PE**		For larger-graft dressing changes, all physicians, advanced practice nurses, and other healthcare professionals participating in the wound care should apply cap, mask, and gown. Smaller-graft changes may require less personal protective equipment. If family is doing dressing changes at home, mask, cap, and gown are not used.
4. Remove bulky, outer dressings and discard. Place a towel or pad under exposed extremity.	Old dressings can contain large amounts of body secretions and blood. A towel allows a place for the patient to rest an extremity during care.	The initial dressing is commonly left in place for 3–5 days, while the bulky, outer dressings are changed and the nonadherent gauze is left in place. Follow provider orders and institutional standards.
5. Remove and discard gloves; perform HH and apply clean gloves.	Examination gloves are contaminated by handling the burn dressing; clean gloves are needed for wound care.	
6. If prescribed, gently lift nonadherent gauze from grafted site, anchoring graft in place as needed. *Note:* The surgeon may have stapled on a dressing that is to remain in place until the skin graft heals (e.g., Biobrane). Follow institutional standards.	Some grafts are not firmly attached to the wound bed and can be pulled loose for up to 5 days after grafting.	Normal saline solution or warm tap water may be used to loosen dressings stuck to the graft area.
7. Gently rinse the graft site and surrounding tissue with normal saline solution or warm tap water with gauze or washcloths.	Cleanses wound of exudate and reduces microorganisms. Use pH-neutral cleansing agents.	Special care is necessary during the cleansing process not to displace the skin graft.
8. Use scissors and forceps to remove loose necrotic tissue. If the graft is a sheet graft, assess for and remove any pockets of fluid under the graft.	Clears debris that can harbor microorganisms. Pockets of fluid separate the graft from the wound bed, which is vital for blood supply, causing graft loss in that area.	If the sheet graft has been in place for <48 hours and the fluid is near the edge of the sheet graft, roll the fluid to the edge and out; otherwise, make a small nick in the sheet graft directly over the area of fluid accumulation and gently express the fluid through the hole. Gently remove exudate with gauze dampened with sterile normal saline solution or sterile water. Follow institutional standard.
9. Remove staples as prescribed that are no longer needed to hold graft or dressing in place.	Prevents embedding of staples, local irritation, infection, and scarring.	Staples can be removed starting 5–7 days after grafting. Removing a large number of staples may be very painful and may necessitate an anesthesia-assisted procedure. Follow institutional standard.
10. Assess the graft for progression of healing and for complications.	Validates the healing process and identifies complications.	

Procedure for Care of Skin Grafts—*Continued*

Steps	Rationale	Special Considerations
11. Apply nonadherent dressing (if interstices are open), cover with secondary dressings, and secure; or apply moisturizer to healed adherent graft areas where interstices are closed and cover with thin secondary dressings to promote mobility.	Protects graft while healing.	A water-based lotion is used to prevent drying and reduce itching when interstices are closed.
12. Remove and discard gloves; perform HH and apply clean gloves.	Reduces transmission of microorganisms.	
13. Apply splints to the appropriate limb and elevate the involved extremity. Hands and arms may be elevated with pillows or elastic net sling. Elevate the head of the bed.	Maintains position of function, prevents contractures, and reduces edema and pain.	If possible, prevent the patient from lying on grafted areas. Consider the use of pressure-reduction mattress for grafts or donor sites on posterior surfaces. After the initial period of immobilization, splints are used only when the patient is unable to participate in range-of-motion exercises or self-care.
14. Remove and discard **PE**.		
15. **HH**		

Expected Outcomes

- Graft take of >90% is attained
- Patient maintains a self-identified acceptable level of pain relief
- Patient attains comfort from measures provided for anxiety and itching
- Patient and family verbalize knowledge of patient condition and plan of care
- An optimal level of function is maintained
- Patient and family response and interactions demonstrate adaptation to injury
- Patient and family collaborate in management of care
- At the time of discharge, patient and family verbalize and demonstrate an understanding of posthospital care

Unexpected Outcomes

- Bleeding
- Infection
- Graft failure

Procedure continues on following page

Patient Monitoring and Care

Steps	Rationale	Reportable Conditions
		These conditions should be reported if they persist despite nursing interventions.
1. Follow institutional standards for assessing pain. Administer analgesia as prescribed. Ask the patient to rate pain on a scale of 0–10 (or other appropriate scale); check the orders for analgesic, sedative, and anxiolytic agents before dressing changes; evaluate the patient's medication requirements with previous dressing changes; and assess the need for more medication throughout the dressing change. Incorporate alternative pain-relief techniques (e.g., relaxation techniques, distraction, massage therapy, music therapy, visual imaging).[9]	Identifies need for pain interventions. The patient with new skin grafts will have some baseline pain that requires pain medication; pain medication requirements may be increased and sedation or anxiolytic agents may also be necessary for the procedural pain involved in graft care.[9] Attention to the patient's pain fosters the patient's trust in healthcare personnel to control pain and promotes cooperation with future graft care.	• Continued pain despite pain interventions • Increased heart rate • Increased or decreased blood pressure • Increased respiratory rate • Verbalization of pain • Nonverbal indications of pain (restlessness, grimacing, teeth clenching) • Inability to cooperate with dressing change
2. Monitor vital signs throughout the procedure, and continue to assess for 30 minutes after procedure is complete.	Changes in vital signs can be an indication that the patient is experiencing pain or anxiety. Decreasing blood pressure, heart rate, and respiratory rate can be complications of pain medication (especially after dressing change is complete and stimulation has stopped).	• Oversedation • Increased or decreased heart rate • Increased or decreased blood pressure • Increased or decreased respiratory rate and depth of respirations • High peak pressures on ventilator
3. Assess graft site for appearance (e.g., color, drainage, bleeding, graft necrosis, graft loss, cellulitis) and progression toward healing (e.g., vascularization of the graft, reepithelialization of the interstices, decreased pain, adherence of the graft).	Observe for usual progression of wound healing versus complications.	• Foul odor • Purulent or increased amounts of drainage • Increased pain • Cellulitis • Hematoma or fluid collection under sheet grafts • Graft necrosis • Sloughing • Bleeding
4. Place the patient in a position of optimal function during the initial period of immobilization of newly grafted areas, with splints used to maintain position. After the first 5 days, encourage exercise, activities of daily living, and range-of-motion exercises during dressing changes. Use pain medication as needed to facilitate mobility.[2] **(Level E*)**	Grafted skin contracts during the healing phase if not correctly splinted and exercised. Loss of function is a complication of immobility. Pain inhibits patients from moving.	• Contractures • Loss of function

*Level E: Multiple case reports, theory-based evidence from expert opinions, or peer-reviewed professional organizational standards without clinical studies to support recommendations.

Patient Monitoring and Care —*Continued*

Steps	Rationale	Reportable Conditions
5. Monitor the patient's tolerance of tube feedings or ingestion of a high-calorie, high-protein diet with supplements[3]; encourage nutritious diet and discourage empty calories. Limit free water.[12,13] **(Level D*)**	Nutrition is necessary for wound healing.[3] Burn patients are hypermetabolic.[12,13]	• Poor wound healing • Graft failure
6. Continue to follow institutional standards for assessing pain. Administer analgesia as prescribed.	Identifies need for pain interventions.	• Continued pain despite pain interventions

*Level D: Peer-reviewed professional and organizational standards with the support of clinical study recommendations.

Documentation

Documentation should include the following:
- Patient and family education
- Date and time of graft care
- Appearance of graft site (e.g., color, drainage, bleeding, graft necrosis, sloughing, cellulitis)
- Progression toward healing (e.g., adherence and vascularization of the graft, reepithelialization of the interstices, decreased pain)
- Dressings and topicals applied
- Pain assessment, interventions, and effectiveness
- Medications given for pain and sedation
- Patient's response to analgesics and sedatives
- Other comfort measures used
- Patient's tolerance of the procedure
- Unexpected outcomes
- Nursing interventions

References and Additional Readings

For a complete list of references and additional readings for this procedure, scan this QR code with any freely available smartphone code reader app, or visit http://booksite.elsevier.com/9780323376624.

PROCEDURE

129

Intracompartmental Pressure AP Monitoring

Julia E. Dunning

PURPOSE: Compartment syndrome can occur within any confined anatomical region when elevations in tissue pressure are sufficient to cause neurovascular compromise of the tissues in that region or compartment. Typically, diagnosis of this syndrome is made with serial clinical examinations of the involved extremity. However, in patients with inconclusive physical findings or with an altered level of consciousness, direct measurement of the intracompartmental pressure is a useful diagnostic adjunct.

PREREQUISITE NURSING KNOWLEDGE

- Nurses performing intracompartmental pressure monitoring (IPM) must have detailed knowledge of the anatomy of the involved limb compartments (Fig. 129-1), including external landmarks associated with each compartment. Compartment syndrome may also develop in the abdomen (abdominal compartment syndrome). Refer to Procedure 112 for information on intraabdominal pressure monitoring.
- All clinicians involved with performing and assisting with the procedure should have knowledge of aseptic techniques.
- Physicians, advanced practice nurses, and other healthcare professionals should be trained and approved by their facilities to perform IPM. This should include supervised training in the techniques used for IPM and opportunities to maintain clinical competence.
- Clinicians should have a high index of suspicion that the patient is at risk for developing compartment syndrome. Etiologies can be divided into internal and external sources. Examples of internal causes include fractures, contusions, and edema formation associated with crush injuries or reperfusion injuries. External sources are generally related to compression of the limb and include such things as eschar from burn injuries, splints, casts, dressings, and immobility.[1,9] Definitive treatment may be as simple as releasing a splint, cast, or dressing. More advanced treatment may require release of the compartment with an escharotomy or fasciotomy.

- The pathophysiology of compartment syndrome is related to compromised perfusion. Blood flow to any tissue or organ requires a sufficient perfusion pressure, which is generally calculated as the mean arterial pressure minus the intracompartmental pressure and should be 70 to 80 mm Hg.[2] Therefore, as the mean arterial pressure decreases or the intracompartmental pressure increases, the perfusion to the tissue is reduced. Compartment syndrome occurs when the pressure within the muscle compartment rises above the capillary perfusion pressure gradient, causing cellular anoxia, muscle ischemia, and death.[4]
- Normal compartment pressure within an unaffected compartment is considered less than 10 mm Hg.[3,5] Clinically significant pressure changes are generally defined in one of two ways:
  - ❖ An absolute value of more than 30 mm Hg in the presence of other signs and symptoms of compartment syndrome. Injury of the area may lead to elevations of the intracompartmental pressure in the absence of actual compartment syndrome.[7] Positioning of the extremity may also cause elevations in intracompartmental pressure, particularly when assessing dependent compartments.
  - ❖ A delta compartment pressure (Δp) of less than 30 mm Hg: the diastolic blood pressure minus the intracompartmental pressure. This measurement may be a more reliable indicator of the risk for development of compartment syndrome because it takes into account blood pressure.[8,10]
- The diagnosis of compartment syndrome based solely on a single intracompartmental pressure measurement has a high false-positive rate and therefore should be used only to confirm clinical suspicion.[12]
- Acute compartment syndrome is a true orthopedic emergency. Signs and symptoms can develop in as little as 2 hours after injury. Ischemic damage to muscles and nerves can start in 4 to 6 hours, with permanent damage occurring in 12 to 24 hours.[3]

AP   This procedure should be performed only by physicians, advanced practice nurses, and other healthcare professionals (including critical care nurses) with additional knowledge, skills, and demonstrated competence per professional licensure or institutional standard.

Compartments of the Calf

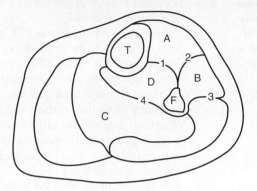

A Anterior compartment
B Lateral (peroneal) compartment
C Superficial posterior compartment
D Deep posterior compartment
T Tibia
F Fibula
1 Interosseous membrane
2 Anterior intermuscular septum
3 Posterior intermuscular septum
4 Intermuscular septum

Compartments of the Forearm

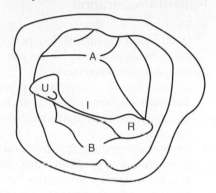

A Volar (anterior) compartment
B Dorsal (posterior) compartment
I Interosseous membrane
R Radius
U Ulna

Compartments of the Thigh

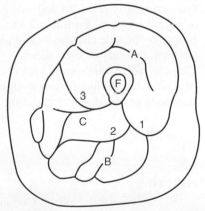

A Anterior compartment
B Postorior compartment
C Medial compartment
F Femur
1 Lateral intermuscular
   septum
2 Posterior intermuscular
   septum
3 Medial intermuscular
   septum

Figure 129-1 Muscle compartments of the calf, forearm, and thigh. *(Tiwari A, Haq AI, Myint F, Hamilton G: Acute compartment syndromes,* Br J Surg *8:397–412, 2002.)*

EQUIPMENT

- Electronic pressure monitoring device (bedside pressure monitor or a handheld monitoring device)
- Prefilled sterile saline solution syringe
- Dedicated disposable tubing with needle
- Chlorhexidine gluconate
- 1% lidocaine without epinephrine
- Sterile gloves
- Sterile dressing
- One roll of hypoallergenic tape

PATIENT AND FAMILY EDUCATION

- Explain the indications and rationale for performing this procedure to the patient and family. *Rationale:* Explanation of the procedure may decrease patient and family anxiety and assist in patient cooperation.

- Explain steps of the procedure to the patient and family (if applicable). Answer any questions as they arise. **Rationale:** Explanation reinforces understanding of previously presented information and may assist in allaying anxiety.
- Inform the patient that pain medication will be given before the procedure is initiated. **Rationale:** This promotes patient comfort.

PATIENT ASSESSMENT AND PREPARATION

Patient Assessment

- Review the patient's history for conditions associated with the development of compartment syndrome. **Rationale:** This review raises the index of suspicion for diagnosis of compartment syndrome leading to early detection and treatment.
- Clinical presentation of compartment syndrome is traditionally listed with a series of "Ps."[1,11] **Rationale:** Presence of these symptoms may be sufficient to diagnose acute compartment syndrome in neurologically intact patients. In patients with an impaired level of consciousness, these symptoms signal the need for IPM. Pain assessment in the setting of compartment syndrome is most useful in the conscious patient due to the ability of the patient to identify quality and location of pain.
  - *Pain:* In addition to being the most sensitive identifier, pain is the most commonly reported and earliest symptom of compartment syndrome.[6] Pain from compartment syndrome is often difficult to differentiate from that which is caused by the primary injury and is described as out of proportion to the injury or minimally responsive to analgesic interventions (e.g., intravenous narcotics). It is also exacerbated by active or passive stretching of the muscle groups involved.
  - *Parasthesia:* This sign precedes loss of motor function and occurs as pressure increases on the affected nerve. Parasthesia and tingling are early *symptoms*. Loss of two-point discrimination may be an early *sign*.
  - *Paresis* or *paralysis:* This sign is a late finding that occurs as a result of pressure on the nerve or necrosis of the affected muscles.
  - *Pulselessness:* Pulselessness is another late finding, from occlusion of the arterioles by the increasing intracompartmental pressure. This sign also results in pallor or coolness of the affected extremity.
  - *Pressure:* Tense edema and firmness in the affected extremity are the earliest and only noninvasive objective findings in early compartment syndrome. It is important to remember that this may be the only initial sign of compartment syndrome in the sedated, unresponsive, or obtunded patient.[9] Pallor may be seen in the affected limb, which could also be mottled or cyanotic. Elevations in intracompartmental pressure are also considered part of the confirmatory diagnosis.

Patient Preparation

- Verify that the patient is the correct patient using two identifiers. **Rationale:** Before performing a procedure, the nurse should ensure the correct identification of the patient for the intended intervention.
- Obtain a formal consent, if the procedure is not emergent. **Rationale:** Informed consent documents that the patient or family understands the explanation and need for the procedure.
- Remove constricting dressings and bandages. Assist with the modification of splints, casts, and other devices on the affected extremity. **Rationale:** Removal reduces external pressure on the tissue of the affected extremity.
- Place the patient in the supine position with the extremity at the level of the heart. **Rationale:** Access to the affected compartment is provided and maintains the extremity in a neutral position. Positioning the extremity above the heart may impede circulation and place it in a dependent position, and may worsen edema.
- Consider administration of a short-acting analgesic and/or anxiolytic. **Rationale:** An analgesic and/or anxiolytic decreases patient discomfort during the procedure.

Procedure	for Intracompartmental Pressure Monitoring	
Steps	Rationale	Special Considerations

Many one-time and continuous intracompartmental pressure-monitoring devices are available in healthcare settings. This procedure assumes the use of the Stryker Intracompartmental Pressure Sensor (Stryker Medical, Kalamazoo, MI; Fig. 129-2).

Steps	Rationale	Special Considerations
1. **HH**		
2. **PE**		
3. Cleanse the insertion site with antiseptic solution.	Reduces bacterial flora on the skin.	Allow the antiseptic solution to dry for maximal effectiveness.
4. Remove gloves and wash hands.		
5. Assemble the disposable needle, prefilled sterile saline solution syringe, and pressure transducer.	Prepares the monitoring system.	

Procedure for Intracompartmental Pressure Monitoring—*Continued*

Steps	Rationale	Special Considerations

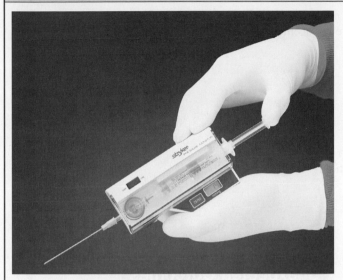

Figure 129-2 Stryker intracompartmental pressure monitor. (*Courtesy Stryker Instruments.*)

Steps	Rationale	Special Considerations
6. Place the assembled disposable system into the pressure-monitoring device. A. Ensure that the system is securely inserted and that the wings of the syringe are flat against the device. B. Close the cover until an audible click is heard. **(Level M*)**	Prepares the monitoring system.	
7. Tilt the device so that the needle is at least 45 degrees upward and purge the system with the saline solution. **(Level M)**	Removes air bubbles and ensures an accurate reading.[10]	
8. Apply nonsterile gloves.		
9. Inject local anesthetic agent at the site.	Increases patient comfort.	Consider concomitant use of intravenous (IV) analgesics or anxiolytics if appropriate for patient's condition.
10. Determine landmarks for insertion.	Place the patient in the supine position and identify landmarks for anterior, deep posterior, superficial posterior, and lateral compartments of the calf.[4]	Differences in needle-insertion location can affect the measured value.
11. A. Estimate the angle of insertion with the pressure-monitoring device. B. Turn the device on and press the "zero" button. C. Wait until the display shows that the device is zeroed. **(Level M)**	Eliminate atmospheric pressure, ensuring accurate reading.	
12. Remove the needle cover and insert 1–3 cm depending on which compartment is being measured.	Depth of needle insertion is dependent on compartment being assessed.	
13. Inject 0.1–0.3 mL of saline solution into the compartment. **(Level M)**	Equilibrates the device to allow for pressure measurement.	
14. Observe the pressure reading displayed on the device.	Allow the device to equilibrate to a constant reading	

*Level M: Manufacturer's recommendations only.

Procedure continues on following page

Procedure for Intracompartmental Pressure Monitoring—*Continued*

Steps	Rationale	Special Considerations
15. Verify placement by manually pressing on the tissue near the insertion site or by flexing and extending the extremity distal to the insertion site (e.g., ankle, wrist, or knee).	Fluctuations in pressure readings verify correct placement of the needle.	Patients with normal compartment physiology have a rapid rise in pressure during palpation or contraction of the muscle, with a rapid return to baseline pressure. Patients with compartment syndrome have a slow return to baseline pressure after relaxation of the muscle.
16. Remove and discard the needle and syringe in appropriate receptacles. Apply an occlusive sterile dressing to the puncture site.	Reduces the risk of contamination.	
17. Discard used supplies.		
18. 🄷🄷		

Expected Outcomes

- Procedure completed without complications in a timely manner
- Minimal patient discomfort
- Pressure readings consistent with clinical presentation of the patient's extremity
- If compartment syndrome is present, a rapid fasciotomy of the involved compartment is required; obtain immediate surgical consultation as necessary

Unexpected Outcomes

- Failure to recognize compartment syndrome, resulting in long-term morbidity for the patient
- Inaccurate pressure readings obtained
- Excessive bleeding from the catheter-insertion site
- Signs and symptoms of procedure-related infection

Patient Monitoring and Care

Steps	Rationale	Reportable Conditions
		These conditions should be reported if they persist despite nursing interventions.
1. Complete a neurovascular assessment of the affected extremity hourly and as necessary.	Documentation and review of serial trends in assessment detect the onset and development of compartment syndrome.	• Onset of pain or worsening of pain despite administration of analgesic agents • Paresthesia or hypoesthesia of the affected extremity • Changes in the extremity skin color (mottling, cyanosis, pallor) and skin temperature • Decrease or loss of peripheral pulses • Paralysis of the affected extremity • Increase in circumference and tenseness of the extremity
2. Assess the insertion site for signs and symptoms of infection.	The needle insertion site may be a source of infection.	• Erythema, swelling, or drainage around the insertion site • Increase in skin warmth surrounding the insertion site • Increased pain and tenderness at the insertion site • Increase in white blood cell count on complete blood count • Fever
3. Follow institutional standards for assessing pain. Administer analgesia as prescribed.	Identifies need for pain interventions.	• Continued pain despite pain interventions

Documentation

Documentation should include the following:

- Consent information for the procedure, including potential complications
- Clinical findings before and after compartment pressure measurement
- Description of the compartment(s) assessed
- Medications administered during the procedure
- Results of the compartment pressure measurement
- The condition of the puncture site and dressing after the needle is removed
- Description of how the patient tolerated the procedure
- Development of unexpected outcomes
- Additional interventions
- Pain assessment and response to interventions

References and Additional Readings

For a complete list of references and additional readings for this procedure, scan this QR code with any freely available smartphone code reader app, or visit http://booksite.elsevier.com/9780323376624.

130 Suture and Staple Removal

Brian D. Schaad

PURPOSE: Sutures and staples are placed to approximate tissues that have been separated. When wound healing is sufficient to maintain closure, sutures and staples are removed.

PREREQUISITE NURSING KNOWLEDGE

- Wound healing is a nonspecific response to injury. It involves the biologic processes of inflammation, collagen metabolism, and contraction in an overlapping, integrated continuum. Wound healing is divided into three phases: inflammatory, fibroblastic, and remodeling. The condition of the tissues and the mechanism of wound closure determine the relative duration of these phases and the end result of the healing process.
- Factors influencing the choice of wound closure method are determined by risk for infection, wound location, need for tension, cosmetic considerations, age and condition of the patient, and cost.
- There are three types of sutures: nonabsorbable, absorbable (which dissolve in as little as 10 days), and slowly absorbable (which take up to 6 months to completely dissolve).[4]
- In addition to conventional metal staples, absorbable staples are available that are placed under the skin by the stapling device and absorb within a few months. The use of the absorbable staple has been found to save both time and cost, with comparable cosmetic outcomes to conventional metal staples.[1]
- Nonabsorbable sutures and staples must be completely removed to avoid further tissue inflammation, possible infection, and unnecessary discomfort to the patient.
- Retention sutures are a special type of suture made of very strong material, with each stitch passing through a larger amount of tissue than conventional sutures. They may be used to reinforce a primarily closed and sutured incision or to aid in the management of the open abdomen. Retention sutures reduce the risk of evisceration, allowing ongoing dressing changes and gradual closure of the abdominal incision.[3]
- Timing of suture and staple removal depends on the following (Table 130-1):
  - Shape, size, and location of the incision
  - Absence of inflammation, drainage, and infection
  - The patient's general condition
  - Type of suture used
- Timing of suture removal may be prolonged in patients with the following risk factors:
  - Steroid use
  - Irradiation treatment
  - Cytotoxic agent use
  - Diabetes
  - Rheumatoid arthritis
  - Trace element imbalance
  - Advanced age

EQUIPMENT

- Nonsterile gloves and mask
- Sterile gloves, towel, or drape
- Sterile swab with antiseptic cleaning solution according to facility's policy (e.g., chlorhexidine)
- 4 × 4 gauze pads
- Suture removal kit with scissors and forceps (if no kit is available, obtain sterile scissor and forceps)

or

- Staple remover
- Skin tape or adhesive skin strips (e.g., Steri-Strips) of appropriate width
- Skin adherent (recommended because it helps with adherence and protects the periwound area)

PATIENT AND FAMILY EDUCATION

- Explain the procedure to the patient and family. Reassure the patient that he or she may feel a pulling or stinging sensation as the sutures or staples are removed. Assure the patient that the wound is healing properly and that removal of the sutures or staples does not weaken the incision. Explain the use of adhesive skin strips if needed. ***Rationale:*** Explanation decreases patient anxiety and encourages patient and family cooperation and understanding of procedure.
- Instruct the patient and family on aftercare: pain medication, wound care, activity restrictions, and observation for signs and symptoms of infection. ***Rationale:*** Education facilitates patient comfort, decreases risk for infection, and encourages prompt follow-up for treatment of possible infection.

PATIENT ASSESSMENT AND PREPARATION

Patient Assessment

- Obtain the history of the present injury and a medical history. ***Rationale:*** This knowledge allows a better

TABLE 130-1	Timing of Suture Removal
Location of Sutures	**Days Before Removal**
Extremities, scalp, and trunk	7–14
Face	3–5
Palms, soles, back, and skin over mobile joints	10–14
Retention sutures	14–21

understanding of the nature of the injury and any factors complicating suture or staple removal.

- Assess patient allergies, especially to adhesive tape and povidone-iodine, chlorhexidine, or other topical solutions or medications. *Rationale:* Further tissue damage can be prevented.
- After determining when sutures or staples were placed, observe the wound for signs of gaping, drainage, inflammation, infection, or embedded sutures. *Rationale:* Findings may delay suture or staple removal.

Patient Preparation

- Ensure that the patient and family understand preprocedural teachings. Answer questions as they arise, and reinforce information as needed. *Rationale:* Understanding of previously taught information is evaluated and reinforced.
- Verify that the patient is the correct patient using two identifiers. *Rationale:* Before performing a procedure, the nurse should ensure the correct identification of the patient for the intended intervention.
- Administer pain medication as prescribed. *Rationale:* Pain medication promotes patient comfort and reduces activity during suture or staple removal to provide a stable field.
- Provide privacy and position the patient for comfort without undue tension on the suture line or staples. *Rationale:* Provides patient comfort and promotes cooperation during procedure.
- Adjust the light to shine directly on the suture line or staples. *Rationale:* Light is used to facilitate visibility.

Procedure for Suture Removal

Steps	Rationale	Special Considerations
1. Check order to confirm exact timing and other relevant information.	Ensures appropriate treatment.	Prescribing physician, advanced practice nurse, or other healthcare professional may want to leave some sutures in place for an additional day or two to support the suture line.
2. **HH**		
3. **PE**		
4. Apply sterile drapes or towels over or under the area as needed.	Provides protective barrier.	
5. Gently tug on the sutures to test the wound line before removal, to be sure the wound does not separate. If any doubt exists to the integrity of the suture line, apply a skin adherent and adhesive skin strips between sutures before removing them. Remove alternate sutures initially, until integrity of the incision is ensured; then remove the remaining sutures.[5] **(Level E*)**	Ensures that the wound is healed sufficiently before removal of all sutures.	If the patient has both retention and regular sutures in place, retention sutures may remain in place for 14–21 days.
6. Clean the suture line with antiseptic skin cleanser. The wound is considered clean, so when cleaning it, wipe from clean to dirty, moving from the inner aspect to the outer margins of the wound.	Decreases the number of microorganisms and reduces the risk for infection.	Be particularly careful to clean the suture line before removing mattress sutures, especially if the visible, contaminated part of the stitch is too small to cut twice for sterile removal. Carefully remove encrusted drainage to allow visualization of all sutures to be removed.

*Level E: Multiple case reports, theory-based evidence from expert opinions, or peer-reviewed professional organizational standards without clinical studies to support recommendations.

Procedure continues on following page

Procedure for Suture Removal—*Continued*

Steps	Rationale	Special Considerations

7. Use sterile techniques to remove running sutures (Fig. 130-1)[2]:
  A. Use sterile forceps to grasp the knot and gently raise it off of the skin.
  B. Use the rounded tip of the sterile suture scissors to cut the suture at the skin edge on one side of the visible part of the suture.
  C. Remove the suture by lifting the visible end of the skin to avoid drawing the contaminated portion through subcutaneous tissue.
	Visible part of suture is exposed to skin bacteria and is considered contaminated.
	
	Prevents pulling it through and contaminating subcutaneous tissue.[6]
		For running sutures, each individual section needs to be cut to prevent the contaminated suture material from being pulled through the subcutaneous tissue.

8. To remove mattress sutures (Fig. 130-2)[6]:
  A. Remove the small visible portion of the suture opposite the knot by cutting it at each visible end and lifting the small piece away from the skin.
  B. Remove the rest of the suture by pulling it out in the direction of the knot.
  C. If the visible portion is too small to cut twice, cut once and pull the entire suture out in the opposite direction.		

9. If the wound dehisces, apply butterfly adhesive strips or paper tape to support and approximate the edges and call the physician or physician extender.	Adhesive strips may be used to reapproximate the wound edges until complete wound closure occurs.	Wound dehiscence is the premature opening of a wound along a suture line.[6]
10. Wipe the incision line gently with gauze soaked in antiseptic skin cleanser or prepackaged swab.[2] **(Level E*)**	Removes serous or bloody drainage from the suture line.	
11. Apply adhesive skin strips or paper tape and a light, sterile gauze dressing, if desired. Leave strips in place for 3–5 days or as ordered.	Holds incision edges together, decreases transmission of microorganisms, and decreases irritation from clothing.	
12. Dispose of gloves and equipment in appropriate receptacles.		
13. **HH**		

---

*Level E: Multiple case reports, theory-based evidence from expert opinions, or peer-reviewed professional organizational standards without clinical studies to support recommendations.

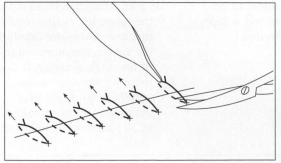

Figure 130-1 Removal of plain interrupted sutures with sterile forceps and scissors.

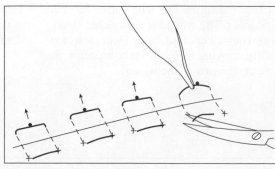

Figure 130-2 Removal of interrupted mattress sutures with sterile forceps and scissors.

Procedure for Staple Removal

Steps	Rationale	Special Considerations
1. Check order to confirm exact timing and other relevant information.	Ensures appropriate treatment.	Prescribing physician, advanced practice nurse, or other healthcare professional may want to leave some staples in place for an additional day or two to support the staple line.
2. **HH**		
3. **PE**		
4. Apply sterile drapes or towels over or under the area as needed.	Provides protective barrier.	
5. Gently test the wound line before removal of the staple to be sure the wound does not separate. If any doubt exists, apply a skin adherent and adhesive skin strips between staples before removing them. Remove alternate staples initially, until integrity of the incision is ensured, then remove the remaining staples.[5] **(Level E*)**	Ensures that wound is healed sufficiently before removal of all staples.	
6. Clean the staple line with antiseptic skin cleanser. The wound is considered clean, so when cleaning it, wipe from clean to dirty, moving from the inner aspect to the outer margins of the wound.	Decreases the number of microorganisms and reduces the risk for infection.	Carefully remove encrusted drainage to allow visualization of all staples to be removed.
7. Use sterile techniques to remove staples (Fig. 130-3). A. Gently place the tip of the staple remover under the staple at its center. B. If the incision line is under tension, gently squeeze the opposite sides together with your free hand as each staple is removed. C. Compress the staple remover until the staple bends in the center and the edges lift out of the skin. D. Discard the staple and proceed to the next staple.		
8. If the wound dehisces, apply butterfly adhesive strips or paper tape to support and approximate the edges and call the prescribing physician, advanced practice nurse, or other healthcare professional.	Provides approximation of wound edges until the physician, advanced practice nurse, or other healthcare professional reassesses the wound.	Monitor wound dehiscence for sign of infection.

**Level E: Multiple case reports, theory-based evidence from expert opinions, or peer-reviewed professional organizational standards without clinical studies to support recommendations.

Procedure continues on following page

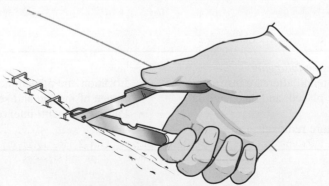

Figure 130-3 Staple removal.

Procedure for Staple Removal—*Continued*

Steps	Rationale	Special Considerations
9. Wipe the incision line gently with the gauze soaked in antiseptic skin cleanser or prepackaged swab.	Removes serous or bloody drainage from the staple line.	
10. Apply adhesive skin strips or paper tape and a light, sterile gauze dressing, if desired. Leave strips in place for 3–5 days or as ordered.	Holds incision edges together, decreases transmission of microorganisms, and decreases irritation from clothing.	
11. Dispose of gloves and equipment in appropriate receptacle.		
12. **HH**		

Expected Outcomes

- Wound remains infection free
- Function is preserved
- Appearance is restored

Unexpected Outcomes

- Wound infection and possible sepsis
- Loss of function
- Abnormal appearance
- Wound dehiscence

Patient Monitoring and Care

Steps	Rationale	Reportable Conditions
		These conditions should be reported if they persist despite nursing interventions.
1. Retest range of motion and sensory perception after suture or staple removal.	Ensures no further damage was imposed.	• Altered range of motion • Change in sensation, paresthesia, tingling
2. Observe for wound discharge or other abnormal changes.	Allows for early treatment and prevents systemic infection.	• Wound that is red, swollen, tender, or warm • Wound that begins to drain or fester • Red streaks around the wound • Tender lumps in the groin or under the arm • Chills or fever • Redness that surrounds the incision and does not gradually disappear or shows only a thin line after a few weeks[2]
3. Provide detailed patient and family education, including wound care, medications, signs and symptoms of infection, when the patient can get the incision wet, and follow-up instructions.	Facilitates patient and family cooperation.	
4. Follow institutional standards for assessing pain. Administer analgesia as prescribed.	Identifies need for pain interventions.	• Continued pain despite pain interventions

Documentation

Documentation should include the following:

- Patient and family education and aftercare instructions
- Date and time sutures were placed, and date and time sutures were removed
- Care of the wound after suture removal
- Location and appearance of wound
- Range of motion and sensory perception
- Pain assessment, interventions, and effectiveness

References and Additional Readings

For a complete list of references and additional readings for this procedure, scan this QR code with any freely available smartphone code reader app, or visit http://booksite.elsevier.com/9780323376624.

131 Wound Closure AP

Joanna C. Ellis

PURPOSE: Wound closure is the process of holding body tissues together to promote wound healing until the body's natural tensile strength is sufficient to maintain closure. In addition, formal wound closure can provide hemostasis, minimize scarring, decrease risk for infection, and aid in maintaining proper positioning of surgically placed tubes and drains.

PREREQUISITE NURSING KNOWLEDGE

- The skin is the largest organ of the body and is responsible for several important functions, including temperature regulation, fluid balance, and soft tissue protection. It consists of two major tissue layers: the outer epidermis and the inner dermis.
  - The epidermis consists of stratified, squamous cells with keratin and melanin. This layer provides thermoregulation, immunological activity, fluid balance, and pigmentation.
  - The dermis consists of fibro-elastic connective tissue with capillaries, lymphatics, and nerve endings. This layer provides energy, nourishment, and strength.
- A wound is any alteration to tissue that causes a disruption in the tissue's integrity, whether it be from trauma or surgery. In some situations, formal wound closure is necessary to promote healing.
- Wound healing occurs in three overlapping phases: inflammation, proliferation, and maturation.
  - *Inflammation:* At the time of injury, there is immediate local vasoconstriction to decrease blood loss, while platelets and thromboplastin are released to aid in clot formation and promote hemostasis. Granulocytes and lymphocytes come to the wound with the express purpose of suppressing bacterial growth and infection.[25,26] Macrophages are released for phagocytosis to clear the wound of any cellular debris and foreign substances. Later, kinins and prostaglandins are released to produce vasodilation and increase vascular permeability to produce inflammatory exudate and promote wound repair. Fibrin formation occurs later to create a protective wound scab if the wound is left open to heal by secondary intention. Wounds left open for 3 hours show a dramatic increase in vascular permeability, which results in thick inflammatory exudate and may limit the therapeutic value of antibiotics.[7,25,28]

Therefore, early definitive closure is essential in infection prevention.
  - *Proliferation and epithelialization:* This phase of wound healing occurs 2 to 3 days after the initial insult and lasts up to 2 to 3 weeks. It is characterized by the regeneration of new tissue, collagen, and blood vessels. Fibroblasts are released to rebuild collagen, fill in the wound defects, and aid in producing new capillaries. Wound edges will begin to contract to decrease the wound defect and epithelialization will occur. Epithelialization occurs when epithelial cells migrate across the new tissue to form a barrier between the wound and the environment.
    - In general, epithelialization times can vary based on wound type and method of closure (if any). Epithelialization in wounds that are formally closed with suture or staple can occur within 18 to 48 hours, whereas wounds that are left open to heal by secondary intention may take longer. The physician, advanced practice nurse, or other healthcare professional needs to be aware that there are multiple factors that can aid or delay epithelialization, and inform the patient accordingly.
  - *Maturation/Remodeling:* This is the final phase in wound healing. New collagen is formed and reorganized to increase strength of the new tissue. This process can take from weeks to years to complete.
- The goals of wound closure include decreasing the amount of time required to heal a wound, decreasing the risk for a wound infection (by minimizing dead space and decreasing vulnerable open surfaces in a timely manner using aseptic technique), minimizing potential loss of function involving the affected area, and minimizing scarring.
- Potential complications include infection and/or tetanus, wound dehiscence, loss of function or structure, scarring, and impaired cosmetic appearance.[4]
- Wound closure occurs via primary intention, secondary intention, or delayed primary closure.
  - Closure via primary intention occurs when a wound is formally closed using sutures or staples. For this method to succeed, the wound must be free from contamination, with limited tissue loss and clean edges that can be easily reapproximated and closed. The goals of primary

AP   This procedure should be performed only by physicians, advanced practice nurses, and other healthcare professionals (including critical care nurses) with additional knowledge, skills, and demonstrated competence per professional licensure or institutional standard.

wound closure are to stop bleeding, prevent infection, preserve function, and restore appearance.

- ❖ Closure via secondary intention occurs when the wound is unable to heal via primary intention. Contributing factors include gross wound contamination and/or infection, traumatic wound with significant tissue loss, or jagged wound edges preventing effective reapproximation.[26,28] In situations such as this, the wound is often left open and allowed to granulate in. Multiple wound-care techniques may be employed at this time to clean the wound and promote wound healing.

- ❖ Closure via delayed primary closure allows a grossly contaminated wound time to be aggressively cleaned and potentially prepped for a formal wound closure in a delayed fashion. These wounds remain open with scheduled dressing changes and débridement over a 3- to 5-day period. In some cases, temporary sutures are preplaced in anticipation of formal closure. If after 3 to 5 days the wound remains clean with good granulation tissue with no signs of infection, the wound will be irrigated and closed. However, if the wound appears infected, it will remain open and left to heal by secondary intention. Wounds that have been contaminated by saliva, feces, or purulent exudate or have been open greater than 8 hours may benefit from delayed closure to decrease the risk for infection.

- Depending on the type of wound and available resources, referral to an appropriate specialist (e.g., vascular, orthopedic, plastic, or general surgeon) may be warranted for wounds with damage to the blood supply, nerves, or joint; wounds on the face; or wounds with extensive tissue damage or infection.

- The wound should be prepared to optimize successful closure and healing. Irrigation of the wound is the first step in wound closure and is essential in minimizing risk for infection. Though not necessary, removal of hair from around the anticipated suture site may be considered if the hair is going to interfere with the wound closure. If hair must be removed, use an electric clipper rather than razors, as razors can cause abrasions and microscopic skin nicks that may increase the risk of infection.[8,16,18,19,24]

- Wound closure is performed employing several traditional methods including the use of sutures, staples, tissue adhesives, and adhesive skin strips. (i.e., Steri-Strips).

- ❖ Sutures and staples are the most commonly used methods for wound closure and provide the sturdiest closure. Staples have a distinct advantage over sutures in that they can be quickly placed with minimal difficulty and are less reactive than sutures, and therefore may cause less scarring and infection. They are most often used for lacerations to the scalp, trunk, and extremities. Alternatively, sutures can be used on hands and feet (overlying joints) and for deeper facial and neck lacerations. Skin adhesive or tape should be considered for straight and superficial lacerations and wounds of the hands, feet, neck, and face, avoiding any surfaces overlying joints, any surface tension, mucosa, or lips.[5] Cosmetically, use of staples or sutures produces minimal scarring (unless the patient is predisposed to developing scar tissue or keloid), and can be slightly uncomfortable upon removal.

- ❖ Adhesive skin-closure strips are ideal in straight superficial lacerations with good skin approximation and minimal to no tension. They are most commonly used in the face, areas of flaps, and on any friable skin not amenable to sutures or stapling (e.g., skin in the elderly or that is immunosuppressed).[22]

- ❖ The use of tissue adhesives is newer than its counterparts in wound closure, having only been approved for use by the Food and Drug Administration in the late 1990s.[26] The most common tissue adhesives in use today are cyanoacrylate polymers such as n-butyl-2-cyanoacrylate (HistoAcryl or PeriAcryl) or 2-octyl-cyanoacrylate (Dermabond or SurgiSeal).[20,26] Again, short, clean wounds with easily approximated wound edges in areas with minimal to no tension are appropriate for tissue adhesives, in addition to any friable skin not amenable to sutures or stapling (i.e., skin in the elderly or immunosuppressed). Adhesives should not be used over joints of the hands and feet, lips, or mucosa; on infected, puncture, or stellate wounds; or in patients with poor circulation or a propensity to form keloids.[8] They are best suited for short (<6 to 8 cm), low-tension, clean-edged, straight to curvilinear wounds that do not cross joints or creases.[2,9,10] Dermabond is a brand of tissue adhesive popular in emergency departments because it is easily applied, reaches maximum strength within minutes of application, and provides a barrier against moisture and bacteria.[26] Though the tensile strength is not equivalent to sutures or staples at the time of application, the healing strength of the wound at the 1 week mark is about equivalent.[20] Overall, tissue adhesives have been found to be comparable in terms of cosmetic appearance and acceptability.[12–14,17]

- Suture needles are curved, and come either tapered or cutting. Tapered needles are used in soft tissues (intestine, blood vessels, muscle, and fascia) and produce minimal tissue damage, whereas cutting needles are used in tougher tissue, such as skin. Reverse cutting needles have a cutting edge on the outside of the curve. Most needles are swaged, or molded, around the suture, providing convenience, safety, and speed during suture placement. Needles should be handled only with a needle driver to prevent damage to surrounding tissue and injury to the user.

- Sutures are absorbable or nonabsorbable and come in varying sizes and materials. Suture selection is based on anatomical location and healing potential. Other factors taken into consideration include tissue reactivity, flexibility, knot-holding ability, wick action, and tensile strength (Table 131-1).

- ❖ Suture size is indicated by "0." The higher the number that precedes "0," the smaller the suture (e.g., 4-0 is smaller than 3-0).

- ❖ Absorbable suture (i.e., natural gut, synthetic polymers) is used for layered closures. Gut suture is broken down via phagocytosis and induces a moderate inflammatory reaction. Chromic gut suture has increased strength and lasts longer in tissue. It is not used in the skin because it can cause a severe tissue reaction. Synthetic absorbable sutures are favored over gut because of decreased infection rates and increased strength and longevity.[3] Synthetic braided absorbable sutures provide the best closure for interrupted dermal sutures and ligation of bleeding vessels.

- ❖ Nonabsorbable sutures are either natural fibers (i.e., silk, cotton, linen) or synthetic fibers (i.e., nylon, Dacron, polyethylene) and are best for superficial lacerations due to their ease of handling and knot construction.

- ❖ Although braided sutures provide more strength than monofilament, they also have small spaces between the braids that may harbor bacteria for infection. Monofilament is best suited for skin closure because it produces less inflammatory response; however, the knots are less dependable.

- • Suture and knotting technique
  - ❖ The preferred knotting technique involves a square knot or double loop followed by a square knot tie. The number of sutures required is purely dependent on the size of the wound, with the goal to only use as many needed to hold the wound edges together without crimping. Tension should be minimized but not eliminated on the wound edges. The more tension on a wound, the closer the sutures should be placed.
  - ❖ When performing a suture repair, the practitioner must remember not to tie sutures too tightly during placement, as injured tissue will become edematous and will automatically tighten around the suture within 12 to 24 hours. If sutures are tied too tightly, there is a risk of developing tissue necrosis.

- • Lacerations are approximated using a variety of suturing techniques.[7]
  - ❖ Simple interrupted dermal suture (Fig. 131-1) can be used when the skin margins are level or slightly everted. The needle should enter and exit the skin surface at a right angle. The stitch should be as wide as the suture is deep and no closer than 2 mm apart. The knot should be tied with an instrument tie and repeated four or five times. The first suture is placed in the midportion of the wound. Additional sutures are placed in bisected portions of the wound until it is appropriately closed.
  - ❖ Subcutaneous sutures with inverted knot or buried stitch (Fig. 131-2) are used for deeper wounds or wounds under tension. Absorbable sutures are used in this setting, with the knot inverted below the skin margin. Begin at the bottom of the wound, come up and go straight across the incision to the base again, and tie. Deep, buried subcutaneous sutures are used to reduce the tension on skin sutures, close dead space beneath a wound, and allow for early suture removal.[11,15]
  - ❖ Vertical mattress sutures (Fig. 131-3) promotes eversion of the skin, which promotes less prominent scarring.[15] Mattress sutures are used when skin tension is present or where the skin is very thick (palms and soles of feet). This suture is identical to a simple suture, but an additional suture is taken very close to the edge of each side of the wound.

TABLE 131-1	Suggested Guidelines for Suture Material and Size for Body Region	
Body Region	**Percutaneous (Skin)**	**Deep (Dermal)**
Scalp	5-0/4-0 monofilament*	4-0 absorbable[†]
Ear	6-0 monofilament	—
Eyelid	7-0/6-0 monofilament	—
Eyebrow	6-0/5-0 monofilament	5-0 absorbable
Nose	6-0 monofilament	5-0 absorbable
Lip	6-0 monofilament	5-0 absorbable
Oral mucosa	—	5-0 absorbable[†]
Other parts of face/forehead	6-0 monofilament	5-0 absorbable
Trunk	5-0/4-0 monofilament	3-0 absorbable
Extremities	5-0/4-0 monofilament	4-0 absorbable
Hand	5-0 monofilament	5-0 absorbable
Extensor tendon	4-0 monofilament	—
Foot/sole	4-0/3-0 monofilament	4-0 absorbable
Vagina	—	4-0 absorbable
Scrotum	—	5-0 absorbable[†]
Penis	5-0 monofilament	—

From Newell K: Wound closure. In Dehn, RW, Aspry DP, editors. Essential clinical procedures, ed 3, St. Louis, MO, 2012, Sanders, Fig 23-3.
*Nonabsorbable monofilaments include nylon (Ethilon, Dermalon), polypropylene (Prolene), and polybutester (Novafil).
[†]Absorbable materials for dermal and fascial closures include polyglycolic acid (Dexon, Dexon Plus), polyglactin 910 (Vicryl), polydioxanone (PDS [monofilament absorbable]), and polyglyconate (Maxon [monofilament absorbable]).

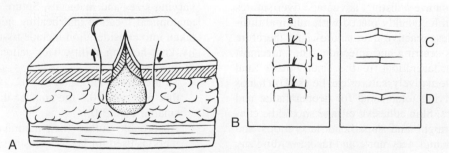

Figure 131-1 Interrupted dermal suture. **A**, Proper depth. **B**, Proper spacing (a = b). **C**, Proper final appearance. **D**, Improper final appearance. (*From Pfenninger JL, Fowler GC, editors:* Pfenninger and Fowler's procedures for primary care, *ed 3, St. Louis, 2011, Mosby.*)

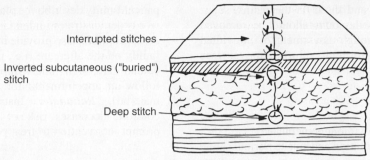

Figure 131-2 Inverted subcutaneous suture. Also shown is layered closure. *(From Pfenninger JL, Fowler GC, editors:* Pfenninger and Fowler's procedures for primary care, *ed 2, St. Louis, 2006, Mosby.)*

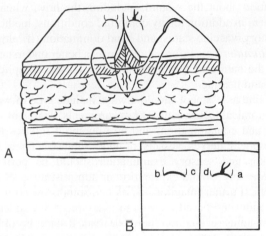

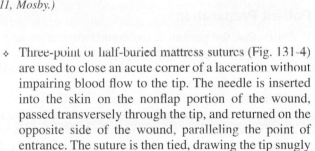

Figure 131-3 Vertical mattress suture. **A,** Cross section. **B,** Overhead view. Begin at *a,* and go under skin to *b.* Come out, go in at *c,* and exit at *d. (From Pfenninger JL, Fowler GC, editors:* Pfenninger and Fowler's procedures for primary care, *ed 3, St. Louis, 2011, Mosby.)*

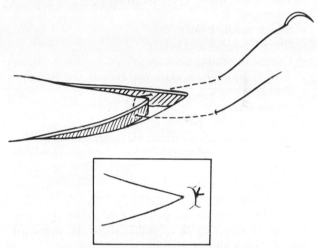

Figure 131-4 Three-point or half-buried mattress. *(From Pfenninger JL, Fowler GC, editors:* Pfenninger and Fowler's procedures for primary care, *ed 2, St. Louis, 2006, Mosby.)*

❖ Three-point or half-buried mattress sutures (Fig. 131-4) are used to close an acute corner of a laceration without impairing blood flow to the tip. The needle is inserted into the skin on the nonflap portion of the wound, passed transversely through the tip, and returned on the opposite side of the wound, paralleling the point of entrance. The suture is then tied, drawing the tip snugly in place.[11,15]

❖ Subcuticular running sutures (Fig. 131-5) are used for linear wounds under little or no tension and allow for edema formation. Wound approximation may not be as meticulous as with an interrupted dermal suture. An anchor suture is placed at one end of the wound, then continuous sutures are placed at right angles to the wound less than 3 mm apart. The wound is pulled together and the other end secured with either another square knot or tape under slight tension.

• Sutures must be completely removed in a timely fashion to avoid further tissue inflammation and possible infection. Sutures on extremities and the trunk should be removed in 7 to 14 days; those on the face should be

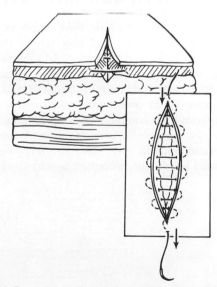

Figure 131-5 Subcuticular running suture. *(From Pfenninger JL, Fowler GC, editors:* Pfenninger and Fowler's procedures for primary care, *ed 3, St. Louis, 2011, Mosby.)*

removed in 3 to 5 days; and those on the palms, soles, back, and skin over mobile joints should be removed in 10 to 14 days. A thorough assessment of individual healing is performed before all suture removal (see Table 130-1).[7,21]

EQUIPMENT

- Local anesthetic (with or without epinephrine)
- Antimicrobial skin prep solution and sterile normal saline solution
- 8 to 10 4 × 4 gauze sponges
- Sterile metal prep basin
- 30- or 60-mL syringe and 18-gauge needle
- Sterile drape
- Fenestrated drape
- Sterile gloves, mask, eye protection
- For suturing
  - ❖ 6-inch needle holder
  - ❖ Suture material and needle
  - ❖ Curved dissecting scissors
  - ❖ Two mosquito hemostats: one curved, one straight
  - ❖ Suture scissors
  - ❖ Tissue forceps
  - ❖ Scalpel handle and No. 15 knife blade
  - ❖ Skin retractors (for atraumatic tissue handling)
- For other wound closures
  - ❖ Staple gun
  - ❖ Skin-closure strips
  - ❖ Skin adhesive
- *Note:* Most hospitals use prepackaged suture kits; thus, it may be unnecessary to assemble all of the items listed here if such a kit is available.

Additional equipment, to have available as needed, includes the following:

- Electric clippers (only if hair removal is necessary)
  - ❖ 27–30-gauge needles

PATIENT AND FAMILY EDUCATION

- Explanation of the procedure, risks involved, potential benefits and alternatives, and expectations during and after the procedure should be included during patient education. *Rationale:* Explanation decreases patient anxiety, encourages patient and family cooperation, and improves understanding of the procedure.
- Once explanation is complete and all patient/family questions have been answered, consent can be obtained. *Rationale:* Suturing is an invasive procedure, so consent should be obtained before the procedure is started. Having the patient/family describe the planned procedure in their own words demonstrates understanding.
- As appropriate, also provide instructions to the patient and family on the aftercare (i.e., pain medication, anticipated wound care, signs and symptoms of infection, and any follow-up appointments for removal of wound-closure material). *Rationale:* Instruction facilitates patient comfort, decreases risk of infection, and encourages prompt intervention to treat possible infection.

PATIENT ASSESSMENT AND PREPARATION

Patient Assessment

- Assess the patient's current medical history, medications (prescribed and over the counter), and any pertinent information about the wound, including the how, when, and where in addition to any comorbid conditions, medication history, vaccine status, and hand domination (if relevant). *Rationale:* This information allows a better understanding of the nature of the injury and any factors complicating wound healing.
- Wound assessment should always include type of wound, anatomical location, exact measurements, degree of severity and contamination, and any potential injuries to the peripheral nerves, vessels, or underlying structures. A full motor and sensory examination should be performed before any wound exploration or administration of anesthetic. Further imaging studies or specialist referrals may be indicated based on wound assessment. Consideration for tetanus vaccination should be made if status is unknown or expired. Administer vaccination if criteria are met (see http://www.cdc.gov/tetanus/index.html). *Rationale:* Provides baseline data. The possibility of tetanus from an unclean wound is a preventable complication.

Patient Preparation

- Verify that the patient is the correct patient using two identifiers. *Rationale:* Before performing a procedure, the nurse should ensure the correct identification of the patient for the intended intervention.
- Administer pain medication as necessary. Consider moderate procedural sedation for deep wounds and laceration requiring repair.[17,22] Consider use of LET (lidocaine, 4%; epinephrine, 0.1%; and tetracaine, 0.5%) topically for local pain relief.[17,22] *Rationale:* Adequate pain control is essential to gain cooperation during the procedure and will provide the best opportunity for a successful wound closure.

Procedure for Wound Closure

Steps	Rationale	Special Considerations
1. Prepare all necessary equipment and supplies.	Prepares for the procedure.	
2. ▉HH▉		
3. ▉PE▉		
4. Anesthetize the wound. Infiltrate the area with local anesthetic. May proceed with LET applied topically. Use local anesthetic with or without epinephrine and a 27- to 30-gauge needle to infiltrate the area.[1,23,27] **(Level C*)**	Provides for maximal patient comfort and cooperation during suturing.	Immobilization of the site also aids in decreasing pain.
5. Examine the wound thoroughly for foreign bodies, deep tissue layer damage, joint involvement, and injury to nerve, vessel, or tendon.	Prevents further damage. Assesses need for referral.	Use aseptic techniques to decrease contamination of wound. Radiographic imaging may be necessary to rule out a retained foreign body before wound closure.
6. Clean the wound.	Removes foreign substances and bacteria, and reduces risk for infection.	
A. Mechanical: wiping, brushing, and irrigating with copious amounts of saline solution; use a 30- or 60-mL syringe with 18-gauge needle to generate pressure to remove debris as needed.	Mechanical cleaning is important for prevention of infection. The wound must be properly cleaned and irrigated before wound closure.	Aggressive cleansing of the wound can cause further trauma. A pressure of 8–12 psi is considered effective for cleansing and avoiding damage to the tissues.
B. Chemical: antiseptic solution. Apply in concentric circles, moving toward the periphery.[16] **(Level A*)**	Reduces bacterial colony counts.[3,16]	Use a cleansing solution that is nontoxic to tissues.
C. Only if necessary, remove any hair in the area with an electric clipper.[16,18] **(Level A)**	Do not remove hair at or around the suture site unless it interferes with the procedure.[6,8] Electric clippers (rather than razors) have been associated with significantly fewer infections.[6,8]	Consider use of hair-apposition techniques with longer hair to avoid shaving and promote wound closure without suturing.[13]
7. Remove nonsterile gloves, wash hands, and apply sterile gloves.		
8. Apply sterile drapes over and under the area as necessary.	Creates a sterile field. Reduces risk for infection.	
9. Examine the wound again for devitalized tissue that needs removal or débridement (see Procedure 133). Use a scalpel or sharp tissue scissors if necessary.	Débridement reduces contamination and optimizes wound-healing potential.	Débridement should be conservative and limited to removal of devitalized tissue that could act as a medium promoting bacterial growth.
10. If needed, loosen the wound from the subcutaneous tissue beneath the dermis with the scissors or scalpel. *Note:* For wound-closure methods other than suturing, **skip to Step 22.**	Promotes approximation of skin edges.	

*Level A: Meta-analysis of quantitative studies or metasynthesis of qualitative studies with results that consistently support a specific action, intervention, or treatment (including systematic review of randomized controlled trials).

*Level C: Qualitative studies, descriptive or correlational studies, integrative reviews, systematic reviews, or randomized controlled trials with inconsistent results.

Procedure continues on following page

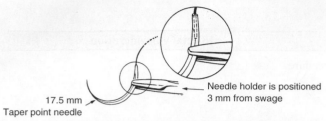

17.5 mm
Taper point needle

Needle holder is positioned
3 mm from swage

Figure 131-6   Because the laser-drilled hole is 15 mm long, this needle can be grasped by the needle holder 3 mm from the swage *(insert)*. Needle holder grasps the needle 3 mm from its swage. *(Copyright © 1996, 2010, Covidien. All rights reserved. Used with permission of Covidien.)*

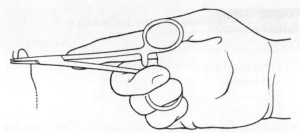

Figure 131-7   Thumb-ring finger grip of needle holder. *(Copyright © 1996, 2010, Covidien. All rights reserved. Used with permission of Covidien.)*

Procedure	**for Wound Closure—*Continued***	
Steps	**Rationale**	**Special Considerations**
11. Select the appropriate needle and suture material according to the type of wound.	Provides maximal support with the least amount of tissue trauma and encourages the best cosmetic outcome.	
12. Arm the needle between the jaws of the needle holder (Fig. 131-6).	Prevents needle bending and provides for guided insertion.	The needle holder should be perpendicular to the needle and should grasp the needle 3 mm beyond the swaghole. The handle of the needle holder should be closed to the first or second ratchet.
13. Grasp the needle holder (Fig. 131-7).	Correct grasp ensures smooth entry of needle and proper stitch placement with minimal manipulation.	
14. Position the free end of the suture away from the operator.	Allows optimal visualization of the free end of the suture and ensures that it does not become entangled during knot construction.	
15. Pass the needle through the tissue until the needle point is visualized.	Allows visualization of the needle.	Hand should start prone; supination of the wrist passes needle in a direction toward the person suturing and in the direction of the curvature of the needle.
16. Using tissue forceps to grasp the needle point, unclamp the needle holder jaws.	Stabilizes the needle to maintain its position in the tissue.	
17. Regrasp the needle between the needle holder jaws and pull the desired length of the suture through the wound.	Prepares for tying a knot.	Keep the wrist in the prone position.
18. Tie the suture knot. Edges should be slightly everted.		Secure the precise approximation of the wound edges without strangulating the tissue. The suture should be tied snugly, but gently.
A. Form suture loop: wrap the fixed suture end over and around the needle holder twice.	Double wrap provides increased strength.	Keep the length of free suture end <2 cm.
B. Pass the free end of the suture through the loop to create a throw.		Has a figure-eight shape.

Procedure	**for Wound Closure—*Continued***	
Steps	**Rationale**	**Special Considerations**
C. Advance the throw to the wound surface by applying tension perpendicular to the wound.		
D. Repeat four or five times.		With each throw, your hands must reverse positions and apply equal and opposing tension to the suture ends in the same plane.
19. Cut the suture by holding the scissor blades perpendicular to the suture and keeping the knot in view between the blades, allowing 3-mm tails to remain.	Tails allow for easy identification of sutures upon removal. The perpendicular positioning is helpful in preventing accidental cutting of the knot.	
20. Reposition the knot away from the wound edges.	Facilitates suture line care.	
21. **Repeat Steps 11–20** until the wound is appropriately closed. Dress the wound appropriately. **Go to Step 24.**		
22. Other wound-closure techniques: select the wound-closure technique to be used.		
A. Staples: use fingers or forceps to approximate the edges. Apply firm pressure with the stapler and dispense staples as directed. Place staples 0.5–1 cm apart. An assistant can help evert the wound edges while the primary operator uses the stapler.	Keep constant pressure and wound approximation to assist with even staple placement for wound closure.	
B. Adhesive skin strips: ensure that the skin is not oily or hairy and that the wound has minimal drainage. The strips should overlap the wound about 2–3 cm on each side of the wound. Start at the midpoint of the wound to approximate the sides and work out to the ends of the wound. Strips should be placed about 2–3 cm apart. Additional strips can be placed over the cross tapes to prevent the ends from coming loose.[1]	Clean, smooth skin surfaces is optimal for best adherence of skin-closure strips.	Should not be used for large wounds or on patients who may remove them (confused, uncooperative, very young patients). Skin adherent (i.e., tincture of benzoin or Mastisol liquid adhesive) may be applied to the area to increase adhesion of skin strips. Although these adherents are widely used, their application should be limited only to intact skin, avoiding contact with the wound bed.
C. Skin adhesive: apply to dry, well-approximated wound edges. Open the product, saturate the porous applicator tip, and paint the edges of the wound with short brush strokes in a multilayering process. Allow 15 seconds between layers. Usually four layers are applied. Hold edges together for 30–60 seconds.[5]	Precise application is important to avoid contaminating the wound with adhesive.	Avoid skin adhesive getting into the wound. If skin adhesive gets into the wound, it is ineffective, impairs healing, and increases the potential for foreign-body reaction.

Procedure continues on following page

Procedure for Wound Closure—*Continued*

Steps	Rationale	Special Considerations
23. After applying staples and adhesive skin strips, cover the wound with nonadherent dressing for the first 24–48 hours. Depending on institutional protocol, a topical antimicrobial ointment may be added before dressing application. Skin adhesive: dressing is unnecessary, but a dry gauze pad may be used. Do not use ointments, creams, or tape strips. Do not soak, scrub, or expose to prolonged wetness. Patient may shower or gently bathe.[1]	Protects the wound from further injury; discourages microbial invsion[2]; minimizes bleeding, edema, and potential dead space; provides a physiological environment that is conducive to epithelial migration and scab formation; takes tension off the wound edges; cushions the wound from extraneous trauma; and restricts motion, which decreases lymphatic flow and minimizes the spread of wound microflora.[7]	For continued oozing, consider applying a pressure dressing. First assess for local perfusion to avoid dressing-related ischemia.
24. Dispose of equipment in appropriate receptacles.	Standard Precautions.	
25. 🅷🅷		

Expected Outcomes

- Bleeding ceases or is controlled
- Wound remains infection free
- Function is preserved
- Appearance is restored

Unexpected Outcomes

- Continued bleeding from the wound site or hematoma
- Wound infection and possible sepsis
- Skin necrosis
- Loss of function
- Abnormal appearance
- Wound dehiscence

Patient Monitoring and Care

Steps	Rationale	Reportable Conditions
		These conditions should be reported if they persist despite nursing interventions.
1. Serial examination of the wound.	Allows for early treatment and prevents systemic infection. Frequency of serial examination will depend on patient and wound history.	• Wound that is red, swollen, tender, or warm • Suppurative wound • Red streaks surrounding the wound • Tender lumps in the groin or under the arm • Chills or fever
2. Administer prophylactic antibiotics if A. Contamination of trauma site is suspected. B. Animal or human bite wounds exist. C. Preexisting medical conditions subject the patient to increased risk for infection (e.g., valvular heart disease, diabetes).	Prevents wound infection.	

Patient Monitoring and Care —*Continued*

Steps	Rationale	Reportable Conditions
3. Follow institutional standards for assessing pain. Administer analgesia as prescribed (agent and dose are determined by the extent of the trauma, the pain perception and threshold of the patient, age, and the concerns of the patient).	Identifies need for pain interventions.	• Continued pain despite pain interventions
4. Provide appropriate support to wounds under considerable tension (i.e., rigid splints, adhesive strips, or retention sutures, as clinically indicated).	Decreases lymphatic flow, thereby decreasing the spread of wound bacteria. Provides support and limitation of movement to allow for proper wound healing and patient comfort.	
5. Keep the wound and dressing clean and dry. If the dressing becomes wet, use sterile techniques to remove it, blot dry with gauze pad, and reapply a clean, dry dressing.[14]	Decreases opportunity for infection from wicking action of a wet dressing.	
6. Keep dressed for 24–48 hours. If needed, clean with nontoxic cleaning solution, blot dry, apply triple antibiotic ointment (unless contraindicated), and reapply a sterile, nonadherent dressing.[7] Avoid the use of triple antibiotic ointments or topicals, if the patient has a drug sensitivity or develops symptoms consistent with sensitivity.	Decreases risk for wound contamination and infection. Beyond 48 hours, whether an incision must be covered by a dressing or whether showering or bathing is detrimental to healing is unclear.[16]	

7. Remove sutures or staples[7,21] (see Procedure 130).
   A. Facial wounds in 3–5 days.
   B. Scalp and extremity wounds in 7–14 days.
   C. Palms, soles, back, and skin over mobile joints in 10–14 days.
	Prevents infection, enhances proper healing, and decreases risk for undesirable scar formation.	

8. Provide detailed patient and family education, including wound care, medications, signs and symptoms of infection, and follow-up appointments.	Facilitates patient and family cooperation.	

Documentation

Documentation should include the following:

- Informed consent
- Patient and family education
- Location and appearance of wound
- Time since injury
- The procedure used to clean wound
- The procedure and technique used to close wound
- How the patient tolerated the procedure

- Care of the wound after closure
- Instructions given to patient and family
- Pain assessment and medication given
- Antibiotics given
- Tetanus status, if given
- Unexpected outcomes
- Nursing interventions

References and Additional Readings

For a complete list of references and additional readings for this procedure, scan this QR code with any freely available smartphone code reader app, or visit http://booksite.elsevier.com/9780323376624.

PROCEDURE

132 Cleaning, Irrigating, Culturing, and Dressing an Open Wound

Marylou V. Robinson

PURPOSE: Cleaning, irrigating, culturing, and dressing open wounds are performed to optimize healing. Wound culturing may be necessary to isolate and allow for treatment of organisms.

PREREQUISITE NURSING KNOWLEDGE

- Goals of wound care must be clearly outlined so that proper wound care products are used.
- Wound care products should be matched to the patient and wound conditions. Although no specific dressing is considered superior to others,[13,18] properties of dressing products are different and should be assessed relative to wound treatment goals.[1,16]
  - Dressings may be categorized as semiocclusive or occlusive. Semiocclusive dressings are semipermeable to gases (O_2, CO_2, moisture) and are impermeable to liquids; they provide the moist wound healing environment that optimizes wound healing. Occlusive dressings lack permeability to gases and liquids.
  - Coarse gauze, used in a wet-to-dry dressing, nonselectively débrides the wound bed mechanically and absorbs wound fluid.
  - Dressings such as calcium alginates, foams, and hydrofibers enhance wound exudate absorption; hydrogels, hydrocolloids, and transparent films provide moisture to nondraining wounds with minimal absorption.
  - Wounds with excessive wound drainage also require protection of periwound skin (i.e., skin barrier wipes).
- Wounds heal by primary, secondary, or tertiary intention (Fig. 132-1).
  - Normal wound healing is often described as a progressive process that involves three overlapping phases: inflammation, proliferation, and maturation. The inflammatory phase is marked for hemostasis, increased vasodilation, and migration of neutrophils and macrophages to the area. The proliferation phase begins 2 to 4 days after injury and is the healing phase of the wound process in which epithelialization, angiogenesis, and collagen synthesis predominate.[9,13] The maturation phase involves the body remodeling collagen fiber and increasing tissue tensile strength.[9,13]

- Most clean wounds heal by primary intention. Suturing each layer of tissue approximates the wound edges. These wounds typically heal quickly and require minimal wound care.
  - Open wounds heal by secondary intention by granulating from the base of the wound to the skin surfaces and contracting and epithelializing from the wound edges; care must be taken to allow for uniform granulation and prevention of open pockets or tunneling.
  - Tertiary intention involves a period of secondary healing to achieve edema reduction and decreased exudate production, followed by surgical closure for primary healing.
- Clean, moist wound beds allow for effective wound healing under the support of a dressing.
  - Openly granulating wounds heal more slowly, may result in drying of granulating tissue and tissue death, and may be more painful for the patient.[20]
  - The presence of exudate is not synonymous with infection but is the natural result of the inflammatory response to maintain moisture and allow movement and replication of epithelial cells necessary for healing. A change in volume, color, or consistency of exudate may indicate impending infection.[1,5,17]
- Wound cleansing should be accomplished with minimal chemical or mechanical trauma.
  - Cytotoxic cleaning agents (i.e., chlorhexidine, iodine, hydrogen peroxide) should be limited because they can delay healing.[5,10,13,17]
  - Wound cleaning solutions should be pH neutral.
  - Normal saline (NS) solution is the cleaning agent of choice; however, tap water is safe and effective for cleaning of most acute and chronic wounds if the water is potable and from a known safe source including water system contaminants such as Listeria and amoeboid populations.[4,6,19] The practice of using tap water is mostly used in remote and resource-restricted situations.

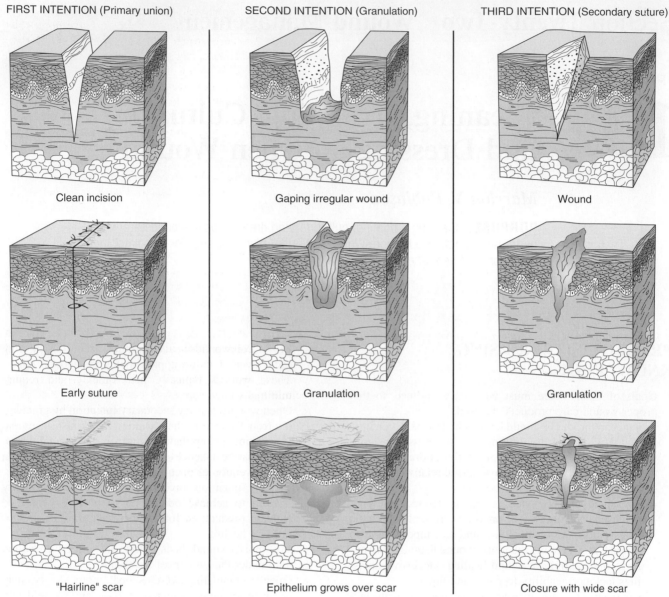

FIRST INTENTION (Primary union)   SECOND INTENTION (Granulation)   THIRD INTENTION (Secondary suture)

Clean incision   Gaping irregular wound   Wound

Early suture   Granulation   Granulation

"Hairline" scar   Epithelium grows over scar   Closure with wide scar

Figure 132-1   Wound healing by primary, secondary, and tertiary intention.

- All wounds should be cleansed to remove adherent and infectious material from the wound surface. Infected and deeper wounds typically require irrigation.
  - ❖ The irrigating solution must be delivered with enough force to physically loosen foreign materials and bacteria without injuring the tissue. Effective wound irrigation is best achieved when solution is delivered at 8 to 13 psi (Fig. 132-2). A 35-mL syringe attached to an 18-gauge angiocatheter tip only delivers fluid at 8 psi. A 12-mL syringe with a 22-gauge angiocatheter tip provides 13 psi. A 20-mL syringe with an 18-gauge angiocatheter tip provides 10 psi. (Increasing syringe size decreases the pressure of the stream, and increasing the bore of the catheter tip increases the pressure.) Pressures greater than 15 psi may actually force bacteria and debris deeper into the wound bed.[1,9,13,17] The exception is first cleaning of heavily contaminated or debris-filled wounds in an emergent or operative setting where the benefits are deemed to outweigh the risks.[2]

  - ❖ The volume of isotonic irrigation fluid required is 50 to 100 mL per centimeter of wound size.
- Wound infections delay wound healing. Wound cultures (obtained before antibiotic therapy) may isolate organisms and differentiate between colonization and active infection.
  - ❖ Wound contamination is the presence of bacteria on the wound surface that are not actively multiplying. Signs and symptoms of infection are not present, and healing is not impaired.[20,21]
  - ❖ Colonization is the presence of bacteria in the wound that are actively multiplying or forming colonies. Colonization can delay healing but may not elicit signs of infection.
  - ❖ Wound infection is present if organisms are present and have attached at $>10^5$ colony-forming units per milliliter in conjunction with clinical findings such as erythema, edema, pain, purulence, fever, and leukocytosis.

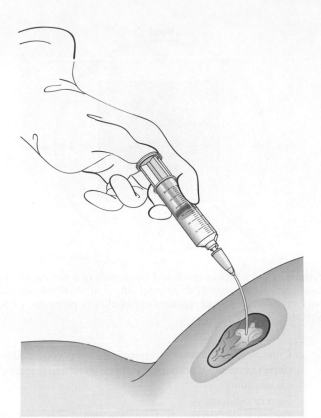

Figure 132-2   Irrigation of a wound.

❖ With the proliferation of organisms like methicillin-resistant *Staphylococcus aureus* and aggressive bacteria that cause necrotizing soft tissue infections (e.g., group A *Streptococci* and *Streptococcus pyogenes),* the standard of empirically implementing antibiotic treatment without wound culture is being questioned. Knowledge of whether resistant strains of bacteria are present at the onset of treatment is critical to provide the optimal situation for healing and rapid intervention.[16–18,21]

• Rapid 1-hour polymerase chain reaction tests are becoming available to speed correct antibiotic selection and/or to aid in determining that these medications are not required.[11]

❖ Bacterial invasion of wounds is managed with cleansing (see Procedure 132), débridement, and antibiotic therapy (local or systemic). Soaking can macerate the wound and periwound tissues, and may not improve bacterial counts.[19]

❖ Biofilms, a polymicrobial structure that includes microorganisms (fungi protozoa as well as bacteria), proteins, polysaccharides, and lipids, prevent wound healing by forming a physical barrier preventing access to topical treatments and proper granulation. They form within 24 hours of wound development and must be removed frequently to promote healing.[21]

❖ Critically ill patients commonly encounter factors that impair adequate wound healing, compounding the risks for poor patient outcomes. Nursing care should focus on early recognition and correction of underlying systemic disorders and patient-specific comorbidities that can impede wound healing goals.[1,8,9,13,14,17,18]

• Frequent comorbidities that can compromise optimal healing trajectories are diabetes mellitus, cardiovascular disease, chronic obstructive pulmonary disease, peripheral vascular disease, cancer, endocrine imbalances, renal failure, cerebral vascular accident, nicotine addiction, alcohol abuse, neurovascular deficit, obesity, and ascites.

• Trauma-associated wound considerations include penetrating injuries that create anaerobic pockets and deep tissue injury; reperfusion of previously ischemic injuries that can trigger paradoxical injury extension; and possible contamination with organic and inorganic bodies that can inhibit effective wound healing, including feces, saliva, soils, and environmental vectors such as metal, rock, and glass.

• Sometimes medications and treatment interventions may jeopardize wound healing goals. Medications that impair tissue perfusion (i.e., vasoconstrictors) or the immune response (i.e., steroids, immunomodulators, antirejection drugs, antineoplastics), and treatments that impair tissue hydration (diuretics and fluid restrictions), may adversely affect wound healing.

• Poor nutritional status includes low serum protein, vitamin C, zinc, copper, and magnesium, and uncontrolled glucose.[5]

• Other factors that compound effective wound healing include hypothermia or hyperthermia, extended surgical procedures, intraoperative hypotension, immobility, hypoxemia, anemia, poor tissue oxygenation, sepsis, extremes of age, inadequate sleep or rest, uncontrolled pain,[20] clotting abnormalities, mechanical friction on the wound, and the development of adhesions or hypertrophic or keloid scars.

• Clean technique is used for most chronic wounds. Sterile technique is used for acute wounds and compromised host patients.[8]

• No evidence is found to support use of sterile techniques when changing dressings on chronic wounds.[8,9] The evidence for use of tap water irrigation has generally been limited to acute wounds and open fractures (specifically excluding patients with a history of diabetes)[6]

• Some intensive care units include wounds in their surveillance culture programs. There is no firm evidence whether this is cost effective, nor contributory to individual patient outcomes. Care priorities are made more complex when the culture results are not directly associated with the wound in question.[15]

• Ultrasound can play a role in diagnostic accuracy of the development of necrotizing fasciitis and abscess.[12]

EQUIPMENT

• Nonsterile and/or sterile gloves (two pairs); sterile field (depending on type and age of wound)
• Two or three sterile cotton-tipped applicators
• NS solution or ordered commercial irrigation solution per institutional protocol
• Sterile basins
• Waterproof barriers
• Sterile 35-mL slip-tip syringe and 18-gauge angiocatheter sheath for irrigation (if necessary; other syringe selection

to keep within the 8–13-psi recommendations may be used in place of the 35-mL syringe).

- Sterile gauze (4 × 4); possibly, ABD dressings (if the wound has excessive drainage, an absorptive dressing may be necessary; if the wound has minimal drainage, a moisture-enhancing dressing may be needed)
- Liquid skin barrier or wafer; apply around the wound edge to protect periwound tissue
- Hypoallergenic tape; tubular mesh bandage or one set of Montgomery straps

Additional equipment, to have available as needed, includes the following:

- Swab culture: two sterile serum-tipped swabs and culturettes
- Tissue biopsy: sterile field, scalpel, forceps, gauze for hemostasis, and container
- Needle aspiration: 10-mL syringe, 22-gauge needle, and syringe cap

PATIENT AND FAMILY EDUCATION

- Explain the procedure and rationale that supports wound cleaning and dressing management. *Rationale:* Patient anxiety and discomfort are decreased.[20]
- Discuss patient's role in the procedure. *Rationale:* Patient cooperation is elicited; patient is prepared for wound management on discharge (as appropriate).
- Explain the reason for obtaining a wound culture (if planning on obtaining one). *Rationale:* Patient anxiety is decreased.[1,20]
- Discuss signs and symptoms of local and systemic wound infection (erythema, pain, increased wound drainage, odor, fever) and inform the patient when to consult a physician, advanced practice nurse, or other healthcare professional. *Rationale:* The patient is prepared for wound management on discharge.

PATIENT ASSESSMENT AND PREPARATION

Patient Assessment

- Assess the following. *Rationale:* Assessment provides information about the healing process and assists in early identification of wound infection. True wound bed assessment cannot be completed until after the wound bed has been cleansed. Inadequate long-term glycemic control as well as major swings in glucose levels in diabetics is linked with three times the number of wound complications.[5] Traditional swabs may not capture the full bioload, especially when wounds have developed a biofilm.[20]
  - Wound drainage (amount, consistency, color, and possible odor)
  - Size, shape, length, width, and depth of wound bed, including pockets (Fig. 132-3)
  - Appearance of wound bed (color, presence of debris, i.e., necrotic or darkened areas on tissue bed are black, slough is green or cream yellow, and healthy tissue is red)

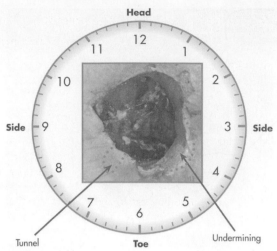

Figure 132-3   Measurement and assessment of a wound. (*From Lewis SL, Heitkemper MM, Dirksen SR, et al: Medical-surgical nursing: Assessment and management of clinical problems, ed 9, St. Louis, 2014, Mosby.*)

- Condition of wound margins and periwound skin (intact versus maceration or xerosis; abnormal textures/undermining)
- Pain or tenderness
- Presence of erythema (blanches with pressure) or ecchymosis (does not blanch with pressure)
- Elevated temperature or localized warmth at wound site
- White blood cell count; may be elevated or show a change from baseline
- Altered blood chemistries, especially hypokalemia and hyperglycemia (>200 mg/dL) and acid-base disturbances
- With advance age, subtle changes in activity and cognition may be the only indications of infection[1,7]
- Nutrition assessment including long-term glycemic control[5]

Patient Preparation

- Verify that the patient is the correct patient using two identifiers. *Rationale:* Before performing a procedure, the nurse should ensure the correct identification of the patient for the intended intervention.
- Ensure that the patient understands preprocedural teachings. Answer questions as they arise, and reinforce information as needed. *Rationale:* Understanding of previously taught information is evaluated and reinforced.
- Place patient in position of optimal comfort and visualization for wound care procedures. *Rationale:* Proper positioning provides for effective wound visualization and enhances patient tolerance of procedure.
- Optimize lighting in the room and provide privacy for the patient. *Rationale:* Lighting facilitates visualization.
- Administer premedication with prescribed analgesic, if indicated. *Rationale:* Medication decreases patient anxiety and increases comfort. Pain and stress are recognized deterrents for healing.[18,20]

Procedure for Cleaning, Irrigating, Culturing, and Dressing an Open Wound		
Steps	**Rationale**	**Special Considerations**

Cleaning and Irrigating Wounds

Steps	Rationale	Special Considerations
1. **HH**		
2. **PE**		
3. Place a waterproof barrier under the wound area to collect drainage.	Controls flow of cleansing solution and minimizes solution contact with intact skin.	
4. Position the wound-cleaning materials and soiled contamination container within reach of the practitioner; conform to the principles of aseptic techniques.	Decreases cross contamination during the wound-cleaning process; enhances body mechanics for the practitioner.	
5. **HH**		
6. **PE**		Face and eye barriers are strongly suggested with irrigation of wounds to protect the physician, advanced practice nurse, or other healthcare professional against splash contaminate.[15,17]
7. Remove soiled dressing, noting any change in drainage and frequency of needed change. Discard in appropriate containers.	Increasing drainage and frequency of change may indicate impending infection.[1,13,17,18]	
8. Assess condition of periwound skin and wound bed for shape and size, odor, and amount and consistency of drainage. Gently probe with cotton swab to note depth of tunnels and undermining. Remove soiled gloves.	Assesses for indications of healing or deterioration (see Fig. 132-3).	True wound bed assessment cannot be completed until after the wound bed has been cleansed. Measurements or photographs should be taken intermittently to document progression.
9. For wounds requiring sterile technique: A. **HH** B. Don sterile gloves. C. Establish sterile field. D. Open sterile drape gauze. E. Place sterile water or NS cleaning solution in a sterile container. For clean techniques, set up supplies per protocol to prevent cross-contamination. Use clean gloves.[13]	Decreases cross contamination during the wound-cleaning process. Cleansing solution should not be cytotoxic.[10,13,17]	No evidence is found to support the use of sterile techniques when changing dressings on chronic wounds.[8,9,14] The evidence for use of tap water irrigation has generally been limited to acute wounds and open fractures (specifically excluding patients with a history of diabetes).[6]
10. If irrigation (see Fig. 132-2) is necessary, attach an angiocatheter sleeve to the syringe for irrigation. A. **HH** B. Apply gloves. C. Draw solution up into the syringe. D. Maintain a 1- to 3-cm distance from wound surface. E. Direct solution onto the wound bed from area of least contamination to greatest. F. Continue with irrigation until return solution is clear.[6,13]	Irrigation reduces the bacterial population and removes excess debris to enhance healing. A 35-mL syringe with an 18-gauge needle provides approximately 8 psi, which is sufficient force to remove debris without creating wound bed damage. The smaller the syringe, the greater the psi.[17] Too great a force during irrigation can create tissue damage, drive bacteria deeper into the tissues, reinitiate the inflammatory process, and delay wound healing.[1,2,9,13,17]	Research does not support scrubbing or swabbing wounds.[19] Bulb syringes do not create enough psi to be effective.[13,19] Not all open wound beds need irrigation.

Procedure continues on following page

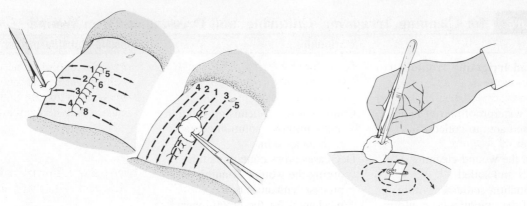

Figure 132-4   Cleaning of a wound. (*From Potter PA, Perry AG, Stockert PA, Hall A:* Fundamentals of nursing, *ed 9, St. Louis, 2017, Mosby.*)

Procedure	**for Cleaning, Irrigating, Culturing, and Dressing an Open Wound—Continued**	
Steps	**Rationale**	**Special Considerations**
11. Cleaning a closed wound: A. 🖐 B. Apply nonsterile gloves. C. With moistened gauze, cleanse from top of the wound to the base (or the center of the wound to edges). D. Discard gauze. E. Clean from area of least contamination to greatest (Fig. 132-4).	Prevents wound contamination during the cleaning process.	If cleaning around a drain, clean from drain site outward in a circular motion; discard gauze with each circle.
12. Dry intact skin surrounding the wound with gauze.	Limits maceration of healthy skin surrounding the wound.	
13. Apply dressing as prescribed.	Protects wound.	
14. Discard uses supplies.		
15. 🖐		
Culturing Wounds		
Swab Culture		
1. 🖐		
2. Apply new gloves after cleansing and remove swab from the culturette tube; maintain sterile techniques.	Must clean wound before obtaining culture to ensure that debris contamination is not cultured.[15]	Sterile gloves may decrease inadvertent contamination to a statistically significant degree, but typically not a clinically significant rate.[3]
3. Swab firmly across the central surface of the wound in a zigzag manner, simultaneously rotating the swab between finger and thumb with gentle pressure to extract any tissue fluid. **(Level D*)**	Tissue fluid, not superficial exudate, is desired for proper results. Swabbing the center of the wound and not the wound edges ensures collection of an adequate specimen.[17,19]	Culturing of wound edges may result in contamination from skin flora and wound debris.[1,17]
4. Carefully place the saturated swab into the culturette tube without touching the swab or inside of the container.	Enables adequate sample collection and prevents contamination.	

*Level D: Peer-reviewed professional and organizational standards with the support of clinical study recommendations.

Procedure for Cleaning, Irrigating, Culturing, and Dressing an Open Wound—*Continued*		
Steps	**Rationale**	**Special Considerations**
5. Crush the ampule of the medium in the culturette and close securely; observe that culture medium surrounds the swab.	Keeps specimen from drying and provides growth-supporting medium for culture.	With collection of an anaerobic culture, ensure the tube is maintained upright to prevent carbon dioxide from escaping.
6. Apply dressing as prescribed.	Protects wound.	
7. Discard used supplies.		
8. **HH**		
9. Label the specimen with the patient's name, date, and wound site; transport to laboratory as soon as possible.	Delays in culture transport increase the risk of invalid testing from exposure to temperature changes.	Bacterial overgrowth occurs with delays in plating and analysis.[1,17,20]
Tissue Biopsy		
1. **HH**		
2. Set sterile field. Apply sterile gloves; with sterile scalpel and forceps, curette, or punch biopsy, obtain a tissue sample approximately 1–2 mm in size (width and depth); apply pressure with sterile gauze to tissue sampling site. **(Level D*)**	Ensures site markings have been made where appropriate. Ensures good tissue sample size free of necrotic tissue; provides for homeostasis of tissue bed. Curette can obtain full biofilm organisms that can be missed by swabs.[21]	Caution must be exercised in obtaining a tissue biopsy; consider local anesthetic to the site before the procedure; assess for excessive bleeding and damage to underlying and surrounding structures. Advanced training is required for nurses who perform this skill.
3. Place tissue sample in sterile container and close tightly; sample may be placed on an agar plate, if indicated.	Prevents contamination of sample.	
4. Apply dressing as prescribed.	Protects wound.	
5. Discard used supplies.		
6. **HH**		
7. Label specimen with patient name, date, wound site; transport to laboratory as soon as possible. **Proceed to Dressing Open Wounds.**		
Needle Aspiration		
1. **HH**		
2. A. Cleanse the skin. B. Apply sterile gloves. C. Insert sterile needle on 10-mL syringe filled with 0.5 mL air into intact periwound tissue. D. Aspirate fluid from several vectors with a fan technique approach and pull plunger rapidly to draw tissue fluid into the syringe.[1]	Ensures good specimen collection if two to four angles of aspiration are used.[10,17]	Goal is to obtain tissue fluid, not wound exudate. Caution required not to reinject fluid back into tissues.[1]
3. Express excess air out of the syringe.		
4. With sterile technique, remove needle and replace with a blunt end cap.	Maintains Standard Precautions; prevents contamination.	
5. Apply dressing as prescribed.	Protects wound.	
6. Discard used supplies.		
7. **HH**		

*Level D: Peer-reviewed professional and organizational standards with the support of clinical study recommendations.

Procedure continues on following page

Procedure for Cleaning, Irrigating, Culturing, and Dressing an Open Wound—*Continued*

Steps	Rationale	Special Considerations
8. Label specimen with the patient's name, date, and wound site; transport to laboratory as soon as possible.		
Dressing Open Wounds	Apply dressing appropriate to wound type and patient condition. Moisture-retentive dressings facilitate wound healing.	
1. **HH**		
2. **PE**		
3. Apply wet dressing: A. Open sterile gauze 4 × 4 pads. B. Place in bowl and saturate with NS solution. C. Wring out excessive moisture. D. Apply 4 × 4s loosely over wound bed. E. Gently pack gauze to the wound edge but do not exceed wound edge.	Saturating gauze on packet greatly increases risk of contamination unless wrapping is coated to prevent bleed through of fluids. Open, moist gauze protects wound bed and allows for placement of dressing without creating open areas or pockets; dressing must be moist but not wet to allow for absorption.[10]	Moist dressing must stay within parameters of the wound bed to prevent surrounding skin maceration. Dressings packed too firmly into the wound compromise perfusion and wound healing. Wound care dressing products that absorb drainage or provide moisture may also be used. Gauze dressing may not control excessive wound exudate; alternative dressings to control exudate should be considered.
4. Place dry gauze 4 × 4s and ABDs over moist dressing.	Provides protection and absorption.	
5. Secure dressing. A. Tubular mesh dressings: sized to secure loose dressings underneath.	Conforming mesh dressings reduces the skin friction associated with tape removal and adhesive irritation. They allow airflow and increase security of coverage without added bulk.	
B. Tape: apply tape across the wound dressing, extending approximately 2 inches beyond the dressing onto skin.	Hypoallergenic tape is less traumatic to noninjured skin and secures dressing in place.	
C. Montgomery straps (Fig. 132-5): i. Apply a liquid or hydrocolloid barrier to surround skin where straps will be applied. ii. Peel paper backing off straps and apply to skin surface with gentle, even pressure. iii. Lace the disposable ties (twill/trach tape; large rubber bands) through the holes in the straps in a crisscross fashion.	Alternative if nonlatex mesh is unavailable for sensitive clients. 1. Assists with providing a protective skin barrier and more effective anchoring of Montgomery straps. 2. Secures Montgomery straps to skin. 3. Secures dressing in place beneath the Montgomery strap.	The straps, tapes, or twill used must be replaced if they become soiled or moist because they become a reservoir for contamination.
6. Discard uses supplies.		
7. **HH**		

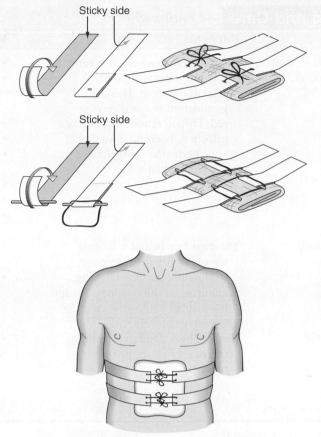

Sticky side

Sticky side

Figure 132-5 Montgomery straps.

Expected Outcomes

- Healed wound
- Wound bed is free of devitalized tissue
- Wound culture specimen obtained confirms and identifies causative organism of infection
- Wound heals uniformly without tunneling, abscess formation, or tracking
- Surrounding skin is free of maceration and erosion
- Wound is free of signs of infection or compromised perfusion

Unexpected Outcomes

- Cross contamination of wound
- Damage to wound bed (hemorrhage, dehiscence) from excessive force during irrigation
- Maceration or inflammation of surrounding skin
- Hemorrhage from tissue biopsy culture technique
- Signs of infection; changes in amount and character of wound drainage
- Wound healing (granulation and contraction) not noticeably progressing on a weekly basis
- Development of wound tunneling, abscess, or tracking

Patient Monitoring and Care

Steps	Rationale	Reportable Conditions
		These conditions should be reported if they persist despite nursing interventions.
1. Follow institutional standards for assessing pain. Administer analgesia as prescribed.	Identifies need for pain interventions.	• Continued pain despite pain interventions

Procedure continues on following page

Patient Monitoring and Care —*Continued*

Steps	Rationale	Reportable Conditions
2. Assess patient, wound bed, and skin surrounding wound.	Continued assessment is essential; wounds must be free of infection to heal. Healthy granulation tissue is pink or red. Discoloration may indicate infection, necrotic tissue, or poor perfusion or hypoxemia at the wound bed site.	• Foul drainage or odor • Darkened or pale areas on tissue bed; red, green, or yellow tissue bed • Erythema; new ecchymosis • Pain • Change in wound drainage (amount, color, odor) • Elevated temperature • Elevated white blood cell count • Hyperglycemia in a patient with diabetes
3. Monitor the wound dressing site for bleeding.	The capillary bed of a healing wound is fragile. Excessive stimulation during cleansing, culturing, or biopsy may disrupt the capillary integrity, creating excessive bleeding.	• Bleeding that does not stop with mild pressure to the wound bed • Excessive bleeding
4. Assess the wound bed and edges for undermining, pockets, or tunnels.	Healing by secondary intention increases risk for pockets or tunnels.	• Presence and depth of undermining, pocket, or tunnel

Documentation

Documentation should include the following:
- Patient and family education
- Pain assessment, premedication given, patient tolerance of procedure, and response to pain medication
- Wound cleaning and irrigation procedure completed; date; time including whether clean or sterile techniques were used.
- Description of wound bed before and after cleaning or irritation; drainage and odors if appropriate; presence of necrotic and granulation tissue
- Description of surrounding skin (color, moisture, integrity)
- Weekly measurements of wound size (measure or trace wound area and depth when appropriate)

- Progression of difficult-to-heal or complex wounds (consider use of digital photography to document)
- Wound culture completed, date, time; type of culture obtained (swab, aerobic, anaerobic, needle aspiration, tissue biopsy)
- Description of approximate site where wound culture was obtained
- Description of wound drains, surrounding skin, and characteristics of wound drainage
- Type of dressing applied after wound care
- Unexpected outcomes
- Nursing interventions

References and Additional Readings

For a complete list of references and additional readings for this procedure, scan this QR code with any freely available smartphone code reader app, or visit http://booksite.elsevier.com/9780323376624.

133 Débridement: Pressure Ulcers, Burns, and Wounds

Julie Lynn Henderson

PURPOSE: Wound débridement is the removal of necrotic nonviable tissue to promote wound healing.

PREREQUISITE NURSING KNOWLEDGE

- Before wound débridement, the patient and wound should be assessed for underlying causes or contributing factors, such as the patient's physical condition, nutritional status, and current healthcare treatment plan, including medications.[3]
- Normal wound healing progresses through an orderly sequence of three overlapping phases: inflammation, proliferation, and reepithelialization and remodeling (see Procedure 130 for pathophysiology of wound healing).
- The presence of necrotic tissue or debris interrupts the normal sequence of wound healing, retards healing processes, and provides a medium that promotes bacterial growth.[4]
- Acute wounds may be classified as either partial-thickness or full-thickness wounds. Partial-thickness wounds penetrate the epidermis and part of the dermis; partial-thickness wounds can be further described as superficial or deep partial-thickness wounds. Full-thickness wounds extend to all skin layers, the epidermis and dermis, and may penetrate subcutaneous tissues.[3]
- Pressure ulcers are defined as localized injury to the skin or underlying tissue usually over a bony prominence as a result of pressure.[7] The National Pressure Ulcer Advisory Panel staging system is used to describe pressure ulcers.[1,7]
  - ❖ Stage I: Intact skin with nonblanchable redness of a localized area usually over a bony prominence. Darkly pigmented skin may not have visible blanching, but the area may differ in color from surrounding tissues.[7]
  - ❖ Stage II: Presents as partial-thickness loss of dermis as a shallow open ulcer with a red-pink wound bed, without slough. May also present as an intact or open/ruptured serum-filled blister.[7]
  - ❖ Stage III: Is described as full-thickness tissue loss. Subcutaneous fat may be visible; however, bone, tendon, and muscle are not exposed. Undermining and tunneling may also be present, as well as slough.[7]
  - ❖ Stage IV: Presents as a full-thickness tissue injury to include exposed bone, tendon, or muscle. Slough or eschar may be present on some parts of the wound bed.
  - ❖ Unstageable: tissue injury that cannot be adequately assessed because of the slough or eschar covering the wound base. Wound débridement should occur before staging the tissue injury.[7]
  - ❖ Suspected deep tissue injury: a purple or maroon localized area of discolored intact skin or blood-filled blister from damage of underlying soft tissue from pressure or shear. The area may be painful, boggy, warmer, or cooler compared with adjacent tissue.[7]
- Necrotic tissue is nonviable tissue and may range in color from whitish gray, tan, yellow, and finally progressing to black. Necrotic tissue nourishes bacteria and slows healing by retarding the inflammatory phase.[4] It may lead to deeper penetration of bacteria into tissues, resulting in cellulites, osteomyelitis, and possible limb loss.[5]
- Débridement provides a mechanism of removal of necrotic tissue and converts chronic wounds into acute wounds. This allows healing to continue until epithelialization is achieved.[15] Biofilm is the adherence of microorganism cells on a surface. This can lead to a prolonged inflammatory state of the wound and possible chronic infection.[16] Débridement allows removal of biofilm from the wound surface. Frequent débridements help to suppress biofilm and accelerate healing.[16]
- Vascular evaluation is essential before nonburn wound débridement. Inadequate perfusion may result in the wound extending into a deeper dermal or full-thickness wound after débridement.[9] Pressure ulcers, burns, and chronic wounds may develop necrotic tissue that requires débridement for wound healing to progress.
- Newer evidence suggests biologic therapy using sterile maggots is effective in achieving débridement in chronic wounds.[14]
- Débridement may be achieved with several methods[2]:
- Surgical débridement: effective means of removal of devitalized tissue. Requires sedation, use of sterile instruments, and conditions and availability of a qualified clinician.[2,9] Large amounts of necrotic tissue may be removed. This may be considered in burn patients with large amounts of eschar or with necrotizing soft tissue infections (i.e., necrotizing fasciitis).[5] Surgical débridement

---

requires a trained surgeon, anesthesia, and hospital admission. As a result, this method is more costly.[13]

- Sharp débridement: similar to surgical débridement, but local anesthesia may or may not be administered. Sharp débridement procedures should be performed only by qualified physicians, advanced practice nurses, and other healthcare providers (including critical care nurses) with additional knowledge, skills, and demonstrated competence per professional licensure or institutional standard.[2,9] This kind of débridement may be performed at the hospital bedside, clinic, or office. Scalpels, scissors, and forceps may be used.[13] Sharp débridement is best for adherent dry eschar with or without infection present. The bacterial count is rapidly reduced.[4] Sharp débridement may be difficult on hard, dry wounds. Consider enzymatic débridement as a first option.[9] Sharp débridement should be discontinued in the presence of pain, bleeding, or exposure of underlying structures. A key to successful safe sharp débridement is assessment and knowledge of anatomy.[5]
- Chemical (enzymatic) débridement: highly selective method of removal of necrotic tissue. Relies on naturally occurring enzymes that are exogenously applied to the wound surface to degrade tissue. This is a slower process that requires a moist wound bed with an adequate secondary dressing to absorb wound exudate. Enzymatic debriding agents may be selective or nonselective to viable tissues. Nonselective agents may be best for thick, leathery, adherent eschar. Selective agents may be best when excess protein buildup is present.[6] Examples of wounds that may benefit from chemical débridement are a partial-thickness burn wound, unstageable pressure ulcer, or patients that are not surgical candidates.
- Mechanical débridement: method of physical removal of debris from the wound. Methods range from wet-to-dry gauze dressings, irrigation, pulsatile lavage, and whirlpool therapy. Débridement is nonselective, and healthy tissue and necrotic tissue and debris may be removed in the process, causing bleeding and pain.
- Autolytic débridement: uses the properties of moisture-interactive dressings to facilitate digestion of devitalized tissue by the body's own enzymes. Typically, if tissue autolysis does not begin to appear in the wound in 24 to 72 hours, another method of débridement should be considered.[2]
- Wound care procedures should adhere to principles of aseptic techniques.
- Clinical judgment should be used in determining whether clean or sterile techniques are indicated in the wound dressing procedure. Generally speaking, acute wounds may be cared for with sterile techniques and chronic wounds may be cared for with clean techniques.[1] The clinician must assess the patient, type, or stage of wound, and type of procedure in deciding which technique should be used in wound care.

EQUIPMENT

- Sharp débridement
  - Personal protective equipment (gown, goggles, mask)
  - Sterile gloves and field
  - Normal saline (NS) solution
  - Gauze 4 × 4 pads
  - Sterile instrument set (scissors, forceps, No. 10 scalpel)
  - Wound dressing
  - Tape
- Chemical débridement
  - NS solution or water to clean wound
  - Clean gloves or sterile gloves (depending on type and age of wound)
  - Enzymatic preparation or solution (prescribed)
  - Tongue blade
  - Filler dressing if needed; secondary absorptive dressing
  - Tape
- Mechanical débridement (wet-to-dry gauze dressing)
  - Clean or sterile gloves (depending on type and age of wound)
  - NS solution
  - Gauze (rolled or 4 × 4 pads)
  - Secondary absorptive dressing
  - Tape
- Autolytic débridement
  - Clean gloves
  - NS solution or water to clean wound
  - Moisture-retentive dressing (transparent film, hydrocolloid dressing, hydrogels)
  - Secondary absorptive dressing as indicated
  - Tape

PATIENT AND FAMILY EDUCATION

- Explain the procedure and the reason for wound débridement; educate the patient and family regarding potential complications such as bleeding if sharp débridement is the prescribed procedure. ***Rationale:*** Explanation decreases patient anxiety and comfort and informs the patient.
- Discuss the patient's role during the procedure. ***Rationale:*** Patient cooperation is elicited.

PATIENT ASSESSMENT AND PREPARATION
Patient Assessment

- Vascular assessment should be completed before débridement. ***Rationale:*** Poor perfusion may result in the extension of the wound after débridement.
- Assess tissues or underlying structures before sharp débridement. ***Rationale:*** Sharp débridement is contraindicated if underlying structures such as muscle, bone, tendon, and blood vessels may be exposed.
- Assess for signs and symptoms of local and systemic infection. ***Rationale:*** Débridement may seed bacteria into systemic circulation; appropriate antibiotics should be considered before débridement in at-risk patient populations.[8] Surgical débridement, the most aggressive type of débridement, is the method of choice when signs of severe cellulitis or sepsis are present.[1]
- Ensure that coagulation parameters are within normal limits. ***Rationale:*** Coagulation abnormalities may result

in unwanted bleeding complications from the débridement process.

- Assess the patient for pain or anxiety and consider premedication. **Rationale:** Medication decreases patient discomfort. Patients with neuropathy may still experience significant preprocedural anxiety

Patient Preparation

- Ensure that the patient understands preprocedural instructions. Answer questions as they arise, and reinforce information as needed. Fully review known risks, benefits, and alternatives. **Rationale:** Understanding of previously taught information is evaluated and reinforced.
- Verify that the patient is the correct patient using two identifiers. **Rationale:** Before performing a procedure, ensure the correct identification of the patient for the intended intervention.
- Obtain informed consent for surgical and sharp débridement.[2,11] **Rationale:** Informed consent ensures patient knowledge of procedure.
- Before the procedure, comply with Universal Protocol requirements.[11] Ensure all relevant studies and documents, including informed consent, are available. Ensure site

markings have been made where appropriate. Before surgical or sharp débridement, perform a preprocedure verification and time out, if nonemergent. **Rationale:** Ensures patient safety.

- Premedicate patient with prescribed analgesia and/or sedation, if needed. Assess the patient's response to the analgesic before start of procedure. Reassess patient's need for additional analgesic agents throughout the débridement procedure. Consider topical lidocaine. This will not be effective in the face of infection and should not be used on burns. **Rationale:** Patient anxiety and discomfort are decreased. Pain results in vasoconstriction of the cutaneous tissues from the increase in adrenergic activity. Adequate pain control improves tissue perfusion and results in improved healing.[3]
- Place the patient in a position of optimal comfort and visualization for dressing the wound. Keep the patient warm while the wound is exposed. **Rationale:** Positioning provides for effective wound visualization and enhances patient tolerance of the procedure. Keeping the patient warm prevents vasoconstriction that impairs wound healing.[12]
- Optimize lighting in the room and provide privacy for the patient. **Rationale:** Facilitates visualization.

Procedure for Débridement: Pressure Ulcers, Burns, and Wounds

Steps	Rationale	Special Considerations
Sharp Débridement	Fast and effective means of selective removal of devitalized tissue; should be performed by a qualified physician, advanced practice nurse, or other healthcare professional.	The sharp débridement procedure should be performed only by physicians, advanced practice nurses, and other healthcare professionals (including critical care nurses) with additional knowledge, skills, and demonstrated competence per professional licensure or institutional standards.
1. Premedicate the patient for pain.	Systemic analgesic may be administered before and throughout the procedure as needed for patient tolerance and compliance.	Assess patient response to analgesia.
2. **HH**		
3. **PE**	Reduces transmission of microorganisms; Standard Precautions.	
4. Prepare sterile drape and field of instruments, NS solution, gauze, and secondary dressing.	Maintains aseptic techniques.	Gauze may be needed to provide hemostasis during procedure.
5. Discard nonsterile gloves, HH, and apply sterile gloves.		
6. With forceps, lift eschar and gently cut with sterile scalpel or scissors. Débride tissue to the line of demarcation of the healthy tissue.	Goal of sharp débridement is removal of devitalized tissue without damage to the healthy wound bed.	Pain and bleeding are signs of healthy tissue. Stop the procedure if pain or bleeding is excessive or if there is impending bone, tendon, or proximity to fascial plane.[5]

Procedure continues on following page

Procedure   for Débridement: Pressure Ulcers, Burns, and Wounds—*Continued*

Steps	Rationale	Special Considerations
7. Lavage the wound bed with NS solution.	Allows for removal of loose devitalized tissue and debris.	Reassess wound bed.
8. Apply a moist wound dressing of choice.	Promotes wound healing.	Assess for hemostasis before application of the dressing.
9. Discard used supplies in appropriate receptacles.		
10. 🄷🄷		
Chemical Débridement	Selective débridement technique.	Requires prescription for desired enzyme preparation.
1. Premedicate the patient for pain.	Systemic analgesic may be administered before and throughout the procedure as needed for patient tolerance and compliance.	Assess patient response to analgesia.
2. Perform hand hygiene, apply nonsterile gloves, and clean the wound.	Maintains aseptic techniques.	
3. Discard gloves, perform hand hygiene, and apply a new pair of nonsterile gloves.	Maintains clean technique.	
4. If wound eschar is hard and dry, a No. 10 scalpel may be used to crosshatch necrotic tissue. (**Level C***)	Cross-hatching technique may allow better penetration of the enzymatic agent and enhance enzyme activity.[5]	
5. Discard gloves, perform hand hygiene, and apply nonsterile gloves.	Maintains aseptic technique.	
6. Establish a sterile field with enzymatic agent, NS solution, and a secondary moist healing dressing.	Maintains aseptic technique.	
7. Apply the enzymatic agent with a tongue blade to the eschar in the wound bed.	Assists with even application of the enzymatic agent over the necrotic wound tissue.	Concentrate enzymatic agent over the nonviable tissue.
8. Place a moisture-retentive dressing (typically, gauze moistened with NS solution) over the wound.	Most enzymatic agents require a moist dressing to be applied over the agent for effective action.	Other dressings that promote moist wound healing may be used.
9. Secure a secondary dressing in place.	A secondary dressing is needed to absorb wound exudates.[9]	Assess the periwound for irritation and breakdown from moisture. Consider application of a liquid skin barrier to the periwound edge.
10. Discard used supplies in appropriate receptacles.		
11. 🄷🄷		
Mechanical Débridement: Wet-to-Dry Gauze Dressing	Nonselective débridement technique.	Nonviable and viable tissue may be lost with this method of débridement.
1. Assess patient response to analgesia.		
2. Perform hand hygiene and apply clean gloves.	Maintains clean technique.	
3. Establish sterile field: gauze dressing moistened with NS solution.	Maintains aseptic technique.	

*Level C: Qualitative studies, descriptive or correlational studies, integrative reviews, systematic reviews, or randomized controlled trials with inconsistent results.

Procedure	for Débridement: Pressure Ulcers, Burns, and Wounds—*Continued*	
Steps	**Rationale**	**Special Considerations**
4. Clean the wound.	Wound cleansing is a means of mechanical débridement; also removes nonadherent bacteria.	Remove any gauze particles left in the wound bed with gentle irrigation.
5. Wash hands and apply nonsterile gloves.	Maintains aseptic technique.	
6. Place moistened gauze loosely into the wound bed.	Excessive packing of gauze into the wound bed may compromise perfusion.[7]	If more than one gauze dressing is used, place the ends of two dressings close to each other for easy removal or consider use of a rolled gauze.
7. Cover the wound with a secondary absorptive dressing and secure.	Protects the wound from external contamination and absorbs exudates.	Consider changing the dressing if ≥75% area of the secondary dressing is saturated with wound drainage. Assess the periwound area for maceration; consider use of liquid skin barrier or hydrocolloid to protect the periwound skin.
8. Discard gloves and perform hand hygiene.		
9. After the prescribed time interval, wash hands, apply nonsterile gloves, and remove the dressing to create the mechanical débridement action.	The drying action of the gauze adheres it to the necrotic tissue, which is detached with the dressing removal.	If the dressing is dry and adherent to viable tissue, lightly moisten the gauze to prevent excessive débridement of viable tissue and to minimize pain.[2,12]
10. Apply wound dressing as prescribed.	Protects wound.	
11. Discard used supplies in appropriate receptacles.		
12. **HH**		
Autolytic Débridement		May not be effective for large wound surfaces. Can take several weeks to complete.
1. Perform hand hygiene and apply nonsterile gloves.		
2. Clean the wound bed with NS solution or water.	Wound cleansing is a means of mechanical débridement; also removes nonadherent bacteria.	
3. Apply a moisture-retentive dressing.	Provides moist wound healing environment that enhances autolytic débridement process.	Assess dressing for absorptive properties. Consider changing the dressing if ≥75% area of the secondary dressing is saturated with wound drainage.
4. Apply a secondary dressing as indicated.	Autolytic débridement results in production of wound exudates. Apply a secondary dressing to absorb exudate away from wound bed.	
5. Discard used supplies in appropriate receptacles.		
6. **HH**		

Procedure continues on following page

Expected Outcomes

- Wound bed is free of necrotic tissue and debris
- Inflammatory progressing to proliferation stage of wound healing is reestablished, and wound healing progresses along normal trajectory
- Wound is free of infection or signs of compromised perfusion
- Wound hemostasis is established after sharp débridement

Unexpected Outcomes

- Depth of wound extends, and necrotic tissue recurs
- Normal wound healing process is not reestablished by removal of devitalized tissue, and wound healing fails to progress[1-3]
- Bacterial infection is present; signs of local or systemic infection are present
- Excessive bleeding from lack of wound hemostasis

Patient Monitoring and Care

Steps	Rationale	Reportable Conditions
		These conditions should be reported if they persist despite nursing interventions.
1. Assess patient, wound bed, and surrounding skin for signs of infection. **(Level D*)**	Wound débridement may not effectively remove all bacteria; continued assessment for wound infection is essential for healing.[7,10]	• Erythema and warmth at wound site • Pain and tenderness • Edema • Change in wound drainage amount, color, odor, or consistency • Fever • Elevated white blood cell count
2. Monitor dressing for signs of bleeding.	Wound débridement may disturb newly formed, fragile blood vessels and established blood vessels and cause bleeding.	• Bleeding that does not stop with mild pressure to wound bed • Excessive bleeding
3. Assess wound for signs of healing after débridement. **(Level D)**	Goal of necrotic tissue débridement is to establish wound healing in the form of granulation tissue and wound contracture.[2,7,10]	• Discoloration of wound bed noted (i.e., ecchymosis, ischemia) • Development of necrotic tissue in wound bed • Changed, diminished, or absent pulses distal to wound bed
4. Follow institutional standards for assessing pain. Administer analgesia as prescribed.	Identifies need for pain interventions.	• Continued pain despite pain interventions

*Level D: Peer-reviewed professional and organizational standards with the support of clinical study recommendations.

Documentation

Documentation should include the following:
- Patient and family education
- Description of wound bed before and after débridement
- Description of periwound skin assessment (color, maceration, integrity, evidence of infection, etc.)
- Size of wound after wound débridement procedure
- Description of dressing applied to wound bed (primary and secondary dressings as appropriate)
- Pain assessment, interventions, and effectiveness
- Premedication given, patient tolerance of procedure, and response to pain medication
- Description of wound débridement process and any unexpected complications
- Vascular assessment
- Description of established wound hemostasis obtained at completion of procedure
- Digital photography is recommended to document progression of wound healing[1]
- Obtain patient consent per institutional standards

References and Additional Readings

For a complete list of references and additional readings for this procedure, scan this QR code with any freely available smartphone code reader app, or visit http://booksite.elsevier.com/9780323376624.

134 Drain Removal

Brian D. Schaad and Mary Beth Flynn Makic

PURPOSE: Drain removal is performed when the drain is no longer needed for wound management.

PREREQUISITE NURSING KNOWLEDGE

- Goals of wound care should be clearly outlined so that proper wound care products are used after drain removal. The wound care products selected are based on the size, location, and care of the wound bed needs and include continued moisture management.
- Drains are placed in wounds to facilitate healing by providing an exit for excessive fluid accumulation in or near the wound bed (e.g., seromas and hematomas).[7] Drains may be removed when drainage is considered to be minimal, approximately 30 to 70 mL/24 hours.[1,5,8,10]
- Type of drain, location, and how the drain is secured should be known before drain removal. Competence should be demonstrated by the clinician performing drain removal because significant tissue injury may result from an improperly removed drain.[1,8] Never force removal of the drain. If resistance is felt, stop and notify the physician, advanced practice nurse, or other healthcare professional.
- Common surgically placed wound drains include Hemovac (Zimmer Inc., Warsaw, IN), bulb suction drain (e.g., Jackson-Pratt or JP drain), and Penrose. Negative-pressure wound therapy devices may also be placed to assist with wound drainage.[2]
- Apply appropriate dressings after drain removal. Coarse gauze absorbs wound fluid but may adhere to the wound bed; calcium alginates, foams, and hydrofiber dressings enhance wound absorption; hydrogels provide moisture to nondraining wounds; hydrocolloids provide wound moisture with minimal absorption; and film dressings are for nonexudating wounds.[3,4,6,9,10]
- Continue to monitor the wound bed after drain removal; mark the dressing for the presence of leakage after drain removal and continue to monitor.

EQUIPMENT

- Nonsterile gloves
- Gowns, face shield
- Sterile gauze 4 × 4 pads
- Dressing for exit site based on characteristics of the wound
- Suture removal kit or sterile scissors
- Hypoallergenic tape

PATIENT AND FAMILY EDUCATION

- Verify that the patient is the correct patient using two identifiers. *Rationale:* Before performing a procedure, the nurse should ensure the correct identification of the patient for the intended intervention.
- Explain the procedure and the reason for drain removal. *Rationale:* Patient anxiety and discomfort may be decreased.
- Discuss the patient's role in drain removal. *Rationale:* Patient cooperation is elicited.
- Provide patient and family education regarding monitoring the wound for drainage. *Rationale:* Patient is engaged in care of the wound site in preparation for discharge.

PATIENT ASSESSMENT AND PREPARATION

Patient Assessment

- Signs of wound infection at drain site include the following. *Rationale:* Drains are placed to remove excessive wound fluid and decrease the risk for infection. Changes in wound drainage may indicate presence of infection; early detection of infection facilitates prompt and appropriate interventions.
  - ❖ Change in the amount, odor, or characteristics of wound drainage
  - ❖ Erythema
  - ❖ Pain
  - ❖ Elevated temperature
  - ❖ Elevated white blood count
  - ❖ Foul drainage from exit site
  - ❖ Pressure or tenderness at drain exit site

Patient Preparation

- Ensure that the patient understands preprocedural teachings. Answer questions as they arise, and reinforce information as needed. *Rationale:* Understanding of previously taught information is evaluated and reinforced.

- Premedicate the patient with prescribed analgesic, if needed. *Rationale:* Patients may not need premedication for drain removal; however, the patient's pain and need for analgesia should be assessed before the procedure and treated appropriately.

- Optimize lighting in the room and provide privacy for the patient. *Rationale:* These measures allow for optimal assessment and patient comfort.

Procedure for Drain Removal

Steps	Rationale	Special Considerations
1. **HH**		
2. **PE**		
3. Check order to confirm drain removal procedure.	Ensures appropriate treatment.	Prescribing physician, advanced practice nurse, or other healthcare professional may want to review the drain volume and drainage characteristics in the previous 24 hours before removing the drain from the wound bed.[5,8]
4. Open sterile scissors; cut any sutures, if present.	Releases the drain from tissue suture anchors.	
5. Open gauze 4 × 4; place gauze close to drain skin exit site; instruct patient to take a deep, easy breath; withdraw the drain swiftly and evenly. **(Level D*)**	Gauze is used to capture body fluids as the drain is removed. Deep breathing may decrease the pain the patient feels with drain removal.[9,10]	Do not force removal of the drain. If resistance is felt, stop and notify the prescribing physician, advanced practice nurse, or other healthcare professional.
6. Place a sterile dressing over the drain exit site and secure with tape.	Provides protection for open wound site; prevents entrance of microorganisms.	Monitor dressing for wound drainage.
7. Discard materials, drain, and personal protective equipment in appropriate receptacles.	Maintains infection control practices and decreases contamination; Standard Precautions.	
8. Perform hand hygiene.	Maintains infection control practices and decreases contamination; Standard Precautions.	

Expected Outcomes

- Intact drain is removed without resistance
- Wound drainage is minimal from exit site
- Drain exit site is free of signs of fluid accumulation, inflammation, or infection
- Wound healing continues to progress without presence of excessive wound fluid

Unexpected Outcomes

- Resistance is felt on drain removal, creating tissue trauma beneath the skin surface
- Wound fluid accumulates beneath skin and drain exit site[1]
- Infection or inflammation occurs at drain exit site
- Poor approximation of skin edges occurs at drain exit site, requiring wound healing by secondary intention
- A portion of the drain remains in the wound tract

Patient Monitoring and Care

Steps	Rationale	Reportable Conditions
		These conditions should be reported if they persist despite nursing interventions.
1. Assess for presence of drainage from drain exit site.	Drainage should be minimal and cease within 24 hours. Continued drainage from drain exit site may indicate accumulation of wound fluid beneath the skin that needs to be evacuated.	- Continued drainage - Edema or pain at drain exit site

*Level D: Peer-reviewed professional and organizational standards with the support of clinical study recommendations.

Procedure continues on following page

Patient Monitoring and Care —*Continued*

Steps	Rationale	Reportable Conditions
2. Monitor for signs of infection.	Drains are placed to remove excessive wound fluid and to decrease the risk for infection.	• Erythema • Pain • Elevated temperature and white blood cell count • Change in wound drainage amount, color, odor • Pressure or tenderness at drain exit site
3. Follow institutional standard for assessing pain. Administer analgesia as prescribed.	Identifies the need for pain interventions.	• Continued pain despite pain interventions

Documentation

Documentation should include the following:

- Patient and family education
- Type of drain removed, placement, date, time, and condition of the drain (i.e., intact drain)
- Amount of wound drainage documented in the last 24 hours before drain removal[5]
- Premedication given, patient tolerance of procedure, and response to pain medication

- Type of dressing applied after drain removal
- Appearance of exit site
- Unexpected outcomes (i.e., resistance, nonintact drain on removal)
- Pain assessment, interventions, and effectiveness
- Nursing interventions

References and Additional Readings

For a complete list of references and additional readings for this procedure, scan this QR code with any freely available smartphone code reader app, or visit http://booksite.elsevier.com/9780323376624.

135 Fecal Containment Devices and Bowel Management Systems

Jane V. Arndt

PURPOSE: Fecal containment devices and bowel management systems (BMS) may be used to divert liquid fecal matter associated with acute diarrhea. Containment of feces may assist with the prevention or treatment of incontinence-associated dermatitis, pressure ulcers, contamination of perineal wounds, and infection. Use of BMS may result in increased patient comfort and cost savings. BMS do not replace appropriate skin care and should be considered when skin protection measures have failed to prevent initial skin breakdown or worsening of skin breakdown.

PREREQUISITE NURSING KNOWLEDGE

- Critically ill patients have multiple risk factors that increase the chance of pressure ulcer development. A valid and reliable pressure ulcer risk assessment tool should be used to assess a patient's risk on admission and consistently throughout the hospitalization.[1]
- Patients with fecal incontinence and immobility are considered to be at increased risk of pressure ulcers.[13,20,22,27]
- Acutely ill patients are at high risk of fecal incontinence related to administration of a variety of medications (i.e., antimicrobial, cardiovascular, central nervous system, and gastrointestinal agents), enteral feedings, disease processes (e.g., gastrointestinal, hepatic disease, spinal cord trauma, etc.), and enterotoxins (e.g., *Clostridium difficile*).[24,28]
- *C. difficile* infections have high mortality and a high economic burden.[11] Personal protective equipment should be used to avoid the possible spread of highly infectious organisms. Use of BMS may reduce cross contamination in incontinent patients with *C. difficile*.[9,11,18,21]
- BMS may result in cost savings due to less use of linens, less nursing time requirements, and fewer patient complications, including skin breakdown and infection.[13]
- BMS may increase nursing satisfaction with incontinence care.[21]
- BMS may have a special port for obtaining fecal samples, which also helps prevent cross contamination.[2,4,10]
- Urinary and fecal incontinence results in skin breakdown.[7,28,29] Excessive moisture changes the skin's protective pH and increases the permeability of the skin, decreasing its protective function. Fecal content is more irritating than urine because digestive enzymes in feces contribute to erosion of skin.[12]
- Perineal skin damage may progress rapidly and ranges in severity, presenting with erythema, edema, weeping, denuded skin, and pain.[7,8,12,28] Other negative outcomes

may include skin ulceration and secondary infection, including bacterial *(Staphylococcus)* and yeast *(Candida albicans)* infections that increase discomfort and treatment costs.[7,12,16]
- Incontinence-associated dermatitis (IAD) is inflammation of the skin that occurs when urine or stool comes into contact with perineal or perigenital skin.[8] IAD is the clinical term used to describe incontinence-associated skin damage. IAD often occurs in conjunction with pressure and shear and friction forces that precipitate pressure ulcers.[8]
- Although it is well established that excessive moisture and incontinence, especially fecal incontinence, significantly increase the patient's risk of IAD and pressure ulcers, the research to guide fecal containment practice is limited.[8,28]
- Management of fecal incontinence should include the following elements:
  - Identification and treatment of the diarrhea. If the source of fecal incontinence cannot be eliminated, drug therapy may be used; however, the efficacy of these drugs is not known because randomized studies have focused on the management of chronic diarrhea in outpatients rather than acute diarrhea in hospitalized patients.[28,29]
  - Meticulous perineal skin care. Maintain clean, healthy skin by cleansing the skin with a pH-balanced no-rinse skin-cleansing solution after each episode of diarrhea. Avoid soap and water. Most soaps are alkaline, and the skin's pH is acidic (5.0 to 6.5); use of soap and water to cleanse the skin can further disrupt the skin's protective properties.[6]
  - Apply a moisturizer with skin protectant. Moisturizers help hydrate intact skin, replace oils in the skin, and soothe skin irritation. Moisturizers that contain petrolatum, lanolin, dimethicone, or zinc can provide a protective barrier to protect and sooth denuded areas.[7,28]
  - Use absorbent underpads that wick effluent away from the skin and allow for circulation of air between the

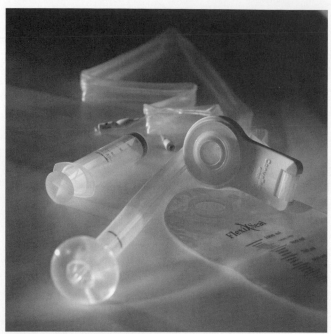

Figure 135-1 Flexi-Seal FMS, ConvaTec, Skillman, NJ. *(Copyright © 1996, 2010 Covidien. All rights reserved. Used with the permission of Covidien.)*

patient's skin and support surface. Avoid use of adult incontinence briefs that trap the moisture against the skin. Change underpads frequently.[17]

❖ Consider application of a fecal containment device or BMS.

- An external fecal containment device adheres directly to the perianal skin, moving feces away from the skin and into a drainage container. The device can remain in place for 1 to 2 days without leaking.[19] If the device is well adhered and not leaking, it may remain in place longer if clinically indicated. Care must be taken during removal of the device to prevent skin trauma or tears.

- The general agreement in the literature is that the perianal incontinence pouch offers many advantages over adult incontinence briefs and balloon rectal catheters and is the least invasive method of fecal containment.[5]

- At times devices not intended for management of fecal incontinence have been used. Adaptation of a device for an unapproved use may be associated with patient injury and concerns of increased liability if a problem arises.[22,29] The clinician should use US Food and Drug Administration (FDA)–approved fecal containment systems rather than adapting devices for management of liquid feces.

- BMS are FDA-approved devices that may be inserted into the rectal vault for up to 29 days for the diversion of stool into a collection system (Figs. 135-1 and 135-2). Early research suggests the devices successfully divert feces, allowing for perineal skin protection and healing.[22]

  ❖ Manufacturer-specific contraindications for BMS include allergies to product components; children; adults with strictured anal canals; and patients with impactions or recent rectal surgery (<6 weeks), severe hemorrhoids, localized inflammatory process or disease, or an incompetent rectal sphincter.[2,4,10]

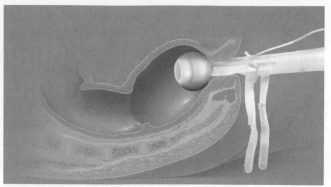

Figure 135-2 ActiFlow Indwelling Bowel Catheter. *(Courtesy of Hollister, Inc., Libertyville, IL.)*

- The BMS may be inserted to manage existing diarrhea or provide fecal diversion away from existing wounds; however, the stool must be liquid or semiliquid.[2,4,10]

- Adverse events reported in the literature include autonomic dysreflexia in a patient with a spinal cord injury. The BMS should be considered as a cause in a patient experiencing autonomic dysreflexia.[23]

  ❖ Use with extreme caution in patients on anticoagulation therapy or with rectal varices, inflammatory bowel disease, low platelet count, or high international normalized ratio. Reports of rectal ulceration, rectal trauma, and gastrointestinal hemorrhage have been documented in the literature.[14,15,25]

- If blood is present in the rectum, ensure there is no evidence of pressure necrosis from the device. Discontinuation of the use of the device is recommended if evident. Notify the physician of any signs of bleeding.[2,4,10]

- Follow manufacturer's guidelines when using ointments or lubricants with petroleum base because they may compromise the integrity of the BMS device.[2,4,10]

- BMS are most commonly used in critical care settings but they may be appropriate in a wider range of acute-care settings.[26]

- Transient fecal incontinence and diarrhea are common among hospitalized patients. Goals of a bowel management program should be clearly discussed among all physicians, advanced practice nurses, other healthcare professionals, patient, and family. Goals should include treatment of the cause of the fecal incontinence if possible and prevention of perineal tissue injury, and may not require a containment device.

EQUIPMENT

- Nonsterile gloves
- Personal protective equipment (e.g., gowns and face protection)
- Water
- Water-soluble lubricant
- BMS
- Underpads
- Skin-cleansing solution

Additional equipment, to have available as needed, includes the following:

- Scissors

Procedure for Fecal Containment Device and Bowel Management System (BMS)—*Continued*

Steps	Rationale	Special Considerations
11. Inflate the BMS balloon with water or normal saline solution per instruction guidelines. **(Level M*)**	Water or normal saline solution may be used to inflate the balloon and hold the device in place.	Manufacturer may include prepackaged syringes. Do not exceed the manufacturer's recommended volume for balloon inflation. Additional fluid volume in the balloon can increase the amount of pressure on intestinal mucosa and contribute to leakage of the device.
12. Gently pull the BMS back to ensure the balloon is in the rectum and positioned against the rectal floor (Fig. 135-3). **(Level M)**	The device should rest on the rectal floor to collect fecal material and provide a seal.	Some BMS manufacturers have a position indicator noted on the drainage tubing that should be visible after insertion.

*Level M: Manufacturer's recommendations only.

Procedure continues on following page

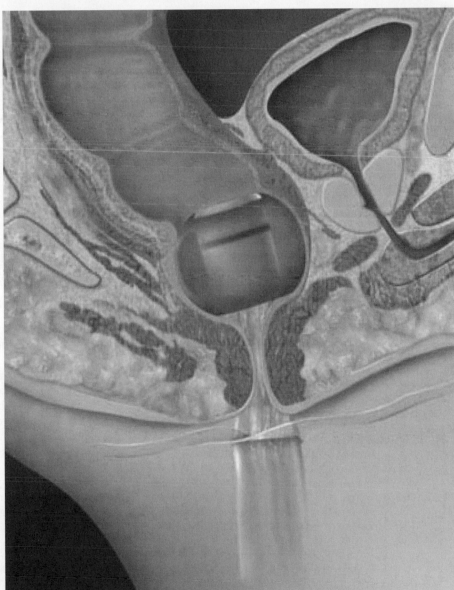

Figure 135-3 Correct placement of a bowel management system in the rectum. (*Courtesy of Hollister, Inc., Libertyville, IL.*)

PATIENT AND FAMILY EDUCATION

- Explain the procedure and rationale for insertion of a BMS. *Rationale:* Patient and family anxiety and discomfort may be decreased.
- Discuss goals of bowel management program and expected benefits of the intervention. *Rationale:* The patient is prepared for placement of the BMS, possible odors, and perineal skin and wound care interventions.

PATIENT ASSESSMENT AND PREPARATION

Patient Assessment

- Review the patient's medical record and discuss medical history with the patient for possible contraindications before placement of a BMS. *Rationale:* Possible complications associated with placement of device are avoided.
- Evaluate consistency of fecal contents; contents must be liquid to semiliquid to flow through the BMS. *Rationale:* Liquid fecal consistency is important to prevent occlusion of the device.[3]

- Assess perineal skin for the presence of open areas and pressure ulcers, and apply moisture barrier creams. *Rationale:* BMS may be used to prevent and treat IAD, and additional skin care products may be indicated to assist in perineal skin healing.[29]
- Evaluate the patient need for analgesia or sedation. *Rationale:* Patient may tolerate the procedure more comfortably.

Patient Preparation

- Verify that the patient is the correct patient using two identifiers. *Rationale:* Before performing a procedure, the nurse should ensure the correct identification of the patient for the intended intervention.
- Ensure that the patient and family understand preprocedural teachings. Answer questions as they arise, and reinforce information as needed. *Rationale:* Understanding of previously taught information is evaluated and reinforced.
- Optimize lighting in the room, and provide privacy for the patient. *Rationale:* These facilitate visualization and enhance patient tolerance of the procedure.[3]

Procedure for Fecal Containment Device and Bowel Management System (BMS)

Steps	Rationale	Special Considerations
Fecal containment devices are commercially available. General principles for placement of the device are consistent between systems; however, the physician, advanced practice nurse, or other healthcare professional should read and follow manufacturer-specific guidelines for placement of the device. Procedure may be most effectively performed with two physicians, advanced practice nurses, or other healthcare professionals.		
Fecal Containment Device		
1. **HH**		
2. **PE**		
3. Position the patient in the left lateral position with the upper knee slightly flexed.[3,28] **(Level D*)**	Assists with visualization and comfort of the patient for placement.[3]	
4. Cleanse the perineal area with no-rinse, pH-balanced cleansing solution. Allow skin to dry thoroughly.[28] **(Level D)**	Evaluate skin for presence of breakdown. Fecal containment device adheres better to clean, dry skin.	Do not apply device if perineal skin is not intact.[28,29] Consider clipping hair to facilitate better adherence.[28]
5. Separate the patient's buttocks. If recommended by the manufacturer, a no-sting skin protectant barrier solution can be applied and allowed to dry.[19,29] **(Level D)**	Application of the containment device usually requires a pair of experienced physicians, advanced practice nurses, or other healthcare professionals to correctly position the patient and apply the device correctly.[19,29]	Avoid use of adhesive products that can cause discomfort or irritation to delicate perineal tissue. See manufacturer's instructions for specifics on application and tips for better adherence.
6. Remove protective wrap and firmly apply the fecal containment device around the anus. **(Level M*)**	Firm pressure and body heat allows the adhesive backing of the fecal containment device to adhere more effectively to the skin.	The opening of the fecal containment device may need to be adjusted by the physician, advanced practice nurse, or other healthcare professional to fit comfortably yet snugly around the anal opening.

*Level D: Peer-reviewed professional and organizational standards with the support of clinical study recommendations.
*Level M: Manufacturer's recommendations only.

Procedure continues on following page

Procedure	for Fecal Containment Device and Bowel Management System (BMS)—*Continued*	
Steps	**Rationale**	**Special Considerations**
7. Attach the collection bag to the distal opening of the fecal containment device and place in a dependent position. **(Level M*)**	The collection device moves the fecal material away from the skin.	Unless contraindicated, position the patient in a side-lying position and avoid placing the patient's weight on the device.
8. Monitor the volume, consistency, and color of fecal material. Fecal output needs to be evaluated as part of the patient's overall output assessment.	If diarrhea is excessive, fluids and electrolytes may be lost in the feces, resulting in dehydration and electrolyte imbalances.	
9. Change the fecal containment device if leaking is noted or if the stool is too thick to pass through the device; if diarrhea has resolved, consider discontinuing use.	An adequate seal is necessary for effective performance of the fecal containment device and protection of perineal skin.	Gently remove the fecal containment device to avoid tearing skin. Use a nonirritating, no-sting adhesive remover to assist with removal of the device.
10. Discard used supplies.	Maintains infection-control practices and decreases contamination.	
11. ⬛		
Bowel Management System (BMS)		
1. Obtain the system prescribed.	Obtains equipment.	Several systems are commercially available. General principles for placement of the device are consistent between systems; however, the physician, advanced practice nurse, or other healthcare professional should read and follow manufacturer-specific guidelines for placement of the device.
2. ⬛		
3. ⬛		
4. Administer prescribed analgesia or sedation agents if ordered.	May assist patient tolerance of the procedure.	
5. Position the patient in the left lateral position with the upper knee slightly flexed.[3,28] **(Level D*)**	Assists with visualization and comfort of the patient for placement.[3]	
6. Apply water-soluble lubricant to a gloved finger and perform a manual digital rectal examination.[3,28] **(Level D)**	Evaluates rectal vault for impacted stool and rectal tone.[3]	Perform digital disimpaction before continuing with placement of the BMS. The device may not be retained if rectal tone is poor.
7. Remove anything else from the rectum, such as temperature probes. **(Level M*)**	Prevents trauma and improper placement of the device.	
8. Cleanse the perineal area with a no-rinse, pH-balanced cleansing solution.	Allows for better visualization of the skin, and thus evaluation for the presence of breakdown.	
9. Open the BMS kit and connect the pieces according to the manufacturer's instructions. **(Level M)**	The functionality of the device should be assessed before placement.[2,4,10]	
10. Apply water-soluble lubricant to the distal end of the BMS. With slow, gentle pressure, advance the balloon through the anal sphincter. **(Level M)**	Lubricant assists with insertion of the device gently through the anus and into the rectal vault.	Do not advance BMS if resistance is felt.

*Level D: Peer-reviewed professional and organizational standards with the support of clinical study recommendations.
*Level M: Manufacturer's recommendations only.

Procedure	for Fecal Containment Device and Bowel Management System (BMS)—*Continued*	
Steps	**Rationale**	**Special Considerations**
13. A. Position the drainage bag in a dependent position.	Allows for effective flow of fecal material.	Unless contraindicated, posi[tion the] patient in a side-lying pos[ition] and avoid placing the pati[ent's] body weight on the device [or] tubing.
B. Ensure there is no traction on the drainage bag or tubing.	Prevents damage to the rectal mucosa (monge).	
C. Secure the tubing and drainage bag.	Prevents traumatic removal and possible damage to the rectal mucosa (sparks).	
14. Evaluate the consistency of the fecal material. Stool should be liquid to semiliquid. The BMS may be irrigated with water as necessary to ensure patency.[4,12] **(Level M*)**	Allows for effective flow of fecal material.	Slight leakage or smear of fe[ces] often unavoidable. Do not [exceed] manufacturer's recommen[dation] for fluid volume in the bal[loon].
15. Discard used supplies and remove protective equipment and gloves and discard.	Maintains infection-control practices.	
16. ⬛		

*Level M: Manufacturer's recommendations only.

Expected Outcomes

- Containment of liquid feces
- Perineal skin remains intact or, if compromised before placement of BMS, healing of skin is evident
- Input and output balance are maintained

Unexpected Outcomes

- Injury to anal sphincter or rectal vault
- Fluid and electrolyte imbalances
- Infection
- Pressure necrosis
- Loss of sphincter tone*
- Perineal skin breakdown

Patient Monitoring and Care

Steps	Rationale	Reportable Conditions
		These conditions should be re[ported] if they persist despite nursi[ng] interventions.
1. Assess patient, perineal skin, and fecal drainage. **(Level C*)**	Continued assessment of patient IAD and possible development of pressure ulcers is essential because they may prolong the patient's hospitalization.[16]	- Foul drainage or odor - Worsening erythema and e[dema] - Pain - Elevated temperature - Elevated white blood cell c[ount]
2. Monitor fluid and electrolyte balances.	If diarrhea is excessive, fluids and electrolytes may be lost in the feces, resulting in dehydration and electrolyte imbalances.	- Output greater than input - Abnormal electrolyte labor[atory] analysis - Signs and symptoms of ele[ctrolyte] imbalances (i.e., cardiac ec[topy,] neuromuscular symptoms, tachycardia, decreased urin[ary] output, thirst, signs and sym[ptoms] of dehydration

*Level C: Qualitative studies, descriptive or correlational studies, integrative reviews, systematic reviews, or randomized controlled trials with inconsistent [results]

PREREQUISITE N[URSING] KNOWLEDGE

- Negative-pressure wound [therapy is a method of] wound care therapy that [uses a sealed,] transparent device-speci[fic or generic] dressing, tubing, and pow[ered suc-]tion canister.[15]
- Other terms found in th[e literature include] topical negative pressure, [vacuum-assisted,] and subatmospheric press[ure.]
- Many different U.S. F[ood and Drug Administration] (FDA)–approved vacuum [devices deliver] NPWT.[8,12,15] The Agency [for Healthcare Research and] Quality (AHRQ) provide[s a comparison of the] manufacturers.[20] The mos[t commonly used in the] acute-care practice setting[s are the V.A.C.] Therapy Systems (KCI Lic[ensing, Inc.), San Antonio, TX;] Fig. 136-1). ActiV.A.C. a[nd others use a reticulated] open-cell foam wound co[ntact layer. Other devices] on the market use either an[timicrobial gauze or a wet-to-moist] pack method with an antim[icrobial solution or dress-]ing. The use of a moisten[ed gauze dressing has] also been reported in the lit[erature as a method] for NPWT.[1,6]
- Most randomized controll[ed trials (RCTs) involving] NPWT have been conducte[d with very] small, randomized controll[ed trials. No RCTs compare alter-]nate NPWT systems to the[devices to date] to be comparable.[1,5,16] Furth[er research into] wound closure outcomes w[ith various devices] is needed.[6,8,12]
- NPWT assists with wound [healing by creating con-]trolled subatmospheric (neg[ative) pressure on the] wound bed. This mechanica[l stress creates a compres-]sive force on the wound b[ed and periwound tissue,] increasing the effectivene[ss of wound closure by] enhancing the proliferation [of granulation tissue.] NPWT enhances lymphatic [drainage and interstitial] fluid, decreasing wound e[dema and removing from] the wound site, further a[ssisting in healing (Fig.] 136-2).[2,3,6,8,10,12,22]

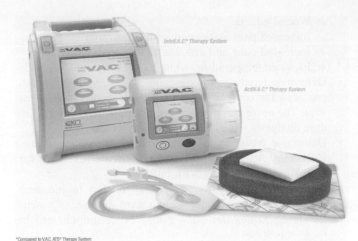

Figure 136-1 Components of the Vacuum-Assisted Closure System: ActiV.A.C. Therapy System and InfoV.A.C. Therapy System. *(Used with permission. Courtesy of KCI, an Acelity Company.)*

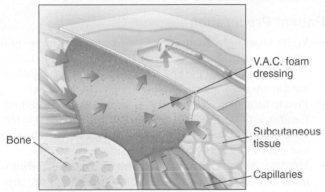

Figure 136-2 V.A.C. Therapy System Illustration. Fluid, exudate, and debris removed from wound bed. *(Used with permission. Courtesy of KCI, an Acelity Company.)*

- Wounds with infections should have systemic antibiotic treatment before initiation of NPWT. If continued deterioration of the wound or infection persists, consider discontinuation of NPWT with possible evaluation for surgical drainage of infection per the physician, advanced practice nurse, or other healthcare professional.
- Wounds treated with NPWT develop a characteristic, beefy red granulation bed. A pale wound bed or friable granulation tissue is a secondary sign of infection and may be more reliable than the traditional indicators of infection.[19]
- Dehisced infected sternal wounds with use of NPWT require effective débridement of infected bone and a specific nonadherent wound contact layer before a NPWT dressing is placed.[6]
- Successful management of enteric fistulae with NPWT with use of special application techniques has been reported in case studies but no clinical trials at this time. See NPWT device manuals for specific techniques in the management of fistulae.
- Rapid formation of granulation tissue with NPWT can lead to the development of abscesses. The surgically

dehisced wound with NPWT should be monitored closely for abscess formation, particularly in patients with large irregular wounds with undermining present.
- Transcutaneous oxygen pressure ($Tcpo_2$) evaluation should be considered before initiation of NPWT to lower extremity or toe wounds because of vascular flow requirements that are needed for optimal wound healing with NPWT.
- Contraindications to the use of NPWT include malignancy disease in the wound, untreated osteomyelitis, non-enteric and unexplored fistulae, and necrotic tissue with eschar present.[6,12,21] See the manufacturer's NPWT manual for special precautions required with exposed blood vessels, organs, tendons, and nerves. Precautions should be used for wounds with active bleeding, for difficult wound hemostasis, and for patients undergoing anticoagulation therapy.[10]
- For significant bleeding, NPWT should be stopped immediately and measures taken to stop bleeding. The dressing should be left in place and the treating physician or surgeon consulted.[21]
- For optimal NPWT with the VAC device, at least 22 hours of daily uninterrupted therapy should be delivered.[21] The newer vacuum units do not have research evidence at this time for the required time duration of uninterrupted therapy for wound healing. NPWT dressings are usually changed every 48 to 72 hours, 2 or 3 times weekly.[12,21] However, infected wound beds may require more frequent dressing changes (every 12 hours), and dressings over grafts may be changed less frequently (every 3 to 7 days).[11,17,21] The wound bed should be free of necrotic tissue and debris before application of the NPWT dressing.
- In highly exudative wounds, drainage from the wound bed may be significant in the first 24 to 48 hours of therapy. Additional fluids may need to be provided for individuals with heavily draining wounds.[14]
- Nutritional requirements for wound healing are great. These needs must be assessed, met, and monitored frequently because poor nutrition can impede successful NPWT wound healing.
- The NPWT units discussed previously (ActiV.A.C. and InfoV.A.C. Therapy Systems) offer home units with increased portability. Smaller size and increased battery life allow for continuation of therapy outside of the acute hospital setting.

EQUIPMENT

The following is generic equipment used for most NPWT units. Device- and wound-specific variations may need to be considered by the physician, advanced practice nurse, or other healthcare professional.

- Sterile and nonsterile gloves, gown, as indicated per institutional policy
- Normal saline or wound cleanser with appropriate psi delivery device (see Procedure 132)
- Protective barrier film/wipe for periwound protection
- NPWT dressing with tubing/transparent drape kit (device specific)

- NPWT vacuum unit/collection chamber (device specific)
- Sterile scissors

PATIENT AND FAMILY EDUCATION

- Assess patient and family readiness to learn and any factors that may affect learning. Identification of the patient's preferred learning strategies (auditory, visualization, return demonstration) is also important. *Rationale:* The nurse can develop the most appropriate teaching strategy for each patient.
- Provide information about NPWT, the procedure, anticipated duration of therapy, and the equipment. *Rationale:* Information may decrease or alleviate anxiety by assisting patient and family to understand the procedure, why it is needed, and the preferred outcomes.
- Explain the procedure and the reason for changing the wound dressing. *Rationale:* May decrease patient anxiety.
- Discuss the patient's role during the dressing change procedure and in maintaining the NPWT system. *Rationale:* Patient cooperation is elicited; the patient is prepared for wound management on discharge.

PATIENT ASSESSMENT AND PREPARATION

Patient Assessment

- Fully assess the wound with documentation of wound measurements, characteristics, and appropriateness for the procedure. *Rationale:* Assessment ensures that use of NPWT is not contraindicated. Data are provided for comparison at successive dressing changes.
- Assess for signs and symptoms of wound infection, including the following.[18] *Rationale:* Although NPWT assists with removal of excessive fluid, thus reducing the potential of bacteria in the wound bed, assessment for signs and symptoms of wound infection is necessary, especially in patients with compromised conditions.
  - ❖ Periwound erythema
  - ❖ Increased periwound warmth
  - ❖ Wound edema
  - ❖ Increased pain associated with the wound
  - ❖ Increased odor and amount of wound exudate
  - ❖ Elevated temperature, white blood cell count, or chills
- Determine baseline pain assessment. *Rationale:* Data are provided for comparison with postprocedure assessment data. The nurse can plan for preprocedure and intraprocedure analgesia.
- Determine baseline nutritional and fluid volume status. *Rationale:* Adequate fluids and protein are necessary for optimal wound healing with NPWT.
- Assess medical history, especially related to bleeding problems, fistula formation, malignant disease, or vascular status. *Rationale:* NPWT may be contraindicated in these conditions.
- Assess current medications specifically related to anticoagulant use. *Rationale:* Possible areas of caution that should be monitored with NPWT use are identified.
- Assess current laboratory values, especially coagulation studies. *Rationale:* Abnormalities possibly associated with risks related to NPWT use are identified.

Patient Preparation

- Verify that the patient is the correct patient using two identifiers. *Rationale:* Before performing a procedure, the nurse should ensure the correct identification of the patient for the intended intervention.
- Ensure patient and family understanding of the procedure. Reinforce teaching points as needed. *Rationale:* Understanding of previously taught information is evaluated, and a conduit for questions is provided.
- Validate the presence of patent intravenous access. *Rationale:* Access may be needed for administration of intravenous analgesic medications.
- Position the patient in a manner that will ensure patient comfort and privacy, and facilitate dressing application. *Rationale:* The patient is prepared to undergo the procedure.
- Administer prescribed analgesics if needed. *Rationale:* Analgesics improve comfort level and tolerance of the procedure and decrease patient anxiety and discomfort.

Procedure	for Negative-Pressure Wound Therapy		
Steps	**Rationale**		**Special Considerations**

Procedure for KCI VAC Therapy for Wounds; VAC Application

Steps	Rationale	Special Considerations
1. Obtain and prepare equipment.	Prepares for the procedure.	General principles of NPWT are consistent across devices; however, wound-specific and device-specific guidelines need to be reviewed before NPWT. **Steps 1–8** are generic to all NPWT applications. This procedure uses a clean technique; however, sterile techniques may be desired per wound characteristics or clinician preference.[21]
2. **HH**		
3. **PE**		
4. Prepare a clean field for a dressing change, then remove gloves. Repeat **HH** and **PE**.	Prevents contamination of supplies and materials.	
5. Position the patient to facilitate wound cleansing with dressing application.	Provides for patient's comfort and allows for visualization and access to the wound.	
6. Assess, measure wound, and assemble supplies as indicated.[5,8,9] **(Level D*)**	Select NPWT dressing type with appropriate size approximating the wound size. Multiple types of VAC-specialty size dressings are available (refer to the manufacturer's manual). VAC-specific dressings: A. Black polyurethane foam (GranuFoam) has larger pores and is considered to be more effective in stimulating granulation tissue formation and wound contraction. It is the most frequently used. B. White polyvinyl chloride foam (WhiteFoam) is more dense, is premoistened, and has increased tensile strength. Because of its higher density, it requires higher pressure to obtain the same granulation rate as black foam. C. Black polyurethane foam, GranuFoam Silver, has antimicrobial silver and may reduce infections in wounds.[5,21]	The black VAC dressing does not hold moisture but allows exudates to pass through the dressing and be removed. Its design results in rapid growth of new granulation. The white VAC dressing holds moisture but also allows exudate to be removed through it. It is nonadherent and can be used in tunnels and shallow undermining because of its higher tensile strength. Additional precautions must be taken when using Granufoam Silver™. Please refer to specific product instructions when using Granufoam Silver™. It should not be used as a replacement for systemic therapy for infection.[5]
7. Cleanse the wound according to orders (see Procedure 132) or institutional protocol.[19]	Wound bed cleansing and irrigation prepare the wound bed for the application of the dressing.[10]	

*Level D: Peer-reviewed professional and organizational standards with the support of clinical study recommendations.

Procedure continues on following page

Procedure   for Negative-Pressure Wound Therapy—*Continued*

Steps	Rationale	Special Considerations
8. The physician, advanced practice nurse, or other healthcare professional may debride (see Procedure 133) necrotic tissue or eschar if applicable.	NPWT assists with autolytic and mechanical débridement of surface slough; it should not be used as a primary means of débridement. Sharp débridement of necrotic tissue should be performed before initiation of therapy for optimal healing with NPWT.[9,10]	If extensive débridement is needed, surgical débridement in the operative suite may be necessary.
9. Prepare the periwound by cleansing with warm solution. Clip the hair around the wound. Dry the skin and prepare the periwound tissue with a barrier protective film.[4,9,14] (**Level D***)	Moisture from perspiration, oil, or body fluids may interfere with the drape's adherence. Barrier films act as a protectant against periwound maceration.	Multiple removals of transparent drape may irritate hair follicles and result in folliculitis.
10. Remove gloves.		
11. 🖐		
12. Apply nonsterile gloves.		
13. Open an intact package and cut the VAC foam with sterile scissors; do not cut the foam directly over the wound.[12,21] (**Level E***)	Prevents small particles of dressing from falling into the wound. The dressing should be cut to fit the size and shape of the wound, including tunnels and undermined areas. Tunneling can result in a cyst or abscess when vacuum pressure or granulation closes the entrance to the tunnel. Bacterial invasion and impaired healing result from unfilled dead space.[18]	Any exposed sutures, tendons, ligaments or nerves should be protected with placement of a layer of nonadherent dressing over them. Foam dressings should not be placed in direct contact with exposed blood vessels, anastomotic sites, organs, or nerves. Any exposed vessels or organs in or near the wound must be fully protected before NPWT is applied.[21] See manufacturer NPWT manual for special precautions required.
14. Gently place foam into the wound, ensuring contact with all wound surfaces. Do not allow foam to overlap onto intact skin. Do not force foam dressing into any area of the wound. Always note total number of foam pieces used with notation on transparent drape and in the patient's chart.[17] (**Level E***)	Capillaries can be compressed if dressings are packed too tightly, and pressure on newly formed granulation tissue may prevent or delay healing.[12] Foam that is placed directly on intact skin may cause skin breakdown.	More than one dressing may be used to fill the wound bed. Foam pieces should be in contact with but not overlapping each other to allow equalization of negative pressure applied to the wound bed by the suction device.[2,21] For small wounds, a larger piece of foam may need to be placed on top of the wound filler foam to provide an adequate surface for the Therapeutic Regulated Accurate Care T.R.A.C. Pad. Protect intact periwound skin with skin prep and drape under the foam.[21]
15. Trim and place the VAC transparent drape to cover the foam dressing and an additional 3–5 cm of intact periwound skin. Avoid stretching the drape over the wound.[21] (**Level M***)	Avoids tension and shearing forces on the surrounding tissue.	Bridging of wounds can be done for more than one wound of similar pathology in close proximity with one vacuum pump. See manufacturer-specific instructions.

*Level D: Peer-reviewed professional and organizational standards with the support of clinical study recommendations.

*Level E: Multiple case reports, theory-based evidence from expert opinions, or peer-reviewed professional organizational standards without clinical studies to support recommendations.

*Level M: Manufacturer's recommendations only.

Procedure	for Negative-Pressure Wound Therapy—*Continued*	
Steps	**Rationale**	**Special Considerations**
16. Cut a 2.5-cm hole in the transparent drape, for fluid to pass through. Cut a hole rather than a slit because a slit may self-seal during therapy. Apply the T.R.A.C. pad with tubing directly over the hole in the transparent drape. Apply gentle pressure around the pad to ensure complete adhesion.[21] **(Level M*)**	The vacuum does not function without an occlusive seal. The drape may also help maintain a moist wound environment. The drape is vapor permeable and allows for gas exchange. It also protects the wound from external contamination.	The foam contracts into the wound bed if seal is obtained. If foam does not contract, reassess the outer dressing for possible leaks in the system or dressing seal.[2,9]
17. Ensure the position of the T.R.A.C. tubing is not over bony prominences.[9,21] **(Level E*)**	Minimizes the risk of pressure related to tubing placement.	Extra foams with drape can be used under the tubing to reduce pressure and stabilize the tubing.
18. Remove the VAC canister from the packaging and insert into the vacuum unit. Connect T.R.A.C. pad tubing to canister tubing and ensure clamps are open.	Closed clamps prevent activation of the negative therapy.	
19. Turn the power on to the vacuum unit and select prescribed therapy setting. Assess the dressing to ensure seal integrity. The dressing should collapse with a wrinkled appearance and no hissing sounds.[21] **(Level M*)**	Setting options include continuous or intermittent negative-pressure therapy. The settings are determined by type of wound, exudate, and goals as ordered by the physician (Table 136-1).	If the dressing does not collapse, check tubing and transparent drape for leaks. Use an additional drape to seal leaks as necessary.
20. Discard used supplies; remove gloves.		
21. 🖐		

*Level E: Multiple case reports, theory-based evidence from expert opinions, or peer-reviewed professional organizational standards without clinical studies to support recommendations.
*Level M: Manufacturer's recommendations only.

Procedure continues on following page

TABLE 136-1	Recommended Therapy Setting for KCI VAC Therapy	
Wound Characteristics	**Continuous Therapy**	**Intermittent Therapy**
Difficult dressing application	X	
Flap	X	
Highly exuding	X	
Grafts	X	
Painful wounds	X	
Tunnels or undermining	X	
Unstable structures	X	
Minimally exuding	X	X
Large wounds	X	X
Small wounds	X	X
Stalled wound healing progress	X	X
VAC white foam dressing	X	X

Responsible physician or advanced practice nurse should be consulted for individual patient conditions. Consult device user manual and manufacturer's recommended guidelines before use.
(Adapted from 2014 V.A.C. Therapy Clinical Guidelines, page 20, Table 1-1: Recommended Therapy Settings. Used with permission. Courtesy of KCI, an Acclity Company.)

Procedure for Negative-Pressure Wound Therapy—*Continued*

Steps	Rationale	Special Considerations
VAC Dressing Removal Procedure 1. Provide analgesia as appropriate for the patient's condition before the procedure.	Patients may experience discomfort during dressing changes or removal.[21]	
2. ▦		
3. ▦		
4. To remove the dressing, raise the tubing connector above the level of the vacuum unit and tighten clamps on the dressing tubing. Disconnect the two tubings at the connection point.	Removes any remaining fluid from the tubing for purposes of infection control, preventing leakage.	
5. Allow the vacuum unit to pull the exudate through the canister tubing into the canister, then tighten the clamp on the canister tube. Turn off the vacuum unit. Remove the canister from the vacuum unit and discard.	Allows exudate to be contained; the canister should be discarded per institutional policy.	
6. Allow foam to decompress. Gently stretch the transparent drape horizontally to release adhesive from the skin. Do not peel vertically. Gently remove foam dressing from wound.[21] **(Level M*)**	Decreases patient discomfort and potential for skin and wound trauma.	
7. Discard used supplies; remove gloves.		
8. ▦		

*Level M: Manufacturer's recommendations only.

Expected Outcomes

- Wound healing or granulation enhanced by consistent negative-pressure therapy; early signs of contraction of wound margins
- Decreased volume of wound exudate (over time) and absence of foul odor or color
- Enhanced wound healing because of effective wound fluid or edema removal
- Decrease in the size of the wound with ability for surgical closure with flap/graft or skin graft; complete healing of the wound
- Decreased time to satisfactory healing (may decrease hospital length of stay and cost)

Unexpected Outcomes

- Infection
- Bleeding
- Fistula formation
- Disruption of underlying tissue or structures
- Pain
- Misplacement over exposed vessel, ligaments, other structures
- Lack of improvement in wound after 1–2 weeks of therapy
- Tissue loss
- Ischemia and necrosis
- Periwound maceration

Patient Monitoring and Care

Steps	Rationale	Reportable Conditions
		These conditions should be reported if they persist despite nursing interventions.
1. Assess location of VAC T.R.A.C. tubing to avoid excessive pressure on surrounding tissue or structures.	Excessive pressure may result in tissue breakdown from tubing over bony prominences.	• Tissue breakdown
2. Assess patency of VAC system; drape has an occlusive seal, tubing is patent, and foam is compressed.	The VAC dressing should be collapsed when the seal is maintained and negative pressure is being delivered in a consistent manner. Alarms on the device indicate loss of seal; raised foam dressing indicates loss of negative-pressure therapy. See manufacturer's clinical guidelines for troubleshooting difficulties with NPWT dressings.	• Loss of seal • Raised foam dressing • Wound drainage suddenly decreasing in amount or stopping
3. Assess the amount and type of the drainage.	Color of drainage can suggest bleeding, and the rate of canister filling can alert the caregiver to wound problems.	• Bright red blood or rapid filling of the canister
4. Monitor condition of the wound bed and periwound skin with dressing changes; observe for signs of wound infection.	Identifies any evidence of wound healing or any changes or abnormalities indicative of complications.	• Periwound erythema • Heat, edema, pain • Elevated temperature and white blood cell count • Cloudy or foul-smelling wound drainage • Increased wound drainage • Excess bleeding • Changes in tissue color within the wound bed • Macerated, broken, or discolored periwound skin • New tunneling or undermining • Stool in the wound bed • Signs or symptoms of infection
5. Change the dressing every 48–72 hours, 2 or 3 times weekly. If infection is present, increase the frequency of dressing change to every 12–24 hours.[17,21] **(Level D*)**	Removes exudate from the wound bed. If the dressing adheres to the wound base, consider interfacing a single layer of nonadherent porous material (e.g., meshed silicone, meshed petroleum impregnated dressings and meshed oil emulsion impregnated dressings),[21] also known as a contact layer, between the dressing and the wound when reapplying the dressing. If previous dressings were difficult to remove and painful, consider instillation into the tubing or dressing of a topical anesthetic agent such as 1% lidocaine without epinephrine ordered by the physician or advanced practice nurse.[5]	

*Level D: Peer-reviewed professional and organizational standards with the support of clinical study recommendations.

Procedure continues on following page

Patient Monitoring and Care —*Continued*

Steps	Rationale	Reportable Conditions
6. Monitor the mode (continuous or intermittent) and level of suction.[4] (**Level E***)	Removal of edema and debris alleviates compressive forces, thus improving perfusion. Suctioning fluid from within the wound may remove wound fluid factors that inhibit healing.[6] Application and release of negative pressure on the wound bed stimulate cell proliferation and protein synthesis.[6] Mechanical stretch on the tissue by the negative pressure draws the wound toward the center, closing the defect.[8,21]	• Patient discomfort • Excess granulation tissue overgrowth into the dressing with removal • Continued edema within wound bed
7. Maintain an airtight seal.[9,21] (**Level E***)	Loss of an airtight seal can result in a decreased amount of drainage removal and in desiccation of the wound.[9] See the manufacturer's clinical guidelines for troubleshooting difficulties with maintaining a seal.	• Problems maintaining an airtight seal
8. Label the dressing with the date and time of application and amount of foam pieces placed in wound.	VAC foam dressings are not bioabsorbable. Ensure all pieces of foam are removed from the wound with each dressing change.	• Foam left in the wound for greater than the recommended time period may foster ingrowth of tissue into the foam and create difficulty in removal of foam pieces from the wound or lead to infection[10,21]
9. Change the canister when full, or at least weekly. Keep canister position level.	Controls odor.	• Increased drainage amounts
10. Monitor the amount of wound drainage.[14] (**Level D***)	If a wound produces excessive fluid, the patient may experience a fluid imbalance, requiring intravenous replacement. Excess drainage may also result in increased protein loss. A nutritional consultation to replace protein loss from wound exudates may be indicated.	• Increased drainage amounts • Wound drainage that is foul-smelling and cloudy
11. Follow institutional standards for assessing pain. Administer analgesia as prescribed. Pain can be associated with application of dressing, initiation of initial therapy, intermittent cycling, or removal of the dressing.	Identifies the need for pain interventions. Use of analgesics at dressing changes can reduce the pain. The use of a wound contact layer may also decrease pain with dressing changes.[5,6] Additionally, lowering the initial amount of negative pressure or maintaining the pressure at continual versus intermittent levels can assist in pain control.[5,21] Some evidence has shown decreased pain with dressing changes when using gauze as a wound filler.[5,6] Pain during treatment may be alleviated through the use of the WhiteFoam rather than black foam.[21] See manufacturer-specific instructions.	• Continued pain despite pain interventions

*Level D: Peer-reviewed professional and organizational standards with the support of clinical study recommendations.
*Level E: Multiple case reports, theory-based evidence from expert opinions, or peer-reviewed professional organizational standards without clinical studies to support recommendations.

Patient Monitoring and Care —*Continued*

Steps	Rationale	Reportable Conditions
12. See the manufacturer's guidelines for discharge considerations for patients with NPWT, and consult appropriate healthcare personnel for assistance when discharging patients with NPWT.	Obtaining NPWT for home use can be complex and there are important safety concerns.	

Documentation

Documentation should include the following:

- Patient and family education
- Patient tolerance of the procedure
- Condition of the wound bed and periwound skin description
- Characteristics of wound drainage
- Mode (continuous or intermittent) and degree (mm Hg) of suction
- Nursing interventions
- Pain medication given and patient's response to the pain medication

- Wound débridement procedure (if applicable); wound cleansing procedure completed, dated, and timed
- Size of the wound measured by length, width, and depth (consider obtaining a photograph of the wound, depending on institutional policy)
- Size and type of foam dressing applied, and **total number of foam pieces placed in the wound**
- Unexpected outcomes, reportable conditions

References and Additional Readings

For a complete list of references and additional readings for this procedure, scan this QR code with any freely available smartphone code reader app, or visit http://booksite.elsevier.com/9780323376624.

137 Wound Management with Excessive Drainage

Justin Burleson

PURPOSE: Management of wound exudate is an essential step in wound healing. Pouching may be used to divert and contain excessive drainage. Suction may be used to remove drainage or used in conjunction with pouching. Drains may be placed in the wound for management of drainage.

PREREQUISITE NURSING KNOWLEDGE

- Wound exudate is produced in response to the inflammatory phase of the healing process. As wounds heal, the amount of exudate should diminish. Chronic, nonhealing wounds may produce exudate for prolonged periods of time, necessitating effective management of the fluid.[2,3,5,8,9,11,12]
- Goals of wound care must be clearly identified so that proper wound care products are used.[10] Wound healing is best achieved through adequate cleansing, débridement, and dressing of the wound bed on the basis of wound characteristics.
- Excessive wound fluid may create pressure in the wound bed and compromise perfusion. Excessive moisture may cause periwound tissue damage and extend the wound or skin injury.[2,7,9,12,13]
- Assessment of wound exudate should include the quantity, color, consistency, and odor of drainage. When changes in wound exudate occur, the cause should be explored. These changes along with other clinical signs and symptoms (i.e., fever) may indicate a possible increase in bacterial burden or infection.
- Drains are placed in wounds to facilitate healing by providing a route for excessive fluid accumulating in or near the wound bed to escape. Most wound drains are surgically placed; drains may or may not be secured with sutures.[7]
- Excessive wound fluid may provide a source for proliferation of microorganisms. Wound drains may be ports of microorganism entry. Microorganisms in the wound bed continue the inflammatory phase of wound healing and delay wound resolution; aseptic techniques must be strictly observed to reduce the risk of infection.
- Pouching is an effective means of collecting wound and fistula drainage.[7] Suction may be used with pouching systems to pull fluid away from the wound bed.[5]
- Excessive wound drainage is removed to allow for wound healing to occur without tissue congestion, microorganism proliferation, and skin maceration.

- Excessive wound drainage may need to be calculated into the assessment of a patient's daily intake and output. At a minimum it is necessary to note how often dressings or pads are being changed to track excessive exudate.
- Negative-pressure wound therapy (see Procedure 136) stimulates tissue growth and promotes wound healing. The closed system also provides active withdrawal of excessive wound fluid to assist in the management of exudating wounds.[4,7–10]
- Assess the patient's nutritional needs, specifically for protein along with consideration of micronutrients such as vitamins A, C, and D and trace elements such as copper, zinc, and selenium, with exudating wounds.[6]
- Excessive wound exudate production may result in the loss of up to 100 g of protein daily in wound exudate.[2,6,11,13] Nutritional supplementation of protein is necessary for wound healing.

EQUIPMENT

- Nonsterile gloves and face mask with eye shield
- Sterile gloves and gowns
- Sterile gauze (4×4 pads); abdominal pad (e.g., ABD) or other absorptive dressings may be needed
- Sterile water or normal saline (NS) solution for cleansing
- Liquid skin barrier, skin barrier wafers, paste, powder and sealant, or hydrocolloid to protect periwound surface
- Drainage bag or pouch: ostomy-type appliance
- Hypoallergenic tape

Additional equipment, to have available as needed, includes the following:

- Clean scissors or forceps
- Desiccant powder

PATIENT AND FAMILY EDUCATION

- Explain the procedure and the reason for changing the wound dressing; educate the patient regarding potential pain and odor during the procedure. *Rationale:* Patient anxiety and discomfort are decreased.

- Discuss the patient's role in the dressing-change procedure and maintenance of wound drains or pouches. ***Rationale:*** Patient cooperation is elicited; patient is prepared for wound management at discharge.

PATIENT ASSESSMENT AND PREPARATION

Patient Assessment

- Monitor for signs and symptoms of wound infection, including the following. ***Rationale:*** Early detection of infection facilitates prompt and appropriate interventions.
  - ❖ Erythema
  - ❖ Edema
  - ❖ Increased pain
  - ❖ Elevated temperature and white blood cell count
  - ❖ Changes in wound drainage: amount, color, odor
  - ❖ Increased pressure or tenderness at wound site
- Assess the patency of the wound drainage system. ***Rationale:*** Drains are frequently soft and pliable and thus can easily become kinked or blocked if wound drainage is fibrous in composition. Pouches with drainage systems may also become blocked with fibrous wound drainage; patency of the system is needed to ensure that the wound drainage system moves exudate away from the wound.

Patient Preparation

- Verify that the patient is the correct patient using two identifiers. ***Rationale:*** Before performing a procedure, the nurse should ensure the correct identification of the patient for the intended intervention.
- Ensure that the patient understands preprocedural teachings. Answer questions as they arise, and reinforce information as needed. ***Rationale:*** Understanding of previously taught information is evaluated and reinforced.
- Follow institutional standards for assessing pain. Administer analgesia as prescribed. ***Rationale:*** Identifies need for pain interventions.
- Place patient in the position of optimal comfort and visualization for dressing the wound. ***Rationale:*** Facilitates visualization and enhances patient tolerance of the procedure.
- Optimize lighting in the room and provide privacy for the patient. ***Rationale:*** These measures allow for optimal wound assessment and patient comfort.

Procedure	for Management of Wound Exudate With Drains and Pouches	
Steps	**Rationale**	**Special Considerations**
Dressing Wounds With Drains		
1. **HH**		
2. **PE**		
3. Remove the old dressing.	Maintains clean technique; Standard Precautions.	Use caution with dressing removal to ensure that drains are not dislodged.
4. Remove nonsterile gloves and wash hands.		
5. Establish a sterile field.	Maintains sterile area for dressing supplies. Procedure for acute wounds should be completed with aseptic technique.	No evidence exists to support use of sterile technique when changing dressings on chronic wounds.
6. Clean and irrigate the wound (see Procedure 132) as indicated.	Removes contaminated drainage and debris from the wound.	Irrigation of wound drains should be performed only if indicated and only by the physician or advanced practice nurse.[2,7]
7. Change gloves; open 4 × 4 gauze pads and apply on top of wound and around drains (Fig. 137-1). If a dry wound bed is desired consider a desiccant powder. Avoid wrapping gauze around drain site.	Gauze absorbs drainage to keep underlying skin dry; wrapping gauze around the drain may result in inadvertent drain removal with future dressing changes.	Drains are placed to remove excessive wound fluid. Apply a wound dressing capable of absorbing wound drainage and preventing moisture accumulation on surrounding healthy skin.[1-4,7]
8. If necessary, apply a secondary absorbent dressing (ABD; 4 × 4 gauze pads, foam dressings, etc.).	A secondary dressing absorbs drainage and protects clothing from drainage.	Wound exudate that leaks from the edges or the outer layer of the dressing (strike-through) creates a portal for bacteria to enter the wound. Dressings should be changed when they are 75% saturated or when strike-through is present.[5]

Procedure continues on following page

Procedure	for Management of Wound Exudate With Drains and Pouches—*Continued*	
Steps	**Rationale**	**Special Considerations**

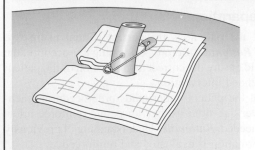

Figure 137-1   Dressing a wound with a drain.

Steps	Rationale	Special Considerations
9. Apply liquid skin barrier to the periwound area and allow to dry. Apply hypoallergenic tape across the wound dressing, extending approximately 2 inches beyond the dressing onto the skin. **(Level E*)**	When tape is used to secure dressings, frequent dressing changes may result in skin irritation or disruption from the adhesive tape. Liquid skin barrier protects periwound tissue from the mechanical irritation of tape.[2,5] Hypoallergenic tape is less traumatic to noninjured skin; extend tape beyond the dressing edges to anchor and secure the dressing well.	Assess periwound edge for chemical and moisture irritation or skin breakdown from wound exudate.

Pouching a Wound With Exudate

1. **HH**
2. **PE**

Steps	Rationale	Special Considerations
3. If the current drainage pouch has an external opening, drain and measure the content volume and discard.	Reduces transmission of microorganisms during dressing change; provides documentation of wound or fistula drainage.	Ensure that all needed supplies are obtained before removing the old pouching system and that adequate time is available to complete the entire procedure.
4. Gently remove the old drainage pouch; support the underlying skin with fingertips while the drainage pouch is being removed; dispose of the pouch in appropriate manner.	Prevents tissue trauma to the underlying skin.	A moist cloth may be applied to loosen the edges of the drainage pouch and assist with the removal process.
5. With wet (i.e., NS) gauze 4 × 4 pads, gently clean the wound site from the area of least contamination to greatest (see Procedure 132); clean and dry the surrounding intact skin.	Maintains clean wound environment; surrounding skin should be free of moisture.	Inspect periwound skin for signs of maceration.
6. If ordered, irrigate wound or fistula (see Procedure 132) as ordered.	Cleans wound bed; decreases microorganism count.	Eye protection should be worn to prevent potential exposure to potential contaminants.

*Level E: Multiple case reports, theory-based evidence from expert opinions, or peer-reviewed professional organizational standards without clinical studies to support recommendations.

Procedure	for Management of Wound Exudate With Drains and Pouches—*Continued*	
Steps	**Rationale**	**Special Considerations**
7. With the wrapper from the wound drainage pouch or wafer, create a template by drawing or measuring the wound or fistula edge onto the wrapper; cut out the center of the pattern on the wound skin barrier and the drainage pouch (cut the pattern slightly larger than the tracing).	Irregular shapes and sizes of draining wounds are difficult to estimate; tracing the wound onto the wrapper allows for a better fit, with less potential for leaking on intact surrounding skin and increasing patient comfort by eliminating unsuccessful application attempts.	
8. Apply skin barrier (wafer, liquid, paste, and sealant). **(Level E*)**	Assists in providing a good seal for the drainage pouch.[5]	A good seal is important to prevent moisture or wound exudate undermining the dressing, creating skin maceration, and creating a pathway for microorganisms.
9. Remove the adhesive paper from the drainage pouch; apply the drainage pouch over the wound, and with gentle, even pressure, secure the pouch edges to the skin barrier (Fig. 137-2).	Gentle, even pressure helps ensure a better seal from the drainage pouch to the skin barrier; care must be taken to avoid development of wrinkles during pouch application; wrinkles in the pouch barrier create a leak, and fluid is not contained within the drainage pouch.[2,5]	If wrinkles are present, sealant paste may be added to the drainage pouch edges to fill spaces created by the wrinkles. Position the pouch to maximize movement of the exudate away from the wound, keeping in mind patient positioning may change after the procedure. Carefully monitor the wound management system for leaks. If leak develops, initiate a wound management change. Trapped effluent can cause denudation within a short period of time.[6]

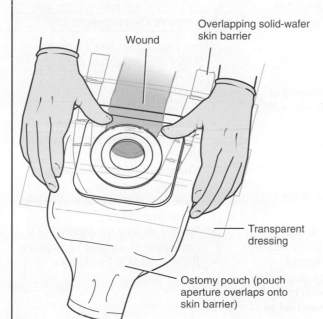

Wound

Overlapping solid-wafer skin barrier

Transparent dressing

Ostomy pouch (pouch aperture overlaps onto skin barrier)

Figure 137-2   Pouching a wound.

*Level E: Multiple case reports, theory-based evidence from expert opinions, or peer-reviewed professional organizational standards without clinical studies to support recommendations.

Procedure continues on following page

Procedure   for Management of Wound Exudate With Drains and Pouches—*Continued*

Steps	Rationale	Special Considerations
10. Close the drainage pouch; wound exudate may be allowed to collect in the pouch, or suction may be attached to the end of the pouch to pull fluid away from the wound into a more distant collection container. **(Level D*)**	The type and amount of drainage coming from a wound determine whether or not suction is added to the drainage pouch.[2]	If suction is not used, empty the appliance regularly. Excessive exudate may create tension within the pouch, causing it to loosen the appliance.

*Level D: Peer-reviewed professional and organizational standards with the support of clinical study recommendations.

Expected Outcomes

- Excessive exudate is removed from the wound bed
- Drains remain intact and patent
- Pouching system effectively collects and directs exudate away from wound bed
- Surrounding skin is dry and free of excessive wound drainage moisture (maceration)
- Wound drainage exit sites are clean and dry, without signs of infection or irritation
- Wound healing is enhanced because of effective wound drainage removal
- Wound drainage decreases in volume (over time) and is absent of foul odor or undesirable color

Unexpected Outcomes

- Wound drain becomes dislodged, blocked, or kinked
- Skin erosion or maceration occurs around wound edges
- Wound drain (if present) is dislodged during dressing or pouching procedure
- Wound is not healing efficiently because management of wound drainage is not effective
- Wound infection is suspected because of inadequate removal of wound drainage that allowed for bacterial growth

Patient Monitoring and Care

Steps	Rationale	Reportable Conditions
		These conditions should be reported if they persist despite nursing interventions.
1. Observe for signs of wound infection.	Drains assist with the removal of excessive fluid but also provide a portal of entry for microorganisms.[7]	• Erythema • Edema • Increase or change in pain • Elevated temperature and white blood cell count • Changes in wound drainage: amount, color, odor • Increased pressure or tenderness at the wound site
2. Assess for patency of the wound drainage system and effective seal of the pouching system.	Drains are frequently soft and pliable and thus can easily become kinked or blocked if wound drainage is fibrous in composition. Leakage from the pouch or secondary dressing may lead to maceration of the periwound skin.	• Wound drainage suddenly decreasing in amount or stopping • Periwound skin breakdown
3. Monitor amount of wound drainage relative to patient intake and output.	Excessive wound drainage may cause a fluid imbalance, necessitating intravenous or oral fluid replacements.	• Tachycardia • Hypotension • Oliguria • Increasing amounts of drainage

Patient Monitoring and Care —*Continued*

Steps	Rationale	Reportable Conditions
4. Monitor caloric and protein intake in the presence of heavily draining wounds. Draining wounds also lose micronutrients and can slow wound healing. Consider supplements and initiate a nutritional consult as needed.	Excessive wound drainage may result in the loss of 100 g of protein a day. Adequate protein needs to be replaced for wound healing.[6]	• Laboratory analysis suggestive of hypoalbuminemia
5. Follow institutional standards for assessing pain. Administer analgesia as prescribed.	Identifies need for pain interventions.	• Continued pain despite pain interventions

Documentation

Documentation should include the following:
- Patient and family education
- Premedication given, patient tolerance of procedure, and response to pain medication
- Wound cleansing, irrigation (if performed), and dressing change completed, with date and time
- Description of wound bed, drains, pouch, (suction pressure if applied), surrounding skin, and characteristics of wound exudate (color, amount, odor)

- Dressing applied
- Unexpected outcomes
- Nursing interventions

References and Additional Readings

For a complete list of references and additional readings for this procedure, scan this QR code with any freely available smartphone code reader app, or visit http://booksite.elsevier.com/9780323376624.

138

Percutaneous Endoscopic Gastrostomy (PEG), Gastrostomy, and Jejunostomy Tube Care

Margaret M. Ecklund

PURPOSE: Gastrostomy, percutaneous endoscopic gastrostomy, and jejunostomy tubes provide long-term access to the gastrointestinal tract for nutrition.

PREREQUISITE NURSING KNOWLEDGE

- Knowledge of the anatomy and physiology of the upper and lower gastrointestinal (GI) system is necessary.
- Patients who cannot have enteral tubes passed orally or nasally because of anatomy or surgery and those who need supplemental enteral nutrition support for longer than 4 weeks should be considered as candidates for long-term enteral access.
- The most commonly used long-term enteral access is the percutaneous endoscopic gastrostomy (PEG) tube. The PEG tube is inserted without general anesthesia. A local anesthetic (i.e., 1% lidocaine injection) is used at the abdominal puncture site. A guidewire is threaded via endoscope through the oropharynx, esophagus, and stomach and brought out through the abdominal wall. The tube is then threaded over the guidewire and passed into the stomach. The tapered end of the tube is brought through a stab wound in the abdominal wall until the mushroomed end of the tube is placed against the stomach wall. An adapter for infusion is attached to the end of the tube, and a disk on the tube is moved up to the abdominal wall to stabilize the tube in place.
- PEG tubes are large-bore catheters that range from 18 to 22 Fr and have a mushroom-shaped, curved end in the stomach and a two-port distal end to instill enteral nutrition, medications, and fluid. Commercial PEG tubes have disks, perpendicular to the tube, to hold the device close to the skin and lessen the shift of the tube in and out of the skin (Fig. 138-1).
- Relative contraindications for PEG placement include the following:
  - ❖ Previous gastric resection
  - ❖ Tumors that block the passage of the endoscope
  - ❖ Ascites
  - ❖ Morbid obesity
  - ❖ Esophageal or gastric varices
  - ❖ Esophageal stricture or narrowing
- Replacement gastrostomy tubes usually have a balloon in the intestinal lumen that is inflated with sterile water. This balloon prevents inadvertent dislocation. The distal end of the tube has an infusion port and a port for the balloon instillation (Fig. 138-2).
- A jejunostomy tube, which does not have a balloon, is indicated in those patients at risk for aspiration or who are unable to tolerate enteral feedings into the stomach. These tubes are routinely sutured in place for stability (Fig. 138-3). They are usually smaller bore, less than 14 Fr, and therefore are more susceptible to occlusion.
- If the tubes are inadvertently removed, reinsertion of the tubes is a routine procedure after the tunnel and stoma are healed (approximately 2 to 6 weeks after insertion).
- Because these tubes all enter through the abdominal wall, skin care at the site of insertion is important for skin integrity and prevention of infection.
- Consult with the multidisciplinary team to individualize nutrition goals. The nutrition plan is developed on the basis of the collaborative assessment of the nurse, dietitian, and physician or advanced practice nurse.

EQUIPMENT

- Nonsterile gloves
- 4 × 4 gauze pads
- Cotton-tipped swabs
- Mild soap
- 4 × 4 gauze pads, drain cut
- Protective skin barrier (e.g., vitamins A and D ointment or other commercial topical moisture barrier products)

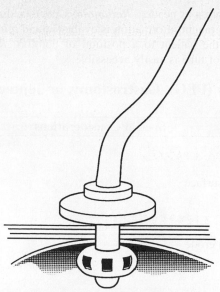

Figure 138-1 Percutaneous endoscopic gastrostomy.

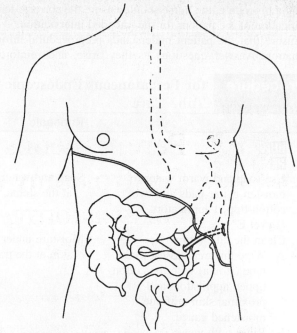

Figure 138-3 Jejunostomy tube placement.

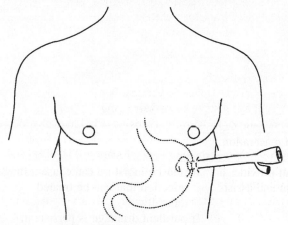

Figure 138-2 Gastrostomy tube.

- Silk tape (or paper tape if patient has a sensitivity to silk tape)

Additional equipment, to have available as needed, includes the following:

- Abdominal binder

PATIENT AND FAMILY EDUCATION

- Explain the purpose for the tube to the patient and family. *Rationale:* This information may decrease patient and family anxiety.
- Explain the reason for skin care assessment and tube maintenance. *Rationale:* This informs the patient and family of what to expect.
- Stress the importance of not pulling on the tube. *Rationale:* Unnecessary pain and skin irritation may be avoided.
- Explain that oral nutrition may be possible even if the patient has a long-term enteral access catheter. *Rationale:* This explanation provides the patient and family with important information.

- Explain that long-term enteral access catheters can be removed when oral intake meets the needs of the individual. *Rationale* This information may serve as a goal for the patient to consume more via the oral route.
- Aspiration is a continued risk when the patient is positioned flat. *Rationale:* Gastric residual volume can reflux and create a risk for pulmonary aspiration.

PATIENT ASSESSMENT AND PREPARATION

Patient Assessment

- Perform a GI assessment. Note the presence of abdominal distension, bowel sounds, flatus, and bowel movements. Determine whether the patient has had diarrhea, constipation, or signs of GI dysfunction. *Rationale:* A patient needs a functional gut to receive enteral nutrition.
- Assess skin condition at the exit site of the feeding tube at the stoma; signs and symptoms of infection include the following:
  Rationale: Intact skin integrity is a defense against infection. Early assessment of signs of infection promotes early, appropriate intervention.
  ❖ Site redness or edema
  ❖ Warmth
  ❖ Purulent drainage
  ❖ Pain or tenderness
  ❖ Fever

Patient Preparation

- Perform a time out and verify that the patient is the correct patient using two identifiers. *Rationale:* Before performing a procedure, the nurse should ensure the correct identification of the patient for the intended intervention.

- Ensure that the patient understands preprocedural information. Answer questions as they arise, and reinforce

information as needed. *Rationale:* Understanding of previously taught information is evaluated and reinforced.

- Assist the patient to a position of comfort. *Rationale:* Stoma of tube is easily accessible.

Procedure for Percutaneous Endoscopic Gastrostomy (PEG), Gastrostomy, or Jejunostomy Tube Care		
Steps	**Rationale**	**Special Considerations**
1. **HH**		
2. **PE**		
3. Use soap and warm water to moisten gauze pads and two cotton-tipped applicators. **(Level E*)**	Soap and water clean the skin surface at the stoma.[1-3]	
4. Clean the tube (stoma) A. Wipe the area closest to the tube (stoma) with the cotton-tipped applicators and proximal skin with the moistened gauze. B. Rinse with water. C. Displace the bumper to ensure cleaning and drying next to the skin at the stoma. D. Verify that the bumper is not too tight against the skin. One finger's breadth should fit between the bumper and the skin. **(Level E*)**	Moisture under the bumper can erode skin at the tract.[1-3]	
5. Dry the skin and stoma thoroughly with a dry gauze pad.	Prevents chafing and skin maceration.	
6. If significant moisture is found on the skin around the stoma, use cotton-tipped applicators to apply a protective skin barrier (e.g., vitamin A and D ointment or other commercial topical moisture barrier products) in a circular motion around stoma. **(Level E*)**	Protective barrier ointment provides a moisture barrier for skin and assists wound healing.	Increased moisture can cause a fungal infection that can be treated topically.[1,3] If purulent drainage is persistent, collaborate with the physician or advanced practice nurse to obtain an order for an antimicrobial ointment and apply it after skin cleansing.[1-3]
7. Apply a 4 × 4 split gauze sponge around the tube and secure it with tape along the edges. Change the gauze every 12 hours or when soiled or moist. **(Level E*)**	Gauze absorbs moisture from the stoma. If no drainage is present, the gauze may be left off.[1-3]	
8. Anchor the tube to the skin at an adjacent area on the abdomen. The bumper (flange) should be rotated to avoid skin damage from repeated taping. **(Level E*)**	Reduces tension on the tube and avoids stoma erosion.[1-3]	
9. Adjust the head of the bed to 30 degrees or higher when feedings are infusing. **(Level C*)**	Minimizes the risk of aspiration.[4]	
10. Remove **PE** and discard used supplies.		

*Level C: Qualitative studies, descriptive or correlational studies, integrative reviews, systematic reviews, or randomized controlled trials with inconsistent results.
*Level E: Multiple case reports, theory-based evidence from expert opinions, or peer-reviewed professional organizational standards without clinical studies to support recommendations.

Expected Outcomes

- Intact skin at stoma of long-term enteral access device
- Long-term enteral access for enteral feeding and fluid administration remains patent

Unexpected Outcomes

- Infection or ulceration at the stoma
- Tube removal by patient or accidental dislodgment with patient movement
- Migration of the tube into the intestinal lumen
- Peritonitis
- Aspiration
- Bleeding
- Gastric outlet obstruction
- Clogged tube
- Degradation of tube

Patient Monitoring and Care

Steps	Rationale	Reportable Conditions
		These conditions should be reported if they persist despite nursing interventions.
1. Assess the integrity of the skin and quality of drainage from the stoma every 4 hours, with any changes or as needed.	Intact skin is the first line of prevention against infection.	• Erosion of the stoma • Signs and symptoms of infection
2. Ensure that the PEG tube has a disk aligned next to the skin without pressure into the skin.	The disk helps prevent excess movement of the tube in and out of the skin. If the disk exerts excess pressure, tissue injury may occur.[1-3]	• Pressure injury adjacent to the stoma • Removal of the tube by the patient • Clogging of the device • Buried bumper • Removal of the enteral access device
3. Ensure that the patient does not remove long-term enteral access device. A loosely applied abdominal binder may help deter a confused patient from pulling on the tube. (**Level E***)	A tube removed before the tract is established is a potential surgical emergency and may necessitate immediate return to the operating room or endoscopy suite for repair and replacement. Inform the physician or advanced practice nurse so he or she can determine the urgency of replacement. The immediate response may be to place a replacement commercial tube or Foley catheter in the tract. Follow institutional standards. Tubes with established tracts can be replaced by the nurse at the bedside with a tube of comparable size and length.[5] Fistula disruption and hemorrhage are the most common complications of device replacement.[6]	

*Level E: Multiple case reports, theory-based evidence from expert opinions, or peer-reviewed professional organizational standards without clinical studies to support recommendations.

Procedure continues on following page

Patient Monitoring and Care —*Continued*

Steps	Rationale	Reportable Conditions
4. Note the distance of the tube from the infusion adapter to the entrance into the skin. Label the tube with the insertion date and the measurement at the entrance to the skin.	Facilitates future assessment for tube migration either inward or outward.	• Length that has deviated significantly
5. Assess for nausea and vomiting.	Nausea and vomiting may indicate pyloric obstruction from a tube migrating inward.[1-3]	• Nausea • Vomiting
6. Evaluate excess wear on the tube caused by ongoing use.	No routine tube change is indicated. The tube is changed when the device fails.[3]	• Tube wear

Documentation

Documentation should include the following:
- Patient and family education
- Condition of the stoma
- Any treatment rendered related to site complications
- Tube patency
- Pain assessment, interventions, and effectiveness

- Type of tube and distance of the tube from the adapter to the entrance into the skin
- Unexpected outcomes
- Nursing interventions

References and Additional Readings

For a complete list of references and additional readings for this procedure, scan this QR code with any freely available smartphone code reader app, or visit http://booksite.elsevier.com/9780323376624.

139 Small-Bore Feeding Tube Insertion and Care

Margaret M. Ecklund

PURPOSE: A small-bore feeding tube is inserted to provide access to the gastrointestinal tract for the patient who is unable to orally consume adequate calories. The tube can be used for administration of nutrients, fluid, and medications.

PREREQUISITE NURSING KNOWLEDGE

- Knowledge of the anatomy and physiology of the upper and lower gastrointestinal (GI) tract is needed.
- The GI tract should be functioning for gastric feedings to be digested and absorbed. Bowel sounds may not be audible, yet the GI tract is functional and enteral nutrition can be instituted safely and effectively and be well tolerated. GI findings that may affect the normal functioning of the tract and preclude gastric feeding are bowel obstruction, paralytic ileus, and some fistulas.
- Small-bore feeding tubes are preferable over larger-bore nasogastric tubes during the course of critical illness because the risk for tissue necrosis in the nares and sinusitis is lower. When small-bore feeding tubes are placed postpylorically, there is a reduced risk of vomiting and pneumonia.[1,7,10]
- The small diameter of the tube allows simultaneous oral intake if the patient is able to consume orally without aspiration.
- Both weighted (tubes with an enlarged tip, filled with tungsten) and unweighted (bolus tip) small-bore nasogastric tubes are available. They typically are packaged with guidewires already in the lumen to assist passage of the tube. After successful placement, the guidewire is removed and discarded. The size of tubes range from 6 to 12 Fr. They are radiopaque along the entire length of the tube. External markings provide accurate insertion depth. Feeding ports are incompatible with IV syringes.[4]
- Weighted-tip tubes are harder for the patient with a compromised condition to swallow; ultimately, the unweighted tube may be a more comfortable choice for the patient.
- Absolute contraindications for insertion of a nasogastric feeding tube are basilar skull fracture, maxillofacial disorders, transsphenoidal surgical approaches, uncorrected coagulation disorders, and some esophageal and gastric abnormalities.[4]
- Small-bore feeding tubes are not designed for drainage of gastric contents. If gastric decompression is desired, the small-bore nasogastric feeding tube should be replaced with a larger-bore nasogastric tube. See Procedure 113 for nasogastric tube placement.

- It is important to review institutional standards regarding insertion of small-bore feeding tubes and complete competency for tube insertion. Some institutions restrict insertion to physicians and advanced practice nurses.

EQUIPMENT

- Small-bore feeding tube
- Irrigation tray
- 50-mL or larger enteral compatible syringe.
- Water (tap or sterile, based on institutional policy)
- Skin preparation agent
- Tape or commercial fixation device
- Nonsterile gloves
- Water-soluble lubricant (if tube is not prelubricated)
- Water-absorbent barrier to protect clothing

Additional equipment, to have available as needed, includes the following:
- Gowns, goggles
- Viscous lidocaine
- Stethoscope
- Capnography
- pH test strips

PATIENT AND FAMILY EDUCATION

- Explain the essential role adequate nutritional status plays in promoting wound healing and recovery from illness. *Rationale:* Explanation may elicit cooperation and allay patient and family anxiety.
- Explain why a feeding tube is needed to ensure adequate nutritional intake. *Rationale:* Explanation may elicit cooperation and facilitate tube insertion.
- Outline the steps of the procedure and the patient's role during feeding tube insertion (e.g., positioning, swallowing as instructed). *Rationale:* Patient cooperation may facilitate insertion.
- Describe the typical sensations experienced during feeding tube insertion. *Rationale:* Explanation may alleviate anxiety and promote patient cooperation.
- Reinforce the importance of using care when changing position or getting out of bed once the tube is placed. *Rationale:* Emphasis may aid in preventing inadvertently dislodging of the tube.

- Explain the reason for the radiograph after insertion. *Rationale:* Knowledge may decrease anxiety and fear of the unknown.
- Discuss reasons for not pulling at the tube once it has been placed and secured. *Rationale:* Leaving the tube in place avoids the need for reinsertion and another radiograph for verification. Reinsertion increases risk for trauma to nasopharyngeal passages. Dislodging the tube can increase the risk of aspiration.

PATIENT ASSESSMENT AND PREPARATION

Patient Assessment

- Assess the patient for the presence of absolute contraindications for nasal placement of small-bore feeding tubes, including recent basilar skull fracture; history of transsphenoidal surgery; facial, nasal, or sinus trauma; or severe clotting abnormalities. *Rationale:* These conditions carry a high risk for complications from passage of the tube through the nasopharyngeal area. Intracranial placement of small-bore feeding tubes has occurred with the nasal approach in patients with basilar skull fracture. The orogastric route is a safer alternative in this situation.
- Evaluate the patient for relative contraindications to nasal or oral placement of small-bore feeding tubes, including esophageal varices with recent bleeding or ligation within 72 hours; esophageal obstruction, recent esophageal surgery or esophageal stent; history of GI surgery with altered anatomical pathways; gastroesophageal reflux; and gastroparesis (unless feeding post pyloric); nasal polyps or other septal abnormalities, sinusitis and minor to moderate clotting abnormalities.[4,6] *Rationale:* These conditions carry a relative risk for complications from passage of the tube through the nasopharyngeal route. Placement of the tube may still be undertaken if the assessment of benefit outweighs risk.
- Assess GI function. *Rationale:* A functional GI tract is essential for safe and effective tube feeding. The integrity and function of the GI tract guides decisions regarding the optimal location for delivery of nutrients (gastric versus postpyloric tip position).

Patient Preparation

- Verify that the patient is the correct patient with two identifiers. *Rationale:* Before performing a procedure, the nurse should ensure the correct identification of the patient for the intended intervention.
- Ensure that the patient and family understand preprocedural information. Answer questions as they arise and reinforce information as needed. *Rationale:* Understanding of previously taught information is evaluated and reinforced.
- Ensure that informed consent has been obtained. *Rationale:* Informed consent protects the rights of the patient and allows the patient to make a competent decision.
- Perform a preprocedure verification and time out, if nonemergent. *Rationale:* Ensures patient safety.
- Assess the need to remove any existing large-bore feeding tube. *Rationale:* In some cases, the large-bore tube may remain in place to allow gastric decompression while delivery of enteral formula takes place in the small intestine. When the large-bore tube is to be replaced by a small-bore tube, the larger tube should be removed before the new tube is passed to avoid dislodging the small-bore tube during removal of the large-bore tube.
- If ordered, administer a prokinetic agent such as metoclopramide or erythromycin 10 minutes before the procedure. Metoclopramide is used with caution because prolonged administration at higher doses is associated with the development of tardive dyskinesia.[9] *Rationale:* Enhanced gastric motility facilitates passage of the tube distal to the pylorus.
- Perform oral care to moisten mucosa. Suction oropharyngeal area of excess secretions.[2] *Rationale:* A moist, cleared oropharyngeal area facilitates patient comfort and passage of the tube.

Procedure	for Small-Bore Feeding Tube Insertion and Care	
Steps	**Rationale**	**Special Considerations**
1. **HH**		
2. **PE**		
3. Sit the patient upright and tip the head forward. Assure patient is in a comfortable position. (Level E*)	Facilitates passage of the tube into the esophagus. If the patient cannot tolerate upright positioning, position laterally to the right side to insert the tube.[3,9,10]	
4. Estimate the depth of tube insertion by measuring the tube from the tip of nose to the ear, then inferior to the stomach. (Level E*)	Approximates the length of the tube to insert. If postpyloric placement is desired, add 10–15 cm to the length of tube measured.[3,9]	

*Level E: Multiple case reports, theory-based evidence from expert opinions, or peer-reviewed professional organizational standards without clinical studies to support recommendations.

Procedure	for Small-Bore Feeding Tube Insertion and Care—*Continued*		

Steps	Rationale	Special Considerations
5. Lubricate the tip of the tube with water. Consider flushing the tube before insertion to lubricate the stylet. **(Level M*)**	Water activates a lubricant on the surface of the tube to facilitate passage through the nares. Flushing the tube eases the removal of the stylet once in place.	If the tube does not have self-lubrication, a water-soluble lubricant can be applied to the tube.
6. Insert the tip of the tube into either naris; advance to the posterior pharynx until resistance is met. **(Level E*)**	Once the tube is advanced through the nares, the oropharynx is reached and the tube meets resistance.	
7. At this point, ask the patient to swallow. If the patient is able to cooperate, give small sips of water to attempt to trigger the swallow reflex and ease tube passage. **(Level E*)**	Swallowing immediately assists passage of the tube into the esophagus. If the patient is unable to swallow, neck positioning may facilitate passage.[3,8,9]	If coughing begins immediately with advancement of the tube, immediately pull back to the nares and allow the patient to recover.
8. As the patient swallows, advance the tube to the desired marking. Remove the guidewire with one hand while holding the tube securely at the nares. **(Level M*)**	The initial swallow gets the tube into the esophagus, and the nurse can advance it to the desired position without repeated swallowing. Removing the guidewire without holding the tube can cause the tube to pull out with the guidewire.	If the patient is unconscious or unable to assist, do not attempt to use water orally to pass the tube. The guidewire may be left in and removed after radiographic verification. Caution is used because the tube may be displaced with stylet removal. The stylet should not be reinserted while the tube is in the patient.
9. Apply skin preparation to the nose and securing surface of the face; allow to dry. **(Level E*)**	Prepares the surface of skin to help with the tape adhering.[4]	
10. Use a commercial tube holder to anchor the tube with minimal pressure on the skin. If tape is used, tape the tube securely to nose, with use of one half of a 3-cm strip. The lower portion of the tape is then split up to the tip of the nose and wrapped around the tube.	The tape needs to hold the tube to prevent slipping it out	Tape the tube so that it does not press against the skin. Excess pressure can cause breakdown.
11. Remove **PE** and discard used supplies.		
12. **HH**		
13. Use two or more of the following methods to predict tube location: Observe for signs of respiratory distress. Use capnography if available Measure pH from aspirate. Observe aspirate.[1] **(Level D*)**	Radiographic verification is the recommended method to ensure correct placement. A lower chest view ensures the tip is in stomach or intestine.[1] **(Level D*)**	Do not use air bolus or water bubbling method to verify tube location.[1] **(Level D*)**

*Level D: Peer-reviewed professional and organizational standards with the support of clinical study recommendations.

*Level E: Multiple case reports, theory-based evidence from expert opinions, or peer-reviewed professional organizational standards without clinical studies to support recommendations.

*Level M: Manufacturer's recommendations only.

Procedure continues on following page

Procedure   for Small-Bore Feeding Tube Insertion and Care—*Continued*

Steps	Rationale	Special Considerations
14. Once radiograph is obtained and tube position is accurately verified, the tube exit site from the nose is marked.[1] (**Level D***)		
15. If postpyloric placement is desired:	The extra length can allow the migration of the tube past the pyloric valve.	
A. Tape additional length with coil in stomach.	Consider use of electromagnetic device if postpyloric location is desired, as accuracy is improved.[5] (**Level C***)	
B. Instill 350 mL of air into the stomach via the tube.[7]	This technique causes the stomach to distend with air and facilitates feeding tube passage through the pyloric sphincter.[7]	Air insufflation is recommended for patients receiving narcotics, as metoclopramide is less effective to facilitate postpyloric placement of feeding tubes.[7] (**Level C***)
C. Position the patient onto the right side.	Assists with peristalsis. If the tube is in the stomach, peristalsis should move it beyond the sphincter.	
D. Ensure that a chest and abdominal radiographs are obtained.	The radiograph should visualize the entire course of the feeding tube to avoid errors.[1] (**Level D***)	Postpyloric placement is verified with radiograph to ensure tip is visualized.
E. If the tube has not migrated postpylorically, continue to position the patient onto the right side and recheck the radiograph.[7] (**Level C***)	Right-side positioning potentially helps pass the tube postpyloric with the aid of peristalsis. The best location is at the beginning of the jejunum, or the fourth portion of the duodenum.[7]	Patients with duodenal feedings may achieve nutritional goals earlier than gastric feedings.[6]
F. If the tube remains in the stomach, consult with the physician or advanced practice nurse, as medication may need to be prescribed.	Promotility agents have shown benefit in moving feeding tubes through the pyloric valve.	Should be used with caution because prolonged administration at higher doses is associated with the development of tardive dyskinesia. Air insufflation is recommended for patients receiving narcotics, as metoclopramide is less effective to facilitate postpyloric placement of feeding tubes.[7]
16. Remove **PE** and discard used supplies.		
17. **HH**		

*Level C: Qualitative studies, descriptive or correlational studies, integrative reviews, systematic reviews, or randomized controlled trials with inconsistent results.
*Level D: Peer-reviewed professional and organizational standards with the support of clinical study recommendations.

Expected Outcomes

- The distal tip of tube is placed in either the stomach or the small bowel.
- A patent tube that accepts enteral feedings, medications, and fluid.
- The patient is able to swallow oral foods and fluids while the small-bore feeding tube is in place, if allowed.

Unexpected Outcomes

- Coughing or dyspnea, indicating potential bronchial placement
- Pneumothorax from inadvertent pleural placement
- Tube coiled in esophagus or posterior pharynx
- Esophageal tear from trauma of tube passing
- Tube dislodging during therapy, necessitating removal and new tube placement. Collaborate with physician, advanced practice nurse, or other healthcare professional, and consider use of bridle technique for securing of tube if patient is agitated and unable to leave tape in place.
- Aspiration of stomach contents despite appropriate placement
- Clogging of enteral tube with medication fragments or enteral formula
- Skin irritation or breakdown at nose

Patient Monitoring and Care

Steps	Rationale	Reportable Conditions
		These conditions should be reported if they persist despite nursing interventions.
1. Monitor tolerance to tube placement.	Agitation may inhibit successful placement. Change in tube length can indicate that the tip of tube may be in an unintended location.[1] Coughing, vomiting, or respiratory symptoms may indicate tube dislodgment or aspiration.	• Inability to tolerate tube placement • Coughing, vomiting, dyspnea, or decrease in oxygen saturation • Patient removal of the tube, requiring reassessment and replacement of tube.
2. Assess the oral cavity and perform oral care per institution standard.[2]	Mouth breathing dries secretions, encouraging bacterial growth and mucosal breakdown.	
3. Ensure that the tube is secured in a way that avoids pressure on the naris. Monitor the insertion site of the tube for pain, redness, swelling, drainage, bleeding, or skin breakdown.	Many critically ill patients have fragile skin and have associated conditions that predispose them to skin breakdown. Frequent monitoring and subsequent repositioning of the tube can prevent serious damage.	• Redness • Swelling • Drainage • Bleeding • Ulceration or signs of skin breakdown at insertion site
4. Follow institutional standard for assessing pain. Administer analgesia as prescribed.	Identifies need for pain interventions.	• Continued pain despite pain interventions.

Documentation

Documentation should include the following:
- The type and size of tube inserted
- Patient response to insertion
- The length of the tube that is external to the patient, measured from nose to the end of the tube
- Radiographic confirmation of the tube position
- Unexpected outcomes
- Nursing interventions
- Medications administered
- Patient and family education

References and Additional Readings

For a complete list of references and additional readings for this procedure, scan this QR code with any freely available smartphone code reader app, or visit http://booksite.elsevier.com/9780323376624.

140 Small-Bore Feeding Tube Insertion Using an Electromagnetic Guidance System (CORTRAK 2 Enteral Access System EAS)

Karen A. Gilbert and Patricia H. Worthington

PURPOSE: The CORTRAK 2 Enteral Access System (EAS; Corpak MedSystems, Buffalo Grove, IL) uses electromagnetic technology to assist with safe bedside placement of small-bore nasoenteric feeding tubes. The guidance system helps to avoid intubation of the pulmonary system and facilitates postpyloric placement of these tubes.[13,15,22]

PREREQUISITE NURSING KNOWLEDGE

- Knowledge of upper respiratory and gastrointestinal anatomy and physiology is necessary.
- An understanding that the correct placement of the receiver unit is required to provide an accurate tracing of the tube path.
- Proficiency in assessing the lungs and abdomen is essential.
- Clinical and technical competence in placement of small-bore feeding tubes and in use of the CORTRAK 2 EAS device.[6,21]
- Recognition of risk factors associated with placement errors during insertion of small-bore feeding tubes including endotracheal intubation, advanced age, altered level of consciousness, and diminished reflexes for airway protection.[23]
- An understanding of the benefits of enteral nutrition for the critically ill, including indications for postpyloric placement, should be understood.[7,20]

EQUIPMENT

- CORTRAK 2 EAS feeding tube placement device (Fig. 140-1)
- CORTRAK 2 EAS feeding tube with transmitting stylet
- Irrigation tray
- 50-mL or larger enteral compatible syringe
- Water (tap water or sterile water based on institutional policy)
- Nonsterile gloves
- Water-soluble lubricant
- Water-absorbent barrier to protect patient's clothing
- Tape or other securing device

Additional equipment, to have available as needed, includes the following:
- Gowns, goggles
- Viscous lidocaine (optional)
- Stethoscope

PATIENT AND FAMILY EDUCATION

- Explain the essential role adequate nutritional status plays in promoting wound healing and recovery from illness. *Rationale:* Explanation may elicit cooperation and allay patient and family anxiety.
- Explain why a feeding tube is needed to ensure adequate nutritional intake. *Rationale:* Explanation may elicit cooperation and facilitate tube insertion.
- Outline the steps of the procedure and the patient's role during feeding tube insertion (e.g., positioning, swallowing as instructed). *Rationale:* Patient cooperation may facilitate insertion.
- Describe the typical sensations experienced during feeding tube insertion. *Rationale:* Explanation may alleviate anxiety and promote patient cooperation.
- Reinforce the importance of using care when changing position or getting out of bed once the tube is placed. *Rationale:* Emphasis may aid in preventing inadvertent dislodgment of the tube.

PATIENT ASSESSMENT AND PREPARATION

Patient Assessment

- Verify that the patient has no implanted medical devices that may be affected by electromagnetic fields. *Rationale:* The CORTRAK 2 EAS system is generally contraindicated for patients with implanted medical devices because of the potential for electromagnetic interference to affect

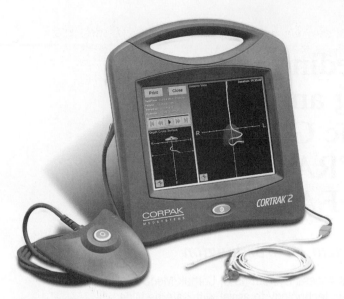

Figure 140-1 The Cortrak 2 Enteral Access System. *(Used with permission from CORPAK, Alpharetta, GA.)*

the function of the implanted device or the CORTRAK 2 EAS. However, no contraindication exists specifically for defibrillators and pacemakers.[11]

- Assess the patient for the presence of absolute contra-indications for nasal placement of small-bore feeding tubes, including recent basilar skull fracture; history of transsphenoidal surgery; facial, nasal, or sinus trauma; or severe clotting abnormalities. *Rationale:* These conditions carry a high risk for complications from passage of the tube through the nasopharyngeal area. Intracranial placement of small-bore feeding tubes has occurred with the nasal approach in patients with basilar skull fracture. The orogastric route is a safer alternative in this situation.[8,17,18]

- Evaluate the patient for relative contraindications to nasal or oral placement of small-bore feeding tubes, including esophageal varices with recent bleeding or ligation within 72 hours; esophageal obstruction, recent esophageal surgery or esophageal stent; history of gastrointestinal surgery with altered anatomical pathways; gastroesophageal reflux; and gastroparesis (unless feeding postpyloric);

nasal polyps or other septal abnormalities, sinusitis and minor to moderate clotting abnormalities. *Rationale:* These conditions carry a relative risk for complications from passage of the tube through the nasopharyngeal route. Placement of the tube may still be undertaken if the assessment of benefit outweighs risk.[8,16–18]

- Assess gastrointestinal function. *Rationale:* A functional gastrointestinal tract is essential for safe and effective tube feeding. The integrity and function of the gastrointestinal tract guides decisions regarding the optimal location for delivery of nutrients (gastric versus postpyloric tip position).[15]

Patient Preparation

- Verify that the patient is the correct patient using two identifiers. *Rationale:* Before performing a procedure, the nurse should ensure the correct identification of the patient for the intended intervention.

- Ensure that the patient and family understand preproce-dural teaching. Answer questions as they arise, and reinforce information as needed. *Rationale:* Understand-ing of previously taught information is evaluated and reinforced.

- Ensure that informed consent has been obtained if required by hospital policy. *Rationale:* Informed consent protects the rights of the patient and allows the patient to make a competent decision.

- Perform a preprocedure verification and time out, if non-emergent. *Rationale:* Ensures patient safety.

- Assess the need to remove any existing large-bore feeding tube. *Rationale:* In some cases, the large-bore tube may remain in place to allow gastric decompression while delivery of enteral formula takes place in the small intes-tine. When the large-bore tube is to be replaced by a small-bore tube, the larger tube should be removed before the new tube is passed to avoid dislodging the small-bore tube during removal of the large-bore tube.

- If ordered, administer a prokinetic agent such as metoclo-pramide or erythromycin 10 minutes before the procedure. Metoclopramide is used with caution because prolonged administration at higher doses is associated with the development of tardive dyskinesia. *Rationale:* Enhanced gastric motility facilitates passage of the tube distal to the pylorus.[2,4]

Procedure	for Small-Bore Feeding Tube Insertion Using an Electromagnetic Guidance System (CORTRAK 2 Enteral Access System [EAS])	
Steps	**Rationale**	**Special Considerations**
1. HH		
2. PE		
3. Place a water-absorbent barrier to protect the patient's clothing.	Prepares for the procedure.	
4. Assist the patient to a supine position with the head of the bed elevated to at least 30 degrees unless contraindicated.[8]	The patient should be as straight as possible for accurate tracking of the feeding tube. This position helps to facilitate the initial advancement of the tube into the esophagus.	
5. Press the orange power button to activate the CORTRAK 2 EAS device.	Provides power.	Hold the button until the power is on.
6. Allow the unit to perform a self-test for about 5 seconds.	Prepares the equipment.	If a fault is detected, the receiver unit will flash red. The fault is cleared and receiver functionality verified by unplugging and replugging the receiver from the monitor.
7. Login by typing username and password.	Prepares the equipment.	Login and Username procedures are determined by organizational policy.
8. Press "New Placement."	Prepares the equipment.	
9. Enter patient information; follow institutional standards.	The device can store a record of the insertion for future reference.	
10. Place the leading foot of the receiver unit over the patient's xiphoid process. The receiver unit cord heads toward the patient's feet (Fig. 140-2).	The receiver unit must be parallel to the spine and centered along the midline to ensure reliable tracking of the tube during placement. Incorrect placement of the receiver alters the appearance of the tracing, making it difficult to interpret the path viewed on the screen.	A weighted band is available to place over the receiver unit for added stability. The receiver can be propped into position with a wedge or cloth to keep the receiver unit parallel to the spine. Do not reposition the receiver unit once it has been correctly placed on the xiphoid process. Movement of the receiver unit alters the alignment and the relationship of the track displayed on the monitor unit.

Procedure continues on following page

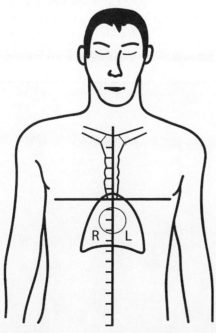

Figure 140-2 Receiver unit placement. *(Used with permission from CORPAK, Alpharetta, GA.)*

Procedure	for Small-Bore Feeding Tube Insertion Using an Electromagnetic Guidance System (CORTRAK 2 Enteral Access System [EAS])—*Continued*	
Steps	**Rationale**	**Special Considerations**
11. Flush the feeding tube with water and dip the tip of the tube in water. Cap the medication port. Move the stylet a few centimeters in and out the tube. Ensure that the stylet is firmly seated in the feeding tube.	If the stylet is moving within the tube during the insertion, the tracing on the monitor is inaccurate. Water activates a lubricant that has been applied to the internal and external surface of the tube. This ensures that the stylet moves freely out of the tube once the desired position is achieved.	Observe for patency or leaks in the tube during flushing.
12. Connect the proximal (orange) end of the feeding tube transmitter stylet to the stylet interconnect cable on the lower right corner of the CORTRAK 2 EAS monitor unit, connecting arrow to arrow.	The CORTRAK 2 EAS feeding tube uses a special stylet that transmits a signal during tube insertion.	Arrows that appear on both the stylet and the cable connectors will only fit together one way, acting as a guide to prevent damage to the equipment during connection.
13. Lubricate the distal end of the tube with water-soluble jelly. Note that viscous lidocaine may be used if prescribed by the physician or advanced practice nurse.[19] **(Level A*)**	Minimizes mucosal injury, facilitates insertion, and promotes patient comfort.	Oil-soluble lubricants should not be used because they are not absorbed by the pulmonary mucosa and may cause complications.
14. Insert the feeding tube into the nares and advance the tube gently along the base of the nostril.		
15. After inserting the feeding tube to the back of the patient's throat (approximately 10 cm), press "Start" either on the CORTRAK 2 EAS monitor unit or on the receiver unit to begin to view the tube tip position.	An "Out of Range" message appears on the screen if the unit is started prematurely. Resistance at approximately 25 cm may indicate contact with the piriform sinus and would require retraction of the tube and gentle readvancement.[8]	If the "Out of Range" message still appears at 30–35 cm, the tube is likely coiled in the mouth or throat. A receiver unit self-test is done, and the monitor indicates the receiver is working before the tube tip is displayed.
16. Ask the patient to swallow if able. Advance the tube to coincide with the swallowing maneuver. If allowed, give the patient sips of water or ice chips.	Swallowing assists passage of the tube into the esophagus.	If the patient is unable to swallow, position the patient's chin to his or her chest if feasible to assist with passage of the tube into the esophagus.

*Level A: Meta-analysis of quantitative studies or metasynthesis of qualitative studies with results that consistently support a specific action, intervention, or treatment (including systematic review of randomized controlled trials).

Procedure	**for Small-Bore Feeding Tube Insertion Using an Electromagnetic Guidance System (CORTRAK 2 Enteral Access System [EAS])—*Continued***	
Steps	**Rationale**	**Special Considerations**
17. Follow the path of the tube tip by the tracing of the illuminated dot on the CORTRAK 2 EAS anterior view screen and the depth tracing on the depth cross-section view (Fig. 140-3). The lateral screen can also be used to monitor depth (Fig. 140-4).[9] **(Level M*)**	The depth cross-section and lateral screens show the distance of the tube tip from the sternum. The relatively posterior anatomical location of the esophagus and the duodenum is reflected by greater depth of these structures in relation to the stomach. A deviation from the expected path may indicate a placement error.[9,10]	During the placement procedure or placement review, the operator is presented with touch screen buttons (toggle buttons) that allow toggling between the major view and the minor view. Before or during the placement process, the operator can press one of the toggle buttons in the major view portion of the screen to toggle the major view between the anterior view (default) and the lateral view. When the lateral view is displayed in the major view pane, the anterior view is displayed in the minor view pane, and the minor toggle button is disabled. When the major view is toggled, the minor view pane returns to the view displayed before the initial toggle of the major view. During placement, while the anterior view is displayed in the major view portion of the screen, the operator can press the toggle button in the minor view portion to toggle the minor view between the depth cross-section and the lateral views.[9,10]

*Level M: Manufacturer's recommendations only.

Procedure continues on following page

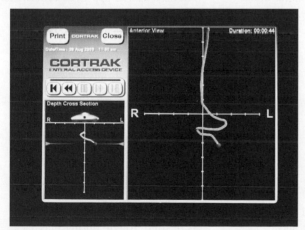

Figure 140-3 CORTRAK screen display, anterior and depth cross-section views. *(Used with permission from CORPAK, Alpharetta, GA.)*

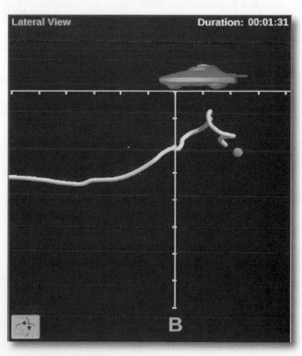

Figure 140-4 Lateral view, major screen. *(Used with permission from CORPAK, Alpharetta, GA.)*

Procedure	for Small-Bore Feeding Tube Insertion Using an Electromagnetic Guidance System (CORTRAK 2 Enteral Access System [EAS])—*Continued*	
Steps	**Rationale**	**Special Considerations**
18. If the patient develops coughing or has signs or symptoms of respiratory distress, or if the tracing veers sharply into the upper right or left quadrant at approximately 35–40 cm, slowly retract the feeding tube to 15 cm to erase the track and continue the placement procedure following the new track.[9,10] **(Level M*)**	This finding may indicate a tube in the bronchus. Slowly pulling back the feeding tube clears the tracing of the placement attempt. A new track is visible as the placement resumes. If resistance is met do not continue to push the tube. Withdraw the feeding tube at this point then continue to advance the feeding tube down the esophagus and into the stomach.	Restarting the device is not necessary. The feeding tube should slide down the esophagus easily. Median distance from the naris to the tracheoesophageal junction is about 20 cm.[8,14] The length of tube needed to reach the stomach is approximately 60 cm; additional length is needed for postpyloric placement.[14]
19. If the feeding tube tip is not moving forward as the tube is inserted, slowly retract the feeding tube until the colored dot begins to move and then proceed with placement.[9,10]	May indicate that the tube is coiling rather than advancing. Coiled loops behind the transmitter are not visible on the monitor. The pathway through the stomach should resemble a backward "C" shape. If gastric placement is desired, the procedure is complete.	Instilling a bolus of air into the tube when the tip is nearing the pylorus may facilitate relaxation of the pylorus and aid in passage into the small bowel.
20. If postpyloric placement is the goal, continue advancing the tube across midline. Assess configuration of the display pattern (pathway and depth) to determine whether the tube is appropriately positioned in the postpyloric region (see Fig. 140-3).[9,10] **(Level M*)**	The pathway through the duodenum often resembles a smaller, forward "C" shape. When the depth indicator is several notches below the horizontal axis, duodenal tube tip location is likely.	A duodenum that is more posterior may show an upward curve in the anterior view before the tube passes farther into the duodenum.
21. Press "End" on the monitor display or the orange button on the receiver. **(Level M*)**	Stops the recording or timing of the insertion procedure.	
22. At this point, the stylet may or may not be removed. Save the stylet in a clean bag (see Step 29).	The feeding tube is well visualized by radiograph with or without the stylet in place; the stylet that comes with the tube may be reinserted to check tube position.	The U.S. Food and Drug Administration approved reinsertion of the transmitting stylet for periodic confirmation of tip location.[9,10]
23. Secure the feeding tube with tape or a commercial fixation device.	Decreases the risk of inadvertent removal or change in position of the tube.	Avoid undue pressure on the naris from the tube to prevent skin breakdown. Consider the use of a nasal bridle system to secure the tube against accidental removal with use of a loop of material through one naris, around the nasal septum, and back out of the other naris. The feeding tube is secured to this bridle.[3]
24. Press "Print" to obtain a tracing of the placement (Fig. 140-5).	The tracing can be used as part of confirming placement and documentation.	If the alternate depth view printout is desired, toggle during playback to allow printing of the depth cross-section or lateral view.
25. Disconnect the transmitting stylet from the interconnect cable.	The procedure is complete.	

*Level M: Manufacturer's recommendations only.

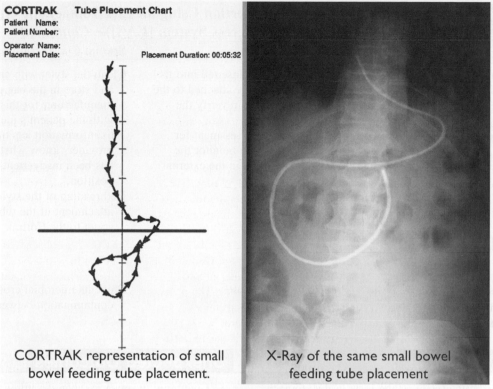

CORTRAK representation of small bowel feeding tube placement.

X-Ray of the same small bowel feeding tube placement

Figure 140-5 Comparison of x-ray with CORTRAK 2 EAS printout. *(Used with permission from CORPAK, Alpharetta, GA.)*

Procedure	for Small-Bore Feeding Tube Insertion Using an Electromagnetic Guidance System (CORTRAK 2 Enteral Access System [EAS])—*Continued*		
Steps	**Rationale**	**Special Considerations**	
26. Press "Close" on the monitor unit; press "Shutdown."	The procedure is complete.	Do not use the orange button to power off.	
27. Obtain a radiographic confirmation of correct placement of the tube before its initial use for feedings or medication administration.[1] (**Level A***)	Radiographic confirmation with abdominal radiograph is the gold standard for determining the exact tube position after insertion.[1,6,21] The tip of the tube usually is not visible on chest radiograph. Some evidence indicates that well-trained and experienced clinicians can achieve a high level of success in placing feeding tubes when a Cortrak device is used. Successful use of this device is dependent on the user's familiarity and dexterity with the device.[6,21]	Gastric auscultation of an air bolus through the tube, aspiration of fluid from the tube, and placement of the proximal end of the feeding tube under water while observing for bubbles are all unreliable methods to confirm placement in the gastrointestinal (GI) tract.[1] Numerous cases have been reported in which clinicians failed to recognize placement of feeding tubes in the respiratory track while using Cortrak guidance; some of these have been associated with fatal outcomes.[1,21]	
28. When proper location of the feeding tube is confirmed, flush with 5–10 mL of water if not flushed before insertion.[9,10] (**Level M***)	Activates internal lubrication to allow easier removal of stylet.	Failure to flush the feeding tube for stylet removal may damage the feeding tube.	

*Level A: Meta-analysis of quantitative studies or metasynthesis of qualitative studies with results that consistently support a specific action, intervention, or treatment (including systematic review of randomized controlled trials).

*Level M: Manufacturer's recommendations only.

Procedure continues on following page

Procedure for Small-Bore Feeding Tube Insertion Using an Electromagnetic Guidance System (CORTRAK 2 Enteral Access System [EAS])—*Continued*

Steps	Rationale	Special Considerations
29. Remove the stylet before administering feedings.[9,10] **(Level M*)**	The stylet can be reinserted into its original tube while attached to the Cortrak system to reverify the tube's position.	Clean the stylet with an alcohol swab and store in the bag provided by the manufacturer for this use. Label with the patient's identification.
30. Note the centimeter marking on the tube at the tip of the patient's nose to identify the depth of tube placement.[4,5]	A simple bedside assessment for displacement is to monitor the tube for a change in the external length.[4,5]	This information lets other healthcare providers know whether the tube has been inadvertently pulled out of position. Rethreading of the stylet requires attachment of the tube transmitter stylet to the Cortrak system.
31. Remove **PE** and discard used supplies.		
32. **HH**		
33. Ensure that the CORTRAK 2 EAS system components are cleaned.[12] **(Level M)**	Prepares for future use.	Prevents microbial cross-contamination between patients.

Expected Outcomes

- The distal tip of the feeding tube rests in the stomach or small intestine
- The patient tolerates enteral feeding at rates that meet established goals
- The patient is able to swallow oral foods and fluids while the small-bore tube is in place, if appropriate
- The small-bore tube accepts enteral feedings, medications, and fluid

Unexpected Outcomes

- Coughing, dyspnea, oxygen desaturation, and restlessness indicate potential pulmonary placement
- Pneumothorax from inadvertent pleural placement
- Pulmonary aspiration of gastric contents
- Epistaxis or esophageal injury during passage of the tube
- Inadvertent tube dislodgment
- Skin irritation or breakdown at the nose
- Occluded feeding tube
- Sinusitis or otitis media

Patient Monitoring and Care

Steps	Rationale	Reportable Conditions
		These conditions should be reported if they persist despite nursing interventions.
1. Monitor the length of the tube in the patient and tolerance to tube placement.[4,5]	Placement may be difficult in agitated patients. Change in tube length can indicate that the tip of the tube may be in an unintended location. Coughing, vomiting, or respiratory symptoms may indicate tube dislodgment or aspiration.[1]	• Inability to tolerate tube placement • Inadvertent removal of the tube (partial or complete) • Coughing, vomiting, dyspnea, or decrease in oxygen saturation
2. Assess the oral cavity and perform oral care per institutional standards.	Mouth breathing dries secretions, encouraging bacterial growth and mucosal breakdown.	
3. Assure that the tube is secured in a way that avoids pressure on the naris. Assess the insertion site for drainage, bleeding, redness, swelling, or ulceration.	Pressure from the tube can compromise blood flow to the tissue and cause skin damage and infection.	• Drainage • Bleeding • Redness • Swelling • Ulceration

*Level M: Manufacturer's recommendations only.

Patient Monitoring and Care —*Continued*

Steps	Rationale	Reportable Conditions
4. Follow institutional standards for assessing pain. Administer analgesia as prescribed.	Identifies need for pain interventions.	• Continued pain despite pain interventions.

Documentation

Documentation should include the following:

- The type and size of the tube inserted
- The length of tube inserted per the tube's measurement marking at the nose
- Patient response to the insertion
- Unexpected outcomes

- Radiographic confirmation of the tube position and printed tracings per institutional requirements
- Nursing interventions
- Medications administered
- Patient and family education

References and Additional Readings

For a complete list of references and additional readings for this procedure, scan this QR code with any freely available smartphone code reader app, or visit http://booksite.elsevier.com/9780323376624.

141

Calculating Doses, Flow Rates, and Administration of Continuous Intravenous Infusions

Shelley Burcat and Maribeth Kelly

PURPOSE: Calculation of doses and flow rates and administration of continuous intravenous (IV) infusions are performed to ensure accurate delivery of medications administered via the IV route. Many of the medications delivered via continuous IV infusion have potent effects and narrow margins of safety; therefore accuracy in calculation and administration of these agents is imperative.

PREREQUISITE NURSING KNOWLEDGE

- Knowledge of aseptic technique is necessary.
- Nurses must be aware of the indications, actions, side effects, dosages, administration/storage, assessment, and evaluation for medications administered.
- Many different types of medications are delivered as continuous IV infusions in acute and critical care settings. These medications include, but are not limited to, vasoactive, inotropic, antidysrhythmic, sedative, and analgesic agents.
- Hemodynamic assessment and electrocardiographic (ECG) monitoring are frequently necessary to evaluate the patient's response to medication infusions. The nurse must be familiar with monitoring equipment such as cardiac monitors, arterial catheters, pulmonary artery catheters, and noninvasive blood pressure cuffs.
- Titration refers to the adjustment of the dose of a medication, either increasing or decreasing, to attain the desired patient response.
- Alterations or interruptions of the flow rate can significantly affect the dose of medication being delivered and adversely affect the patient. For accurate delivery of IV medications, volume-controlled infusion devices are required.
- "Smart technologies" are electronic devices, such as computers, bedside monitors, and infusion pumps, that perform calculations of doses and flow rates after information is entered and programmed by the user. Although these devices are not universally available, their use may reduce medication errors.[4]

- Smart pumps are infusion pumps with comprehensive libraries of medications and dose calculation software that can perform a "test of reasonableness" to check that programming is within preestablished institutional limits before the infusion can begin, which can reduce medication errors, improve workflow, and provide a source of data for continuous quality improvement.[10]
- Use of smart infusion pumps with activated dosage error reduction software alerts the nurse when safe doses and infusion rates have been exceeded.[7] The nurse must use the technology consistently to avoid serious medication infusion errors.[6]
- Be aware that double key bounce and double keying errors may occur when pressing a number key once on an infusion pump, resulting in the unintended consequence of a repeat of that same number. This can result in infusing medications at a higher rate than expected.[5]
- Three factors are involved in the calculations for continuous IV infusions:
  - The concentration is the amount of medication diluted in a given volume of IV solution (e.g., 400 mg dopamine diluted in 250 mL normal saline [NS] solution, resulting in a concentration of 1.6 mg/mL, or 2 g lidocaine diluted in 500 mL 5% dextrose in water [D_5W], yielding a concentration of 4 mg/mL). The concentration is also expressed as amount of medication per milliliter of fluid.
  - The dose of the medication is the amount of medication to be administered over a certain length of time (e.g., dopamine 5 mcg/kg/min, lidocaine 2 mg/min, or diltiazem 5 mg/hr). The units of measure for the dose differ for various medications. The length of time is 1 minute

or 1 hour. If the medication is weight based, the dose of the medication is per kilogram of patient weight.

❖ The flow rate is the rate of delivery of the IV fluid solution expressed as volume of IV fluid delivered per unit of time (e.g., 20 mL/hr). The unit of measure of the flow rate is milliliter per hour.

- All units of measure in the formula must be the same. It frequently is necessary to perform some conversions on the concentration before entering it into the formula. The units of measure of the concentration must be converted to the same units of measure of the dose (e.g., the concentration of dopamine is measured in milligrams, but the dose of dopamine is measured in micrograms).

- The mathematical formula for continuous IV infusions uses three factors (Box 141-1). When two factors are known, the third can be calculated with the basic formula. Therefore when the concentration of the solution and the prescribed dose are known, the flow rate can be determined. When the concentration of the solution and the flow rate are known, the dose can be determined. Variations on the basic formula are used to allow for medications delivered per hour or per minute and for medications that are weight based (Boxes 141-2 and 141-3).

- Calculations for weight-based medications include the patient's weight in the formula. The choice of which weight to use can be challenging. Much disagreement and inconsistency are found in the literature as to which weight to use, ideal body weight, actual body weight, or dry body weight.[2,7] Distribution of specific medications across fat and fluid body compartments varies, thus affecting the therapeutic level. Because most medications are titrated to patient response and a desired clinical endpoint, a consistent approach is to use the patient's admission weight for initial dose calculations. The clinical pharmacist then should be consulted for obese patients and for medications that have potentially dangerous toxicities.

- Central IV access should be used for vasoconstrictive medications and medications that can cause tissue damage when extravasated.[3] Mechanisms and agents that may cause tissue damage include osmotic damage from hyperosmolar solutions, ischemic necrosis caused by vasoconstrictors and certain cation solutions, direct cellular toxicity caused by antineoplastic agents, direct tissue damage from pH strong acids and bases, and direct irritation.[9]

- The Joint Commission goal for medication safety includes standardization and limiting the number of drug concentrations available in organizations.[11] Standardized dosing methods for the same medications reduce IV infusion errors.[7]

- The Institute of Healthcare Improvement (IHI) recommendations for IV medication safety include conducting independent double checks, dose calculation aids on IV solution bag labels, use of IV smart infusion pumps with safety features, and use of premade dose and flow-rate charts.[1]

- A review found there is insufficient evidence to suggest that medication errors are caused by nurses' poor calculation skills. More research and direct observational studies are required to examine calculation errors in practice.[8]

BOX 141-1 **Basic Formula***

1. To determine an unknown flow rate:
$$\frac{\text{Dose (mg/hr or mcg/hr)}}{\text{Concentration (mg/mL or mcg/mL)}} = \text{Flow rate (mL/hr)}$$

2. To determine an unknown dose:
$$\text{Flow rate (mL/hr)} \times \text{Concentration (mg/mL or mcg/mL)}$$
$$= \text{Dose (mg/hr or mcg/hr)}$$

3. To determine the concentration of drug in 1 mL of fluid:
$$\frac{\text{Total amount of drug (mg or mcg)}}{\text{Total volume of fluid (mL)}} = \text{Concentration} \frac{\text{(mg or mcg)}}{\text{(mL)}}$$

Example: When flow rate is unknown, diltiazem 125 mg/125 mL D_5W to be administered at 10 mg/hr.

A. Calculate concentration of drug in 1 mL of fluid:
$$\frac{125\,\text{mg}}{125\,\text{mL}} = \frac{1\,\text{mg}}{\text{mL}}$$

B. Enter known factors into the formula and solve:
$$\text{Flow rate (mL/hr)} \times \text{Concentration (mg or mcg/mL)}$$
$$= \text{Dose (mg or mcg/mL)}$$
$$\frac{10\,\text{mL/hr}}{1\,\text{mg/mL}} = 10\,\text{mL/hr}$$

Example: When dose is unknown, diltiazem 125 mg/125 mL D_5W is infusing at 15 mL/hr.

A. Calculate concentration of drug in 1 mL of fluid:
$$\frac{125\,\text{mg}}{125\,\text{mL}} = \frac{1\,\text{mg}}{\text{mL}}$$

B. Enter known factors into the formula and solve:
$$15\,\text{mL/hr} \times 1\,\text{mg/mL} = 15\,\text{mg/hr}$$

---

*Because there are units on the top of the equation and units on the bottom of the equation, to ensure that the final units are correct, the units on the bottom of the equation must be inverted and multiplied by the units of the top of the equation.

Example: $\dfrac{1800\,\text{mcg/hr}}{200\,\text{mcg/mL}} = \dfrac{9 \times \text{mL}}{\text{hr}} = 9\,\text{mL/hr}$

EQUIPMENT

- Prepared IV solution with medication to be administered
- IV tubing
- IV infusion device
- Nonsterile gloves
- Alcohol pads

Additional equipment, to have available as needed, includes the following:

- Calculator
- Medication compatibility table

PATIENT AND FAMILY EDUCATION

- Explain the indications and expected response to the pharmacological therapy. ***Rationale:*** Patients and families need explanations of the plan of care and interventions.
- Instruct the patient to report adverse symptoms, as indicated. Reportable symptoms include, but are not limited to, pain, burning, itching, or swelling at the IV site; dizziness; shortness of breath; palpitations; and chest pain.

BOX 141-2   Variation for Medication Doses Measured Per Minute (mg/min or mcg/min)*

1. To determine unknown flow rate:

$$\frac{\text{Dose (mg/min or mcg/min)} \times 60 \text{ min/hr}}{\text{Concentration (mg/mL or mcg/mL)}} = \text{Flow rate (mL/hr)}$$

2. To determine unknown dose:

$$\frac{\text{Flow rate (mL/hr)} \times \text{Concentration (mg/mL or mcg/mL)}}{60 \text{ min/hr}}$$
$$= \text{Dose (mg/min or mcg/min)}$$

Example: When flow rate is unknown, nitroglycerin 50 mg/250 mL D$_5$W to be administered at 30 mcg/min.

   A. Convert the concentration to like units of measure:

$$\frac{50 \text{ mg}}{250 \text{ mL}} \times \frac{1000 \text{ mcg}}{1 \text{ mg}} = \frac{50,000 \text{ mcg}}{250 \text{ mL}}$$

   B. Calculate the concentration of medication in 1 mL of fluid:

$$\frac{50,000 \text{ mcg}}{250 \text{ mL}} = \frac{200 \text{ mcg}}{1 \text{ mL}}$$

   C. Enter known factors into the formula and solve:

$$\frac{30 \text{ mcg/min} \times 60 \text{ min/hr}}{200 \text{ mcg/mL}} = 9 \text{ mL/hr}$$

Example: When the dose is unknown, lidocaine 2 g/500 mL D$_5$W is infusing at 30 mL/h.

   A. Convert the concentration to like units of measure:

$$\frac{2 \text{ g}}{500 \text{ mL}} \times \frac{1000 \text{ mg}}{1 \text{ g}} = \frac{2000 \text{ mg}}{500 \text{ mL}}$$

   B. Calculate the concentration of drug in 1 mL of fluid:

$$\frac{2000 \text{ mg}}{500 \text{ mL}} = \frac{4 \text{ mg}}{\text{mL}}$$

   C. Enter known factors into the formula and solve:

$$\frac{30 \text{ mL/hr} \times 4 \text{ mg/mL}}{60 \text{ min/hr}} = 2 \text{ mg/min}$$

*The time factor of 60 min/hr must be added to the basic formula.

BOX 141-3   Variation for Weight-Based Medication Doses Measured Per Minute (mcg/kg/min)*

1. To determine unknown flow rate:

$$\frac{\text{Dose (mcg/kg/min)} \times 60 \text{ min/hr} \times \text{Patient weight (kg)}}{\text{Concentration (mcg/mL)}} = \text{Flow rate (mL/hr)}$$

2. To determine unknown dose:

$$\frac{\text{Flow rate (mL/hr)} \times \text{Concentration (mcg/mL)}}{60 \text{ min/hr} \times \text{Patient weight (kg)}} = \text{Dose (mcg/kg/min)}$$

Example: When flow rate is unknown, dopamine 400 mg/250 mL D$_5$W to infuse at 5 mcg/kg/min. Patient weighs 100 kg.

   A. Convert the concentration to like units of measure:

$$\frac{400 \text{ mg}}{250 \text{ mL}} \times \frac{1000 \text{ mcg}}{1 \text{ mg}} = \frac{400,000 \text{ mcg}}{250 \text{ mL}}$$

   B. Calculate concentration of drug in 1 mL of fluid:

$$\frac{400,000 \text{ mcg}}{250 \text{ mL}} = \frac{1600 \text{ mcg}}{1 \text{ mL}}$$

   C. Enter known factors into the formula and solve:

$$\frac{5 \text{ mcg/kg/min} \times 60 \text{ min/hr} \times 100 \text{ kg}}{1600 \text{ mcg/mL}} = 18.75 \text{ mL/hr}$$

Example: When dose is unknown, dobutamine 500 mg/250 mL D$_5$W is infusing at 15 mL/hr. Patient weighs 70 kg.

   A. Convert the concentration to like units of measure:

$$\frac{500 \text{ mg}}{250 \text{ mL}} \times \frac{1000 \text{ mcg}}{\text{mg}} = \frac{50,000 \text{ mcg}}{250 \text{ mL}}$$

   B. Calculate concentration of drug in 1 mL of fluid:

$$\frac{50,000 \text{ mcg}}{250 \text{ mL}} = \frac{2000 \text{ mcg}}{\text{mL}}$$

   C. Enter known factors into the formula and solve:

$$\frac{15 \text{ mL/hr} \times 2000 \text{ mcg/mL}}{60 \text{ min/hr} \times 70 \text{ kg}} = 7.14 \text{ mcg/kg/min}$$

*The patient's weight in kilograms and the time factor of 60 min/hr must be added to the basic formula.

Rationale: Reporting assists the nurse to evaluate the response to the pharmacological therapy and to identify adverse reactions.

PATIENT ASSESSMENT AND PREPARATION

Patient Assessment

- Assess medication allergies. *Rationale:* Assessment provides identification and prevention of allergic reactions.
- Obtain vital signs and hemodynamic parameters. *Rationale:* The need for vasoactive agents is established, and baseline data are provided to evaluate the response to therapy.
- Assess the patient's cardiac rate and rhythm. *Rationale:* Assessment establishes the need for antidysrhythmic therapy and provides baseline data.
- Obtain other assessments relevant to the medication being administered (e.g., sedation scale for continuous IV sedatives). *Rationale:* Patients are assessed for specific

parameters that are affected by various medications in order to note the efficacy of the medications and to ensure their safe delivery.[2]

Patient Preparation

- Ensure that the patient and family understand information. Answer questions as they arise, and reinforce information as needed. *Rationale:* Understanding of previously taught information is evaluated and reinforced.
- Weigh the patient, if the medication is weight based. *Rationale:* Calculation of the correct dose based on patient weight is permitted. If the patient's weight has changed during hospitalization because of edema or other causes, use of the baseline admission weight is preferable.[12–14]
- Verify patency or obtain patent, appropriate IV access. *Rationale:* Delivery of the medication into the IV space is ensured. Some continuous infusion medications require central line access to prevent irritation or damage to smaller peripheral veins and to reduce the risk for extravasation.

Procedure	for Calculating Doses and Flow Rates and Administering Continuous Intravenous Infusions	
Steps	**Rationale**	**Special Considerations**
1. Verify the prescribed medication order.	Ensures accuracy of medication administration.	A medication order should include the medication, route, dose, and parameters for titration of the medication. The concentration of the solution and the diluent should be indicated in the order or determined by institutional standards.
2. **HH**		
3. **PE**		
4. Verify the five rights of medication administration: right patient, right drug, right dose, right time, and right route. Verify the correct patient with two identifiers.[1-3,11] **(Level E*)**	Reduces the potential for medication administration error.	
5. Connect and flush the IV solution (with prescribed medication) through the tubing system.	Prepares the IV system.	
6. Place the IV infusion in the infusion device. There are two methods to perform the next step; **choose either Step 7 or Step 8 or both** as a double-check. **(Level M*)**	Prepares the infusion system.	Refer to the infusion device user's manual for specific instructions on the use of specific devices.
7. Determine the correct flow rate with manual mathematic calculation method.	Ensures the prescribed dose is administered	Make sure the accurate rate based on the prescribed dose is entered into the infusion pump.
A. Convert the concentration of the solution to the same units of measure as the dose.	All units of measure must be the same to perform the mathematic functions.	
B. Calculate the concentration of the medication per milliliter of fluid.	Necessary for the medication calculation.	
C. Enter the concentration and the dose into the formula and solve for the flow rate.	Necessary for the medication calculation. Entering information into the device is required for the device to infuse at the prescribed rate.	Use alternate formulas if medication dose is a per-minute or weight-based dose (see Boxes 141-1, 141-2, and 141-3).
8. Determine the correct flow rate with electronic devices. **(Level M*)**	Prevents errors in medication administration.	Refer to the manufacturer's user guide for accurate programming of smart pump calculations. Refer to the institutional policy regarding what medications should be infused with smart device capabilities (i.e., Guardrails, Alaris Medical Systems, San Diego, CA).

*Level E: Multiple case reports, theory-based evidence from expert opinions, or peer-reviewed professional organizational standards without clinical studies to support recommendations.
*Level M: Manufacturer's recommendations only.

Procedure continues on following page

Procedure	**for Calculating Doses and Flow Rates and Administering Continuous Intravenous Infusions—*Continued***	
Steps	Rationale	Special Considerations
A. Enter the necessary information into the device, including, but not limited to, patient weight, medication name, concentration of solution, and dose prescribed.	Ensures patient safety. Prevents mathematic errors or data entry and programming errors.	
B. Program the device to electronically calculate the flow rate.		
9. Double-check the flow rate calculations or programming with another qualified individual.	Independent double-checks may reduce errors made when calculating dosages or programming pumps.	
10. Set the flow rate on the infusion pump.	Prepares for medication administration.	
11. Connect the infusion system to the intended IV line or catheter and initiate the infusion.	Initiates the therapy.	Alcohol should always be used to cleanse the IV port (hub) before the infusion is connected.
12. Remove PE and discard used supplies.		
13. HH		

Expected Outcomes

- The desired patient response is achieved
- The correct dose of medication is administered
- The dose is titrated to achieve/maintain the desired patient response

Unexpected Outcomes

- Adverse reactions to the medication occur
- The incorrect dose of medication is administered
- The desired patient response is not achieved or maintained
- Infiltration or extravasation of medication occurs

Patient Monitoring and Care

Steps	Rationale	Reportable Conditions
		These conditions should be reported if they persist despite nursing interventions.
1. Evaluate the patient response by monitoring the indicated parameters for the medication being infused.	Medications given as continuous infusions often have potent effects and potentially serious adverse effects. Most medications given as continuous infusions have a quick onset of action. Frequent monitoring of parameters is necessary during initiation of the infusion.	• Adverse reactions • Hemodynamic instability • Cardiac dysrhythmias • Excessive sedation • Respiratory depression

Patient Monitoring and Care —*Continued*

Steps	Rationale	Reportable Conditions
2. If the patient response is inadequate, titrate the infusion as prescribed following the prescribed parameters.	The patient's response to many continuous infusions is dose-dependent. To achieve the desired response, titration of the dose is necessary.	• Desired response not achieved within an acceptable dosage range
3. Assess the IV access for catheter placement, catheter patency, and signs of infiltration or extravasation every 1–4 hours and as needed.	Ensures delivery of the medication into the venous system. Prevents interruptions in delivery of the medication. Provides early recognition of complications.	• Extravasation of any medication • Intravenous line infiltration

Documentation

Documentation should include the following:
• Name of the medication and the type of solution in which the medication is diluted; concentration of the solution; dose; flow rate; and administration times
• Patient and family education
• Assessment of the IV access and site

• Parameters monitored and patient response
• Adverse reactions and interventions to treat the reaction
• Titration

References and Additional Readings

For a complete list of references and additional readings for this procedure, scan this QR code with any freely available smartphone code reader app, or visit http://booksite.elsevier.com/9780323376624.

Index

Page numbers followed by "*f*" indicate figures, "*t*" indicate tables, and "*b*" indicate boxes.